W9-AHA-332

DATE DUE

JUN 1 2 2001	

GAYLORD   PRINTED IN U.S.A.

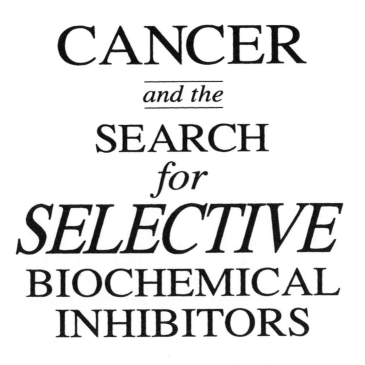

CANCER
and the
SEARCH
for
SELECTIVE
BIOCHEMICAL
INHIBITORS

CANCER

and the

SEARCH
for
SELECTIVE
BIOCHEMICAL
INHIBITORS

E. J. Hoffman

CRC Press
Boca Raton   London   New York   Washington, D.C.

Library of Congress Cataloging-in-Publication Data

Hoffman, E. J. (Edward Jack) 1925–
    Cancer and the search for selective biochemical inhibitors / E.J.
Hoffman.
          p. cm.
    Includes bibliographical references and index.
    ISBN 0-8493-9118-0 (alk. paper)
    1. Carcinogenesis. 2. Enzyme inhibitors--Therapeutic use.
  3. Antineoplastic agents. 4. Materia medica, Vegetable. I. Title.
    [DNLM: 1. Neoplasms--drug therapy. 2. Antineoplastic Agents,
Phytogenic--therapeutic use. 3. Enzyme Inhibitors--therapeutic use.
QZ 267 H699c 1999]
RC268.5.H63   1999
616.99¢4—dc21

                98-49306
                CIP

© 1999 by CRC Press LLC

No claim to original U.S. Government works
International Standard Book Number 0-8493-9118-0
Library of Congress Card Number 98-49306
Printed in the United States of America   2 3 4 5 6 7 8 9 0
Printed on acid-free paper

Preface

In short summary, cancer can be viewed as a metabolic disorder or aberration that occurs in cells. Presumably, it may be caused by or activated by various agents such as viruses, radiation, and chemicals, and may also involve (inherited) genetic malfunctions. Moreover, cancerous cells tend to mimic the cellular source, giving rise to many different kinds of cancers or cancer cells. It may be presumed that the immune system works against the transformation of normal cells into cancerous cells by acting against, for example, invading viruses, but once cancer gains a foothold and proceeds to spread or metastasize, more heroic measures are needed.

These things said, and with the cancer already formed, the question becomes "How can cancer be counteracted?" The standard therapeutic practices of medical orthodoxy, namely surgery, radiation, and cytotoxic chemotherapy—especially the last-mentioned—are coming under increasing scrutiny for their limitations and potentially disastrous side effects or consequences. At best, they may be only an immediacy (for instance, excising the localized mass of cancerous tissue); at worst, they can be deadly in themselves, causing cancer cells to spread or metastasize. For advanced or metastasized cancer, the prognosis is indeed dismal, with cytotoxic chemotherapy the only option at present, and that merely a palliative.

The final resolution or solution may lie in the realm of enzymes and enzyme inhibitors. This is because appropriate enzyme inhibitors provide a means to selectively block cancer cell metabolism. That is to say, enzyme inhibitors may serve as anticancer agents. In further explanation, enzymes are proteinaceous substances that act as catalysts for the biochemical reactions that take place in the body. In the main, each reaction is catalyzed by, and depends on, a specific enzyme. In other words, there are about as many enzymes as there are biochemical reactions.

On the other hand, enzyme inhibitors are also proteinaceous substances, or chemical or biochemical substances, that in various ways control, modulate, regulate, inhibit, deactivate, or block the action of enzymes. In rarer instances, they may serve as enzyme promoters or activators. A given substance may act as an inhibitor for more than one enzyme-catalyzed reaction, which may complicate its use. That is, there may be adverse side effects, expected or unexpected.

Enzyme inhibitors are in fact the basis for modern drug therapy as a means to control or eliminate disease. Thus, antibiotics are enzyme inhibitors that block critical enzyme-catalyzed reactions in bacterial cells but do so without harming human cells—at least for the particular antibiotics and the dosages used. The sulfa drugs are an earlier example. Fluorides used in dental care are said to act as enzyme inhibitors for the vital processes of the cavity-inducing bacteria found in the mouth, and in this way they destroy these bacteria. The subject becomes that of therapeutic chemotherapy, and the use of medicinal drugs can be described in these terms, whether the drug is of natural origins or is a synthetic chemical.

Even the cytotoxic chemotherapy drugs or chemicals used against cancer act as enzyme inhibitors. Unfortunately, these drugs are nonselective, acting against the enzymes involved in cellular DNA/RNA/protein synthesis for both cancerous and normal cells, thus adversely affecting all cells. Hence, the descriptor *cytotoxic* or *cell-toxic* is used. Moreover, these drugs may preferentially act against the faster-growing cells of the immune system and gastrointestinal tract, and only to a lesser degree affect the slower-growing cancer cells—which can also build up an immunity to the drug. (There is the indication also that chemotherapy can cause the cancer to spread or metastasize.) In fact, it is starting to be recognized that conventional cytotoxic chemotherapy is ineffective against solid tumors and works only against blood-related cancers such as leukemia, which are not cancers in the usual sense.

Whereas the DNA/RNA/protein synthesis route denotes the processes for cellular regeneration, there are other cellular processes going on involving still other enzyme-catalyzed reactions, notably those involving what is called *metabolism*. Although the many and varied supportive biochemical reactions occurring in the body may be collectively referred to as *metabolism* or *cell metabolism,* more commonly the term has a special meaning. This meaning pertains to the biochemical reaction sequences or pathways by which cells convert glucose or similar carbohydrate compounds to energy, a process sometimes called *primary metabolism* but more usually referred to as *glycolysis.*

In turn, there are two routes for glycolysis. In the one, which may be referred to as *aerobic glycolysis,* glucose or blood sugar (or its polymer, called *glycogen*) is ultimately converted to carbon dioxide and water, which are the end products from normal cell metabolism. In the other, glucose is eventually converted instead to lactic acid or lactate, the chief end product from cancer cell metabolism. The one involves oxygen, the other does not. Each glycolysis sequence or pathway requires a succession of specific enzymes (and may also involve coreactants and supporting reactions), with some of the slower enzyme-catalyzed reaction steps controlling the overall sequence.*

Although there have been other differences noted, the above distinctions between normal cell and cancer cell metabolism may be central to the treatment of cancer, because these metabolic differences underscore a potential way in which the growth and sustenance of cancer cells can be selectively disarmed without affecting normal cells. The objective is to "starve" the cancer cells, so to speak.

In effect, we are talking about the use of (nontoxic) enzyme inhibitors to selectively inhibit or block cancer cell metabolism without unduly interfering with normal cell metabolism. That is, the idea is that, in the concentrations used at least, these enzyme inhibitors affect cancer cells but not normal cells. Some of these inhibitors evidently exist in the very foods we eat, whereas others occur in so-called medicinal plants—some of which, unfortunately, are also toxic in varying degree. The catchall

---

* For example, the formation of lactic acid or lactate by the enzyme lactate dehydrogenase is a critical step in the anaerobic sequence, and there are a number of known inhibitors that act against this enzyme—with others no doubt in the offing. This affords the possibility for negating the anaerobic sequence or pathway.

term for these plant-derived biologically active (bioactive) substances is *phytochemicals* or *plant-chemicals.* *

These plant-derived substances include such classes of compounds as alkaloids, glycosides or glucosides, flavonoids, saponins, and so on. There is the admonition, however, that "the dosage level is the poison," a saying from medical folklore. The situation is muddied by the fact that the concentration or potency of bioactive substances in a given plant species will vary with the geographic location, with the time of year or season (and even with the time of day), and with the plant part—not to mention such factors as soil makeup or fertility, and climate.

In a manner of speaking, most or all plants or plant substances are bioactive in one way or another and to some extent or another, even if we are speaking of foods or such food components as vitamins and minerals. Thus, more specifically, we must be concerned with the phytochemical or plant-chemical content, including the mineral or inorganic content—that is, both the nature of the compounds present and their concentrations. In effect, toxicity vs. nontoxicity becomes relative, that is, a matter of degree and of how much is consumed or administered.

The necessary reminder is that bioactive plants include what are also called poisonous and medicinal plants, which may include some of the herbals, and caution is the order of the day. A complication is the fact that there are no uniform standards for measuring and monitoring plant bioactivity or even to ensure that the customer is getting the particular plant indicated. However, in some other countries, there are more stringent controls—in Germany, for instance.

To continue, what may be a promising avenue for noninvasive cancer treatment is the use of nontoxic phytochemicals or other nontoxic substances as enzyme inhibitors for anaerobic glycolysis. For, according to the Warburg theory first enunciated back in 1926, cancer cells in the main undergo anaerobic glycolysis to produce lactic acid or lactate, whereas normal cells undergo aerobic glycolysis to ultimately yield carbon dioxide and water. (Warburg later won the Nobel Prize in 1930 for other work.) It is interesting that a number of known enzyme inhibitors for controlling enzyme-catalyzed reactions of anaerobic glycolysis are anticancer agents as found in medical folklore.

While medical research apparently has not picked up on this avenue of investigation, it has at least been noted. Thus, Donald Voet and Judith G. Voet, in their treatise on biochemistry, make the following comment:

> Attempts to understand the metabolic differences between cancer cells and normal cells may one day provide a clue to the treatment of certain forms of this deadly disease. (Voet and Voet, *Biochemistry*, Wiley, New York, 1995, p. 595)

The wide disparity between the glycolysis rate of cancer cells and of normal cells is observed by Robert A. Harris in a chapter in another comprehensive treatise on

---

* Some of these bioactive plants or plant substances are accused of being carcinogenic or cancer-causing in themselves. In fact, a common-enough observation is that a particular plant or plant substance may act as an anticancer agent at lower concentrations, but may be carcinogenic at higher concentrations, or may be toxic in other ways. It may be noted that some of the antibiotics have been found to act as anticancer agents, but are too toxic to use.

biochemistry where, in experiments on rats, the glucose consumption rates under anaerobic conditions were found to be 20 times greater than under aerobic conditions (Harris, in *Textbook of Biochemistry: with Clinical Correlations*, Thomas M. Devlin ed., Wiley, New York, 1982, p. 353).

Admittedly, this is not the entire story, and other things are going on, such as glutaminolysis (the utilization of the amino acid glutamine) as well as a relatively limited aerobic glycolysis, as set forth by E. Eigenbrodt, P. Fisher, and M. Reinacher in their work on carbohydrate metabolism in tumor cells (Eigenbrodt et al., in *Regulation of Carbohydrate Metabolism*, Vol. II, Rivka Beitner, ed., CRC Press, Boca Raton FL, 1985, pp. 141–179). However, anaerobic glycolysis can be perceived as the main metabolic route for cancerous cells.

In consequence, the testing of known or proposed anticancer agents against lactic acid- or lactate-producing enzymes seems like a promising and ultrasimple route of research to pursue—preferably in a clinical setting. But in fact, it is one that the patient might consider pursuing independently, because even common garden variety vegetables and fruits contain bioactive substances such as alkaloids and glycosides, usually in trace amounts, that are potential enzyme inhibitors for anaerobic glycolysis.

As to bodily lactic acid or lactate buildup, prior to its reconversion to glucose or glycogen in the liver, this might provide a simple indicator for cancer—and for monitoring progress made against cancer. A change, up or down, in the concentration of lactate dehydrogenase, the enzyme that produces lactic acid or lactate, may also be an indicator for cancer. There may be better indictors, however.

With regard to the foregoing, adopting a vegetarian diet has sometimes been observed to stop cancer in its tracks. The question is, why don't vegetarian diets work more often, or always? Are we therefore talking of biochemical individuality, or chance, or what? In other words, what are the other factors involved, and how can they be 100 percent accommodated?

What we think of as foods are generally nontoxic in the amounts used—the winnowing of the ages. The use of what may be called poisonous and medicinal plants or plant substances may be otherwise. This latter category may include some of the more common herbs, and the word is to use *extreme caution*.

In fact, what we call poisons act as enzyme inhibitors for certain critical body processes. They may produce respiration failure, for example, or cause cardiac arrest. Interestingly, however, in minute concentrations or dosages, some have historically been used as medicines and are still in use today. There may be, however, a fine line between medicinal doses and toxic doses. A common example is in the use of digitalis for heart disease, which must be taken only in the prescribed therapeutic amounts determined to be safe.

A rule of thumb is that the more poisonous a plant or plant substance may be, the greater its potential usefulness as a medicine. A number of the alkaloids, which are noted for producing pronounced physiological effects, are toxic in the extreme. And in the searching of the rain forests for bioactive plants, the presence of alkaloids is the main criterion used for assessing a plant's possibilities. Among the most deadly substances are proteinaceous toxins found in a very few plants. Other plants or plant components may contain what are called *glycosides* or *glucosides*, some of which may have cyanide-containing chemical structures and can be deadly. A controversial example is laetrile or amygdalin, as found in bitter almonds, apricot pits, and the like. It is thought to release cyanide by the action of an enzyme more prevalent in cancer cells, which is offset by a detoxifying enzyme in normal cells. The *Mycota* or *fungi* may also contain or produce such pharmacologically active compounds as alkaloids and are considered a potential source for effective anticancer agents.

At the same time, it would also be of great interest to know just what substances or foods might favor anaerobic glycolysis—that is, function as enzyme promoters or activators for, say, lactate dehydrogenase. In other words, these substances or foods—although not necessarily cancer causing—could nonetheless stimulate cancer-cell growth.

●　　●　　●

With cancer overtaking heart disease as the leading killer in this country, with nearly 600,000 humans dying of cancer each year (a death every minute), and with some 1.5 million new cases surfacing, the major media nevertheless remain quiescent. There is a resignation to the facts of life, that profit-making enterprises have both an upside and a downside. That is, there is the familiar enigma that profits are the incentive for developing new products, at the same time excluding less-profitable or unprofitable undertakings. And plant or herbal remedies per se are for the most part not of interest to the pharmaceutical industry, if a proprietary position cannot be attained. Only if synthetic derivatives of the natural substances can be developed is a patent position foreseeable and a suitable return on investment guaranteed. Clearly, there is a role for independent government support or participation for unprofitable undertakings in the public interest.

The "war on cancer" has been going on since 1972, with billions upon billions spent—but with no sure-fire cures yet in evidence, either from medical orthodoxy or from alternative medicine. One can wonder if research has become too much a bureaucracy whose perpetuation is assured by the very act of not finding a cure. And if this seems overstated, then where is the cure?

It is informative to note that the further development of penicillin and its clinical use took 12 years for Florey and Chain to perfect, after its discovery by Fleming. But the motivation and the genius of Florey and Chain were there when needed, and their modest operation was for other than profits

Another comparison is with the development of the atomic bomb during WWII, which took only about four years—but the motivation and the genius of Robert Oppenheimer and associates were there, pushed by General Leslie Groves, all for better or worse.

May there be the same for cancer.

MEDICAL ORTHODOXY VS. ALTERNATIVE MEDICINE

There is the speculation that the entire cancer situation needs a vigorous airing. For instance, the appropriate congressional committee or committees should conduct hearings—although we should not hold our breath. Perhaps class action lawsuits are in order, as with the tobacco industry, say over the promotion and routine use of conventional nonselective and cytotoxic chemotherapy drugs, in the context of failures and profits.

If the press has been remiss, investigative (and controversial) TV and radio talk shows are also way overdue for tackling the cancer situation in its entirety (and enormity). Basically, the controversy is about medical orthodoxy vs. alternative medicine (also called *complementary and alternative medicine*, or CAM), and of conventional vs. alternative treatments, and the successes and failures of each—and why. In sum, therefore, outlook, theory, and practice must be reconciled in a cure or cures. So far, medical orthodoxy has reacted against anything that smacks of alternative or naturalistic therapies, when in fact there is as much chemistry in, for example, plant substances as in other chemical substances. The chemistry and pharmacology of the one is every bit as demanding as that of the other, both in the chemical and physical properties and in the synthesis of the compounds.

As to research, although there are perhaps 15,000 to 20,000 publications about cancer appearing each year, mostly about research, and an occasional press release makes the newspapers, no absolute cures are in evidence. Nor is there much criticism about this research and its lack of success. It is as if research were its own justification.

If this judgement seems outrageous, then one may proceed to inspect all of the published (technical) literature—the volumes upon volumes of journals and books on any and all subjects. See how many papers or articles or books actually resolve a practical problem, much less a life-threatening dilemma such as cancer. Most can be viewed as merely high-class prestidigitations—the "busy work" so often found in PhD theses. But cranking out research papers has become the measure of success and esteem, in academic circles called the familiar "publish or perish" syndrome.

Arthur Koestler, in his landmark study *The Act of Creation*, speaks to the scientific mind in its corporate aspect, whereby a particular branch of science becomes controlled by a sort of establishment, which includes universities, learned societies, and the editorial offices of the technical journals (Koestler, *The Act of Creation*, Macmillan, New York, 1964, p. 239). "Corporate orthodoxy has been the curse of genius . . . throughout the centuries its phalanxes have sturdily defended habit against originality." Koestler goes on to cite a few instances from the medical world, in particular the case of Ignas Semmelweiss, circa 1847, who was hounded out of the profession for claiming that the uncleanliness of physicians infected their own patients. Semmelweiss eventually became mad and died in a mental institution.

Princeton psychologist Julian Jaynes once wrote of scientisms or clusters of scientific ideas that "almost surprise themselves into creeds of belief" (Jaynes, *The Origin of Consciousness in the Breakdown of the Bicameral Mind*, Houghton Mifflin, Boston, 1976, p. 441). Even mathematics has its uncertainties, embodied for instance in the title of a book by Morris Klein (Klein, *Mathematics: The Loss of Certainty*, Oxford University Press, New York, 1978).

These brief excursions serve to indicate that medical orthodoxy is not infallible, nor is science, nor are the prevailing attitudes about cancer and its treatment.

ADDENDUM

The full sequence of glycolytic enzymes is available in bacteria cultures such as of the genus *Lactobacillus*, and these enzymes are available commercially. Also available from commercial sources are the several specific enzymes involved, ranging from hexokinase to lactate dehydrogenase. Some of these commercial sources are in fact mentioned in Part 8 of this book. Known (or at least suspected) enzyme inhibitors for the controlling enzymes of anaerobic glycolysis are listed in Appendix A. An update is furnished in Appendix Y. Of these, inhibitors for lactate dehydrogenase may prove the most important. (Some enzyme inhibitors for the CO_2- and H_2O-producing tricarboxylic acid cycle are presented in Appendix B, but these are to be avoided, since they could shut down respiration.)

In Part 1 and Appendix C, it is substantiated that conventional cytotoxic chemotherapy is also based on enzyme inhibitors—unfortunately, by nonselectively killing off all body cells, and especially red and white blood cells, e.g., of the immune system—and is followed by other listings of enzymes and enzyme inhibitors involved in cellular DNA/RNA/protein synthesis, and so forth. Some protease inhibitors are also listed, this being a newer avenue of investigation in cancer research.

In further comment about the contents, which review the available information from a number of books on alternatives, the material is sometimes necessarily technical, with much said about the biochemistry of cancer, enzymes and enzyme inhibitors, bioactive plants and phytochemicals, the biogenesis of cancer, viruses and cancer, and enzyme inhibitors as anticancer agents. There are 26 appendices for documentation.

Among other things, extensive listings are provided of newer information about anticancer plants from around the world. As the benchmark, these listings are compared with the entries in Jonathan L. Hartwell's compendium of about 3,000 bioactive plant species that have been tried against cancer (Hartwell, *Plants Used Against Cancer*, Quarterman Publications, Lawrence MA, 1982). Hartwell's survey ranged worldwide, from the ancients to the present. The degree of duplication between past and present is perhaps not so amazing.

The common denominator is chemical taxonomy, and ultimately in terms of plant-chemicals or phytochemicals. Although not infallible, there is a sometimes striking correlation between certain plant families and bioactivity. In particular, bioactive alkaloids and alkaloid-containing plants are emphasized, and the Mycota or fungi and their chemical makeup are also explored.

Not only are compounds from these several classes found to be anticancer agents, but some of these and other substances have been found to act variously as antibacterial, antiviral, antifungal, and antiparasitic agents. As bacterial infections grow increasingly resistant to antibiotics, and as new viral diseases emerge, these kinds of substances will likely become of great importance. Listings have been furnished.

There seems to be a relationship between what are referred to as *poisonous* or medicinal plants and their action as anticancer agents, which can be explained in terms of enzyme inhibitors.

It may also be noted that the results of *in vitro*, *in vivo*, and clinical tests are sometimes contradictory. The ultimate test is whether cancer remission occurs in the patient without undesirable side effects. Due to the urgency of the situation, it is not necessarily advisable to go through the full retinue of testing, and cancer patients who volunteer should have this option. (For example, a new drug being so tested, called pamidronate disodium or Aredia®, is said to alter the surface properties of metastasized cancer cells such that they do not adhere to other tissue surfaces.)

Prescreening can be used, however, by testing various known or suspected anticancer agents against the specific enzymes involved. These enzymes may be the entire sequence necessary for, say, anaerobic glycolysis, or may be only one or more of the several controlling enzymes involved—for example, lactate dehydrogenase.

The dosage levels used and frequency of dosage will expectedly be critical, and can of course be life threatening. It is suggested therefore that *Cancer Clinical Research Centers (CCRCs)* or their equivalent be set up in new or existing facilities, where such bioactive substances could be administered to so-called *terminal* cancer patients with advanced or metastasized cancer. (It is the intent that the word *terminal* become a misnomer.) The patients (who may be outpatients) would be under the care of MDs and/or DOs who are supported by a pool of specialists in pharmacology; in biochemistry, microbiology, or molecular biology; in botany or ethnobotany; in herbalogy or naturopathy; and in allied subjects. Such will require the monitoring of the patient for vital signs as well as cancer regression.

In using potentially toxic bioactive substances or drugs, or any drug for that matter, there is always the possibility of adverse effects such as cardiac arrest and or respiration failure, and over the longer term such organs as the liver and kidneys may be affected. There is the additional possibility of allergic reactions in a given individual, even unto anaphylactic shock. Such adverse reactions require immediate life-saving measures—for example, that of utilizing antihistamines such as epinephrine or adrenalin.

From all this, patterns of discovery will predictably emerge, establishing the most effective substances and the optimum dosage levels. Undoubtedly, dosage levels should start minuscule (say, at the very low concentrations as used in homeopathy) and should only be increased as warranted by the general health of the patient—and as cancer remission occurs.

Worthy of further mention is that, in the text proper, there are words, phrases, sentences, and passages which seem of special interest, and which are highlighted in *italic*. An alphabetized list of references is furnished at the end of each part, and appendices are provided as an informative convenience at the end of the book.

About the Author

E.J. Hoffman is neither physician, biochemist, nor microbiologist but is another of the legion whose lives have been transfixed by cancer. Rather, his background is in matters of a scientific and engineering nature, and more so with regard to our purported powers of reason. These directions are reflected in two preceding books, *Analytic Thermodynamics: Origins Methods, Limits, and Validity*, and *Power Cycles and Energy Efficiency*. Basic to everything are the abstractions of epistemology—the origins, methods, limits, and validity of knowledge, utilized in the subtitle of *Analytic Thermodynamics*. It is the objective of simplifying all things to their most elemental level.

Thus, Hoffman's first irrefutable injunction of the universe is the maxim that the processes of reason require that we deal either in tautologies or, alternatively, in error—that is, we either state the same *exact* thing, albeit in a different way, or else we do not. And if we do not, then we are in error. And furthermore, who vouches for the original proposition in the first place?

The notion of tautologies vs. error reaches back to the corresponding analytic propositions (*Verstand*) vs. synthetic propositions (*Vernunft*) of Kant, and way before that back to 1 John 4:6 in terms of the spirit of truth vs. the spirit of error, and even before that to Plato's *Phaedo* and his absolute equalities. And Plato declared in the *Meno* that, if we don't know the solution to a problem, then we don't know what the problem is, but if we do know the solution, then there is no problem. The famous mathematician Karl Gauss once said that he had possessed his solutions for a long time but hadn't figured out how to arrive at them. And, speaking of the latter, a solution can't say any more than the original statement or equation, if as much, but is merely a more convenient or useful form.

As has been known almost from the very beginning, in Aristotelian logic the conclusion is buried in the premise. And if not, then any conclusion whatsoever can be reached—and is—whereby "logic" itself must forever remain suspect. As in *Alice*, first the verdict then the trial. As to pure mathematics, supposedly the symbol of logic unfettered, it has been called but a system of tautologies and conventions. Otherwise, any proposed system of logic will always have contradictions and inconsistencies—that is, error.

This is followed by the second injunction, about the explanations of science, that, in the strict sense of the word, what we call *science* signifies only that the experiments or observations are repeatable, and the data or results are reproducible—from which we can formulate "laws," e.g., Kepler's laws of planetary motion. These laws reiterate but do not explain. (The various forms for the laws of motion are at best but tautological with Kepler's laws, including the energy forms and the trajectory, which circle back mathematically to Kepler's laws.) All the rest—the theories, hypotheses, conjectures, or explanations—lies in the aeries of our imagination. And even the most fundamental of concepts—e.g., space, time, and mass—can never be defined absolutely, only measured.

In the case of cancer, the author has conducted an extensive literature review aimed at discerning the underlying features or abstractions of cancer—not only its genesis, particularly by means of the pervasive viral invasion of cell chromosomes, but more importantly its immolation by *selective* biochemical agents. This is most apparent in terms of enzymes, the myriad proteinaceous biochemical catalysts that direct each and all body processes, and in turn leads to the subject of enzyme inhibitors, the chemical or biochemical agents that inhibit, block, regulate, modulate, or control (or even promote) these same enzymes and body processes. Of particular concern are the enzyme inhibitors, which may *selectively* block cancer cell metabolism, the molecular processes by which cancer cells are sustained and proliferate. The usual cytotoxic (cell-toxic) chemotherapy agents are nonselective, destroying both normal cells and cancerous cells.

The literature (and medical folklore) already indicates that there are arrays of such bioactive substances, notably from the plant or herbal world—even food-stuffs—expressible as phytochemicals (plant-chemicals). Many or most of these substances, unfortunately, may have adverse or even life-threatening side effects. Or in another way of saying it, a given bioactive substance usually inhibits more than one enzyme. This potential toxicity can range from the acute extremes of cardiac arrest and respiratory failure to chronic actions against the liver and kidneys or other vital organs—and sometimes the side effects may be largely benign. In other words, the administration can oftentimes be critical, necessitating professional counsel and guidance—the same as with any drug, natural or synthetic, and is the customary trade-off.

In consequence, Hoffman is an advocate for the widespread establishment of Cancer Clinical Research Centers (CCRCs) or their equivalent for the treatment of patients with advanced or metastasized cancer. Biochemical treatments would be administered under strict medical supervision, with adequate technical backup. (In the case of utilizing plants or herbs, for instance, the concentrations of phytochemicals in a given species vary with plant part, geography, climate, season, even time of day, not to mention substitutions, which is an argument for using the pure compounds.) Such therapeutic regimes would be closely monitored for the patient's vital signs, and by rapid and noninvasive tests—mostly yet to be determined—the progression or regression of cancer would be evidenced. The bioactive agent used, mode of treatment, and dosage levels and frequency would be changed or adjusted accordingly, with allowances made for biochemical individuality. Predictably, a pattern of successes would emerge, establishing the preferred therapies.

There is the thought that a biochemical cure or cures for cancer already exist. As with Michelango's philosophy of sculpting, it is a matter of chipping away to find the finished form, which was there all the time. Sometimes referred to as *alternative medicine,* there is the inference that the cure or cures will precede the completed understanding.

For more, much more, consult the pages of *Cancer and the Search for Selective Biochemical Inhibitors.*

To Suzanne

Contents

The Biochemistry of Cancer and Its Treatment

Part 1

The Biochemistry of Cancer and Its Treatment

1.1   INTRODUCTORY REMARKS

The biochemistry of cancer and its treatment may lie in the differences between cancerous cells and normal cells, in what may be called *cell metabolism*. Whatever insights may be evidenced afford the possibility of cures or remissions above and beyond the comparatively few now in evidence. Although by no means fully known, there are a few differences dating back to 1926, when Otto Warburg first noticed that in the main cancer cells undergo anaerobic behavior, whereas normal cells under go aerobic behavior. That is to say, cancer cells in the main do not require oxygen as is the case for normal cells. The fuel or energy source is principally glucose or its equivalent, although amino acids such as glutamine may also serve that purpose, at least to a limited extent. In the terminology followed, the overall process by which glucose is converted or utilized may be called *glycolysis,* whereas the utilization of glutamine, say, is called *glutaminolysis*. With cancerous cells, the main end product from glycolysis is lactic acid, also called *lactate*. With normal cells, the main end products are carbon dioxide and water—the same as for simple combustion.

Generally speaking, *metabolism* can mean any biochemical reaction or reaction sequence, and what are called *metabolites* can be both reactants and reaction products. In a more restrictive usage, however, metabolism or primary metabolism pertains to biochemical reactions or conversions in which energy is produced. That is to say, the reactions are *exothermic,* meaning that heat energy is given off, but which may be converted to, or make an appearance as, still other forms of energy. Kinetic energy is, of course, one form. Chemical or biochemical energy for instance is stored as biomass, for subsequent purposes. Also in a more restrictive fashion, metabolites are generally considered only the reaction products. Primary metabolites, moreover, are those produced from energy-giving biochemical reactions; the products from all other kinds of reactions can be referred to as *secondary metabolites*.

It may be noted that there may be great divergences in the amount of heat energy furnished by different reactions. Thus, in the case of cancer cell metabolism, which is in the main anaerobic, only a small amount of energy is given off. Conversely, in normal cell metabolism, which is aerobic, a large amount of energy is given off—equivalent to the heat of combustion. Glutaminolysis in turn does not give off much energy.

In a nutshell, the problem becomes that of blocking cancer cell metabolism without affecting normal cell metabolism, which enters the realm of enzymes and enzyme inhibitors. The idea is to avoid supporting the existence of cancer cells, or in other words, "starve" the cancer cells. At the same time, the operative word is "selective," such that a particular inhibitor does not block vital body processes such as respiration, produce cardiac arrest, or act against the liver or kidneys—the so-called side effects or adverse effects.

Each biochemical reaction is catalyzed or favored by a particular proteinaceous substance called an *enzyme,* and a sequence of reactions will require a separate enzyme for each individual reaction. (In biochemistry, these reaction sequences are ordinarily called *pathways*.) Some of the enzymes may be more important than others, depending on whether they control the overall conversion rate. That is, the slower reaction or reactions in the sequence will tend to control the overall conversion rate.

There is a growing technical literature about enzymes, and their purposes lie in the realm of biochemical or organic catalysis, as distinguished from inorganic catalysis. A recent addition to the literature is *Comprehensive Biological Catalysis: A Mechanistic Reference*, in four volumes, edited by Michael Sinnott and published in 1998.

In turn, each enzyme-catalyst may be modulated, regulated, controlled, blocked, "poisoned," or inhibited by another proteinaceous substance or other chemical substance that interferes with catalysis. In the parlance of catalysis, these substances may deactivate the active sites, or *receptor sites,* as they are also called. Thus, it is often said that modern drug therapy is based on enzyme inhibitors, antibiotics being the most notable example. Here, the antibiotics act to block vital enzyme-catalyzed pathways in bacterial metabolic processes. What are regarded as poisons act as enzyme inhibitors, severely interfering with a life-sustaining process such as respiration. And the drugs of conventional cytotoxic therapy also act as enzyme inhibitors, in this case interfering with the DNA/RNA/protein synthesis pathway. All cells are affected, however, but mostly fast-growing cells such as comprise the immune system and gastrointestinal tract, with anemia also a side effect.

With regard to cancer and other diseases, it should therefore be of first importance that the enzyme inhibitors used be *selective.* This is generally the case for the antibiotics commonly employed, at least in the dosages used, which attack bacterial cells but not human cells. Unfortunately, as noted, this is not the case for conventional cytotoxic chemotherapy drugs, which attack normal cells as well as cancer cells.

We are therefore critically interested in what substances could interfere with cancer cell processes but not normal cell processes. And the answer may lie in cancer cell metabolism as distinguished from normal cell metabolism.

Thus, the statement of Donald Voet and Judith G. Voet bears repeating (Voet and Voet, *Biochemistry,* p. 595; in first ed., New York, Wiley, 1990, p. 557). "Attempts to understand the metabolic differences between cancer cells and normal cells may one day provide a clue to the treatment of certain forms of this deadly disease." As does the observation of Robert A. Harris that glucose consumption under anaerobic conditions may be 20 times greater than under aerobic conditions (Harris, in *Textbook of Biochemistry,* p. 353).

The foregoing does not necessarily preclude a peripheral interest in the causes of cancer. Thus, we may go along with current thinking that cancers are primarily of genetic origin, inherited or otherwise, and have their basis in our chromosomes and genes. The subject has been explored for example in several articles published by the American Cancer Society in *CA—A Cancer Journal for Clinicians.* The articles are variously by Felix Mitelman, by Avery A. Sandberg, and by Robert A. Weinberg. However, there has been, and is, a school of thought that cancers are viral related as well as radiation and chemical related. As it turns out, there is really no impasse, since it can be advanced that radiation and chemicals, certainly, cause chromosomal/gene damage, and it can be similarly advanced that viruses may also cause chromosome/gene damage. More than this, a virus is only a segment of protein of uncertain makeup and characteristics, and there are even subviruses called *prions.* There is a spectrum of phenomena that can be going on which may never be clearly understood.

In the meantime, we remain most concerned with cures or remissions, not causes, and further proceed on that basis. In anticipation, we therefore add a few comments.

- The biochemistry which relates to cancer cells and their proliferation, and to their treatment and remission, is connected to the twin subjects of enzymes and enzyme inhibitors. This will lead back to the subject of DNA, RNA, and protein synthesis, and the encoding of genetic information. Subliminally, there are such matters as whether genetic codes are time dependent—that is, is the inherited genetic code preprogrammed to initiate cancer at a certain time in a lifespan, or not? Or is there only an inherited genetic weakness, awaiting cause and effect? The questions always seem to outstrip the answers. Nevertheless, some of the factors known or surmised will be examined in terms of the biochemistry for this intricate and complex topic.

- First to be considered are the biochemical reactions connected with cell metabolism, and in particular the differences between normal cell metabolism and cancer cell metabolism. In these differences may lie a cure for cancer—that is, by inhibiting or breaking the enzyme-catalyzed reactions which are most associated with cancer growth. That is, the glycolysis rate for cancer cells is way above and beyond that required for normal cells and their respiration. The difference for the most part is aerobically converted to lactate or lactic acid, which must be recycled via the liver back to glucose or glycogen. In breaking this vicious cycle may lie a cancer cure. This is fundamentally the position taken by Nobel-Prize winner Otto Warburg when he first found this difference between cancer cell and normal cell metabolism. The only things that have changed is that the biochemical reactions occurring in cell metabolism are far more complicated and involved than originally thought. Accordingly, these metabolic processes will be first reviewed.

1.2 A DETAILING OF ENZYME-CATALYZED BIOCHEMICAL REACTIONS INVOLVED IN CELL METABOLISM

The term *metabolism* means the ways by which energy is supplied to cells, from which life and growth are sustained. It is fundamentally related to the processes of respiration and notably to the biochemical conversion of glucose. *Cell respiration* means oxygen intake or uptake—which translates to enzyme-catalyzed oxidation steps ultimately yielding carbon dioxide and water. (By *plant photosynthesis* we mean the opposite, the processes by which carbon dioxide and water are converted to organic material using sunlight as the photochemical energy source—the processes of which, by the way, are also enzyme-catalyzed.) The term *aerobic* is reserved for those conversions that are pronouncedly dependent on oxygen, whereas the term *anaerobic* refers to those conversions that are not overtly dependent on oxygen—though this is a matter of degree, since oxygen may be implicitly involved in one way or another. The term *fermentation* is sometimes employed to denote anaerobic biochemical conversions—but then there are so-called aerobic fermentations as well as anaerobic fermentations.

In any event, the projection is to cancer cells versus normal cells and to anaerobic behavior versus aerobic behavior. Enzymes are the catalysts necessary for all these varied biochemical reactions or conversions, and enzyme inhibitors may be used to affect the outcome. While glucose is regarded as the fundamental fuel, other carbohydrates may serve or be involved, even amines.

Thus, a more recent development concerns the role of glutamine in cancer metabolism. In other words, cancer metabolism is not confined to the conversion of glucose alone but may also involve glutamine, a nonessential amino acid (that is, glutamine can be produced internally by body processes). This aspect is examined for instance in a chapter by E. Eigenbrodt, P. Fister, and M. Reinacher titled "New Perspectives on Carbohydrate Metabolism in Tumor Cells," in Vol. II of *Regulation of Carbohydrate Metabolism*, edited by Rivka Beitner and published in 1985. The phenomenon is called *glutaminolysis,* as distinguished from glycolysis. Detailed flow diagrams are provided distinguishing the metabolic chemistry of tumors from normal cells and incorporating glutaminolysis into the loop.*

For the tricarboxylic acid cycle, the pathway is diagrammed by Karla L. Roehrig, *Carbohydrate Biochemistry and Metabolism*, p. 70; by Merle L. Olson, in *Textbook of Biochemistry with Clinical Correlations*, p. 280; and by Donald and Judith G. Voet, *Biochemistry*, p. 539. The end products from the cycle are carbon dioxide and water. The descriptor "tricarboxylic" is from the fact that successive organic acids are initially involved which contain three carboxyl groups (–COOH), starting with citric acid or a salt of citric acid (citrate).

The anaerobic conversion of pyruvic acid to lactic acid may or may not be included at the end of glycolysis. If so, the overall process may be called *anaerobic glycolysis* as distinguished from aerobic glycolysis. Aerobic glycolysis is completed by the tricarboxylic acid cycle, whereby pyruvic acid or pyruvate is in part converted or oxidized to carbon dioxide and water as the final end products, with the remainder recycled as oxaloacetic acid or oxaloacetate.

For glutaminolysis and its interface with the tricarboxylic acid cycle, a diagram is also furnished by Thomas L. Diamondstone, in *Textbook of Biochemistry with Clinical Correlations*, p. 608, and by Donald and Judith Voet, *Biochemistry*, p. 735. Also by Shank and Aprison in *Glutamine and Glutamate in Mammals*, Vol. II, p. 10; by N.P. Curthoys et al., in *Glutamine Metabolism in Mammalian Tissues*, p. 12; and by Merle L. Olson et al., in *The Regulation of Carbohydrate Formation and Utilization in Mammals*, p. 156. Other amino acids also metabolize, though glutamine is the predominant amino acid. (The subject area is rapidly expanding, and numerous recent references can be found by a computer search in MEDLINE.)

Based on the foregoing references, simplified representations, listing enzymes, are presented in Figs. 1.1 through 1.4 for (1) glycolysis to produce pyruvic acid or pyruvate, (2) the anaerobic conversion of pyruvate to lactate, (3) the interfacing with glutaminolysis, and last but not least (4) the aerobic tricarboxylic acid cycle oxidizing pyruvate. Each forward reaction step is denoted by an arrow ($\downarrow$). If the reaction is reversible, a double arrow ($\uparrow\downarrow$) is used.

We further distinguish between the acid and the "-ate" form. Thus, for example, pyruvic acid is $CH_3COCOOH$, which may dissociate or ionize in aqueous solutions as CH_3COCOO^- and H^+, the former

---

* A sampling of the more readily available technical literature reveals a number of detailed diagrammatic representations for glycolysis: e.g., by Karla L. Roehrig, *Carbohydrate Biochemistry and Metabolism*, pp. 64–65; by Robert A. Harris, in *Textbook of Biochemistry with Clinical Correlations*, p. 334; and by Donald and Judith G. Voet, *Biochemistry*, p. 446.

being the negatively charged pyruvate ion or anion, the latter being the positively charged hydrogen ion or cation. (That is, in the conventions of electric potential in terms of a voltage or emf difference, an anion is attracted to the positively charged anode, and a cation is attracted to the negatively charged cathode.) We may also speak of the salts of pyruvic acid, $CH_3COCOONa$, for instance being the sodium (Na) salt, or sodium pyruvate, which would dissociate in aqueous solutions as $CH_3COOCOO^-$ and Na^+. Consequently, the pyruvate group can be regarded as the more generic form. It would be understood that it carries a negative charge. However, it would be much simpler in some respects to carry the chemical equations through using the acid or –COOH form (which would simply be CH_3COOOH for pyruvic acid) such that the complete molecule is viewed as not carrying a net charge but rather is neutral. This is doubly true for the formation of lactic acid from pyruvic acid, vis à vis lactate from pyruvate, and is particularly so for the succession of compounds involved in the tricarboxylic acid cycle, associated with respiration, which will be examined subsequently.

Thus, each step in a reaction chain or loop involves an enzyme, as has been noted, many of which are indicated in the accompanying representations for glycolysis, pyruvic acid fermentation to form lactic acid or lactate, glutaminolysis, and the tricarboxylic acid cycle. Further specific information is found for instance in *Carbohydrate Metabolism*, edited by Willis A. Wood, and appearing as Vols. IX, XLI, XLII, 89, and 90 of the series *Methods in Enzymology*. Additional information appears in *Glutamate, Glutamine, Glutathione, and Related Compounds*, edited by Alton Meister, which is Vol. 113 in the series *Methods in Enzymology*. The series is up to 262 volumes at this writing. Information is also supplied about inhibitors for the specific enzymes. And speaking of enzyme inhibitors, there are comprehensive compilations extant. One, by Mahenda Kumar Jain, is titled *Handbook of Enzyme Inhibitors* (1967–1977), published in 1982. The other, by Helmward Zollner, first published in 1989, is also titled *Handbook of Enzyme Inhibitors*, with a revised edition published in 1993. J. Leyden Webb's *Enzyme and Metabolic Inhibitors*, in three volumes, was published in 1963 and 1966. A further, more detailed technical description of the phenomena involved is as follows.

It may be commented beforehand that the biochemical reactions displayed, and as complicated as they appear to be, are only stoichiometric conversions or material balances. A further analysis would get involved in such matters as reaction mechanisms, reaction equilibria, and reaction kinetics for each individual stoichiometric reaction or conversion, which may involve other consecutive and simultaneous reactions among the several component species. In turn, there are such matters as intermediate chemical or biochemical complexes and heat transfer and mass transfer rates between component species, including the biochemical catalyst species or enzymes. Ad infinitum. It is for these reasons that empiricism must come first; we simply cannot wait until all the theory is sorted out.

1.2.1 GLYCOLYSIS

Figure 1.1 shows in more detail the pathway for glycolysis to yield pyruvic acid or pyruvate, sometimes called the Embden-Meyerhoff-Parnas pathway. Other substances entering into glycolysis are:

ATP	Adenosine triphosphate
ADP	Adenosine diphosphate
P_i	Orthophosphate ion, in various ionization states
NAD^+	Nicotinamide adenine dinucleotide, oxidized form
NADH	Nicotinamide adenine dinucleotide, reduced form
H^+	Hydrogen, oxidized form, or hydrogen ion

The ions magnesium Mg^{++} and potassium K^+ are also present (Voet and Voet, *Biochemistry*, p. 446). Names used vary, e.g., hexose phosphateisomerase as phosphoglucose or phosphohexose isomerase. The simplified supporting or complementary reactions in Fig. 1.1 are further dealt with as follows.

Adenosine itself has the stoichiometric formula $C_{10}H_{13}N_5O_4$ with a structural formula representable as $H_2N–C_5H_2N_4–CO–C_3H_3(OH)_3$ $–CH_2–O–H$, or R–O–H, where R is defined by the substitution. The combining entity is the hydroxyl group –(OH), here designated –O–H, which may combine or bond with one, two, or three orthophosphate ions, which for the purposes here can be designated as the mono-hydrogen or mono-acid phosphate HPO_4^{2-} or $H–O–(PO_2^-)–O^-$.

Glucose

$$ATP \rightarrow ADP \downarrow \text{hexokinase} \tag{1}$$

Glucose-6-phosphate

$$\uparrow\downarrow \text{hexose phosphateisomerase} \tag{2}$$

Fructose-6-phosphate

$$ATP \rightarrow ADP \downarrow \text{phosphofructokinase} \tag{3}$$

Fructose-1, 6-bisphosphate

$$\uparrow\downarrow \text{adolase} \tag{4}$$

Glyceraldehyde-3-phosphate

$$\uparrow\downarrow \text{triosphosphate isomerase} \tag{5}$$

Dihydroxyacetone phosphate

Glyceraldehyde-3-phosphate

$$P_i + NAD^+ \rightarrow NADH + H^+ \uparrow\downarrow \text{glyceraldenyde-3-phosphate dehydrogenase} \tag{6}$$

1,3-Bisphosphoglycerate

$$ADP \rightarrow ATP \uparrow\downarrow \text{phosphoglycerate kinase} \tag{7}$$

3-Phosphoglycerate

$$\uparrow\downarrow \text{phosphoglyceromutase} \tag{8}$$

2-Phosphoglycerate

$$\uparrow\downarrow \text{enolase} \tag{9}$$

Phosphoenolpyruvate (plus H_2O)

$$ADP \rightarrow ATP \uparrow\downarrow \text{pyruvate kinase} \tag{10}$$

Pyruvate

Figure 1.1 Glycolysis conversion sequence yielding pyruvic acid or pyruvate, with enzymes listed. Based on information from Voet and Voet, *Biochemistry*, p. 446, and Harris, in *Textbook of Biochemistry*, p. 334.

Speaking first, therefore, of phosphates and phosphoric acids, there are three possibilities, with the following formulas: metaphosphoric acid, HPO_3; orthophosphoric acid, H_3PO_4, the commonly recognized, ordinary phosphoric acid of commerce; and pyrophosphoric acid, $H_4P_2O_7$. Considering orthophosphoric acid, the orthophosphate ion can be written as $(PO_4)^{3-}$ or simply as PO_4^{3-}, with a negative charge or valence of three. As the orthophosphoric acid molecule, the structure can be perceived as three hydrogen's linked to three oxygen's which are in turn connected to phosphorus, with the fourth oxygen connected to phosphorus by a double bond. That is, $(H–O–)_3 P=O$.

However, we can also speak of $H_2(HPO_4)$ where the mono-hydrogen or mono-acid orthophosphate ion HPO_4^{2-} has a negative charge of two. Or we can even of speak of $H(H_2PO_4)$, where the di-hydrogen or di-acid orthophosphate ion $H_2PO_4^-$ has a negative charge of unity. These mono-hydrogen and di-hydrogen orthophosphate ions can be regarded as successive oxidized states of the orthophosphate ion proper. The Voet and Voet reference accommodates this contingency, however, by using a generalized symbol P_i to designate the orthophosphate ion, or ions, with the qualification that it can exist in the necessary degree of ionization or oxidation, or ionic state.

In passing, observe furthermore that the metaphosphate ion PO_3^- has a negative charge of unity. And the pyrophosphate ion $P_2O_7^{4-}$ has a negative charge of four and can conceivably be written as the combination $(PO_4^{3-} + PO_3^-)$. Furthermore, the Voet and Voet reference utilizes the generalized symbol PPi for the pyrophosphate ion, again with the qualification that it can also exist in whatever ionization or oxidation state is required.

If adenosine, therefore, is viewed as combined or bonded with a single mono-hydrogen orthophosphate ion HPO_4^{2-}, the result is adenosine monophosphate or AMP, which in actuality denotes the adenosine monophosphate ion R–O– (PO_2^-)–O$^-$, with a total of two negative charges. (In this scenario, H_2O would a coproduct.) The ionic group (PO_2^-) can alternately be viewed as $(O=P–O^-)$ where the second oxygen is the source of the negative ionic charge, and it is the phosphorus which bonds with the oxygen's outside the group. This is in agreement that phosphorus has a valence of bonding capacity of five—that is, phosphorus is pentavalent.

In turn, if adenosine monophosphate is viewed as combined or bonded with a di-hydrogen ortho-phosphate ion $H_2PO_4^-$, the result is ADP, which is the adenosine diphosphate ion R–O–$(PO_2)^-$ –O–$(PO_2)^-$–O$^-$, which has three negative charges. (H_2O again would be a coproduct.)

If adenosine diphosphate is then viewed as combined or bonded with a di-hydrogen orthophosphate ion $H_2PO_4^{2-}$, the result is ATP, representable as the ion R–O–$(PO_2)^-$–O– $(PO_3)^-$–O– $(PO_2)^-$–O$^-$, which has four negative charges. (H_2O is a coproduct.)

By the conventions used,

$$AMP^{2-} + H_2(PO_3^-) \rightarrow ADP^{3-} + H_2O$$

which is in ionic balance. Also,

$$ADP^{3-} + H_2(PO_3^-) \rightarrow ATP^{4-} + H_2O$$

which is in ionic balance. On the other hand, adding to the previous equations,

$$AMP^{2-} + 2\ H_2(PO_3^-) \rightarrow ATP^{4-} + 2\ H_2O$$

As presented in Voet and Voet, the latter two expressions are reversible and read, respectively,

$$ADP + P_i \leftrightarrow ATP + H_2O$$
$$AMP + PP_i \leftrightarrow ATP + H_2O$$

where it should be again emphasized that the Voet and Voet reference stipulates that the symbol P_i can stand for any of the oxidation or ionization states, and similarly for PPi

As may also be noted as per reactions (1) and (3) and reactions (7) and (10) in Fig. 1.1, the ATP/ADP conversion can be viewed as reversible.

The apparently reversible ATP/ADP conversion provides a way to introduce phosphate and retrieve phosphate, and it is of profound metabolic significance. (It is also a way to introduce and retrieve H_2O.) By virtue of its apparent reversibility, the ATP/ADP conversion can be viewed as self-regenerative, internally regenerative, or auto-regenerative, not requiring an external regeneration cycle outside of the glycolysis pathway. (Albeit a different enzyme is required for the reverse reaction, as will be further explained.) In the conventions used, the negatively charged ionic entity involved may be written either as $[(PO_2^-)$–O$^-]$ or as (PO_3^{2-}) and is labeled the *phosphoryl group,* with the conversions called *phosphoryl-transfer reactions.*

Moreover, in Fig. 1.1 there is the supporting or complimentary reaction for reaction (6), which involves the oxidized and reduced form for nicotinamide adenine dinucleotide (NAD). The oxidized and reduced forms can be written as

$$NAD^+ R'–C_6H_4H–(C=O)–NH_2$$
$$NADH\ R'–C_6H_4H_2–(C=O)–NH_2$$

where the symbol R' represents a complicated structure involving adenosine and D-ribose, and the remainder corresponds to nicotinamide. However, the structure of the ring denoted by (C_6H_4H) changes for the conversion to $(C_6H_4H_2)$. If the bonds are covalent, however, then the acronym NAD$^+$ does not necessarily represent a positively charged ion. There has merely been a loss of hydrogen from the reduced form NADH. Be as it may, the conversion between the two forms may be portrayed as

$$NAD^+ + 2[H] \rightarrow NADH + H^+$$

where the hydrogen is furnished from another source. (It can be argued also that the hydrogen H^+ should not be represented in ionic form but in the free-hydrogen form [H]. such that $NAD^+ + [H] \rightarrow NADH$. Either way, it also comes out in the wash if both ionic forms are retained)

At the same time, as presented for reaction (6), there is a reaction involving P_i, which may be included in the totality as

$$P_i + NAD^+ \rightarrow NADH + H^+$$

where the participating orthophosphate ion P_i is so indicated in boldface. In fact, the orthophosphate ion P_i is transferred to the reactant glyceraldehyde-3-phosphate (GAP) to form 1,3-bisphosphoglycerate. (1-3-BPG) plus H_2O. This ionic transfer releases hydrogen for the above-indicated conversion of NAD^+ to NADH. That is, a di-hydrogen orthophosphate ion would convert to say the orthophosphate ion proper, that is $(H_2PO_4{}^{2-}) \rightarrow (PO_4{}^{4-})$. More precisely, we can speak of a further phosphorylation of GAP^-, which has one double negatively-charged phosphoryl group $(PO_3{}^-)$, to yield 1,3 bisphosphoglycerate or 1,3-BPG^{2-}, which has two double negatively-charged phosphoryl groups attached. Thus, it can be written that

$$GAP^{2-} + P_i{}^{2-} + NAD^+ \rightarrow 1,3\text{-}BPG^{4-} + NADH + H^+ + H_2O$$

which is in ionic balance (whether NAD and H are positively charged or not).

To complete the cycle, hydrogen would have to be furnished from another source to regenerate the P_i as di-hydrogen orthophosphate. This source presumably could be material that is dehydrogenated.

In a manner of speaking, therefore, the above becomes a way to retrieve hydrogen from another reaction, that is, to dehydrogenate. At the same time, there is provided a way to further introduce phosphate into the metabolic sequence. Once again, the life-sustaining role of phosphates is revealed.

The foregoing NAD^+/NADH conversion is not reversible nor regenerative within the glycolytic pathway proper. Thus, the NADH must eventually be regenerated, reconverted, or oxidized back to NAD^+ by other means outside the glycolytic pathway that results in pyruvic acid or pyruvate. This outside means or peripheral activity will involve the removal of hydrogen from the NADH. Somewhere, therefore—say in the mitochondria—there must also be oxidation occurring in support of the glycolytic pathway proper, that is, of glycolysis to yield pyruvic acid or pyruvate.

1.2.2 OXIDATION-REDUCTION REACTIONS

In the customary convention followed here, *oxidation* will pertain to the removal of negative charges from an ionic, atomic, or molecular entity, whereas *reduction* will pertain to the addition of negative charges to an ionic, atomic, or molecular entity. That is, with oxidation, the entity becomes less negatively charged; with reduction, the entity becomes more negatively charged.

It may be further generalized that the negative charge may also be carried by an ionic, atomic, or molecular entity itself, which serves as the medium of transfer for the negative charge. The ionic, atomic, or molecular entity is in fact the embodiment for the negative charge. A negative charge embodied as an electron (or electrons) per se needs no carrier for transfer.

The oxidizing agent performing the oxidation can be referred to as an *electron* or *negative-charge receptor* and is thereby in itself reduced. Conversely, the reducing agent performing the reduction is referred to as an *electron* or *negative-charge donor* and is in itself oxidized. Thus, both oxidation and reduction always occur simultaneously, and the collective phenomena are known as *redox reactions*.

The best known examples of simple oxidation involve the reaction of free oxygen with say a metal to form a metallic oxide in an ionic sort of relationship. For simple reduction, hydrogen is regarded as the ubiquitous reducing agent. Thus, hydrogen will reduce a metallic oxide back to the metallic state, forming H_2O in the process.

In, say, a metallic oxide, an ionic bond exists where there is no sharing of orbital electrons between the component species. In organic chemistry, notably, there exist what may be called covalent bonds in which orbital electrons are viewed as shared between the species, say between hydrogen and a carbonaceous entity. Here the connotations of oxidation and reduction become more ambiguous if there is no clear distinction for who is doing what to whom. In a way of looking at it, for example, both hydrogen and the carbonaceous entity would be contributing electrons to be shared.

1.2.3   PHOSPHATE IONS AS OXIDIZING AND REDUCING AGENTS

The di-hydrogen orthophosphate ion ($H_2PO_4^-$) can be viewed as an oxidizing agent, whereby it is itself reduced to form (HPO_4^{2-}) or even (PO_4^{3-}). That is to say, the di-hydrogen orthophosphate ion acquires additional negative electrical charges by making another entity more positive. This latter function can be viewed either as furnishing positively charged hydrogen ions H^+ or as furnishing free hydrogen [H] while making some other atomic or molecular entity positively charged.

On the other hand, di-hydrogen orthophosphate can be viewed as a reducing agent by contributing a negative ionic group to another molecular entity. Thus, AMP^{2-} is reduced to ATP^{3-} by the phosphorylating action of ($H_2PO_4^-$), whereby

$$ADP^{3-} + (H_2PO_4^-) \rightarrow ATP^{4-} + H_2O$$

and it can be said that $H_2(PO_3^-)$ itself is oxidized to H_2O. That is, it loses its negative charge.

Therefore, the addition of a phosphoryl group (PO_3^{2-}) to a molecular entity can be viewed as a reduction of that molecular entity, in that the entity as a whole will then have a greater negative charge. Conversely, the subtraction of a phosphoryl group can be viewed as oxidation, since the molecular entity will then have a smaller negative charge. Another example is that the addition of phosphoryl group reduces GAP to 1,3 GPD, whereas the subtraction of a phosphoryl group oxidizes 1,3-GPD to GAP.

1.2.4   THE TRANSPORT AND BINDING ROLE OF ENZYMES

Described in terms of heterogeneous catalysis, the enzyme itself would serve as the scene for catalytic activity. Heterogeneous catalysis is generally described in terms of the transport of reactants to the catalyst surface, reaction at the surface active sites, and transport of the products away from the surface. When equilibrium is reached, there is a buildup of products such that no net driving forces exist furthering the conversion.

The qualifier may be interjected, however, that if a new heterogeneous catalyst is introduced into the reacting system, the reactions will proceed in other directions, yielding different products (conceivably even in the reverse direction). A new equilibrium condition could eventually be reached, involving different components or constituents. In other words, the total nature of the reacting system has been changed.

On the other hand, although called catalysts or enzyme-catalysts, enzymes may perform a different sort of role—that of transport or transfer. That is, enzymes may serve as carriers for a reactant, e.g., the orthophosphoric ionic entity P_i in one or another of its oxidation states (also designatable as the phosphoryl group). Considering reaction (1) for example, the enzyme hexokinase transports the ion designated P_i from the ATP molecular entity to the glucose molecule, whereby the ATP then becomes ADP. In reaction (10), an entirely different enzyme named pyruvate kinase transports P_i from phosphoenolpyruvate to ADP, which them becomes ATP.

In other instances, a reactant or substrate is perceived as binding to an enzyme at an "active" site whereby a conversion of the reactant occurs. This can be viewed as the case for instance when a so-called supporting or complimentary reaction is not involved. This also corresponds to the idea of a surface reaction in conventional heterogeneous catalysis theory. The Voet and Voet reference provides ample descriptions for these kinds of reactions during glycolysis. In net sum, enzymes may provide both a reactant transport function and a binding/activation function with a reactant.

1.2.5   ENZYME NOMENCLATURE VS. FUNCTION

For the record, the enzymes used are classified by their functions (J. Lyndal York, in *Textbook of Biochemistry*, pp. 139–145). The classes are as follows: oxidoreductases, which include dehydrogenases; transferases, which include kinases; hydrolases; lyases, which include decarboxylases, dehydratases, and synthases; isomerases; and ligases, which include synthetases and carboxylases.

Dehydrogenases, for example, act first to remove hydrogen from one group and transfer it to NAD or, in another way of speaking, transfer electrons from one group to another, whereby NAD^+ is converted to $NADH + H^+$. Kinases involve the transfer of the phosphorylating group, say P_i, from ATP or another nucleotide triphosphate, to various acceptors. At the same time, ATP converts to ADP. Hydrolases involve reaction with H_2O. Decarboxylases remove CO_2 from various organic acids. Dehydratases remove H_2O in a dehydration reaction. Synthases remove a group to form a double bond, that is to form say –HC=CH–.

Isomerases convert one molecular form or structure to another, both having the same stoichiometric formula, being called *isomers* of one another. Synthetases pertains to enzymes which join two molecules at the expense of the ATP *high-energy phosphate bond,* whereby ATP becomes ADP + P_i. Carboxylases add CO_2 to form organic acids and at the same time are supported by the ATP conversion.

The designator polymerase indicates that the enzyme catalyses monomer molecules into forming a polymer, say by removing H_2O or some other molecular entity or group from between molecules, by one or another of the foregoing type reactions. Further and more complete information can be obtained from *Enzyme Nomenclature*, published by Academic Press, or from *Enzymes*, by M. Dixon and E.C. Webb, also published by Academic Press.

For more details on the particular enzymatic actions involved in, say, glycolysis, the Voet and Voet reference may be consulted. Thus, action of the enzyme hexokinase in reaction (1) is to transfer phosphoryl groups from ATP to the metabolite, substrate, or reactant, e.g., glucose. As previously indicated, in this case, the action is not catalysis of chemical reactions in the stricter sense of the word but rather is that of ionic transport. Other catalytic effects involve the binding of a reactant to the enzyme at an active site, accompanied by reaction or conversion at the site. And each successful explanation or answer raises a new question for these complex phenomena.

1.2.6 CLOSING THE BALANCES

The reaction relationships of Fig. 1.1 are not necessarily balanced as they appear, depending on the ionic charge assigned to P_i. An exhaustive analysis is provided in the references previously cited (Voet and Voet, *Biochemistry*, p. 443ff.; Harris, in *Textbook of Biochemistry*, p. 325ff). An overall balance is as follows, which includes all supportive reaction components, with the glucose converted in its entirety to pyruvate (Voet and Voet, *Biochemistry*, p. 445):

$$\text{Glucose } (C_6H_{12}O_6) + 2\,NAD^+ + 2\,ADP^{2-} + 2\,P_i^{2-} \rightarrow 2\,NADH + 2\,\text{Pyruvate } (C_3H_4O_3^-) + 2\,ATP^{4-} + 2\,H_2O + 4\,H^+$$

Inasmuch as each pyruvate ion or anion CH_3COCOO^- carries a negative charge, this will fulfill the ionic balance. The fact that H_2O appears on the right hand side of the equation is an indication that an oxidative source is implicit in the conversion.

Observe that in Fig. 1.1 the reaction stoichiometry is displayed as if half of the glucose is converted only to dihydroxyacetone phosphate (DHAP), and the other half is converted to glyceraldehyde 3-phosphate (GAP), with the GAP further converted to pyruvate ($C_3H_4O_3^-$) or to pyruvic acid ($C_3H_5O_3$).

In a way of speaking, the glucose at least in part has been dehydrogenated to pyruvic acid or pyruvate by the action of the NAD^+ supportive conversion above.

If converted in totality to pyruvate, the overall conversion can be viewed simply as

$$\text{Glucose } (C_6H_{12}O_6) \rightarrow 2\,\text{Pyruvic acid } (C_3H_4O_3) + 4\,[H]$$

where 4 [H] enters into the supportive reactions. In other words, glucose has been dehydrogenated to pyruvate or pyruvic acid.

It is further noted that the oxidizing power of the NAD^+ must be recycled (Voet and Voet, *Biochemistry*, pp. 445–446). That is, the NAD^+ must be regenerated from NADH. This is done in three ways.

1. Under anaerobic conditions in muscle, NADH reduces pyruvate to lactate by homolactic fermentation, and is itself oxidized.
2. In yeast fermentation under anaerobic conditions, the pyruvate is converted to acetaldehyde, then by NADH to ethanol, whereby the NADH is oxidized.
3. At aerobic conditions, each NADH is oxidized directly to yield three ATPs.

The glycotic pathway is affected by such *poisons* as 2-deoxyglucose, sulfhydril reagents, and *fluoride* (Harris, in *Textbook of Biochemistry*, p. 346). Fluoride is a potent inhibitor of enolase, the enzyme for reaction (9) in glycolysis, as per Fig. 1.1.

Overall, the aerobic conversion of glucose to pyruvate and then to CO_2 and H_2O by the mitochondrial processing of pyruvate can be represented as follows—borrowing from the references—where here oxygen is introduced directly into the equation (Harris, in *Textbook of Biochemistry*, p. 328):

$$\text{D-glucose } (C_6H_{12}O_6) + 6\ O_2 + 38\ ADP^{3-} + 38\ P_i^{2-} + 38\ H^+ \rightarrow 6\ CO_2 + 44\ H_2O + 38\ ATP^{4-}$$

where $38\ P_i^{2-} + 38\ H^+ \rightarrow 38\ P_i^-$. Furthermore, $38\ ADP^{3-} + 38\ P_i^- \rightarrow 38\ ATP^{4-} + 38\ H_2O$.

The above equation is in ionic balance. However, it is required that the ATP^{4-} be converted back to $ADP^{3-} + (P_i^{2-} + H^+)$ or $ADP^{3-} + P_i^-$ to sustain the cycle. This is expectedly accomplished by the hydrolysis of ATP^{4-} (Devlin, in *Textbook of Biochemistry*, pp. 245–246):

$$38\ ATP^{4-} + 38\ H_2O \rightarrow 38\ ADP^{3-} + 38\ P_i^-$$

This hydrolysis reaction will require a different enzyme. Also according to the references, Na^+, Mg^{2+}, and K^+ ions are involved.

On the other hand, the anaerobic conversion of glucose to lactate or lactic acid may be represented as follows (Voet and Voet, *Biochemistry*, p. 594):

$$C_6H_{12}O_6 + 2\ ADP^{3-} + 2\ P_i^- \rightarrow 2\ \text{lactate } (C_3H_5O_2^-) + 2\ (H^+) + 2\ H_2O + 2\ ATP^{4-}$$

The equation is in ionic balance.

Aerobic glycolysis to produce CO_2 and H_2O as the final end-products is represented in the Voet and Voet reference as

$$C_6H_{12}O_6 + 38\ ADP^{3-} + 38\ P_i^- + 6\ O_2 \rightarrow 6\ CO_2 + 44\ H_2O + 38\ ATP^{4-}$$

where again $38\ ADP^{3-} + 38\ P_i^- \rightarrow 38\ ATP^{4-} + 38\ H_2O$. The above equation is in ionic balance as represented, provided P_i has a negative charge of unity and agrees with the previously stated result for aerobic glycolysis.

As per the foregoing, it may be noted that there is a great increase in ATP production in going from anaerobic glycolysis to aerobic glycolysis, which is confirmed by the above relations. Furthermore, the activity of phosphofructokinase or phosphofructosekinase (PFK), the enzyme which controls glycolysis by regulating the subsequent citrate- and adenosine nucleotide-steps, decreases sharply when switching from anaerobic to aerobic metabolism. This accounts for the pronounced drop in the glycolysis rate under aerobic conditions.

1.2.7   OVERALL HEAT OF REACTION

The standard heat of reaction or heat of combustion for the complete oxidation of D-glucose, neglecting any supportive reactions, is as follows, in different units:*

- 673 kcal per gram-mole
- 673,000 cal per gram-mole
- 1,211,400 Btu per lb-mole

Or, in other words,

$$C_6H_{12}O_6\ (s) + 9\ O_2 \rightarrow 6\ CO_2 + 6\ H_2O\ (l) \quad \Delta H_o = -673.0 \text{ kcal/g-mole}$$

where the negative value for the standard heat of reaction ΔH_o denotes the fact that the reaction is exothermic, that is, gives off heat. The designators (s) and (l) denote that the substance is in the solid or liquid state, whereas it is understood that both O_2 and CO_2 are in the gaseous (g) state. Since the molecular weight of glucose is 180, the value on a mass or weight basis is about 3.7 kcal/g or 3700 calories per gram, as compared to carbon, which is about 7800 calories per gram (or 14,000 Btu/lb). The above figure will be of further utility in comparing the heat of reaction for aerobic glycolysis with that of anaerobic glycolysis, wherein lactic acid is produced.†

---

* The value is taken from O.A. Hougen, K.M. Watson, and R.A. Ragatz, *Chemical Process Principles, Part I, Material and Energy Balances*, 2d ed., John Wiley & Sons, New York, 1943, 1954, p. 307.

1.2.8 SPONTANEOUS HUMAN COMBUSTION (SHC)

This weird phenomenon is given occasional publicity (e.g., as reported in *Arthur C. Clarke's Mysterious Universe*, shown or reshown on the Discovery Channel, October 22, 1996, and, as noted, is mentioned in Charles Dickens' *Bleak House*). If such does indeed occur, it might be better referred to as spontaneous ignition, followed by combustion. Without passing judgement, the remark can be made that it is at least conceivable for malfunctions to occur among the enzymes involved in the metabolism of glucose or other carbohydrates to CO_2 and H_2O. Normally, the metabolic reaction rates are very slow as compared to combustion or combustive oxidation. If promoters should act on the enzymes, however, or the normal action of enzyme inhibitors or modulators does not control and limit the rate of conversion, then it can be inferred that the metabolic processes may be accelerated, and runaway metabolic reaction rates could occur, as in the ignition and further combustion of combustibles. This would of course be dependent upon an adequate oxygen supply. It can be surmised that there might be enough oxygen already present in the body to initiate ignition; further combustion presumably would require the transport or diffusion of outside air to the ignition site(s). (Combustible hydrogen may also be produced as a reaction intermediate by the steam-reforming of body combustibles.) This is all speculative, but it provides a scenario of sorts.

As a further comment about the spontaneous combustion of organic materials, it is a well known fact that rags soaked in linseed oil, or even paints and varnishes, can spontaneously ignite and combust if the heat from low-grade oxidation (the heat of combustion) is not dissipated. For this reason, such rags are stored in air-tight containers prior to disposal or spread out so that the heat can be dissipated. Low-rank coals, especially, are also prone to spontaneously ignite and combust, and coal storage piles require monitoring. And some of these low-rank coals, when dried in a sized-reduced or pulverized condition, are pyrophoric—that is, will burst into flame when exposed to the air. Brazil nuts, of the Brazil-nut tree, species *Bertholletica excelsa* of the family Lecythidaceae, are prone to spontaneous ignition and combustion when stored. Accordingly, piles of the nuts have to be raked and turned to dissipate the heat. Thus, spontaneous ignition and combustion is not that uncommon.

Returning to the human body system, it is if course a given that the immune response can cause the body temperature to rise, to produce what is otherwise known as a feverous condition. This involves reducing the heat normally dissipated to the surroundings. If one should wish to put numbers on the normal heat dissipation, either directly or indirectly as with kinetic exercise, consider the average daily caloric intake. For each 1000 nutritional calories per day, which is really in thermal kilocalories (kcal), this amounts to 1,000,000 thermal calories per day, or 3.9657(1000/24) = 165.24 Btu/hr of heat that has to be dissipated in one way or another. For 2000 nutritional calories per day, the figure would be double that, or 330.48 Btu/hr.

If this considerable heat rate were not dissipated, the body temperature would rise inordinately. For example, over an hour's time, considering the average specific heat of the body in its entirety to be 0.25 Btu/lb/°F, the hourly energy balance for a 150-pound person, rated at 2000 nutritional calories per day, would be 330.48 = 150(0.25)(ΔT) where ΔT is the hourly rise in temperature produced by the undissipated heat. The value of ΔT calculates to a 0.55° F (degrees Fahrenheit) rise in body temperature per hour. For a 24-hour period, this would produce a 13.2 degree rise, for a body temperature of say 98.6 + 13.2 = 111.8° F, which is already well beyond the fever limit of approximately 105° F. And so forth, with kindling temperatures for some raw organic solids such as low-grade coal or lignite set as low as circa 300° F, depending.

Parenthetically, the concepts of flash point, kindling temperature, and ignition temperature are not necessarily precise and depend on the physical configuration of the system and other factors. Furthermore, the actual constituents that combust are the gases that are evolved during the heating, or thermal degradation or pyrolysis, of the solid or liquid carbonaceous material. The exact nature of the gases evolved—which include hydrocarbons, carbon monoxide and carbon dioxide, and hydrogen—is influenced by the presence of moisture, which favors eminently combustible hydrogen. That is, hydrogen is in part formed by reactions with the carbonaceous constituents via so-called *reforming reactions*. And some of the more volatile gases will have flash points lower even than ambient temperature, the flash point being the temperature at which the gases ignite when a flame—or spark—is introduced. Thus, it

---

† It may be commented in passing the kcal (kilocalorie) is what is ordinarily called a "calorie" in rating the caloric content of foodstuffs. That is, a food calorie is 1000 times as large as a conventional science or engineering calorie.

is at least conceivable for effluxing body gases to be ignited from an external source. Ordinarily, the ignition temperature refers to the temperature at which spontaneous combustion will be sustained—that is, the heat of reaction is greater than the heat of dissipation. The term "kindling temperature" more or less means the ignition temperature, but not necessarily. For these reasons, the American Society of Testing and Materials (ASTM) has instituted standardized tests whereby the configuration and conditions are the same in each test. However, other systems and conditions will expectedly deviate from these kinds of empirical standardized results.

Looking at the situation in another way, for each pound of combustible material in the body—fat, carbohydrate, and protein—let the average heating value or heat of combustion be, say, 7000 Btu/lb—equivalent to wood or low-grade coal—and the specific heat be 0.25 Btu/lb/°F. Accordingly, neglecting heat dissipation entirely, the theoretical energy balance for producing a rise in body temperature via the heat of combustion would be $7000 = 0.25(T - 98.6)$ where T is the final temperature and 98.6° F is the normal body temperature. Clearly, the final theoretical temperature T or temperature difference $T - 98.6$ would reach astronomical proportions, whereby this hypothetical difference so calculates to 28,000° F. This is of course an anomaly, but it illustrates that there is a potential for spontaneous combustion if body heat dissipation falls off and a sufficient oxygen source is available.

1.2.9 LACTIC ACID OR LACTATE

As per Fig. 1.2, pyruvic acid pyruvate may be converted to lactic acid or lactate, a process sometimes called *homolactic fermentation*. The catalyst is the enzyme lactate dehydrogenase, which may exist in several forms. The stoichiometric conversion of pyruvate to lactate is as follows:

$$CH_3COCOO^- + [2H] \rightarrow CH_3CH(OH)COO^-$$

which is supported by (from Voet and Voet, *Biochemistry*, pp. 464, 568)

$$NADH + H^+ \rightarrow NAD^+ + 2\,[H]$$

Interestingly enough, this is the reverse of the supportive reaction for reaction (6) as denoted for glycolysis.

Overall, the conversion can be viewed as

$$CH_3COCOO^- + NADH + H^+ \rightarrow CH_3CH(OH)COO^- + NAD^+$$

where the positive ionic charges balance the negative charges. It may also be noted that

$$P_i + NAD^+ \rightarrow NADH + H^+$$

where P_i is used to denote the fact that hydrogen can be produced via the ADP/ATP conversions as noted previously for glycolysis.

Accordingly, the conversion can alternately be viewed as

$$CH_3COCOO^- + P_i \rightarrow CH_3CH(OH)COO^- + NAD^+$$

where P_i signals an involvement between ADP and ATP, as previously described. Thus, the orthophosphate ion or phosphorylation is also involved, another example of the ubiquity of phosphate.

Pyruvate

$NADH + H^+ \rightarrow NAD^+ + 2[H] \downarrow$ lactate dehydrogenase

Lactate

Figure 1.2 Anaerobic conversion of pyruvic acid or pyruvate to lactic acid or lactate. Based on information from Voet and Voet, *Biochemistry*, p. 464, and Harris, in *Textbook of Biochemistry*, p. 334.

Even though the conversion is considered anaerobic, there must be an oxygen source or an oxidizing source from somewhere, since it is required that an oxygen source drive the conversion.

$$NADH + H^+ + [O] \rightarrow NAD^+ + H_2O$$

A more complete statement of the overall conversion would then be

$$CH_3COCOO^- + NADH + H^+ + [O] \rightarrow CH_3CH(OH)COO^- + NAD^+ + H_2O$$

This oxidative source may be ascribed as involving what are called the mitochondria, the sites of cellular respiration, located in the eukaryotic cells or eukaryotes (Voet and Voet, *Biochemistry*, pp. 9, 464, 569).

Alternately, regeneration can be perceived as occurring in the supporting reaction for reaction (6) in the glycolytic pathway.

With different enzymes (from yeast), aldehyde is first produced (the enzyme is pyruvate decarboxylase), then ethyl alcohol or ethanol (the enzyme is alcohol dehydrogenase), and the process is called *anaerobic alcoholic fermentation* (Voet and Voet, *Biochemistry*, pp. 464–470). If starches are used as the raw material, as in a mash composed of crushed grains, the starches must first be converted to sugars via the enzyme amylase, obtainable from young barley sprouts via what is known as the *malting* process.

Regarding the formation of lactic acid or lactate, a buildup of lactic acid in body tissues is called lactic acidosis (Harris, in *Textbook of Biochemistry*, pp. 357–358). Ordinarily the lactic acid is oxidized to CO_2 and H_2O or else converted back to glucose by gluconeogenesis. Decreased oxygen availability, however, will both increase lactate production and decrease lactate utilization. *Bicarbonate* can be administered to help control the acidosis accompanying lactic acid accumulation.

1.2.10 EUKARYOTIC AND PROKARYOTIC CELLS

The subject of eukaryotic cells has been introduced. In brief review, without trying to dig much deeper into the subject at this time, and based on the exposition presented for instance in Chapter 1 of *Biochemistry* by Voet and Voet, all cells may be divided into prokaryotes and eukaryotes. The former include the bacteria. The latter, which are a thousand to a million times larger in volume, are much more complex. Each such cell is a profusion of membrane-enclosed organelles, each organelle with a special function, and all bound together by a plasma membrane. The organelle that is the eukaryotic cell's nucleus is the repository of its genetic information encoded in the enormous number of DNA molecules that in turn make up the discrete number of chromosomes characteristic of each species. Enter, of course, the matter of "genes" somehow, in an abstract sense, being hereditary units of action or function, about which there is apparently not a complete consensus. In any event, each such unit evidently can be shown to occupy a specific locus in a chromosome, and a gene may change into different forms called *alleles,* the fundamental basis for mutations. And so on, as if we really know what we're talking about.

Nevertheless, it is observed that there is a close connection between what is called gene action and enzyme activity. For example, many mutant genes are related to the disappearance or inactivation of specific enzymes. If the absence of an enzyme causes a biochemical reaction to be blocked, and its absence is inherited, the block is called a *genetic block.* The inference is obvious: there may be a connection favoring enzyme-catalyzed cancer cell metabolism vis à vis enzyme-catalyzed normal cell metabolism.

Another phenomenon that occurs is called *gene amplification,* in which the gene action or activity is reinforced many times over, which may also appear as a reinforcement of enzyme activity.

1.2.11 OVERALL HEAT OF REACTION

The standard heat of reaction for the overall conversion of glucose to lactic acid, neglecting side reactions, is of comparative interest. This may be referred to as *anaerobic glycolysis,* as compared to *aerobic glycolysis* as per the preceding section. The value for the standard heat of reaction for the combustion of lactic acid is as follows, in different units:*

---

* The value is again taken from O.A. Hougen, K.M. Watson, and R.A. Ragatz, *Chemical Process Principles, Part I. Material and Energy Balances*, 2d ed., John Wiley & Sons, New York, 1943, 1954, p. 307.

- 325.8 kcal per gram-mole
- 325,800 calories per gram-mole
- 586,440 Btu per lb-mole

For two moles of lactic acid reacting, the heat of combustion would thus be –651.6 kcalories per gram-mole. Or, in other words,

$$2 \ C_3H_6O_3 \ (s) + 9 \ O_2 \rightarrow 6 \ CO_2 + 6 \ H_2O \ (l) \quad \Delta H_o = -651.6 \ \text{kcal/g-mole}$$

From the previous section, for aerobic glycolysis,

$$C_6H_{12}O_6 \ (s) + 9 \ O_2 \rightarrow 6 \ CO_2 + 6 \ H_2O \ (l) \quad \Delta H_o = -673.0 \ \text{kcal/g-mole}$$

Subtracting the first equation from the second equation, above, will yield

$$C_6H_{12}O_6 \ (s) \rightarrow 2 \ C_3H_6O_3 \ (s) \qquad \Delta H_o = -21.400 \ \text{kcal/g-mole}$$

Thus, ideally at least, the anaerobic conversion of glucose to lactic acid is slightly exothermic. The inference is that not much metabolic energy results, and that the anaerobic glycolysis rate must increase markedly in order to support bodily energy requirements. At the most, the increase could by 673/21.4 = 31 times as much. This would of course be offset by the fact that part (or maybe most) of the lactic acid is recycled through the liver to be reconverted to glucose (or glycogen). It is interesting to note, however, that as cited elsewhere, anaerobic glycolysis rates have been detected which are twenty times aerobic glycolysis rates (Harris, in *Textbook of Biochemistry*, p. 353). An ancillary effect is that the body loses weight as it uses up stored energy reserves in order to meet energy requirements which cannot otherwise be supported by aerobic glycolysis.

1.2.12 GLYCOGEN

Speaking of glycogen and its synthesis and degradation, the regulatory enzymes are glycogen synthase and glycogen phosphorylase, respectively, which are correspondingly activated by glucose 6-phosphate and adenosine monophosphate or AMP (Harris, in *Textbook of Biochemistry*, p. 391ff). These are in turn regulated by cAMP, which stands for 3',5'-cyclic adenosine monophosphate. It is reported, furthermore, that in acting as a hormone regulator, *cAMP also acts as a cancer inhibitor*, which has been verified by *in vitro* and *in vivo* studies (Boik, *Cancer & Natural Medicine*, p. 48). Moreover, arginine was found to assist. The enzyme cAMP phosphodiesterase degenerates cAMP.

It can also be mentioned that the Gold therapy (of the Syracuse Research Institute, Syracuse, NY) advances hydrazine sulfate as an anticancer agent. It is said to inhibit the enzyme responsible for the re-formation of glycogen in the liver, and thereby can be presumed to act against the formation of lactic acid or lactate.

1.2.13 cAMP LEVELS

If there are agents that inhibit cAMP levels, there are also agents that elevate cAMP levels—that is, may act against cancer. Among the natural agents cited in the Boik reference which raise cAMP levels are the species *Andrographis paniculata* (of the plant family Acanthaceae), *Polyporus umbellatus* (of the fungal family Polyporaceae), *Salvia multiorrhiza* (of the plant family Labiatae), *Ziziphus jujuba* (of the plant family Rhamnaceae), *Cnidium monnieri* (of the plant family Umbelliferae), *Actinidia chinensis* (of the plant family Actinidiaceae), *Aconitum carmichaeli* (of the plant family Ranunculaceae), *Cinnamomum cassia* (of the plant family Lauracae), and the alkaloid caffeine. Hartwell's *Plants Used Against Cancer* lists all save for the genera *Andrographis* and *Actinidia* and their corresponding plant families.

1.2.14 GLUTAMINOLYSIS

An abbreviated reaction scenario for glutaminolysis is shown in Fig. 1.3. The subject of glutaminolysis is only part of the more general undertaking of the metabolism of amino acids. The latter topic is covered for instance by Thomas I. Diamondstone in successive chapters titled "Amino Acid Metabolism I: General

Glutamine ($\leftarrow H_2O$ added)

↓ glutaminase

Glutamate ($\rightarrow NH_3$ released)

↓ glutamate dehydrogenase

Oxoglutarate or **α-Ketoglutarate**

↓ 2-oxoglutarate or α-ketoglutarate dehydrogenase

Succinate

↓ succinate dehydrongenase

Malate

↓ malate dehydrogenase

Pyruvate   **Oxaloacetate**

↓   ↓

Lactate   **Aspartate**

Figure 1.3 Glutaminolysis interfacing with tricarboxylic acid cycle. Based on information from Eigenbrodt et al., in *Regulation of Carbohydrate Metabolism*, pp. 145, 153; Voet and Voet, *Biochemistry*, p. 741; and Diamondstone, in *Textbook of Biochemistry*, p. 583. Under carbohydrate or glucose limitation, all lactate will be produced from glutamine rather than from glucose via glycolysis.

Pathways," and "Amino Acid Metabolism II: Metabolism of the Individual Amino Acids," in *Textbook of Biochemistry with Clinical Correlations*, edited by Thomas M. Devlin; and by Donald and Judith G. Voet in a chapter titled "Amino Acid Metabolism," in their volume *Biochemistry*.

That cancer cell metabolism may be supported by glutaminolysis, and aminolysis in general is an additional complication in attempting to suppress cancer growth.

1.2.15 TRICARBOXYLIC ACID CYCLE

The tricarboxylic acid cycle is of course the more desirable way for the utilization of the pyruvic acid or pyruvate obtained from glycolysis in normal cells. Also called the citric acid cycle, or Krebs cycle, organic acids are involved that have three carboxylic groups per molecule, hence the name. The carboxylic group is designated either as $-(C=O)-OH$ or preferably as $-COOH$. An example is citric acid, representable as $HOC(CH_2COOH)_2COOH$.

In the schematic diagram of Fig. 1.4, there is a substance called coenzyme A or CoA that enters into the tricarboxylic acid cycle. Necessary to the initiation of the cycle, it is found in other body processes such as involving fatty acids and so forth. Its makeup is diagrammed in most biochemistry textbooks (for instance, by Merle L. Olson, in *Textbook of Biochemistry*, p. 270; and by Donald and Judith G. Voet, *Biochemistry*, p. 826). It may be regarded as a combination of β-mercaptoethylamine, pantothenic acid, adenine, and D-ribose (Olson, in *Textbook of Biochemistry*, p. 270). It is biosynthesized starting with pantothenic acid with, in a succession of reactions, each catalyzed by the designated enzyme (Diamondstone, in *Textbook of Biochemistry*, p. 671; and Voet and Voet, *Biochemistry*, p. 826). As such, it may be considered as existing also in the thio (–SH) form, that is, with sulfur and hydrogen attached, and be written as CoASH. Replacement of the (H) above with the acetyl group ($CH_3CO–$) yields acetyl-CoA, which could as well be written as acetyl-CoAS or acetyl-SCoA. In other words, the sulfur content is carried through the subsequent reactions.

The foregoing indicates how vital pantothenic acid is to normal aerobic metabolism. More than this, it may conceivably offset the anaerobic metabolism associated with cancer and thereby act as an anticancer agent.

In the presence of the pyruvate dehydrogenase multienzyme complex, pyruvic acid or pyruvate reacts with CoASH to form acetyl-CoA and CO_2, by what is called oxidative decarboxylation (Olson, in *Textbook of Biochemistry*, 269ff). At the same time, NAD^+ is converted to $NADH + H^+$. That is, according to the references, starting with say pyruvic acid,

$$\textbf{Pyruvate} \text{ plus CoASH}$$

$$NAD^+ \rightarrow NADH + H^+ \downarrow \text{pyruvate dehydrogenase (PDH) multienzyme complex}$$

$$\textbf{Acetyl-CoA} \text{ (and } CO_2 \text{ released)}$$

$$\textbf{Oxaloacetate} \text{ (recycled) plus } \textbf{Acetyl-CoA} \text{ plus } H_2O \text{ less CoASH}$$

$$\downarrow \text{citrate synthetase} \tag{1}$$

$$\textbf{Citrate} \text{ (} \rightarrow H_2O \text{ released)}$$

$$\downarrow \text{aconitase (} \rightarrow H_2O \text{ released)} \tag{2}$$

$$\textbf{cis-Aconitrate}$$

$$\downarrow \text{aconitase (} \leftarrow H_2O \text{ added)} \tag{2}$$

$$\textbf{Isocitrate}$$

$$NAD^+ \rightarrow NADH + H^+ \downarrow \text{isocitrate dehydrogenase} \tag{3}$$

$$\textbf{Oxalosuccinate}$$

$$\downarrow \text{isocitrate dehydrogenase (} \rightarrow \textbf{CO}_2 \text{ released)} \tag{3}$$

$$\textbf{α-Ketoglutarate}$$

$$NAD^+ \rightarrow NADH + H^+ \downarrow \text{a-ketoglutarate dehydrogenase (} \leftarrow \text{CoASH; } \rightarrow \textbf{CO}_2\text{)} \tag{4}$$

$$\textbf{Succinyl-CoA} \text{ (} \leftarrow \text{CoASH added)}$$

$$GDP + Pi \rightarrow GTP \downarrow \text{succinyl CoA-synthetase (} \rightarrow \text{CoASH released)} \tag{5}$$

$$\textbf{Succinate}$$

$$FAD \rightarrow FADH2 \downarrow \text{succinate dehydrogenase} \tag{6}$$

$$\textbf{Fumarate}$$

$$\downarrow \text{fumarase (} \leftarrow H_2O \text{ added)} \tag{7}$$

$$\textbf{Malate}$$

$$NAD^+ \rightarrow NADH + H^+ \downarrow \text{malate dehydrogenase} \tag{8}$$

$$\textbf{Oxaloacetate} \text{ (to be recycled)}$$

Figure 1.4 Tricarboxylic acid cycle with enzymes listed. Based on information from Voet and Voet, *Biochemistry*, p. 539, and Olson, in *Textbook of Biochemistry*, p. 280.

$$\text{pyruvic acid} + \text{CoASH} \rightarrow \text{acetyl-CoA(S)} + CO_2$$

where CoA(S) may alternately be written simply as CoA, albeit it is understood that sulfur (S) is present in the molecule, and stays in the molecule. Or, writing the reaction more completely, starting with pyruvic acid,

$$(CH_3CO)COOH + \text{CoASH} \rightarrow (CH_3CO)\text{–CoA(S)} + CO_2 + 2 \text{ [H]}$$

where (CH_3CO) is the acetyl group. Note that the reaction stoichiometry or material balance requires that hydrogen [H] or its equivalent be produced in one form or another, as well as carbon dioxide. Occurring simultaneously with the above reaction is the supporting reaction,

$$NAD^+ + 2 \text{ [H]} \rightarrow NADH + H^+$$

which uses the hydrogen generated, and where the above substances are further defined below. If the two reactions are added together, then the overall conversion would appear as

$$(CH_3CO)COOH + CoASH + NAD^+ \rightarrow (CH_3CO)-CoA(S) + CO_2 + NADH + H^+$$

It is to be understood that there is an oxidative source, representable either as O_2 or [O}, whereby any net hydrogen produced is ultimately converted on to water. That is,

$$2 [H] + [O] \rightarrow H_2O$$

This, it may be observed, is a highly exothermic reaction, that is, gives off a large quantity of energy. Moreover, the very fact that CO_2 is produced also signals that additional exothermicity occurs.

And as previously explained, the generalization is that oxidation may also pertain to the removal of electrons by which a net positive charge or association is created on an ionic, atomic, or molecular entity ion, whereas reduction may pertain to adding electrons and creating a net negative charge. Furthermore, in a manner of speaking, in an oxidation/reduction-type reaction, the oxidizing agent or oxidant is reduced, whereas the reducing agent is oxidized. Thus, in the above reaction for example, the oxygen is the oxidizing agent, which is reduced; the hydrogen is the reducing agent, which is oxidized. The one becomes the inverse of the other.

The other substances entering into the tricarboxylic acid cycle are represented as

NAD^+	Nicotinamide adenine dinucleotide, oxidized form
NADH	Nicotinamide adenine dinucleotide, reduced form
H^+	Hydrogen, oxidized form, or hydrogen ion
GTP	Guanosine triphosphate
GDP	Guanosine diphosphate
P_i	Orthophosphate ion as HPO_4^{2-}
FAD	Flavin adenine dinucleotide
$FADH_2$	Flavin adenine dinucleotide, hydrogen reduced form

The supportive reactions are as follows.

The conversion of NAD^+ occurs also during glycolysis, as previously shown:

$$NAD^+ + 2 [H] \rightarrow NADH + H^+$$

which is a way to dehydrogenate another substance—that is the [H} would come from the source being dehydrogenated. The conversion of GDP is as follows (Olson, in *Textbook of Biochemistry*, p. 285):

$$GDP + P_i \rightarrow GTP + H_2O$$

which provides a way to remove orthophosphate P_i and a way to add H_2O. The conversion of FAD is as follows (Voet and Voet, *Biochemistry*, p. 401):

$$FAD + 2 [H] \rightarrow FADH_2$$

which provides an additional way to dehydrogenate another compound.

The regeneration of NADH to NAD^+ can be regarded as an oxidation step:

$$NADH + H^+ + [O] \rightarrow NAD^+ + H_2O$$

Thus, the supportive reactions that occur—not only with acetyl-CoA formation but with reactions (3), (4), and (8) of Fig. 1.4—must be countered with a regeneration step involving oxidation.

The foregoing oxidation of nicotinamide adenosine dinucleotide in its reduced form (NADH), not overtly stated in Fig. 1.4, utilizes the respiratory oxygen intake or uptake, whereby the oxidized form (NAD$^+$) is regenerated. That is to say, oxygen does not overtly appear during the tricarboxylic acid cycle as represented in Fig. 1.4.

The overall conversion represented in Fig. 1.4 indicates that one mole of pyruvic acid converted should produce a net of three moles of CO_2 and two moles of H_2O, which requires the addition of oxygen as follows:

$$CH_3COCOOH + 5 \, [O] \rightarrow 3 \, CO_2 + 2 \, H_2O$$

Starting with pyruvate instead,

$$CH_3COCOO^- + 9/2 \, [O] \rightarrow 3 \, CO_2 + 3/2 \, H_2O$$

Whereas the CO_2 released is correct, the net H_2O released is deficient as represented, in either case. The side reactions or supportive reactions can be viewed as making up the difference in H_2O as well as contributing oxygen or [O] directly or indirectly, and implementing the net H_2O that has to be produced. Not only this, but there can be a linking with other reaction cycles or sequences, in particular, glycolysis. In short, the situation is even more complicated than represented.

1.2.16 NUCLEOTIDES AND NUCLEOSIDES

It may be remarked in passing that CoA, NAD, and so on are of a class of substances called nucleotides, which are the monomeric units for the polymers that constitute nucleic acids (Voet and Voet, *Biochemistry*, pp. 795–796). ATP and ADP on the other hand are of a class of substances called nucleosides. Specifically, nucleotides are phosphate esters of pentoses (or C_5 sugars) to which a nitrogenous base is linked. If this particular phosphate group is absent, the compound becomes a nucleoside. Thus, ATP or adenosine triphosphate is a nucleoside triphosphate—that is, a nucleoside to which phosphate (or phosphates) has been added—but not in the same place that phosphate occurs in the nucleotide form.

1.3 CANCER CELLS VS. NORMAL CELLS

By way of introduction, on first examination it would seem that the glycolysis sequence producing pyruvic acid or pyruvate should be left alone and not interfered with, and adjustments should be made favoring the tricarboxylic acid cycle over anaerobic fermentation to produce lactic acid. This would presumably favor normal cells over cancer cells. The situation may be much more complicated, however, as follows, in that cancer cells are found to have an extra-high glycolysis rate.

It is found that animals, for instance, can sustain anaerobic glycolysis for only a short time, since the PFK (phosphofructokinase enzyme) cannot function at an acidity much below pH7. The PFK is inhibited by the increased acidity from lactic acid production, marked by lower pH levels. Nevertheless, the enzymes of glycolysis are present in such high concentrations that glycolysis persists (Voet and Voet, *Biochemistry*, p. 595).

Furthermore, as Warburg found in 1926, cancer cells produce much more lactic acid under aerobic conditions than do normal cells (Voet and Voet, *Biochemistry*, p. 595).* *The glycolytic pathway produces pyruvate at rates much faster than the tricarboxylic cycle can use.* The explanations include the possibility that the interlocking controls of the system have been broken down, or that the ATP utilization is too rapid to be replenished by oxidative phosphoration. *Attempts to understand the metabolic differences between cancer cells and normal cells may one day provide a clue to the treatment...of this devastating disease....*

---

* Heart attacks and strokes are caused by oxygen deprivation in portions of the heart and brain. The authors afford an explanation of why this causes cell death rather than a loss of cellular activity. The processes involved apparently cause the cell to swell and become more permeable, leaking its contents.

Allowing for the foregoing, since hexokinase is the enzyme for the first biochemical reaction of the glycolysis sequence, its inhibition nevertheless seems the most logical place to start. That is, if hexokinase is inhibited, and the first reaction is thus inhibited, the remaining reactions in the sequence must also be inhibited. The first reaction is controlling and, if hexokinase is inhibited, the glycolysis rate will be slowed.

The trick would be to inhibit hexokinase for the cancer cells without adversely affecting glycolysis in normal cells. There may even be a fortuitous degree of selectivity among enzyme inhibitors, to be determined for a particular enzyme.

The interlocking effects in glycolysis involve other reactions, however. It has been found, for instance, that hexokinase, phosphofructokinase (PFK), and pyruvate kinase are the controlling enzymes in glycolysis (Voet and Voet, *Biochemistry*, p. 471). That is, they are the enzymes for the slower or controlling reactions in the glycolysis sequence, the other reactions being much faster.

A few inhibitors are provided in the reference. Thus, glucose-6-phosphate is listed as an inhibitor for hexokinase, since it is a reaction product. ATP and citrate are inhibitors for PFK, and ATP is an inhibitor for pyruvate kinase, since it is a conversion product. Many more inhibitors are listed in Appendix A. Interestingly, the above reference also lists some activators or promoters for PFK. These include ADP, fructose 6-phosphate (which is a reactant), fructose 1,6-bisphosphate (which is a product), the ammonium ion, and the orthophosphate ion P_i.

Thus, an enzyme could be inhibited for a controlling reaction farther down in the glycolytic sequence—say, phosphofructokinase or pyruvate kinase. This would cause the products to build up ahead of the particular reaction that is blocked, thereby suppressing the preceding reactions.

Better yet, perhaps the formation of lactate or lactic acid could be blocked using an inhibitor for lactate dehydrogenase. This could result in a buildup of pyruvate and the products of the previous reactions, thereby suppressing glycolysis. A buildup of pyruvate, on the other hand, would favor the normal oxidation of pyruvate via the carboxylic acid cycle. Whether the cancer cells would respond similarly or to the degree that normal cells would respond is an open question. However, cancer cells are known to exhibit aerobic glycolysis to some extent, though the conversion to lactate or lactic acid occurs to a much greater extent—on the order of ten times as great.

There are some other things going on, moreover, in terms of glutaminolysis as well as lactate formation. These other effects have been analyzed as follows.

1.3.1 GLYCOLYSIS IN CANCER CELLS VS. IN NORMAL CELLS

An analysis of the differences in the glycolysis route for cancer cells at high and low glucose concentrations versus that of normal cells has been provided by Eigenbrodt et al. in *Regulation of Carbohydrate Metabolism*, p. 144. The analysis is involved, to say the very least, and is first presented as follows more or less verbatim, then synopsized. As points of reference, the accompanying Figs. 1.5, 1.6, and 1.7 pertain to the corresponding parts A, B, and C of the analysis. The overall objective in this exercise will be to try to determine if the enzyme inhibitors for the particular controlling enzyme reactions can be linked to anticancer agents, known or unknown.

(A) Regulation of Glycolysis by Oxygen in Normal Cells

With sufficient oxygen, normal cells adjust pyruvate production to their level of acetyl-CoA consumption and energy needs. The regulation occurs mainly as a result of the ATP inhibition of phosphofructokinase, the enzyme which catalyzes reaction (3) of Fig. 1.1. Thus, reaction (3) can be said to be controlling.

This in turn leads to a decrease in the conversion rate of fructose 6-phosphate to fructose-1-6-biphosphate, the reactant and product of reaction (3). Moreover, the steady-state levels of fructose-1,6-bisphosphate are further lowered, since this metabolite is rapidly converted to pyruvate (there is a high glycolytic capacity from fructose-1,6 bisphosphate to pyruvate), or by a side reaction to fructose 1,6-phosphate (by the enzyme fructose-1,6-bisphosphatase).

Low levels of fructose-1,6-bisphosphate are not sufficient to overcome the ATP inhibition of phosphofructokinase in reaction (3). Glucose 6-phosphate, which accumulates as a result of the inhibition of phosphofructokinase, in turn blocks its own synthesis by hexokinase.

Therefore, the mitochondrial ATP production governs the glycolytic sequence mainly through phosphofructokinase (PFK) inhibition. [This is related to the Pasteur effect, whereby oxygen indirectly inhibits glycolysis and lactate accumulation by the initiation of respiration. Thus, in the absence of oxygen,

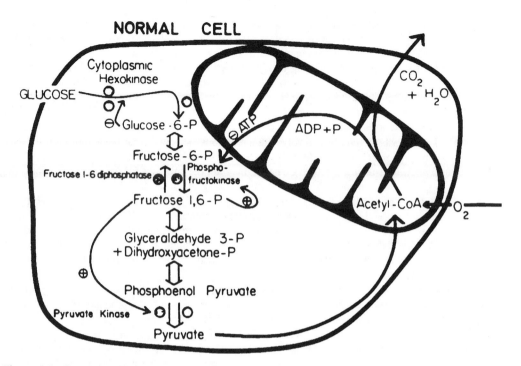

Figure 1.5 Regulation of glycolysis in normal cells. Reproduced with permission from Eigenbrodt, E., Fister, P., and Reinacher, M., "New perspectives on carbohydrate metabolism in tumor cells," in *Regulation of Carbohydrate Metabolism,* Vol. II, Beitner, R., ed., CRC Press, Inc., Boca Raton, FL, 1985, pp. 141–179.

glycolysis may occur at as much as *20 times* the rate in the presence of oxygen (Harris, in *Textbook of Biochemistry*, p. 353).]

Under anaerobic conditions, mitochondrial ATP production by the oxidation of acetyl-CoA is blocked. Hence, ATP levels decrease, phosphofructokinase is deinhibited, and fructose-1,6-bisphosphatase is blocked by the increased AMP levels (not shown). Fructose-1,6-bisphosphate accumulates and further stimulates the phosphofructokinase and pyruvate kinase activities.

The resulting fall in the glucose 6-phosphate levels enhances the hexokinase capacity. The concerted effect of all these mechanisms allows the cell to utilize the total glycolytic capacity for ATP production under anoxic (oxygen-deficient) conditions. Lactate is formed under these conditions from pyruvate in order to reoxidize the NADH formed via the glyceraldehyde 3-phosphate dehydrogenase reaction, reaction (6).

(B) Regulation of Glycolysis by Oxygen in Tumor Cells at High Glucose Concentration

In tumor cells, enhanced activities by the enzyme hexokinase (the mitochondrially bound form) in reaction (1), by the enzyme phosphofructokinase in reaction (3), and the enzyme pyruvate kinase in reaction (10), all ensure a high glycolytic capacity. Pyruvate kinase of the isoenzyme type M_2 (tumor type), in reaction (10) is inhibited by alanine, phenylalanine, and ATP.

The fructose-1,6-bisphosphate formed by reaction (3) is only slowly converted to pyruvate until fructose-1,6-bisphosphate levels exceed a concentration necessary to overcome the ATP inhibition of pyruvate kinase-M_2 in reaction (10). The accumulated fructose-1,6 bisphosphate thereby overthrows the mitochondrial control of glycolysis.

The fully activated hexokinase (not inhibited by the glucose 6-phosphate formed), along with deinhibited phosphofructokinase and pyruvate kinase, leads to a drastic increase of the glycolytic intermediates from glucose 6-phosphate, the product of reaction (1), to glyceraldehyde 3-phosphate, the product of reaction (4). This results in a high aerobic glycolytic rate.

Since the fructose-1,6-bisphosphatase activity is sharply reduced in tumor cells, the fructose-1,6-bisphosphate levels and aerobic glycolysis remain permanently elevated. (The side reaction converting

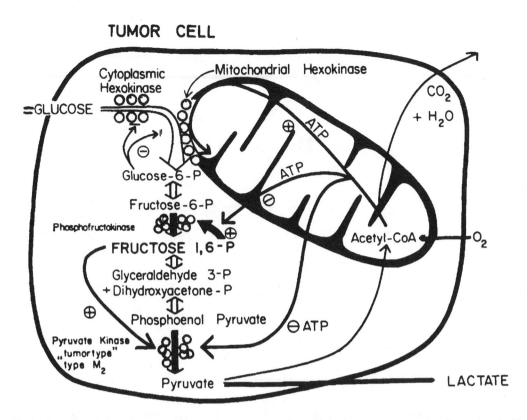

Figure 1.6 Regulation of glycolysis by oxygen in tumor cells at high glucose concentration. Reproduced with permission from Eigenbrodt, E., Fister, P., and Reinacher, M., "New perspectives on carbohydrate metabolism in tumor cells," in *Regulation of Carbohydrate Metabolism*, Vol. II, Beitner, R., ed., CRC Press, Inc., Boca Raton, FL, 1985, pp. 141–179.

fructose-1,6-bisphosphate to fructose 1,6-phosphate by the enzyme fructose-1,6-bisphosphatase is therefore minimized.) Tumor cells, in contrast to normal cells, constantly use almost the total glycolytic capacity regardless of the oxygen tension (pressure or activity).

(C) Regulation of Glycolysis by Oxygen in Tumor Cells at Low Glucose Concentrations or with Alternative Substrates (or Reactants)

At low glucose concentrations (50 µM, or 50 micromolar) or with other substrates or reactants, levels of fructose-1,6-bisphosphate (and P-ribose-PP) are extremely low compared to high glucose conditions (5000 µM). Therefore, the enzyme pyruvate kinase of reaction (10) is functionally inactive. No phosphoenolpyruvate is converted to pyruvate, no ATP is synthesized in the glycolytic pathway, and no pyruvate is available for ATP production by pyruvate oxidation.

When ATP is used by enzymes, it is decomposed to ADP and P_i. The resulting P_i activates the phosphate dependent glutaminase, and glutaminolysis begins, as per Fig. 1.3, yielding 5 ATP + 1 GTP per mole of glutamine under aerobic conditions.

As a result, the ATP levels are restored, and the small amounts of glucose are available for serine, aspartate, and P-ribose-PP synthesis. At this point, proliferation can start.

A synopsis of the foregoing is as follows:

(A) Regulation of Glycolysis by Oxygen in Normal Cells

Reaction (3) of Fig. 1.1 is controlling under normal aerobic conditions and is catalyzed by the enzyme phosphofructokinase, which is inhibited. That is, reaction (3) is slower than the other reactions. This is offset, however, by a high capacity to convert the fructose-1,6-bisphosphate product of reaction (3) on

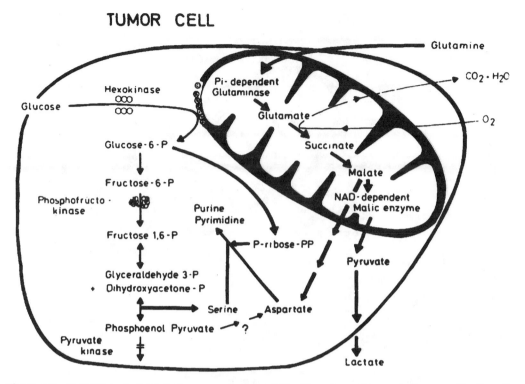

Figure 1.7 Regulation of glycolysis by oxygen in tumor cells at low glucose concentrations or with alternative substrates (or reactants). Reproduced with permission from Eigenbrodt, E., Fister, P., and Reinacher, M., "New perspectives on carbohydrate metabolism in tumor cells," in *Regulation of Carbohydrate Metabolism*, Vol. II, Beitner, R., ed., CRC Press, Inc., Boca Raton, FL, 1985, pp. 141–179.

to pyruvate. Under anaerobic conditions, the phosphofructokinase enzyme of reaction (3) is activated or promoted, increasing the concentration of product fructose-1,6-bisphosphate, which stimulates the conversion of pyruvate to lactate as per Fig.1.3.

(B) Regulation of Glycolysis by Oxygen in Tumor Cells at High Glucose Concentrations

In tumor cells, there is a heightened activity of the enzyme hexokinase in reaction (1), of the enzyme phosphofructokinase in reaction (3), and of the enzyme pyruvate kinase in reaction (10), all of which produce a high glycolytic capacity. The formation of pyruvate by reaction (10) will be decreased, however, by the presence of alanine, phenylalanine, and ATP, which inhibit the enzyme pyruvate kinase.

Nevertheless, as the concentration of fructose-1,6-bisphosphate builds up via reaction (3), it eventually overcomes the inhibition of the enzyme pyruvate kinase in reaction (10). The result is again a high glycolytic rate.

It is commented that tumor cells, as compared to normal cells, use almost the total glycolytic capacity, regardless of the amount of oxygen present. That is, it apparently makes no difference whether an aerobic or anaerobic condition exists.

(C) Regulation of Glycolysis by Oxygen in Tumor Cells at Low Glucose Concentrations or with Alternative Substrates (or Energy Sources, e.g., Glutamine)

It is noted that, for low glucose concentrations, the levels of fructose-1,6-bisphosphate produced by reaction (3) are very much lower than for high glucose conditions. (This can be caused in part by the fact that there is a much lower concentration of glucose to start with.)

This produces a deactivation of the enzyme pyruvate kinase of reaction (10). There is no conversion to pyruvate, no ATP is synthesized. (Furthermore, no pyruvate is available for pyruvate oxidation via the tricarboxylic acid cycle, or for fermentation to lactic acid.)

However, the ATP which has been used up produces the orthophosphate ion P_i, which activates glutaminase for the conversion of glutamine, and glutaminolysis proceeds as per Fig. 1. 3. This then sustains the proliferation of the cancer cells.

1.4 ENZYME INHIBITORS FOR GLYCOLYSIS, LACTATE FORMATION, AND GLUTAMINOLYIS IN TUMOR CELLS

In view of the foregoing, the problem is that of how to suppress cancer cell proliferation via routes (B) and (C) above. Accordingly, inhibitors for the enzymes involved, and which have been listed in Jain's *Handbook of Enzyme Inhibitors* and Zollner's *Handbook of Enzyme Inhibitors*, are shown in Tables A–1 through A–3 of Appendix A. The inhibitors are listed by the enzymes involved, each of which corresponds to a particular reaction. The corresponding reactions may be regarded as if in sequence, although all reactions are occurring simultaneously. Some of the inhibitor sources are listed, as found in the Zollner reference under each enzyme category. For the inhibitor sources in the Jain reference, the particular enzyme inhibitor must be looked up separately.

It has been observed that the metabolic behavior of tumor cells is different from that of normal cells in several ways (Eigenbrodt et al., in *Regulation of Carbohydrate Metabolism*, p. 143). Tumor cells exhibit an enhanced aerobic glycolysis and glucose uptake, enhanced glutaminolysis, enhanced nucleic acid (DNA) synthetic capacity, and enhanced lipid synthesis.*

Tumor cells also show a reduced pyruvate and acetyl-CoA oxidation rate, a lower sensitivity to oxygen, and a lower growth hormone requirement. Thus, as a potential anticancer measure, there is the objective of limiting glycolysis and glutaminolysis and at the same time limiting lactic acid or lactate formation. Concomitantly, there is a need for enhancing respiration or oxygen uptake, thereby favoring the tricarboxylic acid cycle over lactate formation.

In Table A–1a through A–1c for glycolysis, in Table A–2 for lactate formation, and in Table A–3 for glutaminolysis, some of the more common and more simple chemical types of enzyme inhibitors are shown in boldface, as are some of the known anticancer agents. (Enzyme inhibitors that could adversely affect the tricarboxylic cycle or respiration are listed in Appendix B.)

1.4.1 GLYCOLYSIS

Thus, in Table A–1a, A–1b, and A–1c, pertaining to glycolysis per se, certain metallic or mineral substances are listed. Calcium and magnesium (as the cations Ca^{++} and Mg^{++}) are, of course, among the more essential minerals in the diet. Lithium is used in treating depression, notably manic depression. Anions are listed and, in one form or another, the phosphate ion is ubiquitous. Sulphate also makes an appearance.

Chromium occurs as part of an ATP complex. The principal chemical complex in ATP and ADP is adenosine-. Sulfides or disulfides, which are listed, also act as poisons or inhibitors for inorganic catalysts.

The names for various sugars in the listings end in "-ose" whereas the ending "-ine" denotes an amino acid, notably L-alanine and L-phenylalanine. Noting the suffix "pyridox-", it may be commented that pyridoxine or pyridoxin is vitamin B6. Arginine is one of the essential amino acids.

Diethylstilbesterol (DES) is a synthetic hormone used as an estrogen.

Citric acid is, of course, a component of citrus fruits and is an intermediate of the metabolic tricarboxylic acid or citric acid cycle. The appearance of ethanol or ethyl alcohol is a surprise, as is glycerol. As to caffeine, coffee enemas are sometimes used in cancer treatment. Creatine, a nitrogen compound, is a known anticancer agent—in particular as used with urea in a mixture called "Carbatine."

Fatty acids are noted, in particular as lauric acid and unsaturated oleic acid. Flavianic acid is highlighted in that it is used to prepare arginine and tyrosine; arginine for instance has been used in treating cancer, with Moss's *Cancer Therapy* containing a chapter about the subject.

---

* Inhibiting the enhanced DNA synthesis capacity of cancer cells is the objective of conventional cytotoxic chemotherapy drugs, and of chemopreventive substances, to be discussed subsequently. For the record, the molecules called lipids include the fatty acids. Lipids are relatively small molecules as compared to the other kinds of molecules, the macromolecules called proteins, nucleic acids, and polysaccharides (Voet and Voet, *Biochemistry*, pp. 14–16). Proteins, of first importance, are polymers of amino acids, nucleic acids are polymers of what are called nucleotides, and polysaccharides are polymers of sugars.

Quercetin is a known anticancer agent, and it occurs, for example, in chaparral or the creosote bush, itself considered an anticancer agent.

1.4.2 LACTATE OR LACTIC ACID FORMATION

As per Table C–2 of Appendix A, inhibitors working against lactate or lactic acid formation include lactic acid itself. Since it is a reaction product, a buildup would be expected to work against further formation. Albeit pyruvic acid is also listed, being instead a reactant. Other inhibitors include oxalic acid, a component of spinach and rhubarb for instance, and considered toxic in too large a consumption. Interestingly, salicylic acid (aspirin) and urea appear, both known as anticancer agents. Serotonin is a brain neurohormone or neurotransmitter for which the building block is the essential amino acid tryptophan. Serotonin is noted to have a relaxing effect on the mind.

1.4.3 GLUTAMINOLYSIS

With regard to Table C–3 of Appendix A, listing inhibitors for glutaminolysis, bromcresol (or bromocresol) green and purple are dyes derived from sulfonephthalein, starting with meta-cresol. [Phenolphthalein, another organic dye, and also used as a laxative (e.g., in Ex-Lax), is sometimes considered as an anticancer agent.] As to cresols in general, they are kin to phenol or to the mixture that is called creosote, and phenolic-type compounds occur in the chaparral or creosote bush.

Albizzin is an anticancer agent. It is derived from the genus *Albizzia*, a tree of India and Malaysia, and which is listed in Hartwell's compendium (Hartwell, *Plants*).

Interestingly, the metals copper (as Cu^{++}), lead (as Pb^{++}) and mercury (as Hg^{++}) are listed variously as enzyme inhibitors. They may also be viewed as catalyst poisons or inhibitors for inorganic catalysts.

Ammonia (NH_3) is listed as an enzyme inhibitor. It shares kinship with urea and such other inorganic ammoniacal compounds as hydrazine sulfate. All may be considered potential enzyme inhibitors, if not for glutaminolysis, then for other metabolic reactions. Both urea and hydrazine sulfate have been used in cancer treatment, with mixed success—the usual conclusion.

The material called Tris is 2,3-dibromopropanol phosphate. Once used as a fire-retardant for clothing or nightwear, it is now suspected of being carcinogenic.

There are no doubt many other naturally-occurring substances from the plant world that would qualify as enzyme inhibitors and that, in themselves, are considered as anticancer agents. These substances may very well include many of the alkaloids. In fact, every substance known or suspected of being an anticancer agent could be tested for its potential as an enzyme inhibitor for one or more of the enzymes and reactions involved in tumor metabolism.

1.5 TRICARBOXYLIC ACID CYCLE: ENZYME INHIBITORS TO BE AVOIDED

As to the tricarboxylic acid cycle, arsenic poisoning is of special mention. Here, the enzymes affected are pyruvate dehydrogenase and α-ketoglutarate dehydrogenase, as well as other enzymes in other places (Voet and Voet, *Biochemistry*, pp. 547–548; Harris, in *Textbook of Biochemistry*, p. 348, 349). **The result can be overreaction, shutting down respiration.** With a smaller but cumulative dosage, the result is chronic arsenic poisoning. With micro-amounts, it may serve to stimulate the immune system, as used in homeopathy for instance.*

Inasmuch as the two enzymes cited above for the tricarboxylic acid cycle are apparently critical to maintaining respiration, inhibitors are listed in Appendix B as **potentially capable of leading to undesirable and sometimes life-threatening consequences.** Thus, enzyme inhibitors for pyruvate dehydrogenase are listed; only a very few entries of enzyme inhibitors were found for α-ketoglutarate dehydrogenase. There is, however, an extensive list of inhibitors which are noted to act against respiration or respiratory enzymes in general, and which are also presented.

There are some surprises here. While acetaldehyde is generally assumed to be bad news, this is not necessarily so for citric acid. Alkaloids are, of course, undesirables, and anesthetics require close monitoring. Aromatic acids such as phenol would be undesirables, as certainly are arsenate, cyanide, isothiocyanate, and thiocyanate. With cadmium, cobalt, copper, ruthenium, vanadate, and zinc, we are getting into the heavy metals, long known to be detrimental to health.†

---

* Both Jain's *Handbook* and Zollner's *Handbook* show a number of other enzymes which are inhibited by arsenate and arsenite ions. Interestingly, arsenic as such is not listed by either reference as an enzyme inhibitor.

Fatty acids would be unsuspected, as probably would "guaiaretic acid, nordihydro," better known as NDGA or nordihydroguaiaretic acid, the main active ingredient in chaparral or creosote bush.

Progesterone is another one of the hormones, and not much of a surprise. Nor is sucrose, or common table sugar. The alkaloids papaverine and theophylline also show up as enzyme inhibitors.

1.6 COFACTORS, COENZYMES, VITAMINS, AND HORMONES

Sometimes enzymes either do not interact or interact very slowly. This calls for the use of what are called *cofactors*. Thus, enzymes are generally less satisfactory for catalyzing oxidation-reduction type reactions (*redox* reactions), and for this reason they require an association with small molecular entities known as cofactors, which may be said to activate or promote the enzymes (Voet and Voet, *Biochemistry*, pp. 337–338). Some cofactors may consist of a metal ion such as Zn^{++} or may be organic molecules called coenzymes such as NAD^+.

If an organism cannot synthesize the essential cofactors internally, then these cofactors must be present in the diet. They are then called *vitamins,* and vitamins may be regarded as precursors for coenzymes. Many coenzymes were in fact discovered in efforts to relieve nutritional deficiencies. Thus, there is a component of NAD^+ which is known as nicotinamide (or niacinamide); its carboxylic acid analog is called nicotinic acid (or niacin). The use of niacin or niacinamide cures the human vitamin deficiency known as pellagra.

The vitamins in the human diet that are coenzyme precursors are all water-soluble. The others, the fat-soluble vitamins such as vitamin A and vitamin D, are not components of coenzymes, though they are necessary in the diet of many higher animals, including humans.

Technically speaking, vitamin D is said to be a hormone rather than a vitamin. Vitamins are organic compounds necessary for growth, reproduction, and health, but they cannot be synthesized in the body, or if so, not in the amounts for normal needs (Ungar, in *Textbook of Biochemistry*, p. 716). In contrast, hormones are produced within the body and secreted by specific glands. The form of vitamin D called cholecalciferol (D_3) is synthesized in the skin from the ultraviolet irradiation of 7-dehydrocholesterol, a metabolite or metabolic product of cholesterol (Chaney, in *Textbook of Biochemistry*, pp. 1204–1207). The almost identical form called ergocalciferol (D_2) is synthetically prepared by the irradiation of ergesterol from yeast and is the type used in nutritional supplements and fortified foods. Large doses are considered toxic.*

As a matter of record, Table 1.1 is a listing of vitamins, chemical names, and stoichiometric chemical formulas. In most cases, the vitamin structure is too complicated for any kind of simplified structural representation. Enzymes inhibited by various vitamins are listed separately in Appendix Z.

For a recounting of vitamins used against cancer, there is *Modulation and Mediation of Cancer*, by F.L. Meyskens and K. Prasad, published in 1983. Another volume is titled *Vitamins and Cancer*, edited by F.L. Meyskens and K. Prasad and published in 1986. The general subject of vitamins is a proliferating literature, but a couple of noteworthy citations are as follows: *Handbook of Vitamins*, 2d ed., edited by Lawrence J. Machlin and published in 1991, and *The Doctors' Vitamin and Mineral Encyclopedia*, published in 1990 and written by Sheldon Saul Hendler, assisted by a medical advisory board, most or all being MDs. The latter includes other substances such as herbs, amino acids, and so on, with many citations for different kinds of cancers. The remarks are candid, but there are no positive recommendations for cures.

The subject of hormones, along with neurotransmission, has been included under the category biochemical communications (Voet and Voet, *Biochemistry*, p. 1261ff). These chemical messengers, called hormones, communicate intercellular signals, as do nerve-transmitted electrochemical signals in higher animals. Hormones may be divided into polypeptides and amino-acid derivatives, and the reference

---

† Both Jain's *Handbook* and Zollner's *Handbook* have extensive listings for other enzymes that are inhibited or poisoned by the cyanide ion, as well as by the cyanate ion. There are also many entries for copper as Cu^{++}. One of the more famous victims of acute copper poisoning was frontiersman Jesse Chisholm, after whom the Chisholm Trail is named. He died after eating bear grease which had been stored in a copper container.

* As a point of distinction, vitamin C or ascorbic acid is a vitamin in human nutrition, since a necessary enzyme is missing that would convert gluconolactone to ascorbic acid (Ungar, in *Textbook of Biochemistry*, p. 719). However, in such animals as the rat, this enzyme is present, so ascorbic acid would be defined as a hormone.

Table 1.1   Vitamins

Vitamin A	Retinol	$C_{19}H_{24}-CH_2OH$
Vitamin B1	Thiamine hydrochloride; thiamin chloride	$C_{12}H_{18}Cl_2N_4OS$
Vitamin B2	Riboflavin; lactoflavin; vitamin G	$C_{17}H_{22}N_4O_6$
Vitamin B6	Pyridoxin	$C_8H_{11}NO_3$
Vitamin B12	Cobalamine; cyanocobalamin	$C_{63}H_{90}N_{14}O_{14}PCo$
Folic acid	Pteroylglutamic acid (PGA);folacin; vitamin Bc; vitamin M	$C_{14}H_{11}N_6O_2-(C_5H_7NO_3)_n-OH$ where $n = 1 - 7$ $C_{19}H_{19}N_7O_6$ for $n = 1$
Niacin	Nicotinic acid; 3-pyridinecarboxylic acid	$(C_5H_4N)COOH$
Pantothenic acid	or N(α,γ-dihydroxy-β,β dimethylbutyryl)β-alanine	$HOCH_2C(CH_3)_2CH(OH)CO-NHCH_2CH_2COOH$, $C_9H_{17}NO_5$
Vitamin C	Ascorbic acid; Antiscorbutin	$CO(COH)_3CHOHCH_2OH$ $C_6H_8O_6$
Vitamin D	Calciferol	$C_{28}H_{44}O$
Vitamin E	α-Tocopherol; 5,7,8-trimethyltocol	$C_{14}H_{17}O_2(C_5H_{10})_3H$
Vitamin K	Phthiocol; 1,4-naphthoquinone, 2-hydroxy-3-methyl- Vitamin K occurs in several forms, e.g., K_1 (phylloquinone), K_2 (menaquinone), L_3 (menadione), and may itself be inhibited by dicoumarol and warfarin.	$C_{11}H_8O_3$

provides a tabulation (Voet and Voet, *Biochemistry*, p. 1263). In a manner of speaking, therefore, hormones may be regarded as proteins. For a listing of various hormones, also consult Appendix Z.

Hormones as well as vitamins serve as enzyme inhibitors, as presented in Appendix Z, which lists the enzymes inhibited corresponding to the hormone tabulation cited in the previous paragraph above (Voet and Voet, *Biochemistry*, p. 1263).

Hormones are classified by the distance within which they act. Autocrine hormones act on the same cell that releases them. An example is interleukin-2. Paracrine hormones act on cells close to the cell that releases them. Examples are prostaglandins and polypeptide growth hormones. Endocrines act on cells at a distance. Examples are the endocrine hormones insulin and epinephrine, which are released into the bloodstream by endocrine glands. A table of various endocrine hormones is provided in the reference. Most hormones consist of polypeptides, amino acid derivatives, or steroids. Some examples of functions are as follows.

- The pancreas serves as an exocrine gland for producing various digestive enzymes. It also secretes insulin and glucagon, which regulate blood glucose levels, and somatostatin, which regulates the insulin and glucagon secretions.
- The gastrointestinal hormones are secreted into the bloodstream by cells lining the gastrointestinal tract. *These no doubt are affected by the ravages of conventional cytotoxic chemotherapy, which in particular attacks the cells of the gastrointestinal tract.*
- Thyroid hormones regulate metabolism.
- Parathyroid hormone along with vitamin D and calcitonin (a polypeptide hormone) regulate calcium metabolism.
- The adrenal glands, which are divided into the medulla (core) and the cortex (outer layer), furnish catecholamines and steroids, respectively. The catecholamines are hormonally-active, and consist of norepinephrine and epinephrine. Steroids variously affect carbohydrate, protein, and lipid metabolism, regulate the salt/water losses of the kidneys, and affect sexual development and function. Androgens

and estrogens fall in the last-mentioned category. Another adrenal hormone of note is ACTH, or adrenocorticotropic hormone. Cortisol is an adrenal product, which can be converted to cortisone. (Another name for cortisol is hydrocortisone, described as a major glucorticoid produced by the adrenal cortex. It is involved in the "fight or flee" reflex and is associated with the neurobiology of depression, as described by Charles B. Nemeroff in the June 1998 issue of the *Scientific American*. A related and interesting observation by Ohio State virologist Ronald Glasser was previously reported in the *Los Angeles Times*, home edition, November 16, 1996. Glasser indicated that weak immune systems, such as caused by high-stress hormone levels, are prone to infection by "viruses that are linked to cancer.")

- The hypothalamus and the pituitary gland act together to control much of the endocrine system. Included is regulation of the growth-hormone GH, also called somatotropin.

No effects were noted in the reference as pertains to cancer. Two chapters on the biochemistry of hormones are provided by Frank Ungar in *Textbook of Biochemistry*. Again, no direct connection with cancer could be found. There are, however, some interesting inferences which can be made from a section on thyroid hormone functions which deal with thermogenesis and oxygen consumption (Ungar, in *Textbook of Biochemistry*, pp. 753–754). Increased oxygen consumption and heat production go together and correlate with increased thyroid activity. *In comments about the foregoing effect of increased thyroid activity, it is the contention that higher body temperatures (hyperthermia) act against cancer. In turn, this indicates increased capacities for the tricarboxylic acid cycle, also manifested as an increased aerobic glycolysis rate, whereas cancer cells in the main undergo anaerobic glycolysis. Hence, the inhibition of anaerobic glycolysis should favor a marked increase in aerobic glycolysis instead, which presumably could raise body temperatures and act against cancer—the same as when the immune system raises body temperatures to produce a fever and fight off an infection, in this case, cancer cells.*

It may be noted that iodine is related to thyroid activity. The reference observes that obesity is connected with a reduced ATPase enzyme activity.

1.7 CHEMOTHERAPY DRUGS

The drugs used in chemotherapy may take any of several directions, involving biochemical reactions at the DNA/RNA level, and particularly as involves enzymes and enzyme inhibitors. In general, we are talking about metabolism and about metabolites as involved in biochemical reacting systems. Metabolism pertains to the processes of biochemical synthesis, maintenance, and decay, which also involve an energy exchange. Energy may be produced (by exothermic reactions) or consumed (by endothermic reactions), although the former is the usual connotation. Metabolites are the chemical species, constituents, or components undergoing change in biochemical reacting systems. Metabolites may be viewed either as reactants or products but are chiefly thought of in terms of the latter.

Enzymes, as previously noted, are the biochemical catalysts for these reactions or conversions. A specific reaction will require a specific enzyme, except in rare instances. The enzymes may be inhibited or promoted by still other substances, the former case known as inhibitors, in the latter case as promoters or activators.

Basic to any consideration are nucleotides, the basic chemical structures that contribute to cellular functions. Depending upon their chemical makeup, they are divided into two classes, purines and pyrimidines, and are precursors to DNA and RNA. More will be said about the phenomena involved in later sections.

1.7.1 PURINE AND PYRIMIDINE NUCLEOTIDES

The purine and pyrimidine nucleotides are the metabolites upon which many cellular functions are based. The formation and fate of purine and pyrimidine nucleotides is therefore critical to normal cell growth and functions. The subject is addressed for instance by Joseph G. Cory in a chapter on Purine and Pyrimidine Nucleotide Metabolism appearing in *Textbook of Biochemistry*.

These nucleotides called purines and pyrimidines are formed de novo (anew) in the cell from amino acids, ribose, formate, and CO_2. (Cory, in *Textbook of Biochemistry*, p. 628ff.) The diseases or syndromes resulting from deficiencies in the synthesis of these nucleotides include gout, the Lesch-Nyhan syndrome, orotic aciduria, and *immunodeficiency diseases*.

The last category, of course, includes cancer. And since the nucleotides are necessary for DNA and RNA synthesis, the defective metabolic pathways involved are where the cells are cancerous and are the sites at which anticancer agents are directed.

1.7.2 ENZYME INHIBITORS IN CHEMOTHERAPY

Apropos of previous considerations about enzymes and enzyme inhibitors as related to metabolic processes, the applications described here pertain to cancer cell growth and destruction. In consequence, some enzyme inhibitors act as chemotherapeutic agents.

To start with an example, there is a thing about enzymes and enzyme inhibitors in that they are sometimes chemically or structurally similar (Voet and Voet, *Biochemistry*, p. 355ff). For instance, methotrexate (or amethopterin) and hydrofolate are chemically similar, and therefore the former binds to an enzyme called dihydrofolate reductase. This prevents the enzyme from converting dihydrofolate to tetrahydrofolate, the latter being essential in the biosynthesis of the DNA precursor thymidylic acid. The premise is that cancer cells, which are also active in DNA synthesis, are more susceptible than normal cells to the effects of the inhibitor.

Thus, drug therapy in large part rests on the inhibition of specific enzymes (York, in *Textbook of Biochemistry*, p. 165ff.) Inhibitors are classed variously as competitive, noncompetitive, and uncompetitive. It is noted also that enzyme activity will be inhibited by a buildup of product and that enzymes may inhibit or even activate other enzymes.

Competitive enzyme inhibitors are those whose activity is compromised by an increased presence of substrate or reactant. The inhibitor and substrate are enough alike, chemically or structurally, that they compete for the same site on the enzyme, and as the concentration of substrate or reactant increases, the substrate predominates at the expense of the inhibitor. A noncompetitive inhibitor binds at other sites than the substrate binding site and is therefore not affected by increased concentrations of the substrate or reactant. Irreversible inhibitors bond chemically with the substrate or reactant.

Drugs are therefore used to inhibit a specific enzymes in a specific metabolic pathway. These include antiviral and antibacterial drugs as well as antitumor drugs. The attempt, moreover, is to administer these drugs under conditions of limited toxicity. Toxicity is unavoidable, with the exception of cell-wall biosynthesis in bacteria, since "there are no critical metabolic pathways that are unique to tumors, viruses, or bacteria" (York, in *Textbook of Biochemistry*. p. 167). *Hence, drugs that will kill these organisms will also kill the host cell.* The only advantage is that the undesirable organisms may have comparatively short generation times. These organisms are especially sensitive to antimetabolites, and especially to those which inhibit or block enzymes involved in replication.

With regard to the statement above that there are no critical metabolic pathways unique to tumors, it is set forth elsewhere that glycolysis rates are many times greater for cancer cells than for normal cells. This consideration, then, can be construed as an exception. It is in fact the raison d'être for not only slowing down glycolysis but especially for blocking lactate or lactic acid formation and glutaminolysis. This approach was spelled out in previous sections, naming the controlling enzymes involved and listing inhibitors for those enzymes. Inhibition of the particular enzymes involved may in fact be the role played by many unorthodox anticancer agents, both organic or herbal, and inorganic. If so, the objective then becomes that of making the known anticancer agents more effective and of finding other and better anticancer agents.

1.7.3 SULFA DRUGS

The use of sulfa drugs marks the beginnings of modern chemotherapy, that is, of conventional chemotherapy (York, in *Textbook of Biochemistry*, p. 167). These compounds have the general formula $R–SO_2–NHR'$, where R and R' represent arbitrary molecular groups. Sulfanilamide is the simplest and best known, with the formula $H_2N(C_6H_4)–SO_2–NH_2$. It acts as an antibacterial agent by a competitive inhibition with *p*-aminobenzoic acid (PABA), the latter being required for bacterial growth. In fuller explanation, bacteria cannot absorb the necessary vitamin folic acid, but must instead synthesize it, a sequence which requires *p*-aminobenzoic acid. Inasmuch as sulfanilamide is a structural analog of PABA, the enzyme dihydropterate synthetase is "tricked" into using sulfanilamide instead of PABA, which subverts the conversion to folic acid. The bacterium is deprived of folic acid or folate and cannot grow or divide. Inasmuch as humans obtain folic acid or folate from external sources, the sulfanilamide is not harmful at the dosage levels used.

1.7.4 ANTIFOLATE DRUGS

In the biosynthesis of purines and pyrimidines, the heterocyclic bases used in the further synthesis of DNA and RNA, folic acid is required as a coenzyme (York, in *Textbook of Biochemistry*, p. 168). As part of this latter synthesis route, there is involved the conversion of deoxyuridine-5'-phosphate to thymidine-5'-phosphate. This requires the introduction of a methylene derivative of tetrahydrofolate, which is first produced from 7,8-dihydrofolate using dihydrofolate reductase as the enzyme. The compound called methotrexate (4-amino-N^{10}-methyl folic acid) is a structural analog of folate or folic acid, and it competes with dihydrofolate for the enzyme dihydrofolate reductase and is 1000 times more successful. This, in effect, stops the synthesis of thymidine 5'-phosphate, the thymidine nucleotide necessary for cell division. In this way, methotrexate has been successfully used in the treatment of childhood leukemia, since cell division depends upon thymidine in addition to other nucleotides.

Unfortunately, *other rapidly dividing cells, such as in bone marrow, are also sensitive for the same reasons*. Furthermore, *prolonged usage causes the tumor cells to produce larger amounts of the reductase enzyme, thus becoming resistant to the drug*.

1.7.5 IRREVERSIBLE ANTIMETABOLITES

Irreversible inhibitors are also known as *suicide substrates* or *active site directed inhibitors*. An irreversible inhibitor is a compound that not only has an affinity for an active enzyme site but also chemically reacts with the site. In this way, tetrahydrofolate reductase may be deactivated using a compound called a *substituted dihydratriazine*. The latter compound reacts with the site and blocks the access of dihydrofolate to the site. The net effect is similar to that produced by sulfanilamide, above.

1.7.6 OTHER ANTIMETABOLITES

Other analogs to the purines and pyrimidines emphasize the similarity between chemotherapy agents and normal substrates or reactants. The chemotherapy drug 5-fluorouracil (5-FU) is an analog of thymine, in which a methyl group is replaced by fluorine. The deoxynucleotide formed from this compound is an irreversible inhibitor of the enzyme thymidylate synthase, also called thymidylate synthetase, which is necessary in DNA synthesis (Voet and Voet, *Biochemistry*, pp. 812–816; Cory, in *Textbook of Biochemistry*, p. 677). For the purposes of consistency, the first-mentioned version will be used herein. (Strictly speaking, there is a difference between "synthase" and "synthetase.")

Another example is the drug 6-mercaptopurine, which is an analog of hypoxanthine, and in turn of adenine and guanine, two of the basic constituents of nucleotides, and in turn of DNA synthesis. This drug therefore acts as a broad-spectrum antimetabolite in competition with most reactions involving adenine and guanine and their derivatives. Of course, if it acts against cancerous cells, it will also act against normal cells.

1.7.7 LISTINGS OF CYTOTOXIC CHEMOTHERAPY DRUGS

Information about the major cytotoxic chemotherapy drugs is provided by Ralph Moss in the appendices of his book *Questioning Chemotherapy*. The use of the descriptor "cytotoxic," denoting cell-toxic, emphasizes the role of these drugs in destroying not only cancer cells, but normal cells. In plain terms, these drugs are poisons.

Moss provides the chemical names and trade names, along with the manufacturer of each, and the protocols or combinations in common use. This is followed by descriptions of the properties and side effects of the individual drugs. In other parts of the book, cancer types are listed with the particular chemotherapy drugs used, describing the success or lack of success, but mostly the latter, with the few exceptions being blood-related cancers such as leukemia. The overall picture is depressing in the extreme.

As a postscript, a news release dated June 17, 1996 describes the rapid FDA approval of Pharmacia & Upjohn's Camptostar, said to be the first new drug for colorectal cancer in nearly 40 years. A Dr. Leonard Saltz of Memorial-Sloan Kettering gave an enthusiastic recommendation. Reportedly, a follow-up treatment for 5-FU for cancers which have metastasized, there are nevertheless adverse side effects such as a reduction in white blood cells. No mechanism for the action of the drug was furnished. It can be wondered if this is not another cytotoxic drug with effects similar to 5-FU, which would already have debilitated the patient.

1.8   THE DNA/RNA CONNECTION

At the DNA level there are some highly-involved chemical reactions taking place, among a multitude of others, that are related to cell growth and metabolism, including that of cancer cells. The connection is to nucleotides and their synthesis into DNA and RNA.

"Since nucleotides are obligatory for DNA and RNA synthesis in dividing cells, the metabolic pathways involving the synthesis of nucleotides have been the sites at which many antitumor agents have been directed" (Cory, in *Textbook of Biochemistry*, p. 628). Some have already been reviewed. Further details are as follows, in terms of the specific enzymes involved.

1.8.1   THYMIDYLATE SYNTHASE INHIBITION

The component of DNA called deoxythymidine monophosphate (dTMP) may be synthesized from deoxyuridine monophosphate (dUMP) using the enzyme called thymidylate synthase (Voet and Voet, *Biochemistry*, pp. 796, 813ff). The foregoing is presumed more related to cancer cell growth than to normal cell growth—but not exclusively so.

It has been found that the chemical 5-fluorodeoxyuridylate (called FdUMP) irreversibly inhibits thymidylate synthase, thus blocking the synthesis of dTMP. This has led to the use of FdUMP as an antitumor agent, as well as 5-fluorouracil (5-FU) and 5-fluorodeoxyuridine as antitumor agents, since they convert to dUMP. It is commented that most normal mammalian cells are relatively insensitive to dUMP—with the exception of *bone marrow cells, much of the immune system, intestinal mucosa, and hair follicles.* (To which may be added, ultimately, the rest of the body cells.)

1.8.2   DIHYDROFOLATE REDUCTASE INHIBITION

Another reaction sequence going on at the DNA level involves folate or folic acid. (Folic acid, one of the B vitamins, and sometimes written as vitamin Bc or vitamin M, has the chemical name pteroyl-glutamic acid or PGA.) Folate is first reduced to 7,8-dihydrofolate (DHF) and then to tetrahydrofolate (THF). Both the foregoing reactions utilize dihydrofolate reductase (DHFR) as the enzyme (Voet and Voet, *Biochemistry*, pp. 764, 814–815). On the other hand, the oxidation of THF back to DHF is catalyzed by thymidylate synthase.

If the enzyme DHFR is inhibited, then all the cells' THF is converted back to DHF by the enzymatic action of thymidylate synthase. This is regarded as a desirable situation in that it stops cancer growth. It acts against dTMP synthesis, above, and also blocks other THF-dependent biological reactions. DHFR blockage has been accomplished by such antifolate chemotherapeutic agents as methotrexate (ametho-pterin), aminopterin, and trimethoprim.

These antifolates have been used, for example, against childhood leukemia. (A strategy is described in which a lethal dose of methotrexate is introduced, then the patient is "rescued" some hours later by administering massive doses of 5-formyl-THF and/or thymidine). Another comment about using meth-otrexate is that, when administered in a proper dosage, it kills cancer cells *without fatally poisoning* the patient (Voet and Voet, *Biochemistry*, p. 355).

1.8.3   OTHER INHIBITORS

There is of course the probability that less lethal substances can be employed to inhibit or block thymidylate synthase and dihydrofolate reductase. Some possibilities are listed in Appendix C. (Jain's *Handbook* contains only the category Thymidylate Synthetase, whereas Zollner's *Handbook* has only the category Thymidylate Synthase. For the record, both listings are presented in Appendix C, although both names apparently apply to the same enzyme.) An inspection indicates that these substances are not ordinary run-of-the-mill, garden-variety chemicals, either, with the exception say of folic acid. Albeit natural substances are the source for producing some of these chemicals, for instance the much-studied and infamous bacterium *E. coli*, short for *Escherichia coli*.

1.9   GENE THERAPY AND *ESCHERICHIA COLI*

The bacterium *E. coli* is a prokaryote which has been studied intensely for many years, both from a biochemical and a genetic standpoint (Voet and Voet, *Biochemistry*, pp. 4–5). It is found in the colon of higher mammals. (The collective term coliform bacteria is used for the various members of the genus *Escherichia* which live in the colon of higher mammals. Their presence in water supplies is evidence of contaminating fecal matter.) The cell DNA of *E. coli* is thought to encode some 3000 proteins, not all of which have been identified. There are maybe 6000 different kinds of molecules consisting of proteins, nucleic acids, polysaccharides, lipids and other varieties. Of these different kinds, there may be more than 100,000 molecules per cell that metabolize glucose, and as few as 5 per cell that metabolize lactose (Edward Glassman, in *Textbook of Biochemistry*, p. 952). On the other hand, if lactose is present instead of glucose, the necessary enzyme (β-galactosidase) may mobilize a thousandfold.

Prokaryotes or bacteria can meet their nutritional requirements from simple compounds such as H_2O, CO_2, NH_3, and H_2S (Voet and Voet, *Biochemistry*, pp. 4–5). For some bacteria, the necessary energy sources may come from the oxidation of NH_3, H_2S, or even the ferrous ion Fe^{2+}.

For other bacteria, light energy becomes the source, starting with CO_2 and H_2O and yielding carbohydrates $(CH_2O)_n$ in the process, denotable by

$$n\ CO_2 + n\ H_2O \rightarrow (CH_2O)_n + n\ O_2$$

This version of photosynthesis, the most common, is carried out be plants and by what are known as cyanobacteria ("cyano-" meaning the presence of the -CN or cyanide group). These are the green, chlorophyll-containing organisms found growing in water, or at exposed surfaces in water, and were formerly called blue-green algae. Some species of cyanobacteria can convert atmospheric nitrogen into organic nitrogen compounds, as is done by bacteria growing on the roots of legumes.

Another, less-known form of photosynthesis utilizes such sulfur compounds as H_2S and thiosulfates, even hydrogen or organic compounds. The process may be represented by

$$n\ CO_2 + 2n\ H_2S \rightarrow (CH_2O)_n + n\ H_2O + 2n\ S$$

The latter may occur for instance in oxygen-free aqueous environments where the H_2S is generated from the decomposition of organic matter. It also occurs in the ocean at volcanic vents.

Many mammalian genes have been cloned into *E. coli*. The DNA of the desired gene is placed in a vector or vehicle which will carry the DNA into the *E. coli* cells (Glassman, in *Textbook of Biochemistry*, p. 986–995). Gene coding has been performed for insulin, growth hormone, interferon, and other mammalian proteins. The subject becomes that of genetic engineering. The objectives are to produce useful proteins such as insulin, blood-clotting factors, hormones, and so on, and to use cloned normal human genes to replace defective genes such as for diabetes, sickle cell anemia and hemophilia.

The abiding hope, of course, is to use these techniques to subvert cancer. Instead of destroying cell DNA/RNA as in conventional chemotherapy, the object is to replace the DNA/RNA of cancer cells. (Although the cancer cells are presumably targeted, will there be some unexpected side effects for normal cells? That is, will the DNA/RNA of normal cells be similarly affected?) One might say that the efforts are directed toward replacing chemotherapy with biotherapy.

1.10 FOLIC ACID

In a chapter on the B vitamins, folic acid or folate is described in Ralph Moss's *Cancer Therapy* as having been used in cancer treatment, particularly for lung and cervical cancers (Moss, *Cancer Therapy*, pp. 42–44). It is said to increase the white-blood cell count as a defense against cancer. Natural sources include liver, kidney, mushrooms, yeast, spinach, and other leafy green vegetables. Broccoli may be added among the vegetables, and citrus fruits, notably oranges, are a substantial source of folic acid. John Heinerman also gives special mention to folic acid in his book *The Treatment of Cancer with Herbs*.

Along with vitamin B12, it has long been regarded as a preventive and treatment for certain kinds of anemia, e.g., pernicious anemia, and has recently been given renewed attention in the prevention of birth defects. Its role as an enzyme inhibitor has been much less publicized, and remains hidden away in treatises about biochemistry.

A comprehensive account of the subject is provided for instance in *Folate in Health and Disease*, edited by Lynn B. Bailey. Another volume has the unusual title *Apricots and Oncogenes: On Vegetables and Cancer Prevention* by Eileen Jennings. The latter focuses on two vitamins: folic acid and beta-carotene. It is indicated that folic acid deficiency may be a major cause of colon cancer and breast cancer.*
In a study called "Diet, Alcohol, and Smoking in the Occurrence of Hyperplastic Polyps of the Colon

and Rectum," by Kearney et al. of the Department of Nutrition, Harvard School of Public Health, it was found that low folic acid levels correlated with an increase in cancerous polyps, as well as cancer itself.

Folic acid may occur several forms, the simplest being called monopteroylglutamic acid (Stephen G. Chaney, in *Textbook of Biochemistry*, p. 1219ff). It more usually occurs in the form of polyglutamarate derivatives, which are ultimately changed in the intestines into tetrahydrofolate by the action of the enzyme dihydrofolate reductase. Subsequent reactions, with chemical formulas, are described in the reference.

The most pronounced effect of folate deficiency is said to be the inhibition of DNA synthesis, which also slows down the maturation of red blood cells. Special mention is made of folate deficiency during pregnancy, and of drugs which interfere with folate metabolism and cause folate deficiencies.

Thus, many substances have been tested for interference with specific diseased steps in purine and pyrimidine metabolism (Joseph G. Cory, in *Textbook of Biochemistry*, p. 674ff). The substances include compounds synthesized or isolated from plants, bacteria, fungi, and so forth. The substances may be further classed as glutamine antagonists, antifolates, and antimetabolites. Inasmuch as the first-mentioned substances are toxic in the extreme, the latter two classes will be of primary concern—and they are toxic enough.

Interestingly, it may be remarked again that the interfering or enzyme-inhibiting substances disclosed are not ordinary, run-of-the-mill chemicals. No readily-recognizable natural or naturally occurring substances seem to have made the listings of enzyme inhibitors for the particular enzymes involved—with maybe the exception of folic acid and some of its derivatives. If the testing of similar ubiquitous natural substances was always negative, then perhaps the range of natural substances tested was limited.

1.10.1 COMPARISON WITH CONVENTIONAL CHEMOTHERAPY DRUGS

A reiteration of the action of chemotherapy agents is in order (e.g., Cory, in *Textbook of Biochemistry*, p 674ff). Thus, with regard to the formation of tetrahydrofolate from folic acid, antifolates are compounds that inhibit this conversion by blocking dihydrofolate reductase and in turn block the formation of thymidylate. That is, antifolates also block the formation of thymidylate by acting as an inhibitor for thymidylate synthase, as previously mentioned—as well as inhibiting or blocking dihydrofolate reductase. The action is twofold.

Folic acid or folate evidently acts as in this manner, inasmuch as it is listed as an inhibitor for both of these enzymes. It is noted that the chemotherapy drug methotrexate or MTX, previously mentioned, is an antifolate very similar chemically to folic acid.

On the other hand, the action of 5-fluorouracil (5-FU or FUra) becomes that of an antimetabolite. It is described as a pyrimidine analog, with no biological action in itself, but which is converted in the body to other cytotoxic (cell-toxic) agents which are the actual antimetabolites. Specifically, 5-FUra is first converted to fluorodeoxyuridylate (in the references called FdUMP) and to fluorouridine triphosphate (FUTP). FdUMP is in turn a potent inhibitor for thymidylate synthase, but FUTP adversely enters the various RNA species of the cell.*

The use of 5-FU or FUra in cancer therapy is observed to have some serious consequences or side effects due to product FUTP acting on cell RNA, and which are quoted as follows (Cory, in *Textbook of Biochemistry*, p. 677). "...*the incorporation of 5-FUra into RNA has serious effects on normal RNA metabolism and is a factor in the cytotoxicity of this agent....*" In other words, the normal cell RNA is compromised, as well as the tumor cell RNA. (It is further stated that the nucleosides thymidine and uridine may both rescue the FUra-treated cells from the action of the FUra. These nucleosides, therefore, may be regarded as antidotes.)

It is also mentioned that hydroxyurea will inhibit DNA synthesis with very little effect on RNA (Cory, in *Textbook of Biochemistry*, p. 678). That is, according to the reference, it inhibits ribonucleotide reductase, blocking the formation of DNA, although high concentrations are required. The similarity with urea as an anticancer agent is not to be overlooked.

---

* It may be mentioned that folate is commonly used in conjunction with the chemotherapy drug 5-FU, but as a carrier for the drug, although the folate may be of value in itself.

* According to Zollner's *Handbook*, 5-fluoro-dUMP or FdUMP is also an inhibitor for dCMP deaminase (dCMP is apparently deoxycytidine monophosphate), which evidently is important in DNA synthesis. According to Jain's *Handbook*, FUTP—designated uridine-5'-triphosphate—is an inhibitor for many enzymes, including DNA kinase, glucose-6-p-dehydrogenase, protein kinase, PRPP synthetase, and pyruvate carboxylase.

These things considered, then what better way to accomplish the same sort of objectives than to use folic acid (or one of its derivatives)? According to Appendix C, it is an inhibitor for the same enzymes blocked by the customary cytotoxic chemotherapy drugs. It is a substance natural to the body, however, and not some mysterious plant or animal extract from afar. Effective dosage levels would have to be established and may require intravenous injection rather that oral usage. The mental block would have to be overcome, whereby most doctors are reluctant to give even B12 or B-complex shots, much less what may turn out to be megadoses of folic acid, whose side effects have yet to be established. As with other cancer treatment alternatives, the serious patient may have to look toward Mexico or overseas.*

The foregoing is, of course, speculation, but it seems worthy of independent clinical trials, the mark of credibility. Folic acid and some of its derivatives may be the key to the regulation and control of cancer cells, although the biochemical processes involved would without doubt be intricate and inter-connected with other biochemical processes. The trouble is, not much money would be changing hands involved if, say, folic acid treatments should become routine.

1.10.2 CLINICAL TRIALS

A search of MEDLINE yielded a few bits of information about the use of folic acid and potential hazards for supplemental megadoses. For instance, there have in fact been clinical trials conducted at the University of Arizona as part of a Southwest Oncology Group Intergroup study (Childers et al., in *Cancer Epidemiol. Biomarkers Prevention*, March, 1995). These studies tested folic acid against a predisposition to cervical cancer but found no significant difference between the test group and the control group. Oral dosage levels of 5 mg per day were used, which is more than 10 times the level of circa 400 mcg usually found in vitamin supplements. (Doses have been reported elsewhere of as much as one gram per day, or 200 times the experimental dosage used above, or 2500 times as much as usually found in vitamin supplements.) A difficulty in evaluating such investigations, of course, is that the tests did not pertain to actual, developed cervical cancers, and that the control group taking placebos may already have been receiving sufficient folic acid in the diet for their needs. Plus, there is the possibility that perhaps folic acid should be taken intravenously for maximum effectiveness—all of which complicates the investigations.

Another article has addressed the adverse and toxic effects that may occur with such substances as folic acid and its analogs or derivatives, and with quinazolines, also under study as anticancer agents in the context of thymidylate synthase antagonists or inhibitors (Jackman and Judson, in *Cancer Investigation*, Vol. 12, 1994). It is titled "Oncology Drug Discovery and Clinical Trial Testing: Who's Listening?" There evidently can be side effects on the kidneys, for instance, that should be taken into account.†

Still another article, which appeared in the Spring, 1992 issue of *Mol. Neurobiol.*, by S.R. Snodgrass, deals with vitamin neurotoxicity. The concern was that megadoses of certain vitamins could produce neurotoxicity. In tests on animals, it was found that a high dosage of folate directly into the brain or cerebrospinal fluid would cause seizures and excitation. On the other hand, folate toxicity in humans has rarely been reported, although fatal reactions to IV thiamine or thiamin are well known. The article concludes that megadose vitamin therapy is more hazardous to peripheral organs than to the nervous system, and that a high vitamin intake could cause symptoms that may be confused with a disease. Furthermore, direct vitamin administration into the brain, sometimes recommended for certain diseases, is best avoided. The issues are complicated by the fact that individual susceptibilities vary, and even ordinary vitamin dosages may adversely affect an occasional patient with genetic disorders.

1.11 ENZYME CHANGES

The proliferation of cancer cells can be explained in terms of the biochemical changes that occur (Cory, in *Textbook of Biochemistry*, p. 665). There are not only quantitative changes in enzyme levels but qualitative changes—that is, the chemical structure of the enzymes may shift, and the enzymes change

---

* It may be added that folic acid and its analogs and derivatives function as inhibitors for a number of other enzymes. These enzymes are listed in Jain's *Handbook*. Thymidylate synthetase or synthase is listed several times, dihydrofolate reductase once.

† Quinazoline may be regarded as a derivative of quinoline, in turn a derivative of aniline, a coal tar chemical, and the parent of many alkaloids. The medicinal substance known as quinine is a member of this extended family of chemicals.

into corresponding isoenzymes or isozymes. Based on experimental studies, these biochemical changes have been categorized as (1) transformation linked, (2) progression linked, and (3) coincidental alterations. The first of these denotes that tumors show certain increased or decreased enzyme levels regardless of growth rate. The second one denotes alterations that correlate with growth rate. The third category denotes alterations not connected to the malignancy.

For a few examples of the above categories, the levels of thymidylate synthase, ribonucleide reductase, and IMP dehydrogenase increase with the tumor growth rate. The enzymes PRPP amidotransferase, UDP kinase, and uridine kinase are increased in all tumors, regardless of growth rate.

It is commented that, although certain enzymes show fast growth rate in normal tissue, the quantitative and qualitative patterns are different for tumor tissue. If the enzyme growth rates decrease, then some sort of inhibiting action can be presumed.

For the record, the above-cited enzymes pertain to the following reactions or conversions, which are involved in purine and pyrimidine nucleotide metabolism (Cory, in *Textbook of Biochemistry*, pp. 642–644, 653, 661). The role of thymidylate synthase and ribonucleide reductase, and their inhibitors, has been previously discussed.

- The enzyme IMP dehydrogenase catalyzes the conversion of inosine 5'-monophosphate (IMP) to xanthosine 5'-monophosphate (XMP).
- The enzyme PRPP amidotransferase catalyzes the conversion of 5-phosphoribosyl 1-pyrophosphate (PRPP) to 5-phosphoribosylamine, which is in turn converted to IMP in an unregulated step, that is, an enzyme catalyst is not required.
- The enzyme UDP kinase catalyzes the conversion of uridine or uridine 5'-monophosphate (UMP) to uridine 5'-diphosphate (UDP).
- Uridine kinase catalyzes the conversion of uridine to uridine monophosphate (UMP).

All the preceding are among the myriad reactions and corresponding enzymes related to the synthesis and replication of DNA. Enzyme inhibitors for the foregoing enzymes are provided in Appendix D, with the exception of the enzyme UDP kinase.

1.12 DNA, RNA, AND THE SYNTHESIS OF PROTEINS

The acronym DNA stands for deoxyribonucleic acid, where "ribo-" signifies a connection with or derivation from ribose (a five-carbon sugar) with, say, the formula $C_5H_{10}O_5$. In turn, RNA stands for ribonucleic acid. Their main function is directed toward the formation of protein. Necessary to life itself, some of the biochemical characteristics of DNA, RNA, and proteins will be outlined—without attempting to signify from whence the spark of life first comes.

The controlling functions of DNA as related to RNA and proteins can be diagrammed as follows (Stelios Aktipis, in *Textbook of Biochemistry*, p. 796; Voet and Voet, *Biochemistry*, p. 916):

$$DNA \rightarrow RNA \rightarrow protein$$
$$\downarrow$$
$$DNA$$

Biological information flows from DNA to RNA, from one class of nucleic acid to another, and thence to creating protein. The transfer of information from the DNA to RNA is called *transcription*. The RNA translates this information into the creation of protein in a process appropriately called *translation*. Additionally, DNA can reproduce or self-replicate, thus ensuring the hereditary chain of life. DNA makes copies of itself as each cell divides, with these copies transferred to the daughter cells, which then inherit all the properties and characteristics of the original cell. Or, as said in an anonymous quote, "People are DNA's way of making more DNA" (Voet and Voet, *Biochemistry*, p. 1020).

Briefly stated, DNA molecules are polynucleotides—giant chains of subunits called *nucleotides* with the genetic information stored in the sequences of subunits. Nucleotides consist of a carbohydrate residue (deoxyribose) with a heterocyclic base usually of adenine, guanine, cytosine, or thymine, and a connecting phosphate group. Most (99 percent) DNA occurs in the dense protein-DNA complexes called *chromosomes* but also occurs in mitochondria and chloroplasts. The sequences of subunits are unique to an individual, the basis of DNA fingerprinting or typing.

1.12.1 DNA AND ITS FUNCTIONS

DNA is confined almost exclusively to the eukaryotic cell nucleus, whereas the transcribed RNA is transported to the surrounding cytoplasm, to the cytosol, the part of the cytoplasm exclusive of the membrane-bound organelles (e.g., Voet and Voet, *Biochemistry*, p. 8, 918). Moreover, the cytosolic RNA-containing particles are protein rich and are called *ribosomes*. (As noted, the prefix "ribo-" pertains to pentose, a five-carbon sugar inherent in the DNA/RNA structures.) And, speaking of DNA, a given individual has identical DNA molecules throughout the body.

DNA is synthesized from the polymerization of deoxyribonucleotides, which are formed first from precursor ribonucleotides (Cory, in *Textbook of Biochemistry*, p 656). The ribonucleotides are chemically reduced to produce the deoxyribonucleotides using an enzyme called either nucleoside diphosphate reductase or ribonucleotide reductase. (The actual reactants and products are in the form of nucleoside diphosphates) Deoxyadenosine triphosphate (dATP) is a potent inhibitor for ribonucleotide reductase, and explains why deoxyadenosine is toxic for mammalian cells. The pool of deoxyribonucleotides is low except during DNA replication, when the pool increases to support the synthesis of more DNA.

There is a constant turnover of nucleic acids resulting in the release of pyrimidine nucleotides, manifested as a constant synthesis and *degradation*. (Cory, in *Textbook of Biochemistry*, p. 659). Moreover, the synthesis is affected by the presence of the enzyme deoxyuridine triphosphatase (dUTPase), which converts deoxyuridine triphosphate to deoxyuridine monophosphate. "Mammalian cells have a very specific dUTPase in high concentration for the reaction dUTP to dUMP + pyrophosphate, and it is critical for normal DNA replication that dUTP not be present in the nucleotide pool" (Cory, in *Textbook of Biochemistry*, p. 660). In other words, dUTPase serves to prevent the misincorporation of dUMP into the DNA, which would have other major consequences. It may in fact be related to *cancer* proliferation. Polymerization is catalyzed by various enzymes called *nucleases*, which serve in a selective manner (Aktipis, in *Textbook of Biochemistry*, p. 802). Depending on function, some are called *exonucleases*; others are called *endonucleases*. Other names used are the *DNases*. Applied to RNA, there are the RNases. (For a listing of various DNases and RNases and inhibitors see Appendices E and F.)

The DNA macromolecule encodes an enormous quantity of biological information in its polynucleotide structure (Aktipis, in *Textbook of Biochemistry*, p. 798ff). *Structurally, DNA is a polynucleotide.* These polynucleotides that constitute DNA are polymers formed from nucleotides, analogous to proteins being the polymers formed from amino acids. The nucleotides are classified into what are called *pyrimidine* and *purine* chemical structures, the former being a single-ring structure with carbon and nitrogen in the ring, the latter a double-ring structure. The nucleotides so classified in turn provide four principal bases of chemical structures. For pyrimidine, these are cytosine and thymine; for purine, these are adenine and guanine. Modifications may also occur. Thus, other less common bases include uracil (2,4-dioxpyrimidine). These bases will appear variously in the DNA molecule and in the RNA molecule.

It has been found that in DNA there are equal numbers of the adenine and thymine residues, and equal numbers of guanine and cytosine residues (Voet and Voet, *Biochemistry*, p. 849). Called Chargaff's rules, these results may be expressed as A = T and as G = C. Relatively speaking, G + C may range from 39 to 46 percent of the total in mammals, and from roughly 25 to 75 percent in bacteria.

The polynucleotides are formed by the joining of nucleotides by phosphodiester bonds, which are the analog of the peptide bonds in proteins (Aktipis, in *Textbook of Biochemistry*, 798ff). The result may be a linear chain or may have side chains. A polynucleotide bond may be represented by joining a phosphoric acid group [designated $-(P=O)O(OH)$] with a hydroxyl group [designated as HO– or –OH]:

$$R-(P=O)O(OH) + HO-R' \rightarrow R-(P=O)O-O-R' + H_2O$$

where R and R' denote arbitrary residues (that is, the rest of the nucleotide or polynucleotide segment). A bonding may occur at the opposite ends of each nucleotide, or at other points, depending upon the nature of each individual nucleotide.*

For proteins, the peptide bond can be represented say by the joining of a carboxylic acid group [designated as $-(C=O)OH$] with an amino group [here designated as H_2N- or $-NH_2$]:

$$R-(C=O)OH + H_2N-R' \rightarrow R-(C=O)-NH-R' + H_2O$$

---

* The fact that O–O appears signifies a diester. For an ester or monoester, only one oxygen would appear at this location.

where R and R' again denote arbitrary residues (in this case, the rest of the amino acid or protein segment). A bonding again may occur at the opposite ends of each amino acid, or at other points, depending on the nature of each individual amino acid. The fact that H_2O is produced in both cases signifies these bondings are formed from what may be called *condensation reactions*.

The above-described similarity between the structures of polynucleotides and proteins is a factor in transmitting genetic information between the DNA and protein macromolecules (Aktipis, in *Textbook of Biochemistry*, p. 798). RNA serves as the intermediate for transmitting the information. In fact, "all cellular RNA is synthesized on a DNA template and reflects a portion of the DNA base sequence" (Gray, in *Textbook of Biochemistry*, p. 872). That is, DNA sets the pattern for RNA.

1.12.2   RNA AND ITS FUNCTIONS

The primary genetic information is localized in the cell nucleus and encoded in the DNA (cf., Peter N. Gray, in *Textbook of Biochemistry*, p. 872ff). A means is required to transfer this information from the DNA to the protein-synthesizing machinery, located outside the nucleus in the cytoplasm. The macromolecules which transfer this information reflect the sequence of pyrimidines and purines of the DNA, and are called ribonucleic acids or RNA's. (As noted above for DNA, the modifier "ribo-" is derived from the word ribose, signifying a sugar of the pentose class, with five carbons, say $C_5H_{10}O_5$.) The process of transference is called transcription.

There are several distinct molecular forms for RNA, one of which is called messenger RNA, or mRNA. Another is called transfer RNA, or tRNA. Still another is called ribosomal RNA, or rRNA. A table of the different kinds is provided in the reference. It is noted that RNA reflects the DNA base sequence, and therefore all RNA is associated with DNA at some time or another. While RNA functions in the cytoplasm outside the nucleus, some RNA remains inside the nucleus performing structural and regulatory roles.

Thus, RNA is chemically very similar to DNA but is not very stable, being first synthesized, then used, and finally and rapidly degraded (Gray, in *Textbook of Biochemistry*, p. 874). RNA can be described, furthermore, as an unbranched linear polymer with the monomeric units consisting of ribonucleoside 5'-monophosphates.

The single-ring pyridines are cytosine and uracil; the double-ring purines are adenine and guanine. These bases are the same as in DNA except that uracil replaces thymine.

The various monomers which make up the polymer are joined at bonds linking a phosphate group with an OH group in the ring structure. That is,

$$R-(P=O)O(OH) + HO-R' \rightarrow R-(P=O)O-O-R' + H_2O$$

There is a similarity with DNA except that the 5' carbon in one ribose is always linked with the 3'-carbon of the next ribose structure. Thus, the bond or link may be called a 3',5' phosphodiester. Furthermore, the polymers are linear, forming a chain.

Both DNA and RNA are synthesized or involved in reactions with specific enzymes for catalysts, and there are in turn enzyme inhibitors for the catalysts. Enzymes and inhibitors are set forth in Appendix E for DNA, and in Appendix F for RNA. The list of enzymes is extensive, indicating that quite a number of things go on with DNA and RNA.

As to inhibitors, some of the more common compounds or substances are highlighted in bold-face—and many of the antibiotics are represented in italics as enzyme inhibitors. (Antibiotics may variously be recognized by their suffixes: -ycin, -cin, -cline, -icol, -oside, -orin, -yxin, -ampin.) As will be subsequently indicated, the antibiotics are specific to the functions of prokaryotic cells, that is, to bacteria.

A number of alkaloids are listed, usually ending in "-ine." In Appendix E there are acridine derivatives, ellipticine, an ellipticine derivative, spermidine, spermine, fagaronine, theophylline, and papaverine. In Appendix F there are fagaronine, lasiocarpine, a derivative of quinoline, acridine, atropine, emetine, spermine, and vinblastine.

1.12.3   TRANSCRIPTION

As to transcription, the synthetic process transferring genetic information from DNA to RNA, the enzyme responsible is called DNA-dependent RNA polymerase (Gray, in *Textbook of Biochemistry*, p. 889). Also known as DNA-directed RNA polymerase, it is infrequently referred to as transcriptase. Alternatively, the enzyme may be called simply RNA polymerase (Voet and Voet, *Biochemistry*, pp. 919). It occurs in the DNA-containing organelles of all cells, located in the nucleus. The enzyme links the ribonucleoside triphosphates named adenosine triphosphate (ATP), cytosine triphosphate (CTP), guanosine triphosphate (GTP), and uridinetriphosphate (UTP). The process is known as RNA synthesis, and the basic linkages formed are the RNA residues, which constitute the polymer that is RNA.

Transcription is inhibited by substances which block the functions of RNA polymerase (Gray, in *Textbook of Biochemistry*, p. 897ff.) These include actinomycin D, probably the best known. Ethidium bromide is another well known inhibitor. Actinomycin D is also regarded as an antitumor agent, although its toxicity prevents its widespread use (Gray, in *Textbook of Biochemistry*, p. 899). It is noted that the potent toxin α-amanitin, obtained from the poisonous mushroom *Amanita phalloides*, acts as a specific inhibitor for RNA polymerase II.

1.12.4 TRANSLATION

Translation is the biosynthesis of polypeptides or proteins from amino acids, which is directed by messenger RNA or mRNA (Voet and Voet, *Biochemistry*, p. 959). It involves the linking together of the 20 common amino acids to form proteins (Voet and Voet, *Biochemistry*, p. 965ff). The molecules which transfer the amino acids from the soluble amino acid pool are called transfer RNA or tRNA (Gray, in *Textbook of Biochemistry*, p. 892). The amino acids are transferred to the ribosomes, the ribonucleic particles in the cell cytoplasm where protein synthesis takes place.

Translation requires the choice of the correct amino acid for attachment to tRNA and the proper selection of the amino-acid attached tRNA specified by mRNA (Voet and Voet, *Biochemistry*, pp. 971–973). This is accomplished by enzymes known as aminoacyl-tRNA synthetases.

1.12.5 PROTEINS

Proteins are polymers of amino acids. Proteins perform two essential types of functions in mammals: dynamic, and structural or static (Richard M. Schultz, in *Textbook of Biochemistry*, p. 30ff). Enzymes are an example of proteins that perform a dynamic type of function, being the catalysts for biochemical reactions. Another dynamic function is that of transport. Thus, hemoglobin carries oxygen in the blood and myoglobin carries oxygen in the muscle. Transferrin transports iron in the blood. Other proteins move hormones in the blood from one site to another, and many drugs and toxic compounds bind to proteins to be carried throughout the body system. Proteins may act against disease; for instance, immunoglobins and interferon protect the body against bacterial and viral infections. The protein fibrin is formed to protect against blood loss.

Many hormones are in fact proteins, such as insulin, thyrotropin, somatotropin (the growth-hormone), the ovarian luteinizing hormone, and the follicle stimulating hormone. Protein-type hormones of relatively low molecular weight are known as *peptides*. Among the peptide hormones are adrenocorticotropin, antidiuretic hormone, glucagon, and calcitonin. A point of distinction is that the term peptide is used for molecules with less that 50 amino acids, and "protein" for molecules with more that 50 amino acids.

The proteins myosin and actin are involved in muscle contraction. Gene transcription and translation are carried out by proteins. There are variously the histone proteins, repressor proteins, and proteins in the ribosomes.

The structural proteins include collagen and elastin. These proteins form the matrix for bone and ligaments, and give strength and elasticity to the organs and to the vascular system. The protein α-keratin plays a role in the structure of epidermal tissue.

All proteins are initially synthesized in the body from only 20 different amino acids. These are called the common amino acids, which are those which have a specific codon or set of codons in the DNA genetic code, to be further explained in a separate section.

The common amino acids have the general structure R–CH(NH$_2$)COOH where the first carbon is the central or *alpha* carbon, and R is an arbitrary side chain (Schultz, in *Textbook of Biochemistry*, p. 32ff). The side chain R, a hydrogen, the amino group (–NH$_2$) and the carboxylic acid group (–COOH) are all attached to the same central carbon. Alternatively, the representation may be expressed as R–CH(NH$_3^+$)COO$^-$. The nature of the amino acid will depend on the particular side group or side chain R. Structures of the 20 common amino acids are provided in the reference.

It may be noted that some of the side chains or groups may contain nitrogen or sulfur as well as carbon, hydrogen, and oxygen. Thus, methionine and cysteine both contain sulfur. Tryptophan, asparagine, glutamine, lysine, arginine, and histidine contain nitrogen in the side chain or group R.

Polymerization of the common amino acids into polypeptides or proteins within cells is enzyme catalyzed. Dehydration occurs, with H_2O released. The part of the amino acid left over after dehydration is called the residue. According to the above, a residue will have the form R–CH(NH–)COO– where (–) denotes a point of linkage to the next residue. The specific amino acid sequence which occurs in the polymer formed is called the primary structure.

The structure becomes increasingly complicated, however, and is so designated by the terms secondary, tertiary, and quaternary structures (Schultz, in *Textbook of Biochemistry*, p. 58ff).

Cell requirements for protein synthesis vary greatly (Muench, in *Textbook of Biochemistry*, p. 926ff). Mature red blood cells for instance do not have the enzymes and organelles (cellular compartments) necessary for protein synthesis, and die-off after about 120 days. Some cells are able to maintain the status quo, having the necessary and sufficient enzymes for replacing structural proteins as needed. Growing and dividing cells demand higher levels of protein synthesis. And some cells synthesize enough protein for export. The last-mentioned category includes for example pancreatic cells, endocrine cells, and liver cells. These cells contain large quantities of the ribonucleoproteins called ribosomes in the cytoplasm (the part of the cell outside the nucleus), whose function is to biosynthesize proteins. Even the organelles called the mitochondria, which are connected with respiration, have a limited synthetic protein capacity (Devlin, in *Textbook of Biochemistry*, pp. 21–22).

It may be remarked that protein synthesis occurs in the cell endoplasm, the inner part of the cell cytoplasm, the latter being the part of the cell exclusive of the nucleus. There is an extensive membrane that forms a labyrinthine compartment or organelle called the *endoplasmic reticulum* (Voet and Voet, *Biochemistry*, p. 8). Part of this organelle, called the *rough* endoplasmic reticulum, is covered with ribosomes where protein synthesis occurs, with the proteins either remaining membrane bound or else secreted. Another part, called the *smooth* endoplasmic reticulum, and bare of ribosomes, is where lipid synthesis occurs. Synthesis products move on to the Golgi apparatus or Golgi complex, a packet of flattened membrane sacks, for further processing and dissemination.

1.12.6 CHANGES

Deviations in the normal mechanisms that regulate cell growth manifest themselves in several ways, including chromosomal changes that can be detected microscopically. For example, chromosomes may exchange material, a process called *translocation*. The result may be altered genes, called *oncogenes*, which are responsible for abnormal cell proliferation. The subject has been described in depth by Avery A. Sandberg in an article appearing in the May/June, 1994 issue of *CA—A Cancer Journal for Clinicians*. Tabulations are presented for chromosomal changes which occur in a number of tumors.*

The foregoing indicates that genetic changes can lead to serious, life-threatening consequences in the form of cancer. No doubt there are other manifestations. It gives pause to efforts to manipulate the genetic code. And as to tinkering with the genetic code, the warning signs continue. For instance Jane Rissler and Margaret Mellon of the Union of Concerned Scientists, Cambridge MA, have written *The Ecological Risks of Engineered Crops*. It seems that the transplanting of presumably desirable genes from one plant species into another may cause some untoward and unexpected side effects. We may expect more of the same with animals. The big argument of course remains that about genetic manipulations within the human animal.

1.13 THE GENETIC CODE

The makeup of the genetic code comprises permutations of the four purine and pyrimidine base residues (Muench, in *Textbook of Biochemistry*, pp. 918–920). The base residues are adenine, guanine, cytosine, and thymine, designated respectively as A, G, C, and T, but may alternatively include uracil U, say, instead of thymine. These designators are arranged in groups of three, or triplets, in all possible combinations or permutations. In some groups a letter designator may appear three times, in others, twice, in the rest, once. This is a feature of arranging permutations in all possible combinations.

---

* We may wonder at what part enzymes may play in these genetic changes, and what part enzyme inhibitors may also play.

Each triplet is called a "codon." The number of possible permutations is $4^3 = 64$ for groups of three in terms of these four bases. The set or entirety of the 64 codons or triplets is known as the genetic code.

The way the system works is that each triplet is a combination that encodes the genetic instructions for the protein-making machinery to form an amino acid. Sometimes, the order of the sequence may be determining. Thus, consider the code combinations for the genetic instructions to produce adenine, cytosine, and guanine, which may be represented as ACG, AGC, GAC, GCA, CAG, and CGA. These stand, respectively, for codons for threonine, serine, aspartate (aspartic acid), alanine, glutamate (glutamic acid), and arginine. There are other groups or combinations, however, that will encode the same acid.

Thus, some amino acids will be encoded by one codon or triplet, such as tryptophan or methionine. Other amino acids may have as many as six codons that are the codes for producing the acid, for example, arginine, leucine, and serine.

Four of the 64 codons or triplets are used to denote start and stop signals for protein synthesis. The start signal is AUG, which is also signifies the code of genetic instructions for producing methionine. That is, adenine, uracil, and guanine uniquely form the triplet or codon AUG, which is the code for forming methionine. When AUG appears at the beginning of a message, it will signal that methionine is the initial amino acid at the amino terminal of the protein to be synthesized. The stop signals, UAA, UAG, and UGA specify no amino acids, and are designated as nonsense codons. The genetic code is universal, with the exception of unique uses in the mitochondria, the cell organelles or compartments associated with respiration.

It so turns out that 20 different synthetic amino acids may be encoded by the codons. These are the so-called common amino acids. They are alanine (Ala), arginine (Arg), asparagine (Asn), aspartate (Asp), cysteine (Cys), glutamine (Gln), glutamate (Glu), glycine (Gly), histamine (His), isoleucine (Ile), leucine (Leu), lysine (Lys), methionine (Met), phenylalanine (Phe), proline (Pro), serine (Ser), threonine (Thr), tryptophan (Trp), tyrosine (Tyr), and valine (Val).

The combination of codons or triplets forms a synthetic peptide or protein. Aberrations may be viewed as mutations. Some viruses, for instance, may contain aberrations, causing tumors.

Since a human DNA molecule may obtain upward of 5 million nucleotides or subunits, the possible arrangements are nearly infinite, as per DNA fingerprinting. The chances are near zero that two persons could have matching DNA—and if not, then they can't be the same person.

As to concrete uses of genetic engineering in cancer treatment, there is talk of the creation of genetic time bombs within cells, which would be triggered by the presence of cancer proteins. For example, a gene-produced bacterial enzyme called purine nucleoside phosphorylase would be formed, which turns a harmless cellular compound into a toxic cell-killing chemical. Presumably, the effect would be localized in the cancerous cell and thus be selective. Obviously there are hazards—for instance, something else might trigger these genetic time bombs. Genetic engineering is both difficult and uncertain at best and, like so many other things, it may prove to be no ready panacea. More straightforward and simple methods would indeed be welcome.

1.13.1 GENETIC CANCER THERAPY

The systemic treatment of cancer by cytotoxic or hormonally active agents has been reviewed by Irwin H. Krakoff in an article published by the American Cancer Society, with biological agents (bioactive substances) considered the next big step. Beyond this is gene therapy, whereby the introduction of tumor suppressor genes can confer genetic resistance. The subject of oncogenes and tumor suppressor genes had previously been reviewed in an article by Robert A. Weinberg, who supplied a listing of cloned tumor suppressor genes. As an example, the colon cancer model was utilized, where the APC suppressor gene in mutant form permits the outgrowth of early colonic polyps. These mutant APC genes may be random (not inherited) or may be the more rare familial type (inherited from a parent). The latter are thus implanted in all colonic cells—a predisposing resulting in hundreds if not thousands of polyps. In turn, there may be further mutations over a period of years, leading to the uncontrolled growth of colon cancer cells. The problem, of course, is how to turn it all off.

1.14 DIGESTION

The previous considerations about proteins enters into the arena of digestion, which generally involves the salivary glands, the gastric mucosa, and the pancreas, which release enzymes into the gastrointestinal tract (Chaney, in *Textbook of Biochemistry*, p. 1135ff). Additionally, hydrochloric acid is secreted in the gastrointestinal tract, and the electrolytes sodium chloride and sodium bicarbonate are involved. In addition to proteins, the main dietary classes are carbohydrates and fats.

1.14.1   DIETARY PROTEINS

The foregoing synthesized proteins are not necessarily the same as the nutritional or dietary proteins. These dietary proteins are broken down by digestive enzymes into amino acids for further cell protein synthesis, as previously outlined. These synthesized proteins variously become a structural component of all cells, enzymes and hormones, and plasma proteins, which are involved in cellular osmotic balances, in transporting substances through the blood system, and in maintaining immunity (Chaney, in *Textbook of Biochemistry*, p. 1179ff.) Most of the protein consumed in the diet is usually in excess, however, and is used instead as a source of energy, with the glycogenic amino acids converted to glucose or glycogen, and the ketogenic amino acids converted to fatty acids and keto acids. [The prefix "keto-" denotes or relates to ketones, a special class of chemical compounds containing the carbonyl (C=O) group.] The final metabolic products are excreted as urea and ammonia, both nitrogen-containing compounds.*

The overall nitrogen balance is that of dietary protein in (N in), forming an amino acid pool, compared against that used in the body for conversion to tissue protein and for biosynthetic reactions plus energy, and that lost be excretion (N out). Normally, in adults, the nitrogen is in balance. That is, there is a steady-state condition. With growing children, there is a positive balance, with more N going in than goes out. A negative nitrogen balance is caused by injury or illness, when the body catabolizes its protein stores, including that in the tissues. This happens during the ravages of cancer and its chemotherapeutic treatment, for instance, signaled by the wasting-away called cachexia.

The nutritional requirements of mammals require certain amino acids which are divided into essential and nonessential amino acids. The essential amino acids must be obtained from outside the body. The nonessential can be synthesized within the body.

The ten essential amino acids are arginine, histidine, isoleucine, leucine, lysine, methionine, phenylalanine, threonine, tryptophan, and valine. The eleven nonessential amino acids are alanine, asparagine, aspartate, cysteine, glutamine, glutamate, glycine, hydroxyproline, proline, serine, and tyrosine. Hydroxy-proline is not one of the 20 common amino acids.

1.14.2   CARBOHYDRATES

Carbohydrates are the main source for energy, with any excess converted to glycogen and triglycerides or fats, to be stored (Chaney, in *Textbook of Biochemistry*, p. 1189ff). Dietary carbohydrates are the most important energy source, and include mono-, di-, and polysaccharides (Chaney, in *Textbook of Biochemistry*, p. 1156ff). The various saccharides may be regarded as esters formed from glucose and carboxylic acids. Starch is a notable example of a polysaccharide. Other examples of carbohydrates are the sugars, ending in "-ose". The reference supplies a few representative carbohydrates: amylopectin from potatoes, rice, corn, bread; amulose from the same; sucrose; trehalose from mushrooms; lactose from milk; fructose from fruit and honey; glucose from fruit, honey, grapes; raffinose from leguminous seeds. By the processes of digestion, enzymes catalyze the conversion of carbohydrates, notably to glucose. Some carbohydrates are relatively indigestible, since the necessary enzymes are lacking, the main example being leguminous seeds or beans.

1.14.3   FATS

Triglycerides or fats are used as an energy source and as a part of membrane structure. Any excess is stored only as fat or triglyceride (Chaney, in *Textbook of Biochemistry*, p. 1190). A triglyceride—also called a neutral fat, or more properly, a triacylglycerol—is a chemical compound called an ester which is formed from the reaction of glycerol with a fatty acid. Glycerol, a trihydroxy alcohol may be represented as $(HO)CH_2CH(OH)CH_2(OH)$. Fatty acids and glycerol are found in nature in the combined form usually called triglycerides, which are of a class of substances called lipids (Voet and Voet,

---

* Amino acids whose carbonaceous products are first pyruvate, then recycled glucose or glycogen via the Cori cycle, and/or CO_2 and H_2O via the tricarboxylic acid cycle, are called glycogenic. Those which first yield acetyl CoA, acetoacetyl CoA, or free acetoacetate, which is of the keto form, and eventually yield fatty acids and keto acids, are called ketogenic (Diamondstone, in *Textbook of Biochemistry*, pp. 580–581).

Biochemistry, p. 278). Lipids are soluble in organic solvents but sparingly soluble in water. Lipids embrace what are called fats and oils, and also include certain vitamins and hormones. Most nonprotein cell membrane components are lipids. Triacylglycerols or triglycerides are converted to the corresponding fatty acids in the body, which are in turn used for energy or for other biochemical processes (Francis N. LeBaron, in *Textbook of Biochemistry*, p. 440ff). Fatty acids may also be synthesized in the body. Some fatty acids are considered essential, e.g., palmitic, palmitoleic, stearic, oleic, linoleic, linolenic, and arachidonic. The digestion of lipids is initiated by the enzyme lipase, of pancreatic origin, producing hydrolysis (Chaney, in *Textbook of Biochemistry*, p. 1162ff). Further action is by way of liver bile acids. Fatty acids are thus produced, to be absorbed by intestinal cells. The final product is formed as "chylomicrons," which are microglobules. The chylomicrons are released onto intercellular space and eventually move into the blood system or into the lymph vessels, depending upon globule size.

1.15   PROTEASES AND PROTEASE INHIBITORS

Proteases are enzymes involved in the digestion of proteins. Inasmuch as a newly-proposed treatment for AIDS involves the use of protease inhibitors, this particular subject area will be explored further. Because AIDS is an immunodeficiency disease, and cancer is at times described in the same way, there may be a connection. In other words, what works against AIDS may also work against cancer, and vice versa.

The enzymes that are involved in the digestion of proteins are in general called *peptidases* (Ulrich Hopfer, in *Textbook of Biochemistry*, p. 1150ff). These are hydrolases that break the peptide bonds in the protein polymers. This general classification is divided into endopeptidases (which break internal bonds, liberating large peptide fragments) and exopeptidases (which clip off one amino acid at a time from the either the COOH end or the NH_2 end of the peptide fragments). Exopeptidases are further divided into carboxypeptidases and aminopeptidases, depending on whether the carboxy or COOH end is attacked, or the amino or NH_2 end is attacked. The endopeptidases are also called *proteases*. They are formed from precursors called proenzymes.

The digestion of proteins is ordinarily considered to occur in is the gastric, pancreatic, and intestinal phases, depending on the respective sources of the enzymes.

Gastric juices contain hydrochloric acid (HCl) plus proteases of the pepsin family. The acid kills off microorganisms and makes the proteins more easily hydrolyzed by the proteases. The pepsins, incidentally, are active in an acid environment but not at neutral conditions.

Pancreatic juice contains protease enzymes such as trypsin, chymotrypsin, and elastase. These enzymes catalyze reactions involving a "serine" residue and thus may be called *serine* proteases. Still other enzymes furnish carboxypeptidase activity.

It is noted in the reference that compounds that interact with serine will inactivate or inhibit these enzymes. An example furnished is diisopropylphosphofluoridate.

The final digestion phase occurs in the small intestine, where the surface epithelial cells furnish aminopeptidase activity. The end products are free amino acids and di- and tri-peptides, which are absorbed into the epithelial cells. The di- and tri-peptides are for the most part hydrolyzed in the cell cytoplasm, and the end-product amino acids enter the portal blood stream going from the intestine to the liver, for subsequent utilization.*

The serine proteases not only include trypsin, chymotrypsin, and elastase from the pancreas, but various proteases from other sources (Voet and Voet, *Biochemistry*, p. 389ff). A table is provided in the reference. Whereas the pancreas enzymes are associated with digestion, these other proteases have other functions. Some of these other serine protease sources are from blood or serum, from animal cells, from moth larvae, and even from bacteria.

Thus, the protease known as Complement C1, obtained from blood serum, is involved in the immune response. Cocoonase, from moth larvae, is involved in dissolving the cocoon after metamorphosis. The enzyme α-lytic protease is from the bacterium *Bacillus sorangium*; proteases A and B are from *Streptomyces griseus*; the protease subtilisin is from *Bacillus subtilis*. The latter three proteases are assumed to be involved in digestion.

---

* It is this portal blood stream that carries colon cancer cells to the liver. Thus, colon cancer cells unfortunately tend to metastasize to the liver.

An inhibitor for trypsin is named the *bovine pancreatic trypsin inhibitor* or BPTI (Voet and Voet, *Biochemistry*, p. 396ff). Its main purpose is to keep prematurely activated trypsin from digesting the pancreas itself. Apparently, the BPTI structure resembles trypsin, thus binding to trypsin and canceling its enzymatic activity.

The reference further states that protease inhibitors are common in nature, having both protective and regulatory functions. Moreover, protease inhibitors may comprise about 10 percent of the almost 200 proteins found in blood serum.

For one example, α_1-protease inhibitor, secreted by the liver, inhibits leucocyte elastase. In further explanation, leucocytes (or leukocytes) are a form of white blood cells, and the enzymatic action of leucocyte elastase is said to be part of the inflammatory process. *Very possibly, the inhibitory action of α_1-protease inhibitor may stimulate the immune system, although the reference provides no details.*

Another example provided is a variant of what is called the α_1-proteinase inhibitor, and which is associated with pulmonary emphysema, a disease resulting from the hydrolysis of the elastic fibers of the lung. Although unstated, presumably there is excess enzymatic activity of α_1-proteinase, which is ordinarily controlled by the α_1-proteinase inhibitor. Smoking is noted to cause a reduced activity of the α_1-proteinase inhibitor, which is not regained until several hours after smoking.

Natural protease inhibitors such as occur in soybeans and other seeds are said to act as survival agents by preventing the seeds from being digested by proteolytic enzymes in the gastrointestinal tract of animals (Boik, *Cancer & Natural Medicine*, p. 156). More than this, however, protease inhibitors are reported to act against cancer. A particular example is the Bowman-Birk protease inhibitor (BBI), obtained from soybeans, which has been found to act against cancers of the colon, oral cavity, lung, liver, and esophagus, at least in animals. The reference states that soybeans contain other agents that evidently also act against cancer, e.g., isoflavones and lignans.

For the record, a listing of protease inhibitors is given in Appendix G, with the anticipation that these inhibitors and their sources might provide some clues in the treatment of AIDS and of cancer. The listings are from Jain's *Handbook of Enzyme Inhibitors* and Zollner's *Handbook of Enzyme Inhibitors*.

Some of the sources for various protease inhibitors and proteinase inhibitors include black-eyed peas, lima beans, kidney beans, wheat and rye germ, potatoes, bovine cartilage, bee venom, and viper venom. Human bronchial secretions and guinea pig blood are also mentioned.

The various beans (of the plant family Leguminosae) contain not only *cyanoglycosides* (e.g., laetrile or amygdalin) but *alkaloids*. Wheat and rye (of the plant family Gramineae) evidently contain trace amounts of *alkaloids*, and potatoes (of the plant family Solanaceae or Nightshade family) are especially noted for *alkaloids*. These several species are entered in Hartwell's *Plants Used Against Cancer*. Bovine cartilage has been proposed as an anticancer agent, along with shark cartilage, as will be noted elsewhere, and snake venom was once touted as an anticancer agent.

1.16   PROTEIN DEGRADATION

Cells are in the continual process of both synthesizing proteins and degrading them to their component amino acids (Voet and Voet, *Biochemistry*, p. 1010ff). Cell proteins may in fact have lifetimes ranging from a few minutes to weeks or more. The purposes for this turnover are to get rid of abnormal or harmful proteins and to regulate cell metabolism by eliminating unneeded enzymes and regulatory proteins. It is commented, furthermore, that controlling the rate of degradation is as important as controlling the rate of synthesis.

The connection to destroying cancer cells is obvious.

An example provided is that of hemoglobin which is synthesized with the valine analog α-amino-β-chlorobutyrate, which has a half-life of approximately 10 minutes as compared to normal hemoglobin, which lasts over the lifetime of 120 days for red cells (making it probably the cytoplasmic protein with the longest lifetime). The ability to degrade abnormal cell proteins is essential to preventing the buildup of substances that interfere with cell metabolism.

The elimination rate of normal cell proteins varies with identity. For instance, the most rapidly degraded enzymes are those that occupy important metabolic controls.

The protein degradation rate in a cell also depends on nutritional and hormonal conditions. For example, if nutritionally deprived, cells degrade protein more rapidly to furnish nutrients for critical metabolic processes. Increased rates of degradation can be prevented by antibiotics, which block protein synthesis in the first place.

If the above is so, then antibiotics may possibly block the degradation of cancer cells as well as normal cells.

The lifetime of a cytoplasmic or cellular protein depends on the N-terminal residue, that is, upon the identity of an end or terminal group. The lifetimes of cytoplasmic proteins terminating Met, Ser, Ala, Thr, Val, Gly, and Cys residues tend to be stable, with half-lifetimes of approximately 20 hr. Those with Ile, Glu, Tyr, and Gln have half-lifetimes of approximately 10–30 minutes, while those with Phe, Leu, Asp, Lys, and Arg have half-lifetimes of approximately 2–3 minutes. Other factors, enter, however, in that proteins with segments of Pro, Glu, Ser, and Thr (called PEST proteins) are rapidly degraded.

It would be important to know, therefore, whether the proteins in cancer cells are different from those in normal cells.

1.17 ANTIBIOTICS

Antibiotics act as protein synthesis inhibitors (Voet and Voet, *Biochemistry*, pp. 1002–1004). More specifically, "Antibiotics are bacterially or fungally produced substances that inhibit the growth of other organisms." Some are known to inhibit such biologically essential processes as DNA replication (e.g., novabiocin), transcription (e.g., rifamycin B), and bacterial cell wall synthesis (e.g., penicillin). The great majority block translation in prokaryotic cells—that is, in bacteria. Of these, many are medically useful. Some of the best known are streptomycin, chloramphenicol, tetracycline, and diphtheria toxoid. The toxoid, which is formaldehyde-killed toxin, is used for immunization against diphtheria.

At lower concentrations, streptomycin causes the ribosome to misread mRNA. At higher concentrations, it prevents chain initiation, resulting in cell death.

The broad-spectrum antibiotic chloramphenicol inhibits the activity of the enzyme peptidyl transferase. Its side effects are toxic, so its use is limited to severe infections.

Tetracycline and its derivatives inhibit tRNA binding and nucleotide synthesis (a nucleotide called ppGpp). Resistant strains of bacteria have caused serious problems.

Diphtheria toxoid is a formaldehyde-inactivated toxin, an antitoxin prepared from horse serum. It binds with the diphtheria toxin, thereby inactivating the toxin. Diphtheria toxin itself is a protein that works to inhibit eukaryotic protein synthesis in the body. The toxin is the result of a bacterial infection by *Corynebacterium diphtheriae*, which secretes the toxin.

The selectivity of antibiotics lies in the fact that they interfere with prokaryotic protein synthesis rather than eukaryotic protein synthesis (Muench, in *Textbook of Biochemistry*, pp. 936–937)—that is, of the bacteria rather than of the body cells. Some of the antibiotics are too toxic for clinical use but are nevertheless important in studying the steps in protein synthesis.

There is not much emphasis on antibiotics serving as anticancer agents, although they fall under the general category of chemotherapy, e.g., in the section on Drug and Drug Action in the *Encyclopedia Britannica*. At least two have been cited, however, e.g., daunomycin and adriamycin, which are closely related (Voet and Voet, *Biochemistry*, First Edition, Wiley, New York, 1990, pp. 862–863). They have been used in the treatment of certain human cancers and are called valuable chemotherapeutic agents. Their action is to bind to DNA so as to inhibit both transcription and replication. Another antibiotic, called actinomycin D, inhibits nucleic acid synthesis. Perhaps for these and other reasons, some antibiotics are regarded as too toxic to be used for antibiotic purposes.

A considerable number of antibiotics are prominently listed in Appendices E and F as inhibitors for some of the enzymes involved in DNA/RNA processes. A search of MEDLINE for cancer and antibiotics indicates that most antibiotic uses are for fighting infections that may occur during cancer treatment. On occasion, however, certain antibiotics have been studied for their anticancer effects. At the University of Texas M.D. Anderson Cancer Center, for example, there have been investigations on the effect of actinomycin D and doxorubicin, considered anticancer agents, along with the *mitotic* inhibitors vinblastine and Taxol.* According to encyclopedic references, doxorubicin, daunorubicin, bleomycin,

---

* Derived from plant extracts, the latter two inhibit cell division or mitosis. Vinblastine is a *Vinca* alkaloid derived from the Madagascar periwinkle, now more properly named *Catharanthus roseus* (the similar alkaloid vincristine is derived from the same plant, another alkaloid of many). Taxol is derived from the yew tree of the Pacific Northwest.

mitomycin, and dactinomycin are antineoplastic or anticancer agents, albeit too toxic for routine antibiotic use.

1.18   DNA REPLICATION

DNA replication pertains to the synthesis of more DNA. It occurs by virtue of *DNA-directed DNA polymerases* or *DNA-dependent DNA polymerases,* called simply *DNA polymerases* (Voet and Voet, *Biochemistry*, p. 1021). In other words, DNA may be said to direct its own replication (Voet and Voet, *Biochemistry*, p. 854). DNA polymerase plus various other DNA polymerases are listed in Appendix E, along with inhibitors for each. There is also a category called *RNA-directed DNA polymerase* or *RNA-dependent DNA polymerase,* often called *reverse transcriptase,* which is included in Appendix F with its inhibitors. (Reverse transcriptase is a distinguishing feature of *retroviruses* such as HIV and the Marburg and Ebola viruses.) The subject of DNA repair and recombination may be included with DNA replication, but here will treated separately.

Enzymes involved in *DNA replication* include DNA gyrase, DNA polymerases I, II, and III, and such others as helicases and DNA ligases (Voet and Voet, *Biochemistry*, pp. 952–957). While prokaryotic (bacterial) DNA has its own mechanisms for replication (Voet and Voet, *Biochemistry*, pp. 1030–1038), the mechanisms for eukaryotic (animal cell) DNA replication are more complex. Thus, the DNA polymerases involved can in turn be broken down into DNA Polymerase I, DNA Polymerase II, and DNA Polymerase III, as found in the prokaryotic cells of *E. coli*. In turn, there are the DNA polymerase versions α, β, γ, δ, ε as occur in eukaryotic cells. The subject gets increasingly complicated.

1.19   DNA ALTERATIONS

The repairs, recombinations, and other modifications that may occur in DNA can be linked with cancer as follows.

1.19.1   REPAIR

It has been noted that DNA contains the base thymine, whereas RNA contains the base uracil instead. The reasons behind this were discovered in that the base cytosine, also present in DNA and RNA, will convert to uracil (Voet and Voet, *Biochemistry*, pp. 1049–1050). If uracil had originally been a base in DNA, there would then be a mismatch among the bases, and mutations would occur. As it is, any uracil that shows up is converted or excised by the enzyme uracil N-glycosylase, and replaced by cytosine. (Uracyl N-glycosylase is also involved in DNA replication.) In these complex ways does nature correct itself at the DNA level.

The inference here is that if the correction does not occur, will the cells then become mutagenic and cancerous? This may mean that the enzyme uracil N-glycosylase has been inhibited.*

It is observed that agents such as UV radiation, alklyating agents, and cross-linking agents cause DNA damage in *E. coli* (Voet and Voet, *Biochemistry*, p. 1051ff). This in turn produces a cellular changes in *E. coli* called the *SOS response*. The affected cells cease dividing and act instead to repair the DNA damage.

The question, of course, is that if the prokaryotic cells of the bacterium E. coli *act in this way, under what circumstances will damaged or cancerous eukaryotic (animal or human cells) also act to repair themselves in the same manner?*

It is noted in the reference that some *E. coli* with mutant genes have their SOS response permanently turned on. Some very complicated procedures are modeled for controlling the SOS response.

1.19.2   CARCINOGEN IDENTIFICATION

Further information is provided in the reference for identifying chemicals that may be carcinogenic (Voet and Voet, *Biochemistry*, p. 1051). Thus, carcinogens can induce an SOS response in bacteria and cause

---

* An entry for uracil N-glycolase could not be found in either Jain's *Handbook* or Zollner's *Handbook*. The closest similarity was uracil-DNA glycohydrolase in Zollner's *Handbook*. For the record, the four inhibitors listed for the latter enzyme are 6-aminouracil, 5-azauracil, inhibitor protein, and uracil. The last mentioned, uracil, may act as an inhibitor by virtue of being in the particular reaction or else by being chemically similar to a reactant or product, as may the other inhibitors.

mutations, and there is a strong correlation between mutagenesis and carcinogenesis. This is the basis for the Ames test.

The Ames test uses a special strain of the bacterium *Salmonella typhimurium* which cannot synthesize histidine and therefore cannot grow in its absence. The bacteria are placed in a culture medium lacking histidine but which contains a suspected mutagenic or carcinogenic agent. If mutagenesis occurs due to the added agent, some of the bacteria revert and are then able to synthesize histidine and are observed to grow.

Among the carcinogens that have been found by the Ames test is tris (2-3-dibromopropyl) phosphate, commonly called Tris. Formerly used as a fire-retardant on children's sleepwear, it can be absorbed through the skin. At one time in Japan, it was even used as an antibacterial agent in food.

It is mentioned that carcinogens also occur in food, e.g., in alfalfa sprouts. The potent toxin called aflatoxin B_1, produced by a mold which grows in peanuts and corn, is cited as one of the most powerful carcinogens known. Charred or browned foods are another source of carcinogens. The list could no doubt go on. For more, consult Part 6.

1.19.3 DNA RECOMBINATION

DNA genetic recombination is the exchange of segments between DNA molecules (Voet and Voet, *Biochemistry*, p. 1053ff). It provides a way to install foreign DNA in the recipient's chromosome. The segment may originate from another chromosome, a plasmid, or a virus. (A plasmid is a foreign DNA molecule.)

The inferences are obvious. For recombination can be a conduit for the formation of cancerous cells.

In what is called DNA combination repair, the damaged DNA segment is replaced by the corresponding segment from undamaged strand of DNA.

Both of the foregoing types of recombinations have been found to be catalyzed in *E. coli* by an enzyme called RecA protein (further identified as a 38-D nuclease).

1.19.4 DNA METHYLATION

Another aberration that may occur is the introduction of a methyl group into the base residues, i.e., into adenine and cytosine (Voet and Voet, *Biochemistry*, p. 1065ff). The circumstantial evidence is that DNA methylation cuts off eukaryotic gene expression in mammals, although how this is done is not known. Presumably methylation is catalyzed by methylases, and the methyl group is furnished by a methyl donor such as S-adenosinemethionine. Furthermore, the eukaryotic methylation varies with species, tissue, and the position along the chromosome. Also, the methylation sites are palindromic, giving the same pattern forward or backward or, in other words, are symmetric. For various reasons, this will favor the same pattern in daughter cells for succeeding generations.

Again, the inferences are obvious—that methylation could lead to the formation of cancerous cells. Not only this, but the origins of different kinds of cancers can be explained in that methylation varies with species, tissue, and position. And the methylation pattern will be inherited, being maintained in succeeding generations of cells.

1.20 VIRUSES AND SUBVIRUSES

Whereas DNA is the main store of genetic information, other information can also be carried in RNA (Gray, in *Textbook of Biochemistry*, p. 873). This occurs in the sequence of bases that constitute RNA and which serves as the genome in several viruses. (In genetic parlance, a genome can be viewed as the abstraction that represents all the genetic information, whether at the molecular level of for the organism as a whole.) Normally, however, RNA does not serve as the genome in eukaryotic or prokaryotic cells, but rather is found in the *tumor viruses* and other small RNA viruses such as poliovirus and reovirus.

Viruses are defined as infectious particles that consist of a nucleic acid molecule surrounded by a protective coat that is made up of protein (Voet and Voet, *Biochemistry*, pp. 841, 1074). The virus particle is known as a *virion;* the protein coating is called a *capsid*. In more complex viruses, the capsid may be encased by an envelope derived from a host cell membrane.

When adsorbed by a cell, the virus insinuates its nucleic acid, whereby the viral chromosome redirects the cell's metabolism to produce new viruses, which in turn initiate further infection. The virus has no metabolism of its own and can be described as the ultimate parasite. Viruses are not living organisms and, in the absence of the host cell, are biologically inert—the same as any other large molecule. Viruses called bacteriophages, which infect bacteria, have been used to study bacterial genetics as well as viral genetics. And since viruses have no metabolism, their presence is indicated by killing the host cell.

It is noted that mutant or wild-type phages or viruses may occur (Voet and Voet, *Biochemistry*, p. 842). Thus, we may be speaking of genetic crossovers, such as for influenza viruses that invade humans as well as animals, and even of such incidences as of the Ebola and Marburg viruses.

Furthermore, since viruses in a sense "eat" the host cell, and hence may be called "phages," e.g., bacteriophages, there may be a connection to what is called *pleomorphism*, where viruses or microbes are thought to change their form or makeup. That is, if a virus eats or destroys bacteria, then there is nothing left but a virus, or virus particles called virions.

Infecting plants and bacteria as well as animals, viruses are divided into helical viruses and spherical viruses, and their great simplicity as compared to cells aids in the study of gene structure and function, although viral modes of gene replication are more varied (Voet and Voet, *Biochemistry*, p. 1076). No particular mention is made of cancer-causing viruses in the reference.

However, in a section on subviral pathogens, it is commented that our ideas about infectious agents are still evolving (Voet and Voet, *Biochemistry*, p 1113ff). Thus, two types of subviral agents have been discovered that cause infectious diseases. The one is the viroid, composed of a small single-stranded RNA molecule. The other is the prion, which is apparently only a protein molecule.

It is thought that viroids are similar to what are called *introns*. In the language of genetic codes, an intron is the noncoding sequence in mRNA molecules, as compared to the *exon*, which is the coding sequence (Gray, in *Textbook of Biochemistry*, p. 906).

Prions are now thought to be what were formerly called "slow viruses," because the resulting diseases took months or years or decades to develop (Voet and Voet, *Biochemistry*, p. 1116). These particular diseases pertain to the mammalian nervous system. None of the diseases exhibits inflammation or fever, indicating that the immune system is neither activated nor impaired by the disease. The word *prion* stands for "proteinaceous infectious particle," and the protein itself is called PrP (for prion protein).*

The above brief discussions about viroids and prions serve to illustrate that there are many unknowns left to be uncovered. Cancer causes and cures may very well lie in this domain and may tie in with some of the unconventional cancer therapies—e.g., the work of Naessens, Livingston, Rife, and others, whose findings about pleomorphism seem to have upset the conventional wisdom about microorganisms.

As an interesting adjunct, 1974 Nobel Prize cowinner Christian de Duve, e.g., in an article in the April, 1996 issue of the *Scientific American*, advances the idea that human or mammalian eukaryotic cells evolved from bacterial prokaryotic cells. That is to say, tiny, primitive bacteria were transformed into the large, intricately organized cells of humans and other mammals. One can wonder if the processes are ongoing and reversible.

1.20.1 ANTIVIRAL AGENTS

The most pervasive and well known is, of course, the immune system, in terms of the immune response. Certain types of white blood cells, collectively called the lymphocytes (or lymphocites), leave the blood vessels and patrol the intercellular regions looking for foreign invaders (Voet and Voet, *Biochemistry*, p. 1207). The lymphocytes arise from precursor cells in the bone marrow, as do all blood cells. The lymphocytes eventually return to the blood by way of the lymphatic vessels after interacting with such lymphoid tissues as the thymus, lymph nodes, and the spleen.

The two types of immunity recognized are cellular immunity and humoral immunity. The former protects against virally infected cells, fungi, parasites, and foreign tissue. Its functions are carried out by T lymphocytes or T cells, which develop in the thymus. Humoral immunity (*humor* meaning fluid) is most active against bacterial infections and viral infections outside the cell. Its functions are carried out by proteins called antibodies or immunoglobulins. The antibodies are generated by B lymphocytes

---

* While we're at it, we might as well mention that there is something called a *mycoplasma*, which is the smallest microorganism capable of independent replication and growth. These mycoplasmas may be regarded as a cross between a bacterium and a virus. The inference is that there may be an extended spectrum of micro/molecular entities ranging from fungi and bacteria down through viruses to subviruses—even to various molecular-sized particles, pieces, or segments—and back up again.

or B cells in the bone marrow. Another action of the immune system is to raise the body temperature, which is another way to killing off the invader's body.

Vitamin C (ascorbic acid), besides its other purposes, e.g., in preventing scurvy, is a suspected antiviral agent, although the point is controversial and not settled. In other words, the effectiveness of vitamin C as a cure or preventive for the common cold is still argued, regarding the work of Linus Pauling, although recognition has come about that vitamin C at least alleviates its symptoms (Chaney, in *Textbook of Biochemistry*, p. 1227). To this it may be added that the common cold is caused by a virus, and if vitamin C is not always effective, neither is the immune system, or we would never get sick in the first place.

Vitamin C "enhances the utilization of folic acid, either by aiding the conversion of folate to tetrahydrofolate or the formation of polyglutamate derivatives of tetrahydrofolate" (Chaney, in *Textbook of Biochemistry*, p. 1226). Inasmuch as folic acid has a number of roles in body chemistry, including that of an anticancer agent, there may be further connections with the benefits of vitamin C that are yet to be spelled out.

There is another thing about ascorbic acid, $C_6H_8O_6$, in that it is closely related chemically to glucose, $C_6H_{12}O_6$ (Chaney, in *Textbook of Biochemistry*, p. 1225). Whether this chemical resemblance has a desirable effect on some of its properties is fuel for speculation. Its main biochemical role is said to be that of a reducing agent in certain important hydroxylation reactions, e.g., of lysine and proline in protocollagen. It is therefore of importance in maintaining normal connective tissue.

It may be commented also that ascorbic acid or ascorbate or vitamin C serves as an enzyme inhibitor. Jain's *Handbook* lists a number of enzymes or phenomena that may be affected: adenylate cyclase; atpase, Na, K; catalase; catechol o-methyl transferase; ferredoxin-NADP reductase; glucose-6-p dehydrogenase; lipase; oxygenase, fatty acid; peroxidase; phosphodiesterase, cAMP; tyrosinase; urea levels. Zollner's *Handbook* lists the following affected enzymes: o-aminophenol oxidase; catalase; β-glucuronidase; GTP cyclohydrolase I; hydroxymethylglutaryl-CoA reductase; lactoylglutathione lyase. Whether these inhibiting actions by vitamin C in some way involve the immune system and/or cancer repression evidently is not known. The enzyme catalase, incidentally, catalyzes the decomposition of hydrogen peroxides to water and oxygen (Voet and Voet, *Biochemistry*, p. 9). Whether its inhibition would be beneficial under the special circumstances remains to be determined.

As a final note, there is the observation that antiviral agents act to inhibit the replication of nucleic acids. There is a connection with anticancer agents that are enzyme inhibitors for DNA processes. In a way, the connection is obvious, in view of the fact that viruses are but pieces of DNA. A search of MEDLINE indicates that antiviral agents being clinically tested include inhibitors for the enzymes called nucleoside phosphorylases and M-deoxyribosyltransferases.

It does not take long to see why there are dissentions about the complete role of nutrients and foreign substances in body biochemistry, in that it has not all been figured out yet—at least not in commonly-accepted terms and theories. In other words, the completed rationale hasn't made its way into the treatises and texbooks.

1.21 CHEMOPREVENTION

The National Cancer Institute has a program underway in what is unambiguously labeled "chemoprevention." Information about this program is contained in articles here and there. In further comment, an editorial in the September 20, 1990 issue of the *New England Journal of Medicine* described some of the ongoing and future work in these directions. Written by Frank L. Meyskens and titled "Coming of Age—the Chemoprevention of Cancer," it mentions clinical tests on volunteers using beta-carotene and isotretinoin, the latter being a retinoid compound.*

Other chemopreventive agents selected for study include *folic acid,* vitamin C, and vitamin E. It is noted that a vast array of other potential chemopreventive agents from dietary sources await testing. The National Cancer Institute has in fact set up a decision-making protocol to select the most promising, and several large-scale projects are already in progress involving some 100,000 subjects. Decisive results either are not in yet, however, or have not been heavily publicized.

---

* The word *retinoid* ordinarily indicates a resin-like substance. And speaking of resins, such are present in the chaparral or creosote bush. Here, however, it is meant to be a derivative of retinol, more commonly called vitamin A.

As noted above, folic acid is to be included as a potential cancer chemopreventive. Results already in on the use of beta-carotene and isotretinoin were mixed, however. The beta-carotene may have been given in too high a dosage, possibly interfering with other necessary nutrients, though isotretinoin was found to prevent the formation of secondary tumors and may work against primary tumors as well.

Of more than passing interest is the fact that the NCI is to use intermediate markers of genetic, biochemical, and immunological function rather than waiting out the long time period for cancer to develop (or not develop). Even more decisive would be clinical tests applied to patients already suffering with cancer.

Since that time, there has been a succession of articles about work underway. These articles or papers have been published in various journals, as written by NCI staff and as a result of NCI sponsorship and funding at other research institutions. As a sampling, the American Cancer Society published an article on the subject in the January/February, 1995 issue of *CA—A Cancer Journal for Clinicians*, written by Greenwald, Kelloff, Burch-Whitman and Kramer, all of the National Cancer Institute. They observed that the specific chemopreventive agents in *fruits and vegetables* have yet to be established. The authors also outline selected NCI clinical trials with candidate chemopreventive agents and provide a short list of known or suspected oncogenes and tumor suppressor genes.

A further sampling of articles obtained from the NCI is as follows. Thus, a series of introductory articles by Michael B. Sporn and others of the NCI staff were published early on, circa 1991–1993, to be followed by more technical articles as work progressed.

In an article by Sporn titled "Carcinogenesis and Cancer," cancer is described as an evolving molecular and cellular process, rather than a static condition, and should be treated as such. Syphilis and cancer are compared, in that the former is treated when the first lesions or symptoms appear, whereas for cancer early lesions are usually considered to have no significance, and cancer is not treated until more fully developed.

The case is made that vitamin A (here called retinol) and its synthetic analogs (here called retinoids) have an ability to maintain a hormone-like control over cell functions. Furthermore, retinoids have exhibited an ability to arrest or reverse carcinogenesis. Moreover, retinoids act merely as physiological agents rather than cytotoxic agents, the latter being the usual role of chemotherapy drugs.

It is noted that retinol and its esters (which are the forms of vitamin A from the food we eat) have some undesirable toxicological properties (at least at higher intake or supplement levels). Accordingly, many synthetic analogs have been made, some of which so far show promise, notably derivatives of retinoic acid. In particular, a compound called 13-*cis*-retinoic acid has reversed premalignant lesions for certain kinds of cancer.*

In a review article on "Interactions of Retinoids," Michael B. Sporn and Anita B. Roberts describe new information about the effect of retinoids on the transforming growth factor β (TGF-β). The latter comprises a family of genes and peptides (or proteins) that regulate normal cell differentiation (or cellular changes) and proliferation. There is evidently a beneficial connection between retinoids and TGF-β, which infers that retinoids may in turn also act on oncogenes—the cancer-causing genes.

In another article by Sporn, a viewpoint paper titled "Chemoprevention of Cancer," published in 1993, the apparently controversial use of tamoxifen is mentioned. (Tamoxifen citrate is regarded as one of the less toxic chemo drugs, though it has some adverse effects as well. Used for estrogen-related cancers of the breast, blocking the estrogen receptors on cancer cells, it is known to cause eye damage, mental confusion, gastrointestinal problems, skin photosensitivity, bone pain, bleeding, and blood problems, and it may sometimes affect the liver.) It is then stressed that the chemoprevention of cancer is to be defined as the use of *noncytotoxic* nutrients or pharmaceutical agents to enhance the intrinsic physiological mechanisms that protect against cancer. This is contrasted against conventional chemotherapy, which is aimed at killing cancer cells. In contrast, chemoprevention attempts to block the initiation of carcinogenesis, or else to arrest or reverse the further growth of premalignant cells, before they become invasive or metastatic.

Thus, as per the foregoing, by the NCI's own definition of the word, *chemoprevention is not directed at curing cancer after the cancer has developed*. Chemoprevention is to be strictly preventive—as the

---

* Although certain retinoids may prove of value in the treatment of epithelial cancers (cancers in body cavities), the point has been made that vitamin A itself may never be useful since it only slowly converts to retinoic acid and furthermore can accumulate to toxic levels in the liver, a problem that does not exist with retinoic acid (Chaney, in *Textbook of Biochemistry*, p. 1203).

coinage of the word clearly implies—although, admittedly, the theories and therapies may be of use even after the cancer has developed.

In a research paper published in 1994, Anzano et al. use a vitamin D analog (rather than a vitamin A analog) for the inhibition of breast cancer in rats. Rats were first treated with a specific tumor-causing chemical, and the vitamin D analog was then fed in combination with the conventional chemotherapy drug tamoxifen, and as such proved very effective in reducing the tumor burden. The authors furthermore propose that vitamin D analogs be called *deltanoids,* in the manner that vitamin A (or retinol) analogs are called *retinoids.*

In another research paper by Anzano et al., the results are presented for using 9-*cis*-retinoic acid (9cRA) alone or in combination with tamoxifen (TAM) against breast cancer in rats. The rats were treated with a specific tumor-causing chemical and then fed *nontoxic* levels of 9cRA. The dosages were effective in reducing the tumor incidence and tumor burden. Even more effective was the use of 9cRA with *low levels* of TAM.

A review paper by Waun Ki Hong et al. of the University of Texas M.D. Anderson Cancer Center, published in 1995, dealt with retinoid treatments for the chemoprevention of aerodigestive cancers. These are secondary cancers of the aerodigestive tract, arising from primary epithelial cancers. Epithelial cancers are those occurring in the lining of body cavities and are manifested as cancers of the lung, head, and neck, accounting in one way or another for 35 percent of the cancer deaths in the United States. The authors state the case for using retinoids but note that chemoprevention methods are not yet standard clinical practice. Some random test results are provided from the U.S. and abroad that, for the most part, are considered to have a positive outcome. More clinical trials will be necessary, however, in this lengthy line of investigation. A subsequent review article by Peter Greenwald of the NCI appeared in the September, 1996 issue of *Scientific American.*

We may conclude from the foregoing that research on chemoprevention is still in its infancy. In the meantime, folkloric preventives are of renewed interest. Furthermore, chemoprevention is obviously a less difficult and less controversial task than treating read curing fully developed cancers

1.22 COMMENTS

The aforementioned and cited works cover a lot of highly scientific information, but few insights are provided about controlling and curing cancer. As in "pure" science, the application seems of less concern—often embodied in the saying that "further research is needed." Furthermore, if metastasization has not yet occurred, the excision by surgery may suffice, as may radiation and even conventional cytotoxic chemotherapy to a degree. Metastasized or advanced cancer is another proposition, however, calling for selective biochemical inhibition.

As a matter of record, in addition to the works already mentioned, there are such learned journals as *Cancer* (published by the American Cancer Society) and the *Journal of the National Cancer Institute.* There are also *Cancer Research* (published by the American Association for Cancer Research) and the *Proceedings of the American Association of Cancer Research.* In addition, there is *Carcinogenesis* (published by the Oxford University Press). An inspection of *Ulrich's International Periodicals Directory* under the heading Medical Sciences—Oncology will yield many more. The series of monographs *Advances in Cancer Research* is published by Academic Press and is up to 67 volumes at last count. These and the many other articles and books dealing with cancer or oncology provide a formidable literature about cancer—but no sure-fire cures.

It is of concern that relatively few natural-occurring substances are listed—as if they had hardly ever been tried. Outside of *folic acid* and some of its derivatives, few commonly found recognizable substances appear in the listings for the chemotherapy drugs used as enzyme inhibitors—say as listed in Appendix C—and the others may have some unusual primary sources.

The fact remains that no general, systematic, absolute cure for cancer has entered the mainstream of medical treatment—or nonmedical treatment, for that matter. Such may already exist outside the main-stream but, if so, the applications have necessarily been haphazard, the results have been random, and no major substantive clinical evidence has yet been forthcoming. Whether this is by design or by happenstance is debatable, but there is a constant in the equation that no commonly recognized bio-chemical theory has been specified for the treatment, read *cure,* of cancer.

And, although the causes for cancer appear straightforward enough, there remains a pressing need for a unified theory of how biochemical remediation can act against metastasized or advanced cancers and an explanation of why certain empirical or folkloric treatments (read *cures*) do indeed work. Enter, therefore, the domain of enzymes and of enzyme inhibitors, natural or synthetic. This, therefore, is the purpose herein, to generate theory in terms of selective enzyme inhibitors for cancer cell metabolism, and to provide particulars for the myriad possibilities, especially from the plant world.

At the same time, it is acknowledged that this route is also fraught with problems, perceived in terms of side effects or adverse effects. That is, even a single substance or chemical compound will almost without exception inhibit more than one enzyme and in fact, in extreme cases, may block respiration, causing suffocation, or may act to produce cardiac arrest, or otherwise may adversely affect such vital body functions as of the liver and kidneys.

The encompassing descriptor is toxic or poisonous. And with plant or herbal substances, which contain many bioactive plant chemicals or phytochemicals, the possibilities for adverse effects are intensified. Nevertheless, we proceed to investigate the possibilities in the parts to follow.

REFERENCES

Anzano, Mario A., Stephen W. Byers, Joseph M. Smith, Christopher W. Peer, Larry T. Mullen, Charles C. Brown, Anita B. Roberts and Michael B. Sporn, "Prevention of Breast Cancer in the Rat with 9-*cis*-Retinoic Acid as a Single Agent and in Combination with Tamoxifen," *Cancer Research*, **54**, 4614–4617 (September 1, 1994).

Anzano, Mario A., Joseph M. Smith, Milan R. Uskoković, Christopher W. Peer, Larry T. Mullen, John J. Letterio, Marta C. Welsh, Mark W. Shrader, Daniel L. Logsdon, Craig L. Driver, Charles C. Brown, Anita B. Roberts and Michael B. Sporn, "1α, 25-Dihydroxy-16-ene-23-yne-26,27-hexafluorocholecalciferol (Ro24-5531), a New Deltanoid (Vitamin D Analogue) for Prevention of Breast Cancer in the Rat," *Cancer Research*, **54**, 1653–1656 (April 1, 1994).

Boik, John, *Cancer & Natural Medicine: A Textbook of Basic Science and Clinical Research*, Oregon Medical Press, Princeton MN, 1995, 1996.

Carbohydrate Metabolism, Willis A. Wood Ed., Vols. IX, XLI, XLII, 89, and 90 of *Methods in Enzymology*, Sidney P. Colwick and Nathan O. Kaplan, Editors-in Chief, Academic Press, Orlando FL, 1966, 1975, 1982.

Childers, J.M., J. Chu, L.F. Voigt, P. Feigl, H.K. Tamimi, E.W. Franklin, D.S. Alberts and F.L. Meyskens, "Chemoprevention of Cervical Cancer with Folic Acid," *Cancer Epidemiol. Biomarkers Prev.*, **4**(2), 155–159 (March, 1995).

Comprehensive Biological Catalysis: A Mechanistic Reference, in four volumes, Michael Sinnott Ed., Academic Press, San Diego and London, 1998.

Curthoys, N.P., R.A. Shapiro and W.G. Haser, "Enzymes of Renal Glutamine Metabolism," in *Glutamine Metabolism in Mammalian Tissues*, D. Häussinger and H. Sies, eds., Springer-Verlag, Berlin, 1984.

de Duve, Christian, "The Birth of Complex Cells," *Scientific American*, **274**(4), 50–57 (April, 1996).

Eigenbrodt, E., P. Fister and M. Reinacher, "New Perspectives on Carbohydrate Metabolism in Tumor Cells," in *Regulation of Carbohydrate Metabolism*, Vol. II, Rivka Beitner Ed., CRC Press, Boca Raton FL, 1985, pp. 141–179.

Folate in Health and Disease, Lynn. B. Bailey Ed., Marcel Dekker, New York, 199X.

Greenwald, Peter, "Chemoprevention of Cancer," *Scientific American*, **275**(3), 96–99 (September, 1996).

Greenwald, Peter, Gary Kelloff, Cynthia Burch-Whitman and Barnett S. Kramer, "Chemoprevention," *CA—A Cancer Journal for Clinicians*, **45**(1), 31–49 (January/February, 1995).

Handbook of Vitamins, 2d ed. Lawrence J. Machlin Ed., Marcel Dekker, New York, 1991.

Hartwell, Jonathan A., *Plants Used Against Cancer*, Quarterman Publications, Lawrence MA, 1982.

Heinerman, John, *The Treatment of Cancer with Herbs*, B.World, Orem UT, 1984.

Hendler, Sheldon Saul and medical advisors Joe Graedon, Alex Mercandetti, Robert Nagourney, and Deborah U. Waters, *The Doctors' Vitamin and Mineral Encyclopedia*, Simon & Schuster, New York, 1990.

Hong, Waun Ki, Scott M. Lippman, Walter N. Hittelman, and Reuben Lotan, "Retinoid Chemoprevention of Aerodigestive Cancer: From Basic Research to the Clinic," *Clinical Cancer Research*, **1**, 677–686 (July, 1995)

Jackman, A. and I. Judson, "Oncology Drug Discovery and Clinical Trial Testing: Who's Listening?" *Cancer Investigation* (New York), **12**(1), 105–108 (1994).

Jain, Mahenda Kumar, *Handbook of Enzyme Inhibitors* (1965–1977), Wiley, New York, 1982.

Jennings, *Eileen, Apricots and Oncogenes: On Vegetables and Cancer Prevention*, McGuire & Beckley Books, Cleveland OH, 1993.

Kearney, J., E. Giovannucci, E.B. Rimm, M.J. Stampfer, G.A. Colditz, A. Ascherio, R. Bleday, and W.C. Willett, "Diet, Alcohol, and Smoking and the Occurrence of Hyperplastic Polyps of the Colon and Rectum," *Cancer—Causes—Control*, **6**(1) 45–56 (January, 1995). Department of Nutrition, Harvard School of Public Health, Boston MA.

Krakoff, Irwin H., "Systemic Treatment of Cancer," *CA—A Cancer Journal for Clinicians*, **46**(3), 134–141 (May/June, 1996).

Meister, Alton, ed., *Glutamate, Glutamine, Glutathione, and Related Compounds*, Vol. 113 of *Methods in Enzymology*, Sidney P. Colwick and Nathan O. Kaplan, Editors-in Chief, Academic Press, Orlando FL, 1985.

Meyskens, Frank L., "Coming of Age—the Chemoprevention of Cancer," *New England Journal of Medicine*, **323**(12), September 20, 1990.

Meyskens, F.L. and K. Prasad, eds., *Vitamins and Cancer*, Humana Press, Totowa NJ, 1986.

Meyskens, F.L. and K. Prasad, *Modulation and Mediation of Cancer*, S. Karger, Farmington CT, 1983.

Mitelman, Felix, "Chromosomes, Genes, and Cancer," *CA—A Cancer Journal for Clinicians*, 44(3), 133–135 (May/June, 1994).

Moss, Ralph W., *Cancer Therapy: The Independent Consumer's Guide to Non-Toxic Treatment & Prevention*, Equinox Press, New York, 1992.

Moss, Ralph W., *Questioning Chemotherapy*, Equinox Press, Brooklyn NY, 1995.

Olson, Merle S., Roland Scholz, Cynthia Buffington, Steven C. Dennis, A. Padma, Tarun B. Patel, Parvin Waymack, and Michael S. DeBuysere, "Regulation of α-Keto Acid Dehydrogenase Multienzyme Complexes in Isolated Perfused Organs," in *The Regulation of Carbohydrate Formation and Utilization in Mammals*, Carlo M Veneziale, ed., University Park Press, Baltimore, 1981, pp. 153–189. Papers from a symposium held at the Mayo Medical School, Rochester MN, July 9–11, 1981.

Rissler, Jand and Margaret Mellon, *The Ecological Risks of Engineered Crops*, MIT Press, Cambridge MA, 1996.

Roehrig, Karla L., *Carbohydrate Biochemistry and Metabolism*, AVI Publishing Co., Westport CT, 1984.

Sandberg, Avery A., "Cancer Cytogenetics for Clinicians," *CA—A Cancer Journal for Clinicians*, 44(3), 136–158 (May/June, 1994).

Shank, Richard P. and M.H. Aprison, "Glutamate as a Neurotransmitter," in *Glutamine and Glutamate in Mammals*, Vol. II, Elling Kvamme Ed., CRC Press, Boca Raton FL, 1988.

Snodgrass, S.R., "Vitamin Neurotoxicity," *Mol-Neurobiol.*, 6(1), 41–73 (Spring, 1992).

Sporn, Michael B., "Carcinogenesis and Cancer: Different Perspectives on the Same Disease," *Cancer Research*, **51**, 62115–6218 (December 1, 1991).

Sporn, Michael B., "Chemoprevention of Cancer," *Lancet*, *342*, 1211–1213 (November 13, 1993).

Sporn, Michael B. and Anita B. Roberts, "Interactions of Retionoids and Transforming Growth Factor-β in Regulation of Cell Differentiation and Proliferation," *Molecular Endocrinology*, 5(1), 3–7 (1991).

Textbook of Biochemistry with Clinical Correlations, Thomas M. Devlin Ed., Wiley, New York, 1982. Second edition, 1986.

Voet, Donald and Judith G. Voet, *Biochemistry*, 2d ed., Wiley, New York, 1995; 1st ed., Wiley, New York, 1990. For the purposes herein, the second edition will be utilized.

Webb, J. Leyden, *Enzyme and Metabolic Inhibitors*, in three volumes, Academic Press, New York, 1963, 1966.

Weinberg, Robert A., "Oncogens and Tumor Suppressor Genes," *CA—A Cancer Journal for Clinicians*, 44(3), 160–170 (May/June, 1994).

Zollner, Helmward, *Handbook of Enzyme Inhibitors*, VCH Verlagsgesellschaft mbH, Weinheim, FRG, 1989. VCH Publishers, New York.

Zollner, Helmward, *Handbook of Enzyme Inhibitors*, 2d ed. revised and enlarged, in two volumes, VCH Verlagsgesellschaft mbH, Weinheim, FRG, 1993. VCH Publishers, New York.

Plant Biochemistry and Cancer

Part 2

Plant Biochemistry and Cancer

If there are indeed selective anticancer agents that act as enzyme inhibitors for cancer cell metabolism—e.g., blocking or inhibiting a critical enzyme or enzymes in anaerobic glycolysis—then the most likely such substances will originate in the plant world. This, of course, does not preclude the chemical synthesis of similar substances, but naturally occurring plant-chemicals or phytochemicals provide, at the very least, a point of departure often rooted in medical folklore. As a base reference, estimates are that, worldwide, half of all medicines are derived from plants and animals. Even in the U.S., it is sometimes said that perhaps one-fourth of all medicines are so derived.

Accordingly, in Parts 2 through 5, a detailing is furnished of the plant world—its particular biochemistry, its chemical taxonomy, and its more bioactive substances, including alkaloids. Also of interest are the fungi or mycota, which have some unusual characteristics that potentially relate to cancer—both the causes and remediation.

Generally speaking, bioactivity infers toxicity, and such sources are often referred to as poisonous and medicinal plants. It is often, however, a fine line, depending on plant activity and dosage levels, biochemical individuality, and other factors.

Following these significant diversions, a closer look will be taken at the genesis of cancer, and in particular the role of viruses. Last, the role of enzyme inhibitors will be examined in depth, for this very well may not only prove to be the first line of defense against cancer but the means by which cancer itself can be conquered.

2.1 INTRODUCTION

There is a considerable literature on plant biochemistry, and there is a similarity between plant biochemistry and mammalian or human biochemistry. The same nomenclature and terms tend to accommodate each, with the notable exception of photosynthesis, which is exclusive to plant life, and of nutrition, digestion, and assimilation, the processes that mark mammalian life. Even here, however, there are exceptions to the exceptions, the gray areas wherein some very few plants or organisms function by chemosynthesis, deriving their biosynthesis and sustenance from inorganic chemical energy rather than solar energy, and some very few plants have primitive digestive systems. Higher life, meaning mammalian life, derives its energy and sustenance from organic chemical energy, or biochemical energy, although inorganics or minerals are also vital to life processes—the same as for plant life.

Thus, for example, various members of what are called the (Group V) transition metals will show up, possibly even nickel, which in its oxidized and activated (or partially reduced) state is a prominent inorganic catalyst for hydrogenation reactions. Copper, molybdenum, and vanadium are found in enzymes. Vitamin B12 contains cobalt. Chromium is an essential trace element. Iron is a necessary component of blood hemoglobin. And so on. Such other trace elements as selenium have a bad name, with a number of indicator plants showing that there are excessive selenocompounds in the soil. Selenium toxicoses such as the *blind staggers* occur in both animals and humans—but on the other hand, in minute amounts, selenium is said to be an anticancer agent as is another trace element, germanium. Another of the mysteries of trace elements or compounds: they are vital in minute amounts, toxic in excess.

A very few of the more recent books available include the series *Methods in Plant Biochemistry*, in six volumes, edited by P.M. Dey and J.B. Harborne, with individual editors for each volume, and the four volume series *Toxicants of Plant Origin*, edited by Peter R. Cheeke. Another of interest is *Naturally Occurring Carcinogens of Plant Origin: Toxicology, Pathology and Biochemistry*, edited by Iwao Hirono. Reference will be made to various chapters and chapter authors, and the full citations are included in the end-of-chapter references. Mention can also be made of the multivolume set *The Biochemistry of Plants: A Comprehensive Treatise,* published by Academic Press, and of other specialized treatments such as on alkaloids, some of which will be referenced. With regard to alkaloids, there is the continuing series, *The Alkaloids: Chemistry and Pharmacology,* edited by R.H.F. Manske et al. and published by Academic Press, with 46 volumes to date. Also, there is the four-volume set *Alkaloids: Chemical and Biological Perspectives,* edited by S. William Pelletier. A notable single-volume reference is Geoffrey A. Cordell's *Introduction to Alkaloids: A Biogenetic Approach,* as is *Biochemistry of Alkaloids,* edited by K Mothes, H.R. Schütte and M. Luckner.

Bridging biochemical compounds and botany, and including alkaloids, there is Will H. Blackwell's authoritative *Poisonous and Medicinal Plants,* a more technical exposition which goes into the chemistry and which will be further detailed. For color photographs along with technical descriptions, there is *A Colour Atlas of Poisonous Plants,* by Dietrich Frohne and Hans Jürgen Pfänder, translated from the German. About the correlation between plant chemicals and taxonomy, there is *Infraspecific Chemical Taxa of Medicinal Plants,* by Péter Tétényi, which will be further cited in Part 3.

As with Blackwell, another technical authority about the biochemistry of plants who hails from southern Florida is Julia F. Morton. Morton, director of the Morton Collectanea at the University of Miami, wrote *Major Medicinal Plants: Botany, Culture and Uses,* as well as the *Atlas of Medicinal Plants of Middle America: Bahamas to Yucatan,* both of which will be further cited in Part 3. Active chemical agents are named for each species, where known.

Not to be overlooked is James A. Duke, who contributed the *CRC Handbook of Medicinal Herbs.* This reference and several others by Duke will be further utilized in Part 3.

In many of the botanical-type references, very little is said about the active principle or principles involved. In other words, the chemistry is not a consideration—only the plant name or taxonomy. There are outstanding exceptions, however, such as in Blackwell's *Poisonous and Medicinal Plants* and Cordell's *Introduction to Alkaloids: A Biogenetic Approach.* It will be an objective, therefore, to attempt to fill in the biochemistry of bioactive plants and plant substances to the extent known. This will entail a knowledge of the kinds of chemical compounds that occur, including specific examples of compounds, and some of their actions or reactions.

Even here, however, although the chemistry of the compounds may be supplied, the further physiological, biological, or biochemical effects of these substances on the body as, say, *enzyme inhibitors* is not usually set forth. For it is mainly as enzyme inhibitors (or promoters) that these compounds affect the biochemistry of the body.

The trouble with not supplying both the chemistry and the biochemical role is that it is not possible to know how or if a plant or plant substance really functions as an anticancer agent or other agent. Its efficacy is reduced to the vagueness of hearsay, anecdote, and folklore. In other words, there is no way to judge whether the substance actually works.

It may be added that the classification of plants below the level of species is increasingly concerned with the chemical components in the plant as a means of distinction or differentiation, a subject called *infraspecific taxa.* The subject of chemical taxonomy is to be further examined in Part 3, in particular as presented by Tétényi. The difficulties encountered in this sort of non-Linnaean classification are presented by J.G. Hawkes in the introductory chapter to *Infraspecific Classification of Wild and Cultivated Plants.*

In *Plant Taxonomy and Biosystematics,* Clive A. Stace divides the categories of compounds encountered into primary metabolites, secondary metabolites, and semantides (Stace, *Plant Taxonomy,* p. 89). The first category pertains to vital metabolic pathways, and the second to nonvital functions. The third denotes information-carrying molecules. In further respect, DNA is a primary semantide, RNA a secondary semantide, and proteins are tertiary semantides. Examples are furnished in the reference.

In his book on *Plant Taxonomy,* Tod F. Stuessy has a chapter on chemistry in which he discusses the types of compounds of main interest and lists extensive references. He states that the chemistry of plant classification falls under several labels: *chemotaxonomy, chemosystematics, biochemical systematics,* or *taxonomic biochemistry.* Another term used is simply *systematics.* Part 3, to follow, is titled Chemical Taxonomy, and Tétényi speaks of *Infraspecific Chemical Taxa* in the title of his book. The same or similar designators are mentioned in the section on plant chemistry and taxonomy in Part 3.

Of primary interest to Stuessy are the micromolecular compounds designated flavonoids, terpenoids, alkaloids, betalains, and glucosinolates. It is indicated that betalains could be regarded as alkaloids but are treated separately for taxonomic purposes. Also mentioned is that *glucosinolates are sulfur-containing mustard-oil glucosides or glycosides* which, when hydrolyzed with acid or the enzyme myrosinase, yield *isothiocyanate* and glucose. They are most commonly found in the family *Cruciferae*. Very possibly, there is a link here with the *anticancer* action noted in folklore for various species of Cruciferae. The macromolecular compounds are divided by Stuessy into proteins and nucleic acids. There will be the occasion to further discuss these kinds of compounds, with the underlying emphasis directed at cancer and its immolation.

There is the inference, in taking up the subject of plant biochemistry, that a cure for cancer and other intractable diseases may exist in plant substances, known or unknown. For one thing, there is the commonality between plant metabolism and mammalian metabolism and the enzymes involved. And for another thing, only a relatively few of the myriad plant species worldwide have ever been tested for bioactivity. Given the great diversity of plants, and the even greater diversity of complex plant substances, there is the strong indication that anything is possible.

Searching for and assaying plant bioactivity is an Augean undertaking, unfortunately, which is where discernment comes into play. In other words, native folklore is invaluable. There is the comment, however, that given, say, an acre of tropical rain forest, one is as likely to find bioactivity by random selection as from identified known plant species. This, in a way of looking at it, may mean that most plant species are in fact bioactive in one way or another. And if bioactivity is more or less equated with toxicity, this is to say that probably more plants are poisonous than nonpoisonous.

It is this poisonous element that is of special interest, however, for this may be the prime reason that plants can serve as medicines. The problem is to control this toxicity, to play one thing against another so to speak. Thus, minute dosages may serve, as is already done with a certain few plant poisons. Of the many classes of plant toxins, we will here be most concerned with those that are called glycosides, phenolics, and especially alkaloids. Flavonoids, a category of phenolics, will also be of particular interest. There is already evidence that some of these kinds of compounds act as anticancer agents and sometimes as antibiotic or antiviral agents. There expectedly are many, many more, and for the ones that are already identified, it may be more a matter of adjusting the application, the amounts and the proportions, so as to be toxic to cancer cells but not normal cells.

Whereas the plants that will be considered are land plants, a word should also be said about what are called marine plants of various sorts. They are part of the plant kingdom as well, and many display toxicity, some deadly, although very little so far appears about their role in cancer and cancer therapy. In this connection, there is a chapter titled Drugs from Plants of the Sea, by Ara H. Der Marderosian, which appeared in *Plants in the Development of Modern Medicine*, edited by Tony Swain and published in 1972. Since the different phyla and estimated numbers of plant species are always of interest, this information along with the proportions that are marine plants is indicated in Table 2.1, as adapted from the reference. It may be commented that other systems of classification may use other names and divisions for the phyla. Furthermore, the scope of classification may be viewed as somewhat generous, since it includes bacteria and fungi. But, after all, if these entities are not part of the animal kingdom, then they must be included as plants—or else we must introduce an additional kingdom of some sort.

The reference also provides a tabulation for the different phyla which lists genera or species that have toxic properties and encapsulates the medicinal and toxic properties. The text gives further information about antibacterial, antiviral, and antifungal properties, and so forth, and about toxic properties, ranging from the merely innocuous to the deadly.

Inasmuch as cancer is tabulated but once, only this particular species will be mentioned. It is *Nostoc ribulare*, which is classified within the phylum Cyanophyta (blue-green algae). It is cited as being of interest in the study of cancers, which means that it could be either carcinogenic or anticancer, or both, depending on the circumstances. The fact that the phylum is labeled Cyanophyta, which has connotations of cyanide, may be indicative of the sort of bioactivity displayed by this particular marine species.

2.2   CANCER AND ANTICANCER AGENTS

In a chapter titled "Assays Related to Cancer Drug Discovery," in *Methods in Plant Biochemistry*, Vol. 6, Mathew Suffness of the National Cancer Institute (NCI) and John M. Pezzuto of the University of Illinois College of Medicine note that, while systematic chemotherapy is the primary treatment for attacking disseminated disease, new clinically efficacious agents need to be uncovered. Among these

Table 2.1 Phyla and Plant Species (Data from Ara H. Der Marderosian in *Plants in the Development of Modern Medicine,* p. 226.)

Phylum	Estimated number of species	Estimated number of marine species
Schizophyta (bacterial)	1,500	180
Cyanophyta (blue-green algae)	200	150
Rhodophyta (red algae)	4,000	3,900
Phaeophyta (brown algae)	1,500	1,495
Chlorophyta (green algae)	7,000	900
Pyrrophyta (dinoflagellates)	1,100	100
Charophyta (stonewarts)	75	10
Euglenophyta (euglenoids)	400	12
Chrysophyta		
Golden-brown algae	650	130
Coccolithophorids	300	190
Diatoms	10,000	5,000
Xanthophyta		
Vaucheria	60	10
Mycophyta		
Fungi	75,000	300
Lichens	16,000	15
Bryophyta	25,000	0
Liverworts and mosses		
Tracheophyta		
Psilopsida, club mosses, horsetails, ferns, cyads, conifers	10,000	0
Flowering plants	250,000	(sea grasses) 50

possibilities are plants. "Plants are a proven source of antitumor compounds, and it is reasonable to assume that additional agents are in existence that remain to be uncovered." Not only are plants of consideration, but the reference provides a very good summary of the thrust of work on cancer and anticancer agents in general. The authors mention that there are perhaps some *250,000 plant species worldwide,* but there is as yet no definitive method of screening for the desired biological activity.

Although a few plant substances have progressed to clinical trials (e.g., *ellipticine, homoharringtonine,* and *taxol*), there is no guarantee that these will prove successful. A larger number of agents have in fact proved unsuccessful in clinical trials, e.g., acronycine, aristolochic acid, bruceantin, indicine-N-oxide, lapachol, maytansine, nitidine, tylocrebrine. Not only may the substance be excessively toxic in itself, but the supply may be extremely limited. Nevertheless, the studies involving these substances may lead to other valuable information—hence the descriptor "lead" compounds.

Besides *taxol* for instance, other substances studied include *bleomycin, camptothecin, brystatin and phorbol esters,* and *forskolin*. Citations are given in the reference. The reference is further concerned with the criteria for assays or tests which can be used to screen for antitumor agents from natural sources.

Key definitions for biological effects include the descriptors *cytotoxic*, designating toxicity to cells in cultures, which may further described as *cytostatic*, stopping cell growth, or *cytocidal*, killing cells. *No selectivity is implied between cancer cells and normal cells.* The descriptor *antitumor* indicates effectiveness to a model tumor system *in vivo*, that is, outside the test tube or culture dish, and also implies selectivity against the tumor as compared to the host. (*In vivo* involves the living organism or host, whereas *in vitro* means inside the test tube or culture dish.) The descriptor *anticancer* indicates effectiveness against the actual disease state in humans. The determination of anticancer activity per se requires human trials, that is, clinical trials. These definitions are more restrictive than commonly used, to prevent misinformation. Thus, the growth inhibition of a cell line *in vitro* may not be an anticancer effect as such but rather may be a toxic effect, affecting all cells. (Conventional chemotherapy, by affecting all cells, is cell-toxic or *cytotoxic*.)

Cancer refers to the uncontrolled, malignant growth of poorly differentiated cells that can occur in any organ of the body, with the cancer cells tending to resemble the tissue from which they originated (Suffness and Pezzuto, in *Methods*, 6, p. 72ff). For example, lung cancer more closely resembles lung tissue than it would resemble other cancers such as colon cancer or brain cancer. Thus, *cancers of different organs do not resemble each other.* More than this, *cancers within a given organ vary,* and there being many subtypes, depending in part on the different tissues within the organ. There is therefore the classification of cancers by histopathological type ("histo-" meaning tissue), and *each type even within the same organ may respond differently to chemotherapy.* The extension of this means of classification results in more than *100 distinct types of cancer,* with some sources putting the figure as high as 300 and some going as high as 600. In spite of many years of effort, according to the authors, no commonality has been found for the various cancer types. This seems to negate the idea of broad-spectrum anticancer agents, and distinct drugs may be required for each type of cancer.

Inasmuch as cancers are very similar to the tissue from which they originated, there are few differences to be exploited by drugs or anticancer agents. Among the few distinctions is that tumor cells are relatively less differentiated than normal cells. (By *differentiated* is meant that there is a pronounced degree of difference between generalized cells and specialized cells. That is, the cell population varies in its characteristics.) Also, tumor tissue may lack key receptors or antigens that are found in normal tissue. Another distinguishing feature of a tumor is the many slightly subtypes of tissue. (That is, *tumors are heterogeneous.*) Treatment may affect some of these subtypes, leaving other resistant types to grow and repopulate the tumor. Some tumors may require years to develop, while others may occur within a short time, say due to radiation or chemicals. Even though located in the same organ, the fast-growing tumors will not be similar to the spontaneous slow-growing tumors and will not respond in the same way to treatment.

The effective treatment of cancer will require that the drug not only kill or disable a variety of cancerous subtypes or cell populations but do so while neither harming normal tissue of the same origin nor normal tissue throughout the body. In antibacterial chemotherapy, this is selectively accomplished, since there is such a difference between the microbe and the human host. (That is, bacteria are prokaryotic cells, whereas human cells are eukaryotic.)

The known targets for chemotherapy are recognized as:

1. anything to do with *stopping cell growth and division*
2. *stopping angiogenesis,* which pertains to a tumor establishing its own capillary blood-supply network
3. *stopping metastasis,* whereby cancer cells break off the primary tumor and travel to different sites, to produce new tumors.

The only known treatment affecting the primary tumor is the inhibition of cell growth and division.

The problem with targeting cell growth and division is that normal cells are also affected, and cells with a rapid turnover rate are particularly affected. Of the latter, bone marrow and gastrointestinal epithelium are the most prominent targets of chemotherapy drugs and, unfortunately, they yield toxicological responses.

The ideal anticancer drug will not only behave selectively between cancer tissue and normal tissue, but will kill all tumor subpopulations. Some of the drugs tested so far may produce these effects, but the cells tend to revert when the drug is withdrawn. The NCI, however, is continuing this line of research in its *in vitro* screening procedures.

Programs of the National Cancer Institute utilize various human cancer cell cultures toward discovering anticancer agents (Suffness and Pezzuto, in *Methods*, 6, p. 84ff). Among the properties sought is *selectivity,* which would work against a specific type of cancer cell. Another test of interest is the stem cell assay, stem cells being precursor cells within a tumor that will give rise to descendent cells, which will renew the tumor and promote metastasis. Notice is taken of correlating cancer lines with specific genes or oncogenes.

Cell lines standardized by the NCI which have been used for *in vivo* testing include the following (Boik, *Cancer & Natural Medicine*, p. 109):

- B16 melanoma (B1)
- Adenocarcinoma (CA)

- CD8F1 mammary tumor (CD)
- Colon 26 (C6)
- Colon 38 (C8)
- Colon 46 (CY)
- Colon 51 (CZ)
- Dunning leukemia (DL)
- Ehrlich ascites (EA)
- Ependymoblastoma (EM)
- Carcinoma of nasopharynx (KB, *in vitro*)
- L-1210 lymphoid leukemia (LE)
- Lewis lung carcinoma (LL)
- M-5076 ovarian carcinoma (M5)
- Novikoff hepatoma (NH)
- P-1534 leukemia (P-4)
- P-338 Adriamycin resistant (PA)
- P-338 vincristine resistant (PV)
- P-338 L-alanosine resistant (P6)
- P-388 lymphocytic leukemia (PS)
- Sarcoma 180 or S-180 (SA)
- Walker carcinosarcoma 256 (WA)
- Human colon cancer (CX-1 and CX-5)
- Human lung cancer (LX-1)
- Human mammary tumor (MX-1)

Carcinoma denotes a cancer of epithelial tissue, sarcoma of nonepithelial tissue. The largest human cell collection is at the John T. Dorrance, Jr. International Cell Science Center at the Coriell Institute for Medical Research at Camden, NJ.

It is a well known fact that *cancer patients become resistant to anticancer drugs* (Suffness and Pezzuto, *Methods*, 6, p. 88). Although a number of mechanisms may be involved, the most important may be due to the formation of what is called P-glycoprotein, which decreases intercellular drug accumulations. On the other hand, melanoma involves the enzyme tyrosinase, but there are in turn natural products that can be activated or metabolized by tyrosinase to become toxic to melanoma cells.

The cell structure or cytoskeleton is composed of a number of elements including microtubules which are also involved in cell dynamics. In particular, mitosis may be involved—the complex changes that precede cell division. Many chemical compounds work against mitosis, including colchicine, podophyllotoxin, maytansine, vincristine, and taxol. Vincristine is already widely used for blood-related cancers, and taxol is undergoing further clinical testing.*

Whereas a localized primary tumor can often be excised by surgery and radiation surgery, it is the metastasis or spread of cancer by means of the circulatory system that presents the major difficulty (Suffness and Pezzuto, *Methods*, 6, p. 91). In this regard, *in vitro* procedures have been tested. It has been found that metastatic tumor cell lines cause blood platelate aggregation, which at the same time releases substances which favor tumor cell growth. Platelate aggregation has been inhibited by a natural substance, called *forskolin*, derived from the roots of a plant identified as *C. forkohlii*. Forskolin also stimulates the platelate enzyme adenylate cyclase, which correlates with antimetastatic behavior, and other compounds that stimulate this enzyme may also be potential antimetastatic agents. The proteolytic digestive enzyme collagenase is known to be connected with metastasis. Thus, inhibitors for this enzyme are being tested.

Abnormal cell *differentiation* (changes in cell substances or structures) is thought to be related to malignancy (Suffness and Pezzuto, *Methods*, 6, p. 93). A large number of compounds have been classified as differentiating agents, and they are generally low molecular weight substances that cause malignant cells to behave as normal cells. Differentiating agents cause a mediation; that is, cause the cancerous

---

* An update on taxol and associated compounds, or taxoids, is provided by Nicolaou, Guy, and Potier in the June, 1996 issue of the *Scientific American*. Judging from the side effects, such as suppressing the immune system, these compounds are cytotoxic or cell toxic.

cells to be more like normal cells. A number of cancer cell types are affected by differentiating agents, including colon cancer, lung cancer, and melanoma. Citations are provided in the reference.

The elevation of cAMP (cyclic-adenomonophosphate) levels is known to arrest growth and differentiation (Suffness and Pezzuto, *Methods*, 6, p. 94). *Forskolin,* for instance is a natural substance that elevates cAMP concentrations, in addition to being an antihypertension agent and inhibiting platelate aggregation. The synthesis of cAMP requires the enzyme adenylate cyclase, and promoters for this enzyme are also potential anticancer agents. Inasmuch as cAMP is not normally long lived, and its demise is catalyzed by the enzyme cAMP phosphodiesterase, inhibitors for the latter enzyme could potentially serve as anticancer agents. Well known inhibitors include the alkaloids *theophylline* and *papaverine*, and many natural products function in this way. Citations are provided in the reference.

The interaction of antitumor agents with DNA is varied (Suffness and Pezzuto, *Methods*, 6, p. 96). Examples of alkylating agents include chlorambucil, cyclophosphamide, melphalan, and streptozocin. Examples of antitumor antibiotics include bleomycin, doxorubicin, and mithramycin. Another substance is cisplatin. The reference observes that this is all paradoxical, since *modification of the linear sequence of DNA (mutation) by chemical or physical means is generally regarded as a deleterious (carcinogenic) event.* The dose-response has a noticeable effect, however, and the benefits are assumed to outweigh the bad effects. The research continues, especially with relatively small molecular weight substances that are DNA site specific. Agents tested for interaction with DNA and deoxyoligonucleotides include low-molecular weight ligands, a special type of chemical compound or chemical bond.

The standard test for detecting mutagenic response is the Ames test, which monitors a particular strain of bacteria for histidine independence. Other tests include the biochemical induction assay, or BIA.

The stimulation of the immune system is another approach to producing antitumor and antiviral responses (Suffness and Pezzuto, *Methods*, 6, p. 101). Test substances included bestatin and arphamenines A and B. Amastatin levels measured effectiveness. Very interestingly, in tests in lymphocytes, it was found that exceedingly low concentrations of cytotoxic or cytostatic agents stimulated these cells. (This is, of course, a claim of homeopathy.)

Furthermore, *preclinical studies have shown that low doses of the antitumor agents cytosine, arabinoside, adriamycin, and methotrexate may produce immune stimulation.* Not only this, but *toxicity can be circumvented if a therapeutic response could be mediated by the administration of such extremely low doses of active agents.* Citations were provided.

The number of lymphokines or factors related to the immune response continues to increase. Some examples are interferons, interleukins, the interleukin receptor, tumor necrosis factor, and granulocyte/macrophage colony-stimulating factor. The theory is that *low-dose therapy* with an appropriate agent could induce the synthesis of one or more of these substances. Tests are underway on interferon and interleukin induction and also on natural killer (NK) cells.

Enzymes that are involved in biological processes contributing to cancer are the *proteases,* notably serine proteases, thiol proteases, acid proteases, metallo-endopeptidases, aminopeptideases A and B, alkaline phosphotase, esterase, glycosides, and others. Accordingly, the search is on for inhibitors for these enzymes. The last four categories mentioned above are located on the surface of mammalian cells, and are particularly vulnerable to inhibitors.

Antimetabolites may be described as compounds that affect the synthesis of sugars, amino acids, nucleic acid precursors, and so forth (Suffness and Pezzuto, *Methods*, 6, p. 104). (Presumably this also includes the utilization of the sugars and the processes of metabolism.) Microbial systems have been developed that can detect the antimetabolic activity of substances. The methodology used will discriminate against general antibiotic activity, which is not of interest. A number of antimetabolic compounds have been so determined.

Thus, certain *protease inhibitors* will work, as previously presented. Other enzyme inhibitors have been found that act as antitumor agents for the following enzymes: orotidine 5'-phosphate decarboxylase; inosine 5'-phosphate dehydrogenase; carbamyl phosphate synthetase; thymidylate synthetase (an enzyme inhibited by the chemotherapy drug 5-FU); the enzyme for phosphorylation of deoxycytidylic acid; ribonucleotide reductase; phosphoribosyl-1-pyrophosphate amidotransferase; the enzymes variously for *in vitro* RNA formation, DNA formation, or protein biosynthesis; aspartate transcarbamylase; the enzyme for formate incorporation into purines; for (non)histone protein phosphorylation; for oxidative phosphorylation; (deoxy)ribunuclease; DNA or RNA polymerases; deoxythymidylate kinase; deoxythymidylate mono(di)phosphate kinases; S-adenosyl-L-methionine methyl transferase.

Included also are *hexokinase* and *phosphofructokinase*, which are enzymes for two of the controlling reactions in glycolysis, plus *lactate dehydrogenase,* the enzyme for lactate or lactic acid formation. Further enzymes involved are as follows, with those involved in glycolysis highlighted in boldface, and those involved in the tricarboxylic acid cyle in italics. To continue, in the order given in the reference: **glucose-6-phosphate dehydrogenase; fructose-1,6-diphosphatase;** *malic dehydrogenase, succinic dehydrogenase*; adenosine phosphatase; **glyceraldehyde 3-phosphate dehydrogenase; glucose 6-phosphatase**; plus 5'-nucleotidase; enzymes for DNA synthesis and repair with isolated nuclei; the enzyme for oestrogen reception; for partial reactions of protein biosynthesis; for 80S initiation complex formation; for ternary complex formation; for tRNA aminoacetylation; for initiation of protein synthesis; and for elongation of protein synthesis.

Some inhibitors of total protein synthesis show antitumor activity, and the list grows. Citations for all of the above are provided in the reference. An attempt has been made to use the various inhibitors in a therapeutic strategy (G. Weber, in *Cancer Research, 43*, pp. 3466–3492).

Dihydrofolate reductase indirectly catalyzes purine nucleotide synthesis by maintaining intracellular folates in the reduced form (Suffness and Pezzuto, *Methods,* 6, p. 106). *Methotrexate,* for example, is believed to be an inhibitor for dihydrofolate reductase, as has been mentioned elsewhere, and is called an *antifolate*. (Unfortunately, methotrexate is also highly toxic.) Hence, antifolates serve as (nonselective) anticancer agents, and the search continues for new antifolates.

Adenine nucleoside analogs may serve as anticancer agents. They are inactivated, however, by the presence of the enzyme adenosine deaminase, which may be in relatively high concentrations in tumor tissues. In any event, inhibitors for adenosine deaminase are of interest, and several have been isolated or synthesized.

Increasing levels of intracellular calcium produces a binding of the calcium cation Ca^{++} with calmodulin (an eukaryotic protein designated as CaM). In this conformation, calmodulin interacts with certain enzymes, increasing their activity. Among the enzymes that are activated or promoted are phosphodiesterase, adenyl cyclase, and protein kinases and phosphatases. By this means, cell proliferation ensues. A number of antagonists for calmodulin are known, calmodulin being a target for anticancer agents.

Growth factors are produced by malignant cells that further cell proliferation (Suffness and Pezzuto, *Methods,* 6, p. 107). The phenomenon is called autocrine secretion, and an association has been found with several peptides. These peptides include proteins similar or identical with what is called the growth factor-α, with the platelet-derived growth factor, and with bombesin and gastrin. By antagonizing this association, a mechanism is provided to inhibit cancer cell growth. As an alternative, the growth-factor response may be inhibited directly. Thus, the enzyme tyrosine kinase favors autocrine activity, but inhibitors have been isolated and identified. Still other types of reactions or functions are under investigation, such as site-specific interactions with DNA.

It has been found that the phorbol ester 12-O-tetradecanoylphorbol 13-acetate (TPA) binds to and activates the enzyme protein kinase C. This is an important step in the genesis of tumors. Substances are under investigation that would inhibit this TPA binding to and activation of protein kinase C. Also, the source of protein kinase C is itself under investigation, as well as inhibitors for this enzyme.

There is a so-called second messenger system that binds to and activates protein kinase C. Of the several second messengers, the natural second messenger is regarded as 1,2-diacylglycerol (DG). In principle, an agent that inhibits the production of say DG might function as an *anticancer agent.*

It is known that polyamines and polyamine metabolism are related to cancer, and inhibitors of polyamine biosynthesis may be useful anticancer agents. The enzymes involved include ornithine decarboxylase, S-adenosinemethionine decarboxylase, aminopropyltransferases, and the enzyme for polyamine transport. Inhibitors for these enzymes may therefore prove productive against cancer, and a number have been determined. The first irreversible step in the formation of polyamines is the conversion of ornithine to putrescine, from which CO_2 is liberated, and which is catalyzed by ornithine decarboxylase. This enzyme has been extensively studied, and the work continues. Other enzymes are spermidine and spermine synthases, and the search is for inhibitors for these enzymes.

Protease production and activity is associated with cell proliferation, the genesis of tumors, and cell transformations. A protease known as a plasminogen activator cleaves plasminogen to plasmin (plasmin is a proteolytic enzyme which breaks down blood clots). The inhibition of this activity is of concern, since it may be related to cancer. No inhibitor test results were presented in the reference.

Tumor-derived factors have been found to stimulate the proliferation of endothelial cells and induce angiogenesis. (Endothelial pertains to the blood vessels and other cavities of the body, and angiogenesis is the formation of a tumorous blood-vessel system.) The search is for *angiogenesis inhibitors.* No results were presented. It is noted in the reference that *bacteria can be used in the search for anticancer agents.*

Various pitfalls are discussed in evaluating antitumor agents, in that there can be many crossover actions or side effects. For example, *Vinca* alkaloids are thought of as antimitotic agents, preventing the complex biochemical reactions which precede cell division., but there is also an effect on nucleic acid synthesis. Other problems are described with *taxol.* The complexity becomes baffling.

It is further commented that human tumors are *heterogeneous*, meaning a variety of cell populations are present (Suffness and Pezzuto, *Methods*, 6, pp. 115–116). These cell populations vary in their sensitivity to drugs, and cells that were initially sensitive become insensitive. Moreover, some of the cell populations are insensitive to start with.

Resistance acquired during drug therapy is a major cause of treatment failure.

The major cause of resistance is attributed to natural mutations, although some treatments can in themselves produce mutations. Cells resistant to one kind of drug may prove resistant to another. Thus, colchicine-resistant cells were found to be resistant also to puromycin, daunorubicin, taxol, vinblastine, and emetine. On the other hand, cells selected for resistance to daunorubicin also proved resistant to colchicine, puromycin, vinblastine, emetine, and doxorubicin. However, both the colchicine-resistant and daunorubicin-resistant cell lines were more sensitive to acronycine than were the parent cell lines.

Solid tumors have slow growth rates (Suffness and Pezzuto, *Methods*, 6, p. 116.) Many human solid tumors—including most subtypes of major killers such as lung, colon, prostate, and breast cancers—have slow growth rates.

"Given the slow turnover rate of tumor cells in these diseases compared to the rapidly dividing tissues such as bone-marrow and gastro-intestinal epithelium, it is apparent that agents which are essentially antiproliferative and therefore attack cell growth and reproduction targets, are unlikely to be effective. Most of the anticancer drugs discovered to date, with the notable exception of hormonal agents, are primarily active against fast-growing cells, and are unlikely to be useful models for the kinds of new agents sought."

It is difficult to model slow-growing tumors due to the long time period required for testing and evaluation.

The chapter concludes with a section on the types of models used and their evaluation. For the most part, mouse tumor models have been used, although human tumors can be transplanted into mice, as can genes.

No mention was made in the foregoing reference of recognized herbal treatments for cancer, nor of the particular herbs or extracts used, and the biochemicals that may be involved, such as in Essiac tea, chaparral or creosote bush, bloodroot, the Hoxsey mixture, garlic, laetrile or amygdalin, Naessen's 714X, hydrazine sulfate, urea, creatine, and so on, as further described say in Moss's *Cancer Therapy* and Walters' *Options.* None of the alternative cancer therapies spelled out, for instance, by Moss and by Walters receives mention, nor do any of the wide assembly of herbs or plants listed in Hartwell and in Heinerman. Specific anticancer agents are outside the scope of the investigation, which deals mainly with assay methods. Nevertheless, the comments are well taken about cancer and growth rates—and the ineffectiveness of chemotherapy on solid tumors.

Plant or herbal remedies are in fact a touchy subject to mainstream medicine and for the most part remain discredited. It is all complicated by the fact that what may be perceived as harmless or beneficial at one dosage level becomes toxic at other, higher dosage levels. Or as the adage goes, "the dose makes the poison." And what are classed as bioactive or medicinal plants or plant substances can indeed be poisonous, very poisonous, or fatal.

A case in point constitutes a chapter in Volume III of the series *Toxicants of Plant Origin.* The subject of the chapter is *lathyrogens*, which are toxic components from the seeds of certain *Lathyrus* species of the plant family Leguminosae—in particular *Lathyrus sativus.* These toxic components produce lathyrism, an ancient neurological disorder of both animals and humans (Dwijendra N. Roy and Peter S. Spencer, in *Toxicants of Plant Origin*, 3, p. 170ff). The genus *Lathyrus* is a kind of vetch, called chickling or chickeling vetch, whose consumption is brought about by drought conditions, particularly in India. While the seeds may serve as nourishment for a very brief period, over longer periods there is a cumulative toxicity. The causative agents may be classed as osteolathyrogens and neurolathyrogens. A number of components may in fact be causative, but the most likely candidates were found to be β-aminopropion-itrile (BAPN) and β-N-oxalylamino-L-alanine (BOAA). It may be added that the genus *Lathyrus* is listed in Hartwell's *Plants Used Against Cancer.*

May it be said again, therefore, that a plant or plant extract may act as an anticancer agent at one level of dosage and be entirely toxic at higher levels. Furthermore, these criteria can be expected to vary from one individual to another, a matter of biological/biochemical individuality. As the saying goes, our differences lie in our genes. More than this, it lies in the sequences of amino acids that constitute cellular proteins and their functions, whereby a person's immune system or immune response acts in a manner unique to that person, which will be further set forth in Part 7 in the section on immunity. In particular, there is the matter of what is called the *major histocompatibility complex,* or MHC, by which one's immune system distinguishes foreign bodies or antigens or cells—but not one's own cells, even though cancerous.

Speaking further of bioactive plants or plant substances that work against cancer, an extensive listing is provided in Appendix H as selected from James A. Duke's book, the *CRC Handbook of Medicinal Plants.* Worldwide, Duke lists some 365 medicinal plant species, presumably one for each day of the year, of which some 212 are noted as being active against cancer. Most of these appear in Jonathan L. Hartwell's *Plants Used Against Cancer.* With virtually every species, Duke includes an array of chemical compounds noted to occur, many of which are obtained from *Hager's Handbuch der Pharmazeutischen Praxis*, an exhaustive compilation of the results of plant analyses carried out through the years. A few of these compounds are included within Appendix H as being representative. More will be said about these compounds and compound classes in subsequent sections and in Parts 3 and 4. Special mention is made of the presence of alkaloids, being the most bioactive class of chemical compounds found in plants, followed by glycosides. Additional tabulations for anticancer plants by country or geographical region are provided in Appendices M through S.

2.3 ANTIBACTERIAL AND ANTIVIRAL AGENTS

Cancer is not the only topic of concern. Thus, there is a chapter titled "Screening Methods for Antibac-terial and Antiviral Agents from Higher Plants," by D.A. Vanden Berghe and A.J. Vlietinck, which also appears in *Methods in Plant Biochemistry*, Volume 6.

The authors note that, in spite of the wide array of clinically useful antibiotics presently available, the search continues for more. The major antibiotics now in use not only may be for narrow-spectrum applications and/or may have serious side effects, but overuse has led to antibiotic-resistant organisms. In addition, there is the emergence of previously uncommon infections. There is a need for new substances that act against such microorganisms as toxicogenic *Staphylococci*, anaerobes, *Pseudomonas*, *Legionel-lae*, various fungi, and still others. No cross resistance with existing antibiotics would be a desirable criterion.*

The same arguments apply to the discovery and development of new antiviral drugs. The present list is very short and is restricted to only a few specific viruses. Since viruses inhabit the cells that they infect, an agent that kills viruses is very likely also to kill or injure the host cells.†

There is also a need for new topical anti-infective agents, which serve as antiseptics and disinfectants. Such agents should be less toxic to human skin and tissues, should be biodegradable, and should be less harmful to the plant and animal life of the environment. These new drugs should preferably have broad-spectrum germicidal activity, including not only bactericidal, sporicidal, and fungicidal capabilities, but protozoicidal and virucidal capabilities as well. Prophylactic antiseptics that kill pathogens such as *Chlamydia*, papilloma, herpes, and HIV but do not harm normal skin flora would be most welcome for healthcare personnel.

---

* In some parts, a mixture of sulfur and molasses is still taken internally for infections, even boils. Whether the molasses kills the taste of the sulfur or the sulfur kills the taste of the molasses is debatable. In any event, something is going on, and presumably sulfur is the active ingredient, and may be an enzyme inhibitor, among other things

† This sort of problem also exists for cancer cells, in that cancer cells are similar to the cells of the organ from which they are derived, and anticancer agents that destroy the cancer cells are likely to destroy normal cells—not only those particular normal cells, but normal cells from other organs or parts of the body.

A strategy for research into finding new anti-infective drugs could involve chemotherapeutic compounds that are widely different from those in present use. These compounds could come from sources that have not been widely investigated—in particular, from *higher plants*. Plants contain a great diversity of antimicrobial and antiviral constituents, some of which may be of promising value.

A number of tests measure the growth response of microorganisms in the presence of plant tissues or extracts, but the results will vary with method. Most screening studies have been performed using one or two bacteria, notably *Staphylococcus aureus* and *E. coli*. Positive results, however, do not mean that the plant extracts will also be effective against other problem-pathogenic bacteria such as resistant *S. aureus*, *Pseudomonas aeruginosa*, *Proteus vulgaris*, *Klebsiella pneumoniae*, *Neisseria gonorrhoeae*, and *Candida albicans*. The test procedures are presented in some detail in the reference but are not of further interest for the purposes here.

Several studies identify individual plants that contain antimicrobial agents, and citations are provided in the reference. These agents, for the most part, are called *higher plant secondary plant metabolites*. "In many cases, investigation with modern methodology has confirmed folkloric accounts of the use of higher plant preparations for the treatment of infections." However, at least until now, these antimicrobial plant substances have either been too toxic to animals or else cannot compete with the products of microbial origin (antibiotics).

Garlic possess antibacterial properties and has been so used for centuries in folk medicine. Garlic oil consists primarily of diallyldisulfide with small quantities of diallyltrisulfide and diallylpolysulfide (Watt and Breyer-Brandwijk, *Africa*, pp. 675–677). Other constituents are an *alkaloidal* product, vitamins A, B, C, and probably D, plus reserve carbohydrates in the form of sinistrin rather than starch. A component called *alliin* is the source of allicin, a water-soluble, colorless, unstable oil with the chemical formula $C_6H_{10}OS_2$, called S-oxodiallyl disulfide. It is reported that allicin dilutions of 1:125,000 to 1:85,000 are effective against both gram negative and gram positive organisms, including *Staphylococci*, *Streptococci*, *Eberthella typhosa*, *Bacterium dysenteriae*, *Bacterium enteritidis*, *Vibrio cholerae*, and acid-fast bacteria. One milligram of allicin is equivalent to 15 Oxford units of penicillin, with low-temperature products biologically superior to high-temperature products.*

The alliin content varies with the site in which the garlic is grown. Alliin itself is an amino acid with the stoichiometric chemical formula $C_6H_{11}O_3NS_{1/2}H_2O$. A colorless needle-like crystalline material at room temperature, it melts at 163 to 165° C. It also decomposes readily which has hampered its therapeutic use. The cause is the enzyme alliinase, though it is possible to stabilize the alliin. While alliin is not an antibiotic itself, and is odorless, and on decomposition or cleavage it becomes an antibiotic with the characteristic garlic odor. (Presumably, the form of garlic marketed as Kyolic is in a stabilized form.)

The reference, published in 1962, notes that "Experiments of a tentative nature have been made on the effects of alliin on experimentally produced cancers in animals." With respect to allicin, the reference also states that "allicin inhibits sulphydryl (–SH) enzymes, a reaction which suggests that allicin may also have an inhibitory effect on the malignant cell." (This aspect will be discussed further in Part 8, from the standpoint of allicin being an inhibitor for lactate dehydrogenase, the distinguishing enzyme for cancer cell metabolism.)

As to antiviral activity, although vaccines have been very successful in controlling many viral diseases, it may turn out that some diseases can only be controlled by antiviral chemotherapy. Compared to antibiotics, antiviral agents have had many problems, including that of toxicity. Moreover, since viruses have only a very limited intrinsic enzyme system and few structural components, being largely dependent on the host cell, there are relatively few places that a virus can be attacked. The requirements for an antiviral agent are that it display specificity to the virus and that, furthermore, it block viral synthesis so as to stop the viral infection and restore normal cell synthesis. Other desirable characteristics listed are broad-spectrum activity, favorable pharmacodynamic properties, and an absence of immunosuppression. Ideally, the drug checks the infection while the immune system destroys the virus to the last particle. The authors observe that this latter point is critical for patients immunocompromised, say by AIDS, or cancer, or by drug therapy such as used in organ transplants and cancer chemotherapy. It is mentioned that a frequent cause of death in the foregoing circumstances is due to viral infections. It may be commented that there is a similarity between the action of anticancer

---

* Garlic powder is used as an insecticide by the home gardener, which brings to mind that perhaps hospital interiors should be dusted with garlic powder as a way to control runaway staph infections.

agents and the proposed antiviral agents in particular, since cancer is sometimes known to be caused by viruses.

Since may of the present-day antiseptics and disinfectants fail to kill all pathogenic viruses in the allotted time of five minutes at room temperature, there is need for new substance with the extra degree of virucidal activity. In screening antiviral compounds from plants, there is a difference to be noted between true antiviral activity and virucidal activity. In principle, the former presumably is more general, actually suppressing viral activity by blocking the further spread of the virus. Initial *in vitro* screening can be backed up by *in vivo* testing.

The viruses deemed most suitable for *in vitro* testing are adenovirus, herpes simplex, poliomyelitis or coxsackie, measles, Semlica forest, and vesicular stomatitis. Their morphologies are variously double-stranded DNA and single-stranded RNA. The infections induced in the main involve the respiratory system or the nervous system. A table is furnished in the reference, and further information about test procedures is outlined.

In previous decades, much information was gathered by the screening of plant extracts for antibacterial and antifungal activity, but relatively less has been reported for antiviral activity. Nonetheless, many antiviral agents have been isolated and characterized, and several review articles have surfaced, which are cited in the reference. Several substances have either emerged as true antiviral agents or else may lead the way. For example, different 3-methoxyflavones and synthetic derivatives may lead to the development of antirhinovirus drugs. The saponin known as glycyrrhizic acid is highly active against herpes simplex, varicella-zoster, and human immunodeficiency viruses. The clinical potential remains to be seen.

Unfortunately, other active substances interfere with host cell replication while exibiting virucidal properties. These other substances include flavonoids, phenolics, tannins, triterpenes, and alkaloids. Some of the virucidals, notably flavonoids and tannins present in food, may prove valuable, since they are known to inhibit the replication of picorna-, rota-, and arenaviruses in the gastrointestinal tract.

A chapter called "Tropical Plants Used in Chinese Medicine," in the volume *Medicinal and Poisonous Plants of the Tropics*, compiled by A.J.M. Leeuwenberg, has a section on parasitic agents and another on anti-inflammatory and antimicrobial agents. With regard to the former, 1'-acetoxychavicol acetate obtained from the rhizome of *Alpinia galanga* acted as a fungicide against species of *Trichophytron* and *Epidermophyton*. Quisqualic acid from the seeds of *Quisqualis indica* was used to treat ascariasis. Quassinoids from the fruit of Brucea javanica showed *in vitro* and *in vivo* antimalarial activity against *Plasmodia*. The quassinoids used were bruceantinol, bruceines, and brusatol. Artefacts or artifacts (tissue substances or structures) formed on the roots of *Artabotrys hexapetalus* (or *A. uncinatus*) during storage were identified as Yingzhaosu A and B. They produced significant antimalarial activity in mice. The roots of a member of the family Annonaceae, *Polyalthia nemoralis*, contain zincopolyanemine, which shows antiplasmoidal activity.

It is noted that the common tropical species *Dichroa febrifuga* has been used to treat malaria for over two millennia. The active component, febrifugine (dichroine), has an antimalarial activity about *100 to 150 times as great as quinine hydrochloride.*

As to anti-inflammatory and antimicrobial agents, the fruit and the rhizome of *Alpinia galanga* has also been used against ulcers. (Ulcers may be bacteria caused.) The active agents were 1'-acetoxychavicol acetate and 1'-acetoxyeugenol acetate. Curcumin, from the rhizome of *Curcumo longa*, is being used as an anti-inflammatory agent in clinical trials in India.

Andrographis paniculata has been used in various preparations for treating 7,143 different cases of bacterial infection. The total effective rate was 90.5 percent. The active agents were identified as andrographolide, deoxyandrographolide, and neoandrographolide.

A high palmatine content occurs in *Fibraurea recisa*. Preparations of both were used to treat more than 1500 cases of infections, with an effective curative rate of 90 percent.

The foregoing instances suggest that tropical plants may hold the key to treating infections that no longer respond to conventional antibiotics.

Megadoses doses of vitamin C are touted from time to time as acting against viral infections, although a mechanism has apparently not been accorded a consensus. In addition, John Heinerman's *Healing Animals with Herbs* cites instances when herbs have been used to cure *rabies* (Heinerman, *Healing*, p 55, 61–65). This would be antiviral action of the first magnitude. Of particular interest is the herb elecampane (*Inula helenium* of the family Compositae, which is listed in Hartwell). It is thought to be of use even after violent symptoms have appeared. Another herb used against rabies is rue (*Ruta graveolus* of the family Rutaceae, also listed in Hartwell). As if in confirmation, an article titled "Navajo Medicine Man" appeared in the July, 1961 issue of *Arizona Highways*. Written by an MD physician, Dr. Joseph G. Lee, it describes the use of rue against rabies. Earlier, in his explorations of Mexico and the American Southwest during the early 1900s, Carl Lumholtz mentioned a cure using the juice of rue (a woody herb, here called *Ruta* v. *Galego officinalis*), olive oil, deer rennet, grape vinegar, and lemon juice (Lumholtz, *Unknown Mexico*, II, p. 347). In a later expedition, he indicated that the Papago Indians had a secret cure for rabies (Lumholtz, *New Trails*, pp. 184–185). It has also been mentioned that eating dog lichen, *Peltigear canina*, is a folkloric treatment. (Lichens consist of a symbiotic arrangement between a species of fungus and a species of algae.) Notwithstanding, modern rabies victims would no doubt prefer the latest Pasteur treatment.

As to just what the antiviral action above might be, it can be noted that both the plant family Compositae and the family Rutaceae have species which contain alkaloids, according to Geoffrey A. Cordell's *Introduction to Alkaloids*. (And rue itself contains a great many alkaloids, whereby pharmacologists view its use as hazardous.)

As a matter of record, some antibacterial agents are listed in Appendix I, and antiviral agents in Appendix J. Inasmuch as they may also have potential bearing as anticancer agents, they are referenced against plant family, genera, and species that appear or do not appear in Hartwell's *Plants Used Against Cancer*. The several information sources include *Rainforest Remedies* by Rosita Arvigo and Michael Balick, a volume titled, *Some medicinal forest plants of Africa and Latin America*, plus *Medicinal Plants in West Africa* by Bep Oliver-Bever, and *The Pharmacology of Chinese Herbs* by Kee Chang Huang. More Phytomedicinal information is furnished in Part 4, dealing with alkaloids as antibacterial and antiviral agents. For known chemical agents, consult *AHFS Drug Information*, American Hospital Formulary Service.

2.4 ANTIFUNGAL AND MISCELLANEOUS AGENTS

Both plants and humans suffer from fungal diseases. Fungal diseases in humans include athlete's foot, caused by *Trichophyton mentagrophytes*, and the most common of all: aspergillosis and actinomycosis, and histoplasmosis and coccidioidomycosis, which affect an estimated 100 million people in the U.S. alone (Jack D. Paxton, in *Methods in Plant Biochemistry*, 6, p. 35ff). On the other hand, fungal diseases in insects are usually beneficial to man.

The taxonomy of fungi is still in flux, but fungi may in general be divided into the *Myxomycota*, the lower fungi, and the *Eumycota*, the higher fungi. Of the former, the lower fungi, there is presumably a merging with what we think of as bacteria. Of the latter or higher fungi, further classifications can be made, but their overall purpose is that of recycling organic materials of all sorts. Nevertheless, fungi can create problems, and their is a need for their control.

Inasmuch as cancers are from time to time attributed to fungi, a closer look at antifungal agents may be in order. Some of these antifungal compounds are found in plants, and the reference cites as a source a book edited by J.A. Bailey and J.W. Mansfield titled *Phytoalexins*, published by Halstead Press in 1982. These studies have been confined to compounds that act against plant fungi, and little is known about how compounds act against mammalian fungal pathogens.

A listing of some representative antifungal agents in provided in Appendix K, and a miscellany in Appendix L. The miscellany variously includes insecticidal, molluscidal (malacology being the study of mollusks), antiparasitical, antiprotozoal, antimetazoal, and anti-inflammatory agents. The same information sources apply as for antibacterial and antiviral agents. More information is provided in Part 4, dealing with alkaloids as antifungal agents.

Also in Appendix L is a listing for hypoglycaemic or hypoglycemic agents that can be construed as antidiabetic agents (Oliver-Bever, *Medicinal Plants in Tropical West Africa*, p. 245ff.) In a hypoglycemic condition, the metabolism of glucose proceeds at levels below normal, whereas in a hyperglycemic condition glucose metabolism (glycolysis) proceeds at levels above normal. Glucose metabolism is related to the production and availability of insulin, the hormone secreted by the β-cells of the Islets of Langerhans in the pancreas. Under normal conditions, insulin induces glucose oxidation (aerobic glycolysis) and at the same time favors the synthesis of liver glycogen from glucose but inhibits the formation of liver glycogen from protein and fat.

The disease known as diabetes can be traced to an insufficiency of insulin, causing a hypoglycemic condition. Normally, external sources of insulin can be used to correct the situation. If too much of a correction occurs, a hyperglycemic condition will be produced, otherwise known as insulin shock.

There are, however, plants or plant extracts that tend to correct this hypoglycemic condition, and the active constituents can be called antidiabetic agents. The action itself can be referred to as the hyperglycaemic or hyperglycemic principle involved.*

Some of these hypoglycaemic or hypoglycemic plant sources are included in Appendix K, as noted. Most if not all can be administered orally. The active components or constituents can be variously classed as hypoglycaemic phytosterin glycosides, alkaloids or amino acids, organic sulfur compounds, and as anthocyanins, catechols or flavonoids, or their glycols and/or tannins. Beyond these categories are still others. Rather than subdividing by chemical category as in the reference, the subdivision has been made by plant family.

The reference also furnishes a section on sweetening agents (Oliver-Bever, *Medicinal Plants in Tropical West Africa*, p. 265ff). Some of this interesting information is as follows.

The climbing species *Abrus precatorius* of the plant family Papilonaceae is chiefly known for its decorative but poisonous beans or seeds, which are the source of the extremely toxic vegetable protein known as *abrin*. (Abrin is apparently an anticancer agent, although an extremely risky one.) However, the leaves, and to some extent the roots, can be used as a sweetening agent. The saponoside called *glycyrrhizin* is present, which is also found in licorice. It is some 60 times sweeter than saccharose (another name for sucrose, or ordinary table sugar). As a bonus, anti-inflammatory, expectorant, antitussive, and antibiotic properties are included.

The red berries of *Dioscoreophyllin cumminsii* of the family Menispermaceae are said to contain the most potent sweetening agent presently known. The species is described as a high forest climber found from Guinea to the Cameroons. The active principle is a basic protein called monellin. It is rated as about 3000 times sweeter than sucrose on an equivalent weight basis. The sweetness is lost under more alkaline and more acid conditions, and the fact that so very little is required may make this source "completely inoffensive."

The small tree named *Synsepalum dulcificum* of the family Sapotaceae yields small, single-seeded red fruits whose pulp serves as a sweetener. The sweet taste is not instantaneous but follows afterward. The active agent is a glycoprotein called miraculin, which contains the constituent sugars arabinose and xylose. It is said to be an appetite depressant as well—even an anorexic agent. The action evidently modifies the taste receptors of the tongue.

Finally, there is the herb *Thaumatococcus danielli* of the family Maracanthaceae, whose crimson underground fruits are known collectively as miraculous fruit. Palm wine is sweetened using this source. The plant grows up to ten feet tall, and the papery leaves can be used to wrap food (e.g., kola). The sweet substance exists in the jelly-like aril (or appendage) surrounding the seed and has been named thaumatin. It contains two high molecular weight proteins with nearly identical amino acid compositions. At more acidic conditions, the sweetness is lost, as it is when heated. Somewhat similar in taste to licorice, it is said to be from 1600 to 4000 times sweeter than saccharose or sucrose. Polyphenols occur in the sweetener, as do flavonols and flavones. (The taste-alikes licorice and anise are derived, respectively, from *Glycyrrhiza glabra* of the family Leguminosae and *Pimpinella anisum* of the family Umbelliferae. Both are in Hartwell.)

Whereas the earlier volumes of *Hager's Handbuch* detail such topics as plant chemicals or phytochemicals, the 1977 edition includes the chemistry of sweeteners (in *German*, of course)—some conventional, some not so conventional—plus other items more of industrial chemistry.

2.5 PLANT ENZYMES

To read about plant enzymes in plant glycolysis is to note the similarity to glycolysis in mammals. Both involve the overall conversion of a hexose to generate ATP (adenosine triphosphate) and pyruvate. (A hexose is defined as a simple sugar with six oxygen atoms in the molecule—for example, both glucose

---

* We may note that cancer cells in the main do not oxidize glucose but rather convert it to lactic acid, the overall process of anaerobic glycolysis. Whether there is a connection with a diabetic condition can only be questioned at this point. And whether diabetically inclined persons are more prone to cancer seems to be a statistic that is not in evidence.

and fructose have the formula $C_6H_{12}O_6$ and are hexoses.) Plant glycolysis is unique, however, in that the conversion occurs in two subcellular compartments, the cytosol and the plastid (W.C. Plaxton, in *Methods in Plant Biochemistry*, 3, p. 146ff). Furthermore, it is perceived that the conversion of hexose to pyruvate involves isoenzymes, the one set the plastidic isoenzymes and the other set the cytosolic isoenzymes. By isoenzymes or isozymes is meant that the enzymes catalyze the same chemical reaction but have somewhat different chemical structures.

Classical glycolysis assumes that one mole of glucose converts to two moles of pyruvic acid or pyruvate, with the initial step the conversion of glucose to glucose 6-phosphate catalyzed by the enzyme hexokinase. (See Fig. 1.1 in Part 1.) This is followed by the second step, the conversion of glucose 6-phosphate to fructose 6-phosphate catalyzed by the enzyme hexose phosphateisomerase. The third step is the conversion of fructose 6-phosphate to fructose 1,6-bisphosphate catalyzed by phosphofructokinase. It can be argued that, in plant glycolysis, the initial step should be the conversion of fructose 6-phosphate to fructose 1,6-bisphosphate, which is the third step in classical glycolysis.

However argued, the above conversion of fructose 6-phosphate to fructose 1,6-bisphosphate is catalyzed by the same enzyme in both plants and animals, the enzyme phosphofructokinase. (Phosphofructokinase is variously designated PFK or PFP, the latter for phosphate-dependent phosphofructokinase.) Carrot roots are a source of PFK, and potato tubers are a source for PFP.

The next step is the conversion of fructose-1,6-bisphosphate to glyceraldehyde 3-phosphate, and is catalyzed by aldolase, the same for plants as for mammals. Additionally, dihydroxyacetone is formed, the same for plants as for mammals. Spinach leaves are a source for aldolase.

This is followed by the conversion of glyceraldehyde 3-phosphate to 1,3-bisphosphoglycerate, catalyzed by glyceraldehyde 3-phosphate dehydrogenase, the same for plants as for mammals. White mustard seedlings are a source for glyceraldehyde 3-phosphate dehydrogenase.

In turn, 1,3 bisphosphoglycerate is converted to 3-phosphoglycerate, catalyzed by phosphoglycerate kinase, the same for plants as for animals. Silver beet leaves (*Beta vulgaris*) are a source for phosphoglycerate kinase.

The next step is the conversion of 3-phosphoglycerate to 2-phosphoglycerate, catalyzed by phosphoglyceromutase, the same for plants as for mammals. Castor bean endosperm tissue is a source for phosphoglyceromutase. (Note: *Castor beans are highly toxic*. The conversion to castor oil involves detoxification procedures.)

Then, 2-phosphoglycerate converts to phosphoenolpyruvate, catalyzed by enolase, the same for plants as for mammals. Castor bean endosperm tissue is a source for enolase.

Lastly, 2-phosphoenolpyruvate is converted to pyruvate, which is catalyzed by pyruvate kinase, the same for plants as for mammals. Castor bean endosperm tissue is a source for enolase, as noted.

To proceed to the tricarboxylic acid cycle, or respiration, the mitichondrial pyruvate dehydrogenase (PDH) complex is involved (also called PDC), with the peripheral supporting reactions involving CoA and NAD^+ (Douglas D. Randall and Jan A. Miernyk, in *Methods in Plant Biochemistry*, 3, p. 176ff). It is the same for plants as for animal. The mitochondrial complex has been obtained from both broccoli and cauliflower (Randall and Miernyk, *Methods*, p. 183).

Photosynthesis obviously is not a part of mammalian metabolism. Although the subject of photosynthesis or photobiology is included in Volume 4 in the series *Methods in Plant Biochemistry*, it will not be of further concern here. Suffice to say, photosynthesis also involves enzymes.

The fact that these very same enzymes, above—which are vital links in mammalian metabolism—can be obtained from plants underscores the role of diet and nutrition. By isolating or synthesizing these nutritional elements, there is the possibility of enhancing human health and well being. This is only a step away from what we call vitamins, which are sometimes also called coenzymes—that is, promoters or activators for enzymes proper. Introduction into the body might be carried out intravenously if oral dosage is ineffective. By adjusting the enzyme amounts and proportions, there is the intriguing thought that cancer cell growth might be selectively controlled or eliminated. This would assume that cancer cell metabolism is sufficiently different from normal cell metabolism. For after all, enzyme mixtures have even been known to dissolve cancers—albeit the mixtures may be composed mostly of digestive enzymes and may have nothing to do directly with cell metabolism per se.

The above-cited conversions and enzymes are but a few described in the volume *Methods in Plant Biochemistry*, 3, edited by P.M. Dey and J.B. Harborne. The clinical application to human illnesses, including cancer, is the purpose of enzyme therapy, an emerging medical specialty outside the mainstream.

2.6   BIOACTIVE/TOXIC PLANT SUBSTANCES

The plants that act as anticancer agents are bioactive substances, which by and large are also poisonous to a degree. The distinction between poisonous and medicinal plants is sometimes a fine line, depending on the level of dosage. As Will H. Blackwell observes in his book, *Poisonous and Medicinal Plants*, in a chapter called Toxic Plant Substances in Poisonous and Medicinal Plants, a given plant is a veritable warehouse of thousands of kinds of chemicals, of which most are harmless, and some of which are not.

The initial processes of photosynthesis first generate simple compounds of carbon, hydrogen, and oxygen, the carbohydrates known as sugars—e.g., glucose. These sugars are in part further converted by complex chemical reactions to amino acids, which utilize nitrogen and which are the building blocks for proteins. Proteins in turn furnish the basic framework for what is called protoplasm, "the living substance." It is affirmed that some 20 different amino acids are essential for life processes. These life processes involve both sugars (e.g., glucose) and the essential amino acids. The sequences or pathways of enzyme-catalyzed biochemical reactions that so occur are collectively known as primary metabolism, and the products may be referred to as primary metabolites. (In the most general terms, the reactants may also be called metabolites. That is, both reactants and products are the constituents or components of reacting systems.)

In turn, still other (secondary) reaction sequences occur that involve the reaction products, and sometimes the primary reactants, plus other or secondary compounds. The products so produced are generally called secondary metabolites. These secondary compounds are alkaloids, glycosides, and other such substances. Moreover, these secondary compounds include toxic substances or toxins. Blackwell classifies plant-derived toxic substances as falling into several broad categories: alkaloids, glycosides, proteinaceous compounds, organic acids, alcohols, resins and resinoids (including phenolics), and mineral toxins (inorganic compounds).

In somewhat earlier days, the preeminent authority on poisonous or toxic plants was John M. Kingsbury, who wrote *Poisonous Plants of the United States and Canada*, published in 1964, and *Deadly Harvest: A Guide to Common Poisonous Plants*, published in 1965. Kingsbury's efforts can be viewed in considerable degree as directed toward preventing toxicity in livestock. A subsequent and more compact volume, based in part on Kingsbury's work, was *Poisonous Plants of the Central United States*, by H.A. Stephens and published in 1980. The major toxic principles are provided for the various plants described, as then known. Stephens' appendix classifies the toxins as follows: alkaloids; dermatitis and hay fever; glycosides, cardiac; glycosides, coumarin; glycosides, cyanogenetic; glycosides, goitrogenic; glycosides, mustard oils; glycosides; protoanemonin; glycosides, saponin; mechanical; nitrates; oxalates, crystals; oxalates, soluble; photosensitizers; phytotoxins; resinoids; selenium; miscellaneous. The scientific and common names of the corresponding plants are listed, along with the plant part that is toxic. Indexing is by the scientific name of the genus, and also by common names. Not all of the plants in the appendix or index are described in the text entries. Medicinal uses, if any, are not included.

Alkaloids, which will be discussed more fully in a following section and in Part 4, are said to occur in perhaps 20 percent of the higher plant families. In mammals, even a minute amount of some alkaloids can have profound effects on the nervous system. There may also be anticancer effects, to be explored subsequently at length.

Glycosides are second in importance to the alkaloids, and a separate section will further discuss their significance. They vary greatly in structure but are basically a simple sugar like glucose bonded to something else that is not a sugar. The non-sugar part is referred to as the *aglycone* or genin. Interestingly, when joined the glycoside may be relatively inert but, if separated, the aglycone may show pronounced activity or toxicity (as with cyanic aglycones). Furthermore, separation may occur during digestion.

The type of aglycone can be used to characterize glycosides, as follows: cyanogenic (cyanogenetic) glycosides; steroid glycosides, which comprise cardiac glycosides (cardenolides) and saponins (sapogenic glycosides); coumarin glycosides; anthraquinone glycosides; mustard oil (and related) glycosides.

In *cyanoglycosides* or cyanogenic glycosides, as the name implies, the aglycone is cyanide or hydrogen cyanide (HCN), also called prussic acid. Its action is to block the activity of a respiration enzyme called cytochrome oxidase, though it will block others as indicated in Appendix B. Plants or plant parts which contain cyanoglycosides include the hydrangea (genus *Hydrangea*), flax (*Linum*), elderberry (*Sambucus*), and wild cherry (*Prunus*). The cyanoglycoside called amygdalin or laetrile is the most well known, being found in the seeds or pits of certain members of the family Rosaceae or Rose family, notably the *Prunus* species almond, peach, apricot, and wild cherry—plus seeds of the apple (of the genus *Malus*, which may alternately be placed in the family Malaceae). On hydrolysis, the products released are sugar, cyanide, and benzaldehyde, the last mentioned being called the "fragrance of almond." Use of the commercial preparation Laetrile (medicinal form) against cancer is said to be inconclusive, and it has been declared ineffective for the usual reasons. Not only that, but it is cytotoxic—as are such common chemotherapy drugs as 5–FU, it may be added.

In *steroid glycosides* the aglycone is a steroid molecule or nucleus. With an additional lactone ring, the substance becomes a cardiac glycoside, effective against congestive heart failure but also a cause of cardiac arrest. The dosage level is critical. The agent is known as digitoxin from the foxglove (*Digitalis*), convallarin from lily of the valley (*Convallaria*), and ouabain from the genus *Strophanthus*. Other sources include dogbane (*Apocynum*), milkweed (*Asclepias*), and oleander (*Nerium*). Saponins do not have the lactone ring and are not cardioactive, but they have other toxic effects, particularly on the GI tract. Plant sources include corn cockle (*Agrostemma*), tungnut (*Aleurites*), pokeweed (*Phytolacca*), English ivy (*Hedera*), and soapwort or bouncing Bet (*Saponaria*). Mixed with water, the saponins produce a frothing action and can be used as soap substitute. (A tree of the southern Great Plains region is called the soapberry, of the genus *Sapindus* of the family Sapindaceae.)

The genus *Strophanthus* (of the family Apocynaceae or Dogbane family) is a well known source for arrow poisons and is so used in Africa. (The species *Strophanthus omaatwa* appears in Hartwell's *Plants Used Against Cancer.*) In small enough doses, it acts medicinally as a cardiac and vascular stimulant; in larger doses it is a poison. The Bushmen of the Kalahari use it for these latter purposes, and the animal suffers a lingering death ranging from hours for smaller animals to days for larger animals. According to the *Britannica*, among the cardiac glycosides present are digitoxin, digoxin, and ouabain. Interestingly, *Strophanthus* is of the same plant family as the genus *Vinca*, source of the *Vinca* alkaloids.

In *coumarin glycosides,* the aglycone is a phenolic-type molecule called a coumarin. An odor is imparted like that of new-mown hay. Usually nontoxic, under certain conditions dicoumarins are formed that prevent blood from coagulating—but can also be used to control clotting. Compounds called furans are related to coumarins and, sometimes toxic, may also occur in moldy sweet potatoes (*Ipomoea*) and in the wild parsnip (*Pastinaca*). The black mold *Aspergillus flavus* yields furanocoumarin substances better known as *aflatoxins*, as found in spoiled grains, and which are suspected liver carcinogens.

In anthroquinone and mustard oil glycosides, the aglycones are anthroquinones, as the category infers. These are typically laxatives. For instance, the glycosides from senna (*Cassia fistulosa*) and from the genus *Aloe* are used in commercial preparations. Mustard oils contain mustard-oil glycosides or glucosinolates, which convert to thiocyanates or isothiocyanates. These are relatively simple nitrogen compounds with sulfur in the molecule. Black mustard (*Brassica nigra*) seeds are a source. (The glycoside sinigrin yields allyl isothiocyanate by enzymatic action.) Usually causing no more than a mild gastric disturbance, certain related goiterogenic glycosides found in the family Cruciferae or mustard family can block iodine uptake and cause an enlarged thyroid gland (goiter). Cabbage (*Brassica oleracea capitata*) is an unsuspected example.

Proteinaceous compounds are ubiquitous, and while the great majority are beneficial and nontoxic, a few are quite toxic. Containing bound nitrogen always, some proteins contain sulfur as well. As has been described elsewhere, in Part 1, proteins are polymers of amino acids consisting of hundreds to thousands of various amino acids linked together. The smaller polymers are called polypeptides.

The true proteins that are highly toxic were formerly called phytotoxins or toxicoalbumins. Contained in only a few plants, their impact is significant. Of note is abrin, found in the seeds of the rosary pea or precatory bean (*Abrus precatorius*). Also of note is ricin, derived from the seeds of the castor bean (*Ricinus communis*), a plant originally native to India. Both have similar effects and are among the most toxic plant substances known. Although most toxic if injected directly, even a few seeds can be fatal if chewed and swallowed. The toxins are similar to bacterial toxins such as occur in cholera, tetanus, and diphtheria and are also similar to certain snake venoms. Abrin and ricin are readily absorbed in the digestive tract, producing ulceration and being transferred to the circulatory system, with accompanying cell damage notably to the kidneys, liver, and nervous system.

There is also an alkaloid found in the seeds of *Ricinus*. It is called ricinine and is described as being only mildly toxic, ricin instead being the toxic component (Cordell, *Alkaloids*, p. 197). Further particulars about *Ricinus*, ricin, and castor oil may be found in *Medicinal and Poisonous Plants of Southern and Eastern Africa* (Watt and Breyer-Brandwijk, *Africa*, p. 428ff).

Abrin and ricin are cytotoxic, acting as proteolytic (protein-digesting) enzymes. They interfere with cell ribosomes, where amino acids are joined to form enzymes and other proteins. The effect is to negate protein synthesis and produce cell destruction and degeneration. [Other known ribosomal inhibitors are chloramphenicol, cycloheximide, erythromycin, fusidic acid, puromycin, tetracycline, and diphtheria toxin (Voet and Voet, *Biochemistry*, p. 1002).] Abrin and ricin are selectively transported by nerve cells or neurons, affecting the nervous system (which can be used clinically for the denervation of parts of the nervous system). The corresponding plant species are listed in Hartwell.

In comment, if these deadly proteinaceous toxins could be made to act selectively against cancer cells, this would be a significant breakthrough.

Abrin, notably, will agglomerate red blood cells, and plant seed proteins which have this effect are called *lectins*. Some lectins, as from abrin, will stimulate other types of blood cells, namely the white blood cells or lymphocytes, to divide and mature. This process is called *mitosis*, and plant lectins acting in this way on white blood cells are called *mitogens*. Among plant mitogens, the proteins (glycoproteins) from pokeweed (*Phytolacca americana*) are being studied as a tool to stimulate the immune response. And in particular, there is an interest as concerns the type of blood cancer known as Hodgkin's disease. (The initial discovery was made when a child died from pokeweed poisoning, but the child's immune system had been triggered.) Plant mitogens have therefore become of great research and clinical interest, with pokeweed foremost on the list. Other mitogenic lectins have been found in the black locust (*Robina pseudo-acacia*) and the sandbox tree (*Hura crepitans*).

There is the prospect that stimulating the immune system will act against cancer, at least in the formative stages.

Toxic polypeptides occur in several of the fungi of the infamous genus *Amanita*, for instance *A. phalloides* (death cap) and related species. These polypeptides have an assortment of names: amatoxins, phallotoxins, and phalloidin. Their molecular structure consists of seven or eight amino acids in a cyclic or circular arrangement, and they are referred to as cyclic polypeptides. In similar manner to the toxic proteins, these cyclic polypeptides interfere with cellular processes, specifically blocking the enzyme RNA-polymerase. The effect is to inhibit the generation of new and vital proteins, at the same time producing the destruction and degeneration of cells in the intestines, liver, kidney, and even the heart wall. (These effects sound familiar, with reference to the action of the chemotherapy drug 5–FU.) The *Amanita* mushrooms are the most common source of fatal poisoning in humans. Cyclic polypeptides also are found in blue-green algae (cyanobacteria), which grows in farm ponds during late summer and causes livestock poisoning.

Toxic amines occur in the genus *Lathrus*, which comprises such plants as sweet peas and vetches or vetchlings. These compounds are variants of aminopropionitrile, in which the amine group ($-NH_2$) and the nitrile group (an organic group in turn containing the $-CN$ group) both contribute to the toxicity of the molecule. Degeneration in the motor tractscords of the spinal cord is caused by the amines in the seeds, embodied as the disease called lathyrism, previously mentioned. The end result can be paralysis and death. Other sources include the berries from mistletoe (genus *Phoradendron*), which contain tyramine and phenylethylamine. In addition to gastroenteritis, a severe lowering of blood pressure can occur, even cardiovascular collapse. For this reason, mistletoe berry extract was once used in treating high blood pressure—but it is dangerous to use.

Organic acids may be designated as compounds having the carboxylic acid group ($-COOH$), or groups, and which in totality consist of carbon, hydrogen, and oxygen without nitrogen—or in a word, are nonamino acids. Those toxic to animals are few in number, the main one being oxalic acid and its soluble salts. Very few plants contain a high enough concentration to be a problem. A few minor examples include beet tops and the leaves of rhubarb (not the stalks). An introduced species called halogeton (*Halogeton glomeratus*), originally from the steppes of southern Russia, has become a serious problem in the more northern, arid parts of the American West. Entire flocks of sheep have been poisoned and lost, and ranches have gone bankrupt.

A few other sources of minor oxalate concentrations include dock (genus *Rumex*), sorrel (genus *Oxalis*), and garden spinach or *Spinacia oleracea*. (Spinach also contains alkaloids.) Another minor source is the family Araceae, also known as the Aroid or Arum family—e.g., jack in the pulpit (*Arisaema atrorubens*), dumbcane (genus *Dieffenbachia*), and caladium (genus *Caladium*), in which the calcium oxalate salts crystallize out as sharp needles.

Highly toxic *alcohols* are rare, although all alcohols may be regarded as toxic to some degree. (Alcohols are distinguished by the $-OH$ group connected to a carbon atom. No other oxygen is involved. An alcohol therefore is to be distinguished from a carboxylic acid, which contains the carboxyl group

–COOH.) The most notorious example of a toxic plant alcohol occurs in the water hemlock (*Cicuta maculata* and related species of the family Umbelliferae). It has caused many deaths for both animals and humans. Looking like a wild carrot or wild parsnip to the unsuspecting, the underground portion of the stem is significantly different. There is also an oily, yellowish exudate from this part of the plant, a fluid not found in the wild carrot or parsnip. The fluid contains a long straight-chain unsaturated alcohol named cicutoxin. It will rapidly affect the central nervous system, causing violent convulsions in the extreme. Death can occur in a few hours or a few minutes.

The chemical formula for cicutoxin is provided in the reference and may be represented as $HOCH_2CH_2CH_2=C-C\equiv C(CH=CH)_3C(OH)HCH_2CH_2CH_3$. The (OH) group identifies it as an alcohol.

Another, somewhat similar toxic alcohol occurs in the white snakeroot (*Eupatorium rugosum*), a plant found growing at the edge of woods in the eastern United States. The alcohol is named tremetol, and it is not as serious as either a poison or a convulsant, but it affects cattle by causing a disease called the trembles. It is passed on to humans who drink the milk and was once called milk sickness. This disease is a thing of the past, since modern dairy processing practices pool the milk from many sources, diluting the effects present from any particular contaminated source.

Resinous substances consist of complex mixture difficult to categorize. In the main, however, these substances are made up of phenolics, a subject to be further discussed in a subsequent section. In a way, phenolics can be regarded as aromatic alcohols in that the alcohol or hydroxy group (–OH) is connected to an aromatic benzene or phenyl ring.

Among the better known phenolic resins occurring in nature is the compound tetrahydrocannabinol (THC). It and related compounds are found in marijuana or hemp (*Cannabis sativa*). The basic structure is provided in the reference and consists of three phenyl rings connected together, along with several side groups and an implanted oxygen in the central ring. An Asiatic fiber plant, marijuana or hemp was formerly grown mainly to make rope. (There are several species. Manila hemp or Manila rope is a term in common usage.) The last domestic rope factory closed in the mid 1950s, but the plant itself has spread more or less all over the United States.

Another resinous or phenolic or resinoid substances is called urushiol, a mixture of slightly varying content derived from poison ivy, poison oak, and poison sumac, all of the genus *Rhus*. Another is hypericin, derived from St. John's wort, *Hypericum perforatum*. The common effect is dermatitis, with hypericin also causing sensitivity to sunlight. Chemical structures are furnished in the reference.

Another group of resin-like or resinous substances is called the terpenoids. Somewhat resembling phenolics, they have different origins, and may be classed as mono-, sesqui- di-, and tri-terpenes, or terpenoids, or whatever. Mostly harmless and sometimes aromatically fragrant, the monoterpenes are oils derived from species of the family Labiatae or Lamiaceae, or Mint family, and from the family Rutaceae or Citrus family. Diterpenoids occur in the pungent latex of members of the family Euphorbiaceae or Spurge family, for instance in the genus *Euphorbia*, and may be carcinogenic. Sesquiterpenes are found in sagebrush, of the genus *Artemisia* of the family Compositae or Asteraceae (or Sunflower family or Daisy family or Aster family), and can cause dermatitis. Triterpenoid derivatives are found in the Mexican yam (genus *Dioscorea*).

Mineral toxins include nitrates, found in some plant species, and a cause of nitrate poisoning in livestock. Among the weeds which contain nitrates are goosefoot or lamb's quarter (*Chenopodium album*) and pigweed (genus *Amaranthus*). The nitrate is in the form of potassium nitrate (KNO_3). The reference notes the phenomenon that the nitrate uptake from the soil is increased when such herbicides as 2,4-D are applied. In ruminant animals, notably cattle, the nitrate may be converted to nitrite during digestion, and which is ten times as poisonous as nitrate. The nitrate or nitrite will interfere with the oxygen-carrying capacity of the blood, causing asphyxiation. The oxygen deficiency is signaled by a chocolate-brown color to the blood. Although not directly a problem to humans, the storage of silage can result in fermentation reactions that produce the yellowish-brown gases that are oxides of nitrogen. The ensuing lung irritation that may happen with exposure is called "silo-filler's disease." It is commented that even nitrocellulose may form due to the reaction of plant cellulose with the nitrogen oxides, and the result may be a totally unexpected explosion in the silo.

Selenium poisoning is a too-often occurrence in range cattle in parts of the American West, such as in Wyoming. (Inasmuch as selenium and uranium may occur together, this fact has been of interest to geologists looking for the latter.) Evidently, selenium displaces or substitutes for sulfur in protein molecules, disrupting protein synthesis. The effects are most noticeable in the liver and kidneys. The end result is cell degeneration. Some species of plants will selectively concentrate this mineral from selenium-rich soils. (That is to say, they will take up and concentrate the element selenium in the form of some of its more water-soluble compounds or salts.) Such plants are called selenium indicators, and they include species of the genus *Astralagus*, sometimes called poison vetches, and still other plants. A number of symptoms can appear in livestock, for instance, the blind staggers, hoof deformity, and sloughing, and what is called "alkali disease," which, as is said, has nothing to do with alkali. The subject of selenium poisoning will be reintroduced in Part 4 in connection with alkaloid-bearing plants such as locoweeds, also a problem in the American West (as per the publication *Weeds of the West*).

For the record, Table 2.2 is a listing of plant families and their particular genera that have caused fatalities. Nearly all also appear in Hartwell's *Plants Used Against Cancer*. There is sometimes a fine line between therapeutic usefulness and toxicity.

As a footnote to the above, a relevant article appeared in the May 6, 1996 issue of *Newsweek*. Titled "Herbal Warning," by Geoffrey Cowley and others of the *Newsweek* staff, it mentioned a number of herbs to be wary of. These include lobelia (*Lobelia inflata* of the family Lobeliaceae), comfrey (*Symphytum officianale* of the family Boraginaceae), germander (*Teucrium chamaedrys* of the family Labiatae), pennyroyal (*Mentha pulegium* of the family Labiatae), coltsfoot (*Tussilago farfara* of the family Compositae), chaparral (*Larrea indentata—Larrea tridentata* is of the family Zygophyllaceae), sassafras (*Sassafras albidum* of the family Lauraceae), senna (*Cassia acutifolia* of the family Leguminosae or Fabaceae, or Legume family or Pea family), yohimbe (*Corymanthe yohimbe* of the family Rubiaceae), ephedra or "Ma Huang" (*Ephydra sinica* of the family Gnetaceae). Some are described as containing alkaloids, and some can cause liver damage in addition to other adverse side effects. All save the last two species appear in Hartwell's *Plants Used Against Cancer*. Incidentally, the last two are noted for their alkaloid content, e.g., ephedrine and yohimbine, as is comfrey, which contains pyrrolizidine alkaloids. As the saying goes, however, the dosage is the poison.

The foregoing article also notes that, according to the American Association of Poison Control Centers, *for every person killed by an herb, there are roughly 500 fatalities from pharmaceuticals*. And for the 50 or so nonfatal poisonings that occur each year due to plants (which includes the accidental poisoning of kids from trying out jade, holly, or poinsettias), there are about *7000 traceable to pharmaceuticals*.

Varro E. Tyler's *The Honest Herbal* refutes the many unsubstantiated claims for the curative powers of herbs. Tyler also notes that both coltsfoot and comfrey contain pyrrolizidine alkaloids, and that mistletoe and pau d'arco are probably cytotoxic. Adamant against Laetrile, he uses the placebo effect to explain why some herbs seem to work. Theories are in short supply, however, such as plant substances acting as enzyme inhibitors for cancer cell metabolism.

2.7 GLYCOSIDES

Of most interest here are *cyanogenic glycosides*. A chapter of that title by Olumide O. Tewe and Eustace A. Iyayi appears, for instance, in *Toxicants of Plant Origin*, Volume II. Cyanogenic glycosides include *laetrile* and *amygdalin*, which contain organic forms of cyanide, with the names sometimes used synonymously, although there is a slight variation in chemical makeup. Used in both world wars as a military weapon, the pharmacological applications of cyanide itself have been widespread (Tewe and Iyayi, in *Toxicants*, II, p. 56). Cyanide has been given in small doses for medicinal purposes over long periods of time without apparent harm, and even with some benefits. In the form of cherry laurel, it was once given for pulmonary disease and has been used for chest complaints, asthma, catarrh, and coughs. It has been used as a sedative and as palliative for tuberculosis. Preparations from almonds and peach stones were once used for flavoring.*

The cyanide release occurs via hydrolysis, and the reference lists a number of cyanogenic glycosides and their three hydrolytic products. Most release D-glucose, and all release HCN, with the third compound variously consisting of such as benzaldehyde, acetone, and so forth. An enumeration of the cyanogenic glycoside names includes linamarin, lotaustralin, dhurrin, amygdalin, taxiphyllin, vicianin,

---

* Although the terms *glycoside* and *glucoside* are often used somewhat interchangeably, strictly speaking, a glucoside may be viewed as a glycoside where the carbohydrate content is glucose or glucose-derived. The term glycoside can therefore be regarded as the more general descriptor. See, for instance, Chapter 15, by Peter A. Mayes, in *Harper's Biochemistry*, pp. 139–140.

Table 2.2 Genera Involved in Fatalities[a]

Acanthaceae	*Justica*: vrisha
Amaryllidaceae	*Narcissus*: narcissus
Apocynaceae	*Acokanthera**
	Nerium: oleander
	Thevetia: yoyote
Araceae	*Arisaema*: Indian turnip
	Arum: arum, dragon tea
	Caladium: ocumo
	Dieffenbachia: dica, mata del cáncer
Araliaceae	*Hedera*: ivy
Asclepiadaceae	*Calotropis*: mudar, arka
	*Cryptostegia** (or the family Periplocaceae*)
Berberidaceae	*Podophyllum*: mandrake, may apple, polophyllum
Capparidaceae	*Courbonia**
Caprifoliaceae	*Sambucus*: elder
Carophyllaceae	*Agrostemma*: nigella, cokle, raden, lolium
Combretaceae	*Terminalia*: myrohalen
Commelinaceae	*Pilocarpus**
Compositae	*Arnica*: arnica
(Asteraceae)	*Eupatorium*: boneset
	Senecio: groundsel
	Tanacetum: tansy
Connaraceae	*Rourea*: awennade
Cucurbitaceae	*Cucurbita*: gourd, pumpkin
	Momordica: balsam-pear
Cycadaceae*	*Cycas**: sago-palm
Dioscoreaceae	*Tamus*: byrony
Ericaceae	*Azalea**: azalea
	Gaultheria: **cancer wintergreen**, creeping wintergreen
	*Kalmia**: laurel
	*Rhododendron**
Euphorbiaceae	*Alchornea**: Christian bush
	Aleurites
	Croton: croton, sangue de drago
	Euphorbia: euphorbia, spurge, milkweed
	Hippomane: manzanillo

Table 2.2   Genera Involved in Fatalities[a]   *(continued)*

	*Hura**: spurge
	Jatropha: physic-nut
	Manihot: manioc, cassava, tapioca
	Mercurialis: mercury
	*Poinsettia**: poinsettia
	Ricinus: castor bean plant
Fabaceae*	*Albizzia*: çirisha, siris (Indian walnut)
(Leguminosae)	*Andira**: dog almond, wormbark
	Cassia: senna, cassia
	Cytisus: broom
	*Dalbergia**
	*Erythophleum**: red-water tree
	*Laburnum**: laburnum, golden chain
	Phaseolus: bean
	*Robinia**: locust
	*Physostigma**: calabar bean
Gramineae	*Lolium*: lolium, Italian ryegrass, darnel
Guttiferae	*Garcinia*: t'eng-huang, gamboge
Hippocastanaceae	*Aesculus*: castagno d'india
Labiatae	*Hoslundia**
(Lamiaceae)	*Lavandula*: lavender
Liliaceae	*Bowiea**: aloe
	Colchicum: ephemeron
	Convallaria: Solomon's seal
	Gloriosa: dorng-dueng
	Paris: herb Paris
	Urginea: squill
	Veratrum: American hellebore
	*Zigadenus**: death camus
Lobeliaceae	*Lobelia*: lobelia
Loganiaceae	*Gelsemium*: yellow jasmine
	*Spigelia**: pinkroot, wormgrass
	Strychnos: nux vomica, strychine
Loranthaceae	*Phoradendron*
Meliaceae	*Melia*: nimva, margosa, neem-tree
Menispermaceae	*Menispermum**: moonseed

Table 2.2 Genera Involved in Fatalities[a] *(continued)*

Monimiaceae*	*Peumus**: boldo
Oleaceae	*Ligustrum*: privet
Phytolaccaceae	*Phytolacca*: poke
Pinaceae	*Juniperus*: juniper
Piperaceae	*Piper*: pepper
Polygonaceae	*Rheum*: rhubarb
Ranuculaceae	*Helleborus*: hellebore
	Actaea: shang-ma, wolfskraut
	Aquilegia: columbine
	Delphinium: delphinium, larkspur
	Aconitum: monkshood, wolfsbane
	Ranunculus: ranunculus, buttercup, crowfoor, chelidonion, celandine
Rosaceae	*Malus*: apple
	Prunus: almond, cherry, plum, peach, apricot
Sapindaceae	*Blighia*: African akee
Scrophulariaceae	*Digitalis*: foxglove, digitalis
Solanaceae	*Atropa*: belladonna, deadly nightshade
	Datura: thornapple, Jimsonweed, Jamestown weed
	Hyoscyamus: henbane
	Nicotinia: tobacco
	Solanum: nightshade, bittersweet, potato, egg plant
Taxaceae	*Taxus*: tâlâsa, yew
Thymelaeaceae	*Daphne*: gnidian berry, mezeron, laureola
	*Gnidia**: lasiosiphon
Umbelliferae	*Aethusa*: petite ciguë
	Cicuta: water hemlock
	Conium: poison hemlock
	Oenanthe: phellandrio, finocchio, aquatico, water fennel
Verbenaceae	*Duranta**: pigeon berry
	Lantana: lantana
Zamiaceae*	*Zamia**

a. From the Introduction to *CRC Handbook of Medicinal Plants* by James A. Duke. Plant families or genera **not** listed in Hartwell's *Plants Used Against Cancer* are denoted by an asterisk. Examples of common names for representative species are provided where readily obtainable. There are 103 entries, of which 77 appear in Hartwell's compilation.

triglochinin, and prunasin. In a table listing the HCN content of different Nigerian cassava varieties and their products, the HCN content in parts per million (ppm) ranged from 11 ppm up to 1250 ppm.

As to an anticancer agent, it is thought that the cyanide released from cyanogenic glucosides attacks cancer cells, which are characteristically low in the enzyme *rhodanese*. (Rhodanese, also known as thiosulfate sulfurtransferase, does not have the characteristic "-ase" suffix generally associated with enzymes.) Normal cells, which are high in rhodanese,* are presumably not affected, being capable of detoxifying the cyanide. The comment was made in the reference that this treatment has not been widely accepted in the medical profession.

The young seedlings of the sorghum species *Sorghum bicolor,* the traditional cereal crop for large parts of Africa, contain significant concentrations of *cyanogenic glycosides* (Larry G. Butler, in *Toxicants*, IV, p. 96). The mature plants contain diverse chemicals having phenolic hydroxyl groups, or polyphenols. Polyphenols are regarded as secondary metabolites in that they do not participate in the metabolic pathways of growth and reproduction. The roots exude quinones. These chemicals variously discourage herbivores, pathogens, and competitors.

The species *Sorghum vulgare* (of the family Gramineae) is listed in Hartwell as an anticancer agent. It is the most common of the sorghums, of which sweet sorghums, called sorgo's, are used to make molasses. Hartwell lists several species of wheat as anticancer agents. Wheat is of the genus *Triticum*, also of the family Gramineae. *Triticum vulgare* is the most common species, which exists as many subspecies or varieties.

2.8   PHENOLICS

Phenolics are a class of chemical compounds consisting mainly of benzene rings in various arrangements, with hydroxyl (OH) groups attached. They may be referred to as phenols, of which the very simplest is phenol itself, sometimes called carbolic acid, with the formula C_6H_5OH. (Phenolics as compounds are distinguished from phenolic resins, which are polymers formed by reacting a phenol with an acetaldehyde.) Phenolics have some very interesting properties and uses, as set forth in the volume *Toxicants of Plant Origin*, IV, edited by Peter R. Cheeke. Among the different kinds of phenolics are what are called simple phenolics, lignins, flavonoids, and tannins.

The phenolic called *gossypol* is a complex yellow substance found in cotton plants, which are of the genus *Gossypium*, hence the name (Mohamed B. Abou-Donia, in *Toxicants of Plant Origin*, IV, p. 2ff). It has a wide range of toxicological, pharmacological, physiological, and biochemical effects, including action against Chagas' disease, influenza, parainfluenza-3, and the herpes simplex virus (Abou-Donia, in *Toxicants*, pp. 6, 17). It is a general antifungal antibiotic and acts as an antibacterial and antitumor agent. In higher doses it becomes toxic, however, causing loss of appetite, weight loss, diarrhea, anemia, edema in the body cavities, degenerative changes in the liver and spleen, hemorrhaging in the liver, intestines and stomach, and other serious consequences.

Work has been conducted on the relationship of phenolics and cancer (George C. Fahey and Hans-Joachin G. Jung, in *Toxicants*, IV, pp. 154–156). *Simple phenolics found in foodstuffs correlate with a decreased risk for certain types of human cancer.* There are relatively large quantities of numerous phenolics which are ingested daily in a normal diet. These compounds have *antimutagenic and anti-carcinogenic properties,* accounting for the anticancer effects of vegetables. Examples of specific compounds producing anticancer activity in animals are derivatives of cinnamic acid, p-hydroxycinnamic acid, o-hydroxycinnamic acid, caffeic acid, and ferulic acid. These anticancer effects are associated with acting against chemical carcinogens.

In other mutagenic systems, gallic acid, chlorogenic acid, catechin, and tannic acid were found to be antimutagenic for nitrosation reactions. *The inhibitory effect of these phenolics was even greater than that for ascorbic acid, which has been used to prevent nitrosoamine formation* in vitro *and* in vivo.

In that phenolics have short half-lifetimes in the pure form and in food, if they are to be used as blocking agents for carcinogens, they should be consumed fresh. It is preferable that fruits or vegetables be used as the source, since the phenolics are present as protective glycosides.

---

* Rhodanese is an enzyme that catalyzes the conversion of cyanide and thiosulfate or thiosulfonate to thiocyanate and sulfate. The enzyme also occurs in animal tissues and bacteria. Inasmuch as thiosulfate or thiosulfonate is involved in the conversion, the presence of these sulfur compounds may be a necessary adjunct to the therapy as a way to protect normal cells.

Conversely, various *plant phenolics may have the capacity to be toxic at the gene level.* On the other hand, they may exert a beneficial effect in protecting against the generation of superoxide radicals and hydrogen peroxide, which can cause genetic changes. *The research continues toward a resolution of phenolic metabolism in the human body and for ways to increase the concentration of phenolics for anticarcinogenesis.*

The class of phenolic compounds called *lignins* have been shown to have *anticancer,* antiestrogenic, antibacterial, antifungal, and antiviral properties (Fahey and Jung, in *Toxicants,* IV, p. 157). Although effective *in vitro* and *in vivo* against animal tumors, their toxicity causes their use in humans to be limited.

> However, there are examples of lignins which are very nontoxic, such as nordihydroguaiaretic acid (NDGA),* used extensively as an antioxidant in human foods, but which still have antitumor activity, especially in combination with *ascorbic acid.*

Cytotoxic agents are found in any number of plants (D.K. Salunkhe, R.N. Adsule, and K.I. Bhonsle, in *Toxicants,* IV, pp. 69–70). A very few examples include vinblastine, derived from *Catharanthus roseus* (family Apocynaceae), which serves as a known anticancer agent for blood-related cancers. Colchicine and demecolcine are from *Colchicum autumnale* (family Liliaceae). Both are also classed as alkaloids, and the former is a suspected anticancer agent. The genus *Podophyllum* (family Berberidaceae) includes the *mandrake* or *May apple, P. peltatum,* and is widely distributed in the U.S. and Canada. The podophyllum of India, *P. emodi,* is found in Himalayan forests. The bioactive component called podophyllotoxin occurs in the roots and rhizomes of the species. *Podophyllotoxin is an anticancer agent, or at least a cancerostatic agent,* as has been known for some time (Fahey and Jung, in *Toxicants,* IV, p. 157). The compounds podophyllotoxin-β-benzylidine glycoside and podophyllic acid ethyl hydrazide have been tested clinically, as have two derivatives of these compounds. One derivative showed activity against Hodgkin's disease and non-Hodgkin's lymphomas, especially reticulum cell sarcoma. A degree of activity was also shown against bladder carcinoma and brain tumors.

With regard to *flavonoids,* there may be a connection with *ascorbic acid (vitamin C)* in that flavonoids may influence tissue concentrations of ascorbic acid in humans (Fahey and Jung, in *Toxicants,* IV, p. 159). This, in turn, may be related to *anticarcinogenic* action. In fact, flavonoids are found to have antimutagenic and anticarcinogenic effects and to be involved in all sorts of body processes, acting as a broad-spectrum defense system for diseases in both plants and animals (Fahey and Jung, in *Toxicants,* IV, pp. 165–166). Although toxicity has been observed *in vitro,* the *in vivo* tests on animals are mostly negative. The flavonoid *quercetin,* a known anticancer agent, has been found to be noncarcinogenic in itself, possibly due to the inhibition of tumor promoters. *Flavonoids are observed to act against the mutagenic activity of metabolites of certain compounds, evidently by preventing the initiation as well as promotion of chemical carcinogenesis.* Certain of the flavonoids called *flavones are noted to disturb the carcinogenic process,* indicating, for one thing, the importance of flavonoids in the diet. Several mechanisms have been proposed, one of which is the interaction of flavones with DNA.

Although the primary physiological activity of *tannins* is their protein-binding properties, which may have adverse effects, there may also be beneficial consequences (Fahey and Jung, in *Toxicants,* IV, pp. 166–170). These beneficial consequences, curiously, may involve DNA- or DNA-breaking activity. That is, tannins can be chemically associated with such antitumor agents as pyrocatechol, catecholamines, and lignins, which also exhibit DNA- or RNA-breaking activity. On the other hand, such DNA breakage can be associated with carcinogenesis, mutation, or virogenesis. Although single-stranded DNA breaks caused by, say, epinephrine are easily repaired, double-stranded breaks are not so easily repaired and can lead to change in cell function. Another variable is that of whether the breaks further occur in cancerous cells or normal cells, or both.

2.9 FLAVONOIDS

Additional information on flavonoids is presented in a chapter in *Naturally Occurring Carcinogens of Plant Origin,* edited by Iwao Hirona. Although some information items are contradictory, most support the following statements on the subject.

---

* It may be emphasized that NDGA is a component of chaparral or creosote bush.

Flavonoids are regarded as a group of secondary metabolites which have a particular sort of common chemical structure (S. Natori and I. Ueno, in *Naturally Occurring Carcinogens*, p. 53ff). The common structure is that of 1,3-dphenylpropane, with other structures attached. For the record, modifications lead to such compounds or compound types, or subclasses, as phenyalanine, cinnamic acid, chalcones, flavanones, flavanonols, flavones, flavonols, isoflavones, pterocarpans, rotenoids, leucoanthocyanidins, catechins, and anthocyanidins. Further modifications lead to what are called biflavonyls, neoflavones, and non-hydrolizable tannins. The reference provides illustrative examples. Two of the more interesting flavonoid compounds are said to be *quercetin* and *rutin*.

The term *bioflavonoid* is used in a special sort of way to connote flavonoids that have biological activity in mammals. In particular, bioflavonoids are flavonoids with favorable bioactivity in humans. This includes reducing and chelating properties and the beneficial effect on minute blood vessels or capillaries. Bioflavonoids are obtained commercially from citrus fruits, notably from the pulp and inner peel. Such citrus sources include concentrates from fresh lemons, oranges, grapefruits, limes, and tangerines. Bioflavonoids are not ordinarily considered to have direct nutritional functions but rather are supportive, as of vitamin C activity. A vitamin supplement for instance will list a citrus bioflavonoid complex and the flavorones hespiridin, eriocitrin, and naringen and naringenin, plus flavonols and flavones. Rutin is accorded a special category. Quercetin may also be obtained in nutritional supplements, and presumably by the definition, can also be regarded a flavonoid.

Flavonoids occur in the edible parts of food plants. For instance, quercetin glycosides exist in stone and berry fruits, and flavonol glycosides are found in the potato, asparagus, carrot, onion, radish, beet, and cabbage. Another study on onion, lettuce, kale, chive, garlic, leek, horseradish, radish, and red cabbage found that lettuce had the highest concentrations of quercetin.

Flavonoids are not acutely toxic to mammals, having no known toxic effects per se on either humans or animals. They play an important role in insect pollination, in part due to the coloration provided by some of the flavonoid chemical types, and some have a bitter taste, which may act as a repellent. They are noted to play an important role as ecochemicals.

An unexpected finding about flavonoids, however, is that they may produce *mutagenicity*. Quercetin is probably the most reactive. Of further note is the fact that *most chemical carcinogens are mutagenic.*

In mammalian tests on albino rats using quercetin, it was first concluded that flavonoids were neither toxic nor carcinogenic. Subsequent tests challenged this conclusion, but more recent tests again conclude that *such flavonoids as quercetin and rutin are not carcinogenic.* In fact, tests indicate that *quercetin suppresses certain kinds of cancer.* For instance, quercetin serves as an inhibitor for lipoxygenase, an enzyme involved in a particular kind of cancer.

Flavonoids have been proposed as vitamins under the category of vitamin P (Natori and Ueno, in *Naturally Occurring Carcinogens*, p. 62). For instance, it was once observed that the extracts of red pepper and lemon juice had beneficial effects on the circulatory system. These early studies have been followed by many more, and some of the more recent findings about pharmacological activities of flavonoids include the following effects: a vitamin C-sparing effect; an epinephrine-sparing effect; an anti-inflammatory effect; an antianaphylactic effect; an antiallergic effect; an antiasthmatic effect; coronary vasolidation; an antibacterial effect; an antiviral effect; an anti-X-ray effect; an *antineoplastic effect;* an antimutagenic effect, and, conversely, a mutagenic effect.

Interestingly, flavonoids are reported to have both an *antimutagenic effect* and a *pro-mutagenic effect,* as indicated above. Of more interest is that flavonoids are reported, as per the foregoing, to have an *antineoplastic effect,* that is, an anticancer effect. Moreover, there is also an anti-X-ray effect, which may be of value in the treatment of cancer by radiation. Finally, there are the antibacterial and antiviral effects, listed above.

Flavonoids have an inhibiting action on various enzymes, a matter to be discussed subsequently for a few particular enzymes. The reference includes a table of enzymes which are inhibited by flavonoids, listed as follows: aldose reductase, aldehyde reductase, ATPases, cAMP- and cGMP-phosphodiesterases, prostaglandin cyclooxygenase, prostaglandin and soybean lipoxygenases, monooxygenase, NADHP-oxidase, virus *reverse transcriptase,* and RNA polymerase. (Reverse transcriptase is the distinguishing enzyme for retroviruses—e.g., HIV as causing AIDS, and the Marburg and Ebola viruses—and which are also suspect in oncogenesis or carcinogenesis.) These inhibiting effects extend to some of the reactions and enzymes involved in glycolysis, a matter to be further mentioned.

Flavonoids are observed to *chelate* with copper and other metal ions, which may be of value in eliminating *heavy metals* from the body system. It is noted in the reference that flavonoids such as rutin and quercetin enhance the biological activity of vitamin C, possibly by chelating with copper ion, since trace amounts of copper ion catalyze the oxidation of vitamin C. It is also commented that *quercetin mutagenicity is inhibited by metallic compounds* such as $MnCl_2$, $CuCl_2$, $FeSO_4$, and $FeCl_3$, so there may be a synergistic connection between flavonoids and metals.

Flavonoids are potentially reactive with active oxygen species. For instance, the lipid antioxidative properties of quercetin and other flavonoids have long been known. In short, quercetin and other flavonoids serve as antioxidants. (Note: Quercetin is a component of chaparral or creosote bush, as is NDGA. The latter is an established antioxidant, and so, evidently, is quercetin.) In particular, flavonoids react with superoxide radicals (Natori and Ueno, in *Naturally Occurring Carcinogens*, p. 65). Quercetin is observed to react with oxygen and various oxygen-active species to produce carbon monoxide as an end product. This oxygen-reactivity characteristic may be the main reason for the diverse biological activities of flavonoids.

Quercetin has been found to be an inhibitor for certain enzymes (e.g., for the glycolysis sequence). The reference singles out aldose reductase and aldehyde reductase. The former is connected with the complications of diabetes, such as cataracts, neuropathy, and angiopathy. Thus, for example, *certain flavonoids inhibit lens aldose reductase, which delays the onset of cataracts.*

Axillarin and three other flavonoids have been investigated for the effect on adenine-nucleotide-requiring enzymes, including hexokinase, pyruvate kinase, *lactate dehydrogenase,* and glucose-6-phosphate dehydrogenase (Natori and Ueno, in *Naturally Occurring Carcinogens*, p. 67). (These enzymes are variously involved in glycolysis.) Also tested were the effects on glutathione reductase, alcohol dehydrogenase, and aldehyde reductase. Of these, only aldehyde reductase was significantly inhibited by the particular flavonoids used. Alcohol dehydrogenase and aldehyde reductase are enzyme-catalysts involved in the conversion back and forth between alcohols, aldehydes, and organic acids in the liver.

It was found in still other tests that the flavonoids quercetin, morin, quercitrin, rutin, 7-hydroxy-ethylquercetin, and three hydroxyethyl derivatives of rutin, all strongly inhibited aldehyde reductase, although in varying degrees (Natori and Ueno, in *Naturally Occurring Carcinogens*, p. 68). Indications are that quercetin and morin would be particularly effective as anticonvulsant medications.

The high aerobic glycolysis in certain tumor cells was found to be suppressed by the flavonoids quercetin, morin, fisetin, and apigenin (Natori and Ueno, in *Naturally Occurring Carcinogens*, p. 68). On the other hand, the flavonoids kaempferol, rutin, and quercitrin did not act in this manner. (It has been noted in Part 1 that cancer cells have been found to have a high *anaerobic* glycolysis rate, as per the initial work of Otto Warburg, although a much lower rate of aerobic glycolysis may also be involved.)

Flavonoids such as quercetin were noted to inhibit the enzymes Na^+K^+-ATPase and mitochondrial ATPase, but without affecting ion transport or oxidative phosphorylation. In normal cells, the ion flux pathways through cell membranes couple with the ATPase of the membranes. In some tumor cell lines, uncoupling occurs, which causes a high ATP (adenosine triphosphate) consumption, yielding a high concentration of ADP (adenosine diphosphate). The high concentration of ADP has the effect of supporting a high rate of glycolysis.

Quercetin, however, restores the ATPase enzyme activity and suppresses high rates of glycolysis. Quercetin also suppresses lactate transport, especially the excretion of lactate from the tumor cells. As the lactate accumulates, intracellular acidification increases, which also acts against the high glycolysis rate of tumor cells. Bioflavonoids with four or five hydroxy groups in their molecular structure are probably the most effective inhibitors. Another matter of a technical nature, the effectiveness is said to be lessened by the reduction (hydrogenation) of the 2,3-double bond, and glycosidation of the 3-hydroxy group. In further experimental studies on the inhibiting effects of quercetin, it was found to bind irreversibly to the Na^+K^+-ATPase enzyme, which interferes with the action of the enzyme. In the tricarboxylic acid cycle, the reactions involving the ATP-dependent reduction of NAD^+ by succinate is evidently inhibited by quercetin (for the carboxylic acid cycle, consult Part 1 and Fig. 1.4). In comment, this would presumably slow down the aerobic glycolysis of cancer cells. Flavonoids were also noted to inhibit ATPases, however, which is contrary to the effect found for the particular flavonoid quercetin.

Quercetin has been observed to increase the cAMP (adenosine-3',5'-cyclic phosphate) level in certain tumor cells, which may due to the inhibitory action of quercetin on the enzyme cAMP phosphodiesterase, which regulates the cAMP level (Natori and Ueno, in *Naturally Occurring Carcinogens*, p. 69). This presumably works against cancer cell metabolism. The reference furnishes a table listing the inhibitory effects of various flavonoids and related compounds on several enzymes. Quercetin is particularly effective as an inhibitor for the prostaglandin enzymes cyclooxygenase and lipoxygenase, which are involved in lipid or fatty acid metabolism.

In net sum, based in part on the above technical considerations, *it can be concluded that quercetin is an anticancer agent,* a conclusion also reached in other quarters.

2.10 PROTEINS AND AMINO ACIDS

The toxic effect of certain plant proteins and amino acids is related to their role as enzyme inhibitors, notably for the digestive enzymes called *proteinases* or *proteases*. Some of these aspects are explored in *Toxicants of Plant Origin*, III, edited by Peter R. Cheeke. In fact, a major role is in acting as plant proteinase inhibitors, or *protease inhibitors,* which may constitute a defense mechanism against herbivory (J. Xavier-Filho and F.A.P. Campos, in *Toxicants*, III, p. 2). In other words, if the plant is indigestible, grazing animals will avoid it. Our purposes are more specific, however, in that protease inhibitors have been proposed as a treatment for AIDS, and since cancer is sometimes also called an immunodeficiency disease, there may be a connection here as well. We further pursue the subject as follows.

Protease or proteinase inhibitors are found everywhere: in bacteria species and in animals, in fungi such as yeasts, in algae, and in various plant parts, the seeds, fruits, tubers, roots, bulbs, leaves, or stems (Xavier-Filho and Campos, in *Toxicants*, III, p. 2ff). Of the assorted plant families, protease inhibitors are found in species or genera of Leguminosae and Gramineae, and Cucurbitaceae; also in Anonaceae, Apocynaceae, Buxaceae, Compositae, Cruciferae, Euphorbiaceae, Fagaceae, Lauraceae, Moraceae, Rosaceae, Trapaceae, and Vitaceae. They are also found in Solanaceae, as well as in Alismataceae or Alismaceae, Amarantaceae, Cyperaceae, Liliaceae, Marantaceae, Musaceae, Nyctaginaceae, Ranuncal-aceae, and Zingiberaceae; plus Amarillidaceae, Araceae, and Iridaceae; and Chenopodiaceae and Pinaceae. It is a who's who of plant families represented in Hartwell.

The inhibitors show a strong association of the competitive type with the corresponding enzymes and abolish all enzyme activity. Of the several types of inhibitors, there are serine proteinase inhibitors, sulfhydril proteinase inhibitors, acid proteinase inhibitors, and metalloproteinase inhibitors. Of the four, serine proteinase inhibitors have been studied the most. In a particular study, it was shown that *tumors induced in potato and tomato plants do not accumulate the inhibitor* (Xavier-Filho and Campos, in *Toxicants*, III, p. 10). Another phenomenon observed was that *new inhibitor forms occur* (Xavier-Filho and Campos, in *Toxicants*, III, p. 11).

The biological role of proteinase inhibitors in plants apparently involves the control of proteolytic activity in plant tissues (Xavier-Filho and Campos, in *Toxicants*, III, p. 12ff). Not only are the inhibitors a defense against herbivores, but they protect against unwanted proteolysis. Thus, seeds for instance have an extraordinary high concentration of inhibitors. For this reason, the digestion of raw seeds such as soybeans can lead to trouble, even depressing the growth rate. The ingestion of methionine or cysteine is noted to counter the effects. Heat treatment also renders the inhibitors inactive.

These brief things said, there is the question of whether proteolysis or protein digestion can be related to cancer occurrence and growth. And by regulating protein digestion or ingestion by consuming proteinase or protease enzyme inhibitors, can this in turn act against cancer? After all, there is a piece of folklore that says to starve a cancer—not to mention that the plant families listed in Hartwell contain proteinase inhibitors. It may be one more reason why eating plants, vegetables, or fruits may guard against cancer.

The subject of *lectins* is taken up in a succeeding chapter of *Toxicants of Plant Origin*, III. Lectins are defined as proteins or glycoproteins of nonimmune origin (A. Pusztal, in *Toxicants*, III, p. 30ff). They act to agglutinate cells and to precipitate similar compounds called *glyconjugates*. The definition may be extended to include monovalent sugar-binding proteins, notably the highly toxic compounds *ricin* and *abrin*. Accordingly, a more comprehensive definition is that "lectins are proteins of nonimmu-noglobulin nature of specific recognition and reversible binding to carbohydrate moieties of complex carbohydrates without altering the covalent structure of any of the recognized glycosol ligands." It is further stated that lectins occur in virtually all taxonomic groups of the plant kingdom, and particularly in the family Leguminoseae or Leguminosae, but also in Graminaceae or Gramineae. Seeds are the richest source, but lectins are also found in other plant parts.

Parenthetically, *immunogloblulins* are connected to the role of *antibodies* (Richard M. Schultz, in *Textbook of Biochemistry*, p. 107); antibody molecules are defined as immunoglobulins produced by an organism (e.g., the human body system) in its response to an invasion by foreign compounds or molecules. These foreign compounds may, for example, be proteins, carbohydrates, or nucleic acid polymers. The antibody molecules associate with the foreign compound or substance, starting a process that results in the elimination of the foreign substance from the organism. The materials or foreign compounds that initiate the antibody production are called *antigens,* which in turn may contain regions called *antigenic determinants,* which are the specific sources of activity. In the case of a protein antigen, for instance, there may be only a few amino acids out of the total protein molecule to which the antibody molecules bind. Further information about the antibody structure is provided in the reference. Suffice to say here, antibody molecules are composed of units of four polypeptide chains of amino acids and thus in themselves can be classed as proteins.

Lectins act to agglutinate erythrocytic cells of various origins. Some are nonspecific; others may work on only specific animal species or blood groups. Among the more recognizable is soybean lectin, or soyabean lectin, taken as a supplemental protein source. Another is wheat germ lectin.

In further explanation, *blood cells can be divided into reticulocytes, erythrocytes, leukocytes, and platelets* (John F. Van Pilsum, in *Textbook of Biochemistry*, pp 1056–1058). Reticulocytes are the immature red blood cells, which mature to form the erythrocytes. The erythrocytes carry hemoglobin and are fueled by glucose, which is metabolized by glycolysis. The leukocytes possess the enzymes involved variously in the hexose monophosphate shunt, glycolysis, the tricarboxylic acid cycle, and respiration. Their primary purpose is phagocytosis, the engulfing and destruction of particulate matter. It is an energy-intensive process, requiring an increased glycolysis rate and a great increase in the metabolism of glucose by the hexose monophosphate shunt. The role of the hexose monophosphate shunt is the production of *hydrogen peroxide*, H_2O_2, from *superoxide*, O_2^-, which is a necessary reactant in phagocytosis. (Hydrogen peroxide, or peroxide, is sometimes considered an anticancer agent.) The leukocytes carry large amounts of glycogen, which becomes the energy source in the absence of glucose. The platelets consist of about 50 percent protein and contain substances required for blood clotting. They contain a contractile protein similar to muscle actomyosin plus ATP (adenosine triphosphate). The principal energy source is from the glycolysis of glucose.

With regard to the functioning of platelets, under aerobic conditions there is a formation of ATP during glycolysis. Under anaerobic conditions, there is an increase in the rate of glucose utilization and lactate production. *Inasmuch as cancer cells exhibit anaerobic glycolysis, producing lactate, there may be a connection between blood platelet activity and cancer, with both related to anaerobic glycolysis.* The destruction of blood platelets during chemotherapy—not to mention the other blood cells—hardly seems a way to resolve the issue.

A type of lectin studied extensively is that from *Phaseolus vulgaris* (PHA), the common kidney bean (Pusztal, in *Toxicants*, III, p. 42ff). Among other effects, on rats at least, there is an accelerated rate of tissue catabolism (Pusztal, in *Toxicants*, III, p. 51).

It is observed that lectins can distinguish different cell types by sugar specificity (Pusztal, in *Toxicants*, III, p. 37). Thus, they may play a role in fighting off pathogenic organisms. There is support for the idea that lectins provide a protective effect against pathogenic fungi and bacteria.

The ricin type of toxic proteins are of common occurrence in plants (Pusztal, in *Toxicants*, III, pp. 59–60). Since they inactivate eukaryotic cell ribosomes, they are called ribosome-inactivating proteins. Ricin and similar compounds, namely abrin, modeccin, volkensin, and viscumin, have the general structure A-B where A is the toxic subunit and B is the lectin subunit. This type of toxin displays a galactose-specific binding to cell surface receptors and as such will show selectivity toward cells that have these receptors. The thought has emerged that transformed cells have different receptors than the original or normal cells. *This gives hope for selectively killing cancer cells (the magic bullet).* However, the great toxicity of ricin, for example, and its modest selectivity, have ruled it out as a practical anticancer agent. *Further modifications, however, have created new toxins that can be rigorously targeted for specific cells, notably cancer cells.*

A perfunctory search of MEDLINE indicates that modeccin acts to inhibit cellular protein synthesis, as does such other toxic proteins as ricin, abrin, and diphtheria toxin—not to mention conventional chemotherapy drugs, notably 5-FU. That is, these toxic proteins act as enzyme inhibitors for the synthesis of cellular protein. Furthermore, there is the indication that AZT, a drug used in the treatment of AIDS, and less well known as 3'-azido-3'-deoxythymidine, counteracts this protein-inhibiting effect. What role this might play as a control or mediator in cancer chemotherapy remains to be seen. Moreover, there may be a connecting role in AIDS therapy, since both cancer and AIDS are referred to as immunodeficiency diseases and may have similar causes and effects. Furthermore, volkensin is being tried against Alzheimer's disease, and viscumin is being tried against hybridoma cells. The latter are somatic cells—e.g., of the nature of organ and tissue cells—formed from the fusion of normal lymphocytes and tumor cells.

The particular plant or organism sources for modeccin, volkensin, and viscumin were left unstated. Albeit ricin is from *Ricinus communis* of the plant family Euphorbiaceae, and abrin is from *Abrus precatorius* of the family Leguminosae. While the former three are not listed, both the latter two are listed in the *Merck Index*.

So, once again, there are compounds ubiquitous to plants that can act against cancer. No doubt many things are going on at once that, with all the interactions, are probably too complicated ever to be analyzed and described fully. We will settle for a cancer cure, however, no matter how arrived at and how explained.

2.11   ALKALOIDS

Alkaloids may be defined as plant substances that exert powerful physiological and/or psychological effects. Further amplification is furnished in Part 4, particularly as directed against cancer.

Some well known examples of alkaloids are morphine, strychnine, quinine, ephedrine, nicotine, and caffeine. Alkaloids have been used variously in medicines, potions, teas, poultices and poisons for thousands of years, but their introduction into formal medical practice was compromised by their potency and variable toxicity (Cordell, *Alkaloids*, pp. 1–2). Some of the first plants used included aconite, colchicum, stramonium, henbane, and belladonna. A popular medicine for centuries, the analgesic and narcotic properties of opium were well known, so it was the most likely medicinal candidate for the emerging science of chemistry. Accordingly, the first such chemical studies were directed at opium, circa 1800, from which morphine was isolated. In the years following, the compounds strychnine, emetine, brucine, piperine, caffeine, quinine, cinchonine, and colchicine constituted the first generation of alkaloids isolated.

Most alkaloids are nitrogen-heterocyclic compounds and are classified by the ring structure, a listing including, for instance, pyridine, isoquinoline, indole, and pyrrolizidine alkaloids (S. Natori, in *Naturally Occurring Carcinogens*, p. 223). Most exhibit a variety of biological actions and have been widely used in medicines, e.g., morphine and strychnine. Although some are acutely toxic, only those which have the *pyrrolizidine* ring are known to be carcinogenic.

The list of alkaloids discovered or uncovered continues to grow, as embodied in the monograph series *Alkaloids*, and now numbers in the thousands. The alkaloids are therefore many and varied, appearing in unexpected places—and yet not so unexpected, considering that alkaloids are ubiquitous in flowering plants. The alkaloid coniine, which is related to pyridine, was the first to be characterized and synthesized (Cordell, *Alkaloids*, p. 2–3). It is obtained from the poison hemlock plant *Conium maculatum*.*

Other alkaloids are present in common wildflowers. One illustrative example from the many is lobeline, from the ornamental flowers of the genus *Lobelia*, of the family Campanulaceae, listed in Hartwell's *Plants Used Against Cancer*. The simplest quinolizidine alkaloid is lupinine, first isolated from a species of lupine in 1835 (Cordell, *Alkaloids*, p. 154). Lupines are of the genus *Lupinus* (of the family Leguminosae or Fabaceae). Members of the Leguminosae in fact contain a significant number of alkaloids, as noted in the reference—and the garden variety of pea itself is not above suspicion, nor are peanuts. Larkspur or delphinium is of the genus *Delphinium* (of the family Ranunculaceae), and contains delphinine. The coneflowers of the genus *Echinaceae* (of the family Compositae or Heliantheae or Asteraceae, or Sunflower family, or Aster family, and so on) evidently contain echinulin, related to

---

* Species of the genus *Conium*, of the family Umbelliferae, are well represented with numerous entries in Hartwell's *Plants Used Against Cancer*. Species of the genus *Cicuta* from the same family are also listed, including *Cicuta maculata* and *Cicuta virosa*, better known as water hemlock. *Conium* is evidently from the Old World, and *Cicuta* from the New. In any event, species from both genera have been tried against cancer, at least according to medical folklore. Another related species from the same plant family, the wild carrot or *Daucus carota* L., is equally poisonous and has extensive listings in Hartwell. (The wild carrot is to be distinguished from the domesticated garden variety, named *Daucus carota sativa*. The latter is also listed in Hartwell.) Some authorities, incidentally, put these genera and species in the family Apiaceae, or Parsley family.

the indole alkaloids (Cordell, *Alkaloids*, p. 846). The ubiquitous silvery and purplish locoweeds or crazyweeds found in parts of the American West are of the genus *Oxytropis* (also of the family Leguminosae or Fabaceae). Locoweeds are fairly loaded with alkaloids.*

A feature of alkaloids is their amine-like nature, which involves nitrogen in ring structures of all sorts of complexities. They are basic or alkaline compared to acids, hence the name employed. The compositional makeup is of carbon, hydrogen, nitrogen, and oxygen, although other stray elements or atoms may show up, such as sulfur or even chlorine or bromine. Several purposes or functions have been assigned for alkaloids, one of the more interesting being that alkaloid concentrations increase as seeds are formed.

The main source of alkaloids has always been flowering plants, also called the angiosperms, the plants that produce seeds inside an ovary or covering. More recently, occurrences have been found in animals, insects, marine organisms, microorganisms, and the lower plants (Cordell, *Introduction to Alkaloids*, p. 2ff). For example, the alkaloid muscopryridine has been found in the musk deer and castoramine has been obtained form the beaver *Castor canadensis*. A derivative of pyrrole occurs as a sex pheromone in several insects. Saxitoxin is the neurotoxic component of red tide (*Gonaulax catenella*). Pyocananine is found in the bacterium *Pseudomonas aeroginosa*, chanoclavine I in the ergot fungus *Claviceps purpurea*, and lycopodine in the club moss genus *Lycopodium*.

It has been observed that certain groups or chemical classes of alkaloids are found in particular families or genera of plants. Although over 40 percent of all plant families have at least one plant with alkaloids, of the total of more than 10,000 genera, only about 8.7 percent are known to possess alkaloids. (The figure would come to about 870 genera.) The most important alkaloid-bearing families are the Liliaceae, Amaryllidaceae, Compositae, Ranunculaceae, Menispermaceae, Lauraceae, Papaveraceae, Leguminosae, Rutaceae, Loganiaceae, Apocynaceae, Solanaceae, and Rubiaceae. Interestingly, all the genera and species in the family Papaveraceae or Poppy family contain alkaloids, though such is not the case with the other plant families.

All 13 of the aforementioned plant families are represented in Jonathan Hartwell's *Plants Used Against Cancer*. Whether this indicates some sort of correlation is not known, but it can be speculated. All told, Hartwell's compilation contains species from 177 plant families and approximately 1500 genera of about 3000 species. The approximately 1500 genera is about twice as large as the total number of genera which contain alkaloid-bearing species.

The Papaveraceae contain such plants as different species of *poppy*, and in particular, *bloodroot* or *Sanguinaria canadensis*.

Some simple alkaloids such as *nicotine* will occur in plants from different families. More complicated alkaloids such as vindoline or *morphine* will be found in only a single species or a single genus.

The alkaloid content tends to be localized within a plant. Thus, *reserpine* concentrates in the roots of *Rauvolfia*, and *quinine* occurs in the bark but not the leaves of *Cinchona ledgeriana*. Morphine is found in the latex of *Papaver somniferum*. Although the alkaloid concentrates in a particular part of a plant, it may be generated elsewhere. Thus, the alkaloids in *Datura* and *Nicotiana* are formed in the roots but are relocated in the leaves.

The alkaloid concentrations may vary widely between different plant species. For example, *reserpine* may be up to one percent in the roots of *Rauvolfia serpentina*, whereas the leaves of *Catharanthus roseus* may contain *vincristine* to the extent of only 4×10^{-6} percent.

The seeds of alkaloid-containing plants such as *Nicotiana*, *Papaver sominiferum*, and *Catharanthus roseus* may contain little or none of the alkaloid. But the seedlings will start producing alkaloids within a short time after germination.†

The reference groups alkaloids into the following classifications: true alkaloids, protoalkaloids, and pseudoalkaloids. All are usually basic but otherwise differ in their chemical or structural makeup. The true alkaloids are derived from amino acids, albeit they are usually basic and will normally contain nitrogen in a heterocyclic ring. The protoalkaloids are relatively simple amines in which the amino acid

---

* The genus *Lupinus* makes Hartwell, as does *Delphinium*. So does *Echinaceae*, considered an herbal anticancer agent and general all-around tonic. *Oxytropis*, however, does not make the list, but other locoweeds of the genus *Astragalus*, of the family Leguminosae, are listed in Hartwell.

† As per the above, the genera *Cinchona*, *Papaver*, *Datura*, and *Nicotinia* are listed in Hartwell's *Plants Used Against Cancer*. *Rauvalfia*, however, is not listed.

nitrogen does not occur in a heterocyclic ring. Examples include mescaline, ephedrine, and N,N-dimethyltryptamine. The pseudoalkaloids are not derived from amino acids. They consist of the steroidal alkaloids such as conessine and the purines such as caffeine.

It may be oberved that, for pseudoalkaloids, there is a connection with mammalian body functions, at least in name. Thus, steroids are hormones, and purines are elemental to the nucleotides from which DNA is formed. No consistent naming system for alkaloids is possible, given the diversity. About the only commonality is in that the names usually end in the prefix "-ine," but not always—and of course so do some other classes of compounds, such as amines per se.

The common name for an alkaloid may be based on the genus name, such as *atropine* from *Atropa belladonna*, or on the species name, such as *cocaine* from *Erythroxylon coca*. Or it may be based on the common name for the drug, such as ergotamine from ergot, or on the physiological action, such as emetine, which is an emetic. The alkaloid pelletierine is named after a famous chemist. (The genus *Atropa* is listed in Hartwell, as is *Erythroxylon* or *Erythroxylum*.)

2.11.1   THE FUNCTIONS OF ALKALOIDS

Perhaps the main purpose of alkaloids relates to the transmission of chemical signals (D. Schlee, in *Biochemistry of Alkaloids*, p. 57ff). In this way, compounds such as alkaloids protect the organism against predators, competitors, or pathogens. This could account for the diversity of alkaloid structures, the location within the organism, and the rapidity of translocation and transmission. There are, for instance, such matters as allelopathic effects, whereby one species may affect another species, which may involve alkaloids. A few examples are as follows.

Alkaloids may play a role in *pigments,* in addition say to the pigments formed by carotenoids and flavonoids in flower petals. Thus, the yellow, brown, or red pigments called pteridines, are found in the wing scales of butterflies, and the red and yellow pigments called betalains are found in certain flowers.

Alkaloids play a role in plant defense due to their irritant, toxic, and/or unpalatable qualities. While some act as repellents, others may act as attractants. Some insects and animals have special detoxification mechanisms, allowing them to feed where others cannot. The reference states that nearly every type of toxin may serve as a feeding stimulant for a particular insect. Thus, the alkaloid *sparteine* serves as a feeding stimulant for the broom aphid.

The cactus and fruit fly have an unusual synergism, which involves both stimulants and repellents. The attractant is a sterol (in *Senita cactus schottenol*) and the fruit fly uses it to synthesize its molting hormone. Conversely, alkaloids repel some species of the insect genus *Drosophila*. That is, the Senita cactus contains the alkaloids *lophocereine* and *pilocereine*, which act as repellants. In the Saguaro cactus, the alkaloid *carnegeine* acts as a repellent.

Solanine, the main alkaloid in the *potato,* may act as a beetle repellent, as may tomatine, the major alkaloid of the tomato. These steroid alkaloids presumably affect steroid biosynthesis in the beetle. In all 26 species of Amaryllidaceae, the alkaloid *lycorine* will repel locusts.

It is known that about 2000 plant species contain natural insecticides, sometimes in combination with repellent effects. *Nicotine* and *anabasine* are both powerful repellants.

Plant alkaloids also may repel grazing animals. Thus, *Senecio jacobaea* of the family Compositae contains the alkaloid *pyrrolizideine*, and sheep and cattle pass it by. *The common name is ragwort or St. James-wort, and it is listed in Hartwell as an anticancer agent.*

Legumes of the genera *Lupinus, Baptisia, Cytisus,* and *Genista* contain quinolizidine alkaloids and are to be left alone by herbivores. The grasses *Phalaris tuberosa* and *P. arundinacea* contain the deterrent alkaloids gramine and hordenine. The grasses *Lolium* and *Festuca* have the quinoline alkaloid *perloline,* and *Crotolaria spectrabilis* has the pyrrolizidine alkaloid *monocrotaline.*

Even animals use alkaloids for defense. Ants, for example, have an alkaloid similar to *coniine* of the hemlock. *The ant alkaloid solenopsin shows haemolytic, insecticidal, and antibiotic activity.*

Toxins may accumulate in small concentrations in the predators themselves and form a line of defense from other predators. The best known example is that for certain butterflies and moths of the order *Lepidoptera*. Other examples are provided in the reference, for instance the relationship between *Senecio vulgaris* (groundsel) and *S. jacobaea* (ragwort) and the tiger moth and the cinnabar moth. Both of the aforementioned plant species, incidentally, are listed in Hartwell as anticancer agents and are members of the family Compositae. There is evidence that alkaloids from host plants provide sex *pheromones* to attract certain insects, long-distance. Other insects produce their own pheromones.

In addition to plant-animal and animal-animal relationships, alkaloids are involved in plant-plant relationships and the relationships between plants and microorganisms. Plant-plant relationships are categorized under *allelopathy*, an aspect of the competition between plants. Thus, phytotoxic (plant-toxic) substances may be released from a plant species by volatilization, by a washing of the surface, by exudation from the roots, and by plant litter. These substances inhibit the germination, growth, and yield not only of other species, but of different plants of the same species. *Berberine* is one such alkaloid, occurring in the roots of *Mahonia trifloliata*, protecting the plant from the fungus *Phymatotrichum omnivorme*. The alkaloids *hordatine* A and B from *Hordeum vulgare* (barley) furnish a protective function against *Helminthosporium sativum*. (These latter alkaloids are chemically related to *arginine*, an *anti-cancer agent*. Hordeum *or barley is listed in Hartwell as an anticancer agent*.)

While other defense substances such as polyphenols reduce the palatability of plant proteins, alkaloids are only needed in much lower concentrations. It is noted that alkaloids are biosynthesized from such precursors as *tryptophan* (or tryptophane) and *tyrosine*. Due to their toxicity, alkaloids are synthesized and stored in special cell compartments.

The detoxification of alkaloids is relatively easy. Methylation or conjugation with carbohydrates, amino acids, or proteins will serve.

There are seasonal and diurnal, even hourly, variations in the concentrations of alkaloids in an organism. This may be very important in determining the full role of alkaloids as chemical signals.

There are some other side effects of alkaloids in plants. Thus, under environmental stress the cellular compartmentalization of the alkaloids may break down, leading to autotoxic effects. An example provided is that of the toxic indole alkaloid *gramine*, found in barley, which may be released internally under heat stress.

Finally, it should be emphasized that in the human body *alkaloids serve as neurotransmitters*, a subject discussed more fully in Part 4 (Cordell, *Alkaloids*, p. 21; Voet and Voet, *Biochemistry*, p. 1261ff).

2.11.2 TOXICITY AND CANCER

There have been conflicting reports about the effect of alkaloid-bearing plants on cancer. A prime suspect is common comfrey, *Symphatum officinale* (of the plant family Boraginaceae), which is used as an herbal treatment for all sorts of ailments, including cancer. Thus, in John Heinerman's book *Healing Animals with Herbs*, there is a description of a farm animal that cured itself of a tumorous condition around the mouth by grazing a patch of comfrey. Hartwell's compendium lists *Symphatum officinale* as a folklore treatment against various cancers. It so turns out, however, that comfrey contains pyrrolizidine alkaloids or PAs (Ryan J. Huxtable, in *Toxicants of Plant Origin*, I, p. 58). Moreover, comfrey has been found to be carcinogenic to rats, the roots being more toxic than the leaves, causing liver and bladder tumors. The general advice is: don't take anything containing comfrey (Huxtable, in *Toxicants*, I, p. 78).

Many pyrrolizidine alkaloids have been found to be carcinogenic, including alkaloids from the several genera *Senecio, Heliotropium, Amsinckia, Petasites, Tussilago, Crotalaria*, and *Symphytum* (Huxtable, *Toxicants*, I, pp. 49–50). These alkaloids may, in fact, be a primary cause of liver cancer in South Africa. The pyrrole metabolites of pyrrolizidines, which are formed in the liver, are said to be alkylating agents which affect RNA, DNA, and proteins. This may be the basis for their mutagenic activity. (Of course, such conventional chemotherapy drugs as 5-FU also affect RNA, DNA, and proteins.) For the record, Hartwell's *Plants Used Against Cancer* lists species from all the foregoing genera except *Amsinckia* and *Crotalaria*.

Other serious conditions may follow the use of pyrrolizidine alkaloids, termed PA diseases. Pyrrolizidine alkaloids are contained notably in the genus *Crotalaria* (of the family Leguminosae). Some tropical people routinely drink tea prepared from one or another of the species such as *C. fulva, C. incana*, and *C. longirostrata*. Over a sufficient period of time this produces a serious condition, called veno-occlusive disease of the liver (Huxtable, in *Toxicants*, pp. 46, 50).

The genus *Heliotropium* (of the family Boraginaceae) has about 20 species that contain pyrrolizidine alkaloids (Huxtable, in *Toxicants*, I, p. 61). These alkaloids have the same toxic action as *Crotalaria* alkaloids. Long known for producing an old-fashioned kind of fragrant flower, there have been numerous cases of poisoning due to contamination of grains with *Heliotropium* seeds.

Three species of the genus *Trichodesma* (of the family Boraginaceae), found in the tropics, contain hepatoxic PAs. And the well known genus *Senecio* of the family Compositae has well beyond 100 species that contain hepatotoxic PAs. A number of species are listed in Hartwell's compilation as anticancer agents, including *S. jacobaea* or ragwort, and *S. vulgaris* or groundsel. There have been numerous poisonings reported (Huxtable, in *Toxicants*, I, pp. 63–68). What has been said about PAs can no doubt be extended to other kinds of alkaloids

2.12 PLANT CARCINOGENS

Bioactive plants may display carcinogenic activity, as noted for plants containing alkaloids, for instance. Other plants and other classes of compounds are sometimes if not always carcinogenic. Some of this information has been presented in previous sections. Additional information is furnished in the volume *Naturally Occurring Carcinogens of Plant Origin* edited by Iwao Hirono, already cited.

This kind of information about carcinogenicity is of special interest in that it can also mean that the same plants and compounds are also potential anticancer agents. That is, what is toxic or carcinogenic at one dosage level can be anticarcinogenic at another dosage level. This paradox is found for many substances, as has been observed elsewhere in these pages. Plant bioactivity is the main criterion, and it is double edged.

The carcinogenic substances described in the above cited reference start off with a chapter on cycads and cycasin (I. Hirono, in *Naturally Occurring Carcinogens*, p. 3ff). Cycads are gymnospermous plants, intermediate between ferns and palms, or between ferns and flowering plants. (A gymnosperm is a plant having seeds not enclosed in an ovary or pod.) The genus is *Cycas* of the plant family Cicadaceae. Cycads are widely distributed in tropical and subtropical regions around the world, both north and south of the equator, with some species reaching into Florida and into Japan. On some tropical islands, cycads are used as a supplementary starchy food source, and cattle may forage on the plant—sometimes with unwanted results.

A toxic glucoside named cycasin is present in the seeds, trunks, and leaves and has been shown to induce tumors of the liver, kidney, and intestine. Most experiments were conducted on mice, but similar effects show up in rats, hamsters and guinea pigs, monkeys, and even fish. Washing ahead of time minimizes these effects. The cycasin is evidently hydrolyzed to another material, a compound formed from the aglycone, which along with its derivatives is carcinogenic. No statistics were provided on humans, and Hartwell does not list either the genus or the plant family The Hirono reference comments that as a result of studies on cytosin, it was found that *intestinal bacterial flora may play a role in carcinogenesis*. The subject of gut flora and cancer will be discussed in Part 6.

Pyrrolizidine alkaloids (PAs) have been previously discussed as to toxicity, particularly as pertains to the herb comfrey (Huxtable, in *Toxicants*, p. 41ff). It was noted that PAs are found in the following genera and plant families: *Senecio* of the family Compositae, *Heliotropium* of the family Boraginaceae, *Amsinckia* of the family Boraginaceae, *Petasites* of the family Compositae, *Tussilago* of the family Compositae, *Crotalaria* of the family Leguminosae, and *Symphytum* of the family Boraginaceae (Huxtable, in *Toxicants*, I, pp. 49–50). Furthermore, it is suggested that the high rate of primary liver cancer in South Africa may be due to low-level exposure to PAs. However, Hartwell's *Plants Used Against Cancer* lists species from all the foregoing genera except *Amsinckia* and *Crotalaria*.

Additional plant families and genera have been added to the PA list, with a more complete listing in Table 2.3 (T. Furuya, Y. Asada, and H. Mori, in *Naturally Occurring Carcinogens*, p. 25ff). Interestingly, every family listed appears in Hartwell, but not every genus. Still, there is an indication that genera and species that contain *pyrrolizidine alkaloids* have been used as anticancer agents. If so, the dosages and frequency are unknown or unstated.

The reference discusses the *hepatotoxicity of pyrrolizidine alkaloids* and notes that it depends on the species and age of the affected animal, the structure of the alkaloid, and the manner in which the alkaloid is ingested—which presumably extends to humans as well. The toxic effects most frequently occur in the liver. "A typical acute effect in the liver is massive centrilobular hemorrhagic necrosis." This involves the failure of *DNA-mediated RNA synthesis, protein synthesis,* and nucleolar segregation. These statements underscore the hazards of indiscriminate use of plant or herbal therapies. (It may be added, however, that such conventional cytotoxic chemotherapeutic agents as *5-fluorouracil* also attack DNA/RNA/protein synthesis.)

As to carcinogenicity, *Farfugium* is added to the list of cancer-causing genera, above. Species of *Petastites* are a common source of food in Japan but are nevertheless carcinogenic. The carcinogenicity of comfrey is discussed, noting that the roots are more active than the leaves. Carcinogenicity is attributed to at least eight pyrrolizidine alkaloids, including isatidine, retorsine, petasitenine, senkirkine, clivorine, monocrotaline, lasiocarpine, and symphytine. Among the many effects, veno-occlusive disease is another hazard, as has been previously mentioned. Further dangers listed are genotoxicity or mutagenicity.

Table 2.3 Plants Containing Pyrrolizidine Alkaloids[a]

Apocynaceae	*Alafia*, Anonendra*, Parsonia*, Urechtites**
Boraganaceae	*Amsinckia*, Anchusa, Asperugo*, Caccinia*, Cynoglossum, Echium, Ehretia*, Heliotropium, Lappula, Lindelofia*, Lithospermum, Macrotonia*, Messerschmidia*, Myosotis, Paracarum*, Paracynoglossum*, Rindera*, Solenthus*, Symphytum, Tournafortia, Trachelanthus*, Trichodesma*, Ulegbekia**
Celastraceae	*Bhesa**
Compositae	*Adenostyles*, Brachyglottis*, Cacalia*, Doronicum, Emilia, Erechtites*, Eupatorium, Farfugium*, Gynura, Kleinia*, Ligularia*, Petasites, Senecio, Syneilesis*, Tussilago*
Euphorbiaceae	*Phyllanthus, Securinega**
Gramineae	*Festuca, Lolium, Thelepogon**
Leguminosae	*Adenocarpus, Crotalaria, Cytisus**
Orchidaceae	*Chysis*, Doritis*, Hammarbya*, Kingiella*, Liparis, Malaxis*, Phalaenopsis*, Vanda, Vandopsis**
Ranunculaceae	*Caltha*
Rhizophoraceae	*Cassipourea**
Santalaceae	*Thesium*
Sapotaceae	*Mimusops, Planchonella**
Scrophulariaceae	*Castilleja*

a. From T. Furuya, Y. Asada and H. Mori in *Naturally Occurring Carcinogens of Plant Origin: Toxology, Pathology and Biochemistry*, edited by Iwao Hirono. Plant families or genera not appearing in Hartwell's *Plants Used Against Cancer* are denoted by an asterisk.

The *bracken fern, Pteridium aquilinum*, is a common plant in many parts of the world, and in Japan and some other countries it is used as human food (I. Hirono and K. Yamada, in *Naturally Occurring Carcinogens*, p. 87ff). Its toxic effects on livestock are well known, and it is also carcinogenic, not only to animals but to humans. It may, in fact, account for the high incidence of stomach cancer in Japan. Plant toxicity varies with location, and the active agent has been found to be transmitted in cow's milk.

The exact identity of the carcinogen has not definitely been established, although a number of different kinds of compounds have been isolated. The flavonoid quercetin has been a suspect, but the tests are inconsequential, as reported elsewhere (Hirono ad Yamada, in *Naturally Occurring Carcinogens*, p. 101). The glucoside ptaquiloside or PT is probably the most likely candidate.

Carrageenan, an extract from seaweed, in so many words is a sulfated polysaccharide containing various ammonium, calcium, magnesium, and sodium salts of the sulfate esters of galactose and 3,6-anhydroglactose copolymers (I. Hirono, in *Naturally Occurring Carcinogens*, p. 121ff). It is used in food products, cosmetics, pharmaceuticals as an agent to stabilize, emulsify, and thicken or gel. Its principal source is *Eucheuma spinosum*, which is treated with hydrochloric acid to yield the form iota-carrageenan. It is no doubt used in commercial ice cream, although by U.S. law, ice cream does not have to list its ingredients. Carrageenan has been noted to produce toxic effects in the gastrointestinal tract of test animals, including the appearance of intestinal lesions and *colon polyps*.

Carcinogenicity has been documented in animal studies using a form called degraded carrageenan, which produced a higher incidence of *colorectal cancer*. Subsequent tests indicated that degraded carrageenan did not produce genotoxicity, but rather it acts as a tumor promoter.

Although *hydrazines* and their derivatives, hydrazides and hydrazones, have long been known for their bioactivity, not until 1951 was a nitrogen-nitrogen bond found in nature (S. Natori, in *Naturally Occurring Carcinogens*, p. 127ff). A *toxic azoxy compound,* macrozamin, was discovered in the early 1960s, and since that time *more than 40 other compounds have been isolated from bacteria, from actinomycetes (bacterial parasites), and from fungi, mushrooms, and other plants.* Hydrazine itself has been detected in tobacco smoke, probably from the pyrolysis of nitrogen compounds in the tobacco. (Hydrazine sulfate, incidentally, is regarded as an anticancer agent, said to act as an enzyme inhibitor for the conversion of lactate to glycogen in the liver.)

The common cultivated mushroom *Agaricus bisporus* of the family Agaricaceae, eaten in large quantities, was later found to yield a glutamic acid derivative named *agaritine*. It was subsequently found in other mushroom species. Agaritine is an example of what are labeled *mushroom hydrazines* or *mushroom hydrazine derivatives*. Another example occurs in the false morel, *Gyromitra esculenta* of the family Helvellaceae, which must be pretreated by drying and boiling before it is safe to eat.

Mushroom hydrazines came under suspicion in 1962 when *hydrazine sulfate was found to induce lung cancer in mice*. This is most interesting, in that hydrazine sulfate is a proposed anticancer agent, as mentioned above. It serves as another illustration of the fact that some substances may be either carcinogenic or anticarcinogenic, depending upon dosage levels and other factors, known or unknown.

While agaritine itself has not proven carcinogenic, there is evidence that its metabolites or decomposition products are carcinogenic. Although agaritine can be destroyed by cooking, the metabolites are not. The reference notes that it has been proposed that human populations abandon mushroom consumption. More information about fungi will be provided in Part 5.

Safrole is one of many similar compounds that occur naturally in plants and in various vegetables, herbs, and spices (M. Enemoto, in *Naturally Occurring Carcinogens*, p. 139ff). For purposes of documentation, these compounds are classed as allylic and propenylic benzene-derivatives with ring methoxy and/or methylene dioxy substituents. Also called alkenylbenzenes, the natural and synthetic substances have been used as flavoring agents and for perfumes.

It has been long known that the ingestion of large amounts of sassafras oil will cause hepatic or liver toxicity in humans. Its carcinogenic properties were reported in 1960, and the use of safrole as an oil and food additive was banned in the U.S.

Sassafras oil contains about 80 percent safrole. Broadly defined, sassafras is any American tree of the genus *Sassafras*. In particular, it is the dried bark of the root of the species *Sassafras varifolium*, or of another species of the genus, which yields the aromatic oil called sassafras oil, or oil of sassafras. The genus is of the family Laureaceae or Laurel family. As may be anticipated, the genus and plant family are well represented in Hartwell.*

Safrole and its derivatives are relatively weak carcinogens, and no deaths apparently have resulted. The reference makes the comment, however, that low lifetime intakes could conceivably cause cancer in humans with predisposed genetic backgrounds. On the other hand, it could be commented the other way around—given the connection between substances that act both as carcinogens and anticarcinogens, depending on dosage levels, such a substance could act against cancer. This may be the role of common garden vegetables, for instance, as will be examined in Part 4.

A category previously discussed is that of tannin or tannins, also called *tannic acid*. Tannins are a large group of phenolic compounds originally used in the process of tanning, the conversion of animal hides to leather (M. Eneomoto, in *Naturally Occurring Carcinogens*, p. 161ff). Tannins are found in the wood, bark, fruit, twigs, leaves, and roots of many plants, most notably the oaks (genus *Quercus*), but also in eucalyptus, mangrove, hemlock, pine, willow, and even the sumac and palmetto. The vegetable tannins are further divided into hydrolyzable and nonhydrolyzable tannins. Tannic acid itself is also called gallotinic acid or gallotannin, no doubt due to its historic origins from oak gall, a swelling of the plant tissues caused by parasites.

Tannins produce an astringent action on taste and adversely affect the liver, even when applied topically for burns. There has apparently been no evidence of carcinogenicity, however. Hartwell has numerous entries for the genus *Quercus* of the family Fagaceae—which indicates that possibly, given

---

* We distinguish sassafras from *sarsaparilla,* a vine which is any of the genus *Smilax* of the plant family Liliaceae, found in tropical and temperate America. Its dried roots provide the flavor of the carbonated drink of the same name, now more commonly called "root beer." As may be expected, this genus and family are also represented in Hartwell.

the right dosage and frequency, tannins could serve as anticancer agents. The facts remain unknown, however.

Betel nut has long been chewed in central and southeast Asian countries and is evidently related to a high incidence of oral cancer (H. Mori, in *Naturally Occurring Carcinogens*, p. 167ff). The betel nut is the fruit of the betel palm, *Areca catechu* of the family Palmae. It is given a citation in Hartwell. The Sanskrit word for the leaf of the betel vine was "tambula," which remains as the Indian word "tambuli" and as the Arabic and Persian word "tambula." (There is a culinary dish of approximately the same name.) The chew or quid is basically composed of betel nut proper along with betel leaf and lime, and it may include tobacco. Betel nut contains such pyridine alkaloids as arecoline, arecaidine, guvacoline, and guvacine. The most significant is arecoline, which is cholinergic, affecting the nervous system (Mori, in *Naturally Occurring Carcniogens*, p. 175). Although mutagenicity has been proven, the carcinogenicity of these particular alkaloids is in doubt.

Cordell classifies arecoline as a tropane alkaloid, typified by atropine, which acts as an acetylcholine antagonist; it is also an alkaloid derived from nicotinic acid (Cordell, *Alkaloids*, pp. 116, 196). More information is provided in Part 4.

The plant family *Euphorbiaceae* is especially large, consisting of about 290 genera containing about 8000 species, of which the genus *Euphorbia* itself has some 1600 species (Y. Hirata, in *Naturally Occurring Carcinogens*, p. 181ff). As may be expected, an array of toxicity problems occur. The specie member *Croton tiglium*, which is native to Africa, has seeds that are toxic but nevertheless has long been used as a purgative. A beverage is made from the aromatic leaves of another species, *Croton flavens*, and is correlated with a high rate of esophageal cancer on the Caribbean island of Curaçao. The species *Yatropha gossypifolia* is habitually used in folk medicine, with a high incidence of esophageal cancer. In fact, there is a commonality within Euphorbiaceae that can be related to esophageal cancer.

For instance, *croton oil* was found to be carcinogenic and, on further analysis, a sequence of discoveries ensued, establishing that diterpene alkaloids were the bioactive constituents. The active esters of these diterpenes show ornithine decarboxlase-inducing effects and Epstein-Barr Virus-activating effects (Hirata, *Naturally Occurring Carcinogens*, p. 183). These include what are called phorbol diesters, the active components of *Euphorbia tiglium*. It may be noted, however, that antileukemic diterpenes were obtained from *Euphorbia esula, Croton tiglium, Cunria spruceana,* and others, and *Euphorbia milii* is a known wart remover (Hirata, *Naturally Occurring Carcinogens*, p. 185).

In the rural and mountainous areas of Japan, for instance, native wild plants have customarily been used for food and/or folk remedies (M. Haga, in *Naturally Occurring Carcinogens*, p. 207ff). Some of the plant/herbal substances have been examined for carcinogenicity. The foods included the kernels of ginkgo nuts (*Ginkgo biloba* of the family Gingkoaceae), the stems of horsetail (*Equisetum arvense* of the family Equisetaceae), fronds of osmund (*Osmunda japonica* of the family Onagraceae), and young ostrich fern (*Matteuccia struthiopteris* of the family Polypodiaceae). Also included are young shoots of aralia (*Aralia cordata* of the family Araliaceae), cacalia (*Cacalia hastata* of the family Compositae), mugwort (*Artemisia princeps* of the family Compositae), and vicia (*Vicia unijuga* of the family Leguminosae). Among vegetables, there were young shoots of bamboo (*Phyllostachys heterocyclia* of the tribe or subfamily Bambusoideae of the family Poaceae), roots of burdock (*Arctium lappa* of the family Compositae), and rhizomes of lotus (*Nelumbo nucifera* of the family Nymphaeaceae).

Plants examined that are used for herbal medicine included dandelion roots (*Taraxacum platycarpum* of the family Compositae), rhizomes of galangal (*Alpinia officinarum* of the family Zingiberacea), terrestrial parts of lathyrus (*Lathyrus palustris* of the family Leguminosae), and leaves of lycium (*Lycium chinense* of the family Solanaceae).* In the main, in tests on laboratory rats, these plants or plant substances proved to be noncarcinogenic.

---

* Hartwell lists all of these, with the exception of the genera *Matteuccia* and *Phyllostachys*. The plant family Polypodiaceae is represented, and the Grass family or the family Poaceae appears in Hartwell as the family Gramineae, although the genus *Phyllostachys* is not cited. Incidentally, at least according to some dictionaries, what is called bamboo is also classified within the genus *Bambusa* or may be within several related genera such as *Arundinaria* or *Dendrocalamus*. The first-mentioned genus is in Hartwell, listed under the family Gramineae. The closest to the second-mentioned is the genus *Arundo*, composed of reeds, and which is also under Gramineae. The third-mentioned does not appear in Hartwell. All told, there are said to be over 75 genera and presumably more than 1000 species, but probably with some overlapping. The giant bamboo *Phyllostachys-bambusoides* is being test grown in South Carolina.

The more than *one million different living species of all kinds worldwide* proceed to grow, propagate, and evolve by utilizing chemical substances (S. Natori, in *Naturally Occurring Carcinogens*, p. 217ff). Variously involved in these reaction sequences or pathways are the compounds called primary metabolites. These are such compounds as sugars, amino acids, and fatty acids, and include such other polymeric substances such as polysaccharides, lipids, peptides, and proteins, plus nucleic acids. Another category, that of *secondary metabolites,* is said to consist of plant products and antibiotics produced by specific organisms. These secondary metabolites are generally considered to be waste products of metabolism.

There are an enormous number of secondary metabolites, but there is a regularity in their structure that suggests a biogenetic origin. A brief classification is as follows:

1. Acetogenins or polyketides formed from a condensation reaction between a mole of acetyl-CoA and several moles of malonyl-CoA.
2. Phenylpropanoids (in the C_6–C_3 range) and related compounds formed from what is called shikimic acid, $C_6H_6(OH)_3COOH$, which is derived from triose and tetrose.
3. Isoprenoids such as terpenes, steroids, and cartenoids, formed from mevalonic acid.
4. Alkaloids formed from amino acids such as phenylalanine, tyrosine, tryptophan, lysine, and ornithine.

Some secondary metabolites are formed from combinations of the preceding. For instance, flavonoids can be viewed as formed from the phenylpropanoid C_6–C_3 unit and three malonates. Other secondary metabolites are considered direct derivatives of primary metabolites, and still others may be formed from a combination of primary and secondary metabolites. In turn, secondary metabolites may undergo further modifications, leading to a complex array of compounds indeed.

Some secondary metabolites exhibit acute toxicities, as occur in toxic plants, and have been used for centuries as poisons such as for arrow heads and fish poisons. Some have later been used for medicines, for example, alkaloids and cardiac glycosides. In fact, many secondary metabolites are now known to exhibit a diversity of biological actions toward other organisms. This has led to perceiving secondary metabolites as products that do not directly influence the functions of the producer but that play roles as ecochemicals, influencing the environment or surroundings. "Thus, the naturally occurring plant carcinogens may be assumed to be a kind of allomone for mammals." (*Allomone* refers to a hormone or other substance that is produced by one species and has an effect on another.) The reference observes that the majority of secondary metabolites are still unknown, awaiting to be isolated, characterized, and tested. More complete information will provide a better understanding of the biochemical bases for biological phenomena.

Although the number of known natural secondary metabolites is rapidly expanding, the number of natural carcinogenic compounds confirmed by tests numbers only about 40. On the other hand, the number of synthetic carcinogenic compounds is relatively high. Some of the few natural carcinogenic compounds noted are *cyacin* in cyads, *aflatoxins* in *Aspergillus flavus,* and *bracken carcinogens*. These substances were first noted to be toxic and later found to be carcinogenic. On the other hand, *safrole* was discovered to be carcinogenic to animals only after large-scale feeding studies were conducted. It is remarked that, although mutagenicity via the Ames test is routinely used for screening naturally occurring substances, *none of the natural mutagenic compounds found has so far been proved to be carcinogenic in animal experiments.*

Some of the pioneering work on natural carcinogens was the discovery of *mycotoxins,* which include *aflatoxins*. The death of turkeys fed peanut meal was found to be caused by the *Aspergillus flavus* in the feed. The metabolites included aflatoxin B1, which was found to produce hepatocarcinoma in rats. Similar compounds have caused subcutaneous sarcomas at the point of injection. As another example, several antibiotics from *Streptomyces* induce cancers in rats and mice. Carcinogens from higher plants include carrageenan and cycasin.

In further summarizing the structures of various naturally occurring carcinogens, the reference observes that carrageenan is composed mainly of the metal salts of sulfate esters of galactose and various galactose polymers. It is classified as a *polysaccharide*. (Polysaccharides are found in fungi for example, and have anticancer activity as is noted in Part 5.) *Cycasin* is composed of the glucoside of an aliphatic alcohol which contains an azoxy group.

Alkaloids are considered to be one of the most important groups of secondary metabolites, and they show a wide variety of biological activities. Some, such morphine and strychnine, have been used as medicines. For the most part nitrogen-heterocyclic compounds, they are usually classified by heterocyclic rings, giving rising to such classes as pyridine, isoquinoline, and indole. To be emphasized is that while many alkaloids are acutely toxic, only those with the pyrrolizidine ring have proven carcinogenic. The pyrrolizidine ring, incidentally, is derived from the amino acid called ornithine.

Mushroom hydrazines are assumed to be amino acid derivatives.

The large group of *phenolics* can be regarded as derived from shikimic acid and acetate malonates. Safrole, for instance, is derived from shikimic acid. Mutagenic flavonoids have shikimate and polyketide origins and usually exist in the glycoside form, with various sugars such as D-glucose constituting the sugar residue. Tannins are divided into hydrolyzable and nonhydrolyzable groups. The former involves the esterification of sugar residues with phenolic acids of shikimic acid origin, whereas the latter are formed by the polymerization of flavonoid compounds. Isoprenoids are derived from mevalonic acid. Phorbol esters, which are tumor promoters, are fatty acid esters of diterpenes.

It is concluded from the above that there is a great diversity, and that no common structural features, patterns, or origins are evident. "In other words, we cannot predict *a priori* carcinogenicity from the chemical structure."

The reference concludes by proposing criteria that would identify potentially carcinogenic compounds. *A further conclusion is that perhaps 80 percent of human cancers are from environmental causes.* All plants and microorganisms produce secondary metabolites that may be physiologically active. And compounds like flavonoids exhibit a kind of genotoxicity, which may imply carcinogenicity, though the latter is not the case for flavonoids. Protein pyrolysis products from cooking are an example of toxification. The formation of carcinogenic nitrosamines from naturally occurring secondary amines and nitrate ion are a problem. Fortunately, genotoxic compounds, although widely distributed in nature, have not proved to be carcinogenic.

In final comment, *genotoxic compounds are those that produce mutagenicity in bacteria by the Ames test—but not in animals.* It would be a stroke of good fortune if this property could somehow be correlated with anticancer activity.

2.13 SCREENING PLANTS FOR ANTICANCER ACTIVITY

The National Cancer Institute (NCI) at this writing has a data base of roughly some 35,000 plant species that have been screened for anticancer activity, with the list growing. The screening program has been noted to test approximately 20,000 to 30,000 substances each year, of all kinds. The test procedures have been expanded to include *in vitro* testing first which, if warranted, is then followed by *in vivo* testing in animals, which usually means special strains of mice. If the results are sufficiently promising, clinical tests are performed on humans.

Many of the substances tested are obtained from foreign countries, and the results must be held proprietary in case the country wants to pursue patent rights. For these and other reasons, including the sheer volume of the work performed, no systematic presentation has yet been put together and made available, although computer retrieval of the more recent data may become an eventuality.

Thus, since 1957 more than 120,000 plant extracts from the more than 35,000 plant species tested have been screened (Jerry L. McLaughlin, in *Methods in Plant Biochemistry*, 6, pp. 1–4). The several ensuing discoveries of antitumor agents include *vincristine, vinblastine, vindesine, the podophyllotoxin derivatives, 10-hydroxy-camptothecin, taxols, indicine-N-oxide, phyllanthoside,* and *homoharringtonine*. The test methods have evolved into *in vitro* screening for 9KB (human nasopharyngeal carcinoma) cytotoxicity and *in vivo* testing against 3PS (P388), which involves methylcholanthrene-induced leukemia in mice. The *in vitro* tests are conducted at several National Institutes of Health (NIH) grantee institutions, and the *in vivo* tests by various contractors. The *in vitro* results usually take about two weeks; the *in vivo* results may take two months. *Toxicity* in vitro *does not necessarily translate to* in vivo *activity.* For instance, many of the *in vitro* cytotoxic compounds, such as the dozens of sesquiterpene lactones from the plant family Compositae, did not show *in vivo* activity. *In comment, the inverse also may hold true, that positive* in vivo *results may not always translate back to positive* in vitro *results. The same sort of discrepancies may show up in comparing clinical tests with* in vitro *and* in vivo *results.**

The Development Therapeutics Program at the NCI has also initiated an *in vitro* screening program for testing more than 50 human cancer cell lines, notably of lung, colon, breast, melanoma and other refractory solid tumors. There is, moreover, the need for reliable and inexpensive prescreening to cut down on unnecessary *in vitro* and *in vivo* testing. The reference describes the use of a novel bioassay method based on the inhibition of crown gall tumors in plants such as the potato tuber. Some representative antitumor prescreen results are shown in Table 2.4

Table 2.4   Representative Prescreen Results

Assay	Biological activities selected
Astrocytoma	Mitotic inhibition
Phage introduction	DNA damage
Aminopeptidase B	Cell surface changes
Candida	Cell membrane actives
Xanthomonas	Glycosylation inhibitors
Agrobacterium	Plasmid transfer
Protein kinase	Inhibition of cell growth proteins
Typoisomerase	DNA conformation
Strand scission	DNA strand cleavage

In addition to the sort of testing or screening described above, the NCI pursues and sponsors basic studies on the mechanisms of cancer. One promising avenue involves the fact that *a line of normal cells will turn over or replicate approximately 85 to 90 times before dying out*—parent to daughter to daughter to daughter to..., whereas with cancer cells there seems to be an enzyme that kicks in about the halfway point, causing a new line of cells to be initiated. Hence, *the line of cancer cells never dies out.* If the enzyme does indeed exist and can be identified, and an inhibitor or inhibitors found, then a cure for cancer will emerge. It will probably not come as too much of a surprise if some of the enzyme inhibitors turn out to be anticancer agents from medical folklore. The problem then will be to determine how much inhibitor is enough but not too much. This will be followed by the hurdle of getting the cure on the market.

2.14   SOME CONCLUSIONS

The previously stated warnings by Ryan J. Huxtable about the uses and misuses of plants or herbs are well taken in that many or all bioactive plants are indeed poisonous in differing degrees, and that this toxicity unfortunately is either not commonly known or is ignored (Huxtable, in *Toxicants*, I, pp. 75–79). Not emphasized is the fact that *many or most of the drugs used by medical orthodoxy can also be toxic*—the toxicity is euphemistically labeled "side effects." Just where this leaves the patient or victim is not clear, other than it seems to be Catch-22 all the way around. If orthodox treatments don't work, as is so often the case for cancer, then what are the alternatives? Certainly with herbal or plant treatments, the dosage level can be critical, just as with orthodox medicines. There may in fact be a "window," where dosages below or above the window are either ineffective or else toxic. In other words, it is a matter of degree. This is all compounded by the difficulty of maintaining quality control, because plant and herbs vary in their bioactivity with place and with time—not to mention that the wrong plant may be substituted, accidentally or on purpose. In Germany, for instance, there are rigorous requirements for testing and confirming activity.

The dichotomy between dosage levels is everywhere. At one level, a dosage may prove beneficial, as in stimulating the immune system. At another, higher level the dosage may be toxic. It is the same with cancer. *At one level, the treatment may help; at another level the treatment can instead cause cancer.* Then, there is the matter of *cumulative dosages*, whereby even taking small hourly or daily doses

---

* All the substances enumerated in this paragraph may be regarded as *alkaloids or their derivatives or precursors. Camptothecin is in itself a powerful antitumor agent,* especially for gastrointestinal carcinoma, but has some undesirable side effects (Cordell, *Alkaloids*, pp. 671–672). Nevertheless, *it is in clinical use in the People's Republic of China.*

can build up toxicity. In the case of some medicines such as antibiotics, on the other hand, too small an hourly or daily dosage may cause the disease to build up a resistance.

The matter of dosage levels and repetitive dosages can become critical. This is why it is insufficient to say that a certain substance is toxic or nontoxic. It may said with justification that all medicines or drugs are metabolic poisons or antimetabolites.

By *metabolism* we mean, in general, the dynamics or changes occurring in any or all biochemical systems connected with an organism, at any level. Usually, these changes are compositional changes, but these in turn may entail say thermal changes, e.g., heats of reaction or any sort of thermal effects associated with change. In sum, the term *metabolism* applies to biological/biochemical/biophysical processes variously at the macro, the micro, or the molecular level, and by including all effects can be called the *thermodynamics of metabolism.*

The changes may embrace either nonreacting or reacting systems, that is, may be physical, chemical, or (more likely) both. A physical change, say, will involve the transfer of a nonreacting component species from one site, position, or location to another, whereas a chemical or biochemical change will involve a change in specie identity. Furthermore, the several component species involved—whether perceived as nonreacting species or as reactants, as intermediates, or as products, and howsoever identified—are all constituents of whatever metabolic system is being studied. As such, they may be referred to as *metabolites.*

These are dynamic concepts but may be applied to a static biosystem at equilibrium, in anticipation that the system may undergo change. Alternatively, a static system may be viewed as existing in a dynamic state of equilibrium, with the forward changes balanced by the reverse changes.

To continue, medicines or drugs in some way or another interfere with metabolic processes, either for better or for worse. That is to say, medicines interfere with both abnormal and normal metabolic processes. The criterion is that an effective medicine in the proper dosages will interfere more, much more, with abnormal metabolic processes than with normal metabolic processes.

Thus, in identifying say anticancer agents, it is not enough to state that the substance acts against cancer. Nor is it enough to state that the substance is toxic or poisonous. For, in a way of looking at it, both verdicts will be correct. The problem is to determine under what conditions, if any, the agent can function as an anticancer agent with a minimum of other toxic side effects. This is where dosage levels and frequency of dosage come into play. It is an enormous problem unto itself.

Hartwell's remarkable compendium *Plants Used Against Cancer* identifies some 3000 plant species or so which are derived from medical folklore. Many are blatantly poisonous—but bioactive plants by and large are poisonous. It is almost a tautology. Apparently, no information about dosage levels or dosage frequency is known or readily available, an omission that is critical. Folklore, however, provides an invaluable screening process for what might work—if only the dosages and frequency could be established. It provides a point of departure for further investigation.

In following the pursuits of basic research, the problems seem to become more and more complicated, for each answer produces more questions. The enormity of the task appears overwhelming, and no final resolution seems attainable. Indeed, scientist/philosopher Karl Popper once wrote that all our efforts amount to nothing more than driving the piling down deeper into the swamp.

What is needed is a solution first, the spark of inspiration, and then the reasons why can be pursued at leisure. As Plato said in the *Meno* a long time ago, if we don't know the answer to a problem then we don't know what the problem is; and if we do know the answer, then there is no problem.

Medical folklore is an age-old trial-and-error screening process, wherein may lie the answers. And some of the folkloric treatments or cures for cancer may indeed be of value, or at least provide a point of departure. If they don't always work, then it is the domain of science to find out why they don't always work. Thus, the answer to the cancer riddle may lie in sorting out the reasons why folkloric cures don't always work, and then making it so they do always work.

A final comment about scientific research and development, and demonstration and commercialization. There is a continual tension between dragging things out for job security on the one hand, and the push to return a profit on the other. This leaves the cancer victim adrift. Either the research stagnates, or the final product doesn't meet expectations, or both. And after spending, say, 50 billion dollars or whatever in the "War on Cancer" to date, there is very little to show for it in the way of a sure-fire cure. The thought comes to mind, therefore, that the victory over cancer may come from altruistic motives rather than profit motives, and may lie more in folklore than in science.

REFERENCES

Alkaloids: Chemical and Biological Perspectives, in four volumes, S. William Pelletier, ed., Wiley, New York, 1983–1987.

The Alkaloids: Chemistry and Pharmacology, R.H.F. Manske et al., eds., Academic Press, 1950–?. There are 46 volumes to date.

Arvigo, Rosita and Michael Balick, *Rainforest Remedies: One Hundred Healing Herbs of Belize*, Lotus Press, Twin Lakes WI, 1993.

Biochemistry of Alkaloids, K. Mothes, H.R. Schütte and M. Luckner, eds., VCH Verlagsgesellschaft, Berlin, 1985.

The Biochemistry of Plants: A Comprehensive Treatise, Academic Press, New York, 1980–1981. Multivolume set.

Blackwell, Will H., *Poisonous and Medicinal Plants*, Prentice-Hall, Englewood Cliffs NJ, 1990. Chapter 5 written by Martha J. Powell.

Boik, John, *Cancer & Natural Medicine: A Textbook of Basic Science and Clinical Research*, Oregon Medical Press, Princeton MN, 1995, 1996.

Cordell, Geoffrey A., *Introduction to Alkaloids: A Biogenetic Approach*, Wiley, New York, 1981.

Cowley, Geoffrey et al., "Herbal Warning," *Newsweek*, May 6, 1996, pp. 60–68.

Duke, James A., *Handbook of Medicinal Herbs*, CRC Press, Boca Raton FL, 1985.

Frohne, Dietrich and Hans Jürgen Pfänder, *A Colour Atlas of Poisonous Plants: A Handbook for Pharmacists, Doctors, Toxicologists, and Biologists*, Wissenschaftliche Verlagsgesellschaft, Stuttgart, 1983, Wolfe Publishing Ltd., London, 1984. Translated by Norman Grainger Bissett.

Hager, Hermann et al., *Hager's Handbuch der Pharmazeutischen Praxis: fur Apotheker, Arzte, Drogisten, und Medizinalbeamte*, J. Springer, and Springer-Verlag, Berlin, 1900, 1902, 1908, 1910, 1920, 1925, 1930, 1949, 1958, 1967, 1973, 1977, 1990.

Harper's Biochemistry, 24th ed., Robert K. Murray, Daryl A. Granner, Peter A. Mayes and Victor W. Rodwell, eds., Appleton and Lange, Stamford CT, 1996.

Hartwell, Jonathan A., *Plants Used Against Cancer: A Survey*, Quarterman Publications, Lawrence MA, 1982. Foreword by Jim Duke.

Heinerman, John, *Healing Animals with Herbs*, BiWorld, Provo UT, 1977.

Heinerman, John, *The Treatment of Cancer with Herbs*, BiWorld, Orem Ut, 1984. Special Foreword by Robert Mendelsohn. Available from the author, P.O. Box 11471, Salt Lake City UT 84147, (801) 521–8824.

Huang, Kee Chang, *The Pharmacology of Chinese Herbs*, CRC Press, Boca Raton FL, 1993.

Infraspecific Classification of Wild and Cultivated Plants, B.T. Styles, ed., Oxford University Press, Oxford, England, 1986.

Kingsbury, John M., *Deadly Harvest: A Guide to Common Poisonous Plants*, Holt, Rinehart and Winston, New York, 1965.

Kingsbury, John M., *Poisonous Plants of the United States and Canada*, Prentice-Hall, Englewood Cliffs NJ, 1964.

Lee, Dr. Joseph G., "Navajo Medicine Man," *Arizona Highways*, XXXVII(8), 2–7 (August, 1961).

Lumholtz, Carl, *New Trails in Mexico: An Account of One Year's Exploration in North-Western Sonora, Mexico, and South-Western Arizona 1909–1910*. Reproduced by the Rio Grande Press, Glorieta NM, 1971.

Lumholtz, Carl, *Unknown Mexico: A Record of Five Years' Exploration among the Tribes of the Western Sierra Madre; in the Tierra Caliente of Tepic and Jalisco; and among the Tarascos of Michoacan*, in two volumes (1902). Reproduced by the Rio Grande Press, Glorieta NM, 1973.

Medicinal and Poisonous Plants of the Tropics, A.J.M. Leeuwenberg (Compiler), Pudoc Wageningen, Centre for Agricultural Publishing and Documentation, Wageningen, Netherlands, 1987. Proceedings of Symposium 5–35 of the 14th International Botanical Congress, Berlin, 24 July–1 August 1987.

Methods in Plant Biochemistry, P.M. Dey and J.B. Harborne, series eds., Academic Press, London, 1990–1991. Vol. 1. *Plant Phenolics*, J.B. Harborne, ed., 1991. Vol. 2. *Carbohydrates*, P.M. Dey, ed., 1990. Vol. 3. *Enzymes of Primary Metabolism*, P.J. Lea, ed., 1990. Vol. 4. *Lipids, Membranes and Aspects of Photobiology*, J.L. Harwood and J.R. Bowyer, eds., 1990. Vol. 5. *Amino Acids, Proteins and Nucleic Acids*, L.J. Rogers, ed., 1991. Vol. 6. *Assays for Bioactivity*, K. Hostettmann, ed., 1991.

Morton, Julia F., *Atlas of Medicinal Plants of Middle America: Bahamas to Yucatan*, C.C. Thomas, Springfield IL, 1981.

Morton, Julia F., *Major Medicinal Plants: Botany, Culture and Uses*, Charles C Thomas Publisher, Springfield IL, 1977.

Moss, Ralph W., *Cancer Therapy: The Independent Consumer's Guide to Non-Toxic Treatment and Prevention*, Equinox Press, Brooklyn NY, 1993.

Naturally Occurring Carcinogens of Plant Origin: Toxology, Pathology and Biochemistry, Iwao Hirono, ed., Kodansha, Tokyo, Elsevier, Amsterdam, 1987.

Nicolaou, K.C., Rodney K. Guy and Pierre Potier, "Taxoids: New Weapons against Cancer," *Scientific American*, **274**(6), 94–98 (June, 1996)

Oliver-Bever, Bep, *Medicinal Plants in Tropical West Africa*, Cambridge University Press, New York, 1986.

Plant Biochemistry, see *Methods in Plant Biochemistry*.

Plants in the Development of Modern Medicine, Tony Swain, ed., Harvard University Press, Cambridge MA, 1972.

Some medicinal forest plants in Africa and Latin America, Forest Resources Development Branch, Forest Resources Division, FAO Forestry Department, Food and Agriculture Organization of the United Nations, Rome, Italy, 1986.

Stace, Clive A., *Plant Taxonomy and Biosystematics*, 2d ed., Edward Arnold, London, 1989.

Stephens, H.A., *Poisonous Plants of the Central United States*, The Regents Press of Kansas, Lawrence, 1980.

Stuessy, Tod F., *Plant Taxonomy: The Systematic Evaluation of Comparative Data.*, Columbia University Press, New York, 1990.

Tétényi, Péter, *Infraspecific Chemical Taxa of Medicinal Plants*, Chemical Publishing Co., New York, 1970. General part translated by Isván Finály. Special part translated by Péter Tétényi.

Textbook of Biochemistry: with Clinical Correlations, Thomas M. Devlin, ed., Wiley, New York, 1982, 2d ed., Wiley, New York, 1986.

Toxicants of Plant Origin, in four volumes, Peter R. Cheeke, ed., CRC Press, Boca Raton FL. Vol. I. *Alkaloids*, 1989. Vol. II. *Glycosides*, 1989. Vol. III. *Proteins and Amino Acids*, 1989. Vol. IV. *Phenolics*, 1989.

Tyler, Varro E., *The Honest Herbal: A Sensible Guide to the Use of Herbs and Related Remedies*, 3rd ed., Pharmaceutical Products Press, New York, 1992. Haworth Press, Binghamton NY, 1993. Revised edition of *The New Honest Herbal*.

Voet, Donald and Judith G. Voet, *Biochemistry*, 2d ed., Wiley, New York, 1995.

Walters, Richard, *Options: The Alternative Cancer Therapy Book*, Avery Publishing Group, Garden City Park NY, 1993.

Watt, John Mitchell and Maria Gerdina Breyer-Brandwijk, *The Medicinal and Poisonous Plants of Southern and Eastern Africa: Being an Account of Their Medicinal and Other Uses, Chemical Composition, Pharmacological Effects and Toxicology in Man and Animal*, E.&S. Livingstone, Edinburgh and London, 1962.

Weber, G., *Cancer Research*, 43, pp. 3466–3492.

Weeds of the West. Tom D. Whitson, ed. Authors: Larry C. Burrill, Steven A. Dewey, David W. Cudney, B.E. Nelson, Richard D. Lee, Robert Parker. With a list of contributors. Published by the Western Society of Weed Science in cooperation with the Western United States Land Grant Universities Cooperative Extension Services, College of Agriculture, University of Wyoming, Laramie, January, 1991.

Chemical Taxonomy

Part 3

Chemical Taxonomy

3.1 A REVIEW OF MEDICINAL PLANT LITERATURE SOURCES

It will be an objective to furnish further examples of known bioactive plants and their chemical constituents, particularly with regard to their use as anticancer agents. This includes information about the different classes of compounds and instances of each. Unfortunately, the specific role of these plants and compounds as enzyme inhibitors (or promoters) is still largely unknown.

Bioactive plants range over the world, and some plant families, genera, and species do the same. What will be of interest here is whether the same plants or plant species, found in different countries and regions, will be found to exhibit the same sort of activity against cancer. In other words, is there a pattern to plant taxonomy and anticancer effects, and to the chemical substances that exist in the plants? By way of introduction, some of the literature sources for the plants of different countries and regions will be set forth first, along with a few more general references of less interest for the purposes here.

Covering North America and the United States, there is Alma R. Hutchens' *Indian Herbalogy of North America*, one of several citations about Native America mentioned in Part 1. Hutchens spells out the uses and administrations of the various plants and plant substances. Homeopathic clinical uses are set forth, as well as folk medicine applications. Special attention is also given to the Russian experience and to the India and Pakistan experiences with these plants or plant substances.

A convenient and comprehensive reference is *A Field Guide to Medicinal Plants: Eastern and Central North America*, with text by Steven Foster and James A. Duke. Duke had previously written the *Handbook of Northeastern Indian Medicinal Plants*, which is No. 3 in the series *Bioactive Plants* published by Quarterman Publications. The first in the series is Jonathan L. Hartwell's *Plants Used Against Cancer*, and the second is *Medicinal Uses of Plants by Indian Tribes of Nevada* by Percy Train et al.

A number of other works are extant, for instance about plants of the American West—e.g., Michael Moore's *Medicinal Plants of the Mountain West: A Guide to the Identification, Preparation, and Uses of Traditional Medicinal Plants Found in the Mountains, Foothills, and Upland Areas of the American West*. Moore has since written *Medicinal Plants of the Desert and Canyon West: A Guide to Identifying, Preparing, and Using Traditional Medicinal Plants Found in the Deserts and Canyons of the Southwest*, and *Medicinal Plants of the Pacific West*. Additional references pertaining to alkaloid-bearing plants are provided in Part 4, and information about the fungi or mycota are furnished in Part 5. Speaking further of deserts and such, L.C. Chopra and B.K. Abrol have furnished *Medicinal Plants of the Arid Zones*.

In addition to the several references on plants and herbs so far cited, a few more can be mentioned. *A Modern Herbal* by Maud Grieve covers many aspects of the use of herbs, grasses, fungi, shrubs, and trees. (For more on fungi, consult Part 5, as previously noted.) John C. Crellin and Jane Philpott have prepared *Herbal Medicine Past and Present*, based on interviews with Appalachian herbalist A.L. Tommie Bass. Volume II is titled *A Reference Guide to Medicinal Plants*. An earlier compilation is *Potter's New Cyclopedia of Botanical Drugs and Preparations*, by R.C. Wren, first published in 1907. It has been rewritten by Elizabeth M. Williamson and Fred J. Evans and was republished in 1988. There has been a sorting out prepared along the way, by Theodora Andrews with the assistance of William L. Corya and Donald A. Stickel, titled *Bibliography on Herbs, Herbal Medicine, "Natural Foods," and Unconventional Medical Treatment*. The last of these, published in 1982, serves to indicate that a continually updated CD or computer file is a necessity in keeping track of this rapidly expanding field.

John Heinerman, cited in Part 2, has since written the *Healing Power of Herbs*, published in 1995. In particular, Heinerman in most instances names the active substance or substances. Other similar books of note include *Medicinal Plants: An Illustrated Guide to More than 180 Herbal Plants*, Bradford Angier's *Field Guide to Medicinal Wild Plants*, and Douglas B. Elliott's *Roots: An Underground Botany and Forager's Guide*. Also of note is *Medicinal Plants: A Source Guide* and a bibliography titled *Medicinal Plants*, compiled by Judith Robinson and Constance Carter of the Library of Congress.

A comprehensive compilation by Daniel E. Moerman is titled *Medicinal Plants of Native America*, in two volumes. Moerman also wrote *Geraniums for the Iroquois: A Field Guide to American Indian Medicinal Plants*. Another is Charles F. Millspaugh's two-volume *Medicinal Plants: An Illustrated and Descriptive Guide to Plants Indigenous to and Naturalized in the United States Which Are Used in Medicine*.

When speaking of medicinal plants, first thoughts are usually of the Amazonian region of South America, although we can also speak of the dense unexplored forests in parts of the African Congo and of the rain forests in Southeast Asia, notably on the island of Borneo. Starting with the first-mentioned region, there is the *Amazonia Ethnobotanical Dictionary* by James Allen Duke and Rudolfo Vasqeuz. Another is *Medicinal and Poisonous Plants of the Tropics*, compiled by A.J.M. Leeuwenberg. Still others include *Medicinal Resources of the Tropical Forest*, published by Columbia University Press, and *Ethnobotany in the Neotropics*, published by the New York Botanical Garden. In addition, there is *Rainforest Remedies: One Hundred Healing Herbs of Belize*, by Rosita Arvigo and Michael Balick.

Walter B. Mors, Carlos T. Rizzini, and Nuno A. Pereira have written *Medicinal Plants of Brazil*, which is No. 6 in the series *Medicinal Plants of the World*, published by Reference Publications, Algonac MI. Robert A. DeFilipps has in turn written *Medicinal Plants of the Guianas*, which is No. 7 in the series *Medicinal Plants of the World*. Also of the same general territory is *Medicinal Plants of the West Indies*, by Edward S. Ayensu, which is No. 2 in the series *Medicinal Plants of the World*. (Professor Ayensu, of the Smithsonian Institution in Washington DC, served as editor for the folio volume *Jungles*, published in 1980 by Crown Publishers, New York, and issued also as *The Life and Mysteries of the Jungle*.) The Food and Agriculture Organization (FAO) of the United Nations has distributed *Some medicinal forest plants in Africa and Latin America*.

As to Africa, there is the massive volume by John Mitchell Watt and Maria Gerdina Breyer-Brandwijk, *The Medicinal and Poisonous Plants of Southern and Eastern Africa*, published in 1962. A newer volume is the *Handbook of African Medicinal Plants* by Maurice M. Iwu, published in 1993. In addition to extensive descriptions of plant species and their medicinal uses, Dr. Iwu has a chapter on Healing and the African Culture, and another on The African Medicine Man. He is a professor of pharmacognosy at the University of Nigeria, and is also affiliated with the Walter Reed Army Hospital in the United States.

Of similar interest is *Medicinal Plants and Traditional Medicine in Africa* by Abayomi Sofowora. Another is *Medicinal Plants in Tropical West Africa* by Bep Oliver-Bever. Similarly, there is *Medicinal Plants of West Africa* by Edward S. Ayensu, which is No. 1 in the series *Medicinal Plants of the World*. Finally, there is *Medicinal Plants of North Africa* by Loutfy Boulos, which is No. 3 in the series *Medicinal Plants of the World*.

The medicinal plants of India are well represented. For instance there is *Medicinal Plants of Bombay Presidency*, by S.P. Agharkar. (The Bombay Presidency is one of three principal divisions of what was once British India. The other two were Madras and Bengal.) Another reference of note is *Medicinal Plants of India and Pakistan: A Concise Work Describing Plants Used for Drugs and Remedies According to Ayurfedic, Unani and Tibbi Systems and Mentioned in British and American Pharmacopoeias*, written by J.F. Dastur. S.K. Jain and Robert A. DeFilipps have contributed *Medicinal Plants of India*, in two volumes, which is No. 5 in the series *Medicinal Plants of the World*. (M.K. Jain compiled the *Handbook of Enzyme Inhibitors*, cited in Part 1.) Another, one of many others, is *Medicinal Plants of India*, published by the Indian Council of Medical Research. Also there is *Major Medical Plants of India*, by R.S. Thakur of the Central Institute of Medicinal and Aromatic Plants, and *Medicinal Plants of India* by Rasheeduz Zafar. V.M. Pathak is the author of *Medicinal Plants of Gwalior*. (Gwalior is a former state in north central India.) The promise of the unusual is provided by Gyanendra Pandey's *Medicinal Flowers: Puspayurveda Medicinal Flowers of India and Adjacent Regions*, which is No. 14 in the series on *Indian Medical Science*.

There are several monographs or reports of note about plants in regions or countries adjacent to India. One is *Medicinal Plants of Nepal Himalaya*. The other is *Medicinal Plants: Report of Committee on*

Economic and Therapeutic Importance of Medical Plants Initiated by the Ministry of Health, Government of Pakistan, edited by Inamul Haq. Another somewhat obscure report is titled *Survey and Regeneration of Medicinal Plants in West Pakistan* by M.A. Quraishi and Mir Alam Khan, issued by the Pakistan Forest Institute. These serve as examples of the vital and continuing interest about the role of plant medicines in this part of the world.

Continuing on to the rest of Asia, there is *Medicinal Plants of East and Southeast Asia*, by Lily M. Perry with the assistance of Judith Metzger. More specifically, there is *Medicinal Plants of Vietnam, Cambodia and Laos*, written and published by Nguyen Van Duong. Van Duong is a former professor and chairman of the Department of Pharmacognosy, School of Pharmacy, University of Saigon, and who is now located in Santa Monica, CA.

Another compilation is David C. Lewis's *Medicinal Plants of Asia: A Systematic Bibliography*. About future research, there is *Medicinal Plants: New Vistas of Research*, edited by J.N. Govil, V.K. Singh and Shamima Hasmi. Also by V.K. Singh is *Medicinal Plants and Folklores: Strategy Towards Conquest of Human Ailments*. Of note is *Medicinal Plants*, Vol. 1, written by Vimala Ramalingam and edited by N. Singh and H.C. Mital.

Last but not least, and perhaps foremost in the use of herbs, is China. *Medicinal Plants of China* has been published by the World Health Organization. James A. Duke and Edward S. Ayensu have compiled the two-volume set *Medicinal Plants of China*, which is No. 4 in the series *Medicinal Plants of the World*. Of striking interest is *Studies on Chinese Medical Plants and Cancer*, by Wong Kin Keung, published in Hong Kong in 1991. University of Louisville pharmacy professor Kee Chang Huang's *The Pharmacology of Chinese Herbs* may be the final word.

The foregoing references serve to illustrate that Asia is a fertile ground for ongoing research into the further medicinal value of plants—and that a cure for cancer may very likely emanate from here. There is even the thought that such a cure may already be known to exist.

For information about historical origins, there is Edith Grey Wheelwright's *Medicinal Plants and Their History*, Frank J. Anderson's *An Illustrated History of the Herbals*, Richard Le Strange's *A History of Herbal Plants*, and *Medicinal Plants in the Biblical World*, edited by Walter and Irene Jacob. The last mentioned is No. 1 of the series *Horticulture and Technology in the Biblical World*. Irene and Walter Jacob also edited *The Healing Past: Pharmaceuticals in the Biblical and Rabbinic World*. Returning more to the present, consult *Plants in the Development of Modern Medicine*, edited by Tony Swain. The monograph by Douglas B. Elliott titled *Roots: An Underground Botany and Forager's Guide*, previously mentioned, also contains considerable information about the historical background of useful plants, albeit nothing about cancer. Also bearing on the subject is *The Medicinal Plant Industry* by R.O. Wijesekera.

Interestingly, Richard Le Strange's *A History of Medicinal Plants* contains a section about the genus *Marsdenia* of the family Asclepiadaceae or Milkweed family. The principal species is *M. condurango*, also called *Gonolobus condurango* or *Condorango blanco*. (Hartwell also refers to the species as *Equatoria garciana*.) This is the *condor vine* (or condorango or condurango), mentioned courtesy of the herbalist O. Phelps Brown circa 1875. It is noted that clinical tests proved the condurango to be of less value than expected, although it may be useful in the early stages of cancer (Le Strange, *History*, pp. 175–176). No active principles have been determined, though the bark contains tannin, glycosides, and an alkaloid similar to *strychnine*. Overdoses are toxic.

Le Strange also mentions the anticancer alkaloids *vinblastine* and *vincristine* of the species *Catharanthus roseus* of the family Apocynaceae or Dogbane family, with the comment that the *side effects are severe* (Le Strange, *History*, p. 258). As to the genus *Solanum* of the family Solanaceae or Nightshade family, it is observed also courtesy the herbalist O. Phelps Brown that the *leaves have been used against cancer* (Le Strange, *History*, p. 236). The active principle is assumed to be the alkaloid *solanine*. Furthermore, the genus *Hyoscyamus* or henbane of the same family contains the alkaloids atropine, hyoscine, and *hyoscyamine* (Le Strange, *History*, p. 141). Not only this, but the genus *Senecio*, generally called *groundsel* or *ragwort*, and which is of the family Compositae or Asteraceae (or the Sunflower or Daisy or Aster family), contains alkaloids (Le Strange, *History*, p. 232). *The presence of alkaloids, glycosides, and other bioactive compounds in fact tends to be almost ubiquitous in herbs or medicinal plants*, a topic to be further explored, and in particular in Part 4. Moreover, the connection to anticancer activity is of paramount concern, presumably either or both for stimulating the immune system and acting as enzyme inhibitors (or promoters or activators).

A comprehensive bibliography of medicinal plants worldwide has been provided by Siri von Reis Altschul in her compilation *Drugs and Foods from Little-Known Plants: Notes in Harvard University Herbaria*. The scientific names are provided according to plant family, along with a brief descriptive annotation for each plant, giving the source of information, and sometimes the medicinal uses or properties. This effort was subsequently followed by a similar volume written by von Reis and Frank L. Lipp, titled *New Plant Sources for Drugs and Foods from the New York Botanical Garden Herbarium*.

For botanical information per se about the tropical regions of the New World, there is the extensive continuing series of monograph volumes titled *Flora Neotropica*, each devoted to a particular plant family. And there are, of course, the several standard botanical references for the United States, notably *Gray's Manual of Botany*, which deals with the flowering plants and ferns of the central and northeastern United States and adjacent Canada. Plus, there are such other regional reference works as *Flora of the Great Plains* and *Atlas of the Flora of the Great Plains*, which shows county-by-county plant distribution patterns. Also of mention is the classic two-volume set, *Manual of the Trees of North America*, by Charles Sprague Sargent. Whereas plant taxonomy is described in great detail in most of these volumes, very little is said about the uses and medicinal properties.

Plant dictionaries can be of much use in obtaining a bit of information about the more obscure plant species, worldwide, and their plant families and locations. A couple of examples suffice. First, there is J.C. Willis' *A Dictionary of Flowering Plants and Ferns*, which has gone into a number of editions. Another is D.G. Mabberley's *The Plant Book: A Portable Dictionary of the Higher Plants*, based on the system used by Willis. As to other information sources, there is the *Guide to Standard Floras of the World* by D.G. Frodin. All three are published by Cambridge University Press.

About common plant names, there is F.N. Howes' *A Dictionary of Useful and Everyday Plants and Their Common Names*, and the *Index to Common Names of Herbaceous Plants*, compiled by R. Milton Carleton. Of particular note is *A Dictionary of Plant Names*, in two volumes, written by H.L. Gerth Van Wijk, which is most useful in tracking down uncommon plant species and their English, French, and German common names. As to covering edible plants, an extensive compilation is provided in *Tanaka's Cyclopedia of Edible Plants of the World*, by Tyôzaburô Tanaka, and edited by Sasuke Nakao.

With regard to searching the literature for information about ongoing plant research, there is the computer file called AGRICOLA, which provides article citations and abstracts. For information about medical research there is MEDLINE, also mentioned elsewhere.

The Flora of North America Project, Missouri Botanical Garden, P.O. Box 299, St. Louis MO 63166-0299, is in the further process of providing a documented standard for making taxonomic decisions. Information is being compiled on the names, taxonomic relationships, continent-wide distribution, and morphological characteristics of all plants throughout their range in North America north of Mexico.

As to information already assembled. the U.S. Department of Agriculture has an extensive data base embodied as the National Plant Data Center (NPDC). This information can be accessed via the Internet at

http://plants.USDA.gov/plants/qurymen.cgi

There are some 45,000 individual taxon within the database, giving the accepted scientific name, common name, symbol, and family. Information is also furnished on growth habit, duration, and origin. Plant synonyms are provided, and a mapping can be pulled up of the distribution of each species by state and county.

3.2 SOME ANTICANCER PLANTS NOTED IN THE UNITED STATES

This subject may be covered in various ways. For starters, a brief recapitulation is shown in Table 3.1, as obtained from *Herbal Medicine Past and Present*, Vol. II, by John C. Crellin and Jane Philpott, based on interviews with Appalachian herbalist A.L. Tommie Bass. Listing is by family and genus, and sometimes by species, with common names provided. The plant names have a familiar ring, as the same plants recur again and again in different compilations of medical folklore. All the plant families are listed in Hartwell.

In Table 3.2, plant names are furnished as found in Alma R. Hutchens' *Indian Herbalogy of North America*. The listings are again presented according to plant families. Hutchens also provides some other comments of interest. She notes the work of herbalist O.P. Brown, published in 1875 and previously mentioned, in favoring the use of *Solanum dulcamara*, commonly called *bittersweet or woody nightshade*

Table 3.1 Some Anticancer Plants Found in the United States[a]

Apocynaceae	*Vinca minor, V. major*: periwinkle
Aristolochiaceae	*Asarum* spp.: wild ginger
Berberidaceae	*Podophyllum peltatum*: mayapple
Boraginaceae	*Borago officinalis*: borage
Boraginaceae	*Symphatum* spp.: comfrey, hound's tongue
Commelinaceae	*Tradescantia* obiensis*: spiderwort
Compositae	*Arctium lappa*: burdock
Compositae	*Gnaphalium* spp.: rabbit tobacco
Crassulaceae	*Sedum telephium*: stonecrop, houseleek
Cruciferae	*Brassica* spp.: cabbage, collard
Dioscoreaceae	*Dioscorea* spp.: wild yam, sweet potato
Euphorbiaceae	*Euphorbia* spp.: spurge or milkweed
Hamamelidaceae	*Hamamelis virginiana*: witch hazel
Labiatae	*Glechoma* hederacea*: ground ivy
Liliaceae	*Lilium* spp.: lilies
Liliaceae	*Polygonatum biflorum**: Solomon's seal
Loranthaceae	*Viscum album* or *Phoradendron serotinum**: mistletoe
Malvaceae	*Althaea officinalis*: marsh mallow
Orobanchaceae	*Conopholis americana*: squawroot, beechdrops, cancer root
Orobanchaceae	*Epifagus virginiana*: beechdrops, cancer root
Oxalidaceae	*Oxalis* spp.: wood sorrel
Papaveraceae	*Sanguinaria canadensis*: bloodroot (contains sanguinarine)
Polygonaceae	*Rumex* spp.: sheep sorrel
Pyrolaceae	*Pyrola umbellata*: pipsissewa
Ranunculaceae	*Hydrastis canadensis*: goldenseal
Rosaceae	*Prunus* spp: almond, peach, apricot, etc.
Saxafragaceae	*Viburnum**: arrow wood
Solanaceae	*Solanum nigrum*: nightshade
Violaceae	*Viola* spp.: violet, pansy
Vitaceae	*Vitis rotundifloria**: grapevine
Zygophyllaceae	*Larrea tridentata*: chaparral, creosote bush

a. From *Herbal Medicine Past and Present*, Vol. II, by John C. Crellin and Jane Philpott, based on interviews with Appalachian herbalist A.L. Tommie Bass. Plant families, genera, or species **not** appearing in Hartwell's *Plants Used Against Cancer* are indicated by an asterisk. Supplemental information, such as common plant names, is supplied from *Gray's Manual of Botany*.

Table 3.2 Some Anticancer Plants from American Indian Herbalogy[a]

Araceae	*Symplocarpus* foetidus*: skunk cabbage
Berberidaceae	*Podophyllium peltatum*: mandrake, American
Borraginaceae	*Symphatum officianale*: comfrey
Caprifoliaceae	*Viburnum opulus*: crampbark high
Caprifoliaceae	*Viburnum prunifolium**: black haw
Compositae	*Vernonia* spp.: iron weed
Coniferae (Pinaceae)	*Thuja occidentalis*: thuja, arbor-vitae
Hamamelidaceae	*Hamamelis virginica, H. virginiana*: witch hazel
Labiatae	*Glecoma* hederaceae*: ale hoof, ground ivy
Leguminosae	*Trifolium pratense*: red clover
Liliaceae	*Veratrum viride*: hellebore, American
Orobanchaceae	*Epiphegus americanus, O. virginiana*: beechdrop
Papaveraceae	*Chelidonium majus*: celandine
Papaveraceae	*Sanginaria canadensis*: blood root
Phytolaccaceae	*Phytolacca decandra*: poke root
Pinaceae (Coniferae)	*Thuja occidentalis*: thuja, arbor-vitae
Polygonaceae	*Rumex crispus*: yellow dock
Polyporaceae*	*Inonotus* obliquus*: chaga
Ranunculaceae	*Hydrastis canadensis*: golden seal
Rubiaceae	*Galium aparine*: cleavers
Saliceae	*Populus tremuloides*: poplar, aspen
Solanaceae	*Solanum dulcamara*: bitter sweet
Ulmaceae	*Ulmus fulva*: slippery elm
Violaceae	*Viola odorata*: violet
Zygophyllaceae	*Larrea divaricata*: chaparral

a. From *Indian Herbalogy of North America,* by Alma R. Hutchens. Plant families, genera, or species **not** appearing in Hartwell's *Plants Used Against Cancer* are indicated by an asterisk. Supplemental information, such as common plant names, is supplied from *Gray's Manual of Botany.*

(of the family Solanaceae), a usage recommended by others for *tumors, cancers, and warts,* going back to Galen in A.D. 150 (Hutchens, *Indian Herbalogy,* p. 43). *A substance from red milkweed or "cancerillo" has been used for centuries by Central American Indians to treat cancer, and has been demonstrated to inhibit the growth of lab-cultured human cancer tissue.* No further specifications were given, but according to *Gray's Manual of Botany,* the species *Asclepias rubra* (of the family Asclepiadaceae or Milkweed family) is called red milkweed. There is also a similar species named *A. purpurascens* or purple milkweed.

The use of *Echinacea angustifolia*, also called *Echinaceae* or *purple coneflower* (of the family Compositae) is described for many and varied ailments, including *cancerous cachexia,* even hydrophobia, plus snakebites, and septicemia or blood poisoning (Hutchens, *Indian Herbalogy*, p. 113). The herb *Helianthemum canadense* or *frostwort* (of the family Cistaceae) is noted to have been used for *cancerous degenerations.* The species *Daucus carota* or *wild carrot* (of the family Umbelliferae) can be grated and used as a poultice for *cancerous sores* (Hutchens, *Indian Herbalogy*, p. 300). It has also been used against anemia. An extract made from carrots is called doucorin—or should it be spelled "daucorin"?

In describing *Larrea divaricata* or *L. tridentata* (the same species), or *Chaparral* (of the family Zygophyllaceae), Hutchens refers to the plant as belonging to a large group of desert Artemesia stretching across the southwestern United States and Argentina, and in Australia (Hutchens, *Indian Herbalogy*, pp. 82–84). Not only is the particular species found in the American Southwest and Argentina, but a similar species occurs in Australia. Interest in Chaparral (medicinal form) seems to be ongoing, and Hutchens provides additional information as follows. It is stated that the leaves and stems of the plant contain gums, resins, protein, partially characterized esters, acids, alcohols, a small amount of sterols, sucrose, and volatile oils. Presumably no alkaloids have been detected, and the plant is said to be nontoxic—at least in some quarters. The case is recounted of the person who apparently cured himself of melanoma by drinking chaparral tea, a case commonly cited in other accounts of herbal treatments and cancer.

Significantly, Hutchens observes that the mechanism for Chaparral's anticancer action can probably be traced to the presence of nordihydroguaiaretic acid or NDGA. *NDGA is said to be able to convert fermentation processes thought to be out of balance.* We therefore wish to comment as per the anaerobic glycolysis sequence as introduced and examined in Part 1. Anaerobic glycolysis involves as the last step the anaerobic conversion of pyruvic acid or pyruvate to lactic acid. No oxygen is involved, and the process can be described as one of *fermentation.* Furthermore, cancer cells by and large undergo anaerobic glycolysis. *It can consequently be advanced that very possibly NDGA may serve as an enzyme inhibitor for anaerobic glycolysis, and in this way acts as an anticancer agent.*

In this regard, according to Appendix B, *Guiairetic acid, nordihydro-* is listed as a *respiration inhibitor,* which is not exactly encouraging. However, the fact that it is an enzyme inhibitor at all opens up the possibility that it may serve as an inhibitor for other enzymes in other enzyme-catalyzed biochemical reactions. For example, consider the enzyme *lactate dehydrogenase* involved in the formation of lactic acid or lactate, or still other enzymes involved in the anaerobic glycolysis sequence such as hexokinase, phosphofructokinase, and/or pyruvate kinase (a listing of known inhibitors is furnished in Appendix A).

It may be added that if NDGA is indeed an inhibitor for respiration, this action is mild, for the main action associated with NDGA is as an antioxidant, and it was at one time used commercially for this purpose. It has been found to have an adverse effect on the kidneys and liver, however. The dosage levels and cumulative time periods for this latter sort of damaging action are not specified with any exactness.

Michael Moore mostly steers clear of cancer in his *Medicinal Plants of the Desert and Canyon West*, but considerable attention is given to Chaparral, also called creosote bush or greasewood. He states that *it contains 18 distinct flavone and flavonol glycones,* plus a dihydroflavonol and larreic acid. And two guaiaretic acid *lignins* are found, one of which is nordihydroguaiaretic acid or NDGA. Also found are several *quercetin* bioflavonoids. Applied as a tincture, tea, or salve to the skin, Chaparral serves as an *antibiotic.* He comments that Chaparral tea itself is virtually undrinkable, although it is said to have "a strong and beneficial effect on impaired liver metabolism." (This may be contrary to other findings, which indicate that Chaparral tea causes hepatitis or liver damage. Richard Walters, however, has some good things to say about Chaparral in his book *Options*, as noted in Part 1.) It may also improve the blood lipid characteristics, that is, the ratio of high-density to low-density lipids or fats in the blood. It is also said to *inhibit the formation of free radicals* that otherwise damage the liver and lungs. By acting against lipid peroxides, it alleviates joint pain (and in fact is a folklore remedy for arthritis). Finally, Moore gives some space to the oft-mentioned effect on cancer, saying that *Chaparral can both inhibit and stimulate cancer cell growth,* and thereby dismisses it as an anticancer agent. (To which can be added, that this carcinogenic/anticarcinogenic effect is commonly found among other anticancer agents, and may be in large part related to dosage levels.) In any event, Moore ascribes only to small daily doses for the other ailments mentioned.

Daniel E. Moerman supplies plant names under the heading "Cancer Treatment" in a table on Indications (Moerman, *Medicinal Plants*, Vol. Two, pp. 555–556). A listing by plant families is shown in Table 3.3. Many other interesting categories are presented by Moerman, for example, "Snake Bite Remedies."

Table 3.3 Some Anticancer Plants of Native America[a]

Araliaceae	*Aralia nudicaulis* (Iroquois): spikenard
Boraginaceae	*Cynoglossum officianale* (Iroquois): hound's tongue
Boraginaceae	*Cynoglossum virginianum** (Cherokee): wild comfrey
Boriganaceae	*Hackelia virginiana* (Cherokee): stickseed, beggar's lice
Celastraceae	*Celastrus scandens* (Chippewa): bittersweet
Commelinaceae	*Tradescantia** *virginiana* (Cherokee): spiderwort
Compositae	*Artemisia tilesii** (Eskimo): species not in Hartwell or Gray
Compositae	*Cacalia atriplicifolia* (Cherokee): pale Indian plantain
Compositae	*Cirsium vulgare** (Iroquois): bull- or common thistle
Compositae	*Crepis runcinata* (Fox): hawksbeard
Cornaceae	*Cornus alternifolia* (Menominee): alternate-leaved dogwood
Corylaceae*	*Ostrya** *virginiana* (Iroquois): ironwood, hop-hornbeam, leverwood
Euphorbiaceae	*Euphorbia corollata* (Cherokee): milkweed
Haemodoraceae*	*Lachnanthes** *caroliniana* (Cherokee): redroot
Hippocastanaceae	*Aesculus pavia** (Cherokee): red buckeye
Leguminosae	*Trifolium pratense* (Shinnecock): red clover
Liliaceae	*Trilium erectum* (Cherokee): birthroot
Onagraceae	*Epilobium angustiflorium** (Kwakiutl): fireweed, great willow herb
Oxalidaceae	*Oxalis corniculalta* (Cherokee): India sorrel
Oxalidaceae	*Oxalis violacea* (Cherokee): violet wood sorrel
Pyrolaceae	*Chimaphila maculata* (Cherokee): pipsissewa
Pyrolaceae	*Chimaphila umbellata* (Iroquois): wintergreen
Pyrolaceae	*Pyrola elliptica** (Nootka): shinleaf, wild lily of the valley, wild lettuce
Ranunculaceae	*Hydrastis canadensis* (Cherokee): golden seal
Ranunculaceae	*Xanthorhiza** *simplicissima* (Cherokee): shrub-yellowroot
Rosaceae	*Prunus emarginata** (Kwakiutl): species not in Hartwell or Gray
Saxifragaceae	*Hydrangea arborescens* (Cherokee): hydrangea
Scrophulariaceae	*Pedicularis canadensis* (Fox): lousewort

a. From *Medicinal Plants of Native America*, Volume two, pp. 555–556, by Daniel E. Moerman. Plant families, genera, or species **not** appearing in Hartwell's *Plants Used Against Cancer* are indicated by an asterisk. The names of the various Indian tribe-sources are included. Supplemental information, such as common plant names, is supplied from *Gray's Manual of Botany.*

An additional compendium of bioactive plants, with the emphasis on anticancer activity, is shown in Appendix *M*, as extracted from *A Field Guide to Medicinal Plants: Eastern and Central North America*, text by Steven Foster and James A.Duke. It may be noted that some of the species are repeated. The reference contains annotations in the margins about the toxicity of the various plants listed, and some are *poisonous in the extreme*. If these extremely poisonous plants can ever be used at all, it would be only in trace amounts, after pronounced dilution.

It may be observed that the plants used or suggested are not necessarily of native or domestic origins, in that many weeds, wildflowers, and domesticated flowers found in the United States are of Euro-Asian and African origins, either introduced accidentally or on purpose. This can be evidenced, for example, in the plant descriptions supplied in *Weeds of the West* or in *Weeds and Poisonous Plants of Wyoming and Utah*. The main distinguishing feature is that the plants tend to be bioactive, or in another way of saying it, are toxic in varying degrees. Generally speaking, the toxicity occurs all through the plant, although it may be concentrated in a particular part such as in the seeds, leaves, stems, rhizomes, roots, or tubers. The reference indicates which plant or parts are considered the most active, but the distinction is not supplied in Tables 3.1 through 3.3, although this sort of information is furnished in Appendix M.

Additionally, Appendix M provides information about different levels of toxicity. It doesn't take long to get the idea that there is a reason why most plants and herbs are considered either poisonous or medicinal, and that edible plants and their parts are mostly confined to those that have long been tested, which we know as common everyday garden variety vegetables and fruits.

In another book about plants or herbs for the most part native to the United States, Michael Moore's *Medicinal Plants of the Mountain West* mostly steers clear of citations about cancer treatment. Only two plants are mentioned, *cleavers* or *Gallium aparine* (of the family Rubiaceae) and *yellow dock* or *Rumex crispus* (of the family Polygonaceae), in the manner of an afterthought. (These plants both appear in other listings of anticancer agents, ref. the previous citations and tables.) No mention is made of Chaparral in this volume. Moore presents some other interesting features, however. To name a few: elderberry contains the alkaloid sambucine; hops act as an antibiotic in preserving beer; hound's tongue contains the alkaloid heliosupine; jimsonweed contains scopolamine and hyoscyamine; mistletoe has acetylcholine; motherwort has leonurine; the plant called Oshá or *Ligusticum poteri* (of the family Umbelliferae) is antiviral; peonies act against panic attacks; plantain contains a proteolytic (protein-digesting) enzyme in the leaves; St. John's wort serves as an antidepressant, due to its hypericin content; native or wild tobaccos are more active than commercial or cultivated tobaccos, containing a wide range of alkaloids such as anabasine and harmine, with uncured plants having a higher content of the pyridine alkaloids including nicotine; valerian contains the alkaloids valerine and chatinine, which act as sedatives; willows possess the glycosides salicin and populin; wormwood contains the lactone glycosides santonin and artemisin; yellow dock contains chrysophanic acid and emodin, plus tannins.

Whether any of these medicinal plants or plant-derived substances actually works against cancer is not definitively known. There is the opinion, however, that the record is probably dismal—about as dismal overall as treatment by orthodox means. There is the possibility, nevertheless, that substances derived from these very same plants may actually work against cancer, say as immune stimulators and/or as enzyme inhibitors (or as enzyme promoters or activators). The critical clinical testing has simply never been performed in an objective, comprehensive, positive fashion. The orthodox wisdom seems to be that unorthodox therapies don't work and can't work, and had better not work.

The criteria are selectivity and toxicity. That is, the anticancer agent should show a selectivity toward cancer cells, in that the cancer cells would be destroyed without the simultaneous degradation and destruction of normal cells. The latter scenario, unfortunately, occurs using such conventional chemotherapy drugs as 5-FU and methotrexate, as has been stressed in Part 1. That such drugs continue to be used is unfathomable, since other drugs or medicines that show similar toxicities and lack of selectivity are routinely banned.

With regard to alternative plant or herbal treatments, there simply have not been any comprehensive, systematic, clinical tests of record, conducted in an unbiased atmosphere by an objective, impartial medical team. Such would require controlled dosages in varying amounts—which in turn would require that the plant-derived substances be of a known composition or purity. In other words, the goal would be to find the exact and particular conditions or circumstances that would make the substance work (insofar as possible) and which may vary from individual to individual. Given the existing biases within orthodox medicine, such an effort would take new institutions, hospitals, and clinics, and new teams of doctors and researchers—and independent evaluation. The subject of alternative medicine is not of consuming interest to orthodox medicine and medical research, which seemingly already has its mind made up.

3.3 INVESTIGATIONS IN OTHER COUNTRIES

John Heinerman's book, *The Treatment of Cancer with Herbs,* names species and describes plants and herbal treatments that have been used, not only in the United States but in many other countries. Considering this a given, to this can be added brief information as obtained from the *Amazonia Ethnobotanical Dictionary,* by James Allen Duke and Rudolfo Vasquez, and from other miscellaneous sources. Some further accounts are as follows. The most extensive information probably comes from Asian countries, notably India and in particular China, although Africa is well represented.

For the purposes here, it will be assumed that the herbal folklore of Europe parallels that of the United States, or vice versa, and that Russian and/or Siberian sources remain an enigma, being for the most part secretive or scarcely known. Thus some illustrative information is presented in the following sections, with the exclusion of European and Soviet countries, as noted.

3.3.1 NEO TROPICA

Bioactive plants are closely associated with the rain forests of the New World. In the appendices a few citations pertaining to cancer are shown in Table N.1 of Appendix N for the Central American country of Belize. The information is taken from *Rainforest Remedies: One Hundred Healing Herbs of Belize,* by Rosita Arvigo and Michael Balick. The term *cytotoxic* is used in the reference, evidently meaning that the plants or plant substances are not only toxic to cancer cells but to normal cells as well. The tests were variously conducted on cancer cells *in vitro* and *in vivo.* The New York Botanical Garden was involved, along with other specialists. The resulting survey was part of the activities of what is called The Belize Ethnobotany Project, which in turn helped in the formation of The Belize Association of Traditional Healers and the Terra Nova Rainforest Reserve.

Arvigo and Balick comment that there is not only a loss of habitat, but an extinction of the knowledge of native plants, since the newer generations are less interested in preserving this information. The authors note that, thousands of years ago, the native peoples of Central America had learning centers that taught and coded knowledge about plant medicines. With the arrival of the Spanish conquistadors, these teachings were banned, and in fact the great books (codexes) of the Maya were burned. (In this connection, John Heinerman's book *Healing Secrets of the Maya* can be mentioned. It is out of print and apparently next to impossible to locate.)

Another compilation of interest is Julia F. Morton's extensive *Atlas of Medicinal Plants of Middle America: Bahamas to Yucatan.* The plants noted as having anticancer properties have been excerpted and are listed in Table N.2 of Appendix N. The reference lists many local vernacular names for each species and sometimes furnishes names for some of the chemicals present. For the purposes here, only representative common plant names given in Hartwell are listed. Most of the species in fact are listed in Hartwell. The reference makes the breakdown by plant family but, unfortunately, the plant families are not in alphabetical order.

Another compilation of interest is taken from *Medicinal Plants of the West Indies,* by Edward S. Ayensu. This information is shown in Table N.3 of Appendix N. At the time of writing, neither the *Medicinal Plants of Guiana,* by Robert A. DeFilipps, nor the *Medicinal Plants of Brazil,* by Walter B. Mors, Carlos T. Rizzini, and Nuno A. Pereira, had yet been published.

There are 40 plant species described in *Some medicinal forest plants in Africa and Latin America.* Very few are noted to be anticancer agents, however. A concise listing is furnished in Table N.4 of Appendix N.

3.3.2 AFRICA

Africa is covered in the large volume by John Mitchell Watt and Maria Gerdina Breyer-Brandwijk, titled *The Medicinal and Poisonous Plants of Southern and Eastern Africa: Being an Account of Their Medicinal and Other Uses, Chemical Composition, Pharmacological Effects and Toxicology in Man and Animal,* published in 1962. Cancer is not discussed except as pertaining to lung cancer caused by smoking, that is, by nicotine, tars, and so forth. About every other ailment conceivable receives mention, however, either as caused by a plant substance or as treated by a plant substance, with short case histories that mount up to a massive amount of information. Although division is by plant families, the sheer volume is overwhelming and sometimes contradictory. Nevertheless, there are many insights and information items not readily found elsewhere, such as the alkaloid content of some common vegetables. There is no doubt information pertinent to treating or curing cancer buried within the text, but it will take persistence to find it. Moreover, many or most of the accounts for other ailments are from folklore, and it seems to document as many failures as successes, if not more. The remedies seem to have been taken almost at random. Deaths from plant or herbal poisoning in fact appear commonplace, a warning to the unwary and a paean for modern medicine, whatever its faults. (**Hartwell posts a warning.**)

A foray into this volume was evidently made by John Heinerman, who reports on Africa in his book, *The Treatment of Cancer with Herbs,* and cites the foregoing volume. A successful further search of *The Medicinal and Poisonous Plants of Southern and Eastern Africa* should probably start by using the book's index to check out plant species or genera known or suspected to have anticancer properties, followed by using the volume for documentation, in one way or another, successful or unsuccessful.

Additional information is furnished in the more recent volume *Handbook of African Medicinal Plants,* by Maurice M. Iwu, published in 1993. There seems to be an emphasis not on cancer but rather on other illnesses. Also about African plants is Abayomi Sofowora's *Medicinal Plants and Traditional Medicine in Africa,* which supplies the information about **anticancer plants** that is shown in Table O.1 of Appendix O.

Another compilation of interest is *Medicinal Plants of West Africa,* by Edward S. Ayensu. For the record, a listing of *anticancer plants* obtained from this volume is presented in Table O.2 of Appendix O. Similarly, information from *Medicinal Plants in Tropical West Africa* by Bep Oliver-Bever is shown in Table O.3 of Appendix O.

As to North Africa, there is the volume, *Medicinal Plants of North Africa,* by Loutfy Boulos, of which the anticancer plants cited are listed in Table O.4 of Appendix O. It is informative about how *some of the same anticancer species keep recurring in different countries and regions.*

An account has also been prepared about the plant foods, medicinal plants, and remedies that were brought to this country by the African Americans. By William Ed Grimé of the Field Museum in Chicago, and titled *Ethno-Botany of the Black Americans,* the subject of cancer and cancer treatment is apparently not mentioned.

3.3.3 AUSTRALIA

The volume, *Toxic Plants & Animals: A Guide for Australia,* edited by Jeanette Covacevich, Peter Davie, and John Pearn, describes all sorts of bioactive or toxic sources. Not only are plants listed and described, including mushrooms and toadstools, but marine animals and terrestrial animals as well. Uses for cancer treatment are not a concern in the above-cited reference work, but a listing of toxic plant species is nevertheless of interest. Some toxic plant species are enumerated in Appendix P in alphabetical order by plant family and genera. Some have their counterparts in the United States and elsewhere and have already been listed as anticancer agents.

Besides toxic plants and fungi, Australia is well endowed, both offshore and onshore, with toxic marine animals and toxic terrestrial animals. For instance, some 70 percent of Australia's land snakes are venomous. And *snake venom is from time to time considered a potential anticancer agent, albeit an apparent failure.*

Speaking further of the ocean, the purple Pacific rope sponge has been found to contain a molecule called AS-2, which slows or inhibits cell division and thus conceivably could act against cancer. This is but one of dozens of chemicals occurring in sponges, described by Henry Genthe in the August, 1998 issue of the *Smithsonian.*

In the neighboring island of New Guinea, the spectacular *bird of paradise* has been found to carry a *deadly toxin on its feathers.* (This could be any of a number of species of the family Paradisaeidae.) More specifically, birder and ornithologist Laura Erickson states that the flesh, feathers, and skin of the *hooded pitohui of New Guinea* contain a nerve toxin called homobatrachotoxin, which is identical to that found in poison-dart frogs (Laura Erickson, *For the Birds: An Uncommon Guide,* Pfeifer-Hamilton, Duluth MN,1994, July 26 entry). She further observes that the *pink pigeon of Mauritius*—the only surviving native pigeon on this isolated island in the Indian Ocean—has *toxic flesh.* (And the flesh of ruffed grouse will become toxic after they feed on laurel leaf buds.)

Spiders and spider venom are, of course, an anticancer possibility everywhere. The common daddy longlegs or harvestman, for instance, is found worldwide and is said to be the most venomous of the spiders, meaning also the most bioactive. It remains harmless to humans—but not to other spiders—due to its short fangs. Comprising about 3,400 species worldwide in the temperate and tropical zones, with about 150 species in the U.S. and Canada, it is of the class Arachnida of the invertebrate phylum Arthropoda (the anthropods). The class Arachnida (the arachnids) comprises about 65,000 species overall and includes the orders that are the true spiders (Araneida), the daddy longlegs (Opiliones, sometimes called Phalangida), the scorpions (Scorpionida), and the mites and ticks (Acarina), and so on. An example of the daddy longlegs order is the species *Phalangium opilio* of the family Phalangidae, of Europe and North America, whereas the true spiders include the family Pholcidae, for instance.

This relatively small segment of invertebrate life illustrates the immense possibilities which await further investigation as to medicinal properties. If poisonous translates to bioactive to medicinal, Australia and environs will likely be a fertile ground for future medical research into selective anticancer agents—in trace amounts, of course—and similarly with some other parts of the world.

3.3.4 INDIA AND PAKISTAN

India is quite serious about medicinal plants, but with regard to cancer, no definitive cure has yet surfaced. Nevertheless, the potential exists.

Among the several compilations that have been previously cited, anticancer plants are listed in the two-volume *Medicinal Plants of India,* by S.K. Jain and Robert A. DeFilipps. This information is provided in Table Q.1 of Appendix Q.

The concise volume, *Medicinal Plants of India and Pakistan,* by J.F. Dastur has an appendix classifying plants by their therapeutic uses. Unfortunately, no categories appear for cancers or tumors or for anticancer or antitumor, or for such terms as carcinogens or anticarcinogenic, or malignancies or malignant, or antineoplastic or neoplastic—although the word cancer appears in the glossary of terms. An inspection will yield much other useful information, however, even a notation or two about tumors, and in some instances the particular plant-containing alkaloids are specified. An itemization is provided in Table Q.2 of Appendix Q.

The small volume *Survey and Regeneration of Medicinal Plants in West Pakistan* by M.A. Quaraishi and Mir Alam Khan lists the *alkaloids* of a certain few plants, notably of *Berberis* spp. (of the family Berberidaceae), *Paeonia emodi* (of the family Ranunculaceae), and *Datura* spp. (of the family Solanaceae). Also listed are the active contents of *Valeriana wallichii* (of the family Valerianaceae), *Thymus serpyllum* (of the family Labiatae), *Dioscorea deltoida* (of the family Dioscoreaceae), and *Colchicum luteum* (of the family Liliaceae). All of the families and genera are represented in Hartwell.

Although the information is now outdated, the report on *Medicinal Plants*, edited by Inamul Haq and issued by the Government of Pakistan in 1983, contains interesting statistics about the amounts of medicinal plants collected and sold, not only in Pakistan but in other Asian countries. The figures are impressive. Much of the product is sold in the United States. For example, it was estimated that about *25 percent of all new and refilled prescriptions in the U.S. were for drugs derived from plants. In the Soviet Union, about 30 percent of the drugs were of vegetable origins.* An approximately *equal percentage was prescribed in Italy. In developing countries, 60 to 90 percent of all patients are treated by native healers.* The tonnages are unexpected; for instance the *Soviet Union was producing about 20,000 tons of wild medicinal plants each year, and an equal amount of cultivated plants.* Furthermore, these medicinal plants are used in *allopathic medicines* as well as indigenous herbal systems of medicines. *Specifically, drugs like artemisia, ephedra, dioscorea, glycyrrhiza, senna, rauwolfia serpentina, podophyllum, and valeriana are used in allopathic medicines.*

In the appendices to the report a breakdown is provided for some of the better known drugs or species as follows: *Ammi majus*, belladonna, *citronella java*, geranium, *Mentha piperita*, berberine, diosgenin, *Ergot sclerotium*, hyoscine and atropine, hyoscine hydrochloride, mint oil, menthol, palmarosa oil, pyrethrum, *Pyrethrum oleoresin*, *Rauwolfia serpentina* roots, xanthotoxin. These plants and substances are produced on drug farms and processed in drug factories. The annual production and sales in India at the time was at a level of approximately 1500 tons per year.

Further breakdowns by plant species were also provided in the appendices of the report. *One breakdown listed 198 different plant species by their scientific names.* Needless to say, most of the genera, if not the species, appear in Hartwell.

3.3.5 EAST AND SOUTHEAST ASIA

A number of anticancer plants are described in *Medicinal Plants of East and Southeast Asia: Attributed Properties and Uses*, compiled by Lily M. Perry with the assistance of Judith Metzger, a contribution from the Arnold Arboretum of Harvard University. This information is presented in Appendix R.

3.3.6 CHINA

The volume *Medicinal and Poisonous Plants of the Tropics*, compiled by A.J.M. Leeuwenberg, contains a chapter on "Tropical Plants Used in Chinese Medicine," by Paul Pui-Hay But. There is a section on antineoplastic agents, which includes the following summarized information.

Pigment refuse from the leaf of *Baphicacanthus cusia* yielded *indirubin*, which was active against chronic myelocytic leukemia. *In clinical trials the effective remission rate was 87.3 percent.* The action was similar to that of *busulfan* but was less toxic. The minor constituents named *tryptanthrin* and *qingdainone* were active against melanoma B_{16}. Qingdainone also showed activity against Lewis lung carcinoma in mice.

Quassinoids isolated from the fruit of *Brucea javanica* included *bruceolides, bruceantin,* and *bruceantinol*. These demonstrated inhibitory action against P_{388} lymphomatic leukemia, L_{1210} lymphoid leukemia, Lewis lung carcinoma, and B_{16} melanoma.

The root of *Harrisonia perforata* contains *perforatic acid*. This compound was tested against the incorporation of ^{3}H-TdR into mouse ascites hepatoma cells *in vitro*, the inhibition rate being 91.2 percent.

The rhizome of *Curcuma aromatica* has been used in an emulsion for the clinical treatment of cervix cancer. The active components isolated from the rhizome oil were *curcumol, curdione,* and β-*elemene*.

The cytotoxic germacranolides *molephantin* and *phantomolin* plus the sesquiterpene lactone *molephantinin* were isolated from *Elephantopus mollis* (*E. tomentosus*) and tested on Walker 256 carcinsarcoma in rats. Significant inhibition was obtained.

It was noted that the alkaloid *maytensine* (or *maytansine*) has been undergoing clinical trials in the U.S. It is found in many tropical and subtropical species of *Maytensus* (or *maytenus*) in China.

The two compounds *nitidine chloride* and *6-methoxy-5,6-dihydronitidine*, obtained from the root of *Zanthoxylum cathartica*, showed activity against leukemia L_{1210} and P_{388} in mice. These chemicals also inhibited Lewis lung carcinoma.

Other substances exhibiting antileukemic effects in varying degree were *allamandin* from *Allamanda cathartica*, *asperuloside, paederoside* and *deacetyllasperuloside* from *Hedyotis corymbosa*, *oldenllandoside* from *Oldenlandia diffusa*, and *daphnoretin* from *Wikstroemia indica*.

Medicinal Plants of China, a publication sponsored by the World Health Organization, is more or less a field guide containing photographs and plant descriptions. It is remarked in the preface that *there are more than 7,000 medicinal plant species in China*, of which 150 of the more common have been selected for this volume. Many of the species have their counterpart in the U.S., for instance. The ailments for which each species is used are included. *Cancer is conspicuously absent, at least as such.* The only possible exceptions found are *Brucea javanica* (of the family Simarubaceae) and *Coix lachryma-jobi* (of the family Gramineae) for warts, and *Phytolacca acinosa* (of the family Phytolaccaceae) for malignant boils. (All three of these plant families are represented in Hartwell's *Plants Used Against Cancer*, with the first two species also listed. The genus *Phytolacca* appears, but not the particular species.)

The comprehensive two-volume set *Medicinal Plants of China*, by James A. Duke and Edward S. Ayensu, contains many plant entries for *anticancer agents and cancer*. A listing is provided in Appendix S by plant family and species. Some of the species have their counterparts in other parts of the world. The reference names many of the active chemicals involved, some of which are mentioned in the tabulation.

Additional information about Chinese anticancer agents is furnished in Appendix S, as noted in *The Pharmacology of Chinese Herbs* by Kee Chang Huang, and in *Cancer & Natural Medicine*, by John Boik.

As ever, one has to be impressed with the musical sound, cadence, and rhythm to the scientific names used for the various families, genera, and species. The parties doing the naming certainly had an ear for it.

3.4 PLANT CHEMISTRY AND TAXONOMY

As previously noted in Part 2, and with varying degrees of success, there have been efforts to categorize medicinal plants by the classes of chemical compounds that occur in the different plant families. In particular, Will H. Blackwell has provided a rundown in his book, *Poisonous and Medicinal Plants*, which was reviewed in Part 2. Some of these classifications were further discussed in Part 2, ref. under the subsequent section headings Glycosides, Phenolics, Flavonoids, Proteins and Amino Acids, and Alkaloids.

For classifications below the level of species, the term "infaspecific" is employed, as previously mentioned in Part 2. Thus, Clive A. Stace, in his book *Plant Taxonomy and Biosystematics*, the second edition published in 1989, has a chapter titled "Chemical Information," in which he first speaks synonymously of plant chemotaxonomy, chemosystematics, chemical plant taxonomy, systematics, or phytochemistry. He adds that this is a rapidly expanding field, one that "seeks to utilize chemical information to improve the classification of plants." A related volume is titled *Infraspecific Classification of Wild and Cultivated Plants*, edited by B.T. Styles and published in 1985, a publication which was also noted in Part 2. It is further labeled Special Volume No. 29 of the Systematics Association. The first chapter, by J.G. Hawkes, is on "Infraspecific classification—the problems." Here, we are not so much interested in the problems as how these schemes for chemical classification can be utilized to predict bioactive plants, their selective behavior toward diseases (notably cancer), and their medicinal components.

In this latter context, another and previous effort worthy of mention is by Péter Tétényi, published in English in 1970 as *Infraspecific Chemical Taxa of Medicinal Plants*. (In this work, as has been previously emphasized, "infraspecific" refers to plant classifications below the levels of species, with the chemical compositions as yet imperfectly utilized for the distinguishing or differentiating criteria.) There will be the occasion to refer to Tétényi's work in considerable detail.

Under "General Remarks" in the latter half of his book, Tétényi presents the following scheme for bioactive agents:

1. Terpenes and related compounds
    1.1 Terpene compounds; sesquiterpene lactones
    1.2 Terpenoids (triterpenes, steroids, saponins, cardenoids)
    1.3 Pseudoalkaloids
2. Other compounds connected with acetate metabolism
    2.1 Derivatives of resorcin, of orcellanic acid; phloroglucins; ranunculin
    2.2 Quinones
3. Derivatives of phenylpropane and flavonoids
    3.1 Simple phenolics; phenylpropane compounds; coumarins; stilbenes; amidic acrids
    3.2 Flavonoids
4. Alkaloids
    4.1 Protoalkaloids
    4.2 Alkaloids proper
5. Isorhodoanidogenes

Tétényi was able to match these classes of compounds with plant families and species. The listing of the particular plant families for each phyla are shown in Table 3.4 for the six phyla involved, a phylum being a major division of the vegetable (or animal) kingdom. The table is labeled "Taxa with Infraspecific Chemical Differentiation," meaning that these plant families can also be distinguished or differentiated from one another by the classes of compounds which occur within each plant family as well as by the purely botanical characteristics.

The plant families of Table 3.4 which do **not** appear in Jonathan L. Hartwell's *Plants Used Against Cancer* are denoted by an asterisk. It may be observed that most of Hartwell's listings occur in the angiosperms, and in turn angiosperms are generally associated with the occurrence of alkaloids or vice versa.

As to specific plant families and species for each chemical classification, a breakdown is provided in Appendix T based on the presentation in Tétényi's book. Particular examples of compounds are furnished for each species.

Another advocacy for the role of chemical taxa is embodied in the book *Plants in the Development of Modern Medicine*, edited by Tony Swain and published in 1972. It was the result of a symposium sponsored by the Botanical Museum of Harvard University and the American Academy of Arts and Sciences, previously held in 1968. As acknowledged by Paul C. Mangelsdorf in the Introduction, instead of declining in importance, drugs derived from plants are of renewed and continuing interest. In a chapter on "Plants as Sources of Biodynamic Compounds," Richard Evans Schultes commented at the time that

Table 3.4 Taxa with Infraspecific Chemical Differentiation[a]

Mycophyta

Agraricaceae* Sphaerioldaceae*	Aspergillaceae*	Clavicipitaceae*

Lichenophyta

Cladoniaceae* Lecanoraceae* Parmeliaceae*	Peltigeraceae* Rocellaceae* Strictaceae*	Usneaceae*

Bryophyta

Grimaldiaceae*	Mniaceae*

Pteridophyta

Aspidiaceae* Aspleniaceae*	Equisetaceae Lycopodiaceae	Polypodiaceae

Gymnospermatophyta

Cupressaceae* Ephedraceae*	Pinaceae Podocarpaceae*	Taxodiaceae*

Angiospermatophyta

Agavaceae*	Ericaceae	Mimosaceae* (Leguminosae)
Amaranthaceae	Erythoxylaceae	Monimiaceae*
Amaryllidaceae	Euphorbiaceae	Moraceae
Apiaceae*	Eupomatiaceae*	Myoporaceae*
Apocynaceae	Eupteleaceae*	Myristicaceae
Araceae	Fabaceae* (Leguminosae)	Myrsinaceae
Aristolochiceae	Fumariaceae*	Myrtaceae
Asclepiadaceae	Geraniaceae	Nyctaginaceae
Asteraceae* (Compositae)	Gramineae	Oxalidaceae
Berberidaceae	Grossulariaceae*	Papaveraceae
Betulaceae	Hamamelidaceae	Piperaceae
Brassicaceae* (Cruciferae)	Helleboraceae*	Polemoniaceae
Burseraceae	Hernandiaceae	Polygonaceae
Buxaceae	Himantandraceae*	Ranunculaceae
Caesalpiniaceae*	Hypericaceae*	Rosaceae
Cannabiaceae* (Moraceae)	Juglandiaceae	Rubiaceae
Capparidaceae	Lamiaceae*	Rutaceae
Caryophyllaceae	Lardizabalaceae	Sapindaceae
Celastraceae	Lauraceae	Scrophulariaceae
Chenopodiaceae	Lemnaceae	Simaroubaceae
Convolvulaceae	Liliaceae	Solanaceae
Corynocarpaceae*	Limanthaceae*	Theaceae
Crassulaceae	Lobeliaceae	Valerianaceae
Cucurbitaceae	Loganiaceae	Verbenaceae
Cyperaceae	Magnoliaceae	Winteraceae
Dioscoreaeceae	Malvaceae	Zingiberaceae
Dipsacaceae	Meliaceae	Zygophyllaceae
Dipterocarpaceae	Menispermaceae	

a. From *Infraspecific Chemical Taxa of Medicinal Plants,* by Péter Tétényi, pp. 192–193. There are six phyla with 106 plant families containing about 750 species. Plant families **not** appearing in Hartwell's *Plants Used Against Cancer* are denoted by an asterisk. Incidentally, Hartwell lists 214 families, comprising 1430 genera and approx. 3000 species.

the "plant kingdom may have as many as 250,000 to 350,000 species," with the following approximate distribution (Schultes, in *Plants in the Development of Modern Medicine*, p. 106ff.):

Algae	18,000 species
Bacteria and fungi	90,000
Bryophytes	20,000
Pteridophytes	9,000
Gymnosperms	675 species in 63 genera
Angiosperms	200,000 species in some 10,000 genera and 300 families

As a comparison, Hartwell's *Plants Used Against Cancer* lists 214 families (mostly angiosperms) containing 1,430 genera, but only about 3,000 species. Tétényi, cited above, lists 106 plant families and about 750 species. As Tétényi noted in his conclusions, there is a long way to go in providing the full range of chemical taxa.

Schultes believed these estimates are low, subsequently revised the figures upward, and mentioned a number more like *500,000 species for the angiosperms alone,* a resource with tremendous phytochemical potential. At the same time, he indicates that the principal drug-yielding families of the angiosperms had been obtained from a survey of one billion prescriptions written in 1967. This information is shown in Table 3.5 in decreasing order. Incidentally, all of these plant families are represented in Hartwell's *Plants Used Against Cancer.*

Table 3.5   Principal Drug-Yielding Families of Angiosperms[a]

Dioscoriaceae	Rutaceae	Rhamnaceae	Gramineae
Papaveraceae	Rubiaceae	Caricaceae	Leguminosae
Solanaceae	Liliaceae	Plantaginaceae	Umbelliferae
Scrophulariaceae	Bromeliaceae	Sterculiaceae	Ericaceae

a. From Richard Evans Schultes in *Plants in the Development of Modern Medicine*, p. 109. The listing is in decreasing order of importance. All these plant families are listed in Hartwell's *Plants Used Against Cancer.*

Schultes was particularly keen on the phytochemical research being directed toward alkaloids in the angiosperms. He noted that about *94 percent of the alkaloids occur in the angiosperms,* with the remaining 6 percent in all other plant groups. For the record, these other nonangiospermous plant groups are the Agaricaceae, Hypocreaceae, Fungi, Algae, Cycadaceae, Equisetaceae, Lycopodiaceae, Pinaceae, Gnetaceae, and Taxaceae.

The angiosperms, in turn, are divided into the *monocotyledons* and the *dicotyledons* (a cotyledon is the first leaf, or one in the first pair of leaves, in a whorl). The monocotyledon families richest in *alkaloids* are the related Amaryllidaceae and Liliaceae. There is a greater distribution of *alkaloids* among the dicotyledons, a distribution which will assuredly increase as more plants are studied and analyzed.

Next in importance to the alkaloids as biodynamic or bioactive compounds, or toxic compounds, are the several classes of *glycosides.* They may, in fact, prove even more widespread than the alkaloids, with the *cardiac glycosides* and *genins* perhaps the most valuable, and which are concentrated mostly in Apocynaceae, Asclepiadaceae, Liliaceae, Moraceae, Ranunculaceae, and Scrophulariaceae. The classes and subclasses include such designators as *cardenolides,* used as arrow poisons and ordeal poisons, and steroidal *sapogenins.* The latter are most conspicuous in the genera *Agave, Yucca,* and *Discorea. Flavonoids* are another group or class of interest, of which *rutin* is the most important example, with antiviral and cytotoxic effects also occurring within this group of compounds.

The reference notes that *many other categories of bioactive plants exist within the angiosperms.* For instance, at the time of writing, there were considerably *more than 2,000 known organic structure categories exclusive of the alkaloid-glycoside classification.* These include what are known as *terpenoids, coumarins, anthraquinones, phenolics such as tannins, essential oils,* and so on.

The search and the work continue in what is referred to as ethnobotany and ethnopharmacology, although anthropology, linguistics, history, sociology, comparative and religion also enter—as well as a mix of botany, chemistry, and pharmacology. Surveys have been conducted in Australia and New Zealand, Borneo and Papua, Malaya, Hawaii, Taiwan, Brazil, Colombia, and Russia, not to mention the United

States and Europe. Some of the specific results relating chemical compounds to cancer will be further presented in the next sections.

Tony Swain, the editor of *Plants in the Development of Modern Medicine*, has a chapter on "The Significance of Comparative Phytochemistry." Swain's treatment of the subject observes that phytochemistry or plant chemistry, also called chemotaxonomy, *chemical taxonomy,* or biological systematics as well as chemical taxa, is further explained as *the study of the distribution of chemical compounds in plants.* In turn, it involves the biochemical operations that occur in the biosynthesis and metabolism of these compounds. (Metabolism here meaning the bioreactions in which these compounds take part.) Although ancillary to other more fundamental subjects, it is nevertheless of importance in a consideration of drugs or medicines as well as foods. As to the former, folklore ascribes to many, many more plants as drugs than as foods.

The reference makes the point that these *medicinal substances are secondary metabolites;* that is, they are not major reactants or metabolites in the fundamental processes of glycolysis and the carboxylic acid cycle in the manner that say glucose is involved. Nevertheless, they can be said to play a regulatory role in that they serve to control the (enzyme-catalyzed) conversions of primary metabolism as well as other body functions. (In other words, these secondary metabolites function as enzyme inhibitors or promoters.)

The well known fact is also mentioned that *plants of the same species may contain widely differing amounts of bioactive substances* (Swain, in *Plants in the Development of Modern Medicine*, p. 139). Thus, for example, *Rauvolfia vomitoria* grown in the Congo may have ten times as much reserpine as plants that grow in neighboring Uganda.

It is noted that the main groups of simple secondary compounds can be regarded as derived from only four elementary precursors (Swain, in *Plants in the Development of Modern Medicine*, p. 142ff). These four precursors are *acetate, shikimate,* and the two diamino acids *lysine* and *ornithine. Acetate* is the progenitor of such classes of compounds as antibiotics, flavonoids, terpenoids, sterols, sapogenins, steroidal alkaloids, and cardiac glycosides. *Shikimate* leads to the amino acids phenylalanine, tyrosine, and tryptophan, and in turn to hordenine and mescaline, or to such isoquinoline alkaloids as papaverine, berberine, morphine, and cochine—and by different routes, to indole alkaloids such as psilocybin and yohimbine, or to cinnamic acids, coumarins, and lignin, or to flavonoids, or to gallic acid and tannic acid or tannins.

The diamino acids *lysine* and *ornithine* are precursors to a number of simple *alkaloids*. Ornithine gives rise to nicotine, cocaine, and the necine alkaloids; lysine results in such alkaloids as anabasine, pseudopelletierine, and the lupinine and sparteine alkaloids.

Although these classes of compounds are found in various plant families, and may be so correlated, the present knowledge of comparative phytochemistry is of little predictive value (Swain, in *Plants in the Development of Modern Medicine*, p. 155). And although general compound classes may be assigned to one family or another, a minor structural difference can render the substance either ineffective or else toxic. However, an example of a success story is the isolation of the *anticancer agent aristolochic acid* from *Asarum canadense* of the family Aristolochiaceae, in that this compound had previously been found in several species of the genus *Aristolochia* of the same family.

Rudolf Hänsel, in a chapter on "Medicinal Plants and Empirical Research" in *Plants in the Development of Modern Medicine*, offers a few specific examples of drugs that have their origins in natural plants.

Foxglove, Digitalis purpurea of the family Scrophulariaceae, was introduced into modern medicine on account of its prior use as a heart stimulant in medical folklore.

Snakeroot, Rauwolfa serpentina or *Rauvolfa serpentina* of the family Apocynaceae, was a source of long-standing use as a hypotensive agent. But when it appeared that the whole of India could not supply the demand for the roots, and the Indian government banned its export, there was a search for new supplies of the alkaloids. It turned out that the African species *R. vomitoria* served equally well.

The search for steroidal *sapogenins* furnishes another example. Widely distributed in the plant kingdom, there are two types of sapogenins. The one type consists of the triterpene sapogenins, which have a C-30 compound as the aglycone part of the structure. The other type consists of steroidal sapogenins, which have a C-27 skeleton as the genin part of the structure. The latter, the steroidal sapogenins, are extensively used as the starting point in the synthesis of certain hormones, mostly of the cortisone type. At first, these steroidal sapogenins were found in only a very few plant families, but phytochemical screening extended the list of sources for both triterpene and steroidal sapogenins. It was found, for instance, that steroidal sapogenins occur in several families of the monocotyledons, whereas their occurrence is only within the genus *Digitalis* in the dicotyledons.

A further example concerns the distribution of *alkaloids* and *cardenolides* within a single plant family.* The plant family *Apocynaceae* is a notable case, containing the genera *Rauwolfa* and *Catharanthius*, which have *alkaloids*, and the genera *Strophanthus*, *Thevetia*, and *Nerium*, which have *cardenolides*. (Only *Rauwolfa* or *Rauvolfa* is not listed in Hartwell.) A taxonomic examination provides an indication of which family members may be most productive, based on such morphological characteristics as the type of fruit, and so on.

The *Aponynaceae* can be further divided into the subfamilies of the Cerberoideae, the Echitoideae, and the Plumerioideae, each having its own distinctive tribes and genera. The reference observes that *cardioglycosides* occur only in species of the Echitoideae, *indole alkaloids* occur only in species of the Plumerioideae, and *piperidine-derived* nitrogenous compounds occur only in species of the Cerboideae. Since many of the members of the Apocynaceae tend to be toxic, the taxonomic characteristics can be used to determine the source of the toxicity—that is, whether by nitrogen-containing indole bases or by glycosidic cardenolides. At the time of writing, nearly 600 different alkaloids had been found in the Plumerioideae, with about 300 identified with certainty, and which were all indole bases of a certain kind. These 300 or so alkaloids can in turn be classed into eight different types. Thus, it can be said that the alkaloids within the subfamily Plumerioideae fit into eight different classifications. The reference notes, however, that the division within the lower echelons—among the tribes, genera, and species—is not so obliging.

Also taken up in the reference is the subject of the correlation between pharmacological activity and physical (and chemical) properties. These physical (and chemical) properties may include basicity, lipophilic nature, bitter taste, anomalies in chemical composition, and so forth. The indication of *basicity or alkalinity* (as opposed to *acidity*) is of notable interest in that it is a property particularly of alkaloids, and in fact was involved in the original discovery of morphine. The reference provides the comment that the theoretical reason for this correlation between basicity and pharmacological action is not known; it is merely an empirical conclusion. However, the observation is further provided that *alkaloids are soluble in both water and lipids (fats),* and this is a fundamental physicochemical requirement for the transport of alkaloids to places of action within the body. This *solubility may be a factor in why alkaloids are so physiologically active.*

Speaking further of solubility, plant constituents or compounds ordinarily display different degrees of solubility between water and lipids, which may be measured in terms of a distribution coefficient, the one to the other. This, in turn, may be related to the excretion of metabolic end products. One such mechanism proposed is where a metabolic end product couples with a sugar (e.g., glucose) residue, making it more soluble in the cellular fluids, thereby aiding in its removal. Another mechanism is that in which a metabolic product dissolves in lipids and is stored in special excretory organelles for ultimate expulsion. Some metabolites will favor the first route and may be referred to as being more strongly hydrophilic; some will favor the latter route and can be called more strongly lipophilic. *Substances that are more strongly lipophilic tend to be more pharmacologically active.* The reference furnishes a few examples.

The class of compounds called *coumarins* occur in plants as either hydroxy- and methoxy-derivatives or their corresponding glycosides. In these states, they tend to be hydrophilic. In the form of nonglycosidic compounds, however, and substituted with lipophilic groups such as isoprene residues and furano-linked rings, they are instead lipophilic. (The peculiarly smelling compound furan, C_4H_4O, was originally obtained from wood tar.) Furano-coumarins cause photosensitivity, whereas lipiphilic coumarins stimulate the central nervous system (CNS). Coumarin itself, however, has a sedating action. It is noted that, at the time, more than 100 coumarin derivatives had been prepared synthetically.

There is a well known Polynesian drug called *kawa* which has active compounds called kawa lactones, with such names as methysticin, dihydromethysticin, and kawain. These compounds belong to a group

---

* For the record, a *cardenolide* is a digitaloid lactone, related to cholesterol, a lactone being an anhydro cyclic ester formed by the elimination of water from a hydroxy acid molecule. The Sigma catalog lists cardenolides as being obtained from the species *Calotropis procera*. This species is of the family Asclepiadaceae, is native to southern Asia and Africa, and was later introduced into South America and the Caribbean islands. The seed floss is downy and fibrous and sometimes called akund floss or calotropis floss. It has been used for upholstery stuffing, sometimes along with the seed fibers called kapok.

of plant constituents called the α-pyrones, which are localized in plant lipoidal cells (fat-like cells). The kawa-lactones act on the CNS, as might be expected.

Flavonoids, discussed in Part 2, occur in plants as hydrophilic or water-soluble glycosides in the cells or as alkylated lipophilic derivatives. (An alkyl group is a hydrocarbon group, that is, is composed of carbon and hydrogen.) The juice from *citrus fruit flesh contains flavonoids* in the form of glycosides of a kind called hesperedin-eriodictyol type. There is also a volatile oil present as a separate phase or lipophilic fraction which contains excretory cells. This oily phase yields a different kind of flavonoid, being of the nobiletin-tangerine type. Both groups of flavonoids have been found to act as a vitamin P factor, producing an anti-inflammatory action. Glycosides per se show no such activity, but *lipophilic flavonoids achieve the activity of hydrocortisone.* There is a apparently correlation between the lipoic or lipophilic nature of these compounds and their pharmacological activity. A similar correlation exists with regard to toxicity, the lipophilic substance being the more toxic. In fact the *lipophilic compounds regarded as what are called chalkones and flavones serve as insecticides and fish poisons.* If, however, hydroxy groups are attached to the molecule, the chalkones and flavones then become water soluble—and are then harmless.

The *Colchicum* species of the family Liliaceae contain the alkaloid *colchicine.* Among other things it has been used in the treatment of *gout* but unfortunately has a high general toxicity. If a methoxy group in the molecular structure is replaced by a hydroxy group, however, the toxicity is reduced. If the hydroxy group is then linked to a sugar molecule, a compound named *colchicoside* is produced, which is *less toxic* still, being only slightly poisonous. (The reference does not comment on whether the bioactivity is also reduced.)

The reference concludes that the number of compounds isolated from plants is much smaller the number of synthetic compounds, possibly of the order of 1/100. Nevertheless, continuing discoveries suggest that the pharmacological studies of the plant kingdom are nowhere at an end. And although many scientists would prefer to put drug research on a more theoretical basis, the empirical mode must suffice in the meantime.

For an encyclopedic compilation of plant species and their chemicals or phytochemicals, there is James A. Duke's *Handbook of Phytochemical Constituents of GRAS Herbs and Their Activities,* which will be referred to further in Part 4, in connection with alkaloids. (The acronym GRAS denotes *generally recommended as safe.*) Also of interest is Duke's *Handbook of Biologically Active Phytochemicals and Their Activities,* which will be referenced in Part 8. And there is, of course, *Hager's Handbuch der Pharmazeutischen Praxis* in its many editions.

3.5 TOXIC/MEDICINAL SUBSTANCES AND CANCER

For starters, an inspection of Julia F. Morton's *Major Medicinal Plants* yields the information presented in Table 3.6, with some of the plant compounds included. In fact, most of the popular herbs have at one time or another been viewed as anticancer agents, as indicated in Table 3.7. Not only this, but some few of what we think of as edible weeds also have anticancer properties. This sort of information has been assembled by James A. Duke in the *Handbook of Edible Weeds* and is presented in Table 3.8.

An informative booklet about some common herbal remedies and their principal bioactive chemical components is Daniel B. Mowery's *Proven Herbal Blends,* condensed from his *The Scientific Validation of Herbal Medicine,* with references furnished. Described as acting against cancer are burdock root (*Arctium lappa* of the family Compositae), kelp (genus *Laminaria* of the algae family Laminariaceae, plus *Macrocytes* and *Ascophyllum*), alfalfa (*Medicago sativa* of the family Leguminosae), chamomile flowers (*Matricaria chamomilla* of the family Compositae), and chaparral (*Larrea divaricata* of the family Zygophyllaceae) for skin cancers as well as other cancers (Mowery, *Proven Herbal Blends*, pp. 7, 9, 12, 16, 19, 31, 37). All are listed in Hartwell.

For the record, Mrs. M. Grieve's comprehensive *A Modern Herbal* may also be consulted. In the nature of a systems approach, further comprehensive information has been provided by S. Morris Kupchan in a chapter on "Recent Advances in the Chemistry of Tumor Inhibitors of Plant Origin," in *Plants and the Development of Modern Medicine,* published in 1972. Although now dated, Kupchan, furnishes some of the initial results gained courtesy of the Cancer Chemotherapy National Service Center (CCNSC) of the National Institutes of Health. Even then, the work had been underway for two decades. Kupchan in particular stresses the work performed at his laboratory at the University of Virginia, which was supported by grants from the National Cancer Institute. His program at the Department of Chemistry at the University of Virginia started in 1959.

The work and results are systematically categorized by classes of compounds and are summarized in Table 3.9. Chemical structural formulas are provided for many of the compounds tested or involved, but they will not be reproduced here.

Table 3.6   Some Major Medicinal Plants as Anticancer Agents[a]

Apocynaceae	*Catharantheus* roseus*: periwinkle. Said to contains 73 alkaloids including reserpine, alstonine, and an alkaloid called ajmalicine, vincein, or vincaine, found mainly in the root, and said to be identical to δ-yohimbine. Contains the alkaloid vincaleukoblastine or vinblastine ($C_{46}H_{58}N_4O_9$) and the alkaloid leukocristine or vincristine ($C_{46}H_{56}N_4O_{10}$). Both are used in the sulfate form as chemotherapy drugs (presumably a patentable form, whereas the naturally occurring substance isn't). The former compound is used for Hodgkin's disease and choriocarcinoma. The latter is used mainly for childhood leukemia and breast cancer. In addition to alkaloids, the leaves produce an oil which contains a variety of other compounds, namely aldehydes, sesquiterpenes, furfurals, sulfurous compounds, an alcohol called lochnerol, monoterpene glycosides such as adenosine and roseoside, and deoxyloganin and loganin. *The reference notes that the prolongued chemotherapeutic administration of Catharanthus alkaloids has the usual noticeable side effects such as hair loss, nausea, dermatitis, and depression, plus blood platelet damage. Excessive dosage will damage the central nervous system (CNS), and can lead to death.*
Caricaceae	*Carica papaya*: papaya. Latex contains apain, which in turn contains the enzymes amylase, lipase, pectase, etc. Used to remove skin cancers.
Dioscoreaceae	*Dioscorea compositae* *: Mexican yam. Contains a saponin from which is derived the sapogenin known as diosgenin, which in turn is used to derive steroid drugs such as esterogens (used for prostate cancer).
Liliaceae	*Colchicum speciosum**: a different species of autumn crocus. Native to Asia Minor, Syria, Lebanon, and Iran. Contains the alkaloids colchicine, demecoline, and 3-desmethylcolchicine. The last-mentioned alkaloid is antileukemic and is cytotoxic.
Podophyllaceae*	*Podophyllum peltatum*: may apple, mandrake. Contains the resin called (Berberidaceae) podophyllum, which contains lignan glycosides such as podophyllotoxin, which yields podophyllic acid and picropodophyllin. Toxic, anticancer.

a. From *Major Medicinal Plants,* by Julia F. Morton. Plant families, general, or species **not** in Hartwell's *Plants Used Against Cancer* are denoted by an asterisk.

Regarding the genus *Catharanthus*, the anticancer properties of members of theis well known genus of the family Apocynaceae have been reported upon elsewhere. Additional information has been furnished by Norman R. Farnsworth in a chapter titled The Phytochemistry and Biological Activity of *Catharanthus lanceus*, which appears in *Plants in the Development of Modern Medicine*, published in 1972.

It is stated that there are six distinct species, listed as *C. roseus, C. lanceus, C. trichophyllus, C. longifolius, C. pusillus*, and *C. scitulus*. Although the genus is sometimes called *Vinca* or *Lochnera*, the name *Catharanthus* is now considered the more correct nomenclature. The species *C. roseus* is pantropical, the species *C. pusillus* is native to India, and the remaining species all occur in Madagascar.

Medicinal activity is attributed mainly to vincaleukoblastine (also called vinblastine or VLB) and to leurocristine (also called vincristine or VCR). These alkaloids are found in *C. roseus*. There are, however, four other alkaloids that show anticancer activity, out of the many which have been found in this same species (a reported 66 at the time of publication, but now expanded). These other alkaloids are variously named leurosine (also called vinleurosine or VLR), leurosidine (also called vinrosidine), leurosivine, and rovidine.

Farnsworth attempts to expand this base of knowledge to the alkaloids occurring in the species *C. lanceus*. Although he notes that folklore does not attribute any anticancer properties to this particular species, the species is given a try. Although *C. lanceus* contains nonalkaloids such as choline, the alkaloids

Table 3.7 Twenty-Five Most Popular Herbs[a]

Aquifoliaceae	*Ilex paraguensis**: **mate** or **maté**. Contains caffeine.
Araliaceae	*Panax schinseng* or *P. ginseng* (China) or *P. quinquefolium** (North America): **ginseng**. May cause the gensing abuse syndrome.
Asteraceae (Compositae)	*Anthemis nobilis*: **camomile** or **chamomile**. May affect those hypersensitive to ragweed pollen.
Boraginaceae	*Symphytum officinale*: **comfrey**. Contains lasiocarpine (a pyrrolizidine alkaloid), etc.
Caesalpiniaceae*	*Ceratonia* siliqua*: **carob**.
Chichoriaceae*	*Chichorium* intybus*: **chicory**.
Fabaceae* (Leguminosae)	*Glycyrrhiza glabra*: **licorice**. Raises blood pressure. (Licorice root contains glycyrrhizin, which is said to be fifty tines sweeter than sucrose or ordinary table sugar. Unfortunately, glycyrrhizin is also a cardioglucoside. Licorice-flavored candy either uses anise as flavoring or artificial flavors.) *Medicago sativa*: **alfalfa**. Contains saponins. *Trifolium pratense*: **red clover tops**. Contains estrogens. *Trigonella foenum-graecum*: **fenugreek**. Contains coumarins.
Gramineae (or Poaceae)	*Cymbopogon* citratus* or *C.* flexuosus*: **lemongrass**. (What is called lemon balm is derived from *C. nardus*.)
Labiatae (or Lamiaceae)	*Mentha piperita*: **peppermint**. *Mentha spicata*: **spearmint**. *Salvia officinalis*: **sage**. *Thymus vulgaris*: **thyme**.
Liliaceae	*Allium sativa*: **garlic**. Lowers blood pressure. *Smilax*: **sarsaparilla**.
Malvaceae	*Hibiscus*: **hibiscus**.
Rosaceae	*Prunus pennsylvanica** or *P. emarginata**: **wild cherry bark**. Contains cyanogenic glucosides. *Rosa*: **rose hips**. *Rubus strigosus**: **raspberry leaves**.
Rutaceae	*Citrus sinensis*: **orange peel**.
Solanaceae	*Capsicum annuum*: **cayenne**.
Umbelliferae	*Foeniculum vulgare*: **fennel seed**. *Petroselinum crispum*: **parsley**. Contains the alkaloid myristicine.

a. From the Introduction of *CRC Handbook of Medicinal Herb,* by James A. Duke. Taken from figures once supplied by the former Herb Trade Association. As fashions change, so no doubt will the popularity. Plant families, genera, or species **not** listed in Hartwell's *Plants Used Against Cancer* are denoted by an asterisk.

present are of primary interest. Some 21 alkaloids were isolated, including leurosine, which is recognized for having anticancer activity as reported above.*

---

* Under the family Apocynaceae, Hartwell lists both *Vinca major* and *Vinca minor* without any further distinction. Whether, say, one is *C. roseus* and the other *C. lanceus*, or vice versa, is not indicated. The genus *Catharanthus* is not represented as such. Cordell, published in 1981, speaks of the genus *Vinca* as different from the genus *Catharanthus* (Cordell, *Introduction to Alkaloids*, pp. 790–791). Moreover, Cordell attributes six species to the genus *Vinca*, the same number as for the genus *Catharanthus*. Furthermore, the *Vinca* alkaloids are said to exhibit no anticancer activity and have such names as vincamine, hervine, reserpinine, sarpagine, vincamajine, strictamine, tabersonine, and vincadine. None is dimeric as is the case for *Catharanthus* alkaloids.

Table 3.8 Edible Weeds as Anticancer Agents[a]

Asteraceae* (Compositae)	*Arctium minus*: common burdock. *Chrysanthemum leucanthemum*: oxeye daisy. *Cichorium* intypus*: chicory. *Cirsium* spp.: thistles.
Brassicaceae* (Cruciferae)	*Nasturtium officinale*: watercress.
Cyperaceae	*Cyperus* spp.: nutgrass, rush, papyrus.
Ebenaceae	*Diosporos virginiana*: common persimmon.
Fabaceae* (Leguminosae)	*Medicago lupulina**: black medis, nonesuch. *Trifolium pratense*: red clover.
Lamiaceae* (Labiatae)	*Prunella vulgaris*: healall.
Liliaceae	*Hemerocallis fulva**: tawny daylily.
Nymphaeaceae	*Nymphaea odorata*: fragrant waterlily.
Oxalidaceae	*Oxalis* spp.: wood sorrel, sourgrass.
Plantaginaceae	*Plantago major*: plantain.
Poaceae* (Gramineae)	*Agropyron repens*: quackgrass. *Arundo donax*: giant reed. *Echinochloa crus-galli*: barnyard grass. *Hordeum jubatum**: foxtail barley, squirreltail. *Phragmites communis*: common reed.

a. From *Handbook of Edible Weeds,* by James A. Duke. Plant families, genera, or species **not** listed in Hartwell's *Plants Used Against Cancer* are denoted by an asterisk.

In the antitumor tests performed by Farnsworth at the time, the results were a mixed bag. The source of activity was considered to be the alkaloids present in the leaves, as is the case for *C. roseus*. However, the leaf extract fractions showed varied activity, acting against some cancers but not others. In particular, the known anticancer agent leurosine was in high concentrations in the fraction tested, and yohimbine was also present, yet this fraction did not exhibit anticancer activity. Thus, Farnsworth reports, "We are unable to explain with any degree of certainty *how an active antitumor alkaloid can be isolated from a crude fraction which has been shown to be devoid of activity.*"

Of the 21 alkaloids isolated, 19 were monomeric indoles, and two were dimeric indoles. Ordinarily, only the latter display anticancer activity. However, all the leaf extract fractions showed cytotoxic activity, which is an indication of sorts for anticancer activity. But such are the inconsistencies in the test results obtained that anything may be possible. It was observed, furthermore, that some of the alkaloids proved to be antiviral.

If anything, the foregoing exercise indicates how imperfect or capricious testing can be. For instance, though leurosine tested out as having anticancer properties, clinical tests were said to be disappointing. And in other instances, the situation may be the other way around.

3.6 A CHINESE PROTOCOL

There is a small but interesting volume from Chinese sources titled *Studies on Chinese Medical Plants and Cancer,* by Wong Kin Keung, and published in Hong Kong in 1991. It observes that Chinese medicines are divided into two main classes, those from *inorganic ingredients,* and those from *organic ingredients.*

The inorganic substances consist mainly of, or are derived from, sulfuric acid (H_2SO_4), phosphoric acid (H_3PO_4), silicic acid (H_2SiO_3), hydrochloric acid (HCl), sodium (Na), potassium (K), calcium (Ca),

Table 3.9   Some Tumor Inhibitors of Plant Origin[a]

Steroidal Derivatives	
Buxaceae	*Buxus sempervirens*: box. *In vitro* cytotoxic and *in vivo* antitumor properties were shown in laboratory animals. The plant contained 3,20-diamines such as cycloprotobuxine-C which showed both kinds of activity, whereas monoamines such as cyclobuxoxine showed only cytotoxic activity.
Cucurbitaceae	*Marah* oreganus*: western wild cucumber. The specimens tested were from California, and contained four previously known cucurbitans.
Solanaceae	*Acnistus arborescens*: belladonna. The plants tested were forwarded from Costa Rica. The active principle turned out to be witheraferin A, the prototype for a novel class of polyfunctional steroid lactones.
Solanaceae	*Solanum dulcamara*: bittersweet, cancer plant. This species, collected near Madison WI, was one of the first studied. The tumor inhibitory principle is the steroid alkaloid glycoside β-solamarine. It is noted that this plant has been used to treat cancers, tumors, and warts since the time of Galen (circa A.D. 180), and references appear in the literature of many countries.
Isoquinoline and Other Alkaloids	
Menispermaceae	*Cyclea* peltata*. Contains the alkaloid tetrandine, which acts against the Walker carcinoma 256.
Ranunculaceae	*Thalictrum dasycarpum**: purple meadow rue. The specimens were collected in Wisconsin and contained the alkaloid thalicarpine. Thalicarpine shows significant action against the Walker intramuscular carcinoma 256 in rats. Also contains thalidasine, a bisbenzylisoquinoline alkaloid.
Solanaceae	*Solanum tripartitum**. An extract from Bolivia yielded the novel liquid alkaloids solapalmitine and solapalmitenine. The extract was tumor inhibiting.
Sesquiterpenoid Lactones and Other Compounds	
Compositae	*Elephantopus elatus**. The antitumor principles are elephantin and elephantopin, which have sesquiterpene dilactone structures.
Compositae	*Eupatorium rotundifolium**. Contains the anticancer agents euparotin and euparotin acetate. Further studies yielded eupachlorin acetate and five other cytotoxic sesquiterpene lactones.
Compositae	*Vernonia hymenolepsis**. Contains tumor-inhibiting vernolepin, a sesquiterpene dilactone. It also inhibits plant growth.
Euphorbiaceae	*Croton macrostachys**. The anticancer principle proved to be crotepoxide, a compound which exhibits the cyclohexane diepoxide structure.
Cardenolides	
Apocynaceae	*Apocynum cannabinum**. Contains the cytotoxic cardenolide glycosides apocannoside and cymarin. It was noted that the activity of cardenolides as cytotoxic agents, cardiotonic agents, and ATPase inhibitors was due to what is called Ring A in the chemical structure.
Asclepiadaceae	*Asclepias currassavica**. Contains cytotoxic calotropin, plus the cardenolide glycosides apocannoside and cymarin.
	Bersama* abyssinica: This plant, from Ethiopia, contains hellebrigenin 3-acetate and hellebrigenin 3,5-diacetate, which function as the antitumor agents. Derivatives of these compounds are strong inhibitors for the enzyme ATPase.

a. From S. Morris Kupchan in *Plants and the Development of Modern Chemistry*, edited by Tony Swain. Plant families, general, or species **not** in Hartwell's *Plants Used Against Cancer* are denoted by an asterisk.

magnesium (Mg), iron (Fe), mercury (Hg), copper (Cu), and lead (Pb), and so on. The biggest surprises are probably mercury and lead, since these two elements and their compounds are ordinarily regarded as toxic.

The organic substances in plants are divided into the following classes of compounds, some of which are considered toxic and some not. The particular parts of the plant where these tend to occur is included.

Alkaloids—leaves, stems, rhizomes, peels, juices of cells

Glucosides or glycosides—roots, green leaves, stems, peels, flowers, seeds

Saponins—roots, aerial stems, green leaves, seeds

Flavones—consists of coloring matter in aerial stems, subterranean stems, leaves, flowers, seeds, fruits

Emodin (a glucoside)—leaves, seeds, roots

Organic acids—flowers, serial stems, raw fruits, roots, peels

Tannins/tannic acids—peels, aerial stems, rhizomes, leaves, tea leaves

Bitter substances—aerial stems, peels, flowers, seeds

Volatile oils—flowers, leaves, fruits, peels, aerial stems, roots

Resins—produced by oxidation of essential oils, found in stems and branches

Oleo-resins—found in seeds, stems, branches

Balsam—found in plant body, seeds, little fruits

Gum—stems, raw fruits, juices, e.g., pectin

Gum-resins—stems, branches

Hormones—found in plant body

Vitamins—fruits, vegetables, tea leaves

Specific plant examples of the foregoing classes are listed in Table 3.10. Ingredients made up into medical pills as a prescription for cancer include the plant species and their compounds or components, as provided in Table 3.11. Note the presence of *alkaloids,* usually signified by the "-ine" ending but sometimes by an "-in" ending, as well as other bioactive compounds.

3.7   OTHER INFORMATION ABOUT CHINESE ANTICANCER AGENTS

The volume, *Cancer & Natural Medicine,* by John Boik contains much information about Chinese plant or herbal medicines used against cancer, which also includes an occasional reference to insects or other unusual sources. This information is encapsulated in Table 3.12 by chemical compound type, and Table 3.13 provides a brief rundown of some of the agents that have been investigated *in vitro* and *in vivo* experiments. Note that Table 3.12 uses the descriptor "cytotoxic" in the heading. Further particulars about Chinese anticancer agents are presented in Appendix S.

Observe in particular that in Table 3.13, chemical compounds called *polysaccharides* are prominently listed, e.g., under the genus *Aloe* of the family Liliaceae. This is of continuing interest in the further use of *Aloe vera* as a source for plant-derived medicines. A company called Mannatech Inc. has been studying fresh *Aloe vera* extracts, or phyto-aloe compounds and has come up with a polysaccharide complex called Mannapol (Mannatech Inc., 2010 N. Highway 360, Grand Prairie TX 75050.) Of particular interest is a patented substance named Acemannan, which is also a *polysaccharide.* Among other things, it is reported that *in vitro* and *in vivo* studies indicate that *this substance causes the destruction of malignant tumor cells and leukemia cells.* Clinical trials are proceeding. Another type of substance derived from the Mexican yam has been found to be a hormone precursor.* The same company also produces flash-dried vegetables, which can be taken in capsule form, or mixed in with "Gummi Bear" candy for children and called "Phyto-Bears."

The above paragraph is a further manifestation of what may be called "nutriceuticals" or "nutraceuticals," corresponding to pharmaceuticals. Whereas pharmaceuticals are usually regarded as synthetic or man made, the former designator denotes plant-derived substances that have been scientifically documented to have proven, reproducible, and beneficial medicinal effects.

---

* The Mexican yam, *Discorea alata* or *D. bulbifera* (or *D. sativa*) of the family Dioscoreaceae, is listed as an anticancer agent in Hartwell. *Discorea* also contains plant sterols—e.g., beta-sitosterol—and saponins. Both classes are observed to act against cancer (Boik, *Cancer & Natural Medicine*, p. 149).

Table 3.10 Examples of Chinese Medical Plants [a]

Plants with Alkaloids

Ephedraceae*	*Ephedra* *sinica*: Chinese jointfir, Narc Wong. Contains 1-ephedrin $C_{10}H_{15}NO$, a-pseudoephedrin $C_{10}H_{15}NO$, a-nor-pseudoephedrin $C_9H_{13}NO$, 1-methyhedrin $C_{11}H_{19}NO$, a-methyl-pseudoephedrin $C_{11}H_{17}NO$, etc.
Rutaceae	*Phellodendron amurense*: Amur cork tree, Wong Parck. **Alkaloids** not specified.
Ranunculaceae	*Coptis chinensis**: chinese clematis, Chinese goldthread, Wong Ling. Contains alkaloid **berberine** $C_{20}H_{17}NO_5$ plus falmitin $C_{21}H_{23}NO_5$, coptisin $C_{19}H_{15}NO_5$, worenin $C_{21}H_{15}NO_4$, etc.
Papaveraceae	*Corydalis ambigua**: yuen woo sok. Contains protopin $C_{20}H_{19}NO_4$, d-tetrahydropalmation $C_{21}H_{25}NO_4$, etc.
Palmae	*Areca catechu**: betelnut palm, areca nut, Pinge Longe. Contains the **alkaloid** arecolin (or arecoline) and arecaidin, arecaine, guwacolin, guwacin. Plus philocarpine.
Stemonaceae	*Stemona japonica** (*Stemona tuberosa*): Park Poo. Contains stemonidin $C_{17}H_{35}NO_4$, hodorin $C_{19}H_{35}NO_5$, sinostemonine, paipuinine, biaknunin, sessilin, etc.
Liliaceae	*Fitillaria verticillata*: fritillary, Poy Mu. Contains **alkaloids** fritillin $C_{25}H_{41}NO_3$, fritillarin $C_{19}H_{33}NO_2$, verticine $C_{18}H_{33}NO_2$, vericillin $C_{19}H_{33}NO_2$, peimine, etc.
Ranunculaceae	*Aconitum sinense**: aconite, Foo Doo. Contains **aconitine** $C_{32}H_4NO_{11}$, hypaconitine $C_{33}H_{45}NO_{10}$, jesaconitine $C_{35}H_{49}NO_{19}$, etc. **Anticancer.**
Solanaceae	*Hyoscyamus agrestia**: belladonna, Lang Garm, Hing Sene Doo. Contains **alkaloids** hyoscamine, atrophine, scopolamine, etc. Very toxic.
Theaceae	*Thea sinensis*: Chinese tea, Chare. Contains **caffeine** $C_8H_{10}N_4O_2$, xanthin $C_5H_4N_4O_2$, theophyllin $C_7H_8N_4O_2$, tannic acid.

Plants with Glycosides

Rosaceae	*Agrimonia viscidala**: agrinomy, Sene Hok Chor. Contains a glycoside, an essential oil, tannin, agrimonin, pectin.
Liliaceae	*Rohdea japonica*: lily of China, Marn Ning Ching. Contains the glycoside rohdein $C_{30}H_{44}O_{10} \cdot 2\text{-}1/2\ H_2O$.
Rosaceae	*Prunus armenica*: **bitter almond**, Foo Ham Yin. Contains the glycoside **amygdalin** $C_{20}H_{27}NO_{11}$. **(Not mentioned as anticancer.)**
Rosaceae	*Prunus armenica*: **sweet almond**, Tem Ham Yin. Contains a glycoside, a fatty oil, albumin, glue, etc. **Does not contain amygdalin.**
Plantaginaceae	*Plantago major* var. *asiation*: plantain, Chaire Chang. Whole herb contains the glycosides aucubin $C_{15}H_{24}N_{10}$ and plantagin $C_5H_8O_3$, and plantenolsaure. Seeds contain glycosides, glue, an amber acid, adenin, choline, and plantenolsaure, etc.
Leguminosae	*Glycyrrhiza glabra*: licorice, Garm Chor. Contains glycosides glycyrrhizin $C_{44}H_{64}O_{19}$ and glycyrrhiyin plus glucuronic acid, mannite, asparagin, glucose, protein, saccharase, urease, resins, etc. **Anticancer.**

Plants with Saponins

Campanulaceae	*Platycodon grandiflorum*: kikio root, baloonflower, Kaat Goun. Contains kikyoosaponin $C_{27}H_{48}O_{11}$, plus insulin and phytosterol $C_{27}H_{46}O$, etc.
Compositae	*Aster tataricus**: aster, Doo Yon. Contains saponin astersaponin $C_{23}H_{44}O_{10}$, shionon $C_{34}H_{50}O$, and **quercetin**. Antitubercular.
Polygalaceae	*Polygala tenuifolia*: Chinese senega, polygala, Yuen Cha. Contains the saponins tenuigenin A $C_{27}H_{40}O_8$ and tenuigenin B $C_{30}H_{40}O_8$.
Liliaceae	*Anemarrhena** *asphodeloides*: Che Moo. Contains unspecified saponins.
Leguminosae	*Phaseolus mungo*: red little bean, Chak Shu Dout. Saponin II $C_{47\text{-}48}H_{48\text{-}92}O_{61}$ and hydrolysis product $C_{27}H_{44\text{-}46}O_3$. Sapogenin plus glucose, rhamnose, arabinose, etc.

Table 3.10   Examples of Chinese Medical Plants *(continued)*[a]

Plants with Flavones (coloring matter)

Thymelaeaceae	*Daphne genkwa*: Yuen Farr. Flavone genkwanin, apigenin $C_{15}H_{10}O_5$, sitosterol $C_{27}H_{46}O$, benzoic cid, etc.
Rosaceae	*Rosa multifolia*: tea rose, multiflora rose,Wing Shit. Flavone multiflorin $C_{27}H_{35}O_{15}$, **kaempferol** $C_{15}H_{10}O_6$, rhamnose $C_6H_{12}O_5$, quercetin $C_{15}H_{10}O_7$, etc.
Typhaceae	*Typha latifolia*: cattail, Poo Wong. Contains a flavone, a fatty oil, and isorhamnetin $C_{16}H_{12}O_7$, etc.
Labiatae	*Scutellaria baicalensis*: Chinese skullcap, Baical skullcap, Wong Som. Contains woogonin $C_{16}H_{12}O_4$ and baicalin $C_{21}H_{18}O_{11}$.
Leguminosae	*Sophora japonica**: Japanese pagoda tree, Wi Farr. Contains a flavone and **rutin**, which hydrolyzes to **quercetin** and glucose.
Rubiaceae	*Gardenia augusta*: cape jasmine (?). Contains gardenin, a-crocetin, essential oils, mannit, chlorogenin, etc.
Rutaceae	*Poncirus* trifoliata*: trifoliate orange, Ja Shit. Contains limonen, linalool, linalylacetat, anthranilsauremethylester.

Plants with Emodin (emodin belongs to a class of glycosides/glucosides)

Polygonaceae	*Rheum officinale*: rhubarb, Tai Wong. Emodin $C_{15}H_{10}O_5$, chrysophan saure, rhein, etc. Germicidal.
Leguminosae	*Cassia acutifolia*: Fan Sair Yip. Contains emodin, Kathartinsaure, kathar ommanit, chrysoretin, sennapikrin, etc.
Liliaceae	*Aloe vera (Aloe vulgaris)*: aloe, Loo Woy. Contains emodin, aloe emodin, aloin, alocemodin, resins, etc.

Plants with Organic Acids

Compositae	*Taraxacum mongolicum*: dandelion, Poo Gong Yin. Contains an organic acid, inulin, laevulin, cluytianol, taraxcin, taraxacerin, inosite, resin, asparagin, p-hydroxyphenyl acetic acid, 3,4-dioxy cinnamicaid, homotaraxasterol, taraxasterol, xanthophyil, cholin, and Vitamins A, B, C, etc. Anticancer. Snakebites.
Umbelliferae	*Conioselinum unvittatum**: Chaun Kown. Contains an organic acid and a volatile oil, which consists of cnidiumlacton $C_{12}H_{17}OH$, cnidium saure $C_{12}H_{20}O_3$, cnidium saure fat $C_{12}H_{19}C_2O-C_{10}H_{17}$, and pure $C_{10}H_{17}OH$, plus sedanon saure $C_{12}H_{18}C_3$, etc.
Ranunculaceae	*Paeonia suffruticosa (Paeonia moutan)*: peels of peony, Mout Darn Pee. Ingredients not specified.
Umbelliferae	*Angelica glabra (Angelica anomala)*: Parck Cha. Contains an organic acid, oxypentadecyclic saure, and angelicotoxin, volatile oil, resin, plus hydrocarotin and angelic acid $C_5H_8O_2$, etc. **Anticancer.** Snakebite.
Oxalidaceae	*Oxalis corniculata*: oxalis, Jare Cheung Chor. Contains an organic acid, the oxalate, and other unkown ingredients. **Anticancer.**

Plants with Tannins

Nymphaeaceae	*Nelumbo nucifera*: lotus, Ling. All parts contain tannin/tannic acid. Seeds contain vitamin C, nelumbine, protein, carbohydrates, raffinose, fat, ash: Cu, Mn, Ti. Leaves contain vitamin C and nelumbine.
Punicaceae	*Punica granatum*: peel of pomegranate, Seack Lu Pee. Contains tannin/tannic acid, pelletierin $C_9H_{15}NO$, isopelletierin $C_9H_{15}NO$, methylpelletierin $C_{10}H_{17}NO$, pseudopelletierin, and vitamin C, etc.
Anacardiaceae	*Rhus javanica**: sumac, nutgall, Ng Poy Doo. Contains tannin/tannic acid of nutgall, fat, resin, vegetable wax, etc.
Rosaceae	*Sanguisorba officinalis*: burnet, Da Yee. Contains tannin/tannic acid, sanguisorbin $C_{27}H_{42}O_3$. **Anticancer.**

Table 3.10 Examples of Chinese Medical Plants *(continued)*[a]

Combretaceae	*Terminalia chebula*: myrobalan, Hor Dood. Contains tannin/tannic acid, chebulic acid, fatty oil, ellagic acid $C_1(?)H_{16}O_8$, ash, etc.

Plants with Bitter Substances

Gentianaceae	*Gentiana scabra**: gentian, Loon Arme Chor. Contains the bitter substance gentiopicrin $C_{16}H_{25}O_9$ • H_2O and gentianose $C_{18}H_{32}O_{16}$, etc.
Scrophulariaceae	*Picrorrhiza kurroa*: Woo Wong Ling. Contains picrrorhizin and cathartic saure, etc.
Compositae	*Tussilago farfara*: coltsfoot, Fone Tung Farr. Leaves contain an organic acid plus gallussaure, destrin, inulin, phytotern, palmitine. Flowers contain a bitter substance plus phytosterin, gerbstoff, and faradiol, etc.

Plants with Oils

Lauraceae	*Cinnamomum loureirii*: cinnamon, Yok Kee. The essential oil is in the peel and contains cinnamicaldehyde, camphene, cineol, linalool, engenol and zimmtsaure, cassiaol, etc. Germicidal. Gout.
Rutaceae	*Citrus nobilis (Citrus aurantium)*: orange, Chin Pee. The peel contains a volatile oil with d-limonen and hesperidin $C_{28}H_{21}O_{15}$ plus vitamin C. Antitubercular.
Myristaceae	*Myristica fragrans*: nutmeg, Yok dout Kout. Contains oil of myristice, starch, tannin/tannic acid, resin, coloring matter, 1-a-pinen, dipenten, olein, fat, etc.
Zingiberaceae	*Hedychium coronarium*: ammonium globosum, Lour. Contains an essential oil, borneol, bornylacetate, 1-camphor, **linalool**, nerolidol, fat, carbohydrates.
Labiatae	*Mentha arvensis*: peppermint, Pok Hoo Yip. Contains a volatile oil, menthon, menthol, pinen, menthylacetate, etc. Colds.
Cyperaceae	*Cyperus rotundus*: rush, Hong Foo. contains an essential oil, cyperene $C_5H_2(?)$, cyperol $C5H_{26}$, etc. **Anticancer.**
Labiatae	*Nepeta japonica*: catmint or catnip, King Ki. Contains an essential oil, d-menthone, **d-limonene**, etc. **Lockjaw.**
Compositae	*Atractylis ovata*: Chong Sote. Contains volatile oil, $C_{15}H_{26}O$ plus atractylene $C_{15}H_{24}O$ and sesquiterpenalkohol, etc.

Plants with Resins

Anarcadiaceae	*Pistacia lenticus*: mastic, Yee Hong. Contains resin, tannin, essential oil, sterines, etc. Anticancer.
Burseraceae	*Commiphora myrrha* (Thymelaeaceae, *Aquilaria agallocha*: aloe-wood): myrrh, Mod Yak. Contains resin, gum, ash, myrrhol C10H14O, myrrhin, yomniphoric acid, myrrholic acid, arabinose, oxydase, galactose, xylose, etc. **Anticancer.**

Plants of the Ginseng Type

Araliaceae	*Panax ginseng*: ginseng, Yin Som. Contains panaquilon $C_{20}H_{50}O_{40}$ and panaxsapogenol $C_{24}H_{48}O_3$, etc. Also glycosides, saponin, vitamins B1 and B2, starch, etc. Anticancer.
Polygonaceae	Polygonum multiflorum: Hoo Su Wo. Contains osymethylanthraquinone, lecithin, starch, fat, ash, etc. **Anticancer.**
Umbelliferae	*Ligusticum acutilobum (Angelica polymorpha* var. *sinensis)*: Dhong Kee Hout. Root stock has essential oils containing n-butyliden n-valerohenon-o-carbonsaure.
Compositae	*Artemesia vulgaris*: mugwort, leaves of wormwood, Ay Yip. Contains cineol, thujon $C_{10}H_{16}O$. sesquiterpenalkohol, sesquiterpen, etc. Also gerbsaures kalim and chlorkali, essential oil, cholie, adenie, vitamin B1 and C, inulin, resin, tannin, etc.

a. From *Studies on Chinese Medical Plants and Cancer,* by Wong Kin Keung. Listings are in the order presented in the reference. In the reference, some of the alkaloids for instance are written with either an "-ine" or "-in" as the ending, and other slight discrepancies for other classes of compounds may occur. Plant families, genera, or species **not** listed in Hartwell's *Plants Used Against Cancer* are denoted with an asterisk.

Table 3.11 Chinese Medical Plants for Cancer[a]

Leguminosae	*Sophora flavescens**. Root contains **matrine** $C_{15}H_{24}N_2O$. Seeds contain a fatty oil and **cytisine** $C_{11}H_{14}N_2O$, etc.
Liliaceae	*Tulipa edulis*: tulip. Contains tulipin and starch, etc.
Anacardiaceae	*Pistacia lenticus*: mastic. Contains resin, tannin, pistacin, essential oils and sterines, etc.
Bursieraceae	*Commiphora myrrha*: myrrh. Resin, gum, ash, myrrhol, yomniphoric acid, myrrholic acid, arabinose oxydase, glactose, xylose, etc.
Oleaceae	*Ligustrum lucidum**: privet. Contains the ingredient $C_{17}H_{24}O_9$ of syringin and invertin, etc.
Umbelliferae	*Ligusticum acutilobum*. Contains essential oil in the root; the rhizome contains n-butuliden and n-valerophenon-o-carbonsaure.
Ephedraceae*	*Ephedra** *sinica*: Chinese jointfir. Contains 1-ephedrin $C_{10}H_{15}NO$, a-pseudoephedrin $C_{10}H_{15}NO$, a-nor-pseudoephedrin $C_9H_{13}NO$, 1-methyhedrin $C_{11}H_{19}NO$, a-methyl-pseudoephedrin $C_{11}H_{17}NO$, etc.
Ranunculaceae	*Aconitum sinense** Contains **aconitine** $C_{32}H_4NO_{11}$, **hypaconitine** $C_{33}H_{45}NO_{10}$, **jesaconitine** $C_{35}H_{49}NO_{19}$, etc.
Zingiberaceae	*Zingiber officinale*: ginger. Contains zingeron $C_{11}H_{14}O_3$, shogaol $C_{17}H_{24}O_3$, etc.
Papaveraceae	*Corydalis ambigua**. Contains protopin $C_{20}H_{19}NO_4$, d-tetrahydropalmation $C_{21}H_{25}NO_4$, etc.
Campanulaceae	*Codonopsis tangshen*: bellflower. Contains starch, saponin, sugar, etc.
Polyporacae	*Poria cocos* (*Pachyma cocos*). A **fungus**. Contains pachymose, cellulose, glucose, fructose, ash.
Compositae	*Atractylis ovata*. Contains atractylol $C_{15}H_{26}O$, atractylene $C_{15}H_{24}$, etc.
Ranunculaceae	*Paeonia albiflora*. Contains asparagin, etc.
Umbelliferae	*Conioselinum unvittatum**. Contains essential oil, conidiumlacton $C_{12}H_{18}O_2$, conidium saure $C_{12}H_{20}O_3$, conidium saure fat $C_{12}H_{19}O_2O$-$C_{12}H_{17}$, sedanon saure $C_{12}H_{18}O_3$, etc.
Cruciferae	*Sinapsis alba* (*Brassica alba*): mustard. Contains sinigrin, myrosin, allyl senfol erucasaure $C_{21}H_{11}COOH$, arachinsaure $C_{19}H_{39}COOH$, etc.
Ophidia	(Evidently not a genus or species). Contains pholesterine, palmitic acid, stearic acid, taurine, etc.

a. From *Studies on Chinese Medical Plants and Cancer* by Wong Kin Keung. Listings are in the order presented in the reference. Plant families, genera, or species **not** listed in Hartwell's *Plants Used Against Cancer* are denoted with an asterisk.

3.8 SYNTHETIC VS. NATURAL COMPOUNDS

Rudolf Hänsel, author of the chapter on "Medicinal Plants and Empirical Research" in *Plants in the Development of Modern Medicine*, notes the controversy between drug firms who systematically examine exotic flora for compounds of potential pharmacological interest, and those who don't. This said, the case for looking into medicinal plants exists at three levels.

1. There are plant constituents that can be used directly as therapeutic agents.
2. Plant constituents can be used as the starting materials for synthesizing new and useful drugs.
3. Plant constituents can serve as models for synthesizing new and useful drugs from scratch.

With regard to the latter two avenues of synthesis, the comment is made that, without naturally occurring active principles to go by, the biochemist would not have a clue of where to start or to end up. Synthesis must therefore proceed by analogy with whatever is already known. It becomes the point of departure. *More than this, however, the annotation can be made that the latter avenues afford the possibility of obtaining patent protection, whereas the first-mentioned avenue does not.*

Table 3.12   Listing of Cytotoxic Chinese Anticancer Plants[a]

Aliphatic Compounds

Alcohols

Berberidaceae	*Podophyllum pleianthum**: **mandrake**. Contains podophyllotoxin, deoxypodophyllotoxin.
Berberidaceae	*Podophyllum versipelle**: **mandrake**. Contains podophyllotoxin, deoxypodophyllotoxin.
Hernandiaceae	*Hernandia ovigera*: **mirobolan**. Contains deoxypodophyllotoxin.
Unidentified	*Dysosma* pleaintha*. Contains podophyllotoxin, deoxypodophyllotoxin.

Acids, Esters, Lactones

| Gramineae | *Coix lachryma-jobi*: **coix grain**, hatomugi. Contains coixenolide. |

Aromatic Compounds

Napthoquinones

| Iridaceae | Iris pollasii*: **iris**. Contains irisquinone. |

Anthraquinones

Polygonaceae	*Rheum coreanum**. Contains rhein, emodin.
	R. palmatum: rawend, **rhubarb**. Contains rhein, emodin.
	*R. tanguticum**. Contains rhein, emodin.
Leguminosae	*Cassia acutifolia*: **senna**. Contains rhein, emodin.
	C. angustifolia: **senna**. Contains rhein, emodin.
	C. fistula: cassia fistula, **purging cassia**. Contains rhein, emodin.
	*C. obtusifolia**. Contains rhein, emodin.
	C. tora: **foetid cassia**, penitora. Contains rhein, emodin.

Benzo-a-Pyrone derivatives

Leguminosae	*Psoralea corylifolia*. Contains psoralen, bavachinin, corylifolinin.
Moraceae	*Ficus carica*: **fig**. Contains psoralen.
Umbelliferae	*Angelica dahurica**: **angelica**. Contains psoralen.
	*A. japonica**. Contains psoralen.
	*A. pubescens**. Contains psoralen.
	Glehnia littoralis*. Contains psoralen.
	Ledebouriella seseloides*. Contains psoralen.

Flavonoids: flavones, flavonols, flavanones, flavanonols, etc.

Leguminosae	*Glycyrrhiza uralensis**: **licorice**. Contains liquiritin.
	Sophora flavescens. Contains trifolirhizin.
	*Sophora subprostata**. Contains trifolirhizin, maackiain, sophoraponicin.
	Trifolium pratense: **red clover**. Contains trifolirhizin, maackiain.

Alicyclic Compounds

Monoterpenoids

Rubiaceae	*Asperula odorata*: **asperula, woodroof, hepâtica**. Contains asperuloside.
	Galium verum: common **cleavers**, bedstraw. Contains asperuloside.
	*Heydotis corymbosa**. Contains asperuloside.

Table 3.12 Listing of Cytotoxic Chinese Anticancer Plants[a] *(continued)*

	Oldenlandia diffusa*. Contains asperuloside.
	Paederia scandens*. Contains asperuloside.
Unidentified	*Daphniphyllum* macropodum*. Contains asperuloside.

Sesquiterpenoids

Compositae	*Elephantopus* elatus*: **elephant's foot**. Contains molephantinin, elephantopin.
Compositae	*E. mollis*. Contains molephatinin, elephantopin.
Zingiberaceae	*Curcuma zedoaria**: **seduer**. Contains curcumenol, curcumol, curdione.

Diterpenoids

Celastraceae	*Tripterygium* wilfordii*. Contains triptolide, triptolide A, tripdiolide, triptonide.
Simarubaceae	*Ailanthus altissima*: **glandulosa**. Contains quassin.
Simarubaceae	*Picrasma quassoides**. Contains quassin.

Triterpenoids

Leguminosae	*Glycyrrhiza uralensis**: **licorice**. Contains glyccyrrhizin, glycyrrhetinic acid and derivatives.

Alkaloids

Apocynaceae	*Strophanthus* spp.: vegetable silk. Contains trigonelline.
Celastraceae	*Maytenus serrata**. Contains maytansine.
	Tripterygium wilfordii. Contains celacemine.
Combretaceae	*Quisqualis* indica*. Contains trigonelline.
Labiatae	*Rabdosia* rubescens*. Contains rubescensine B.
Leguminosae	*Abrus precatorius*: **jequirity**. Contains trigonelline.
	Sophora flavescens. Contains tetrandine, matrine, osymatrine.
	Sophora subprostrata*. Contains matrine, oxymatrine, dauricine, anygyrine, pterocarpine.
	Thermopsis* lanceolata. Contains anagyrine.
	Trigonella foenum-graecum: **fenugreek**. Contains trigonelline.
Menispermaceae	*Menispermum* dauricum*. Contains dauricine.
	Sinomenium* acutum. Contains tetrandine.
	Stephania tetrandra*. Contains tetrandine, fangchinoline.
Moraceae	*Cannabis sativa*: marijuana, **hemp**, hashish. Contains trigonelline.
Rubiaceae	*Coffea* arabica*: **coffee**. Contains trigonelline, nicotine.
Rutaceae	*Zanthoxylum ailanthoides**: **prickly ash**. Contains nitidine chloride.
	Z. avicennae*. Contains nitidine chloride.
	Z. cuspidatum*. Contains nitidine chloride.
	Z. nitidum*. Contains nitidine chloride.
Saxifragaceae	*Dichroa febrifuga*: ch'ang shan. Contains beta-dichroine/febrifugine.
Unidentified	*Arabacia* pustulosa*. Contains trigonelline.
	Velella* spirans. Contains trigonelline. (*Vellea* is in Umbelliferae. *Velleia* is in Goodeniaceae*.)

a. From *Cancer & Natural Medicine: A Textbook of Basic Science and Clinical Research,* by John Boik, Oregon Medical Press, Princeton MN, 1995, 1996, pp. 217–219. Plant families, genera, or species **not** listed in Hartwell's *Plants Used Against Cancer* are denoted by an asterisk.

Table 3.13 Some Chinese Herbs Tested for Antitumor Effects[a]

Actinidiaceae*	*Actinidia* chinensis* (Teng Li). Polysaccharides are active agent.
Araliaceae	*Acanthopanax* spp., A, giraldi, A. senticosua, A. obovatus* (Wu Jia Pi, Ci Wu Jia). Polysaccharides are active agent.
	Panax ginseng (Ren Shen): **ginseng**. Acts to enhance chemotherapy.
Carophyllaceae	*Pseudostellaria* heterophylla* (Tai Zi Shen). Acts to stimulate immune system; **no cytotoxic effects**.
Compositae	*Arctium lappa*: **burdock** root.
	*Atractylodes macrocephala** (Bai Zhu).
Hypocreaceae*	*Cordyceps* sinensis* (Dong Chong Xia Cao): caterpillar **fungus. No cytotoxic effects**, apparently the immune system is modulated.
Iridaceae	Crocus sativus: **saffron. Cytotoxic.**
Labiatae	*Scutellaria baicalensis* (Huang Qin): **skullcap. Inhibits cytotoxicity of chemotherapy agents**.
Lauraceae	*Cinnamon or Cinnamomum cassia* (Rou Gui): cassia, **cinnamon**.
Leguminosae	*Astragalus membranaceus** (Huang Qi): **gum traganth, milk vetch**.
	Astragalus capillaris (Yin Chen Hao): **gum traganth, milk vetch. Cytotoxic**.
Liliaceae	*Aloe vahombe**: **aloe**. Polysaccharides are active agent. Also antibacterial, antiparasitic, antifungal.
	Aloe vera: **aloe**. Polysaccharides are active agent.
Loranthaceae	*Viscum album* (Sang Ji Sheng): **mistletoe**. Used in Europe on thousands of patients for over 60 years. Results uncertain.
Oleaceae	*Ligustrum lucidum** (Nu Zhen Zi): **privet**.
Polyporaceae	*Ganoderma* lucidum* (Ling Zhi): **fungus**. Polysaccharides are active agent.
Rosaceae	*Agrimonia pilosa* (Xian He Cao): **agrimony, harvest lice**.
Rubiaceae	*Rubia cordifolia* (Qian Cao Gen): **madder. Peptides** are active agent.
Schisandraceae*	*Schisandra* chinensis* (Wu Wei Zi). Schizophyllan is active agent.
Solanaceae	*Solanum indicum* (Huang Shui Qie): **nightshade. Cytotoxic.**
Umbelliferae	*Angelica sinensis, A. acutibola* (Dang Gui): **angelica**. Polysaccharides are active agent.
	*Bupleurum chinense** (Chai Hu): **thoroughwax**.
Zingiberaceae	*Curcuma aromatica* (Yu Jin or E Zhu): **seduer**. Volatile oil contains coucurcumin as the active agent.

a. From *Cancer & Natural Medicine: A Textbook of Basic Science and Clinical Research,* by John Boik, Oregon Medical Press, Princeton MN, 1995, 1996, pp. 121–124. Plant families, genera, or species **not** in Hartwell's *Plants Used Against Cancer* are denoted by an asterisk.

The volume *Some medicinal forest plants in Africa and Latin America* has some interesting insights in the introduction. To wit, there has been the synthesis of many hundreds of chemical variants of known classes of cancer therapeutic agents. The improvements have been relatively small, although studies of tumor inhibitors of plant origin continue and are yielding a fascinating array of novel types of growth-inhibiting compounds. However, once bioactivity has been established, the tendency is for the pharmaceutical companies to use the chemical structure as a template for modifications that hopefully will have a greater activity than the natural parent compound.* About this practice, a further comment is provided as follows:

"History shows that it is exceptionally rare that a naturally occurring chemical compound which has found utility as a drug in man will yield a derivative on structure modification that exceeds the value of the parent compound in drug efficacy."

3.9 SOME COMMON POSSIBILITIES FOR ANTICANCER AGENTS

An examination of the various listings of anticancer agents from plant sources in instances will reveal a commonality among different countries or geographical regions. Although these listings for the most part are derived from folklore, there is nevertheless the indication from this commonality that these particular plant species or genera may in fact be out of the ordinary. In fact, as has been observed, some plant families are more bioactive than others, particularly with regard to their alkaloid content.

A case in point is *Catharanthus roseus* of the plant family Apocynaceae, a species that crops up time and again among the various listings. *Some of its many alkaloids* are well known anticancer agents for blood-related cancers—albeit cytotoxic to other cells as well, as evidenced by the severe side effects. Evidently, blood-type cancers are more susceptible to toxicity than are solid tumors, since blood-related cancers can be cured by this version of conventional chemotherapy, whereas it is ineffective on solid tumors.

Continuing with this line of thought, a computer search, say, could be made of the different listings to determine the frequency of occurrence for the different species, genera, and families. Such would provide a relative indication of potential worthiness. (By allowing the data or information to speak for itself, the touchy subject of specific recommendations can be avoided.)

And, in fact, the entire subject of screening, testing, and evaluation has been covered in Abayomi Sofowora's *Medicinal Plants and Traditional Medicine in Africa*. (The term "traditional medicine" denotes Native or nonwestern medicine.) Starting with his Chapter 4, an enumeration of chapter titles is indicative:

4. Standardization of Herbal Potions
5. Scientific Evidence Supporting Some Remedies or Practices Used in Traditional Medicine
6. Relationships Between Traditional Medicine and Modern Drugs
7. Advantages and Disadvantages of Traditional Medicine
8. Integration or Co-recognition of Traditional and Modern Medicine
9. Methods of Obtaining Information on Medicinal Plants
10. Screening Plants for Bioactive Agents
11. Guidelines for Research on Medicinal Plants for Local Drug Production
12. Research Trends on Medicinal Plants in Africa
13. Some Common Medicinal Plants

In Sofowora's Chapter 9, he provides some insights on how to obtain information about native plants and treatments. In Chapter 11, he presents a strong case for further developing and producing medicinal plants or herbs. It is a role well suited for agricultural economies. Although not stressing anticancer plants, the inference is nevertheless there.

Abayomi Sofowora's Chapter 10 has a subsection on "Screening from computer reports" (Sofowora, *Medicinal Plants*, p. 132). He mentions the work of Hartwell and also of N.R. Farnsworth et al., which has appeared in a number of publications, some of which are cited in the references. Following this, there is a section on "Biological Screening" and a section on "Phytochemical Screening." The latter section outlines tests for alkaloids, saponins, tannins, phlobatannins, anthraquinones, and cardiac glycosides.

In the appendices of John Boik's *Cancer & Natural Medicine*, there is a section titled "Overview of Common Research Designs," which can be used as an outline for systematically gathering information about anticancer agents.

Finally, it may be mentioned that certain plants or organisms, or bioactive substances, have in fact been selected for further investigations by the National Cancer Institute, and in China (Boik, *Cancer & Natural Medicine*, pp. 111, 112). This information is provided in Tables 3.14 and 3.15. There is evidently

---

* Left unstated is the need to synthesize new compounds or variations that can be patented, whereas the naturally occurring compound cannot.

Table 3.14 Plant Sources and Compounds Selected for Advanced Development via the NCI Screening Program[a]

Amaryllidaceae	*Pancratium littorale**: **spider lily**. Contains the alkaloid **pancrastatin**.
Apocynaceae	*Ochrosia* moorei*. Contains the alkaloid **ellipticine**.
Aristolochiaceae	*Aristolochia* spp.: aristolochia, clematitis, birthwort Contains the alcohol-like compound aristolochic acid. (Used in Chinese herbal medicine.)
Berberidaceae	*Podophyllum* spp.: **mandrake**. Contains lignans in the form of podophyllotoxin derivatives. (Used in Chinese herbal medicine.)
Bignoniaceae	*Tabebuia* spp.: **pau d'arco**. Contains the quinone **lapachol**.
Boraginaceae	*Heliotropium indicum*: **hekiotrope**, borrajon. Contains the pyrrolizidine alkaloid **indicine-N-oxide**. (Used in Chinese herbal medicine.)
Celastraceae	*Maytenus ovatus*. Contains the alkaloid **maytansine**.
Cephalotaxaceae*	*Cephalotaxus* harringtonia*: **plum-yew**. Contains the alkaloids **harringtonine**, **homoharringtonine**.
Compositae	*Baccharis megapotamica**: **groundsel tree**. Contains the tricothecanes baccharin, isobaccharin.
	Eriophyllum* confertiflorum: eriophyllum. Contains the sesquiterpene lactone eriofertopin.
Euphorbiaceae	*Phyllanthus brasiliensis**. Contains the sesquiterpene phyllanthoside.
Guttiferae	*Psorospermum* febrifugum*. Contains the xanthone psorospermin.
Moraceae	*Ficus* spp.: **fig**. Contains the alkaloid **tylocrebrine**. (Used in Chinese herbal medicine.)
Mucedinaceae*	*Cephalosporium* aphidicola*. Contains the diterpene aphidicolin glycinate.
Nyssaceae*	*Camptotheca* acuminata*: **tree of joy**. Contains the alkaloids **camptothecine, 10-hydrocamptothecine**. **Cytotoxic**. (Used in Chinese herbal medicine.)
Rutaceae	*Acronychia* baueri*. Contains the alkaloid **acronycine**.
	Fagara macrophylla. Contains the alkaloid **fagaronine**.
	Zanthoxylum nitidum*: **prickly ash**. Contains the alkaloid **nitidine**. (Used in Chinese herbal medicine.)
Simarubaceae	*Brucea* spp.: brucea. Contains the diterpine bruceantin. (Used in Chinese herbal medicine.)
Solanaceae	*Withania* spp.: **winter cherry**. Contains the triterpene 4-beta-hydroxy-withanolide E.
Taxaceae	*Taxus brevifolia**: **yew**. Contains the diterpene (taxane-type) **taxol**.
Unidentified	*Ansa macrolide**

a. From *Cancer & Natural Medicine: A Textbook of Basic Science and Clinical Research,* by John Boik, Oregon Medical Press, Princeton MN, 1995, 1996, p. 111. Plant families, genera, or species **not** listed in Hartwell's *Plants Used Against Cancer* are denoted by an asterisk.

also considerable interest in the substances *berberine, indirubin, limonene* and perillyl alcohol, *matrine* and oxymatrine, psoralen, *rhein* and *emodin* as anticancer agents (Boik, *Cancer & Natural Medicine,* pp. 112–120). A brief listing of plant sources is provided in Table 3.16.

Table 3.15 Plant/Organism Sources and Compounds Selected for Advanced Development in China[a]

Apocynaceae	*Catharanthus* roseus* (Chang Chun Hua): **periwinkle.** Contains the alkaloids **vinblastine, vincristine, vindesine. Cytotoxic.** (Listed as *Vinca* in Hartwell)
Cephalotaxaceae *	*Cephalotaxus* harringtonia*: **plum yew** Contains the alkaloids **harringtonine, homoharringtonine.**
Cruciferae	*Isatis tinctoria* (Da Qing Ye or Qing Dai): **indigo,** isatis, woad. Contains the alkaloid **indirubin.**
Labiatae	*Isodon** spp. Contains the diterpenes oridonin, ponicidin.
Leguminosae	*Crotalaria* sessiflora* (Ye Bai He): **rattlebox.** Contains the alkaloid **monocrotaline.**
Nyssaceae*	*Camptotheca* acuminata* (Xi Shu): **tree of joy.** Contains the alkaloids **camptothecine, 10-hydroxycamptothecine. Cytotoxic.**
Stylopsidae	*Mylabris phalerata* (the **beetle** Ban Mao of the order Coloptera). Contains cantharidin.

a. From *Cancer & Natural Medicine: A Textbook of Basic Science and Clinical Research* by John Boik, Oregon Medical Press, Princeton MN, 1995, 1996, p. 112. Plant families, genera, or species **not** in Hartwell's *Plants Used Against Cancer* are denoted by an asterisk.

Table 3.16 Plant Sources for the Anticancer Agents Berberine, Indirubin, Limonene and Perillyl Alcohol, Matrine and Oxymatrine, Psoralen, Rhein, and Emodin[a]

Berberidaceae	*Berberis aquifolium**: Oregon grape, **barberry.** Contains the alkaloid **berberine**
Compositae	*Angelica dahurica** (Bai Zhi): **angelica.** Contains the furocoumarin **psoralen.**
	A. pubescens* (Du Huo): **angelica.** Contains the furocoumarin **psoralen.**
Cruciferae	*Isatis tinctoria* (Da Qing Ye or Qing Dai): **indigo,** isatis, woad. Contains **indirubin.** (Cytotoxic)
Leguminosae	*Cassia angustifolia* and *C. acutifolia* (Fan Xie Ye): **senna.** Contain the anthraquinones **rhein** and **emodin.**
	C. tora and *C. obtusifolia* (Jue Ming Zi): foetid cassia. Contain the anthraquinones **rhein** and **emodin.**
	Psoralea coryfolia (Bu Gu Zhi). Contains the furocoumarin **psoralen.**
	Sophora flavescens (Ku Shen). Contains the alkaloids **matrine** and **oxymatrine.**
	S. subprostata* (Shan Dou Gen). Contains the alkaloids **matrine** and **oxymatrine.**
Moraceae	*Ficus carica*: **fig.** Contains the furocoumarin **psoralen.**
Polygonaceae	*Polygonum multiflorum* (He Shou Wu) and *P. cuspidatum** (Hu Chang). Contain the anthraquinones **rhein** and **emodin.**
	Rheum palmatum and *Rheum* spp. (Da Huang): **rhubarb.** Contain the anthraquinones **rhein** and **emodin.**
	Rumex crispus: **yellow dock.** Contains the anthraquinones **rhein** and **emodin.**
Ranunculaceae	*Coptis chinensis** (Huang Lian). Contains the alkaloid **berberine.**
	Hydrastis canadensis: **goldenseal.** Contains the alkaloid **berberine.**
Rhamnaceae	*Rhamnus frangula*: **buckthorn.** Contains the anthraquinones **rhein** and **emodin.**
	R. purshiana: **cascara sagrada.** Contains the anthraquinones **rhein** and **emodin.**
Rutaceae	*Citrus reticulata*: **orange oil., mandarin orange.** Contains the monoterpene **limonene** and its analog **perillyl alcohol.**
Umbelliferae	*Glehnia* littoralis* (Sha Shen). Contains the furocoumarin **psoralen.**
Umbelliferae	*Ledebouriella* seseloides* (Fang Feng). Contains the furocoumarin **psoralen.**

a. From *Cancer & Natural Medicine: A Textbook of Basic Science and Clinical Research,* by John Boik, Oregon Medical Press, Princeton MN, 1995, 1996, p. 112. Plant families, genera, or species **not** in Hartwell's *Plants Used Against Cancer* are denoted by an asterisk.

REFERENCES

A Field Guide to Medicinal Plants: Eastern and Central North America, Houghton Mifflin, Boston, 1990. Text by Steven Foster and James A. Duke. Line drawings by Roger Tory Peterson, Jim Blackfeather Rose and Lee Allen Peterson. Photographs by Steven Foster.

Agharkar, S.P., *Medicinal Plants of Bombay Presidency*, State Mutual Book & Periodical Service, New York, 1991.

Anderson, Frank J., *An Illustrated History of the Herbals*, Columbia University Press, New York, 1977.

Andrews, Theodora with the assistance of William L. Corya and Donald A. Stickel, *A Bibliography on Herbs, Herbal Medicine, "Natural Foods," and Unconventional Medical Treatment*, Libraries Unlimited, Littleton CO, 1982.

Angier, Bradford, *Field Guide to Medicinal Wild Plants*, Stackpole Books, Harrisburg PA, 1978.

Arvigo, Rosita and Michael Balick, *Rainforest Remedies: One Hundred Healing Herbs of Belize*, Lotus Press, Twin Lakes WI, 1993.

Atlas of the Flora of the Great Plains, R.L. McGregor, Coordinator, T.M. Barkley, Editor, The Great Plains Flora Association, Iowa State University Press, Ames, 1977. Contributors: William T. Barker, Ralph E. Brooks, Steven P. Churchill, Robert B. Kaul, Ole A. Kolstad, David M. Sutherland, Theodore Van Bruggen, Ronald R. Weedon, James S. Wilson.

Ayensu, Edward S., *Medicinal Plants of West Africa*, Reference Publications, Algonac MI, 1978. Introduction by R.E. Schultes. Edited by Keith Irvine. No. 1 of *Medicinal Plants of the World*.

Ayensu, Edward S., *Medicinal Plants of the West Indies*, Reference Publications, Algonac MI, 1981. No. 2 of *Medicinal Plants of the World*.

Blackwell, Will H., *Poisonous and Medicinal Plants*, Prentice Hall, Englewood Cliffs NJ, 1990. Chapter 5, by Martha J. Powell.

Boik, John, *Cancer & Natural Medicine: A Textbook of Basic Science and Clinical Research*, Oregon Medical Press, Princeton MN, 1995, 1996.

Boulos, Loutfy, *Medicinal Plants of North Africa*, Reference Publications, Algonac MI, 1983. Edited by Edward S. Ayensu. No. 3 of *Medicinal Plants of the World*.

Brown, Dr. O. Phelps, *The Complete Herbalist: Or, the People Their Own Physicians, By the Use of Nature's Remedies; Describing the Great Curative Powers Found in the Herbal Kingdom*, Published by the author, Jersey City NJ, 1875.

Chopra, L.C. and B.K. Abrol, *Medicinal Plants of the Arid Zones*, Scholarly Publications, Houston TX, 1983.

Cordell, Geoffrey A., *Introduction to Alkaloids: A Biogenetic Approach*, Wiley, New York, 1981.

Crellin, J.K. and Jane Philpott, *Herbal Medicine Past and Present*, Duke University Press, Durham NC, 1990. Vol. I. *Trying to Give Ease*. Vol. II. *A Reference Guide to Medicinal Plants*.

Dastur, J.F., *Medicinal Plants of India and Pakistan: A Concise Work Describing Plants Used for Drugs and Remedies According to Ayurvedic, Unani and Tibbi Systems and Mentioned in British and American Pharmacopoeias*, D.B. Taraporevala Sons, Bombay, 1962. Asia Book Corporation of America, 1977. State Mutual Book & Periodical Service, New York, 1988. Meyerbooks, Glenwood IL.

DeFilipps, Robert A., *Medicinal Plants of the Guianas*, Reference Publications, Algonac MI, 1996. No. 7 of *Medicinal Plants of the World*.

Duke, James A., *Handbook of Edible Weeds*, CRC Press, Boca Raton FL, 1992.

Duke, James A., *CRC Handbook of Medicinal Herbs*, CRC Press, Boca Raton FL, 1985.

Duke, James A., *Handbook of Biologically Active Phytochemicals and Their Activities*, CRC Press, Boca Raton FL, 1992.

Duke, James A., *Handbook of Northeastern Indian Medicinal Plants*, Quarterman Publications, Lincoln MA, 1986. No. 3 of *Bioactive Plants*.

Duke, James A., *Handbook of Phytochemical Constituents of GRAS Herbs and Other Economic Plants*, CRC Press, Boca Raton FL, 1992.

Duke, James A. and Edward S. Ayensu, *Medicinal Plants of China*, in two volumes, Reference Publications, Algonac MI, 1985. No. 4 of *Medicinal Plants of the World*.

Duke, James Allen and Rudolfo Vasquez, *Amazonia Ethnobotanical Dictionary*, CRC Press, Boca Raton FL, 1994.

Elliott, Douglas B., *Roots: An Underground Botany and Forager's Guide*, Chatham Press, Old Greenwich CT, 1976.

Ethnobotany in the Neotropics, New York Botanical Garden, Bronx NY, 1984. Proceedings of a symposium held at Oxford OH, 1983.

Farnsworth, N.R. and A.S. Bingel, "Problems and Prospects of Discovering New Drugs from Higher Plants by Pharmacological Screening," in *New Natural Products and Plant Drugs with Pharmacological, Biological or Therapeutical Activity*, H. Wagner and P. Wolff Eds., Springer-Verlag, Berlin, 1977, pp. 1–22.

Farnsworth, N.R. and C.J. Kass, "An Approach Utilizing Information from Traditional Medicine to Identify Tumor-Inhibiting Plants," *Journal of Ethnopharmacology*, 3, pp. 85–90.

Fernald, Merritt Lyndon, see *Gray's Manual of Botany*

Flora Neotropica. Published for the Organization for Flora Neotropica by the New York Botanical Garden, New York, 1968–. As of 1994, there were 65 monographs, mainly by plant families.

Flora of the Great Plains, by the Great Plains Flora Association, University Press of Kansas, Lawrence, 1986.

Frodin, D.G., *Guide to Standard Floras of the World: An annotated, geographically arranged systematic bibliography of the principal floras, enumerations, checklists, and chorological atlases of different areas*, Cambridge University Press, Cambridge, England, 1984.

Genthe, Henry, "The Incredible Sponge," *Smithsonian,* 29(5), 50–58 (August 1998).

Gray's Manual of Botany: A Handbook of the Flowering Plants and Ferns of the Central and Northeastern United States and Adjacent Canada, Eighth (Centennial) Edition, D. Van Nostrand, New York, 1950, 1970. Largely rewritten and expanded by Merritt Lyndon Fernald.

Grieve, Mrs. M. (Maud), *A Modern Herbal: The Medicinal, Culinary, Cosmetic and Economic Properties, Cultivation and Folk-Lore of Herbs, Grasses, Fungi, Shrubs & Trees with All Their Modern Scientific Uses,* with a New Service Index, Hafner, New Haven CT, 1970. In two volumes, Dover, New York, 1971, 1982. Originally published by Harcourt, Brace & Company in 1931.

Grimé, William Ed, *Ethno-Botany of the Black Americans,* Reference Publications, Algonquin MI, 1979.

Hager, Hermann et al., *Hager's Handbuch der Pharmazeutischen Praxis: fur Apotheker, Arzte, Drogisten, und Medizinal-beamte,* J. Springer, and Springer-Verlag, Berlin, 1900, 1902, 1908, 1910, 1920, 1925, 1930, 1949, 1958, 1967, 1973, 1977, 1990.

Hartwell, Jonathan A., *Plants Used Against Cancer: A Survey,* Quarterman Publications, Lawrence MA, 1982. Foreword by Jim Duke.

The Healing Past: Pharmaceuticals in the Biblical and Rabbinic World, Irene and Walter Jacob Eds., Leiden, New York, 1993.

Heinerman, John, *Healing Power of Herbs,* Globe Communications, Boca Raton FL, 1995.

Heinerman, John, *Healing Secrets of the Maya: Health Wisdom from an Ancient Empire,* Human Energy Press, Foster City CA, 1989. Edited by Laurance E. Badgley.

Heinerman, John, *The Treatment of Cancer with Herbs,* BiWorld, Orem UT, 1984. Special Foreword by Robert Mendelsohn. Available from the author, P.O. Box 11471, Salt Lake City UT 84147, (801)521–8824.

Howes, F.N., *A Dictionary of Useful and Everyday Plants and Their Common Names:* Based on Material Contained in J.C. Willis: *A Dictionary of Flowering Plants and Herbs* (6th Edition, 1931), Cambridge University Press, Cambridge, England, 1974.

Huang, Kee Chang, *The Pharmacology of Chinese Herbs,* CRC Press, Boca Raton FL, 1993.

Hutchens, Alma R., *Indian Herbalogy of North America,* Shambhala, Boston, 1991.

Index to Common Plant Names of Herbaceous Plants, compiled by R. Milton Carleton, G.K. Hall, Boston, 1959.

Infraspecific Classification of Wild and Cultivated Plants, B.T. Styles Ed., Oxford University Press, Oxford, England. Published for the Systematics Association.

Iwu, Maurice M., *Handbook of African Medicinal Plants,* CRC Press, Boca Raton FL, 1993.

Jain, S.K. and Robert A. DeFilipps, *Medicinal Plants of India,* in two volumes, Reference Publications, Algonac MI, 1991. No. 5 of *Medicinal Plants of the World.*

Keung, Wong Kin, *Studies on Chinese Medical Plants and Cancer,* Elerich Development Limited, Hong Kong, March, 1991. Printed in Hong Kong by Allegiance Printing Press Ltd.

Le Strange, Richard, *A History of Herbal Plants,* Arco Publishing Co., New York, 1977. Foreword by Anthony Huxley.

Lewis, David C., *Medicinal Plants of Asia: A Systematic Bibliography,* Asia Books, San Jose CA, 1987.

Mabberley, D.G., *The Plant-Book: A portable dictionary of the higher plants, utilising Cronquist's* An Integrated System of Classification of Flowering Plants *(1981) and current botanical literature arranged largely on the principles of edition 1–6 (1896/97–1934) of Willis's* A Dictionary of the Flowering Plants and Ferns, Cambridge University Press, Cambridge, England, 1987.

Medicinal and Poisonous Plants of the Tropics, A.J.M. Leeuwenberg (Compiler), Pudoc Wageningen, Centre for Agricultural Publishing and Documentation, Wageningen, Netherlands, 1987. Proceedings of Symposium 5–35 of the 14th International Botanical Congress, Berlin, 24 July–1 August 1987.

Medicinal Plants, compiled by Judith Robinson and Constance Carter, Science Reference Section, Science and Technology Division, Library of Congress, Washington DC, 1981, 1991.

Medicinal Plants, in four volumes, G. Bentley Ed., State Mutual Book & Periodical Service, New York, 1982, 1992.

Medicinal Plants: A Source Guide, Gordon Press, New York, 1991.

Medicinal Plants: An Illustrated Guide to More Than 180 Herbal Plants, Random House Value Publishing, Avenal NJ, 1991.

Medicinal Plants: New Vistas of Research, J.N. Govil, V.K. Singh and Shamima Hasmi Eds., Scholarly Publications, Houston TX, 1992.

Medicinal Plants: Report of Committee on Economic and Therapeutic Importance of Medicinal Plants Initiated by the Ministry of Health, Government of Pakistan, Inamul Haq Ed., Hamdard Foundation Press, Karachi, Pakistan, 1983.

Medicinal Plants in the Biblical World, Walter and Irene Jacob Eds., Rodef Shalom Press, Pittsburgh PA, 1990. No. I of *Horticulture and Technology in the Biblical World.*

Medicinal Plants of China, The Institute of Chinese Materia Medica, China Academy of Traditional Chinese Medicine, World Health Organization, Manila, 1989.

Medicinal Plants of India, Indian Council of Medical Research, New Delhi, 1987.

Medicinal Plants of Nepal Himalaya, State Mutual Book & Periodical Service, New York, 1980.

Medicinal Resources of the Tropical Forest: Biodiversity and Its Importance to Human Health, Columbia University Press, New York. Edited by Michael J. Balick, Elaine Elisabetsky and Sarah A. Laird.

Millspaugh, Charles F., *Medicinal Plants: An Illustrated and Descriptive Guide to Plants Indigenous to and Naturalized in the United States Which Are Used in Medicine,* in two volumes, Gordon Press, New York, 1980.

Moerman, Daniel E., *Geraniums for the Iroquois: A Field Guide to American Indian Medicinal Plants*, Reference Publications, Algonac MI, 1982. Edited by Keith Irvine.

Moerman, Daniel E., *Medicinal Plants of Native America*, in two volumes, Museum of Anthropolgy, University of Michigan, Ann Arbor, 1986. Foreword by Richard I. Ford.

Moore, Michael, *Medicinal Plants of the Desert and Canyon West: A guide to identifying, preparing, and using traditional medicinal plants found in the deserts and canyons of the West and Southwest*, Museum of New Mexico Press, Santa Fe, 1989.

Moore, Michael, *Medicinal Plants of the Mountain West: A guide to the identification, preparation, and uses of traditional medicinal plants found in the mountains, foothills, and upland areas of the American West*, Museum of New Mexico Press, Santa Fe NM, 1979.

Moore, Michael, *Medicinal Plants of the Pacific West*, Red Crane Books, Santa Fe NM, 1993.

Mors, Walter B., Carlos T. Rizzini and Nuno A. Pereira, *Medicinal Plants of Brazil*, Reference Publications, Algonac MI, 1996. Edited by Robert A. DeFilipps. No. 6 of *Medicinal Plants of the World*.

Morton, Julia F., *Atlas of Medicinal Plants of Middle America: Bahamas to Yucatan*, C.C. Thomas, Springfield IL, 1981.

Morton, Julia F., *Major Medicinal Plants: Botany, Culture and Uses*, Charles C Thomas Publisher, Springfield IL, 1977.

Mowery, Daniel B., *Proven Herbal Blends: A Rational Approach to Prevention and Remedy*, Cormorant Books, P.O. Box 386, Lehi UT 84043, 1986.

Mowery, Daniel B., *The Scientific Validation of Herbal Medicine: How to Remedy and Prevent Disease with Herbs, Vitamins, Minerals, and Other Nutrients*, Cormorant Books, P.O. Box 386, Lehi UT, 1986. Also published as *The Scientific Validation of Herbal Medicine*, Keats Publishing, New Canaan CT, 1986, 1990.

Oliver-Bever, Bep, *Medicinal Plants in Tropical West Africa*, Cambridge University Press, New York, 1986.

Pandey, Gyanendra, *Medicinal Flowers: Puspayurveda Medicinal Flowers of India and Adjacent Regions*, South Asia Books, Columbia MO, 1992. No. 14 of *Indian Medical Science*.

Pathak, V.M., *Medicinal Plants of Gwalior*, State Mutual Book & Periodical Service, New York, 1987.

Perry, Lily M. with the assistance of Judith Metzger, *Medicinal Plants of East and Southeast Asia*, MIT Press, Cambridge MA, 1980.

Plants in the Development of Modern Medicine, Tony Swain Ed., Harvard University Press, Cambridge MA, 1972.

Quraishi, M.A. and Mir Alam Khan, *Survey and Regeneration of Medicinal Plants in West Pakistan*, Final Technical Report under PL-480 Programme of U.S.A., Pakistan Forest Institute, Peshawar, 1973.

Ramalingam, Vimala, *Medicinal Plants*, Vol. 1, Irvington Publishers, New York, 1974. Edited by N. Singh and H.C. Mital.

Sargent, Charles Sprague, *Manual of the Trees of North America*, in two volumes, Houghton Mifflin, Boston, 1905, 1922, 1949. Republished by Dover Publications, New York, 1961.

Sigma catalog, *Biochemicals, Organic Compounds, and Diagnostic Reagents*, Sigma Chemical Company, St. Louis, 1996–.

Singh, V.K., *Medicinal Plants and Folklores: Strategy Towards Conquest of Human Ailments*, Scholarly Publications, Houston TX, 1989.

Sofowora, Abayomi, *Medicinal Plants and Traditional Medicine in Africa*, Wiley, Chichester, West Sussex and New York, 1982. Waking Light Press, Ann Arbor MI.

Some medicinal gorest plants in Africa and Latin America, Forest Resources Development Branch, Forest Resources Division, FAO Forestry Department, Food and Agriculture Organization of the United Nations, Rome, Italy, 1986.

Stace, Clive A., *Plant Taxonomy and Biosystematics*, Second Edition, Edward Arnold, London, 1980, 1989.

Tanaka, Tyôzaburô, *Tanaka's Cyclopedia of Edible Plants of the World*, Sasuke Nakao Ed., Keigaku Publishing Co., Tokyo, 1976.

Tétényi, Péter, *Infraspecific Chemical Taxa of Medicinal Plants*, Chemical Publishing Co., New York, 1970. General part translated by Isván Finály. Special part translated by Péter Tétényi.

Thakur, R.S., *Major Medicinal Plants of India*, Central Institute of Medicinal and Aromatic Plants, Lucknow, India, 1989.

Toxic Plants & Animals: A Guide for Australia, Jeanette Covacevich, Peter Davie and John Pearn Eds., Queensland Museum, Brisbane, 1987.

Train, Percy, James R. Henrichs and W. Andrew Archer, *Medicinal Uses of Plants by Indian Tribes of Nevada*, Quarterman Publications, Lincoln MA, 1981. No. 1 of *Bioactive Plants*.

Van Duong, Nguyen, *Medicinal Plants of Vietnam, Cambodia and Laos*, published by N. Van Duong, 938 26th St., Santa Monica CA 90403, (310)828–6649, 1993.

Van Wijk, H.L. Gerth, *A Dictionary of Plant Names*, in two volumes, A. Asher & Co., Vaals-Amsterdam, 1971. Introduction by F.A. Safleu.

von Reis Altschul, Siri, *Drugs and Foods from Little-Known Plants: Notes in Harvard University Herbaria*, Harvard University Press, Cambridge MA, 1973.

von Reis, Siri and Frank L. Lipp, *New Plant Sources for Drugs and Foods from the New York Botanical Garden Herbarium*, Harvard University Press, Cambridge MA, 1982.

Walters, Richard, *Options: The Alternative Cancer Therapy Book*, Avery Publishing Group, Garden City Park NY, 1993.

Watt, John Mitchell and Maria Gerdina Breyer-Brandwijk, *The Medicinal and Poisonous Plants of Southern and Eastern Africa: Being an Account of Their Medicinal and Other Uses, Chemical Composition, Pharmacological Effects and Toxicology in Man and Animal*, E.&S. Livingstone, Edinburgh and London, 1962.

Weeds and Poisonous Plants of Wyoming and Utah. Tom D. Whitson, Editor. Contributors: Roy Reichembach, Mark A. Ferrell, Stephen D. Miller, Steven A. Dewey, John D. Evans, Richard D. Shaw. Published by Cooperative Extension Service, College of Agriculture, University of Wyoming, Laramie, April, 1987.

Wheelwright, Edith Grey, *Medicinal Plants and Their History*, Dover, New York, 1974. Originally published as *The Physick Garden: Medicinal Plants and their History*, Houghton Mifflin, Boston, 1935,

Wijesekera, R.O., *The Medicinal Plant Industry*, CRC Press, Boca Raton FL, 1991.

Willis, J.C., revised by H.K. Airy Shaw, *A Dictionary of the Flowering Plants and Ferns*, Eighth Edition, Cambridge University Press, Cambridge, England, 1973.

Wren, R.C., rewritten by Elizabeth M. Williamson and Fred J. Evans, *Potter's New Cyclopedia of Botanical Drugs and Preparations*, The C.W. Daniel Company Ltd., Saffron Walden, Essex, England, 1988. First published in 1907.

Zafar, Rasheeduz, *Medicinal Plants of India*, CBS Publishers, Delhi, India, 1994.

Alkaloids as Medicines

Part 4

Alkaloids as Medicines

4.1 INTRODUCTION

Alkaloids are among the most interesting classes of chemical compounds, due principally to their biochemical effects, most of which no doubt have yet to be determined. In other words, what are the main purposes and functions of alkaloids in the great scheme of life? Touched upon to some extent in Parts 2 and 3, the subject will be further explored as follows. Among the references are those already cited in Part 2, including Geoffrey A. Cordell's *Introduction to Alkaloids: A Biogenetic Approach*, and *Biochemistry of Alkaloids*, edited by K. Mothes, H.R. Schütte and M. Luckner, as well as Will H. Blackwell's *Poisonous and Medicinal Plants*. Also to be mentioned in passing, there is the four-volume *Alkaloids: Chemical and Biological Perspectives*, edited by S. William Pelletier, and the approximately 46-volume continuing set, *The Alkaloids: Chemistry and Pharmacology*, edited by R.H.F. Manske et al. In particular, and for the purposes here, there will be the occasion to refer to the first three cited.

Given that alkaloids are poisonous to one degree or another almost by definition, and some are carcinogenic, the question is, do they perform any useful purposes for humans? Thus, K. Mothes and M. Luckner, at the end of the introductory chapter to the *Biochemistry of Alkaloids*, note that alkaloidal substances with a general high toxicity occur only in very small concentrations in the plant, but these are the very alkaloids that have *antitumor* activity and may inhibit DNA/RNA/protein biosynthesis. (Hopefully, alkaloids can be found that will act selectively, that is, against cancer cells but not normal cells. Such may also be a matter of dosage levels.)

The numbers and possibilities for alkaloids are steadily increasing, augmented by new discoveries in the rain forests. A computer compilation and printout by Robert F. Raffauf, published in 1970 as *A Handbook of Alkaloids and Alkaloid-Containing Plants*, listed approximately 5,000 different alkaloids. (A newer book by Raffauf is titled *Plant Alkaloids: A Guide to Their Discovery and Distribution*, published in 1996.) Categorizations included plant family versus alkaloid, genus, stoichiometric molecular formula, molecular weight, melting point, and alpha solvent temperature; also discussed are alkaloid names versus plant family, and genus versus alkaloid. Among the better represented plant families are the Amaryllidaceae, Apocynaceae, Buxaceae, Compositae, Lauraceae, Leguminosae, Liliaceae, Loganaceae, Lycopodiaceae, Magnoliaceae, Menispermaceae, Papaveraceae, Ranunculaceae, Rubiaceae, Rutaceae, and Solanaceae. Notable among these are the Apocynaceae, Leguminosae, Papaveraceae, and Rutaceae. Expectedly, the number of known alkaloids has since expanded.

A later reference assigned a value of 7000 or more alkaloids known (Mothes and Luckner, in *Alkaloids*, p. 16; re *The Alkaloids: Chemistry and Pharmacology*, edited by R.H.F. Manske et al.). A more likely number of known alkaloids today is approximately 10,000. Assuredly, some if not many will be *anticancer agents* as well agents for other purposes, including alkaloids which display antibiotic, antiviral, or antifungal activity. For one example, the alkaloid *colchicine* has been used not only against *gout* and tried against *cancer* but has been used against *myasthenia gravis*,* as has the alkaloid *galanthamine* (Cordell, *Alkaloids*, pp. 526–527, 551–552).

___

* As compared to using dangerous toxic alkaloids or other toxic substances, Adelle Davis's nutritional regimen against myasthenia gravis appears benign indeed. (Adelle Davis, *Let's Get Well*, Harcourt, Brace & World, New York, 1965, pp. 295–298). She notes that this illness involves some defect or another in the production of a compound that transmits nerve impulses to the muscles. This compound is known as acetylcholin (or acetylcholine). She reports on the use of vitamin E, all the B vitamins, and manganese for a short time; and/or cholin (or choline), pantothenic acid, and vitamins B1, B2, B6, C and E; plus potassium.

Unfortunately, colchicine is nonspecific against cancer, affecting both normal cells and cancerous cells—but this is the case with other anticancer drugs such as 5-FU (5-fluorouracil), whose fluorine content is an added and unnatural toxicity.

Nor are alkaloids always as poisonous as their reputation. Take *strychnine* for instance. Although widely known as a poison, in reality it is said to be only moderately toxic, relatively speaking at least. (A necessary reminder: The dosage is the poison.) The source is the genus *Strychnos* (of the family Loganiaceae), species of small trees or climbing shrubs native to Africa, Asia, and South America (Cordell, *Alkaloids*, p. 721). Species of the genus are listed in Hartwell as *anticancer agents*. The Asian species are sources of *strychnine* and *brucine*, whereas the South American species yields the mixture known as *curare*.

In his book *Poisonous and Medicinal Plants*, Will H. Blackwell devotes a section to alkaloids, noting their premier importance among potentially toxic plant compounds (Blackwell, *Plants*, p. 35ff). He notes that there is no uniform model, although alkaloid molecules generally have a ring-like structure (single or multiple rings), contain nitrogen, and are basic rather than acidic, but these features do not necessarily distinguish alkaloids from other compounds.

Only a small part of the alkaloids are *psychoactive*, such as *morphine* (from the opium poppy), *cocaine* (from the leaves of the coca plant *Erythroxylum coca*), *hyoscyamine* and *scopolamine* (from henbane and belladonna), plus *mescaline* (from peyote), the alkaloidal substance *LSD* (from the ergot fungus), and *psilocybin* or *psilocin* (from the magic mushroom *Psilocybe*). Other examples of psycho-active alkaloids occur for instance in the *locoweeds* or *crazyweeds* of the American West.

The remainder and vast majority of the alkaloids are not psychoactive, although affecting the nervous system to a greater or lesser extent, and with some certainly more toxic than others. Perhaps most familiar are the alkaloids *caffeine* (in coffee), *theobromine* (in chocolate), *ephedrine* (in nasal sprays), *nicotine* (in tobacco), *lobeline* (in Indian tobacco), *coniine* (in poison hemlock), *quinine* (for malaria), *strychnine* (here described as a powerful convulsant poison), the *curare* alkaloids (as relaxants), and *solanine* (from the green parts of potatoes and tomatoes).

As to anticancer action, whenever or wherever it occurs, this may be presumed to be either by stimulating the immune system and/or by acting as an enzyme inhibitor. There is also the less likely probability that the substance could act as an enzyme promoter or activator. Finally, there is the possibility that the perceived anticancer activity may be due to wishful thinking, the reason for substantiation by laboratory and clinical trials. On the other hand, medical folklore may merely be trying to tell us something.

4.2 CLASSIFICATION OF ALKALOIDS

The alkaloids may be divided into several major types or configurations. (Example chemical structures are provided in the Blackwell reference.) These types are as follows, along with examples, with the genus and plant family in parentheses. Genera or families **not** listed or represented in Hartwell are supplied with an asterisk (*).

- **Belladonna type (tropane or atropine alkaloids):** belladona (*Atropa* of the family Solanaceae), jimson weed (*Datura* of the family Solanaceae), henbane (*Hyoscyamus* of the family Solanaceae), mandrake (*Mandragora* of the family Solanaceae), coca tree (*Erythroxylum* of the family Erythroxylaceae)
- **Groundsel type (pyrrolizidine alkaloids):** groundsel (*Senecio* of the family Compositae), blue devil (*Echium* of the family Boraginaceae), heliotrope (*Heliotropum* of the family Boraginaceae)
- **Hemlock type (pyridine or piperidine alkaloids):** poison hemlock (*Conium* of the family Umbelliferae), Indian tobacco (*Lobelia* of the family Lobeliaceae)
- **Nicotine or tobacco type (pyrrolidine-pyridine alkaloids):** tobacco (*Nicotinia* of the family Solanaceae), horsetail (*Equisetum* of the family Equisetaceae)
- **Coffee or caffeine type (purine alkaloids):** coffee (*Coffea** of the family Rubiaceae), chocolate and cocoa (*Theobroma** of the family Sterculiaceae*), tea (*Camellia* of the family Theaceae)
- **Quinine type (quinoline alkaloids):** quinine tree (*Cinchona* of the family Rubiaceae), globe thistle (*Echinops* of the family Compositae)
- **Opium or morphine type (isoquinoline alkaloids):** opium poppy (*Papaver* of the family Papaveraceae), bloodroot (*Sanguinaria* of the family Papaveraceae), Dutchman's britches and squirrel corn

(*Dicentra* of the family Papaveraceae), golden seal (*Hydrastis* of the family Ranunculaceae), fumatory (*Corydalis* of the family Papaveraceae)

- **Ergot type (indole alkaloids):** ergot (*Claviceps* of the family Gramineae), magic mushroom (*Psilocybe**), locoweed (*Astragalus* of the family Leguminosae), Carolina jasmine (*Gelsemium*) of the family Loganiaceae), Strychnine (*Strychnos* of the family Loganiaceae)
- **Lupine type (quinolizidine alkaloids):** lupines (*Lupinus* of the family Leguminosae), golden chain (*Laburnum** of the family Leguminosae), false indigo (*Baptisia* of the family Leguminosae), Scotch broom (*Cytisus* of the family Leguminosae), Kentucky coffee tree (*Gymnocladus* of the family Leguminosae)
- **Tomato or Solanine type (steroidal alkaloids, glycoalkaloids):** tomato (*Lycopersicon* of the family Solanaceae), Irish potato (*Solanum* of the family Solanaceae), nightshades (*Solanum* of the family Solanaceae)
- **Veratrum type (steroid alkaloids):** false hellebore (*Veratrum* of the family Liliaceae), death camus (*Zigadenus** of the family Liliaceae)
- **Larkspur type (diterpenoid alkaloids):** larkspur (*Delphinium*)of the family Ranunculaceae, monkshood (*Aconitum* of the family Ranunculaceae)
- **Mescaline type (phenylamine alkaloids):** peyote (*Lophophora*of the family Cactaceae), ephedra (*Ephedra** of the family Gnetaceae)

Of more than passing interest, above, is Indian tobacco, *Lobelia inflata* of the family Lobeliaceae, which contains hemlock-type alkaloids, that is, pyridine or piperidine alkaloids. This may account for a nicotine-like affect. Another example is the Kentucky coffee tree, *Gymnocladus dioica*, of the family Leguminosae, which grows across the American Midwest and out onto the Great Plains, e.g., western Kansas. Its beans contain lupine-type alkaloids, that is, quinolizidine alkaloids, which may account for their having a caffeine-like effect.

The species *Ephedra equisetina* of the family Gnetaceae is the natural source for ephedrine or Ma Huang, an alkaloid of importance known to the Chinese for over 5,000 years (Cordell, *Alkaloids*, pp. 284–286). Among its uses is that of a nasal decongestant.

It would be fortunate indeed if each type of alkaloid above would always correspond to a particular plant family, and vice versa. But such is not in general the case; there is a considerable mixing of alkaloid types and plant families.

In his *Introduction to Alkaloids: A Biogenetic Approach*, Geoffrey A Cordell uses a somewhat different, more involved chemical means of classification, as follows, presented in his table of contents.

- **Alkaloids derived from Ornithine:** simple pyrrolidine alkaloids, nicotine, tropane alkaloids, pyrrolizidine alkaloids
- **Alkaloids derived from Lysine:** pelletierine and related alkaloids, anabasine and related alkaloids, *Sedum* alkaloids, alkaloids of *Lobelia inflata*, simple piperidine alkaloids, Lythraceae alkaloids, quinolizidine alkaloids, *Lycopodium* alkaloids
- **Alkaloids derived from Nicotinic Acid:** arecoline, ricinine, anatabine, dioscorine
- **Alkaloids derived from a Polyacetate Precursor:** shihunine, piperidine alkaloids with short aliphatic side chains, piperidine alkaloids with long aliphatic side chains, 9b-azaphenalene alkaloids, naphthalene-isoquinoline alkaloids, *Elaeocarpus* alkaloids, *Galbulimima* alkaloids, cytochalasans
- **Alkaloids derived from Anthranic Acid:** simple derivatives, simple quinoline derivatives, furoquinoline derivatives, quinazoline derivatives, acridine derivatives, 1,4-benzoxazin alkaloids, benzodiazepine alkaloids, cryptolepine
- **Alkaloids derived from Phenylalanine and Tyrosine:** simple tyramine derivatives, peyote and mescaline, ephedrine, khat, cinnamic acid amide derivatives, diketopipierazines derived from phenylalanine, securinine and related compounds, ***melanin, betalains,*** tetrahydroisoquinoline alkaloids, 1-phenyltetrahydroisoquinoline alkaloids, benzylisoquinoline alkaloids, cularine and related alkaloids, dibenzopyrrocoline alkaloids, pavine and isopavine alkaloids, proaporphine alkaloids, aporphine alkaloids, aporphine dimers, oxoaporphine alkaloids, dioxyaporphine alkaloids, aristolactams, and aristolochic acids, azafluoranthene alkaloids, taspine, morphinandienone alkaloids, *Erythrina* alkaloids, protostephanine and erybidine, hasubanan alkaloids, proterberberine alkaloids, protopine alkaloids, rhoeadine alkaloids, phthalideisoquinoline alkaloids, ochotensane alkaloids, benzo[c]phenanthridine alkaloids, phenethylisoquinoline alkaloids, colchicine, *Cephalotaxus* and homoerythrina alkaloids, Amarylli-

daceae alkaloids, mesembrine and related alkaloids, ipecac alkaloids, phenanthroindolizidine alkaloids, phenanthroquinolizidine alkaloids. Amarylladaceae alkaloids which specifically display anticancer activity include narciclasine, and an oxidation product of lycorine; the alkaloid pretazettine has been used with other agents against Rauscher leukemia virus (Cordell, *Alkaloids*, p. 552).

- **Alkaloids derived from Tryptophan:** the simple bases, simple tryptamine derivatives, pyrrolnitrin, physostigmine and related compounds, the oligomers of tryptamine, diketopiperazines derived from tryptophan, *harmala alkaloids, carbizole alkaloids,* cantin-6-ones, *ergot alkaloids,* monoterpenoid-derived indole alkaloids, nitrogenous glycosides and related compounds, *camptothecine,* coryanthe alkaloids, ajmalicine and related compounds, oxindole alkaloids, *yohimbine* and related alkaloids, *Rauvolfia alkaloids,* ajmaline-sarpagine alkaloids, *Cinchona alkaloids, Strychnos alkaloids,* secodine alkaloids, *Aspidosperma* alkaloids, *Melodinus* alkaloids, iboga alkaloids, biogenetic interconversion of monoterpenoid indole alkaloids, pandoline and related compounds, *Catharanthus alkaloids, Vinca alkaloids,* monoterpenoid indole alkaloids lacking the tryptamine bridge
- **Alkaloids derived from Histidine:** casimiroedine, *pilocarpine,* alkaloids related to pilocarpine, miscellaneous alkaloids
- **Alkaloids derived by the Isoprenoid Pathway:** hemiterpenoid alkaloids, monoterpenoid alkaloids, sesquiterpene alkaloids, diterpene alkaloids, *Daphniphyllum* alkaloids, steroidal alkaloids
- **Miscellaneous Alkaloids:** *toxins from the frog family Dendrobatidae,* saxitoxin, *spermidine* and related alkaloids, macrocyclic peptide alkaloids, *mushroom toxins* other than peptide alkaloids, *maytensinoids,* purine alkaloids

The foregoing illustrates the complexity of classifying alkaloids by their chemical makeup. And sometimes what may be viewed as an alkaloid by one criterion may be perceived as a different class of compound by another criterion. Resolution may require adopting both criteria.

As to the *frog family Dendrobatidae,* mentioned above, three toxins have been isolated from skin secretions of the tropical species *Dendrobates pumilio* and *D. Auratus* (Cordell, *Alkaloids,* p. 925). The toxins have been given such names as pumiliotoxin C and histrionicotoxin. A compound called *gephyrotoxin* and related alkaloids have been isolated from the Colombian frog *D. histronicus.*

With regard to *saxitoxin,* also mentioned above, this is an alkaloid that occurs in the *red tide,* the massive bloom of the marine organisms *Gonyaulix catenella* and *G. tamarensis* (Cordell, *Alkaloids,* p. 927). Called *flagellates* due to their whip-like shape, periodic concentrations occur along parts of the east and west coasts of North America, and which can have serious health consequences. Saxitoxin is also found in a few crustaceans such as the Alaska butter clam, *Saxidamus giganteus,* and a mussel named *Mytilus californianus.* The alkaloid is said to be among the most toxic substances ever found. There are also two related toxins called gonyautoxins that occur in the soft-shell clam *Mya arenaria,* due to the presence of *G. tamarensis.*

As to *mushroom toxins,* above, besides peptide alkaloids, there is the toxin gyromitrin from the genus *Helvella* (Cordell, *Alkaloids,* p. 944). In particular, the alkaloid *muscarine* is cited, along with what are labeled isoxazole derivatives, as obtained from *Amanita muscaria,* and from species of the genera *Inocybe* and *Clitocybe.* Further information is provided in Part 5.

The alkaloids termed *maytensoids* (or *maytansoids*) require special mention, as obtained from the fruits of various species of *Maytensus* (or *Maytenus*)from the plant family Celastraceae, which have antileukemic activity (Cordell, *Alkaloids,* p. 948). The chief alkaloid is *maytensine,* mentioned elsewhere, but maysine and maysenine also occur, although the latter two do not show antileukemic activity. It is noted that the Celastraceae of South Africa and Kenya are not the only sources. Maytensoids may also be obtained from *Colubrina texenes* of the family Rhamnaceae, and from the fungi *Nocardia.*

Another alkaloid source from the family Celastraceae is the species *Catha edulis,* which yields sesquiterpene alkaloids, though the stimulatory action is due to norpseudoephedrine (Cordell, *Alkaloids,* pp. 287, 864). More familiarly known as *khat* (or *kat,* or *qat,* or sometimes *privet*), the leaves of the shrub are most usually chewed. It is commonly used in the Mideast, in Arabia and East Africa, notably in Yemen and Ethiopia. Continued use leads to intellectual deterioration, gastrointestinal problems, and impotency. Psychological dependency is noted, but no withdrawal symptoms. It is not listed in Hartwell's *Plants Used Against Cancer,* but another family member, *Celastrus scandens* or bittersweet, is listed.

Purine alkaloids are derived from the xanthine nucleus, a fundamental base unit in nucleotide structures (Cordell, *Alkaloids,* p. 952). Although xanthine per se has not been found naturally, its derivatives include *caffeine,* which can be called 1,3,7-trimethylxanthine, whereas *theophylline* is 1,3-

dimethylxanthine, and *theobromine* is 3,7-dimethylxanthine. This leads to a consideration that these kinds of stimulatory alkaloids may have other effects, in that coffee and tea for instance are sometimes regarded as folkloric anticancer agents.* More information is provided, for instance, in Appendix M under the several plant families Aquifoliaceae, Rubiaceae, Sterculiaceae, and Theaceae.

Whether more of these other kinds of alkaloids will ever prove useful in cancer treatment has to remain conjectural, for there are obviously so many different alkaloids to choose from, and there are so many variables such as concentrations to use and the biochemical individuality of patients. The resolution of this problem demands severely more efficient means of screening and testing.

More about anticancer activity is set forth as follows.

4.3 ALKALOIDS AS ANTICANCER AGENTS

Cordell's *Alkaloids* lists and describes a fair number of alkaloids for their anticancer activity. For the record, these alkaloids which show anticancer activity are set forth in Table 4–1, with Cordell's page numbers in parentheses. Cordell observes that maytansine is one of the most potent plant anticancer agents found and that it inhibits DNA synthesis but not RNA synthesis and protein synthesis (Cordell, *Alkaloids*, p. 951). It displays a degree of neurotoxicity and hepatotoxicity, but its more severe gastrointestinal toxicity has curtailed further clinical tests. (Albeit the same adverse effect happens with conventional cytotoxic chemotherapy drugs such as 5-FU.)

Of the bisindole alkaloids, the genus *Catharanthus* contains the species *Catharanthus roseus*, more familiarly known as the *Madagascar periwinkle*. (*Catharanthus* as such is not listed in Hartwell, though it is prominently mentioned in Heinerman's *The Treatment of Cancer with Herbs*. Hartwell lists *Vinca* instead, there being a slight confusion in terminology.) Two of the major alkaloids of *Catharanthus roseus* are vindoline and catharanthine (Cordell, *Alkaloids*, p. 788).

Several of the bisindole alkaloids display antileukemic activity, although only two are in present-day clinical use (Cordell, *Alkaloids*, pp. 789–790). One is vincaleukoblastine (VLB), and the other is vincaleurocristine (VCR), also called leurocristine. The latter has proven particularly valuable in the treatment of various forms of human cancer. The alkaloid VLB has been used in the treatment of Hodgkin's disease, and in combination with the antibiotics bleomycin and actinomycin, has been effective against testicular cancer. The alkaloid VCR is highly active against childhood leukemia (ACL) and is used in several combinations both for ACL and non-Hodgkin's lymphomas. It is a component of the well known MOPP (for mechlorethamine, oncovin, procarbazine, and prednisone) treatment for Hodgkin's disease.

The common name periwinkle also overlaps into the origins of what are called the *Vinca* alkaloids, derived from two different species, *Vinca major* and *Vinca minor* (Cordell, *Alkaloids*, p. 790). The genus *Vinca* contains six species native to the Mediterranean area of Europe and on into western Asia and evidently ranging down into eastern Africa. *Vinca major* is sometimes called the large periwinkle, whereas *Vinca minor* is a trailing evergreen herb with blue or white flowers. The U.S. version is called myrtle. The woody plant named *Vinca roseus* has large white or pinkish-purple flowers and is called the red or Cape or Madagascar periwinkle. The genus *Vinca* is a member of the plant family Apocynaceae. Hartwell has listings for *Vinca herbacea*, *Vinca major* L., *Vinca minor* L., and *Vinca* sp. According to Hartwell, the common names for the first-mentioned are variously vicapervica, vincapervinca, and chamaedaphne. The last-mentioned is called *vinca pervinca* or *periwinkle*.

4.4 ALKALOIDS AS ANTIBACTERIAL AGENTS

Alkaloids showing antibacterial activity are listed in Table 4.2. The corresponding page number in Cordell is provided.

Interestingly, although not listed in Table 4.2, penicillin can be classed as an alkaloid due to its molecular makeup, as can some other fungal-derived antibiotics, as will be mentioned in Part 5 in the section on Antibiotics.

---

* The reference notes that these alkaloids are catabolized to uric acid and urea (Cordell, *Alkaloids*, p. 958). Since urea is sometimes listed as an anticancer agent, maybe there is a connection.

Table 4.1 Alkaloids Showing Anticancer
Activity (page citations from Cordell, *Introduction
to Alkaloids*)

Acronycine (p. 267, 269)

Berberine (p. 483)

Bisindole *Catharanthus* alkaloids (pp. 785, 788–790)

Camptothecine (pp. 565, 665, 671–672)

Chelerythrine (p. 515)

1,2-Dehydrodroemetine (p. 566)

2,6-Dimethyl-9-hydroxyellipticine (p. 806)

Fagaronine (pp. 515–516)

9-Hydroxy ellipticine (p. 806)

Indicine-N-oxide (p. 136)

Leurocristine (pp. 656, 785, 789–790)

Maysenine (p. 949)

Maysine (p. 949)

Maytansine (p. 951)

Maytanbutine (p. 951)

Maytansinoids (p. 951)

Maytansinol (p. 949)

2-Methyl-9-hydroxy ellipticine (p. 806)

Narciclasine (p. 552)

Nitidine (p. 515)

Plants in Amaryllidaceae (p. 536)

Pretazettine (p. 552)

Pyrido [4,3–6] carbazole alkaloids (p. 800)

Sanguinarine (p. 515)

Tetrandrine (p. 357)

Tylocrebrine (p. 572)

Tylophorine (p. 412)

Vincaleukophorine (pp. 656, 789–790)

Table 4.2 Alkaloids showing Antibacterial
Activity (page citations from Cordell, *Introduction
to Alkaloids*)

Chelerythrine (p. 515)

Dehydroglaucine (p. 406)

Dibromophakellin (p. 844)

Dimeric *Nuphar* alkaloids (p. 863)

Monobromophakellin (p. 844)

Quinine (p. 720)

Sanguinarine (p. 515)

Spermine (p. 935)

Sporidesmin E (p. 605)

Tomatine (p. 903)

4.5 ALKALOIDS AS ANTIVIRAL AGENTS

Alkaloids showing antiviral activity are listed in Table 4.3. The corresponding page numbers from Cordell are included.

Table 4.3 Alkaloids showing Antiviral Activity (page citations from Cordell, *Introduction to Alkaloids*)

N-alkyl dregamine derivatives (p. 706)

Aranotin (p. 296)

Camptothecine (p. 672)

One of the most dreaded viral disease is **rabies or hydrophobia**. According to John Heinerman's *Healing Animals with Herbs*, cited in Part 2, there have been several herbal treatments mentioned in the folkloric herbal literature, including rue (*Ruta gravolens*, of the family Rutaceae), elecampane (*Inula helenium*, of the family Compositae), and yarrow (*Achillea millefolium*, of the family Compositae) with calamint (of the genus *Calamintha*, of the family Labiatae) All are listed in Hartwell. Furthermore, all these plant families appear in Cordell as containing alkaloids.

This much said about folkloric herbal/alkaloid cures for rabies, there is little doubt that most or all rabies victims would opt for the latest version of the Pasteur treatment. Nevertheless, the particular alkaloids involved in the foregoing herbal treatments could be researched for effectiveness against other viral diseases.

From the above, it can be seen that there may be some unexpected ways for treating AIDS and for counteracting the Marbutg and Ebola viruses, and so on. These are *retroviruses* which have the unfortunate property of producing mutations or other intrinsic changes, so that the established methodologies for immunization do not work. In the search for alternative methods of treatment, plant alkaloids and other plant substances may prove a key to curing all sorts of diseases.

4.6 ALKALOIDS AS ANTIFUNGAL AGENTS

Alkaloids showing antifungal activity are listed in Table 4.4, with the corresponding page numbers in Cordell provided.

Table 4.4 Alkaloids showing Antifungal Activity (page citations from Cordell, *Introduction to Alkaloids*)

Chelerythrine (p. 515)

Sanguinarine (p. 515)

Tomatine (p. 903)

While the foregoing introduces the topic of antifungal agents, there is much more information about the fungi or mycota and their toxins—and their uses as medicines, in particular as anticancer agents. This is the subject of Part 5. It is an old subject, newly discovered.

4.7 OTHER MEDICINAL USES FOR ALKALOIDS

Other more specific uses of alkaloids include antimalarial activity, antitubercular activity as indicated in Table 4.5, with the corresponding page numbers from Cordell given.

In *Poisonous and Medicinal Plants*, Will H. Blackwell has a chapter on Significant Medical Plants. Most contain alkaloids, but some do not. In addition to some of the previous topics already mentioned, there is other instructive information. The subjects are placed in alphabetical order by plant family, followed by genera or species, as follows. All the plant families are represented in Hartwell, but not all the genera or species.

Table 4.5   Some Other Uses for Alkaloids (page citations from Cordell, *Introduction to Alkaloids*)

Antimalarial activity

Chinchona species (707)

Dichroa febrifuga (p. 257)

Hydrangea species (p. 257)

Quinine (pp. 656, 720)

Antitubercular activity

Buxus alkaloids (p. 908)

Cepharanthine (p. 364)

Thalidasine (p. 364)

- **(Apocynaceae)** *Rauwolfia serpentina.* The small shrub called *snakeroot* belongs to the Dogbane family. The powdered taproot was used for centuries in India for the treatment of *lunacy,* the "moon disease," and for snakebites and insect bites. About 50 alkaloids have so far been isolated from the root. These include the indole alkaloid *reserpine,* the most famous, plus deserpidine and rescinnamine. Reserpine has been used in the treatment of schizophrenia, where its sedative action permits the patient to lead sort of a semi-normal life. Its effectiveness on the central nervous system is probably due to the fact that it is *chemically similar to the neurotransmitter serotonin* (and even to *LSD*). A side effect is that it lowers blood pressure, so it is used to counteract high blood pressure or hypertension. *Rauwolfia serpentina* is native to northern India, but other species grow in central Africa and in Central America and the Caribbean. (Neither the genus nor the species is listed in Hartwell.)

- **(Apocynaceae)** *Strophanthus gratus.* Known as *sawai* or smooth strophanus, this evergreen species is a member of the Dogbane family. Natives of Africa mashed the seeds into a thick fluid and used it for arrow poison. The end result is quick cardiac arrest. The active agent is the glycoside G-strophanthin, called *ouabain.* Conversely, in the correct dosage—as is often the case—it will serve as a *heart stimulant,* especially in situations of rapid and acute heart failure. It must be introduced intravenously or intra-muscularly, since the drug is but poorly absorbed in the digestive tract. (The genus but not the species is listed in Hartwell.)

- **(Apocynaceae)** *Catharanthus roseus.* The species is called the *Madagascar periwinkle,* an herb with striking white or rose-colored flowers. Two alkaloid extracts, *vinblastine* and *vincristine,* have proved effective against certain kinds of blood-related cancers. Other species of periwinkle have not proved successful against cancer. (The genus is listed in Hartwell as *Vinca.*) Uses against other diseases are apparently in abeyance.

- **(Erythroxylaceae)** *Erythroxylum coca.* Known as *coca,* this species is a small tree or shrub found on the Amazonia side of the Andes. The leaves are chewed by the Andean natives as a means to lessen fatigue at high altitudes. It made its way to Europe where it was used as a local anesthetic in the latter 1800s. The active ingredient was found to be the tropane alkaloid *cocaine.* The rest is history. As with other drugs, an overdose can occur, leading to heart and respiratory failure. Less dangerous pharma-ceuticals have been modeled on the cocaine structure, such as novocaine and xylocaine. (The genus but not the species is listed in Hartwell.)

- **(Leguminosae)** *Physostigma venenosum.* West tropical Africa produces the *Calabar bean,* or *ordeal bean,* a large woody vine. It was once used as the means for "truth by ordeal," where survival meant that the accused was not guilty. The seeds contain toxic alkaloids, including *physostigmine,* also called *eserine.* The poisonous effect is to paralyze the respiratory system, producing respiratory failure or respiratory arrest. In medicine, the so-called ordeal bean has been used as a muscle contractant for *glaucoma* and *myasthenia gravis,* as a counteractant for the muscle relaxing properties of atropine and curare, and even as an antidote for strychnine. (Neither the genus nor the species is listed in Hartwell).

A chapter titled "The Ordeal Bean of Old Calabar," by Bo Holmstead, appears in *Plants in the Development of Modern Medicine*, edited by Tony Swain and published in 1972. Considerable historical background is furnished, including the case of an English doctor who tried it out on himself—and survived. The term *Old Calabar* refers to an area on the West African Coast, originally settled by the Dutch, who had moved in on the Portuguese. It was located near the Niger River delta, south of which there entered the Old Calabar River in what is now Nigeria. A native African people called the Efik used the bean in their ceremonial proceedings, which were conducted by the Egbo or Leopard Society, an association of prominent male members of the Efik. Some of the early accounts are documented in the reference, along with the later influence of the United Presbyterian Mission and the British Consul, who at one time was the famous explorer Sir Richard Burton.

The scientific background is provided as well, which started in the late nineteenth century. The successes of these earlier investigations were followed by determining the role of the principal alkaloid physostigmine (sometimes called *eserine*) in neurohumoral transmission. Eserine or physostigmine was found to act as an enzyme inhibitor for cholinesterase, which is involved in the transmission of impulses from a nerve to an organ by means of the hormone acetylcholine. In so many words, physostigmine serves as a regulator. Its use in treating myasthenia gravis is fully described, as is its unexpected part in the development of carbamates as insecticides.

- **(Liliaceae)** *Aloe* **spp.** The healing power of the aloe leaf sap is attributed to chrysophanic acid, an anthraquinone molecule. It also contains anthraquinone glycosides collectively called *aloin,* including *barbaloin,* which yields *aloe-emodin,* a cathartic. (*Aloe* is listed in Hartwell.)

- **(Liliaceae)** *Colchicum autumnale.* Called the *autumn crocus,* this species is not a true crocus, the latter belonging to the Iris family. It has been used historically for the treatment of gout. The active agent is the alkaloid *colchicine.* Colchicine is very toxic, however, and must be used with care. It is also active in halting cell division and is used in botany to manipulate plant chromosomes to produce variants or mutations. It would serve in the same way to prevent division of blood cancer cells but is too toxic to use in this way, though a similar alkaloid from another species has had limited success against leukemia. (*C. autumnale* is in Hartwell.)

- **(Menispermaceae)** *Chondrodendron tomentosum.* Along with *Strychnos toxifera, Chondrodendron tomentosum* is a principal source of *curare.* The active components are several different alkaloids, unspecified. [Cordell mentions that they are bisbenzylisoquinoline alkaloids, notably *tubocarine* (Cordell, *Alkaloids*, p. 356)] Curare has been used as a muscle relaxant during surgery, for countering the effect of tetanus, in the treatment of cerebral palsy, during the setting of broken bones, and for myasthenia gravis. Synthetic drugs have partially replaced the natural substance. (Hartwell lists the plant family but not the particular genus. *Strychnos* is prominently listed, however.) *Considering the adverse side effects, above, myasthenia gravis deserves a nontoxic nutritional trial, such as set forth by Adelle Davis, previously mentioned.*

- **(Papaveraceae)** *Papaver somniferum.* The opium poppy is the source for the white latex called *opium.* This crude substance was found to contain some twenty different alkaloids, of which the most famous is the alkaloid *morphine.* Morphine, along with cocaine, has been used as a pain reliever in terminal illnesses. A milder drug called *codeine,* which is methylated morphine, acts as a cough suppressant. Another drug known as *thebaine,* which is dimethylmorphine, acts as a convulsant, illustrating the fact that *similar drugs can act oppositely.* Heroin is synthesized as acetylated morphine and is more addictive and dangerous than morphine itself, having a direct action on the part of the brain that governs respiration. (The species is listed in Hartwell.)

- **(Rubiaceae)** *Cephaelis ipecacuanha.* Ipecac is a shade-loving perennial herb found in the forests of Brazil and Bolivia. The alkaloids *emetine, cephaeline,* and *psochotrine* occur in the underground stem and roots. Extracts are used to treat amoebic dysentery. Emetine serves as an expectorant. Syrup of Ipecac is used as a life-saving emetic to induce vomiting in children who have taken poisons. (The species is listed in Hartwell.)

- **(Rubiaceae)** *Cinchona* **spp.** Variously referred to as Peruvian bark, fever tree, Jesuit's bark, and quinine tree, species of the genus *Cinchona* are the natural commercial source for *quinine.* The bark of several species contains quinoline alkaloids, in particular the alkaloid named quinine. It is highly effective against the multiplication of *protozoa which cause malaria,* in particular the protozoan genus *Plasmodium,* which is carried by the *Anopheles* mosquito. Synthetic quinoline alkaloids have largely replaced the natural product. (*Cinchona* is listed in Hartwell.)

- **(Rutaceae)** *Pilocarpus pennatifolius.* Commonly called *jaborandi,* the species *Pilocarpus pennatiflo-rius* and *P. jaborandi* are small trees or shrubs of the Citrus family (or Rue family). The leaves contain the simple alkaloid *pilocarpine.* It is used for the treatment of glaucoma more so than physostig-mine—the latter being derived from the West African climbing plant *Physostigma venenosum* of the family Leguminosae (Cordell, *Alkaloids,* p. 584), and previously described above. (Neither the genus nor the species is listed in Hartwell.)
- **(Scrophulariaceae)** *Digitalis* **spp.** Several species of the plant *foxglove* or *digitalis* have been used medicinally, although the two main species used are *Digitalis purpurea* and *D. lanata.* The powdered digitalis leaf was an English folklore remedy for *dropsy,* an accumulation of fluid in the extremities, the symptoms of what is now known as congestive heart failure. In this case, rather than alkaloids, the active constituents turned out to be the *cardiac glycosides* digoxin, digitoxin, deslanoside, and lanato-side. The effect is to strengthen the heartbeat, at the same time slowing it down. The action is through the nervous system. It is noted that, like with many drugs, *there is not a great deal of difference between a therapeutic dose and a toxic dose,* and the dosage must be monitored carefully. Fortunately, however, in this case an antidote has been developed in the form of digitoxin-specific antibodies from immunized sheep. (*Digitalis purpurea* has a number of entries in Hartwell.)
- **(Solanaceae)** *Atropa belladonna.* Three tropane type alkaloids are found: *hyoscyamine, scopolamine,* and *atropine.* They act as antispasmadics and muscle relaxers. (The species is listed in Hartwell.)

Blackwell concludes at the end of the chapter that the recent track record of using plant medicines has been limited. This fact was pointed out in an article by Varro E. Tyler, published in a 1986 issue of *Economic Botany.* For example, it was noted that *25 years of testing some 40,000 plant species by the National Cancer Institute failed to yield "a single agent of general use in the treatment of human cancer."* Tyler noted that there were mitigating circumstances, however, in that *there was a lack of interdisciplinary cooperation, an unfavorable federal regulatory atmosphere, and the present-day requirement that every-thing be cost-effective.**

Nevertheless, both Blackwell (published in 1990) and Tyler (published in 1986) concur that there are reasons to be optimistic about future findings, for there have been breakthroughs in other countries in developing plant drugs—which, however, are not available in the United States. Examples include antiviral creams prepared from plants. Furthermore, important plant discoveries are very likely as additional tropical exploration proceeds. This will be accompanied by new methods of drug analysis and development, improved bioassay techniques, and refined methods for growing and commercializing rare plant tissue cultures. It will be propelled by a resurgence of interest in a public demanding "green medicine."

Some new discoveries, already commonplace, include new skin creams (especially for acne) that contain vitamin A and other retinoids, which are based on beta-carotene from plants. This trend in plant research and development is predicted to continue, with the twenty-first century introducing a new boom in medical botany.

4.8 TOXICITY VERSUS MEDICAL BENEFITS

Whether a given alkaloid or alkaloid-containing plant or herb is toxic or beneficial may depend almost entirely on dosage levels and frequency, and the biological individuality of the patient. The one must be played against the other—the same as for other medicines. This is why close monitoring is so vital and why the assembly-line practices of modern medicine are not adapted to this kind of special care. It may be that only the patient can tell when a medication is working or not working, and the patient may have to go it alone. The trouble is, alkaloid-containing substances are nothing to trifle with, and some sort of expert close supervision is imperative.

One may conclude that, from the list of anticancer alkaloid substances already known, others will surely be found. Not only this, but the ones already known may work sufficiently well if used in the dosage levels and frequency required—a process of optimization that may have to be tailor made for each patient. One may also speculate that Hartwell's compilation, *Plants Used Against Cancer,* is for

---

* Blackwell also furnishes some other pertinent references, including *Economic and Medicinal Plant Research,* Volume 1, by Wagner, Hiking, and Farnsworth, published in 1985 by Academic Press. Although somewhat dated, apparently not much has changed.

the most part a compendium of alkaloid-containing plants. If one were so bold, it might be projected that many or most alkaloids act against cancer in some way or another and to some degree, if only the dosage level and frequency were established.

Furthermore, it is critical that the nature of the alkaloid and its concentration be known with certainty. For this reason, the isolated or pure alkaloid is preferable to using plants or herbs whose alkaloid content is so variable and sometimes may be nonexistent. In other words, quality control can be maintained with pure substances but not necessarily with the alkaloid-containing plant or herb itself.

An extract from the deadly monkshood is mentioned in Alexander Solzhenitsyn's novel *Cancer Ward*, and this fact is noted in James A. Duke's *CRC Handbook of Medicinal Herbs* (Solzhenitsyn, *Cancer Ward*, pp. 228–233; Duke, *CRC Handbook*, p. 12). Monkshood or aconite is the species *Aconitum columbianum* or *A. napellus* of the family Ranunculeae, and has been previously cited. The principal alkaloid is *aconitine,* which occurs notably in the roots. Solzhenitsyn describes the preparation and use of aconite in a chapter titled "The Root from Issyk Kul." Evidently illegal in the Soviet Union, the roots had been extracted with alcohol (vodka). Of unknown concentration, the extract was contained in a small vial. The extract dosage used was described as a graduated system, from one drop up to ten drops, presumably on succeeding days, then back again down to one drop, with a ten-day interval between courses (Solzhenitsyn, *Cancer Ward*, p. 230). The complete cycle therefore encompassed a 30-day period. The treatment was in turn described as dark superstition and a game with death (Solzhenitsyn, *Cancer Ward*, p. 231), although there is the hint that it had worked.*

Mention is made of *Aconitum* in Plutarch's *Lives*. In the last paragraph of "The Life of Crassus," the cruelty of the Parthian king Hyrodes is revenged. Hyrodes had fallen "into a disease that became a dropsy" and was given "drink of the juice of aconitum" but recovered.

> The dropsy received the poison and one drave the other out of Hyrodes' body, and set him afoot again.

Whereby he was murdered by other means. (The translation of this particular segment is emphasized in Paul Turner's *Selected Lives from the Lives of the Noble Grecians and Romans*, Vol. I, pp. xv, 280.) Dropsy is another name for edema, the retention of fluids in the body, and presumably it is a symptom of more serious ailments. (Dropsy more specifically is referred to as *ascites,* the accumulation of fluid in the peritoneal cavity, a condition that occurs between the membrane lining the abdominal wall and the membrane covering the abdominal walls. Common causes are said to be liver failure, in which the liver blood circulation is impaired causing an elevation of blood pressure levels in the portal vein, heart failure, tumor invasion, and the escape of lymph fluids into the peritoneal cavity.) Apparently, the juice of aconitum, in the dosage used, cured whatever disease it was—which could have even been cancer, since cancer itself can result in dropsy, say due to cancer-caused liver failure. In any event, we have an isolated instance of the curative powers of *Aconitum*, albeit its usual usage is intended as a poison.

4.9 SCREENING PLANTS FOR ALKALOIDS

The word is that, in canvassing the rain forests for bioactive plants, alkaloid activity is the criterion used. If a species does not show alkaloid activity, it is passed by.

The methods for testing are of interest. There are two principal tests which provide a simple and rapid means for the screening of potential alkaloid-containing plants (Cordell, *Alkaloids*, p. 10). The Wall test extracts about 20 grams of dried plant material with boiling 80 percent ethanol. The filtrate is evaporated, and the recovered solids are acidified with 1 percent hydrochloric acid. Mayer's reagent or silicotungstic acid is added, and any alkaloids present will show up as a precipitate. In the Kiang-Douglas test, the dried plant material is moistened with a dilute ammonia solution. This converts the alkaloids—which normally exist as alkaloidal salts in the form of citrates, tartrates, or lactates—to an alkaline

---

* The "Issyk-Kul root" is referred to in George St. George's Time-Life book titled *Soviet Deserts and Mountains* (St. George, *Soviet Deserts*, p. 167), as again described in Part 8 within the section "Enzymes and Inhibitors for Anaerobic Glycolysis." He was traveling near Lake Issyk-Kul in the Tien Shen Mountains, which separate southwestern Siberia and western China. There is a Siberian species named *Aconitium sibiricum*, called a "terrible plant," which is similar to *Aconitum columbianum*, the wild monkshood or wolfsbane as found in the Rocky Mountains. The surreptitious claim is that the root, properly used, is a miracle drug for arthritis. Cancer was not mentioned.

or basic composition. The mixture is extracted with chloroform, the extract is concentrated by partial evaporation, and dilute hydrochloric acid is added. The filtrate is treated with Mayer's, Dragendorff's, or Bouchardat's reagent. A precipitate indicates the presence of alkaloids, as before. The precipitating agents are based on the fact that alkaloids will combine with heavy metals such as mercury, bismuth, silicon, or tungsten, and with iodine. Thus, Mayer's reagent, the least sensitive, contains potassium iodide and mercuric chloride.

4.10 COMMON GARDEN VEGETABLES AND ALKALOIDS

A list of most of the common garden vegetables is furnished in Table 4.6, in some cases with the particular alkaloids that the plant families are known to contain. The extension to all members of the same plant family is only an inference, for all members of the same alkaloid-bearing plant family do not necessarily contain alkaloids, or the same alkaloids (with the possible exception of the family Papaveraceae). However, there are specific alkaloids that are attributed to a particular species or genus, and an attempt is also made to show some of these. It may be considered that the various alkaloids occur in minute or trace amounts, if they occur at all, inasmuch as none of these vegetables are considered toxic, at least in the amounts normally consumed. In other words, *alkaloids possibly may serve as micronutrients,* in the manner of vitamins and trace minerals. It is a topic for further investigation since the alkaloid content, minute though it may be, may in part be responsible for the therapeutic value of these vegetables.

The different parts of these various vegetables contain all sorts of compound classes and compounds, in part of which *nitrogen is ubiquitous.* The nitrogen chain is spelled out in technical detail in successive chapters of the *Biochemistry of Alkaloids.* Thus, in green plants, there is an assimilation of carbon dioxide, nitrate, and sulfate (H. Reinbothe and J. Miersch, in *Biochemistry of Alkaloids,* p. 65ff). Furthermore, several plant-microbe systems, such as in the case of legumes, can assimilate atmospheric nitrogen. *Nitrate as well as nitrogen is reduced to ammonia via the reactions of photosynthesis.* These conversions are enzyme catalyzed, and it is stated that the special protein catalysts used, the enzymes called glutamine synthetase (GS) and ribose-1,5-biphosphate carboxylase, are fundamental to life on earth. The further result is the formation of amino acids, which are precursors for plant proteins and alkaloids.

Several thousand N-heterocyclic ring structures are known to occur in higher plants, animals, and microorganisms (H.W. Liebisch, in *Biochemistry of Alkaloids,* p. 88ff). These are formed from a very few precursors, notably amino acids, but also mevalonate and acetate. *Once formed, the basic N-ring structure may undergo all sorts of further reactions, to create the numerous alkaloids.* This may be referred to as *alkaloid biosynthesis.*

At the same time, there exist the myriad other compounds present, notably the glycosides or glucosides, some of which may combine with alkaloids in still other structures. (An alkaloid can serve as the aglycone or genin part of the glycoside or glucoside molecule, combining with the sugar part of the molecule.) There are, moreover, the *cyanoglycosides,* which contain the cyanide (–CN) group. Add to this what we call *vitamins,* some of which contain nitrogen. Thus, *nicotinic acid or niacin can be viewed as a precursor to a number of alkaloids:* arecoline, ricinine, anatabine, dioscorine, nicotine, and guvacine (Cordell, *Alkaloids,* p. 196ff).

The circumstance becomes tremendously involved, with interrelationships of all sorts existing among the myriad components. Not only will the plant species itself be determining, but also the soil makeup and fertility and the conditions of growth. Hence, any attempt to be definitive will be but a primitive simplification. Nevertheless, we make a few observations in a listing of common vegetables.

The listing in Table 4.6 is according to plant families, with the corresponding page numbers in Cordell cited (designated C), as well as from *Biochemistry of Alkaloids* (designated B), and from *Africa* by Watt and Breyer-Brandwijk (designated A). It is noted that all of these plant families appear in Hartwell. A few other bits of information are included where warranted.

As an additional comment, there are alkaloids and there are alkaloids. Some are poisonous in the extreme, at least above a certain minuscule threshold amount, depending on the alkaloid, the mammalian species, and the particular individual. Others are more benign and presumably can be beneficial, if not vital, in trace amounts. Again, it is a topic for further research.

Moreover, it is sometimes difficult to say just what constitutes an alkaloid, as previously commented. For instance, consider the fabia bean *Vicia fabia* of the family Leguminosae. It is an important pulse or

Table 4.6 Common Garden Vegetables that May Contain Alkaloids[a]

Chenopodiaceae (Cordell, pp. 147, 207, 143, 577): the piperidine alkaloids girgenshonine and pinidine, the lysine-derived alkaloid anabasine, the tryptophan-derived alkaloid dipterine.

Beta vulgaris: **red beet.** Contains betalains or betalain alkaloids (B-255), saponin-betaine alkaloids (A-185).

Spinacia oleracea: **spinach.** Contains phenylalanine/tyrosine alkaloids (C- 275).

Compositae (Cordell, pp. 4, 868, 118, 237): diterpine alkaloids in *Inula*, diterpene alkaloids in *Senecio* and *Petasites*, the simple quinoline alkaloid echinopsine in *Echinops*.

Lactuca sativa: **lettuce.** Alkaloid content 0.02%, narcotic properties (A-243).

Cruciferae or Brassicaceae (Cordell, p. 931): spermidine alkaloids.

Brassica oleracea: **cabbage,** Contains nitrate precursors (B-69), carotenoids (A-328).

Brassica rapa or *B. napobrassica*: **turnip.** Contains carotenoids (A-329).

Raphanus sativus: **radish.** Anticancer (A-334), contains S-glycosides (A-336).

Cucurbitaceae (not in Cordell): variously includes cucumber, melons, gourds, squash, pumpkin, zucchini, and the genera *Cucumis* and *Cucurbita*.

Cucumus sativus: **cucumber.** Contains putrescine (B-100).

Gramineae (Cordell, pp. 269, 622, 955, 276): gramine, 1,4-benzoxyazin-3-one alkaloids, ergot alkaloids, purine alkaloids, the tyramine derivative hordenine.

Hordeum spp.: **barley.** Contains hordenine, gramine, putrescine (C-276, 575, 933)

Oryza sativa: **rice.**

Panicum miliaceum: **millet.**

Secale cereale: **rye.** Contains 1,4-benzoxazin-3-one alkaloids (C-269).

Triticm vulgare: **wheat.** Same as above.

Zea mays: **corn** or maize (or mealie). Same as above plus **HCN** (A-491,492).

Leguminosae (Cordell, pp. 4, 157, 169, 584): N-cinnamoyl piperidinealkaloids, diterpine alkaloids, *Erythrina* alkaloids, harmala alkaloids, monoterpene alkaloids, *Ormosia* alkaloids, piperidine alkaloids, purine alkaloids, pyrrolizidine alkaloids, quinolizidine alkaloids, tryptamine derivatives, tetrahydroisoqinoline alkaloids.

Phaseolus vulgaris: **bean.** Contains piperidine alkaloid precursors (B-130), glycosides to alkaloids (B-166), and **HCN**, which is eliminated when cooked (A-639).

Pisum sativum: **pea.** Contains alkaloid precursors (C-70, 71), and homoserine and methionine (B-79).

Liliaceae (Cordell, p. 4): colchicine-type alkaloids, homoerythrina alkaloids, phenethylisoquinoline alkaloids, steroidal alkaloids, linearisine, crotonosine.

Allium cepa: **onion.** Contains quercetin, alliin, allicin, is antibiotic (A-672, 676, 675).

Allium sativum: **garlic.** Same as above, plus alkaloidal product (A-676).

Asparagus officianalis: **asparagus.** Contains rutin, glycosides, saponins (A-689).

Malvaceae (Cordell, p. 253): quinazoline alkaloids.

Abelmoschus esculentus or *Malva esculentus*: **okra.**

Solanaceae (Cordell, pp. 4, 80, 199, 900): *Solanum* alkaloids.

Capsicum annuum: **Cayenne pepper.** Contains capsaicanoids, related to leucine and valine (B-195).

Lycopersicon esculentum: **tomato.** Contains tomatidine, tomatine (C-900).

Solanum melongena or *S. esculentum*: **egg plant.** Contains solanaceous alkaloids (C-900).

Solanum tuberosum: **potato.** Contains solanidine, solanine (C-903).

Umbelliferae (Cordell, p. 208): piperidine alkaloids

Apium graveolins: **celery.** Contains carotenoids (A-1033).

Daucus carota sativa: **carrot.** Contains pyrrolidine alkaloids, daucine (A-1037).

Note: In a section on "Spermidine and Related Alkaloids," Cordell asserts that *these compounds occur in almost all animals and microorganisms, and probably in most higher plants* (Cordell, *Alkaloids*, pp. 930–931) It is observed that the two polyamines *spermidine* and *spermine* are analogs of another amine, the diamine *putrescine. (All are also considered to be alkaloids.)* Putrescine itself can be regarded as derived from the reductive decarboxylation of the amino acid lysine.

It is further mentioned that these alkaloids or alkaloidal compounds have been detected and/or isolated from higher plants used as foodstuffs. These vegetable sources include **cabbage leaves, tomato juice, apples, and spinach.** Also listed are the **leaves of wheat, maize, pea, black current, and tobacco.**

a. All plant families, genera, and species are listed in Hartwell's *Plants Used Against Cancer.* The plant families in Cordell are cited, giving the page number and the corresponding alkaloid types. The specific genus or species alkaloids are entered as follows: those that appear in Cordell are designated by C; in *Biochemistry of Alkaloids*, designated by B; and in Watt and Breyer-Brandwijk's *Africa*, designated by A. Each designator is followed by the page number.

bean crop in regions of the Near East, Far East, and North Africa. Yet it contains vicine and convicine glycosides, which by their formulas may alternately be construed as alkaloids (Ronald R. Marquardt, in *Toxicants*, II, p 162). The *carotenoids*, the pigments akin to vitamin A, do not contain nitrogen, having a stoichiometric formula of say $C_{32}H_{48}O_8$. On the other hand, the *betalains*, also pigments, have alkaloid structures. The action of the one can be perceived as similar to the action of the other—and vitamin A is presently being tested as an anticancer agent. The hot-tasting, edible peppers of the genus *Capsicum* of the family Solanaceae contain *capsaicinoids*, which are related to alkaloids and are responsible for their unique qualities—and *Capsicum* is, of course, prominently listed in Hartwell.

It may be noted that some plant sprouts or seedlings will have an extra-high alkaloid content, possibly as a protection against grazing animals. Barley sprouts are an example. On the other hand, this may also have bearing on the growth-requirement biochemistry for the seedlings.

Most usually the alkaloids will show up in all the parts of a plant, although they may be more concentrated in some parts as compared to others. And it should again be remarked that, although alkaloids will occur in some of the genera or species of a plant family, this does not mean that all members of the family will contain alkaloids. The sole exception is evidently that of the family Papaveraceae or Poppy family. Taxonomic classification is by criteria other than alkaloid content.

As a cross check, an inspection of Robert F. Raffauf's *A Handbook of Alkaloids and Alkaloid-Containing Plants*, published in 1970, shows that the common garden variety of vegetables each contain the following number of alkaloids, corresponding to the plant families and genera of Table 4.6: *Beta* (2), *Spinacia* (4), *Lactuca* (0), *Brassica* (5), *Raphanus* (1), *Cucumus* (1), *Hordeus* (9), *Oryza* (1), *Secale* (1), *Triticum* (1), *Zea* (1), *Phaseolas* (1), *Pisum* (5), *Allium* (1), *Asparagus* (0), *Abelmochus* (0), *Solanum* (22), *Lycopersicon* (11), *Capsicum* (4), *Daucus* (2), *Apium* (0). These results do not necessarily agree with other findings but are indicative of the prevalence of alkaloids.

An additional survey of alkaloids that occur, or may occur, in common fruits and vegetables is presented in Table 4.7 It is based on data presented in James A. Duke's comprehensive undertaking titled *Handbook of Phytochemical Constituents of GRAS Herbs and Other Economic Plants*. It is a companion volume to Duke's *Handbook of Biologically Active Phytochemicals and Their Activities*. Both are published by the CRC Press. The acronym GRAS stands for Generally Recommended As Safe, as opposed to the acronym GRAP, for Generally Recommended As Poisonous. There is also the acronym GRAF, which stands for Generally Recommended As Food. As Duke points out in the Introduction to both books, the distinction is not always clear cut. (Duke also notes that, unfortunately, there is no acronym GRAM or corresponding category for Generally Recommended As Medicinal.)

It should be emphasized that the information presented in Table 4.7 is only cursory, as selected and extracted from the long list of phytochemicals or plant chemicals that may have been identified for each particular species. For more detailed information, the original reference can be consulted. Another reference which may be consulted is *Hager's Handbuch der Pharmazeutischen Praxis* in its many editions.

As a general comment, many or most of the plant species contain an array of amino acids, both essential and nonessential. These include such essential amino acids as phenylalanine, arginine, histidine, leucine, isoleucine, lysine, methionine, phenylalinine, threonine, and valine, and such nonessential amino acids as alanine, asparaganine, cysteine, glutamine, glycine, proline, serine, and tyrosine. This is interesting, in that *vegetables and fruits are not ordinarily thought of as significant protein sources, but the amino acids, the building blocks for protein, are there.* Proteins per se, however, may be conspicuously absent. The different vitamins are often included in the analyses appearing in the reference, as are, say, fats. Alpha-tocopherol (vitamin E) and ascorbic acid (vitamin C) show up, as do some of the B-vitamins such as pyridoxine and inositol.

Nucleic acid bases and nucleosides are variously represented, notably in the form of adenine or adenosine, guanine or guanosine, cytosine or cytidine, uracyl or uridine, and thymine or deoxythymidine. The adenine derivative inosine shows up fairly regularly. It sometimes seems like a fine line whether to classify a compound as a nucleic acid base or nucleoside, or their kin, or say as an alkaloid, since all contain nitrogen in a ring structure.

Alkaloids are a notable presence, and show up at times—maybe unexpectedly—in some of the more common herbs. As a striking instance, consider *rue* (*Ruta graveolens* of the family Rutaceae). Tried for everything from cancer to rabies, rue is fairly loaded with alkaloids—and is suspected of being toxic in its own right.

Table 4.7 Some Alkaloids and Other Compounds Found in Common Vegetables and Fruits or Medicinal Herbs[a]

Araliaceae
 Panax ginseng: **Chinese ginseng**. Contains ginsenosides.
 Panax quinquefolius*: **American ginseng**. Ginsenosides.

Bignoniaceae
 Tabebuia heptaphylla: **pau d'arco**. Contains chrysophanic acid, β-sitosterol, selenium.

Chenopodiaceae
 Spinacia oleacea: **spinach**. Contains acetylcholine, kaempferol, quercetin.

Compositae
 Cynara scolymus: **artichoke**. Contains eugenol, inulin, tannin.
 Echinaceae spp.: **coneflower**. Contains **betaine**, flavonoids, kaempferol, quercetin, rutin.
 Lactuca sativa: **lettuce**. Contains **hyoscyamine**.
 Taraxacum officinale: **dandelion**. Contains caffeic acid, inulin, saponin, tannin, **taraxacerine, taraxacine**.

Convolvulaceae
 Ipomoea batatas: **sweet potato**. Contains **ipomoeanine**, quercetin.

Cruciferae
 Armoracia rusticana: **horseradish**. Contains kaempferol, quercetin.
 Brassica oleracea: **broccoli**. Contains quercetin, rutin.
 Brassica oleracea var. *capitata*: **cabbage**. Contains cyano compounds, cyanidin-, kaempferol, quercetin.
 Brassica rapa: **turnip**.
 Raphanus sativus: **radish**. Contains diallylsulfide, -cyanide, **sperminidine, spermine**.

Cucurbitaceae
 Citrullus lanatus* or *C. vulgaris*: **watermelon**. Contains **citrulline**.
 Cucumis melo: **cantaloupe**. Contains **citrulline**, rutin, **trigonelline**.
 Cucumis sativus: **cucumber**. Contains **citrulline**.
 Cucurbita spp.: **squash**.
 Cucurbita mavina: **pumpkin**.

Euphorbiaceae
 Acalypha indica: **cancer herb**. Contains **acalyphine, triacetonamine**.

Gnetaceae*
 Ephedra* spp.: **Ma-Huang**. Contains **alkaloids** including **L-ephedrine** and **ephedradine**.

Gramineae
 Avena sativa: **oats**. Contains **colamine, graminine**, β-sitosterol, **spermidine, spermine**.
 Hordeum vulgare: **barley**. Contains **betaine, glaucentrine, hordenine, hordatine**, β-sitosterol, **trigonelline, tyramine**.
 Oryza sativa: **rice**. Contains cyanidin-.
 Triticum aestivum: **wheat**. Contains **betaine, gramine**, quercetin, **trigonelline**, uracil.
 Zea mays: **corn**. Contains **betaine, hordenine**.

Guttiferae
 Hypericum perforatum: **St. John's wort**. contains flavonoids, quercetin, saponin, tannin.

Leguminosae
 Arachis hypogaea: **peanut**. Contains quercetin.
 Medicago sativa: **alfalfa**. Contains **betaine**, β-sitosterol, **trigonelline**.
 Phaesolus lunatus: **lima bean**. Contains **S-methylcysteine**.
 Phaesolus vulgaris: **green bean**. Contains kaempferol, quercetin.
 Pisum sativum: **pea**. Contains **betaine**, cyanidin-, kaempferol, **trigonelline**.
 Trifolium pratense: **red clover**. Contains **L-asparagine**, cyanidin, β-sitosterol.

Table 4.7   Some Alkaloids and Other Compounds Found in Common Vegetables and Fruits or Medicinal Herbs[a] *(continued)*

Liliaceae
Allium cepa: **onion**. Contains cystine, kaempferol, pyruvic acid, quercetin, **trigonelline**.
Allium sativum: **garlic**. Contains diallyl sulfide, quercetin, etc.
Asparagus officinalis: **asparagus**. Contains **asparagine**, inositol, quercetin.
Yucca* baccata: **yucca**. Contains tannin.

Malvaceae
Abelmoschus esculentus or *Hibiscus esculentus*: **okra**.

Musaceae
Musa x paradisiaca: **banana**. Contains kaempferol, quercetin, rutin, shikimic acid, pyruvic acid.

Papaveraceae
Sangunaria candensis: **bloodroot**. Contains many **alkaloids**.

Polygonaceae
Rheum rhabarbarum* or *R. rhaponticum*: **rhubarb**. Contains caffeic acid, cyanidin-, emodin, gallic acid.

Ranunculaceae
Aconitum napellus: **monkshood**. Contains many **alkaloids**.

Rosaceae
Malus domestica*: **apple**. Contains carotenoids, cyanidin-, quercetin, pyruvic acid.
Prunus dulcis or *Amygdalus dulcis*: **almond**. Contains cyanidin, **HCN**, quercetin.
Prunus persica: **peach**. Contains campesterol, cyanidin, flavonol-glycosides, **HCN**, kaempferol, quercetin, β-sitosterol.
Pyrus communis: **pear**. Contains kaempferol, quercetin, shikimic acid.

Rubiaceae
Coffea* arabica: **coffee**. Contains **caffeine, spermidine, spermine, theobromine, theophylline**.

Rutaceae
Citrus sinensis: **orange**. Contains **betaine, caffeine, citrusinine, hordenine**, linalool, rutin, β-sitosterol, **stachydrine**.
Ruta graveolens: **rue**. Contains **arborinine, gergerine, graveoline, marmesine, marmesinine, 6-methoxyamnine, 6-quinoline, phaliosidine, ribalinidine, rutacridine, rutamine, savinine, skimmianine**.

Solanaceae
Capsicum annuum: **bell pepper**. Contains **betaine**, eugenol, **solamine**.
Lycopersicon lycopersicum: **tomato**. Contains **betaine, narcotine, nicotianamine**, pyruvic acid, rutin, **solanine, tomatidine, tomatine, trigonelline**.
Solanum melongena: **egg plant**. Contains **solamargine, solanidine, solanine, solasodine, solasonine, trigonelline**.
Solanum tuberosum: **potato**. Contains campesterol, **cuscohygrine**, cyanoside, cyanonin, kaempferol, **nicotine**, quercetin, **solamine, solanidine, solanine**, tannin, **tomatidine, tomatine, trigonelline**.

Taxaceae
Taxus baccata: **common yew**. Contains baccatins, *cephalomanine*, *taxacitine*, **taxine-A,B**, **(R)-taxiphylline**, taxol, taxol-A,B, **triglochinine**.

Umbelliferae
Apium graveolens: **celery**. Contains linalool, **piperidine, pyrrolidine**, quercetin derivatives, rutin, **sedanoline, toluidine**.
Daucus carota: **carrot**. Contains acetylcholine, benzylamine, borneol, carotoxin, cyanidin-, **daucine**, eugenol, kaempferol, linalool, **putrescine, pyrrolidine**, quercetin.

Vitaceae
Vitis vinifera: **grape**. Contains **betaine**, caffeic acid, flavonoids, kaempferol, linalool, quercetin, shikimic acid, tannin.

Zygophyllaceae
Larrea tridentata: **creosote bush, chaparral, greasewood**. Contains borneol, camphor (not to mention nordihydroguaiaretic acid or NDGA, and quercetin).

a. From *Handbook of Phytochemical Constituents of GRAS Herbs and Other Economic Plants,* by James A. Duke, CRC Press, Boca Raton FL, 1992. Plant families, genera, or species not appearing in Hartwell's Plants Used Against Cancer are denoted by an asterisk. Alkaloids, for the most part, are highlighted in boldface.

The foregoing gives rise to the thought that alkaloids may be involved in the most fundamental of biological processes, and may affect these same processes for better or worse. *It is conceivable, therefore, that alkaloids could integrate into genetic structures and modify the genetic code—again for better or worse.* For example, in this way alkaloids could cause unrestrained cell growth—or selectively act against unrestrained cell growth. The role of alkaloids therefore may be other than, or in addition to, that of enzyme inhibitors. (*Viruses*—which may viewed as nitrogenous pieces of protein—do in fact integrate into the genetic structure to produce oncogenes.)

Another thought is about the role of growth hormone (GH) as related to cancer cell growth. For instance there is a growth hormone-releasing factor (GRF) and the substance called *somatostatin* or growth hormone release-inhibiting factor (GRIF), which may stimulate or inhibit the release of growth hormone (Voet and Voet, *Biochemistry*, p. 1271). Although growth hormone or GH, also called *somatropin*, stimulates general growth, it also *stimulates growth in a variety of special tissues.* For instance, its other activities include causing the liver to produce polypeptide growth factors called *somatomedins*, which in turn stimulate cartilage growth and have insulin-like properties.

The above brings to mind that there may be other compounds that act as growth hormone release-inhibiting factors or GRIFs, which could act selectively against whatever growth hormones, if any, may propel cancer cell growth. Indeed, certain alkaloids might function in this manner.

Incidentally, human growth hormones can be and are synthesized, a fact described in biochemistry or microbiology texts and references. For the record, a structural picturization comprises 191 amino acids with two disulfide bridges (Frank Ungar, in *Textbook of Biochemistry*, pp. 786–787). Also observed is that *somatostatin* (also called SRIF in the reference rather than GRIF, above) is involved in regulating the release of growth hormone, and that the growth hormone GH affects soft tissues as well as organs and bones (Ungar, in *Textbook of Biochemistry*, pp. 784–785). It is further stated that there are several *somatomedins*, which not only regulate cartilage growth but stimulate protein synthesis and amino acid and glucose uptake.

The full inquiry is evidently not complete, but it follows that there is the inference that these regulatory growth systems could be affected by outside agents—which conceivably might be alkaloids or other bioactive substances. For example, pyrrolizidine alkaloids are notorious for affecting human growth patterns as has been indicated in Part 2. Whether it should follow that other, less toxic alkaloids might selectively disrupt cancer cell growth patterns is a matter for serious consideration—and at the least is conceivable. Mention is made in the reference of the neurotransmitters dopamine and norepinephrine being involved, to which can be added that alkaloids are also known to function in the role of chemical neurotransmitters or messengers. What with approximately 10,000 or so known alkaloids to choose from, and the myriad other bioactive plant substances, there are nearly limitless possibilities for coming up with general as well as specific nontoxic anticancer agents.

With regard to the foregoing, there is a similarity to hormones, which also act as chemical messengers (Voet and Voet, *Biochemistry*, p. 1261ff.) and which consist of nitrogen-bearing polypeptides and amino-acid derivatives (Voet and Voet, *Biochemistry*, p. 1263).

Minerals or inorganic compounds are also present in plants and are denoted in the listings by their elemental names such as calcium, potassium, zinc, and so on. Of particular note is the almost ubiquitous presence of selenium, regarded as an anticancer agent in minor or trace concentrations, but which becomes a poison in greater concentrations. It serves as an enzyme inhibitor, as has been noted, e.g., in Part 1 and Appendix A, especially for certain glycolytic reactions.

In addition to alkaloids, which are highlighted in boldface, glycosides or glucosides are conspicuous by their presence, but are not listed here. Occasionally there are *flavonoids*. *Stigmasterol*, sometimes thought of as an anticancer agent, is often present, but it is not included here in the brief listings. Two other substances which are regarded as anticancer agents, *quercetin* and β-sitosterol, are sometimes included in the listings of Table 4.7. *Chrysophanic acid* shows up occasionally, as do some other compounds sometimes thought of as anticancer agents such as *kaempferol* and *linalool*. *Cyano-* or *cyanidin-type compounds* may show up, an indication for the –CN or cyanide group in one form or another.

It may be remarked that each analysis may pertain only to a particular plant, obtained in a particular locale, at a particular time or season, and sampled in a given way. This qualification is advisable since it is a well known fact that *plant compositions for the same species may vary widely. Compositions vary with locality, with the season, and even with the time of day. Compositions also vary markedly with the plant part—e.g., root, rhizome, stem, leaves, flower, and fruit.* Not only do variations occur for organic compounds but for inorganics as well. For instance, plant selenium content can expectedly vary with the soils in which the plant grows, and so on. Thus, growth is in a particular soil under particular but varying climatic conditions. Moreover, there is variation in naming the species itself. That is, the species in one part of the world, although called by the same scientific name, is not necessarily the exact same species in another part of the world. (Accommodation can be made by inserting the qualifier "var.")

This all said, it seems simply incredible that plants can produce such large arrays of chemicals, sometimes diverse, sometimes the same. In the Duke reference, the list of chemicals sometimes runs to several pages—and it may be surmised that this is only the beginning.

It is entirely possibly that our most common plants contain chemicals that can counteract cancers of all types and, in the most general sense, are chemotherapy agents, acting as enzyme inhibitors or regulators for critical biochemical reactions that otherwise support cancer cell growth. It becomes a question of which is which, and how much?

Here, we merely note some of the alkaloids that are or may be present in representative common foods, and also in a representative few of what we think of as herbs or plant medicines. It is entirely possible that the bioactive anticancer ingredients are from classes of compounds heretofore unsuspected, say glycosides or flavonoids, and so on, or some combination. And the distinction between classes is not always sharp, e.g., there are *glycoalkaloids* for instance.

It may be assumed that the samples analyzed are in the raw state, that is, have not been cooked or heated or otherwise treated, which may alter the chemical compositions.

We add that *with foods or foodstuffs we are pretty sure of what we're getting*—that is, *foodstuffs by definition are for the most part nontoxic* when consumed in reasonable amounts, as has been demonstrated amply throughout the course of history. On the other hand, what we think of as herbs or plant medicines may or may not be toxic, depending on dosage levels. And if, say, we purchase a medicinal root or substance of some species or another, how can we ever be sure of what we're getting, or getting into? What manner of certification can in fact be instituted to ensure credibility?

Hence the need to look instead into the plant chemicals or phytochemicals known to be present. But here as well, there can be a question of purity, as witness the trouble with tryptophan a few years back. Vigilance, obviously, is the key—but the problems are not always simple. It is an endeavor that needs the active support and participation of medical professionals rather than their opposition and objections.

It may be added that monitoring the alkaloid content of foods is not ordinarily pursued. Probably the only exception is with potatoes, where the U.S. Department of Agriculture keeps an eye on things, particularly with regard to the introduction of new subspecies or varieties.

4.11 PLANTS AND PLANT FAMILIES CONTAINING POTENTIAL ANTICANCER AGENTS, NOTABLY ALKALOIDS

The plant families appearing in Hartwell contain species that, according to medical folklore, are anticancer agents. For the record, all the families listed in Hartwell are enumerated in Appendix M. The plant families in boldface appear in Cordell, with page numbers provided. These plant families contain species with alkaloids.

Representative common names for some of the plant species as obtained from Hartwell's compilation are furnished for each plant family. These various species are anticancer agents, at least according to medical folklore, but do not necessarily contain alkaloids.

Common names containing the word "cancer" are highlighted, for instance cancer weed or cancerweed, *Salvia lyrata* of the family Labiatae, also called the lyre-leaved sage. It has been long known as a folk remedy for cancer and warts (*A Field Guide to Medicinal Plants*, p. 192). Incidentally, Labiatae is a plant family some of whose members contain alkaloids.

A monograph presenting some of the aspects of certain alkaloid-bearing plants and their alkaloids, previously cited, is *Toxicants of Plant Origin. Volume I. Alkaloids*. Additional information is contained in Geoffrey A. Cordell's *Alkaloids*, in *Weeds and Poisonous Plants of Wyoming and Utah* and *Weeds of the West*, in Ruth Ashton Nelson's *Handbook of Rocky Mountain Plants*, and in *Poisonous Grassland Plants*.

4.11.1 TOBACCO

In speaking about some of the more widely known alkaloid-containing plants, there is notably tobacco, which is of the genus *Nicotiana* of the family Solanaceae, and in particular there is the species known as *Nicotiana tabacum* (L.P. Bush and M.W. Crowe, in *Toxicants*, I, p. 88ff). Expectedly, species of the genus are listed in Hartwell as anticancer agents. There are in fact more than 60 species of *Nicotiana*, with most of the alkaloids appearing as 3-pyridyl derivatives. Nicotine is no doubt the most prominent alkaloid in commercial tobaccos (*N. tabacum* and *N. rustica*). Besides nicotine, the major alkaloids include nornicotine, anatabine, and anabasine. There are also minor alkaloids, for the most part derived from the major alkaloids. Both leaves and roots contain alkaloids, with the greater concentrations in the roots. At low dosages, nicotine stimulates the autonomic ganglia, but at high doses it acts oppositely, blocking the autonomic ganglia. (The ganglia are the masses of nervous tissue containing nerve cells in the autonomic nervous system along the spine, and as are connected to the brain.) As dosage levels increase, there are many other adverse physiological effects listed in the reference. Although nicotine has been used as an insecticide, not all insects are affected.

As to cancer, it is noted that *Nicotiana* alkaloids can produce N-nitrosamines, which are definitely carcinogenic (Bush and Crowe, in *Toxicants*, I, p. 98). In fact the term tobacco-specific N-nitrosamines, or TSNA, is commonly used. TSNA occurs in small amounts in young plants and increases with maturity and "curing." The carcinogenic effects on lung tissue are well publicized, but whether minute injections of *Nicotiana* alkaloids would act against cancer has probably never been addressed. However, nicotine, nornicotine, and anabasine, respectively, have pyridine, pyrrolidine, and piperidine rings (Bush and Crowe, in *Toxicants*, I, p. 101). There is the possibility, therefore, of a connection with other anticancer agents which have these structures.

4.11.2 HEMLOCK

Piperidine alkaloids are of a type that appears in the notorious poison hemlock, namely the species *Conium maculatum* of the family Umbelliferae (K.E.Painter and R.F. Keeler, in *Toxicants*, I, p. 109ff.) The piperidine ring is common to a wide variety of alkaloids occurring not only in plants but in animals and microorganisms. Piperidine alkaloids are regarded as derived from lysine, acetate, or mevalonate. Lysine-derived piperidine alkaloids are found for instance in the following species or genera:

- pelletierene—in the **pomegranate tree** (*Punica granatum* of the family Punicaceae)
- piperine—in **pepper** (genus *Piper* of the family Piperaceae)
- hystrine and lupinine—in **lupine** (genus *Lupinus* of the family Leguminosae)
- sedamine—in **sedum or stonecrop** (genus *Sedum* of the family Crassulaceae
- anabasine—in **tobacco** (genus *Nicotiana* of the family Solanaceae)
- lobeline—in **lobelia** (genus *Lobelia* of the family Campanulaceae)
- securinine—in the genus *Lycopodium* of the family Lycopdiaceae

All of the above are found in Hartwell. Acetate-derived piperidine alkaloids include **coniine** and others, as follows:

- coniine—in the genus *Conium* of the family Umbelliferae
- pinidine—in the genus *Pinus* of the family Pinaceae
- cassine—in the genus *Cassia* of the family Leguminosae
- julioprosopine—in the genus *Prosopis* of the family Leguminosae

All the above genera are listed in Hartwell.

Acetate-derived piperidine alkaloids are found in animals. Anabasine, which is a tobacco alkaloid, is found in ants of the genus *Aphaenogaster*. Various 2,6-disubstituted piperidine alkaloids are found in the fire ant, *Solenopsis saevissima*. More than a hundred different alkaloids have been isolated from neotropical frogs of the family Dendrobatidae, most of which are piperidine alkaloids.

Acetate-derived piperidine alkaloids occur in microorganisms. Thus, the antibiotic cycloheximide, a product of *Streptomyces noursei*, has a piperidine nucleus. Strains of *Streptomyces* and *Actinomyces* contain 2-pentydienyl-Δ'-piperidine and nigrifactin, which are similar to alkaloids found in *Conium macalatum* or poison hemlock.

Mevalonate-derived piperidine alkaloids include the following:

- skytanthine—in *Skytanthus acutus* of the family Apocynaceae
- nupharidine—in the **water lily** (*Nuphar japonicum* of the family Nymphaeaceae)
- solanidine—in the genus *Solanum* of the family Solanaceae
- secodine—in the genus *Rhazya* of the family Apocynaceae

Species of the genera *Nuphar* and *Solanum* are listed in Hartwell.

At all dosage levels tested on animals, *Conium* alkaloids are extremely toxic. In fact the descriptor *teratogenic* is also used, indicating that the plants cause monstrous malformations in the newborn. Nevertheless, many entries for *Conium* appear in Hartwell. Since medical folklore indicates that it has been tried as a cancer treatment, it must have been used only in trace amounts—if that much—and even then is a practice that must have been dangerous in the extreme.

4.11.3 LUPINES

The genus *Lupinus* of the family Leguminosae (or Fabaceae or Pea family) includes species that contain quinolizidine alkaloids (Richard F. Keeler, in *Toxicants*, I, p. 134ff). Some of the species of *Lupinus* are ornamental, some are useful for forage, and some are poisonous due to the presence of high concentrations of quinolizidine alkaloids. Not only are quinolizidine alkaloids found in member species of *Lupinus*, but they are also found in several other genera of Leguminosae. They are found as well in the families Chenopodiaceae, Berberidaceae, and Solanaceae. Needless to say, all these plant families are represented in Hartwell. A listing of alkaloids found in *Lupinus* includes the following: anagyrine, sparteine, lupanine, thermopsine, α-isolupanine, α-isosparteine, β-isosparteine. The alkaloid content not only varies among the different species (*Texas bluebonnets,* for instance, are not considered very toxic) but varies with the plant parts and time of growth (Keeler, in *Toxicants*, I, pp. 138–139). For example, during growth the alkaloids concentrate in the green parts, but *after the flowering period the alkaloids concentrate in the seeds and seed pods.*

More than 100 lupine species grow in the western U.S., and some are grazed by livestock, with the lupine species in general noted for having a high protein content. Unfortunately, this leads to toxicosis and teratogenesis if the plants are grazed extensively. In humans, these alkaloids can induce malaise, nausea, mydriasis, respiratory arrest, visual disturbances, ataxia, diaphoresis, progressive weakness, and coma (Keeler, in *Toxicants*, I, p. 145). The alkaloid sparteine is noted to have been used as an oxytoxic agent (for the hastening of birth or parturation, or as a muscle stimulant). No mention is made in the reference of these alkaloids as anticancer agents but, as previously indicated, the corresponding plant families are represented in Hartwell.

Indole alkaloids or protoalkaloids occur in the genus *Phalarus* and still other members of the family Gramineae (Luis J. Corcuera, in *Toxicants*, I, p.170ff). This is the plant family containing the cereal grains, in this case, notably barley. Since the heterocyclic nitrogen only occurs in the indole ring, the simple indole protoalkaloids are not considered to be true alkaloids. The most common of these alkaloids is named *gramine*. It is noted to concentrate in the leaves during early growth, as in barley seedlings. *Tryptophan,* interestingly, is a precursor to the biosynthesis of gramine. Although used for forage, *Phalarus* species have caused poisoning, even collapse and death.

It is observed that gramine may stimulate biochemical and biological processes at low concentrations but will inhibit the same or other processes at higher concentrations (Corcuera, in *Toxicants*, I, p. 174). The stimulatory effects are possibly due to a similarity with indole-3-acetic acid and tryptophan. Another explanation may be that gramine is catabolyzed, and the indole nucleus is recycled to form tryptophan. In any event, no commentary is provided in the reference about anticancer effects.

Phalarus is not listed in Hartwell as such, but other genera and species of the family Gramineae are listed. Hartwell evidently uses the genus name *Hordeum* for barley species instead of *Phalarus*.

4.11.4 POTATO

The family Solanaceae has plants that contain a variety of *glycoalkaloids* (R.P. Sharma and D.K. Salunkhe, in *Toxicants*, I, p. 180ff). These are distinguished from ordinary alkaloids by the presence of hydroxyl or (OH) groups in the molecular structure. Most investigations have been concerned with the potato, *Solanum tuberosum*, which contains the glycoalkaloids α-solanine and α-chaconine, which only differ slightly in their molecular makeup. Although normally present in only trace amounts, *under certain conditions the concentrations will increase. Potatoes contain high-quality protein,* ranking second only to soybeans in protein production per acre.

Light exposure or mechanical damage will sometimes induce synthesis of these poisonous alkaloids, also called *glycosidic steroidal alkaloids*. Normally in only insignificant amounts, light exposure causes a "greening" of the potato and a change in the taste. The alkaloids are present in most tissues of the potato plant, including the leaves, shoots, stems, blossoms, tubers, tuber eyes, peels and sprouts. The levels in various parts of the plant change as growth proceeds. At flowering, it is highest in the flowers. In the tuber the levels are highest in the eyes, peels, and sprouts. Cooking seems not to change the alkaloid content (Sharma and Salunkhe, in *Toxicants*, I, p.189).

Accidental poisoning from eating potatoes high in alkaloid content has resulted in severe illness, even death (Sharma and Salunkhe, in *Toxicants*, I, pp. 218–219). No mention was made of potential anticancer activity.

4.11.5 LOCOWEEDS

The locoweeds are found abundantly in the American West and consist of a number of species. For example, there is the silky or silvery locoweed or crazyweed, *Oxytropis sericea*, which is of the family Leguminosae or Fabaceae, or Pea family (*Weeds of the West*). Another species, which has purplish-pink blossoms, is *O. lamberti*. The species *O. lagopus* has especially attractive magenta flowers. Livestock are poisoned by locoweeds, and horses are said never to recover. (This particular plant family is represented in Hartwell as Leguminosae instead of Fabaceae, but the genus *Oxytropis* is not listed.)

Locoweeds, as the name implies, are a source of certain toxic alkaloids (P.R. Dorling, S.M. Colgate and C.R. Huxtable, in *Toxicants*, I, p. 238ff). The principal toxicant is named *swainsonine*, an indolizidine alkaloid. Originally isolated from the Australian legume *Swainsona canescens*, it has since been found in the locoweeds of North America and in two different molds. The various plants are of the genera *Swainsona*, *Astragalus*, and *Oxytropis*. The genus *Astragulus* is for instance also found in China and is of the family Leguminosae. In the American West, *Astragalus* is represented by *milkvetch*, as described in *Weeds of the West*. The genus *Oxytropis* includes the well known locoweeds or crazyweeds of the American West, as already mentioned.

The confusion in nomenclature apparently lies in the fact that the plant family designators Leguminosae and Fabaceae are used interchangeably. Hartwell uses Leguminosae, whereas *Weeds of the West* uses Fabaceae. Ruth Ashton Nelson's *Handbook of Rocky Mountain Plants* prefers Leguminosae or Pea family. This is not the only difference in usage. For instance, sunflowers may be found in either the family Compositae, in Hartwell and in Nelson, or in the family Asteraceae or Sunflower family, in *Weeds of the West*. Both versions denote the same family. The common sunflower, incidentally, is of the genus *Helianthus* and specifically is the species *Helianthus annuus*. It makes Hartwell, by the way, with a single citation—from Venezuela. Also in Hartwell, the Grass family is presented as the family Gramineae instead of the family Poaceae. Interestingly, the American West now has an undesirable import called *Swainsonpea*, *Sphaerophysa salsusa*, also of the family Legumonosae or Fabaceae, an import from Asia (cf. *Weeds of the West*). While *Astragalus* appears in Hartwell, neither *Swainsona* nor *Oxyropis* are listed. *Sphaerophysa* doesn't make Hartwell, although there are a few alliterative close calls: *Sphaeralcea* (of the family Malvaceae), *Sphaeranthus* (of the family Compositae), and *Sphaeroccocus* (of the algae family Rhodomelaceae).

Swainsonine has been used as a specific and potent enzyme inhibitor for α-D-mannosidase in glycoprotein research (Dorling, Colgate and Huxtable, in *Toxicants*, I, p. 241). Whether it serves as an inhibitor for other enzyme-catalyzed reactions was not indicated in the reference.

Among the many other toxic effects of livestock ingesting *swainsonine* is that of *neurological damage*, which may not appear until several weeks later. The reference provides a full accounting. It is particularly damaging to pregnant animals. Whether or not this particular alkaloid could ever have any medicinal purposes would seem doubtful in view of its great toxicity, although Hartwell lists the genus *Astragalus*. However, read on.

In a section titled "Swainsonine as a Therapeutic Agent," it is noted in the reference that swainsonine will enhance the immune system *in vitro* (Dorling, Colgate and Huxtable, in *Toxicants*, I, p. 253). Furthermore, swainsonine serves as an immunomodulator *in vivo*.

> The administration of swainsonine restored the capacity of immunodeficient mice to produce antibodies to injected foreign material and completely inhibited the growth of sarcoma ascites cells and reduced lung metastases of B19 melanoma in mice. Swainsonine has no effect on the immune response of normal mice.

The final paragraph of the reference cites the fact that the use of swainsonine as a pharmaceutical is covered by a patent owned by the Fujisawa Pharmaceutical Co., Ltd., of Japan. The patent pertains to the treatment of "diseases caused by the depression of immunoinsufficiency, such as *tumor,* infection, allergy, autoimmune, and steroid-dependent diseases." The reference, published in 1989, concludes that only time will tell whether swainsonine is a useful drug compound.

4.11.6 RED CLOVER

Research into what is called *salivary syndrome* or *the slobbers* in livestock has led to some unexpected findings about alkaloids from red clover and some other legumes (Winston M. Hagler and Warren James Croom, in *Toxicants*, I, p. 257ff.) It was found that slobbers is a mycotoxicosis ("myco-" meaning fungus) produced by the ingestion of red clover (*Trifolium pratense*) and maybe a few other legumes which are infected with the fungus *Rhizoctonia leguminicola*. The causative factor turned out to be the alkaloid *slaframine*. It is an idolizidine alkaloid that the fungus produces from lysine.

There may also be a connection with *swainsonine,* which is a closely related indolizidine. Swainsonine was in fact found along with slaframine in a batch of red clover which caused an outbreak of slobbers, but the issue has not been resolved. The reference comments that, aside from its role in sporadic outbreaks of slobbers, *the major importance of slaframine is in its potential use as a therapeutic agent with high affinity and specificity for the gastrointestinal tract.* Thus, pancreatic flow is increased by the administration of slaframine. Moreover, it has been found that slaframine is associated with the release of growth hormone, at least in cattle and chickens. Talking of animals, by increasing salivation, there is the possibility for correcting digestion inefficiencies. We may extend the inference to humans.

For the record, the pharmacological properties of slaframine are encompassed in the technical classification called a "parasympathomimetic cholinergic antagonist with an affinity for muscarinic receptors" (Hagler and Croom, in *Toxicants*, I, p. 269). In other words, its action opposes salivation antagonists such as atropine. Toxic side effects are noted, which can be counteracted by histamine receptor antagonists such as promethazine hydrochloride.

It is mentioned that the action of slaframine on circulating regulatory hormones may be useful in a number of therapeutic applications, e.g., on the gastrointestinal and endocrine systems. (Hagler and Croom, in *Toxicants*, I, p. 274.) Its action on the exocrine glands of the digestive tract may be of benefit in the treatment of cystic fibrosis.

This much said, there may be a useful connection in the treatment of cancer, at least for cancers of the GI tract. We note that there are many entries for *Trifolium* in Hartwell. Slaframine is briefly described in Cordell (Cordell, *Alkaloids*, p. 148). Whether this reported anticancer action in Hartwell has to do with the fungus, above, or with some other plant substance, is not known.

4.11.7 FESCUE

The grass called *tall fescue* (*Festica arundinacea* of the family Poaceae or family Gramineae) is grown in the north-south transition zone across mid America and is used variously for pasture, lawns, turf, and conservation purposes (R.W. Hemken and L.P. Bush, in *Toxicants*, I, p. 282ff). There are some problems with grazing livestock, however, which are related to a toxic factor present. There are also two other problems not related to the toxic factor. The one is ergot toxicity from the ergot fungus *Claviceps purpurea*; the other is called hypermagnesemia.

The fescue toxicity symptoms, notably with cattle, include what are called fescue foot, summer syndrome, fat necrosis, poor reproductive performance, and a disease called *agalactia*. Not all pastures are affected, however.

The toxicity problem has been traced to an endophytic fungus that sometimes infests fescue. The fungus was originally identified as *Sphacelia typhina*, derived from *Epichloe typhina*, but was renamed *Acremonium coenophialum*. It is estimated that 90 percent of all fescue pastures are infected with *Acremonium*. The fungus infection apparently is passed via fescue seeds.

The alkaloid fraction from tall fescue has been analyzed, and it is found that some of the alkaloids present are not related to the fungus, and some are. All the alkaloids evidently contribute to toxicity in some way or another. The diazophenanthrene alkaloid content is independent of the fungus, is inheritable in certain strains of fescue, and increases with nitrogen fertilization. Another type of alkaloid, of the pyrrolizidine alkaloids, is connected to the fungus but has not been positively identified as causing the toxicity symptoms. The class of alkaloids called *ergot alkaloids* are more likely suspects and can be derived from *Epichloe typhina* or *Acremonium coenophialum*, whichever name is to be used. These alkaloids include ergosine, ergosinine, and chanoclavine.

4.11.8 ERGOT ALKALOIDS

Whether any of the above alkaloids may have other uses in human disease control did not come up. Cordell has an extensive section on Ergot Alkaloids, which are connected to *hallucinogenic properties* (Cordell, *Alkaloids*, p. 623ff). Specifically mentioned are the peptide ergot alkaloids *ergosine* and *ergosinine* as being obtained from the seeds of *Ipomoea argyrophylla* of the family Convolvulaceae (Cordell, *Alkaloids*, p. 631). Entries for this family and genus occur in Hartwell as anticancer agents, with some of the more common names of species being *wild potato* and *goat's foot*. Several chemical variations of chanoclavine appear in Cordell and may be regarded as derivatives of clavine. Although no clavine alkaloids as such were cited as prescription products, it is noted that some have useful properties such as prolactin release (Cordell, *Alkaloids*, pp. 650–651).

Ergot alkaloids in general have three main actions, designated as *peripheral, neurohormonal,* and *adrenergic blockage.* The principal peripheral effects are in promoting smooth muscle tone, as in obstetrics. The neurohormonal effects include to serotonin and adrenaline antagonism. Ergot alkaloids are described as sympathicolytic agents because of their adrenolytic action (inhibiting the response to adrenaline).

As to *prolactin*, mentioned above, it is a mammalian hormone responsible for mammary growth and milk production (Cordell, *Alkaloids*, pp. 353–354). There is evidence, however, that prolactin is involved in the growth of mammary tumors, at least as chemically induced in mice. Thus, prolactin inhibition may be of consequence, and certain of the ergot alkaloids have this effect. Also noted is the remission of pituitary gland tumors with certain of the ergot alkaloids.

4.11.9 LARKSPUR OR DELPHINIUM

The colorful flowering larkspur or delphinium (genus *Delphinium* of the family Ranunculaceae) is known for containing toxic alkaloids. These alkaloids are classed as diterpenoid alkaloids, and at least *111 different alkaloids* have been identified and characterized (John H. Olsen and Gary D. Manners, in *Toxicants*, I, p. 292ff). By no means have all the species yet been examined for alkaloids, but those which have include *D. andersonii, D. barbeyi, D. bicolor, D. geyeru, D. glaucescens, D. glaucum, D. nuttallianum, D. occidentale, D. tricorne,* and *D. virescens.* (Hartwell lists only the species *Delphinium staphisogria.*) *Delphinium glaucescens* is noted to cause considerable livestock loss in parts of the Rocky Mountain West at certain stages of plant growth. Among the alkaloids identified in *D. bicolor* is *methyllycaconitine,* which displays *neuromuscular blocking activity.*

The principal diterpene alkaloids in *Delphinium* are further divided into C_{19}-diterpene alkaloids, C_{20}-diterpene alkaloids, and bis-diterpene alkaloids. The first-mentioned can be subdivided into the alkaloid types *aconitine,* lycoctonine, pyrodelphine, and heteratisine. The first two types occur naturally in *Delphinium,* and all four types are found in the genus *Aconitum,* which is of the same plant family. The species *Aconitum columbianum* is the wild *monkshood* or *wolfsbane* found in the Rocky Mountain West. *A. napellus* is the domesticated version.

The reference provides an extensive tabulation of lycoctonine-type C_{19} diterpenoid alkaloids which have been located in various *Delphinium* species. The list comprises 57 different alkaloids from some 22 different species. Another table is of 7,8-methylenedioxy lycoctonine-type C_{19}-diterpenoid alkaloids, listing 25 different alkaloids from 15 of the same species. Still another tabulation is of C_{20}-diterpenoid alkaloids, 9 in number, from 9 species. There is clearly no shortage of alkaloids in *Delphinium* species.

Of the many alkaloids, *36 different alkaloids from 9 different species are said to be poisonous to cattle* (Olsen and Manners, in *Toxicants*, I, p. 305). A tabulation is provided in the reference, and the effects on cattle are documented. An enumeration of some of the more active diterpenoid alkaloids includes the following: delphinine, methyllcaconitine, elatine, delsemine, lappoconitine, anthroyllycoctonine, condelphine, karakoline, delcosine, delsoline, lycoctonine, deltaline, tricornine, browniine, browniine 14-acetate, and denudatine. Although pharmacological effects for each are furnished in the reference, no anticancer action was noted.

Cordell has a section on the chemistry of diterpene alkaloids, however, noting in particular the genera *Aconitum* and *Delphinium* (Cordell, *Alkaloids*, p. 868ff). It is observed that diterpene alkaloids also are found in the genera *Garrya* of the family Garryaceae, *Inula* of the family Compositae, *Spivaea* of the family Rosaceae, and *Anopterus* of the family Escalloniaceae.

All the above plant families are represented in Hartwell save Escalloniaceae. The genus *Spivaea* does not appear, however, although *Spiraea* is listed, with the common name *ninebark* given. This is not the ninebark of the Rocky Mountain foothills, however, according to Ruth Ashton Nelson's *Handbook of Rocky Mountain Plants*. The latter is the species *Physocarpus monogynus*, which is also of the family Rosaceae or Rose family. It is a bush that flames red and orange in Autumn to provide dots of color on the hillsides and in the draws. Hartwell does not list the genus *Physocarpus*, although there are numerous other entries for the family Rosaceae.

The roots and leaves of *Aconitum* have been used in native remedies for gout, hypertension, neuralgia, rheumatism, and as a local anesthetic. This is in spite of the fact that *Aconitum* species include some of the most poisonous plants known. Additionally, since a considerable number of entries appear in Hartwell, *Aconitum* species have been used against cancer, e.g., as described by Solzhenitsyn in *Cancer Ward*.

4.11.10 SELENIUM INDICATORS

The C_{20}-diterpene alkaloids are relatively nontoxic (Cordell, *Alkaloids*, pp. 868–869). The two principal skeleton structures are the veatchine and the atisine types, the former produced by the *Garrya* species, and the latter occurring in the alkaloids of *Aconitum* and *Delphinium*. It is noted that atisine, the principal alkaloid found in *Aconitum heterophyllum* (a species found for instance in India, according to Hartwell), is isomeric with both veatchine and garryine, having the same stoichiometric chemical formula.

The reason for bringing up the particulars of the foregoing paragraph is that the reference further states that "The main differences in chemical reaction are the products of *selenium* dehydrogenation…" (emphasis added). *The fact that selenium can be involved in reactions occurring with these alkaloidal compounds is an intriguing coincidence*—there are parts of the Rocky Mountain West where larkspur or delphinium are native and where the soil has a relatively high selenium content. More than this, the toxic action of locoweed in part is sometimes thought to involve selenium.

The *woodyaster*, the species *Xylorhiza glabriuscula* of the family Compositae or Asteraceae, or Sunflower or Daisy or Aster family, is a known selenium concentrator or indicator (*Weeds of the West*), and is sometimes found in the same region as alkaloid-containing plants. For this reason, it is toxic to livestock if consumed over an extended period. For that matter, the toxic effects of woodyaster may be in part due to alkaloids.

Milkvetches of the genus *Astragalus*, of the family Fabaceae or Leguminosae, are also considered to be selenium indicators. Milkvetch is noted to be poisonous to livestock throughout the entire growing season (*Weeds of the West*). Besides taking up selenium from the soil, milkvetches contain glucosides or glycosides, not to mention the possibility of alkaloids.

A listing of selenium indicator plants includes the plant families and genera as shown in Table 4.8 (P.D. Whanger, in *Toxicants*, III, p. 144). About half the plant genera are not represented in Hartwell. The reference provides additional information about the occurrence of selenium, its plant and physiological chemistries, and its soil–plant–animal relationships.

4.11.11 JIMSONWEED

Jimsonweed, *Datura stramonium*, is of the family Solanaceae or Nightshade family. It contains the alkaloid *hyoscyamine*, which has been used as a sedative and a hypnotic. The entire plant is toxic: seeds, flowers, and leaves. Hyoscyamine is a tropane alkaloid and is also found in *Atropa belladonna* and *Scopolia tangutica*, as is another tropane alkaloid, *scopolamine* (Cordell, *Alkaloids*, p. 115).

4.11.12 NIGHTSHADE

The species *Atropa belladonna* or nightshade has many entries in Hartwell. The genus *Scopolia* is represented in Hartwell by *Scopolia japonica*, called lang-tang in China. The most typical or well known tropane alkaloid is probably *atropine*, which is antagonistic to muscarinic receptors, an effect called parasympathetic inhibition. *These receptors are variously responsible for regulating heartbeat, constricting the pupil of the eye, vasodilation, and the stimulation of secretions*. Some compounds that exert these regulatory effects are acetylcholine, pilocarpine, physostigmine, and arecoline. Atropine, however, functions as an antagonist to these regulatory effects.

In further explanation, *acetylcholine is a neurotransmitter, as are noradrenaline, dopamine, and serotonin* (Cordell, *Alkaloids*, p. 21ff). *All may be viewed as alkaloids*. The reactive site for these chemicals on an adjacent neuron is designated a receptor. (A neuron is a nerve cell.) The neurons that release acetylcholine are called *cholinergic*, and those that release the others are respectively termed *adrenergic, dopaminergic*, and *serotonergic*. A drug may mimic, facilitate, or antagonize these processes

Table 4.8   North American Plants Serving as Selenium Indicators[a]

Primary Indicators		
Compositae	*Xylorhiza**: woody aster
Compositae	*Oonopsis**: goldenweed
Cruciferae	*Stanleya**: prince's plume
Leguminosae	*Astragalus*: milkvetch
Secondary Indicators		
Chenopodiaceae	*Atriplex*: salt bush
Chenopoduaceae	*Grayia**
Compositae	*Aster*: wild aster
Compositae	*Grindelia*: gum plant
Compositae	*Gutierrezia**: snakeweed or matchweed
Compositae	*Machaeranthera**
Compositae	*Sideranthus**
Santalaceae	*Comandra*: toad-flax
Scrophulariaceae	*Castilleja*: paintbrush

a. From P.D. Whanger, in *Toxicants*, III, p. 144. Plant families or genera not listed in Hartwell's *Plants Used Against Cancer* are denoted by an asterisk.

involving the nervous system. The nervous system itself is composed of two independent parts, the central nervous system and the autonomic nervous system, the latter connecting the spinal cord at the vertebrae.

The neurotransmitter acetylcholine is formed by the action of the enzyme choline acetyl transferase, a synthesis which may be blocked by enzyme inhibitors. Cholinergic drugs mimic the action of acetylcholine and include pilocarpine, physostigmine, and arecoline, above. On the other hand, cholinergic blocking agents oppose these actions, by inhibiting the enzyme-catalyzed production of acetylcholine. Atropine-like compounds act as enzyme inhibitors, and therefore *atropine is called an acetylcholine antagonist*.

The principal effect of atropine is to alter the rate of heartbeat. Interestingly, low doses will slow the heart rate, whereas large doses will increase the heart rate. This is another manifestation of how high- and low-dosage levels of a drug will act oppositely.

4.12   A REVIEW OF BIOACTIVE PLANTS AND PLANT FAMILIES

A listing of all the plant families in Hartwell's *Plants Used Against Cancer* has been provided in Appendix U, including the common name for some of the species. The alkaloid-containing plant families that appear in Cordell's *Introduction to Alkaloids* are highlighted in boldface. Some of the alkaloids associated with these particular plant families are also highlighted.

Bioactive plant families and species more specific to the United States are listed in Appendix V. Some poisonous wild plants that grow in the western United States are listed in Table V-1 of Appendix V. The information is from the publication *Weeds of the West*, some of which also appears in *Weeds and Poisonous Plants of Wyoming and Utah*. Table V-2 contains information from *Poisonous Grassland Plants*, which takes in the Tallgrass Prairie of Oklahoma and Kansas, but duplicates considerable of the information in Table V-1. Plants of the eastern United States which are poisonous are listed in Table V-3, from Will H. Blackwell's *Poisonous and Medicinal Plants*. Again, as would be expected, there is a degree of overlap among Table V-3 and the other tables. For some species are distributed widely. Plants containing significant concentrations of alkaloids apparently constitute a minority.

Blackwell's *Poisonous and Medicinal Plants* has a chapter on Flowering Plant Families of Toxic Significance. Inasmuch as alkaloids occur in these kinds of plants, a closer look is in order. A brief rundown is as follows, based on plant families and genera. This information is included in an alternate form in Appendix V, Table V-3.

- **Amaryllidaceae or Amaryllis Family.** Somewhat similar in appearance to the family Liliaceae, the underground parts or bulbs may contain alkaloids. Potentially toxic are *Amaryllis* (amaryllis), *Galanthus* (snowdrops), and *Narcissus* (daffodils and jonquils). Along with the Iris and Lily families, the Amaryllis family should be regarded with suspicion.

- **Apocynaceae or Dogbane Family.** The members consist of herbs, shrubs, trees, or woody vines. The toxic substances are cardiac glycosides, which affect the heart, or alkaloids, which affect the blood and blood pressure, and the central nervous system. Genera and species include: *Apocynum* (Indian hemp), *Strophanthus* (sawai), *Catharanthus* or *Vinca* (periwinkles), *Rauwolfia* (snakeroot), *Nerium* (oleander). Sawai is the source of the precisely-administered heart medicine *ouabain* (oleander has been tried as a heart medicine, in the manner of digitalis, but the toxic risk is too great).

- **Araceae or Aroid Family.** The aroids contain crystals of calcium oxalate in the leaves and corms (the bulbous upright stems). Genera and species include: *Anthurium*, *Arisaema* (jack-in-the-pulpit), *Caladium*, *Dieffenbachia* (dumbcane).

- **Asclepiadaceae or Milkweed Family.** Not all genera are toxic, but species of the *Asclepias* spp. contain cardiac glycosides and probably toxic resinoids.

- **Campanulaceae or Bellflower Family.** The most prominent genera are *Campanula* and *Lobelia*, both with blue flowers. The latter are likely to be toxic, containing the *emetic lobelia alkaloids*—that is, emetine alkaloids—that affect the nervous system in the manner of nicotine or even poison hemlock.

- **Caryophyllaceae or Pink (Carnation) Family.** Most genera and species are nonpoisonous, though two contain saponins: *Agrostemma* (corn cockle) and *Saponaria* (soapwort).

- **Compositae (Asteraceae) or Sunflower (Aster, Daisy) Family.** Probably the largest family of flowering plants, there are an estimated 20,000 to 30,000 species. The plants are mostly herbaceous, with the head, called the inflorescence, composed of many flowers or florets (which may be rays or discs) and which are to be distinguished from the surrounding petals. The totality appears as if a single flower, but multiple "seeds" or *achenes* are produced. *Most sunflowers are not toxic, although there are a few exceptions.* A species of *Eupatorium* (snakeroot) contains a toxic alcohol that will affect the nervous system. Species of *Senecio* (groundsel) have alkaloids which can damage the liver. *Xanthium* (cocklebur) seedlings are said to be toxic. Other family members include *Ambrosia* (ragweed), *Artemisia* (sagebrush), and *Cirsium* (thistles).

- **Convolvulaceae or Morning Glory Family.** Seeds of species of the genera *Ipomoea* (morning glories) and *Convolvulus* (bindweeds) may contain *LSD-like substances.*

- **Cruciferae (Brassicaceae) or the Mustard Family.** The plants usually have a pungent taste and contain toxic mustard oils, which are glycoside derivatives. A representative genus and species is *Brassica* (wild mustard).

- **Ericaceae or Heath Family.** The members of this family are mostly evergreen shrubs found on acidic soils. The toxic substance is suspected of being a resinoid and probably is a terpenoid substance or terpenoid alkaloid, which is called andromedotoxin or grayanotoxin. Toxic genera and species include: *Andromeda* (bog rosemary), *Kalmia* (mountain laurel), *Leucothoe* (dog laurel), *Peris* (Japanese andromeda), *Rhododendron* (rhododendrons and azaleas).

- **Euphorbiaceae or Spurge Family.** The toxic substances found include diterpenoids (notably in species that produce a milky latex), toxic proteins, and saponins. The more poisonous genera and species include: *Aleurites* (tung nut), *Cnidoscolus* (tread-softly), *Euphorbia* (snow-on-the-mountain, cypress spurge, wartweed), *Hippomane* (manchineel), *Ricunus* (castor bean). Poinsettias, of the genus *Poinsettia,* are only mildly poisonous if at all.

- **Iridaceae or Iris Family.** There is a resemblance to the family Liliaceae and the family Amaryllidaceae. The underground parts or bulbs should therefore be considered potentially toxic, possibly containing alkaloids. However, *the genus Crocus, predominantly made up of spring-flowering species, is not usually regarded as toxic.* However, *Colchium,* the autumn crocus and a member of Liliaceae, is considered to be toxic. There is the suspicion, however, that the Iris family, along with the Lily and

Amaryllis families, should be avoided as a food item. Moreover, even the condiment saffron (which is made from the stigmas of *Crocus sativus*) is to be avoided in excess.

- **Labiatae (Lamicaceae) or Mint Family.** These square-stemmed herbs are generally considered more medicinal than toxic. However, *Glechoma* (ground ivy) is known to be toxic. Mint oils of the genus *Mentha* (mints) are used for digestion, colds, and congestion. Interestingly, mint oils are terpenoids, which are alkaloid precursors (Cordell, *Alkaloids*, pp. 59–60).

- **Leguminosae (Fabaceae) or Legume (Pea) Family.** These plants variously comprise herbs, shrubs, trees, and vines. The toxic substance is either a particular type of alkaloid, which causes digestive upset and which may affect the nervous system, or else is a poisonous protein, affecting the blood and the cell metabolism. The toxic members of the family include: *Abrus* (precatory bean or rosary pea), *Astragalus* (locoweeds), *Baptisa* (false indigo), *Cassia* (senna), *Gymnocladus* (Kentucky coffee tree), *Laburnum* (golden chain), *Lathrus* (vetchlings and sweet peas), *Lupinus* (lupines), *Robina* (black locust), *Wisteria* (wisteria).

- **Liliaceae or Lily Family.** The toxic substances include both cardiac glycosides and alkaloids. The latter are noted to cause gastric distress, affect cell division, produce low blood pressure, and possibly cause birth defects. On the other hand, there may be positive medicinal effects from some of the species. Representative genera and species include: *Aloe* (aloe), *Colchicum* (autumn crocus), *Convallaria* (lily-of-the-valley), *Hyacinthus* (garden hyacinth), *Melanthium* (bunch flower), *Scilla* and *Urginea* (squill), *Ornithogalum* (star-of-Bethlehem), *Veratrum* (false hellebore), *Zigadenus* (death camus).

- **Papaveraceae or Poppy Family.** The alkaloids are of the opium or morphine type, which act to depress the nervous system. The genera and species include: *Papaver* (poppies), *Sanguinaria* (bloodroot), *Chelidronium* (European poppy).

- **Ranunculaceae or Crowfoot (Buttercup) Family.** The toxic substances are two different types of alkaloids and/or toxic glycosides, with other toxic substances still unknown. The genera and the common names of representative species include the following: *Aconitum* (monkshood), *Actaea* (baneberry), *Anemone* (windflower), *Caltha* (marsh marigold), *Clematis* (virgin's bower), *Delphinium* (larkspur), *Helleborus* (Christmas rose), *Hydrastis* (golden seal), *Ranunculus* (buttercup).

- **Rosaceae or Rose Family.** Several members of this family contain amygdalin or similar compounds which can release cyanide following ingestion. Sometimes called laetrile, or Laetrile (there is a slight difference from amygdalin), this substance is referred to as an *alleged* cure for certain kinds of cancer. (The subject is further discussed in Part 8 in the section "Laetrile Again?") Obtained from the pits of apricots and present in peach pits and apple seeds, the substance is also present in the leaves of *Prunus, e.g.,* wild black cherry. The fruits or stones of some species of *Cotoneaster* have a small cyanide content. The species of the genus *Roseus* (roses), on the other hand, are free from cyanogenic compounds.

- **Scrophulariaceae or Foxglove (Figwort) Family.** Though most members of this family are nontoxic, *Digitalis* (foxglove) is an exception. It contains the cardiac glycoside called *digitalis* in the leaves and other parts. Digitalis requires administration in minute or trace amounts, otherwise an overdose will cause cardiac arrhythmias.

- **Solanaceae or Nightshade Family.** A number of toxic alkaloids are found causing a variety of symptoms. Some have been used for medicinal purposes. Toxic genera and species include: *Atropa* (belladonna), *Datura* (jimsonweed), *Hyoscymus* (henbane), *Lycopersicon* (tomato). *Mandragora* (mandrake), *Nicotinia* (tobacco), *Physalis* (ground cherry), *Solanum tuberosum* (Irish potato), *Solanum* spp (various nightshades).

- **Umbelliferae (Apiaceae) or Carrot Family.** Although a sizeable and mostly harmless family, there are at least two deadly exceptions, *Conium* (poison hemlock) and *Cicuta* (water hemlock). The former contains a simple alkaloid, the latter a long-chain alcohol, both affecting the nervous system but otherwise displaying dissimilar symptoms. Although another look-alike family member of the genus *Daucus* (wild carrot) is edible, still another of the genus *Pastinacea* (wild parsnip) contains a substance that sensitizes the skin to sunlight, sometimes called photodermatitis.

- **Urticaceae or Nettle Family.** The stinging hairs or nettles evidently contain a variety of substances, including *histamine* and *acetylcholine*. Representative genera and species include: *Uritica* (stinging nettle) and *Laportea* (wood nettle).

In one way or another the foregoing plant families, genera, and species are found in many different parts of the world. Previous information has been provided in Parts 2 and 3 and in the appendices. Part 8 will further address the curative issues, notably in terms of enzyme inhibitors.

REFERENCES

A Field Guide to Medicinal Plants: Eastern and Central North America, Houghton Mifflin, Boston, 1990. Text by Steven Foster and James A. Duke. Line drawings by Roger Tory Peterson, Jim Blackfeather Rose and Lee Allen Peterson. Photographs by Steven Foster.

Alkaloids: Chemical and Biological Perspectives, in four volumes, S. William Pelletier, Ed., Wiley, New York, 1983–1987.

The Alkaloids: Chemistry and Pharmacology, R.H.F. Manske et al., Eds., Academic Press, New York and Orlando FL, 1950–. There are 46 volumes to date.

Biochemistry of Alkaloids, K. Mothes, H.R. Schütte and M. Luckner, Eds., VCH Verlagsgesellschaft, Weinheim FRG, 1985.

Blackwell, Will H., *Poisonous and Medicinal Plants*, Prentice Hall, Englewood Cliffs NJ, 1990. Chapter 5 written by Martha J. Powell.

Cordell, Geoffrey A., *Introduction to Alkaloids: A Biogenetic Approach*, Wiley, New York, 1981.

Duke, James A., *CRC Handbook of Medicinal Herbs*, CRC Press, Boca Raton FL, 1985.

Duke, James A., *Handbook of Biologically Active Phytochemicals and Their Activities*, CRC Press, Boca Raton FL, 1992.

Duke, James A., *Handbook of Phytochemical Constituents of GRAS Herbs and Other Economic Plants*, CRC Press, Boca Raton FL, 1992.

Hager, Hermann et al., *Hager's Handbuch der Pharmazeutischen Praxis: fur Apotheker, Arzneimittsteller, Drogisten, Arzte und Medizinalbeamte*, J. Springer, Springer-Verlag, Berlin, 1900, 1908, 1910, 1920, 1925, 1930, 1949, 1958, 1967, 1973, 1977, 1990.

Hartwell, Jonathan A., *Plants Used Against Cancer*, Quarterman Publications, Lawrence MA, 1982.

Heinerman, John, *Healing Animals with Herbs*, BiWorld Publishers, Provo UT, 1977.

Heinerman, John, *The Treatment of Cancer with Herbs*, BiWorld Publishers, Orem UT, 1984. Special Foreword by Robert Mendelsohn.

Nelson, Ruth Ashton, *Handbook of Rocky Mountain Plants*, Roberts Rinehart, Niwot CO, 1992. Revised edition by Roger L. Williams.

Plants in the Development of Modern Medicine, Tony Swain, Ed., Harvard University Press, Cambridge MA, 1972.

Poisonous Grassland Plants, Section 4 of a series Pasture and Range Plants, published by the Phillips Petroleum Company, Bartlesville OK, 1957, 1959.

Raffauf, Robert F., *A Handbook of Alkaloids and Alkaloid-Containing Plants*, Wiley-Interscience, New York, 1970.

Raffauf, Robert F., *Plant Alkaloids: A Guide to Their Discovery and Distribution*, Haworth Press, Binghamton NY, 1996.

St. George, George and the editors of Time-Life Books, *Soviet Deserts and Mountains*, Time-Life Books, Amsterdam, 1974.

Solzhenitsyn, Alexander, *Cancer Ward*, Farrar, Straus and Giroux, New York, 1969, pp. 228–233. Translated from the Russian by Nicholas Bethell and David Burg.

Textbook of Biochemistry: With Clinical Correlations, Thomas M. Devlin, Ed., Wiley, New York, 1982.

Toxicants of Plant Origin, in four volumes, Peter R. Cheeke, Ed., CRC Press, Boca Raton FL. Vol. I. *Alkaloids*, 1989. Vol. II. *Glycosides*, 1989. Vol. III. *Proteins and Amino Acids*, 1989. Vol. IV. *Phenolics*, 1989.

Turner, Paul, *Selected Lives from the Lives of the Noble Grecians and Romans*, in two volumes, Southern Illinois University Press, Carbondale, 1963. First published in 1963 by the Centaur Press, Ltd., Fontwell, Sussex, England. Compared together by that grave learned Philosopher and Historiographer Plutarch of Chaeronea: translated out of Greek into French by James Amyot and out of French into English by Thomas North. Now selected, edited and introduced by Paul Turner.

Tyler, Varro E., "Plant Drugs in the Twenty-first Century," *Economic Botany*, 40(3), 279–288 (1986).

Voet, Donald and Judith G. Voet, *Biochemistry*, Second Edition, Wiley, New York, 1995.

Wagner, H., Hiroshi Hiking and Norman R. Farnsworth, *Economic and Medicinal Plant Research*, Volume1, Academic Press, New York, 1985.

Watt, John Mitchell and Maria Gerdina Breyer-Brandwijk, *The Medicinal and Poisonous Plants of Southern and Eastern Africa: Being an Account of Their Medicinal and Other Uses, Chemical Composition, Pharmacological Effects and Toxicity in Man and Animal*, E.&S. Livingstone, Edinburgh and London, 1962.

Weeds and Poisonous Plants of Wyoming and Utah. Tom D. Whitson, Editor. Contributors: Roy Reichembach, Mark A. Ferrell, Stephen D. Miller, Steven A. Dewey, John D. Evans, Richard D. Shaw. Published by Cooperative Extension Service, College of Agriculture, University of Wyoming, Laramie, April, 1987.

Weeds of the West. Tom D. Whitson, Editor. Authors: Larry C. Burrill, Steven A. Dewey, David W. Cudney, B.E. Nelson, Richard D. Lee, Robert Parker. With a list of Contributors. Published by the Western Society of Weed Science in cooperation with the Western United States Land Grant Universities Cooperative Extension Services, College of Agriculture, University of Wyoming, Laramie, January, 1991.

Medicinal Uses of Fungi

Part 5

Medicinal Uses of Fungi

5.1 THE MYCOTA OR FUNGI

Neither fish nor fowl, the Mycota or fungi, as with bacteria, are no longer classified within the Plant Kingdom, albeit neither are they necessarily of the Animal Kingdom. (The term Mycota is capitalized, for instance, in the *Encyclopedia Britannica*, whereas fungi occurs in lower case—except where it signifies the kingdom Fungi.) In other words, there are always exceptions to the rule. Some authorities have proposed a separate kingdom, possibly called the Protista Kingdom, or kingdom Protista, consisting of unicellular organisms, which would include animal-like protozoans on the one hand and unicellular plants on the other. Moreover, *fungi cells are eukaryotic,* with a nucleus, as distinguished from the prokaryotic cells of bacteria. Furthermore, fungi have *chitin* in their structure, the hard substance forming the outer shell or surface of insects, crustaceans, and others.

The issue has since been accommodated, as set forth in the PROPAEDIA: The Outline of Knowledge, an additional volume in the recent editions of the *Encyclopedia Britannica*. Here, life forms have been divided into six kingdoms: Viruses, Monerans (bacteria and other prokaryotes), Protists (algae, proto-zoans, and slime molds), Fungi, Plants, and Animals (with 25 categories). Thus, fungi or Mycota now have their own kingdom—the kingdom Fungi or the kingdom Mycota.

Although most fungi are not poisonous and are not of medicinal value, the exceptions are significant. In fact, fungi comprise the second largest group of organisms in terms of their poisonous and medicinal properties, exceeded only by the flowering plants (Will H. Blackwell, *Poisonous and Medicinal Plants*, pp. 58–59). These poisonous and medicinal properties are oftentimes interrelated, displaying the quality of bioactivity that also occurs in plants, and in particular as concerns *alkaloids*.

The common white button mushroom (*Agaricus bisporus*) is an important *food source* although, as will be seen, it contains a compound identified as causing cancer in test animals. On the other hand, the crude product called *reishi* is from the fungus *Guanoderma luciderm* and is considered to be a cure-all for many ailments, including cancer. Moreover, still other mushrooms, such as the popular shitake or forest mushroom (*Lentinus edodes*), are increasingly mentioned as potential anticancer agents. *In fact, a compound extracted from the shitake mushroom has been found to act against cancer in laboratory studies and in Japan has been approved as an anticancer agent.* Thus, the subject of fungi is of increasing interest, in several directions.

The fungi or Mycota can be described alternatively as *plant-like organisms ranging from the lower or more primitive fungi (yeasts, molds, smuts, and mildews) to the higher fungi (mushrooms or toadstools, puffballs, and the like). Lichens are included but exist symbiotically with algae.* (The dog lichen, *Peltigear canina*, is a folkloric cure for rabies, as indicated elsewhere.) The main distinguishing feature is that *fungi do not produce chlorophyll as do plants, nor do fungi have the usual well defined structures associated with plants such as leaves, stems, and roots.* (What is called *moss*, for instance, is a *plant*.) *At the very lowest end of the scale, bacteria were once classified as fungi, and bacteria are sometimes viewed as spores.* Apart from the others, *slime molds are considered both animal-like and plant-like*—bridging the gap.

Since *fungi contain no chlorophyll and cannot carry out photosynthesis,* their carbohydrate growth sources must be from other materials. These growth sources are compounds of carbon, oxygen, and hydrogen as the name implies. *The carbohydrates for fungal metabolism are variously in the form of sugars, starches, celluloses, hemicelluloses, and lignins—and occur principally in the makeup of plants. Saprobic fungi* or saprobes feed on dead organic material, the process of saprobiosis. *Parasitic fungi* or parasites feed on living organisms, the process of parasitism. *Enzymes are secreted that digest the food source, to be absorbed by the fungus.*

Parasitic fungi invade the host, obtaining nourishment from cell plasma or cytoplasm, which can produce disease and even the death of the host organism. *Pathogenic or disease-causing fungi are most often plant parasites, but a few cause diseases in animals and humans.* Entry is gained through a natural opening or a cut or wound. The relatively few human pathogens include such fungi as *Candida albacans,* universally distributed, and *Paracoccidioides brasiliensis* of Central and South America. Increased international travel has caused fungi to spread.

Some *fungi will attack and capture microorganisms* such as amoebas and roundworms (or nematodes). This can be viewed as a means of counteracting, say, bacterial diseases.

For the record, the division Mycota (fungi) may be divided into the subdivisions Myxomycotina (true slime molds) and Eumycotina (true fungi). These, in turn, are separated into various classes, subclasses, and orders.

The fungus structure is essentially that of a collection of filaments (*hyphae*) which bear spores that are the reproductive agents. The collection of filaments constitutes the *mycelium* and makes up the body, called the *thallus.* A higher fungus such as a mushroom will consist of a fruiting body or *sporophore* above ground in the form of a stem and cap, with gills underneath. This assembly is connected to a large network of hyphae below ground, which are interwoven to form a *mycelium,* the vegetative portion of the thallus.

The fruiting body of fungi may vary from microscopic size to the enormous size of some species of mushrooms and puffballs. In certain of the higher mushrooms, a compact mass of mycelia forms that is called the *sclerotium.* It may occur underground or above ground. *The sclerotium constitutes a food storage reservoir and contains chemicals of interest as well (such as alkaloids), as will be noted.*

Fungi may also be classed as to the way they bear spores. The lower fungi produce spores in sac-like sporophores called *sporangia.* The entire contents burst forth and are called *sporangiospores.* The spores of the lower fungi may be disseminated on the wind or in the water, as the case may be.

The higher fungi—known as the Ascomycetes, Deuteromycetes, and Basidiomycetes—do not produce and distribute spores in such a motile (and mobile) manner. The first-mentioned bears spores in a spore sac or ascus (plural, asci). The last-mentioned produces spores in a club-like structure or organ called a *basidium* (plural, basidia). The asci and basidia are formed directly on the hyphae or in special sporophores called ascocarps or basidiocarps, depending. Thus, this kind of a propagation system produces new fungal "sprouts" in the manner that some plants or trees send up new growth from the roots. This phenomenon can be seen as the *fairy ring.* The ascocarp fungi include the morels, cup fungi, and truffles, whereas basidiocarp fungi include mushrooms, puffballs, stinkhorns, and bird's nest fungi.

These few things said, the main interest here is in the *anticancer* properties of fungi and their in-house chemicals. There is a considerable literature on fungi, and a few sources are cited, although most do not cover the subject of interest, namely cancer and anticancer agents. The multivolume work by G.C. Ainsworth, *The Fungi,* remains a standard reference, although published in the 1960s and 1970s. A newer volume by Michael J. Carlile and Sarah Watkinson, also titled *The Fungi,* was published in 1994. Other works of interest include *Indigenous Medicinal Plants Including Microbes and Fungi,* first published in India, and *Icons of Medicinal Fungi from China,* by Jianzhe Ying and Xiaolan Mao. Another monograph originating in China is *Fungi Pharmacopeia (Sinica)* by Po Liu. More of a layman's guide is William H. Lee's *The Medicinal Benefits of Mushrooms.*

A chapter on Poisonous and Medicinal Fungi by Martha J. Powell is presented in Will H. Blackwell's *Poisonous and Medicinal Plants.* There will be the occasion to refer to this material in some detail in the following sections. It is noted that, like plants, fungi can be either friends or foes. One kind of fungus yields penicillin, effective against most bacterial infections; another, ingested in the form of a deadly mushroom, will be fatal. As previously mentioned, what are referred to as *molds* and *yeasts* are *fungi,* as are, for example, the black spots covering leaves and many other manifestations.

The *molds* in fact are the fungi which, for the most part, *produce either toxic or medically important compounds.* However, *fleshy-type fungi such as mushrooms can also be toxic,* as is well known, producing a kind of poisoning called *mycetismus.* Molds produce a kind of poisoning referred to as *mycotoxicosis.* Some of the molds growing on grains and nuts in storage yield a variety of secondary products known as *mycotoxins.*

5.2 MYCETISMUS

Poisoning from fleshy-type mushrooms is called mycetismus. There are several classes of poisons involved. Of these, what are called protoplasmic poisons consist of the *amatoxins* and *gyrotoxins*. The former include toxins from the genus *Amanita*, which are *cyclopeptides*, ring-shaped molecules of amino acids. The amino acid *tryptophan* is involved, as is a sulfur linkage. The term *amanitin* is variously used for the toxin. Liver cells are the main target of attack. Amanitin acts as an inhibitor for the enzyme RNA polymerase II. This blocks messenger RNA transcription from DNA, and no more protein is produced. The effects continue into the kidneys. Death is from liver or kidney failure.

The gyrotoxins, as from the false morel, occur due to a hydrazine-type compound called *gyromitrin*. The gyromitrin is converted to monomethylhydrazine (MMH), which inhibits the enzyme system requiring the coenzyme pyridoxal phosphate (vitamin B6).

Other mushrooms produce *neurotoxins*, notably the alkaloid *muscarine*, first derived from *Amanita muscaria*, or *fly agaric*, because it attracts and kills flies. It is present in this species in only low concentrations but is in much higher concentrations in other species. Muscarine is a cholinergic activator, stimulating the parasympathetic nervous system.

The neurotoxins *psilocybin* and *psilocin* are found in still other mushroom species. Psilocybin is an indole alkaloid which is hydrolyzed in the body to produce *psilocin*, the active agent. The mind is affected, with euphoria or depression ensuing. Hallucinations appear. These particular hallucinogenic mushrooms are used in Indian religious ceremonies in the remote regions of southern Mexico.

Ibotenic acid and muscimol are body products formed when *Aminita muscaria* is consumed. The result is a form of *hallucinogenic intoxication* that is sometimes fatal.

The mushroom genus *Coprinus* contains the alkaloid *coprine*, which blocks the enzyme aldehyde dehydrogenase in the liver. This prevents the oxidation of ethanol to acetic acid, and toxic aldehydes accumulate. The consumption of alcohol will accordingly make a person very sick. Its action is similar to that of *Antabuse*®, the disulfiram compound employed against alcoholism, and it therefore can be used as an agent to discourage drinking alcoholic beverages. Still other mushrooms can cause gastrointestinal (GI) trouble, especially when consumed along with alcohol.

Knowledge about cancer-causing compounds in fungi is limited, mostly due to the long time interval for the onset of the disease. Most information has come from screening programs and studies on animals. A few carcinogens have been found in mushrooms, however. An example is the phenylhydrazine compound called *agaritine*, found in the common edible mushroom *Agaricus bisporus*.

Although lichens are generally nonpoisonous, there are exceptions. For example, two alpine lichens, *Letharia vulpina* and *Cetraria pinastri*, have been used to poison wolves. The active agent is not specified.

It is noted that mushroom poisoning can be offset by inducing vomiting and by ingesting activated charcoal to absorb the poison. This is not effective with protoplasmic poisons, since the symptoms appear too long afterward. Here, only life-supportive measures can be undertaken. There are, however, antidotes for a few specific kinds of poisoning. Thus, *Amanitin* poisoning may be controlled by thioctic acid. Atropine sulfate, an alkaloid, counters the cholinergenic effects from muscarine poisoning. (It should not be used for *Amanitin muscaria* intoxication, however.) Pyridoxine injections counter the effects of gyromitrin.

5.3 MYCOTOXICOSIS

As to mycotoxicosis, or poisoning from eating foods contaminated with toxic fungi or fungal metabolites, the effects are questionable. For there is the problem of controlling the experimental conditions. "Symptoms of mycotoxicoses are variable and are influenced by dosage levels." Low dosages producing chronic poisoning may be masked by other factors, such as nutrition and disease. High dosage levels causing acute poisoning are more observable and correlatable.

Toxicogenic molds grow on grains, seeds, and on the surfaces of cheeses and cured meats. Temperature and humidity influence growth.

Aflatoxins are by far the most studied mycotoxins. The name comes from *Aspergillus flavus*, the first fungal species shown to produce these toxins. It was called the "turkey X disease," a mystery disease which in one notable incident killed thousands of turkeys in England—and was subsequently traced to the feed used. The aflatoxins are classified by their respective order of absorption on thin plates. Of these, what is designated as aflatoxin B_1 is the most toxic.

Aflatoxins are considered among the most potent carcinogens in naturally occurring substances. They are also mutagenic, even to malformations in embryos. Acute poisoning results in subcutaneous hemorrhaging, liver and kidney damage, and lung congestion. Chronic poisoning stunts appetite and growth. Acute poisoning causes liver cancer to develop, followed by death. Thus, aflatoxin-contaminated feed is a major problem in the livestock industry.

The action of aflatoxins is to bind to DNA and block the transcription of RNA, negating protein synthesis. Protein-deficient diets compound the difficulty. Aflatoxins also compete with hormones for cellular binding sites and interfere with the immune system. Vaccinations are offset by the aflatoxins. In net sum, *aflatoxins are carcinogenic* because of their interactions with DNA.*

Aflatoxins are monitored globally, and in the United States there "safe" levels for different uses of grains. *In the United States, for each batch of, for example, raw, shelled peanuts, an analysis and certification is required for aflatoxin content.* The U.S. Department of Agriculture (USDA) and the Food and Drug Administration (FDA) are the monitoring agencies. The cutoff is 50 parts per billion for human consumption. *If dairy cows are fed with feed containing aflatoxins, the contamination is passed on to the milk.* Thus, here, the cutoff is even lower: 0.5 parts per billion in the feed.

A definitive correlation of aflatoxins with human cancers has not been proven, although *a high incidence of liver cancer is associated with regions having higher rates of food contamination with aflatoxins.* In India, in 1974, about 400 people became ill from eating aflatoxin-contaminated corn, of which more than 100 died.

A *nephrotoxin* ("nephro-" pertaining to the kidneys) named *citrinin* is a product of *Penicillium citrinum* and other molds that grow on barley, oats, and corn. Although an effective antibiotic, it is too toxic to animals be used, damaging the kidneys and liver.

The alkaloidal *fumigaclavines* are produced by the fungus *Aspergillus fumigatus*, a mold found in corn silage. These compounds are neurotoxins, causing cattle to become uncoordinated, in turn followed by muscle tremor and paralysis. Similar symptoms are caused by eating grass contaminated with the ergot fungus *Claviceps paspalum*.

Molds such as *Aspergillus ochraceus* produce a group of isocoumarin derivatives called *ochratoxins*, which are linked to *phenylalanine*. These molds are found on such foods as rice, oats, wheat, chili peppers, legumes, sorghum, dried fish, fermented sausage, and cured ham. Although presumably confined to animals, a similar kidney disease in humans is named *Balkan nephropathy*.

The diphenyl derivative *patulin* is a mycotoxin with antibiotic properties. Since it inhibits mitosis (cell division), it is too toxic to use on animals. Patulin was first isolated from *Penicillum patulum* but is found in other molds. Acute poisoning produces lung hemorrhaging and congestion. Although carcinogenic, this is only in the tissue surrounding the injection. (On the other hand, *if it would locally and selectively inhibit the mitosis of cancer cells, patulin could conceivably serve as an anticancer agent.* Perhaps it is the old story that, at one dosage, a substance is carcinogenic; at another, lower dosage, it is anticarcinogenic.)

The fungus *Pithomyces chartarum* sometimes grows in grass and, when eaten, will attack the liver of sheep and cattle. Phylloerythrin, the active agent, is derived from the chlorophyll in the grass and, if not broken down by the liver, will cause photosensitivity by altering the permeability of the capillaries under the animal's skin.

The sesquiterpenoid structure is common to a large group of toxins called *trichlorenes*. (Terpenoids are precursors to alkaloids.) They inhibit the synthesis of DNA and proteins and have other toxic effects. One type produced from *Fusarium tricinctum* was linked to the Soviets during the wars in Southeast Asia and Afghanistan. Vomitoxin is a similar toxin, an emetic produced from the fungus *Giberella zeae*. The same fungus produces another toxin called zearalenone, an estrogenic factor. Stored wheat and corn are a primary source.

Endophytic toxins are sometimes produced in grass, notably from the ascomycete *Acremonium coenophialum*, which grows in tall fescue, a topic discussed elsewhere. (Ascomycetes are higher fungi with their spores formed in asci or spore sacs. They include the yeasts, molds, mildews, truffles, morels, and others.)

---

* This is the same conclusion that can be reached for the use of conventional chemotherapy drugs such as 5-FU that block DNA/RNA processes. Furthermore, there is the inference that, since chemo drugs interact with DNA, they may also be carcinogenic, as claimed in some quarters. At least it is ventured that chemo drugs may make the cancer spread.

The most famous mycotoxin poisoning is from *ergot*. Open-pollinated grains such as rye are host to the fungus *Claviceps purpurea*, which infects the flower and replaces it with a hard, brittle, banana-shaped, black *sclerotium* (a hard mass stored as food). The sclerotium contains many alkaloids, some toxic, some medicinally valuable. When the infected rye is harvested and ground into flour, so are the sclerotia.

In chronic poisoning, the ergot alkaloids constrict the vascular system, setting up a gangrenous condition. The end result is a loss of extremities. Nervous disorders occur with acute poisoning. The muscles will begin to twitch and go into spasms, and *hallucinations and convulsions appear.* Between convulsions, the victims have a voracious appetite. Death may follow or, if the victim survives, it is with mental impairment.

Ergotism was responsible for thousands of deaths during the Middle Ages. During the gangrenous stage, the extremities burn as if aflame. St. Anthony was made the patron saint for the disease, and it became known as *St. Anthony's Fire.* Peter the Great, of Russia, led an expedition down the Volga River valley in 1720 to capture an ice-free port from the Turkish Empire, but he never made it. His troops and horses ate ergotized grains along the way and became ill. The hysteria that led to the witch trials in seventeenth-century Salem MA was very likely brought on by ergot poisoning. The victims weren't bewitched but were convulsed and felled by ergot poisoning—in particular children, who are more susceptible.

5.4 MEDICINAL FUNGI AND CANCER

Medicinal fungi are of great importance, being the source of modern antibiotics—although, presumably, native peoples were familiar with the basics of primitive treatment. Oriental medicine, for instance, has preserved some of the more ancient ways, using fungi with herbal medicines for a synergistic effect. An example is the polypore fungus *Wolfporia extensa*, which is known by many common names such as hoelen, China root, Indian bread, Virginia truffle, or tuckahoe. The fruiting body forms a white crust on trees, whereas the large potato-like sclerotium forms underground, and is of most medical interest. Tuckahoe is said to be included in over one-third of blended oriental medical recipes, extending back to circa A.D. 25. The position of the compounds within the sclerotium is thought to determine their role in medicine. Thus, the central portion is used for ailments of the central nervous system and so on. Of special interest, in Chinese medicine, extracts of tuckahoe are used to treat breast and uterine cancer and have a clinical basis.

Another polypore cure-all fungus is *Guanoderma lucidum*, which in a crude drug form is called *reishi*. The source is the fruiting body. The applications range from malaise, anorexia, and insomnia through heart disease and extend to the lowering of serum cholesterol and blood sugar. Significantly, *G. lucidum* is one of the many fleshy fungi containing carbohydrates that have been observed to inhibit tumor growth.

The jelly fungi have gelatinous fruiting bodies. Examples are the ear fungus (*Auricularia auricula*) and the black tree fungus (*A. polytricha*). The ear fungus, shaped like an ear, inhibits blood platelet aggregation and therefore serves as a blood anticoagulant in the circulatory system. Another benefit is that it lowers cholesterol levels. Besides all this, it is edible and may contribute to a healthful diet. The reference quotes the Chinese proverb that "Nature cures the disease, the doctor collects the fee."

Various species of the ascomycete genus *Cordyceps* infect insect larvae such as grubs and caterpillars and leave them mummified. A short fungus stalk with cap grows from the insect body. The entire assembly, insect body and fungus, often with herbs, constitutes an all-purpose tonic. Research indicates that there are anticancer agents in the Cordyceps fungi, particularly against lung cancer.

Iceland moss is a misnamed lichen (*Cetraria islandica*) used as a general tonic. The carbohydrate lichenin is one of many compounds present, and the lichen serves as a human food staple in some parts of the world. Besides its other uses as a tonic, *anticancer compounds have been found.*

A number of fungi have been used against hemorrhages and inflammations. These include the puffball group in the genera *Calvatia* and *Lycoperdon*. Puffballs range from ping-pong ball to beanbag chair size and at maturity contain spores within the body. The American Indians used the flesh of the fruiting body in various ways to control bleeding and as a dressing for sores, burns, and swellings. Corn smut is used similarly. It is noted that the ergot fungus *Claviceps purpurea* also contains alkaloids that can stop bleeding.

The underground sclerotium of the polypore fungus *Polyporus mylittae* will kill intestinal worms. It contains significant amounts of the protein-destroying enzyme protease which, in this case, is called *mylittine*. (Protease inhibitors have been proposed as a treatment for AIDS. There may be a connection to cancer as well.)

Another polypore fungus, *Famitopsis officianalis*, is used in small amounts in India variously for controlling lactation, for controlling the night-sweats, and as a purgative. The Ojibway Indians have used it against pneumonia, but it is noted that an overdose can cause paralysis and even death. *This fungus is also said to be used to treat cancer, particularly malignant ulcers.*

In addition to their role in controlling bleeding, puffballs can be used against other ailments, internally and externally. Spores mixed with water and honey act to soothe sore throat, laryngitis, tonsillitis, and throat infections and also serve as an expectorant. Puffball spores and a related fungus called *earth stars* have been used to heal ear and eye infections, and boils.*

The toothed fungi that are Basidiomycetes include the reddish-colored *Echinodontium tinctorium*, found in western North America, a source of red dye. It is called the "Indian paint fungus." Ground up and mixed with animal fats or tree saps, it serves as a barrier for insect bites.

The reference observes that clinical studies are needed to separate the facts from the folkloric accounts of medicinal properties. The work has started. An example provided is the current widespread therapeutic use of natural alkaloids from the ergot fungus, which extends to the use of the synthetic derivatives. Although ergotamine, for instance, produces vasoconstriction and will cause gangrene in the extremities when taken in excess, controlled dosages will control bleeding after childbirth. Ergotamine tartrate has been used against migraine headaches. Another fungal product, D-lysergic acid diethyl amide (LSD) has been tried in psychotherapy but, as is well known, has unpredictable and sometimes disastrous side effects. The alkaloid ergotoxine produces vasodilation and is therefore has been used to treat high blood pressure and cerebral circulation difficulties.

The reference observes that many exciting applications are being uncovered in the use of fungal compounds. A notable example comprises the investigations based on folkloric traditions for using fungi to treat cancer. *"A whole group of complex carbohydrates has been discovered from several fleshy fungi that may help control cancerous tumor growth."* It is further noted that the causes of cancer are many and complex, and that there are biological along with chemical and environmental interactions which affect mammalian molecular processes. The end result may be cancer. *Among the biological causes of cancer are viruses.*

There is a history of fungi or fungal compounds as antiviral agents. The extension is against *viral-induced cancers.* Thus, the milky latex from the mushroom *Lactarius piperatus* has been used against viral warts, as have decoctions from species of the lichen genus *Usnea.* Furthermore, it has been found that fungi can also stimulate the immune system so as to act against cancer. Along the way, some of these same anticancer compounds lower cholesterol levels and aid in controlling cardiovascular diseases.†

To continue, fungal compounds and their metabolites have shown strong *anticancer activity against tumors* transplanted in animals and in tumor cell cultures. These include several different *polysaccharides* or complex carbohydrates which are not cytotoxic in themselves but which stimulate the immune system. This, in turn, is said to fight off the cancer cells. It has been found that different carbohydrates activate different parts of the immune system but are nevertheless classified overall as nonspecific immunostim-ulants. Inasmuch as this kind of immunity does not affect the "immunological memory" of organisms, the compounds must be *administered repeatedly to control the cancer.* Clinical testing has proceeded slowly due to human safety precautions. For example, a potent antitumor glycoprotein called *cavacin,* extracted from the giant puffball *Calvatia gigantea,* showed great promise but was found to be too toxic when tested on animals. Nevertheless, the quest continues, with the possibilities ever increasing.

Among the other fungus-derived anticancer agents are the following.

- *Schizophyllan* is a *glucan* (a *polysaccharide* composed of linked glucose sugars) obtained from the split gill fungus *Schizophyllum commune.* It stimulates the complementary system in blood plasma so

---

* It has been reported in another reference that the giant puffball, *Calvatia gigantea* of the family Gastromycetes, was once a candidate as an anticancer agent (Nelson Coon, *Using Plants for Healing,* p. 78).

† As already noted, dog lichen, *Peltigear canina,* is a folkloric remedy for rabies.

as to increase protective proteins. Highly viscous and difficult to administer, it may be broken up into a less dense phase without losing its anticancer properties.

- The shelf fungus *Coriolus versicolor* yields a complex *glycoprotein* (proteins bound to a polysaccharide) known as *PSK*. (The fungus itself is sometimes called "turkey tail" due to its appearance.) The glucan that is released stimulates the macrophages and other cells in the immune system, in turn to increase the phagocytosis of foreign material and ward off invading organisms and viruses. There are few side effects.
- A glucan similar to schizophyllan, already mentioned, the compound *lentinan* is derived from the popular edible mushroom, the forest mushroom or shitake (*Lentinus edodes*). In experiments on mice with transplanted tumors, injections of lentinan produced a 50 percent total regression of solid tumors. Apparently, the compound activates the T-lymphocyte cells.
- A glucan named *pachyman* is derived from *tackahoe* (*Wolfiporia extensa*), which can be chemically changed to a form called *pachymaran. The latter acts against tumor cells, notably of the lung, even if metastasized.*
- The *cup fungus,* the ascomycete *Peziza vesiculosa*, yields the compound *vesiculogen*. This compound serves as an immunoadjuvant, increasing the production of antibodies but without acting as an antigen or foreign body itself.

A search of MEDLINE for fungi and antineoplastins indicates that further research is ongoing. For instance, *polysaccharides or glucans* from the Chinese mushroom called *Songshan lingahi*, the fruiting body of *Ganoderma tsugae*, are under study. Also under study are polysaccharides or glucans from the fruiting bodies of the well known *Amanita muscaria.*

As a wrap-up, Jonathan L. Hartwell's *Plants Used Against Cancer* has a number of fungal families and species entered toward the end of the book. Some have been mentioned or cited previously. This information is summarized in Table 5.1. As a further note, Hartwell even lists a species of bacteria as an anticancer agent, the well known and ubiquitous *Escherichia coli* or *E. coli* of the family Enterobacteriaceae (Hartwell, *Plants*, p. 698). Families and species of mosses, liverworts, algae, and lichens are also listed (Hartwell, *Plants*, pp. 683–688).

5.5 ANTIBIOTICS

Many fungi are noted to produce compounds or metabolites that act as toxins or antibiotics against other microorganisms. It is a way of competing for space. These toxins will kill microbes; some will not hurt mammals, but others will. In fact, *only a limited few antibiotics have been proven safe for animals or humans.* The most notable is *penicillin,* from the genus *Penicillium*. The original source was the airborne species *Penicillium notatum*, but the species *Penicillium chrysogenum* as found on moldy cantaloupes proved many times more productive.*

Adjustments in the growth media and chemical modifications have broadened the base of application. An important discovery was a form that is not broken down by the digestive system and thus can be administered orally rather than by shots. Further details are provided in the reference.†

---

* In the foregoing connection it may be mentioned that the antibiotic activity of fungi was known long ago by the ancient Chinese. For example, *an orange would be cut in half, allowed to mold, and then the moldy cut surface would be applied to a skin infection*. In a story by the old horse trader Ben K. Green, titled *A Thousand Miles of Mustangin'* and published by the Northland Press of Flagstaff Arizona in 1972, the author describes how his arm became infected after a wild horse bit him. This was on an expedition into Mexico to gather some wild horses, back before penicillin made its appearance known. An elderly Indian woman cured his infected arm using *moldy bread*, grown in the sun under a glass cover. And in Amazonia, for instance, the natives wander barefoot along the trails and through the rain forest growth itself without fear of foot infections. The fungi on the forest floor are their natural protection.

† As these things go, penicillin as a chemical compound has a relatively simple formula (Voet and Voet, *Biochemistry*, p. 270). For the record it consists of a thiazolidine ring (containing nitrogen and sulfur) fused to what is called a β-lactam ring. A variable R group is connected to the β-lactam ring via a peptide link. In benzyl penicillin (penicillin G) for example, the R group is the benzyl group. In the semisynthetic derivative ampicillin, R is the aminobenzyl group. In a way of speaking, therefore, in view of its nitrogen-containing ring structure, *penicillin itself can be regarded as an alkaloid, as can some other antibiotics*. In fact, the formation of alkaloids in *Penicillium* species is a subject treated in several references (M. Luckner, in *Biochemistry of Alkaloids*, pp. 37–40); W. Roos, *Ibid.*, pp. 44–46; R. Schütte and H.W. Liebisch, *Ibid.*, pp. 191, 249; M. Luckner and S. Johne, *Ibid.*, p. 315). It is noted in particular that benzodiazapine alkaloids are formed (Cordell, *Alkaloids*, p. 270).

Table 5.1   Anticancer Fungal Families and Species (from Plants Used Against Cancer: A Survey, by Jonathn L. Hartwell, Quarterman Publications, Lawrence MA, 1982, pp. 688–697)

Agaricaceae	*Agaricus* spp.: mushrooms
	Amanita muscaria or *Agaricus muscarius:* fly agaric
	Lactarius acris or *Agaricus acris* or A. giganteus: agaric
	Lactarius piperatus
	Pleurotus dryinus: toadstool
Boletaceae	*Boletus edulis:* herrenpilz, steinpilz
	Boletus laricis: agaric of Dioscoridies
Helvellaceae	*Helvella acaulis*
Hypocreaceae	*Claviceps purpurea:* ergot, spurred rye
Lycoperdaceae	*Podoxis pistillaris* or *Lycoperdon* **carcinomale** or *Scleroderma* **carcinomale**
Melanconiaceae	No scientific name provided: pestalozzia
Moniliaceae	*Aspergillus* flavus
	Oidium spp.
	Penicillium notatum
Mucoraceae	Mucor, Rhizopus, and several strains of *Pennicillium*
Pezizaceae	*Peziza auricula*
Phallaceae	*Lysurus mokusin* or *Phallus mokusin*
	Phallus indusiatus or *Phallus daemonium* or *Hymenophallus daemonium:* puto-seyton
Polyporaceae	*Fomes annosus* or *Polyporus annosus*
	Fomes applanatus: kinoko
	Fomes fomentarius or *Polyporus fomentarius:* agaric, amadou
	Fomes ignarius or *Polyporus ignarius* or *Boletus ignarius:* agaric, amadou, yesca
	Fomes nigricans or *Polyporus nigricans*
	Fomes officinalis or *Polyporus officinalis:* araricum, acaricum, agaric, etc.
	Poria cocos or *Pachyma cocos:* fungus
	Poria obliqua or *Inonotus obliquus* or *Polyporus nigricans:* chaga
Rhodotorulaceae	*Rhodotorula rubra*
Saccaromycetaceae	*Saccharomyces cerevisiae:* yeast
Torulopsidaceae	*Cryptococcus albidus*
Tremellaceae	*Tremella nostoc:* ratchon-d'lune
Tuberaceae	*Terfezia leonis:* misy
Unknown	Fungus from a species of oak tree (Sweden)

Of interest is the fact that medicinally significant ergot alkaloids are produced from the fungal genus *Penicillium,* as well as from *Aspergillus* and *Rhizopus* (D. Groger, in *Biochemistry of Alkaloids*, p. 295). *Ergot alkaloids,* incidentally, can be classified as derived from *tryptophan.* (Ergot alkaloids have even been found in some genera of bindweed, e.g., genus *Convolvulus* of the plant family Convolvulaceae.) The foregoing are filamentous fungi, containing ergot alkaloids of the clavine type, and are ordinarily derived from the fungal genus *Claviceps.* A special type, called peptide ergot alkaloids, has a unique structure as represented by ergosine, ergosinine, and cycloclavine. These alkaloids have not been found in fungi.

Other antibiotics in the order mentioned in the reference are cephalosporins, griseofulvin, and fusidic acid. It is commented that the activity of still other antibiotics is based on a sesquiterpene structure and an orsellinate group, albeit of no commercial importance.

Mentioned elsewhere are several antibiotics that act against cancer, only their side effects have proven to be too toxic. Some of these act as DNA/RNA enzyme inhibitors, as listed in Appendices E and F. Representative names of anticancer antibiotics include *actinomycin D, bleomycin,* and *daunomycin.* Given the right conditions and dosages, whether any of these antibiotics might display sufficient selectivity between cancer cells and normal cells evidently is not known.

A chapter by Nestor Bohonos titled Biodynamic Agents from Microorganisms appears in *Plants in the Development of Modern Medicine*, edited by Tony Swain, and published in 1972. At the time of writing, it was noted that drugs produced by microbial processes accounted for about 16 percent of all pharmaceuticals in the United States. *These microbial-made drugs consisted of antibiotics, corticoids, and vitamin B12.* Since antibiotics are overwhelmingly the main products produced by microbial processes, the word has become almost synonymous with microbial products, although, strictly speaking, this of course is not the case.

Screening and testing programs involve the following criteria:

- the physical and chemical properties of the compounds produced
- the effects on growth stimulation, inhibition, and toxicity for various organisms ranging from bacteria to higher plants and animals
- the effects variously on glucose, protein, nucleic acid, or fat metabolism, including the inhibition of specific enzyme activities
- pharmacological activities related to the central nervous system (CNS), anti-inflammatory effects, sedation, contraction or relaxation of muscles, diuretic action, and the effect on blood pressure and blood clotting, etc.
- the toxic principles such as they may occur
- folkloric information.

These evaluation programs are complicated by the fact that *a given microorganism may produce different chemicals in wholesale lots.* For instance, *Streptomyces* has been found to yield more than 1,000 antibiotic compounds.

The reference provides examples of the variations that can occur, whereby compounds may be structurally related and will differ in only slight degree, with these differences predicated by different preparation procedures. And sometimes different microorganisms may yield the same compound or compounds.

It is noted that the first microbial bioactive agents discovered were the macromolecular toxins, referred to as *endotoxins* and *exotoxins*. Although much is known about these compounds, they are of limited use.

The first microbially produced bioactive agents of importance were *vitamins,* also called growth factors. It was found that factors required for the growth of certain kinds of microorganisms were often the same as some of the water-soluble vitamins necessary for animal growth. Furthermore, it was found that some microorganisms that did not require these growth factors would instead produce these very same growth factors. In consequence, they could be used for the preparation of nutritional supplements or even pure vitamins. In fact, in this way some vitamins were discovered (Bohonos, in *Plants in the Development of Modern Medicine*, p. 181). For example, microbial studies have played an important role in the discovery of ascorbic acid (vitamin C), biotin, β-carotene, cobalamin (B12), folic acid, nicotinamide, pantothenic acid, pyridoxine (B6), riboflavin (B2), thiamin (B1), vitamin D, and vitamin K. Commercial fermentation processes produce riboflavin and β-carotene, and all commercial cobalamin (B12) is microbiologically produced. It is remarked as well that a fermentation step is involved in producing L-sorbose for the further production of ascorbic acid.

A paragraph is given to *folic acid.* After determining that *Corynebacterium* would produce high yields of this vitamin, extensive testing could proceed. It turned out that there was a series of folic acid or folic acid-derived compounds, the first of which had been isolated from liver and was called pteroylglutamic acid. A similar product produced by *Corynebacterium* was pteroyltriglutamic acid. Inasmuch as it had previously been determined that there was a *larger increase of folic acid in malignant tumors than in normal tissues,* the decision was made to test these different kinds of folic acids or folates against tumors. It was found out from *in vivo* tests that pteroyltriglutamic acid *inhibited malignant tumor growth,* whereas pteroylglutamic acid had no effect. This led to the synthesis of the chemicals *aminopterin* and *methotrexate* (amethopterin) as the first clinically successful anticancer agents.*

The presumption was that folic acid would be preferentially absorbed by cancer cells, and that the pteroyltriglutamic acid content would then act against the cells. But, instead of pteroyltriglutamic acid, the commercial product aminopterin or methotrexate was substituted—but these latter chemotherapy drugs

---

* It may be added that, since the chemicals aminopterin and methotrexate are synthetically produced, they are patentable, whereas pteroyltriglutamic acid itself is no doubt not patentable.

have toxic side effects and can have serious consequences, as previously indicated, e.g., in Part 1. It would be an informative circumstance to try reverting to pteroyl**tri**glutamic acid itself as an anticancer agent.

Also mentioned is the development of the iron scavenging agent "desferrioxamine B" from the growth factor *coprogen* (Bohonos, in *Plants in the Development of Modern Medicine*, p. 181). This and similar agents are used in the treatment of hematochromatosis and acute iron poisoning. (The term *coprogen* is not in common everyday use but will show up in a few references on MEDLINE.)

The subject of antibiotics per se is reviewed in the reference, as of the date of publication (1972). It was observed in passing that the scale-up of the aerobic fermentation processes used was an achievement that permitted wide-scale application. Moreover, improvements in the cultures likewise permitted increased capacities. Beyond this, new antibiotics were being produced, and the cultures and fermentation processes were further refined for selectivity to produce a particular antibiotic.

However, *even then it was commented that the emergence of antibiotic-resistant bacterial strains was starting to be a problem.* The treadmill continues to this day, with science hopefully staying one jump ahead in developing new antibiotics. (Some view the emergence of resistant bacterial strains as a natural phenomenon, wherein some members of a naturally occurring distribution are simply more resistant to start with and are able to survive and proliferate, whereas the less-resistant members are killed off early.)

Chemical formulas are provided for a few of the synthetic or semisynthetic antibiotics, with the notation that some of these have other beneficial effects, for instance, a chelating capacity which leads to the treatment of other diseases. A form of *penicillamine* has even been tried for *schizophrenia,* and for influencing the immune response. *Unfortunately, the side effects were severe.* As to broad-spectrum antibiotics, the tetracyclines are the most widely used. A general structural comparison is furnished in the reference for the different variants.

An antifungal antibiotic named *griseofulvin* resulted from finding that conifers would not grow in a certain kind of heath soil. One thing led to another, and the antibiotic has even been tried on gout. Unfortunately there are undesirable side effects, including *hepatocarcinogenicity.*

Azomycin is an antibiotic of high nitrogen content which has significant antitrichomonal activity (antiparasitic activity). This led to the development of the drug *metroniadazole,* which is similarly active but less toxic.

5.5.1 ANTICANCER ACTIVITY

The Bohonos reference in *Plants in the Development of Modern Medicine* further observes that a great amount of work has been done on screening cytotoxic antibiotics for antineoplastic or anticancer activity. It was noted that animal tumor testing had turned up a number of antibiotics with antitumor activity. These anticancer antibiotics included the *actinomycins, adriamycin, bleomycin(s), chromomycin(s), daunomycin, diasomycins, mithramycin,* the *mytomycins, nogalomycin, olivomycin, puromycin, streptonigrin,* plus *steroid hormones, asparaginases, polysaccharides,* and other *macromolecules.* (Note that *polysaccharides* are included in the above listing of antibiotics.)

The antibiotic *actinomycin D* was the first to be clinically accepted as an anticancer agent. It has so far not been possible, however, to relate this compound and other actinomycins to anticancer activity due to chemical/structural characteristics. Other potential anticancer agents tested include 8-azaguanine and 5-azacytidine, but these have turned out to have only antibiotic action. Guanine and cytidine, incidentally, are fundamental nucleic acid bases or nucleotides (as set forth in Part 1). Derivatives of the nucleotides cytidine and uridine have also been obtained via fermentation.

The reference stresses that the *activities of the antitumor antibiotics is related to their effect on deoxyribonucleic acid (DNA), ribonucleic acid (RNA), and protein metabolism (or synthesis).* In short, *they block DNA/RNA/protein synthesis,* the same as conventional cytotoxic chemotherapy agents, albeit not in the same exact way. In this regard, however, they may also be expected to have *antiviral* and *antifungal* activity.

Actinmycin D, puromycin, and mitomycin C are antitumor antibiotics which have been found to act against the immune response. The antibiotics actinomycin D, puromycin, chloramphenicol, and cyclo-heximide are commonly used (enzyme) inhibitors in biochemical metabolism (for instance see Appendices E and F). Puromycin and cycloheximide have been used in studies on memory processes. Certain antibiotic compounds (not specified) may also affect neuromuscular activity, lipolysis, liver regeneration, muscular contraction, and vascular permeability.

The bacterial enzymes called asparaginases show anticancer activity in the treatment of some kinds of malignancies. Other possibilities include such microbial enzymes as *amylases, cellulases, hemicellulases, pectinases, pentonases, invertases, lactases, glucose oxidases, dextranases, catalases, peroxidases,* and *proteases.* (The last mentioned, *proteases,* is of particular present interest.) A further breakdown includes *streptokinase, fibrinolytic enzymes, keratinase,* and *kininase.* Also of interest are *lipase* and *uricase.*

The subject of medicinal fungi remains of paramount interest, in spite of a few bad experiences with mushroom species, as per an interview in the June, 1998 issue of the *Townsend Letter for Doctors & Patients: The Examiner of Medical Alternatives.* The interview was confined to medicinal mushrooms, as per the experiences of Paul Stamets, of Fungi Perfecti, Olympia Washington, who furnishes descriptive information about several different species and a list of doctors who are up to date on the subject. The information is taken from a publication titled *MycoMedicinals,* coauthored with C. Dusty Wu Yao. A list of references is also furnished. Stamets indicates that a problem with using mushrooms is that of contamination, notably by myriad microorganisms—another argument for utilizing only the pure compounds. Stamets further documents the fact that there are bioactive mushroom-derived chemicals that display *antitumor* activity.

5.6 ANTIFUNGAL VIS À VIS ANTICANCER AGENTS

Maybe not so surprisingly, as per the previous section, antibiotics derived from fungi can also serve as *antifungal agents* (or, "it takes one to know one"). A search of MEDLINE, for instance, indicates that amphotericin-B is an antifungal agent, as is an antibiotic derived from *Streptomyces* spp. Other antifungal agents include such varied compounds as flucytosine, miconazole, itraconazole, and magainins (which are peptides). What is of compelling interest is whether there is a relationship between or among antifungal and antibacterial and anticancer, not necessarily in that order. In another way of looking at it, if a simple test such as an antifungal test could be used to screen potential anticancer agents and be correlated to clinical results, this could both simplify and strengthen the screening process. The final objective, of course, is to determine what will work as a selective anticancer agent, a substance that will kill or immolate cancer cells without also destroying normal cells.

There are also some harrowing overtones in that aflatoxin, botulinum toxin (the agent for botulism), and anthrax (caused by the microorganism *Bacillus anthracis*) are potential means for *biological warfare* and reportedly have been produced and stored for that very purpose.* A defense against these and other toxic fungal or biological agents is in the interests of national security and the welfare of nations. If this defense could also act against cancer, the benefits would be multiplied. And conceivably national defense could be the impetus needed to nail down a cure for cancer, albeit indirectly.

5.7 MICROBIAL TOXINS

Nestor Bohonos, in *Plants in the Development of Modern Medicine,* describes a number of microbial toxins. First on the list is *ergot,* which is a mixture of peptide-type alkaloids and which was probably the first fungal toxin to be used medicinally. The ergot alkaloids are now produced by fermentation rather than from the dried sclerotia of the fungus *Claviceps purpurea* grown on rye plants.†

Another toxin mentioned by Bohonos is the anticoagulant agent *dicoumarol* which was discovered in spoiled hay. Still others are listed and briefly described as follows. Some may be alkaloidal and some may not. The reference in a number of instances supplies the structural formulas.

The *aflatoxins* are mycotoxins which have been detected in many food and feed products including peanuts and corn, as previously mentioned. The most widely known and most toxic compound, Aflatoxin B_1, is derived from the fungus *Aspergillus flavus.* Being *highly carcinogenic,* these toxins may prove of use in studying the conditions for the formation of cancers.

---

* In order of toxicity, plutonium is ranked first, botulism is second, and ricin from the castor bean is ranked third.

† In addition to the previously presented material, a chapter titled Ergot—A Rich Source of Pharmacologically Active Substances appears in *Plants in the Development of Modern Medicine.* Written by Albert Hofman, a brief history is first provided, followed by the chemistry of the ergot alkaloids. It has been found for instance that *ergot alkaloids are also found in higher plants as well as in fungi.*

The toxin *zearalenone* occurs in feeds contaminated with *Gibberella zeae*. It has estrogenic and *anabolic* properties. (The term *anabolic* pertains to constructive metabolism as opposed to destructive or catabolic metabolism).

Slaframine, a product of *Rhizoctonia leguminocola* in red clover, and previously mentioned, causes excess salivation in cattle. It also increases pancreatic flow, and may be of use in cystic fibrosis.

The toxin *decumbin,* first found in contaminated corn and also known as cyanein and brefeldin A, acts variously as an *antifungal and antiviral agent* and as an *antimitotic agent*. These properties may be related to an α,β-unsaturated lactone structure. *The property of antimitosis is that of acting against cell division, and may be potentially useful against cancer.*

Sporidesmin, similar to gliotoxin, is a product of the fungus *Pithomyces chartarum*, which occurs on pasture grasses. It is *hepatotoxic* to grazing animals.

The compounds 8-methoxypsoralen and 4,5',8-trimentylpsoralen are formed by *Sclerotia scleriotrum* has been observed to cause *dermatosis* in celery workers. (Apparently the fungus grows on celery plants.)

A listing of *hepatotoxins* includes the amatoxins, the phallotoxins, islandotoxin, luteoskyrin, ipomeamorone, and xanthocillin. The toxins citrinin and citreimycetin produce *nephrotoxicity*, whereas citreoviriodin produces paralysis and *respiratory failure*. A further listing of other names of mycotoxins is supplied in the reference, with all sorts of toxic manifestations, and includes such compounds as *muscarine*—which is a well known alkaloid.

Another category for toxins is that of *phytotoxins* and *plant-growth regulators*. These are toxins produced by what are called *phytopathogens*, or *plant-pathogens*. A number of instances are supplied in the reference. Some toxins are converted to growth stimulators, and may be regarded as growth hormones. *Of particular interest here is gibberellic acid, which enhances mammalian resistance to ascites tumors (abdominal tumors).*

The foregoing reference provides many other examples of miscellaneous microbial activity ranging from performing as *insecticides*, to producing *serotonin*, to acting as the *catalysts for microbial transformations*. Just where most of this may fit into anticancer activity remains to be seen.

REFERENCES

Ainsworth, G.C., *The Fungi: An Advanced Treatise*, four volumes in five, Academic Press, New York, 1965–73.

Biochemistry of Alkaloids, K. Mothes, H.R. Schütte and M. Luckner, eds., VCH Verlagsgesellschaft, Weinheim, Germany, 1985.

Blackwell, Will H., *Poisonous and Medicinal Plants*, Prentice Hall, Englewood Cliffs NJ, 1990. Chapter 5 by Martha J. Powell.

Carlile, Michael J. and Sarah Watkinson, *The Fungi*, Academic Press, Orlando FL, 1994.

Coon, Nelson, *Using Plants for Healing: An American Herbal*, Rodale Press, Emmaus PA, 1963, 1979.

Cordell, Geoffrey A., *Introduction to Alkaloids: A Biogenic Approach*, Wiley, New York, 1981.

Hartwell, Jonathan L., *Plants Used Against Cancer: A Survey*, Quarterman Publications, Lawrence MA, 1982.

Indigenous Medicinal Plants Including Microbes and Fungi, Purshotam Kaushik, ed., Today and Tomorrow's Printers and Publishers, New Delhi, India and Houston TX, 1988. Distributed by Scholarly Publications, Houston TX.

Lee, William H., *The Medicinal Benefits of Mushrooms: The Benefits of Rare Mushrooms in the Treatment of Hypertension, Allergies, Atherosclerosis and the Maintenance of a Healthy Circulatory System*, Keats, New Canaan CT, 1985.

Liu, Po, *Fungi Pharmacopia (Sinica)*, Kinoco Co., Oakland CA, 1980.

Plants in the Development of Modern Medicine, Tony Swain, ed., Harvard University Press, Cambridge MA, 1972.

Powell, Martha J., "Poisonous and Medicinal Fungi," Chapter 5 in *Poisonous and Medicinal Plants*, by Will H. Blackwell, Prentice Hall, Englewood Cliffs NJ, 1990.

Voet, Donald and Judith G. Voet, *Biochemistry*, Second Edition, Wiley, NY, 1995.

Ying, Jianzhe and Xiaolan Mao, *Icons of Medicinal Fungi from China*, Science Press, Beijing, China, 1987. Lubrecht & Cramer, Forestburgh NY, 1987. Translated by Xu Yuchan.

Biogenesis of Cancer

Part 6

Biogenesis of Cancer

6.1 INTRODUCTORY REMARKS

The causes of cancer can appear in strange ways—take melanoma for instance. Although the primary cause of melanoma is generally considered to be excessive solar radiation, the word is that such anomalies as bee stings have developed into melanoma sites, and there may be other unsuspected causes as well. (For one thing, melanoma may show up on parts of the body not exposed to direct sunlight.) Other potential causes include viruses, and some insects, for instance, may carry large numbers of viruses—e.g., the connection with bee stings, although the toxins in the venom may also be suspect.

As to toxins in bee stings, the venom has been characterized as containing histamine and at least eight other components or fractions (Arnold Mallis, *Handbook of Pest Control*, in a revised chapter by Stanley G. Green). It is noted that the venom will cause the victim's body tissues to produce even more histamine. Of the venom fractions, two are very active. The fraction designated F_1, and called *melitin*, contains 13 amino acids. It is mainly responsible for the localized pain and inflammation, at the same time causing a lowering of blood pressure and a paralyzing effect. The fraction designated F_2 contains 18 amino acids as well as two enzymes, hyaluronidase and phospholipase. It acts similarly to melitin and in addition destroys red blood cells. It may be only a coincidence, but the word *melitin* bears a resemblance to *melanin* and *melanoma*.

Mallis's book also mentions the brown recluse or fiddleback, or violin spider (*Loxosceles reclusa* of the family Loxoscelidae or Brown Spider family), whose venom or toxin has the unusual property of causing a sloughing off of the tissue at and around the site of the bite. The toxins are by no means fully identified, but the recognized authorities include biochemist Collis Geren of the University of Arkansas and Gary W. Tamkin, MD of the Highland General Hosptial, Alameda Medical Center, Oakland CA, and of the University of California, San Francisco.

This particular symptom of sloughing off is remindful of one of the effects of the coastal marine dinoflaggelate subsequently named *Pfiesteria*, described in Rodney Barker's *And the Waters Turned to Blood: The Ultimate Biological Threat* (Simon & Schuster, New York, 1997). This is both the common name used and the genus, and the species name is *Pfiesteria piscicida* (Barker, *Waters*, p. 323). Barker's book is also about the trials and travails of the organism's discoverer, JoAnn Burkholder of North Carolina State University, and is an indictment of a considerable part of the scientific and bureaucratic communities. Although mainly colorless, *Pfiesteria* is of same general family as the "red tides" occurring off the coast of Florida and the Gulf states, which consist of the dinoflagellate named *Gemnodinium breve*, from which nine toxins have been identified whose compositions have been found to change with conditions—but the neurotoxins in *Pfiesteria* still have not been identified (Barker, *Waters*, pp. 189, 301). Red tides date back to Biblical records (Exodus 7:20–21) and, interestingly, a phosphorescent dinoflagellate found off the coast of British Columbia contains a highly toxic **alkaloid** (Barker, *Waters*, p. 33).

In any event, not only do the *Pfiesteria* toxins produce lesions on contact, but they are also airborne, can cause short-term memory loss and confusion in humans, and very possibly could prove fatal, indirectly or directly. To fish and shellfish, *Pfiesteria* is deadly for sure, having caused large fish kills in the North Carolina estuaries, and has now been found along Florida and the Gulf coast. Most probably, it has been there all the time but only proliferates when the water conditions are right, a condition evidently favored by nutrient-laden waters from, say, agricultural runoff, e.g., chemical fertilizers and animal wastes. (Hog farm wastes, for one example, can be a problem in North Carolina, especially when the waste lagoons are breached or overflow due to heavy rainfall.) The organism exists in more than one metamorphic state, being more like a plant or alga when dormant on the estuary bottom, and then more like an animal in propelling itself through the water and attacking its victims. That is, it is *pleomorphic* and may be 10 times its original size after a feeding frenzy.

In further fact, generalizing, there is the question of to what extent do various venoms, toxins, and drug chemicals induce cancer, and by what means? Thus, chemotherapy drugs may be suspect in the further spread of cancer. Albeit the testing of substances for carcinogenicity is an ongoing activity (e.g., the Ames test for mutagenicity), this may not be the entire story. Thus, for instance, if the test is positive, the substance can be labeled a carcinogen and is described as having carcinogenic activity.

However, carcinogenicity may be perceived as a more immediate and direct manifestation, whereas we can speak of oncogenicity as perhaps a more long-term and indirect phenomenon—albeit it can also be stated that carcinogenicity means oncogenicity. This latter phenomenon, more precisely, pertains to the transformation of normal genetic material into cancer-causing genes or what are called *oncogenes*. That is, there are substances that may act as oncogens (as distinguished from "oncogenes") and have oncogenic activity.

Clearly, there is more to the story, which will be further explored in Part 7. For viruses sometimes function as oncogenic agents, not only invading the cell but also the chromosomes, altering the genetic makeup or genome itself. Viruses are ubiquitous, may act in ways as yet unsuspected, and may be the cause of diseases and symptoms not yet understood.

The foregoing brings to mind questions about the presence and availability of bioactive constituents in meat products, seemingly the staple of the American diet. Do these necessary nutritional adjuncts in fact exist in meat, or at least in feedlot beef as distinguished from the grass-fed or range product? The plains Indians consumed a buffalo meat diet apparently without ill effects—although this was supplemented with fruits or berries, and various plants and plant roots were eaten in season. (There is, of course, an herbal tradition among American Indians.) In winter, the diet was mostly in the form of pemmican (pounded or pulverized dried meat and berries mixed and stored in parfleche or animal skin bags). And the Eskimos of the Far North had to survive on a diet practically of meat alone (mostly seal), albeit the arctic lands also have plant life during the brief summers. A further study of these native American diets would be informative.

Besides the above, there are other factors to consider. For instance, Jeremy Rifkin in particular has written the polemic titled *Beyond Beef: The Rise and Fall of the Cattle Culture,* which among other things observes that diseases lurk in cattle. Thus, there is not only the bovine leukemia virus (BLV) but the bovine immunodeficiency virus, which is related to HIV (Rifkin, *Beyond Beef,* pp. 143–144). Also noted is the fact that the Danish death rate fell by 34 percent during WWI when meat was not available, and that there is a correlation between meat consumption and both colon cancer and breast cancer (Rifkin, *Beyond Beef,* pp. 170–173). The discussion will be continued in Part 7.

6.2 CANCER INITIATION, ENZYMES, AND ENZYME INHIBITORS

There is the consideration of how enzymes and inhibitors (or promoters) may affect the very processes of cancer initiation or genesis in the first place. In particular, there are the microorganisms or submicroorganisms as related to cancer formation, appropriate subjects in textbooks or treatises on microbiology. Thus, we are not only interested in these microentities per se, which are variously called viruses or virions, viroids, and prions, or whatever, but in their role if any in cancer formation. Not only this, but are enzymes involved, and if so, what might be the inhibitors? As an aside, at the submicroscopic level, enzymes themselves are of the same relative size as some of the microorganisms that may be involved. In other words, we are talking of macromolecules or molecules, and of bits and pieces of molecules.*

Briefly reviewed, a *virus* consists of a protein coat called a *capsid,* which surrounds a central genetic nucleic acid core, and its replication or assembly of parts occurs within the host cell, with the completed virus called a *virion particle* or simply a *virion,* which is then released from the cell (Atlas, *Microbiology,* pp. 237, 244).

---

* Noted in passing is that, in some quarters, viruses are perceived as the primary cause of cancer, period. That is to say, radiation and chemicals can be viewed as secondary causes that may affect, alter, or activate the primary cause, namely viruses.

A *viroid* consists only of an RNA macromolecule which is transmitted to cells and is reproduced using host cell *enzymes* (Atlas, *Microbiology*, p. 237, 243). As such, it carries a set of genetic information, called an *RNA genome*. Furthermore, viroids are bioactive and have been found to cause infectious diseases in higher organisms.

A *prion* can be described as composed of protein only, and of subviral size but which somehow carries a genetic code for replication (Atlas, *Microbiology*, pp. 237, 244). In other words, the genetic code seems to be stored in protein molecules. It has been suggested that Alzheimer's disease, for instance, might be caused by a prion. Other diseases thought to be caused by prions include kuru and Gerstmann-Straussler syndrome. Kuru is a neurological disease perpetuated via cannibalistic rituals in New Guinea; it is passed along by eating infected human brains. Scrapie is a disease of infected sheep, and now of cattle. Another is Creutzfeldt-Jakob disease (CJD), the human equivalent. These diseases were originally thought to be caused by what were called *slow viruses,* due to the slow development of the disease. Since no viruses could ever be found, the causes have instead been attributed to prions.

Originally found only in sheep, the disease called scrapie was evidently passed on to cows who ate feed pellets fortified with sheep's brains. It reinforces the enigmatic problem of prions, first discovered in 1983—and has raised doubts about the wisdom of eating beef (or sheep), at least in Britain. Also known as bovine spongiform encephalopathy (BSE) or "mad cow disease," it has been taken up by the media and has precipitated a crisis in Britain, which is faced with destroying its cattle herds to eliminate the disease. For example, a summary article titled "Of cows and men, and unfortunate mice" appeared in the Dec. 23–Jan. 5, 1996 issue of the British publication *The Economist, 337*(7946), pp. 101–102.*

Interestingly, there is a little-known but similar disease that occurs in deer and elk, especially as may have been confined in game farms. Called "chronic wasting disease," it has been around at least since 1981, according to the Colorado Division of Wildlife. Noticed mainly in the foothills of northern and northeastern Colorado, the Wyoming Game and Fish Department has observed occurrences in southern Wyoming, and the Wyoming State Veterinary Lab is studying the disease. Apparently, no scientific name has yet been attached, and the disease is known simply as *chronic wasting disease.* No cases of transmission to humans have been found, however, and at this writing the disease is not considered to be a problem.

Viruses themselves have been separated into animal viruses, plant viruses, and bacteriophages or bacterial viruses (Atlas, *Bacteriology,* 257ff.) The designator denotes whether they replicate within animal cells, plants cells, or bacterial cells and correspondingly infect the host organism. (The list may be extended to fungal viruses and protozoan viruses, as will be presented in Part 7.)

In turn, viruses have been divided into families, called the *viridae.* In some, the nucleic acid is DNA, in others RNA. Both types are found in animals. It is noted that the Poxviridae or poxviruses are large viruses that may contain *enzymes* such as RNA polymerase within the viral particle (Atlas, *Microbiology*, p. 260). The virus or virion diameter may range from approximately 20 nanometers for the virus family Parvoviridae up to 300 nm for the Poxviridae, a nanometer being a millionth of a meter. (As will be subsequently noted in Part 7, and based on information from the volume *Vaccination Strategies of Tropical Diseases,* the vaccinia virus, which is closely related to the chickenpox and smallpox viruses, is a potential source for new synthetic vaccines for other diseases, potentially including cancer.)

It may be added that the enzyme known as *DNA-dependent RNA polymerase* (or DNA-directed RNA polymerase) which, as the name implies, is involved in polymerization, has been implicated in the formation of cancerous cells through the medium of viruses. The subject is further encountered in Part 7. On the other hand, *RNA-dependent DNA polymerase* (or RNA-directed DNA polymerase), also known as *reverse transcriptase,* is a distinguishing feature for *retroviruses* such as cause AIDS or other immunodeficiency diseases.

Some inhibitors for RNA polymerases are listed in Appendix F. Some inhibitors for DNA polymerases are listed in Appendix E. Inhibitors for RNA-dependent or RNA-directed DNA polymerases are listed in both Appendices F and E. *Many of the inhibitors for both kinds of enzymes are antibiotics.* It may be noted in fact that, in a few instances, some of the same antibiotics or inhibitors work against both DNA polymerase, or DNA synthesis, and RNA polymerase. *There is the concluding thought that these*

---

* An unintended side effect, as Britons tend to eliminate beef from their diet, is the occasion to study what effect this may have on their general state of health, and in particular on cancer rates. If the general health improves and cancer rates go down, some inferences will be drawn.

antibiotics or other inhibitors are potential agents against immunodeficiency diseases—with the additional thought that, in some quarters, cancer is viewed as an immunodeficiency disease.

The diseases associated with various virus families are noted in the Atlas reference. Thus, for example, there is the family *Rhabdoviridae,* which contains single-stranded, rod-shaped RNA viruses, one of whose members causes rabies.

The *Retroviridae* contain RNA that has to be transcribed to DNA, rather than the other way around, carry the enzyme called *reverse transcriptase,* and contain tRNAs (Atlas, *Microbiology,* p 261ff). It is commented that one subfamily, called the Oncovirinae , causes cell transformations, and the members were at one time known as *RNA tumor viruses.* Another subfamily, called the Lentivirinae, produces slowly lethal diseases. This subfamily includes the *human immunodeficiency viruses* called HIVs which cause the acquired immunodeficiency syndrome called AIDS. Other related viruses of this subfamily include the *simian immunodeficiency virus* or SIV, and the *African green monkey immunodeficiency virus* or AGMIV. (It is not difficult to see why there is talk about HIV and AIDS originating in African monkey populations, and it brings up thoughts about the Marburg and Ebola viruses and so on, or other yet-to-be-encountered Level-4 virus diseases. Especially so when retroviruses and other viruses have the capability of jumping or *mutating from animal populations to humans,* the case notably for influenzas.)

The reference provides a short section on the Transformation of Animal Cells (Atlas, *Microbiology,* p. 257). Thus, the DNA produced during the replication of retroviruses, along with the DNA from some other viruses—such as from herpes viruses—may also enter into the chromosomes of the host cell. The viral genome (code) is thus introduced into the host cell, and this modification results in "virus-specific RNA and viral proteins." *The nature of the host cell genome is therefore changed* and, moreover, this change can be passes to succeeding generations of animal cells. It has been observed *in vitro* that such *transformed cells will have altered surface properties* and will grow even when in contact with a neighboring cell. It is further noted that *infections that induce virus-derived DNA can produce a tumor.* Such viruses are called *oncogenic viruses.* (However, not all host cells will be permissive; some are nonpermissive.) Examples of cancer-causing RNA retroviruses and DNA viruses are provided in the reference. In particular, *cervical cancer may be caused by the transformation of cells by certain papillomaviruses.* *

Cancer has been described in another reference as a cellular phenomenon of uncontrolled growth that may be caused by a *viral infection* (Brock and Madigan, *Microorganisms,* p. 187). Growth inhibition or regulation has been negated, and the cells reproduce uncontrollably, whereas most cells in a mature animal do not divide extensively, apparently due to the presence of growth-inhibiting factors. In fact, ordinarily, cells cease growing when they come in contact with one another, which is called *contact inhibition.* The tumorigenic or cancer-causing properties of viruses can be experimentally observed in an infected cell culture where, starting from a monolayer, cancerous cells continue to pile up as a *focus of growth.* This focus of growth becomes the tumor. (The foregoing brings up the matter of growth-inhibiting enzymes or hormones, or inhibitors for growth enzymes.)

While a virus may destroy a cell—a process called a *lytic infection*—the cell may also stay alive and continue to produce viruses in what are called *persistent infections.* Or the virus may lie dormant for a period, called a *latent infection.* There is also the possibility of a normal cell being transformed to a cancerous cell (Brock and Madigan, *Microorganisms,* p. 214ff). The reference lists the possibilities as indicated in Table 6.1. A normal cell is said to undergo genetic changes that may be initiated by chemicals, by radiation, or by viruses. A statement to be emphasized is that *retroviruses cause cancer* (Brock and Madigan, *Microorganisms,* pp. 225, 229).

In a special highlighted section titled "Virus Surprises," Brock and Madigan comment that the virus picture keeps changing as new discoveries further complicate matters (Brock and Madigan, *Microorganisms,* p. 227). Viruses were originally thought to be like other living organisms, only too small to be seen with an optical microscope. A subsequent discovery, using the *tobacco mosaic virus* or TMV, showed that viruses were composed of protein, in the manner of enzymes. But this was followed by another discovery—that RNA was also present and could act as the infectious agent by itself. Bacterial viruses or bacteriophages (bacteria-eating viruses) were in turn shown to have DNA instead of RNA, as supposedly was the case for plant viruses, e.g., TMV—only to be contradicted when RNA was found

---

* It may be commented that this *alteration of surface properties may in part be the cause of cancer cells metastasizing. The cancerous cells more readily break loose and then adhere in other parts of the body.*

Table 6.1 Human Cancers Possibly Caused by Viruses (From *Biology of Microorganisms*, 6th ed., by Thomas D. Brock and Michael T. Madigan, Prentice Hall, Englewood Cliffs NJ, 1991, p. 216.)

Cancer	Virus	Family	Genome
Adult T-cell leukemia virus (Type 1)	Human T-cell leukemia	Retrovirus	RNA
Burkett's lymphoma	Epstein-Barr virus	Herpes	DNA
Nasopharyngeal carcinoma	Epstein-Barr virus	Herpes	DNA
Hepatocellular carcinoma (liver cancer)	Hepatitis B virus	Not classified	DNA
Cervical cancer (?) (type 2)	Herpes simplex virus (?)	Herpes	DNA
Skin and cervical cancers	Papilloma virus	Papova	DNA

in a bacteriophage and DNA was found in a plant virus. Finally, viruses were found that had both DNA and RNA, namely the retroviruses such as HIV in which genetic information is transferred from RNA to DNA.

But then viroids and prions were discovered, which are simpler than viruses. *Viroids are composed of RNAs without protein,* whereas *prions are small protein molecules only.* In fact, one prion in particular contains only about 250 amino acids and is 100 times smaller than the smallest virus, or approximately 0.2 nanometers. Published in 1991, the authors conclude by asking, "Are there still *more* fundamental surprises awaiting discovery out there in the world of virology?"

A further question can be asked. Do viruses conceivably disintegrate into viroids and prions, and vice versa? After all, a viroid consists of RNA or DNA, and the prion consists of protein. Together maybe they constitute a virus. Stranger things could happen. This notion, of course, merges with the observations, say, of Naessens, Livingston, and Rife, discussed in Moss's *Cancer Therapy* and Walters' *Options*, where cancer-causing submicroscopic entities are perceived as a dynamic system undergoing change. What are called viruses are known to display a wide range of sizes and complexities, and conceivably at the lower end of the range there may exist prions or viroids, and at the upper end there may exist something approaching the notion of a bacterium. Moreover, mutations are found to occur, otherwise describable as changes.

The subject enters the realm of *pleomorphism* versus monomorphism, as suggested in the previous paragraph. It is therefore informative to note that in Volume II of the *CRC Handbook of Microbiology*, the topic of *pleomorphic viruses* is listed. The section or chapter, by H.W. Ackerman, is titled "Natural Groups of Bacteriophages" (Ackerman, in *CRC Handbook of Microbiology*, II, pp. 739, 641). *Pleomorphic viruses are further described as "enveloped, double-stranded-DNA-containing particles without apparent capsid; they may be compared to arenaviruses."* In turn, an *arenavirus* may be broadly defined as a member of a genus of viruses that infect both vertically and horizontally, replicate in a wide variety of mammals, and will result in a persistent infection if there is an insufficient immune response. This is as distinguished from an adenavirus of the virus family Adenoviridae, and which is associated with respiratory and eye diseases in both humans and animals. The question, of course, is, are we also talking of cancer causes and precursors?

It can be asked, therefore, does not this *initiation* or genetic change as described above also involve certain specific enzymes or enzyme catalysts, and do inhibitors exist for these enzymes? This seems like a ready enough experiment to carry out *in vitro*, to test the cancer-associated enzymes in the presence of potential (nontoxic) inhibiting substances. The many bioactive plants or plant substances used or tried against cancer is a pool of possibilities—not only the plants or plant substances per se, but the array of chemicals that exist in each plant. As to carrying out experiments in humans, this is a different proposition, as the reference comments (Brock and Madigan, *Microorganisms*, p. 217). Still, if the substances to be tried are otherwise nontoxic, at least in the dosages employed, where is the harm? And especially so if by *nontoxic* is meant that respiration and the nervous system are not to be adversely affected, nor is the substance to be cytotoxic—that is, not intended to kill normal cells.

Inasmuch as the Centers for Disease Control (CDC) *do not consider cancer to be a communicable disease,* no records are kept, nor is an accounting made, of treatments versus successes and failures, as in the case of other (communicable) diseases. The very fact that *cancer can be virus induced,* however, should cast a different light on the subject—the same as for the more rapidly acting diseases. In its slower-acting mode, cancer has company, namely AIDS and presumably prion-caused diseases, formerly thought caused by "slow viruses." Moreover, cancers can be more explicitly divided into *blood-related cancers* and *solid tumors* or *solid cancers,* with the idea that the former may not be a cancer in the usual sense but should be referred to as something else. In other words, leukemia, say, should retain its own classification apart from solid tumors, and the differences should be further established, with the notation that treatments for blood-related cancer do not work on solid tumors, since different phenomena are apparently involved. There is the judgment call that the diseases are simply not the same.

It may be further added that *cancer cells mimic normal cells,* which is why the body's own immune system does not ordinarily recognize and destroy cancerous cells. However, *the injection of cancerous cells from another person results in their quick destruction*—which is why organ transplants require that the immune system be suppressed. And the fact that cancerous cells mimic normal cells indicates that *there are many possibilities for different kinds of cancer cells,* with some estimates over 100, some as much as 300, and some even as high as approximately 600.

Also, solid malignancies have been divided into *sarcomas* and *carcinomas.* Sarcomas pertain to malignancies of nonepithelial cells or tissues, that is, of connective tissue, lymphoid tissue, cartilage, bone, and so on. Carcinomas occur in epitheleal cells or tissue—that which lines free surfaces or body cavities and is made up of one or more layers of cells with little intercellular substance.

6.2.1 MELANOMA

Still another category of cancer is that of melanomas, which presumably are initiated or activated by radiation, although there may be the suspicion that viruses are somehow involved, if only indirectly. Melanomas may or may not be malignant, and a succinct introduction to the subject is provided by M.W. Wick in a chapter titled "The Relevance of Pigment Cell Biology to Melanoma," which appeared in the volume *Cutaneous Melanoma,* edited by U. Veronesi, N. Cascinelli, and M. Santinami. While the differences in chemotherapeutical agents are prima facie evidence that melanomas constitute a separate category of cancers, more specifically, *pigment cell biology* is involved. It so turns out that cells known as *melanocytes,* which are the source for the manufacture of the pigment called *melanin,* are the place of origin for melanoma. Involved is the conversion of the amino acid *tyrosine* to *levadopa,* which is selectively catalyzed by an enzyme called *tyrosinase.* In turn, the levadopa is oxidized to melanin. *It has been found that melanoma cells will have much more tyrosinase than normal melanocytes.*

It can be concluded that the metabolism or biochemistry for malignant melanoma is therefore uniquely different from that of other cancer cells, which by and large involves anaerobic glycolysis and the conversion of pyruvate or pyruvic acid to lactate or lactic acid, as catalyzed by lactate dehydrogenase. The control of enzyme levels is, of course, a purpose of enzyme inhibitors.

6.2.2 OTHER DEVELOPMENTS

Among the more recent publicized developments involves an enzyme called human *telomerase* (with the accent on the second syllable). It has been discovered that this enzyme contains in its core a long-sought protein which is thought to be the fundamental, molecular-level cause of virtually every kind of cancer. At the same time, it may be central to the aging process.

In further explanation, the normal function of human telomerase is to maintain cell health during cell division—in other words, to keep the cells "young," but not too much so. If this enzyme is overactive, however, the effect is to cause the cells to be overly "young"—that is, to proliferate, unchecked, this being the cancerous condition. There is evidently a balance: *too active an enzyme leads to cancer; too inactive an enzyme leads to premature aging.**

Presumably, the above-mentioned protein determines the enzyme activity, which brings up the point of what substances might serve as inhibitors or promoters, regulators, or modulators. (It may be mentioned that telomerase is not listed in the Sigma catalog. That is, it is not routinely available for testing against various substances as enzyme inhibitors or promoters.)

---

* Investigations conducted at the Whitehead Institute for Biomedical Research in Boston, by researcher Matthew Meyerson, indicate that a gene named human Ever Shorter Telomeres 2, or hEST2, is responsible for making a component of telomerase. Consequently, it may very likely be a key agent in producing uncontrolled cancer cell growth.

A peripheral discovery is that *telomerase shares a chemical similarity with reverse transcriptase,* also called RNA-dependent DNA polymerase (or RNA-directed DNA polymerase). As has been noted, this latter enzyme is a distinguishing feature of *retroviruses,* which cause AIDS and other immunodeficiency diseases. (Interestingly, however, as has also been previously indicated, the polymerization enzyme denoted as DNA-dependent RNA polymerase, or DNA-directed RNA polymerase, has also been implicated in cancer formation.) It is said that the telomerase enzyme maintains the health of dividing cells by continuously rejuvenating the chromosome tips or telomeres, which become frayed from cell division. There may, in fact, be a biochemical connection with the action of such drugs as AZT, used against AIDS, which may result in anticancer drugs. That is, these drugs possibly could also act against overactive human telomerase.

On the other hand, with insufficient or inactive telomerase, the telomeres tend to shrink and break down, causing the cell eventually to die. The problem, in any sort of treatment, will be to maintain a proper balance. That is, telomerase that is too active leads to cancer; telomerase that is too inactive leads to premature aging. It becomes another example of Catch-22.

A review of the cancer situation as per the medical establishment was carried, for instance, in the November 7, 1997 issue of *Science,* published by the American Academy for the Advancement of Science or AAAS. It is mostly a review of the same, as indicated on the editorial page. A criticism leveled in the review is that there has not been a sufficient emphasis on chemoprevention.

One particular highlight, furnished in the series of news items and articles, involves the *disablement of p53, which is the tumor suppressor gene which prevents viral DNA replication (Science,* Nov. 7, p. 1057). In other words, the disablement of p53 would allow viral infection and replication in the tumor, presumably inactivating the tumor. *Disablement is by means of adenovirus, which is a human respiratory virus.* This is turned to an advantage by removing the viral gene which disables p53. Consequently, it was reasoned that the virus would selectively infect only cells in which the p53 was nonfunctional—that is, cancer cells. There have been some encouraging clinical trials, but it is required that the virus be injected directly into the tumor, since if injected into the bloodstream, the immune system would eliminate the virus. The application therefore will be of only limited use for cancers that have already metastasized.

It is apparent, on reading the series of news items and articles, that the investigations are mostly limited to *synthetic chemicals* as distinguished from plant-derived substances, and that the pharmaceutical companies are the most heavily involved. In other words, it is more a business proposition—but a *risky* one. Thus, from the 1400 biotechnology companies located in North America, fewer than 50 products have been successfully commercialized (*Science,* Nov. 7, 1997, p. 1039). *The quote is furnished that biotech is "one of the worst investments on the street."*

In another news item, it is repeated that *animal studies are of limited value, since humans and animal react differently to drugs (Science,* Nov. 7, 1997, p. 1041). A conclusion reached is that *animal studies resulted in "good mouse drugs rather than good human drugs."* Even *xenografts are not reliable, where human tumor cells are transplanted into mice.**

The remainder of the articles are concerned variously with origins, genetic testing for risk, detection by nucleic-based acid methods, oncogenic transcription factors, genetic approaches in the discovery of anticancer drugs, environment and cancer, and chemoprevention. These are the sorts of subjects found within the vast data base on cancer called MEDLINE.

Of special interest here is the article by David Sidransky of the Johns Hopkins School of Medicine, titled "Nucleic Acid-Based Methods for the Detection of Cancer" (*Science,* Nov. 7, 1997, pp. 1054–1058). Among the topics covered is the use of these methods as *markers* for the assessment of tumor burden in cancer patients. Briefly stated, the thesis is that cancer involves the clonal evolution of transformed cells in which there is an accumulation of mutations, which are either inherited (germline) or acquired (somatic). These mutations occur in critical proto-oncogenes and tumor suppressor genes. The genetic alterations that ensue can be used for the detection of cancer cells in samples taken and are based on DNA as the substrate or reactant. DNA is ideal in that it survives under adverse conditions, and its concentrations can be amplified by polymerase chain reaction (PCR) techniques, minimizing the amount of sample required. Aside from using mutations in oncogenes and tumor suppressor genes, *DNA changes*

---

* At this writing, there is a renewed interest in the drugs angiostatin and endostatin for blocking blood supplies to solid tumors. Although successful with mice, the extrapolation to humans is something else again, as has been repeatedly pointed out by specialists in the field. More on the subject is presented in Part 8 in the section on "Anticancer Agents and Angiogenesis."

can be used as markers, a phenomenon which involves changes in DNA repeat sequences called *microsatellites.* In short, what is involved is microsatellite analysis, which is the detection of microsatellite instability—and are simple names for complicated procedures.

It is mentioned also that *the presence of reverse transcriptase* (or RNA-directed DNA polymerase, the enzyme distinguishing retroviruses) may serve in providing a marker. This involves the conversion of isolated RNA to cDNA accompanied by amplification, a process designated as reverse transcriptase (RT)-PCR, or simply RT-PCR. *Telomerase,* the ribonucleoprotein enzyme that extends the sequences at the chromosomal ends (telomeres), is another strong possibility for a marker. *Telomerase is active in over 90 percent of primary human tumors but, for the most part, is inactive in normal cells.**

In a section on sensitivity and specificity, it is stated that a difficulty in looking for cancerous cells in a clinical sample is the fact that *cancer cells are far outnumbered by normal cells.* Moreover, the ratio or concentration will vary among organs and among individuals. Thus, a test for identifying bladder cancer cells in urine—where 50 percent of the DNA may be from sloughed off tumor cells—may not be transferable to the identification of lung cancer in sputum, where less than 0.2 percent of the DNA may be from tumor cells.

In a subsection on *Early detection,* it was indicated that oncogene or tumor suppressor gene mutations—namely *ras* or *p53—occur in many of the drained body fluids of cancer patients.* (The acronym *ras,* as in *ras* genes, stands for rat sarcoma, i.e., rat sarcoma genes, the transforming principle in retroviruses causing rat sarcomas. Known as a family of transforming genes, H-ras pertains to the Harvey sarcoma virus, and *K-ras* pertains to the Kirsten sarcoma virus.) It is noted that *ras* mutations occur early on in colon cancer tumorigenesis, whereas *p53* mutations are usually found in invasive tumors. There is also the possibility that what are called *APC* mutations could serve as *markers.* (The acronym *APC* stands for antigen-presenting cell). These are found in approximately 70 percent of colon adenomas, which are the precursors to colon cancer. In one set of tests on urine samples, *microsatellite markers* detected over 90 percent of bladder tumors.

Additionally, as has been indicated previously, since *telomerase* is expressed selectively in almost all primary cancers, it is viewed as a promising *molecular marker* for detecting cancer.

In a subsection titled "Tumor Burden," the reference states that, in addition to early detection, molecular markers can assess the migration of tumor cells, both locally and into the bloodstream. As a particular application, it is noted that surgery tumor cells often spread beyond the surgical margins and may not be detectable by light microscopy methods. A study is cited based on *p53* mutations, where tumor cells migrated beyond the surgical borders in approximately half of the patients. Even after follow-up radiation treatments, about one-third of the patents had recurrence, often developing new tumors next to or within the area testing positive. It is further stated that, for colorectal and lung cancer patients, even apparently disease-free lymph nodes have exhibited tumor cells by these methods of analysis.

The reference further mentions the fact that, in addition to local spread, malignant cells can also spread by the processes of *metastasis;* that is, the cells enter the blood stream and end up growing in other organs. *Inasmuch as the serum and blood of cancer patients have been found to contain large amounts of circulating DNA, blood samples can be analyzed for mutations and alterations.* The information is furnished that, in the case if patients with head and neck squamous cell carcinomas (HNSCC), 29 percent of the 21 patients tested had these DNA mutations or alterations in serum or plasma. In the case of small-cell lung cancer patients (SCLC), 71 percent of another 21 patients tested showed alterations or mutations.

In a tabulation, the following cancer types were set forth, giving the clinical sample and the corresponding genetic marker:

Head and neck	saliva	*p53*; telomerase
Lung	sputum	*ras/p53*; ras, microsatellites
Colon	stool	*ras*; telomerase
Pancreas	stool; juice	*ras*; *ras*
Bladder	urine	*p53*; microsatellites, telomerase

---

* Telomerase also controls aging, as has been noted. If too inactive, the cells age too fast. If overly active, cancer develops; that is, the cells grow too fast.

In the case of chronic myelogenous leukemia, whole blood and bone marrow (BM) are routinely analyzed for *abnormal transcripts* derived from cancerous or neoplastic cells. This provides a marker for the progress or regress of the disease. In other work, application has been made to patients having solid tumors. Thus, *tyrosine hydroxylase transcripts* correlate with micrometastatic bone marrow disease in neuroblastoma, and *tyrosine transcript levels* relate to the progression (or regression) of melanoma. Among the other substances detectable are *prostrate-specific markers,* notably the *prostrate-specific antigen* (PSA). The detection of micrometastatic disease has as yet proved inconclusive for such tumor types as primary breast, gastric, colorectal, lung, and prostrate cancer.

The reference contains an additional subsection titled *"Adjuncts to cytology and histopathology."* It is first mentioned that *needle aspirates are often used to furnish cancer diagnosis in suspected masses located in various organs. There is a difficulty, however, in distinguishing benign or preneoplastic lesions from overt cancer. Telomerase may furnish the criterion for such needle biopsies.* Thus, for example, telomerase was detected in all of 11 follicular carcinomas of the thyroid but was detected in only 8 out of 33 benign follicular tumors and was never found in normal thyroid tissue. The same procedure has been applied to breast cancer. Work has also been done in substituting for the Pap smear in detecting cervical cancer, which is almost entirely associated with the human papilloma virus (HPV) infections. Other work has been concerned with identifying the primary tumor when a patient exhibits only a metastatic lymph node.

Although these tests using *serum nucleic acid markers* may not yet be satisfactory for early tumor detection, they "may provide useful information on tumor burden and response to therapy."

In further comment, *the fact that the presence of the enzyme telomerase as associated with tumors may suggest a means for treating cancer by utilizing inhibitors for telomerase. The case is similar for the enzyme tyrosinase, as associated with melanoma,* and as indicated elsewhere. *Very possibly, the inhibition of reverse transcriptase (RNA-directed DNA polymerase) could act against cancer as well as retroviruses such as HIV (the AIDS virus), and the Marburg and Ebola viruses.* This is speculation, of course.*

In conclusion, not only should cancer and its causes be looked at differently, with fewer preconceived notions, but its cure (and prevention) should be approached in a different manner. That is, the subject should be approached from the standpoint of enzymes and enzyme inhibitors, inhibitors that *selectively* act against cancer cells—all cancer cells. Very possibly, it will prove sufficient to block anaerobic glycolysis in cancer cells by suitable inhibitors in nontoxic dosages.

6.3 STRESS PROTEINS OR HEAT SHOCK PROTEINS AND MOLECULAR CHAPERONES

A search of MEDLINE under Lactate Dehydrogenase Inhibitors uncovered an article by Taguchi and Yoshida in which chaperonins were mentioned as a protector for lactate dehydrogenase from heat denaturation. This, in turn, brings up the subject of shock proteins or heat shock proteins and how they may be potentially related either or both to cancer initiation and to cancer treatment. *For not only are these kinds of shock-induced proteins connected with the stimulation of the immune system, but it may be asked whether they can act as enzyme inhibitors in themselves, and in particular for, say, lactate dehydrogenase. These kinds of proteins being akin to polypeptides, which are known enzyme inhibitors, there is at least the latent possibility.* This newly emerging and highly specialized subject is further examined as follows.

In so many words, a *chaperonin* or *molecular chaperone* has been described as bringing about nucleosome assemblies in which histones and DNA are connected together in a controlled fashion (Voet and Voet, *Biochemistry,* p. 1130). In further explanation, the chromosomes of eukaryotic cells (human cells) consist of a complex of DNA, RNA, and protein referred to as chromatin (Voet and Voet, *Biochemistry,* pp. 8, 1124–1130). About half of the mass of chromatin consists of proteins called *histones,* divided into five major classes, four of which as a whole exhibit remarkable evolutionary stability,

---

* Telomerase has not yet made the enzyme/enzyme inhibitor handbooks. A number of inhibitors are listed in the handbooks of enzyme inhibitors for RNA-directed DNA polymerase, or reverse transcriptase, and these are listed in Appendix F, including such antibiotics as actinomycin.

although their synthesis may be switched on and off during specific stages of development. The fifth histone, labeled H1, is more variable and may be involved in cell differentiation read cell changes. Physically, chromatin is composed of particles connected by thin strands of DNA. The particles, called *nucleosomes,* consist of an octomer of the four stable histones in association with DNA. The fifth histone, H1, may be associated with the outside of the nucleosome. It has been shown *in vitro* that, at high salt concentrations, nucleosomes will self-assemble, but assembly is much slower at the lower, physiological salt concentrations that occur in the human body. However, in the presence of an acid protein named *nucleoplasmin,* assembly proceeds much more rapidly. *Accordingly, the nucleoplasmin is said to act as a chaperonin or "molecular chaperone."*

There are, in fact, two volumes devoted to the esoterica of the subject, published in 1990 and 1994 by the Cold Spring Harbor Laboratory Press, two out of the many books and monographs published. (Cold Spring Harbor NY is located on the north shore of Long Island.) The first volume is titled *Stress Proteins in Biology and Medicine,* edited by Richard I. Morimoto, Alfred Tissiéres, and Costa Georgopoulos. The second is titled *The Biology of Heat Shock Proteins and Molecular Chaperones,* also edited by Richard I. Morimoto, Alfred Tissiéres, and Costa Georgopoulos.

Heat shock proteins, designated *Hsp* or *hsp,* are described as highly conserved proteins occurring in all organisms, and whose synthesis may be induced by environmental stress such as *heat* (Voet and Voet, *Biochemistry,* 1st ed., Wiley, New York, 1990, p. 303). Moreover, the insertion or transport of proteins into or across a membrane is facilitated by still other specific proteins in an ATP-driven process, and in particular by heat shock proteins such as occur in yeast. Synthesis of the protective heat shock proteins produced by eukaryotic cells in response to high temperatures is regulated by what is called the *heat-shock transcription factor* or HSTF, itself a protein of various sorts (Voet and Voet, *Biochemistry,* 1st ed., Wiley, New York, 1990, p. 1061).

The high concentrations of intracellular proteins will cause an acute problem of *protein aggregation* in all cellular compartments (Morimoto et al., in *The Biology of Heat Shock Proteins,* p. 4). Aggregation is produced by hydrophobic interactions and is more pronounced at higher temperatures. *This aggregation is counteracted, however, by the set of universally conserved proteins, the molecular chaperones.* By minimizing aggregation, the transport and activity of the proteins is assured, expressed in terms of the proper folding and unfolding of the proteins. A further comment provided is that the classification "stress proteins" or "heat shock proteins" is somewhat misleading, in that *most of these proteins are essential for cell growth* over all temperature ranges and conditions. At times, molecular chaperones and heat shock proteins are considered to be one and the same. In this respect, it has been pointed out that not all molecular chaperones belong to the heat shock class of proteins, nor do all heat shock proteins function as molecular chaperones,

Heat shock proteins are classified by size into four main protein families as follows (Morimoto et al., in *Stress Proteins,* pp. 3–5): (1) the large-molecular-weight proteins hsp, designated as hsp83-90, (2) the hsp70 family, ranging from circa hsp66 to hsp78, (3) the hsp60 family—present in bacteria, mitochondria, and chloroplasts (a plastid or specialized cellular unit of plants or protozoa which contains chlorophyll)—and which have been designated as *chaperonins,* and (4) the small heat shock proteins, which are described as a diverse group ranging from circa hsp15 to over hsp30, which include a single form found in yeast and human cells and include more than 30 different forms found in higher plants Moreover, there are some even larger heat shock proteins in the range of hsp100 to hsp110 that are found in mammalian cells. A table is provided in the reference.

The Index of *The Biology of Heat Shock Proteins* lists the following numbers: hsp10, hsp 26, hsp 27/28, hsp27, hsp30, hsp40, hsp56, hsp58, hsp, 60, hsp70, hsp72, hsp73, hsp90, hsp100, and hsp104.

The numerical values above are in kD or *kilodaltons,* which signifies molecular mass. That is, the molecular mass of a particle can be expressed in daltons, a dalton being one-twelfth of the atomic mass of carbon in atomic mass units or amu (Voet and Voet, *Biochemixtry,* p. 4).*

---

* By way of explanation, the atomic mass of the Carbon 12 isotope of mass number 12 is set at 12.00000 atomic mass units or amu, and its atomic weight is nominally 12, or more exactly 12.01115. The atomic mass unit or amu is by definition a unit of mass equal to one-sixteenth or 1/16 of the mass of an atom of oxygen 16, whose mass number is 16, and whose atomic weight was assigned a value of exactly 16, but which has since been adjusted. (On the other hand, the atomic number Z or z, the number of protons within the atomic nucleus, is 6 for carbon and 8 for oxygen.) In terms of actual inertial mass, one amu has a handbook value of 1.65970×10^{-24} grams.

There are also what are called *heat shock cognate proteins* (hsc) with still other functions (Jeffrey L. Brodsky and Randy Schekman, in *The Biology of Heat Shock Proteins*, p. 85ff). These have been categorized, for instance, as hsc70 and hsc73. There are still other versions. For instance, it may be noted that what are called GroEL proteins are hsp60 proteins found in the *cytosol* of bacteria (D.A. Parsell and S. Lindquist, in *The Biology of Heat Shock Proteins*, p 471). (The *cytosol* is the cytoplasm exclusive of its membrane-bound organelles, whereas the *cytoplasm* is the cell exclusive of the nucleus.) GroES is the hsp10 analog, and so forth.

The stress response or heat shock response is universal and is observed in all forms of organisms ranging from bacteria types to vertebrates, although its quality and magnitude vary widely in nature (Morimoto et al., in *Stress Proteins*, pp. 6, 8). Circumstantial evidence indicates that *the function of these proteins is to protect cells from the ill effects of stress,* and the stress response may be activated in various ways. (Morimoto et al., in *Stress Proteins*, pp. 2–3). *Although stress activates stress or heat-shock genes, the expression or manifestation of most other genes is inhibited by stress.* The induction of the stress response can be achieved by means other than heat or thermal shock. Thus, it is observed that a release from anoxia or oxygen deprivation can induce the stress response, as can the addition of sodium azide (a poison or inhibitor for cellular respiration) or the addition of 2,4-dinitrophenol (described as an uncoupler of oxidative phosphorylation). Other inducers of the stress response include sodium arsenate, *ethanol,* sulfhydril agents, *hydrogen peroxide, transition series metals,* amino acid analogs, and *viral infections.* (It may be commented that some of these substances are known *enzyme inhibitors.*)

During bacterial and parasitic infections, there is a synthesis of stress proteins which appear as antigens, and they are potential candidates for vaccines (Morimoto et al., in *Stress Proteins*, p. 25). *Moreover, there may be a relation between stress proteins and neoplasia, that is, the formation of tumors or cancers* (Morimoto et al, in *Stress Proteins*, pp. 25–27). For instance, there is an activation of heat shock genes via DNA and RNA viruses, which occurs through the action of certain oncogenes. Thus, *members of the hsp70 family are associated with the production of a specific cellular oncogene. Viral or chemically transformed cells for example are noted to express high levels of stress proteins.* Another example is the appearance of *estrogen-induced hsp24 in breast cancer cells.* In fact, *the monitoring of stress protein levels may be a diagnostic tool for many diseases, including cancer.*

The role of *fever* is covered in Chapter 3 of *Stress Proteins* and is called the *febrile response. True fever is distinguished from hypothermia* in that the former involves an elevation of a person's thermoregulatory "set point," whereby heat production increases, while at the same time heat losses decrease (Matthew J. Kluger, in *Stress Proteins*, p. 61ff). The *four categories of body temperature* have been defined as normothermia, hypothermia, hyperthermia, and fever. In the first, the set point and actual body temperature coincide. In the second, the actual body temperature is below the set point, and in the third, the actual body temperature is higher than the set point. In the fourth, called fever, the set point is raised, and the body temperature may or may not be raised to the same level.

Fever can be induced by the action of certain known *exogenous pyrogens*—for example by an *endotoxin, which is any of a class of poisonous substances present in certain bacteria* such as the typhoid bacillus, or by other agents or mediators. (The term *exogenous* signifies "from without"; *a pyrogen is a fever-inducing substance.*) Similarly, *fever can also be induced by purified lipopolysaccharides,* denoted as LPS, or by still other agents. (Note that, as mentioned in Part 3, in the section on Other Information About Chinese Anticancer Agents, *polysaccharides are considered to be anticancer agents.*)

Exclusive of the action of exogenous pyrogens, fever was formerly thought to be the response to small proteins called *endogenous pyrogens* or EP released into the bloodstream from activated *macrophages,* which constitute a type of white blood cell. (The term *endogenous* signifies "from within.") The circulating EP was assumed to act on the central nervous system (CNS).

This was succeeded by the idea that other routes and agents are responsible. Such agents or mediators include *interleukin-1* α and β, which are *peptides* said to be equivalent to EP. These peptides are produced by a variety of *phagocytic cells* (cell-destroying cells) which are believed to influence the stereotyped *acute phase response* to infection and inflammation. Also called *cytokines* (cell-produced protein factors that regulate cellular growth and function), *they are thought to stimulate T cells and to lower the plasma concentrations of iron and zinc, but to raise that of copper.* They are thought to affect sleep, cause many of the aches and pains that occur with infections, suppress food appetite, stimulate the production of acute-phase proteins, and produce still other actions. *Other cytokines have been found to be involved as well, including the tumor necrosis factor (TNF), interferon α and interferon γ, and interferon* β$_2$ *(now known as interleukin-6 or IL-6).* In fact, there is work that indicates that the production and release of IL-6, a supposedly endogenous pyrogen or EP, is due to stimulation by IL-1, TNF, and other mediators (Kluger, in *Stress Proteins*, p. 63). The reported actions of IL-1 and TNF are tabulated in the reference. (Note that most of the foregoing items are buzzwords as *anticancer agents.*)

Among the acute-phase responses is *fever. The fever that follows the injection of any of these exogenous pyrogens or cytokines is presumed to be ameliorated by the release of prostaglandins at or near the hypothalamus* (Kluger, in *Stress Proteins*, p. 63). *Antipyretic (fever-reducing) drugs such as aspirin may acting as enzyme inhibitors, blocking the synthesis of prostaglandins, and returning the set point to its original level.* (Aspirin, incidentally, is sometimes regarded as an anticancer agent.)

There is no direct evidence, however, that any of the aforecited and so-called endogenous pyrogens actually account for a fever equal to that caused by the exogenous pyrogens (Kluger, in *Stress Proteins*, pp. 67, 68). "Although many cytokines can induce fever when injected or infused into experimental animals, it is still unclear which, if any, of the supposed or putative endogenous pyrogens actually play a role in infection-induced fever."

In asking the question of whether hypothermia is a fever, it is reported that *a person's body temperature will rise in response to psychological stress* (Kluger, in *Stress Proteins*, pp. 68–69). *In rats, stress-induced hypothermia can be blocked by naloxone (an antinarcotic agent), indicating perhaps that endogenous opioids may cause part of this rise in body temperature. (Note that some alkaloids—opioids, for instance, are alkaloids—serve as anticancer agents.)*

As to fever being beneficial, there is the observation that fever results in—or accompanies—an enhancement of the immune response (Kluger, in *Stress Proteins*, pp. 71, 72). It is further noted that the *interferons exert potent antiviral and antitumor effects as well as antibacterial effects—all of which are enhanced by febrile (feverish) temperatures.* Not only this, but the *in vivo* production of interferon is also increased at febrile temperatures—and the interferon itself seems to be pyrogenic. Moreover, the action of IL-1 on T lymphocytes or T cells seems to be fever facilitated, or at least the T cells proliferate.

In net sum, studies have proven that moderate fever has a beneficial effect on bacterial and viral infections.

As may be anticipated, and which will be further developed subsequently, stress proteins relate to infectious disease (Douglas B. Young, Angela Mehlert, and Deborah F. Smith, in *Stress Proteins*, p. 131ff). The humoral immune response involves binding an antibody to a pathogen, followed by killing the pathogen. The pathogen in fact becomes the antigen. (Young et al. in *Stress Proteins*, p. 133). The cell-mediated immune response involves antigen recognition by T lymphocytes, which activate phago-cytic cells that destroy the pathogen. Here, stress proteins also serve as antigens, activating the immune response to destroy the pathogen. The reference furnishes a tabulation of prominent antigens from a wide variety of infectious agents that have been identified as members of stress protein or heat shock protein families. A partial description is made of some of the stress proteins in terms of amino acid sequences. Additional information is furnished in other parts of the reference (Young et al, in *Stress Proteins*, pp. 143, 148).

Mammalian stress proteins have been further divided into two groups, the heat shock proteins (hsp) and the glucose-regulated proteins (grp), both of which are structurally related (W.J. Welch, in *Stress Proteins*, pp. 239, 242). The reference further divides them into sizes and provides detailed information about each. The glucose-regulated proteins contain phosphate and may involve ADP or ATP (Welch, in *Stress Proteins*, pp. 254–255). The connection to cell metabolism is obvious, and the reference is concerned with differences in the functions of stress proteins in both normal and stressed cells, partic-ularly with regard to hsp70 proteins (Welch, in *Stress Proteins*, p. 264ff). A tabulation is given for these and other stress proteins ranging from size 28 to 100, and under "remarks" there is a mention of nucleotides, RNA, fatty acids, and DNA synthesis. The overall view is that there are many things going on, and there is the inference (unstated) that there may be a relationship not only to cancer cell formation and proliferation but to cancer cell necrosis. The extreme complexity of the system raises more questions than can be answered.

Of most interest here, however, is the role of hyperthermia in cancer therapy. This is explored in Chapter 5 and 6 of *Stress Proteins*, as of the publication date 1990. As of 1984, nearly 11,000 patients had been treated for cancer using hyperthermia (Mark W. Dewhirst, in *Stress Proteins*, p. 101ff). In a study of several hundred cancer patients with the same type of tumor, response rates (but not cure rates) for local hyperthermia combined with radiation were about double that for radiation alone (around 60 percent versus about 30 percent). Despite the optimism, there are still some questions. More specifics are needed on temperature levels and on session length and frequency of treatment. For one thing, temperature distributions in heated tissues are not uniform, and thermotolerance varies. That is, cells develop a level of thermal tolerance.

The rationale for using hyperthermia alone or in combination is said to rest on the following experimental findings (Abe Mitsuyuki and Masahiro Hiraoka, in *Stress Proteins*, p. 117ff.):

1. Heat kills cells at a rate exponential with time at temperatures greater than 42° C or 107.6° F.
2. Hypoxic (anaerobic) cells are at least as heat sensitive as oxic (aerobic) cells.
3. Tumors may contain nutritionally deficient cells with low pH, making them more heat sensitive.
4. Tumors tend to become hotter than surrounding normal tissue due to impaired blood flow.
5. The vascular system of tumors is preferentially damaged with increasing temperature.
6. Radiation-resistant cells developed during radiation are more sensitive to heat.
7. Heat may act synergistically with radiation, a result of the inhibition of damage repair—in particular, in cancerous cells.
8. Heat may intensify the cytotoxic effects of some chemotherapy drugs either by increasing the drug uptake or by increasing the sensitivity to the drug.

Regarding item 2 above, *it is acknowledged that cancer cells are hypoxic (read anaerobic), whereas normal cells are oxic (read aerobic).* There is also the germ of the thought in item 2 that normal cells are heat sensitive as are cancerous cells, although the subsequent items indicate that there is a degree of selectivity toward cancers and cancer cells.

The authors treated patients with superficial and subsurface tumors and mention an average complete regression in 49 percent (66.7 percent in superficial, 39.7 percent in subsurface).

The treatment of deep-seated tumors is more complicated. The treatment depends on the equipment, and the methods developed so far are labeled external, intraluminal, and interstitial heating.

External methods include focused *ultrasound,* but it is difficult to apply, since it is reflected or attenuated by other tissues and by bone. *Regional heating* may use what is called an annular phased array system (APAS) or radio frequency (RF) capacity heating. *Radio frequency (RF) capacity heating has proved more successful,* being applied to the patient who lies between two electrodes. *(Could RF capacity heating in any way be similar to the Rife method presented in Walters' book?)*

Intraluminal or *intracavity methods* for deep heating use a hot fluid, *microwaves,* or *RF.* The use of a hot fluid has been confined mostly to bladder cancer and to the peritoneal dissemination of various cancers. Intraluminal heating is accomplished by inserting a microwave or RF applicator into body lumens (tubular passageways) such as the esophagus, rectum, vagina, uterine canal, and biliary tract. The heating is very localized.

Interstitial heating consists of *RF* current heating, *microwave* heating, and *ferromagnetic* heating. As the name implies, the method consists of heating in the spaces or interstices between tissues. Disadvantages include invasiveness, difficulty in repeating the treatment, and few applicable sites.

Although deep-seated tumors may not regress with hyperthermia, it has also been found that they may not regrow.

Heat shock responses are a familiar manifestation in the way vertebrates regulate their body temperature as a disease-control measure, and they are connected to various infectious diseases (Morimoto et al., in *The Biology of Heat Shock Proteins*, pp. 2, 20). The majority of heat shock proteins play a fundamental role as molecular chaperones or components of proteolytic systems (Morimoto et al., in *The Biology of Heat Shock Proteins*, p. 4). Heat shock proteins are noted to be involved variously in the regulation of protein folding, protein translocation, the assembly and disassembly of protein complexes, and gene regulation.

As previously noted, *the formation of heat shock proteins relates to hyperthermia, as in the treatment of cancer* (Morimoto et al., in *The Biology of Heat Shock Proteins*, p. 3.) This latter reference, *The Biology of Heat Shock Proteins*, was published in 1994, and supplies the statement that, *although hyperthermia has been used in tumor treatment for many years, there still remains no clear consensus,* with some experiments supporting the conjecture, but with some more recent experiments supporting the opposite (D.A. Parsell and S. Lindquist in *The Biology of Heat Shock Proteins*, p. 482).

In a chapter on Chaperoning Mitochondrial Biogenesis, it is emphasized that protein transport across cellular membranes into various cellular compartments is important to understanding cellular processes

(Thomas Langer and Walter Neupert, in *The Biology of Heat Shock Proteins*, p. 53). For instance, *polypeptide chains* apparently make the traverse or translocation through proteinaceous pores. (Polypeptides, incidentally, have been recognized as *anticancer agents*—or enzyme inhibitors, if you please.) In order to translocate, the chains must be in a partially folded or in an unfolded conformation, but they must refold after crossing the lipid membrane bilayer. It has been found that *molecular chaperones*, which are proteins and were originally identified as heat shock proteins, *modulate the folding state of polypeptide chains* in the cellular compartments.

A polypeptide chain exists in a three-dimensional structure or folded configuration in its native state (Voet and Voet, *Biochemistry*, p. 141ff). These structures are many and varied as shown in the reference. As indicated, these structures must be unfolded for translocation or transport across the mitochondrial membrane, an expectedly intricate process (Jerry L. Brodsky and Randy Schekman, in *The Biology of Heat Shock Proteins*, p. 85ff.) Refolding after translocation is equally intricate (Judith Frydman and Franz-Ulrich Harti, in *The Biology of Heat Shock Proteins*, p. 251ff). Both unfolding and refolding depend on heat shock cognate proteins (hsc) or heat shock proteins (hsp) as molecular chaperones to shepherd the changes. Examples include hsc70 for the one, and hsp70 and hsp60 for the other.

The *mitochondria* ("mitochondrion" is the singular) *are the cellular sites or organelles for eukaryotic oxidative metabolism* (Voet and Voet, *Biochemistry*, pp. 8, 564). *Here are located the enzymes that mediate metabolism:* the gycolytic enzymes such as pyruvate dehydrogenase, the tricarboxylic acid cycle enzymes, the enzymes catalyzing fatty acid oxidation, and the enzymes and redox proteins involved in electron transport and oxidative phosphorylation. (Here also, expectedly, will exist *lactate dehydrogenase* for cancerous cells undergoing anaerobic glycolysis or metabolism.) About the size of a bacterium, a mitochondrion is described as having a smooth outer membrane and an extensively invaginated (infolded, or folded) inner membrane, to provide additional surface area. The number of *invaginations,* called *cristae,* will vary with the respiratory activity of the particular cell, in that the mediating proteins are bound to the inner membrane surface, such that the respiration rate varies with surface area. The liver, which has a low respiration rate, has mitochondria with relatively few invaginations or cristae; the heart mitochondria have many invaginations. The *outer membrane contains porin,* a protein that forms pores that permit the transport or diffusion of molecules up to a certain size (e.g., presumably glucose or glycogen, saccharides or polysaccharides, peptides or polypeptides, proteins and heat shock proteins, etc.). In contrast, *the inner membrane is freely permeable only to O_2, CO_2, and H_2O, and controls the passage of such metabolites as ATP, ADP, pyruvate, calcium ion, and phosphate.*

After translocation, newly imported peptides must attain their original or native conformation or active state (Langer and Neuport, *The Biology of Heat Shock Proteins*, p. 68ff). This seems to be an assisted process and may be a function notably of molecular chaperone hsp60.

It appears increasingly evident that cancer cell metabolism will also occur in the mitochondria and may be either assisted, inhibited, or modulated by the transport of various agents into the mitochondria. These agents may include substances that act as enzyme inhibitors to the processes of anaerobic glycolysis, and other processes, and potentially include what are called chaperonins and/or heat shock proteins. Heat shock proteins are also vitally connected with the immune system, and with infectious diseases, about which more follows.

There is a relationship between hsp and human immune response, developed in a chapter of the cited reference titled "Heat Shock Proteins as Antigens in Immunity against Infection and Self" (Stefan H.E. Kaufmann and Bernd Schoel, in *The Biology of Heat Shock Proteins*, pp. 495–531). The cited chapter includes a short tabulation under the heading "Heat Shock Proteins as Major Targets of Infectious Agents." The diseases and their infectious agents include malaria, canadiasis, filariasis, tuberculosis, leprosy, Lyme disease, syphilis, Legionaire's disease, trachoma, brucellosis, pertussis (whooping cough), gastritis, ulcers, and so on. (Neither cancer nor AIDS was mentioned.)

In further discussing the role and purposes of heat shock proteins, authors Kaufmann and Schoel, cited above, provide a particularly lucid review of the immune system and its functions. It is recognized that the immune system continuously encounters a nearly infinite variety of pathogens and deals with this diversity by producing an equally high number of receptors that differentiate one pathogen from another. The receptors are of two types. One consists of antibodies produced by B lymphocytes and is able to recognize their pathogenic counterparts directly. The other consists of T-cell receptors that are expressed on the surface of T lymphocytes and recognize their counterparts indirectly. The molecular entities, which are recognized by these two kinds of receptors, constitute what are called *antigens*. As noted, antibodies are able to recognize "their" antigens directly, "comprising a stretch of six to seven amino acids or five to six carbohydrate residues on proteins or carbohydrates, respectively." Antibodies are specially adapted to contest microbes and microbial secretory products, as occur in extracellular space.

On the other hand, T cells recognize their antigens indirectly, by interacting with oligopeptides ("oligo-" meaning few, a little, scant) of about nine amino acids in length, as presented by cell structures. Antigen recognition by T cells requires intracellular processing by molecules from the major histocompatibility complex or MHC ("histo-" signifying tissue). As a result, T cells are particularly able to oppose microbes living inside host cells.

It is mentioned by the authors that the immune system will encounter certain invaders more frequently than others, and consequently a memory system is developed to focus the immune response on these more frequent encounters. With each successive encounter, the immune response is enhanced. "This so-called booster effect is also the principal mechanism underlying vaccination."

Further complicating matters is the fact that microbial invaders and mammalian host cells will have many components that are virtually the same at the molecular level. Accordingly, the immune system has inactivated those lymphocytes that express receptors for self-structures. Occasionally, however, this self-structure recognition fails, due to the presence of self-antigens and to malfunction in the development of some the T cells. The result may be an autoimmune disease.

Furthermore, heat shock proteins (hsp) pose some special obstacles to the immune system. Described as among the most abundant proteins in the biosphere, the ubiquity of hsp is further elevated under stress. Microbes may also cause an increase, and the hsp, in any event, are highly conserved. Their very abundance and homology (similarity) among various microbes causes the hsp also to be targets for the immune response. Not only this, but there is a similarity with mammalian host cells, which can produce an autoimmune response. If the immune system does not recognize and disregard those regions of hsp shared by microbial predators and mammalian prey, the result can be autoimmune disease. On the other hand, if the immune system ignores the entirety of the hsp, then this will favor the microbial invader, since the major target antigens would be excluded from the immune reaction.

The authors distinguish the major types of infectious agents that are attacked by antibodies. Some microbes reside in extracellular spaces and may secrete toxic components. It is the role of the antibodies to come to the attack and also to neutralize toxic secretions. Other bacteria and protozoa enter host cells and are shielded from antibody recognition and instead must be countered by T lymphocytes. A corollary is increased hsp levels, which are also targeted by the immune response.

Viruses do not grow by themselves but grow by replication in host cells. Although free viral particles are targets for antibodies, once in the cell they are protected from antibodies. Nevertheless, virus-infected host cells are detected by T cells. Although the viral genome (complement of genetic information) itself does not seem to have genes that encode hsp, it has been found that prions will elevate host hsp synthesis. In this way, viral infections can produce immune responses against both viral-caused hsp and self-generated hsp.

This all gets back around to the fact that infectious diseases cause increased levels of hsp, which in turn produce an immune response to hsp. The list of infectious diseases in which immune responses to hsp has been found and is reproduced in the tabulation noted in the last-mentioned reference titled "Heat Shock Proteins as Major Targets of Infectious Agents." That is, infectious agents induce high levels of hsp as antigens and, in turn, high levels of antibodies. This tabulation and other findings "have been taken as evidence that hsp are dominant antigens of infections with various pathogens ranging from bacteria to protozoa to helminths as well as of antimicrobial vaccines." The authors observe that the vaccination of young children with the trivalent vaccine against tetanus, diphtheria, and pertussis (whooping cough) induces high anti-hsp antibody titers (high antibody strengths or concentrations).

The relationship between heat shock proteins and autoimmunity is given as a separate section in the reference. It is commented that the recognition and disposal of senescent or *aberrant* cells would be beneficial for the host. However, an abnormal attack on physiologically active cells would be detrimental.

It is stated that hsp expression caused by various cellular insults could serve as a unique and universal indicator of stressed cells independently from causative insult, including inflammation, transformation, infection, and trauma. (It is this notation that may link hsp to cancer, assuming that cancer cells are stressed cells. Not only could hsp levels be an indication of cancer cells, but they could be projected as initiating action against cancer cells by stimulating an autoimmune response.)

Finally, the authors comment that, based on prior work by one of the authors, hsp are induced by cell activation and participate in protein neosynthesis in activated cells. (Thus, at the same time, hsp could induce cancer cell growth, while initiating action against cancer cells, as noted in the previous paragraph. This could be an explanation for the mixed results obtained by hyperthermia.)

The authors provide the following information about tumors. "In the tumor system, immunization with hsp 96, hsp90, or hsp70 isolated from distinct tumors, causes a specific immune response against the homologous tumor." The reason for this was subsequently found to be due to an association of antigenic tumor-specific peptides with these hsp cognates (of the same or a similar nature). In other words, the talk is of an autogenous cancer vaccine.

In a concluding section titled "Heat Shock Proteins and Autoimmune Disease," the authors state that the general role of hsp in the development of autoimmune diseases is as yet unresolved. For instance, the original enthusiasm about hsp being responsible antigens for rheumatoid arthritis (an inflammation disease) has become more subdued.

The final chapter in *The Biology of Heat Shock Proteins* is titled "Heat Shock Protein Gene Expression in Response to Physiologic Stress and Aging." In this regard, a cellular response to stress has been linked to neuro-hormonal stress responses in animals (Nikki J. Holbrook and Robert Udelsman, in *The Biology of Heat Shock Proteins*, pp. 590–591). (It can, of course, be asked, "Is cancer not also a cellular response to stress?")

Inasmuch as the hsp are proteins, one can further ask, "Do the hsp ever serve as enzymes or enzyme inhibitors?" This was a topic not specifically covered in the aforecited volume, although it was stated that heat shock proteins may function as proteases or unfolded polypeptide-binding proteins (Morimoto et al., in *The Biology of Heat Shock Proteins*, pp. 2, 6, 10). Moreover, hsp90 was found to suppress the function of certain protein kinases (Moritoto, in *The Biology of Heat Shock Proteins*, p. 7). In this context, presumably hsp90 is an enzyme inhibitor. It is also mentioned that polypeptides that are to be degraded are attached to ubiquitin, a highly conserved heat shock protein, and many of the ubiquitin-conjugating enzymes are under heat shock or stress regulation (Morimoto et al., in *The Biology of Heat Shock Proteins*, p. 11). Furthermore, some of the ubiquitin-conjugating enzymes can distinguish between polypeptides that have been damaged by elevated temperatures and those damaged by heavy metals. In this regard, the hsp104 protein found in yeast can protect cells from high temperatures and high concentrations of ethanol, but not from damage by cadmium (Morimoto et al., in *The Biology of Heat Shock Proteins*, p. 6).

As a footnote, some proteins are synthesized as segments of polyproteins, which are polypeptides containing the sequences of two or more identifiable proteins (Voet and Voet, *Biochemistry*, p. 1009). Examples of polyproteins include most polypeptide hormones and the proteins synthesized by many viruses, including those viruses causing polio and AIDS. Additionally, there is ubiquitin, already mentioned and described as a highly conserved eukaryotic protein involved in protein degradation. In this context, ubiquitin can be regarded as an enzyme. (Moreover, ubiquitin shares a word-kinship with "ubiquitous.")

It has been previously mentioned that heat shock proteins act to unfold polypeptides or proteins so that they can enter the mitochondria as well as serving as major dominant antigens that stimulate antibodies against a wide range of infectious agents, including viruses (Morimoto et al., in *The Biology of Shock Proteins*, pp. 4, 22).

In some instances, the peptides occurring in heat shock proteins have been identified and are found to be recognized by T cells; furthermore, heat shock proteins may dramatically enhance the antigenicity of peptides or oligosaccharides, introducing the possibility of better vaccines for infections (Morimoto et al., in *The Biology of Heat Shock Proteins*, p. 22).

6.4 METASTASIS AND GLYCOPROTEINS

It has been noted that oligosaccharide chains ("oligo-" meaning, of course, few or short chains) may have an effect on the adhesive interaction between cancer cells and their normal parent tissue cells (Robert K. Murray, in *Harper's Biochemistry*, p. 660). The phenomenon is related to metastasis.

That is, cancerous cells tend to lose adhesion and break away from the normal cells from which they originate, and stick elsewhere (Hasselberger, *Uses of Enzymes*, pp. 143–144). Thus, cancer cells show a low level of adhesion but much stickiness, whereas normal cells behave oppositely. Moreover, there are enzymes which may reduce the stickiness, but radiation and X-rays may increase the stickiness and contribute to metastasis

To continue, cancer cells may contain patterns of the enzymes called *glycosyltransferases* that differ from those the corresponding noncancerous normal cells (Murray, in *Harper's Biochemistry*, p. 660). The reference calls for an investigation into drugs that may act as enzyme inhibitors for the particular glycosyltransferases that occur in cancerous cells and result in metastasis. (The enzyme glycosyltransferase is not listed in either Jain's or Zollner's *Handbook of Enzyme Inhibitors*.)

Returning to the subject of *oligosaccharides*, these also occur in what are known as *glycoproteins*. Glycoproteins are defined as proteins which have oligosaccharide (glycan) chains attached covalently to a polypeptide backbone (Murray, in *Harper's Biochemistry*, p. 648). The entirety comprises the glycoprotein, which may also be called a *complex carbohydrate*.

In further explanation, for the record, an oligosaccharide consists of a few monosaccharide units joined together by glycosidic bonds (Voet and Voet, *Biochemistry*, pp. 251, 608).

Saccharides in general are equivalently referred to as *carbohydrates*. In fact, the name carbohydrate stands for "carbon hydrate," indicating their composition to be approximately $(CH_2O)_n$, where $n \geq 3$. Monosaccharides, also called *simple sugars,* therefore contain at least three carbon atoms. Examples are D-glucose and D-ribulose, with many more provided in the reference. They may be further classified as hexoses, pentoses, and so on, depending on the number of carbon atoms and other compositional characteristics.

Polysaccharides, on the other hand, consist of many covalently linked monosaccharide units. They are most conspicuous in plants, where cellulose is their principal structural material. Starch in plants and glycogen in animals are polysaccharides serving as important nutritional reservoirs.

In a glycosidic bond, the first carbon of one monosaccharide unit is joined to an OH group of a second unit to build up the polymer either as an oligosaccharide or as a polysaccharide.

Although some 200 occur in nature, *only eight monosaccharides commonly occur in the oligosaccharide chains of the glycoproteins found in humans* (Murray, in *Harper's Biochemistry*, pp. 649, 650). These principal simple sugars or monosaccharides and their abbreviations are as follows:

- galactose (Gal)
- glucose (Glc)
- mannose (Man)
- n-acetylneuraminic acid (NeuAc)
- fucose (Fuc)
- n-acetylgalactosamine (GalNAc)
- n-acetylglucosamine (GlcNAc)
- xylose (Xyl)

Some of the functions served by several of the glycoproteins are as indicated in Table 6.2. It is noted that the carbohydrate content of glycoproteins may range from 1 to over 85 percent by weight.

Mucins, listed in the accompanying Table 6.2, are noted to both lubricate and form a physical barrier on epithelial surfaces (Murray, in *Harper's Biochemistry*, p. 654). (The term *epithelium* is defined as a cellular membrane-like tissue that covers a free surface or lines a cavity and consists of one or more layers of cells with little cellular substance.) Mucins bound to membranes are involved in cell-to-cell interactions. It is further noted that mucins are resistant to the action of proteases (proteolytic or protein-digesting enzymes), an effect produced by the high density of the oligosaccharide chains present in the glycoproteins. This effect may mask or counter surface antigens, thus shielding the cell from immune surveillance. *It is commented that cancer cells form excessive amounts of mucins. In this way, cancer cells may protect themselves from the anticancer action of the immune system.*

It is also noted that the oligosaccharide chains per se, as exist in glycoproteins, may in themselves serve certain useful functions (Murray, in *Harper's Biochemistry*, p. 649). Some of these functions are enumerated as follows, as taken from the reference:

1. Modulation of certain physicochemical properties such as solubility, viscosity, ionic charge, and denaturation.
2. Protection against proteolysis (decomposition of protein), both inside and outside the cell.
3. Affecting the proteolytic processing of precursor proteins to smaller products.

Table 6.2   Some Glycoproteins and Their Functions

Glycoproteins	Function
Collagens	Structural molecule
Mucins	Lubricant and protective agent
Transferrin, ceruloplasmin	Transport molecule
Immunoglobulins, histocompatibility antigens	Immunologic molecule
Chorionic gonadotropin, thyroid-stimulating hormone (TSH)	Hormone
Various enzymes, e.g., alkaline phosphatase	Enzyme
Various proteins involved in cellular interactions: cell–cell (e.g., sperm–ocyte), virus–cell, bacterium–cell, hormone–cell	Cell attachment–recognition site
Certain plasma proteins of cold-water fish	Antifreeze
Some lectins	Interact with specific carbohydrates

Source: Data from *Harper's Biochemistry* by Robert K. Murray et al., 24th ed., Appleton & Lange, Stamford CT, 1990, 1993, 1996. Lange Medical Publications, 1988, p. 648.

4. Involvement in biological activity such as of human chorionic gonadotropin (hCG).
5. Affecting the insertion of substances into membranes, intracellular migration, sorting and secretion.
6. Affecting embryonic development and differentiation.
7. Possibly affecting sites for metastasis as selected by cancer cells.

Note that Item 5 is related to the function of stress or heat shock proteins, or molecular chaperones. Thus, we may infer that these substances are not only proteins but may be glycoproteins, where the activity is provided by the oligosaccharide content. Item 7 suggests a relationship with the *stickiness of migrating cancer cells,* as mentioned previously. If this stickiness is mitigated rather than promoted, then the oligosaccharide content of the glycoprotein could serve as an *anticancer agent.*

Lectins are described as sugar-binding proteins that agglutinate cells or precipitate glycoconjugates, and some are glycoproteins in themselves (Murray, in *Harper's Biochemistry,* pp. 651–652). *More importantly, it has been found that smaller amounts of certain lectins result in the agglutination of tumor cells, as compared to normal cells.* The inference is that the structural or organizational patterns for the glycoproteins occurring on the surfaces of tumor cells may be different from those for normal cells. This has been previously indicated as potentially relating to metastasis.

Glycoproteins may be further divided into three different types (Murray, in *Harper's Biochemistry,* p. 652ff). This and other compositional particulars are not of primary interest here.

The reference next discusses the synthesis and reactions of glycoproteins and the enzymes involved, and in particular of *high-mannose glycoproteins* (Murray, in *Harper's Biochemistry,* pp. 665, 657). In these complicated sequences, some of the enzymes are destined for entry into *lysosomes.* Lysosomes, in further explanation, are defined as single, membrane-bounded organelles of varying size and morphology, being essentially membrane bags containing hydrolytic enzymes that function to digest ingested materials (Voet and Voet, *Biochemistry,* p. 9). What is called mannose 6-P (or Man 6-P) functions as a chemical marker to target certain lyosomal enzymes to lysosomes (Murray, *Harper's Biochemistry,* p. 664). If faulty targeting occurs, what is called *I-cell (inclusion cell) disease* results. The inference is that this may be related to still other diseases, including cancer. The further inference is that sufficient levels of mannose glycoproteins are necessary for the proper functioning of the body.

A number of diseases cited in the reference result from abnormalities in the biosynthesis of proteins (Murray, in *Harper's Biochemistry,* p. 663.) Prominently mentioned is that an increased branching of cell surface glycans (oligosaccharides) may be an important facet in producing *metastasis.*

Furthermore, *glycoproteins are apparently involved in a wide variety of biological processes and diseases* (Murray, in *Harper's Biochemistry,* p. 665). Examples include the influenza virus, HIV-1, and rheumatoid arthritis. For the foregoing reasons, the isolation, synthesis, and utilization of oligosaccharides and glycoproteins is becoming of increasing interest, particularly as involving the eight principal monosaccharides found in the human body. This interest and involvement is signaled, for instance, by Mannatech Inc., of Grand Prairie TX, mentioned in Part 8 within the section "Phytochemicals That May Act Against Cancer," in the subsection "Other Bioactive Substances and Miscellaneous Agents," and whose appellation signifies mannose, one of the eight monosaccharides found in oligosaccharides and glycoproteins as occurring in humans.

In Table 6.2, thyroid-stimulating hormone (TSH) is mentioned, and this introduces the possibility that it might serve as an antidote to cancer. That is to say, *a sub-par thyroid produces the condition known as hypothyroidism*—as opposed to hyperthyroidism—*and may be associated with cancer.* (The thyroid or thyroid gland is the source of the hormone thyroxine, which mainly affects growth.) And according to Broda O. Barnes, MD, and Lawrence Galton, in *Hypothyroidism: The Unsuspected Illness*, this may well be the case. In a chapter titled "The Thyroid, Lung Cancer, and Emphysema," Dr. Barnes states that of the thousands of his patients placed on thyroid-enhancing therapy, *not one developed lung cancer.* The death rate from other malignancies was also markedly lowered. In other chapters, the vital role of thyroid is displayed, notably against infectious diseases—in other words, *thyroid serves to stimulate the immune system. Proper thyroid levels also correlate against diabetes,* and as noted elsewhere, *diabetes incidence can be correlated with cancer incidence*—e.g., as noted by Arctic explorer Valhjalmur Stefansson in his book about cancer and civilization, to be cited subsequently—and seems to play an active role. (As to treatment, consult the *Townsend Letter,* December 1998, p. 122.)

The subject of cancer and diabetes (and insulin) is further presented in Part 8, in the section on "Enzymes and Enzyme Inhibitors for Anaerobic Glycolysis," and in the section on "An Update on Plants and Other Substances as Enzyme Inhibitors." (A diabetic condition indicating that insufficient insulin is being produced.) For instance, it is mentioned that the production of the enzyme pyruvate kinase, which is involved in the formation of pyruvic acid or pyruvate during glycolysis (as per Figure 1.1 in Part 1), is regulated or modulated by the pancreatic hormones glucagon and insulin. Glucagon serves as an inhibitor and insulin as a promoter, to strike a balance. In other words, insulin favors the formation of pyruvic acid or pyruvate, and an insulin deficiency would also suggest a pyruvate-deficiency—denoting, in turn, the incomplete metabolism of carbohydrates or glucose, the usual diabetic condition accompanied by the rejection of sugar in the urine. Or, in other words, aerobic glycolysis becomes incomplete, as does oxygen utilization, and anaerobic glycolysis is to a degree favored. Anaerobic glycolysis, however, is associated with the production of lactic acid or lactate, the signature end product for cancer cell metabolism. (Further details about glycolytic pathways are furnished in Part 1.)

Incidentally, the nonessential amino acid *alanine has been found to enhance the inhibition of pyruvate kinase by glucagon,* which would further decrease aerobic glycolysis in favor of anaerobic glycolysis. This would have the same effect as an insulin deficiency. It has been noted, therefore, that *alanine is a biomarker for anaerobic glycolysis.* That is, the more alanine present, the more likely that anaerobic glycolysis is occurring, and the less so for normal aerobic glycolysis—and anaerobic glycolysis is the principal pathway for cancer cell metabolism.

6.5 INTESTINAL FLORA AND CANCER

In spite of the increasing interest in oncogenes as the source of cancer, there is also an interest in the intestinal or gut microflora in carcinogenesis. This is set forth in a book titled *Role of the Gut Flora in Toxicity and Cancer,* edited by I.R. Rowland and published in 1988. Many of the contributors are from the U.K., although other countries are also represented, including the U.S.

The scope of the book is embedded in its chapter titles:

Methodological Considerations for the Study of Bacterial Metabolism

The Bacterial Flora of the Intestine

Alimentary Tract Physiology: Interactions Between the Host and its Microbial Flora

Deconjugation of Biliary Metabolites by Microflora, β-Glucuronidases, Suphatases and Cysteine
　　　Conjugate β-Lyases and their Subsequent Enterohepatic Circulation

Hydrolysis of Glycosides and Esters

Metabolism of Nitro Compounds

Nitrate, Nitrite and Nitroso Compounds: The Role of the Gut Microflora

Intense Sweeteners and the Gut Microflora

Metabolism of Toxic Metals

Bacterial Metabolism of Protein and Endogenous Nitrogen Compounds

Metabolism of Fats, Bile Acids and Steroids

Metabolism of Carbohydrates

The Effects of Dietary Fibre Utilization on the Colonic Microflora

Mammalian Lignans and Phyto-oestrogens: Recent Studies on Their Formation, Metabolism and
   Biological Role in Health and Disease

Factors Affecting the Gut Microflora

Caecal Enlargement

Mutagens in Human Faeces and Cancer of the Large Bowel

Gut Flora and Cancer in Humans and Laboratory Animal*

The term *gut flora* in the main has bacteriological connotations but may also refer to biochemical and toxicological aspects (Coates et al., in *Role of the Gut Flora*, p. 1; B.S. Draser, in *Role of the Gut Flora*, p. 23). Additionally, *fungi* and *protozoa* may be involved. The comment has been made, therefore, that two oversimplifications occur in the published work on the metabolic effect of alimentary flora (O.M. Wrong, in *Role of the Gut Flora*, p. 227). The first simplification is that research in humans has concentrated on the large intestine which, admittedly, is the most densely populated part of the alimentary tract with bacterial populations numbering circa 10^{11} microorganisms per gram of contents. *"Second is the emphasis on bacteria to the almost total neglect of the fungal and protozoal denizens of the large intestine."* The reference adds that studies on the rumen of herbivorous animals suggests that human alimentary flora might also have some interesting biochemical properties. Furthermore, the ruminal flora include a *protozoal population* that participates in some of the major metabolic processes of that organ.

As to *bacterial flora,* these have been characterized as belonging to the genera *Bacteroides, Eubacteria, Peptococcaceae, Bifidobacteria,* **Lactobacilli,** *Clostridia, Fusobacteria, Enterobacteriaceae,* and *Streptococci* (Drysar, in *Role of the Gut Flora*, pp. 26–36). **The microorganism genera in boldface are known to produce the enzymes for the formation of lactic acid or lactate, the chief metabolic product of cancer cells.** The reference further identifies some 234 specific bacteria species, mostly belonging to the above genera. Overall, there are said to over 400 different bacteria species in the GI tract, most of which are anaerobic, and the individual bacteria organisms are greater in number than the totality of the cells of the whole of the host, constituting a mass similar to that of other mammalian organs (G.L. Larsen, in *Role of the Gut Flora*, p. 80).

6.5.1 BACTERIAL METABOLISM AND CARCINOGENS

"It has been estimated that 80 to 90 percent of cancers are caused by environmental agents." This statement is provided by Michael Hill, in a chapter titled "Gut Flora and Cancer in Humans and Laboratory Animals" (Hill, in *Role of the Gut Flora*, p. 461). A figure of 80 percent is supplied in another reference (Robert K. Murray, in *Harper's Biochemistry*, p. 758). This preponderance is in spite of the importance of genetic factors. Even in inbred strains of laboratory animals, where the genetic factors are more pronounced, "a high proportion of cancers have an environmental etiology rather than an inherited cause." That is, the origins or etiology of cancer is more likely environmental agents rather than genetic factors.

It can be assumed, as a matter of course, that ingested agents or their metabolic products are absorbed in the gut to enter the bloodstream and thus to be carried to cellular sites (which for one reason or another are especially receptive to the particular agent) and there be absorbed into the cellular mechanism. The action can even be perceived as random—the luck of the draw. In the case of cancer formation or etiology, there may be presumed an alteration in the genetic machinery whereby the cell no longer functions normally but takes on the attributes of cancer cells. In the case of cancers of the alimentary

---

* Precisely speaking, the intestine or *gut* does not include the stomach. Speaking more encompassingly, however, microflora exist throughout the entire alimentary canal, from the oral cavity on down, but most resident populations occur at the opposite ends—in the mouth and in the large intestine, or colon, with some action noted even in the appendix or caecum (James B. Heneghan, in *Role of the Gut Flora*, pp. 39, 41). Thus, there is also reference to bacterial flora of the stomach and to gastrointestinal microflora in general (e.g., B.S. Drysar, in *Role of the Gut Flora*, pp. 24–27; AK. Mallett, in *Role of the Gut Flora*, p. 152).

canal—i.e., oral and esophageal cancers, gastric cancers, and colorectal cancers—the action can be viewed as more direct. The action is similar for invasion of the lungs by outside agents, of course, and for skin cancers of topical chemical origins. (As to metastasis, this may sometimes be the case where the *cancer-inducing agents themselves have migrated and taken hold to more than one site.*)

Hill goes on to say, "Since all body surfaces are colonized by bacteria, the normal flora is in a unique position to mediate between the host and its environment.... "This mediation is performed variously by "degrading, releasing, or forming genotoxic agents." (The term *genotoxic* or gene-toxic contains the germ of the thought that there are agents that can cause malfunctions in the genetic machinery of cells and therefore function as the primary cause of cancer.) In further fact, *the normal bacterial flora are noted to produce carcinogens, mutagens, and other agents.* Thus, bacteria can produce carcinogens or tumor promoters from various substances or substrates that enter the gut either from food intake or from liver bile.

In particular, Hill is concerned with the substrates that are dietary β-glucosides, biliary β-glucuronides (in bile); the amino acids known as methionine, tryptophan, and tyrosine; the nitrosatable amines; the bile acids; and cholesterol.

β-Glucosides

Of the many β-glucosides (or glycosides) found in plants, and which produce *carcinogenic aglycones,* the most widely studied is the glucoside *cycasin* (Hill, in *Role of the Gut Flora*, p. 462). It is a component in the cycad nuts of the evergreen cycad plant (genus *Cycas* of the family Cycadiaceae). This plant is native to many Pacific islands and to parts of southeast Asia. It is further noted that cycasin is the β-glucoside of methylazoxymethanol and is highly *hepatotoxic* to humans (and to rodents).

If cycasin is given orally to rodents at levels insufficient to produce hepatotoxic death, the rodents will nevertheless for the most part develop tumors of the intestinal tract. On the other hand, when introduced intravenously, or given to germ-free rats by any method, the cycasin is both nontoxic and noncarcinogenic. The inference is clear. The toxicity and carcinogenicity of cycasin depends on the presence of gut bacterial flora.

The extension of carcinogenicity to humans has not yet been demonstrated. Although cycad nuts have been used in the past as a starch source, a prior water extraction removes the cycasin. Following hurricanes and food shortages, some of the native population has eaten cycad nuts without extracting the cycasin. Although hepatotoxic effects have been experienced, so far there has been no evidence of excessive colorectal cancer incidence.

Polycyclic Hydrocarbons

Polycyclic aromatic hydrocarbons (PAHs) are carcinogenic and are formed by the pyrolysis of organic matter (Hill, in *Role of the Gut Flora*, p. 463). *Grilled, fried, or roasted foods contain these kinds of compounds, as does cigarette smoke* and, in fact, all products of (incomplete) combustion, from fires to motor exhaust fumes. These compounds are lipid (fat) soluble and are absorbed from the GI tract to be carried to the liver, where hydroxylation and conjugation occurs to form what are called β-glucoronides. These conjugates so formed are not carcinogenic per se, but when secreted in the bile for excretion in feces (or faeces), they may be hydrolyzed by the action of bacterial enzyme β-glucuronidase. The hydrolysis products are hydroxylated PAHs, which are still not carcinogenic as such. However, bacterial dehydroxylases may, in turn, act to form the PAHs per se in this complicated sequence. The bacterial hydroxylases are primarily produced by the bacteria genus *Clostridia*.

A further ramification is that a reaction intermediate formed during the hydrolysis step (which is catalyzed by the bacterial enzyme β-glucuronidase) is potentially carcinogenic. This reaction intermediate binds to DNA.

Methionine and Ethionine

The amino acid ethionine is described as the S-ethyl analog of methionine (Hill, in *Role of the Gut Flora*, p. 464). Ethionine is strongly hepatotoxic in many animals and acts as a powerful carcinogen in rodents. It is produced by certain bacterial species when grown in a medium containing mineral salts, sulfate, methionine, and glucose. (One of the ethionine-producing bacteria is the ubiquitous *E. coli*.) The ethionine is noted not to affect the bacteria—only the host animal. Extension has not yet been made to human carcinogenesis, although, presumably, all the ingredients are in the gut.

Tryptophan

Tryptophan is metabolized by the action of gut bacteria flora (Hill, in *Role of the Gut Flora*, p. 465). The principal metabolic pathway is catalyzed by the enzyme tryptophanase, producing ammonia, indole (C_8H_7N), and pyruvate. Indole is considered carcinogenic in itself—as is tryptophan, for that matter. Additionally, simple deamination and decarbozylation occur. Another pathway yields kynurenine, which is described as a tumor promoter. Kynurenine in turn is converted to still other tumor promoters. Tryptophan metabolites have been implicated in human bladder cancer. The reference provides a table of the carcinogenic effect of tryptophan and its metabolites and also furnishes a diagram for the several metabolic pathways due to bacterial action.

Tyrosine

The amino acid tyrosine is converted by gut bacteria to produce phenolic compounds, notably phenol and *p*-cresol (Hill, in *Role of the Gut Flora*, p. 466). These compounds are normally absorbed from the colcn and excreted in the urine in the form of sulfate or glucuronide conjugates, measured as urinary volatile phenol (UVP). Higher UVP levels correspond to a higher amount of protein in the diet; lower levels ensue if the bowel flora have been disturbed. It has been shown that many phenolic compounds are tumor promoters, including phenol and *p*-cresol, at least with regard to mouse skin activated by dimethylbenzeneanthracene. It has been observed, moreover, that germ-free rats do not show any UVP and only rarely have hepatomas—but these are common otherwise.

N-Nitroso Compounds

The N-nitroso compounds are potent carcinogens (Hill, in *Role of the Gut Flora*, p. 467). Some, in fact, are locally acting, such as N-nitrosamides and N-nitrosoureas, whereas others are target-organ specific, such as N-nitrosamines. N-nitroso compounds are formed by the action of nitrate on certain nitrogen compounds, for example on secondary amines, amides, or a urea group, and so on. The *N-nitrosation reactions,* as they are called, are catalyzed or favored by acidic conditions and can be catalyzed by bacteria under neutral conditions.

Documentation is tabulated in the reference for the action of gut bacteria in forming N-nitroso compounds, and a number of bacteria species and genera are listed that are active in nitrosation, in particular *Pseudomonas aeruginosa, Bacillus licheniformis,* and *Neisseria* spp. The species *E. coli is* much less active, whereas *Clostridium* spp. and *Streptoccoccus* spp., for instance, are not active at all. It is commented that bacterial nitrosation can occur at any body site that has all the necessary ingredients: the necessary bacteria, nitrate or nitrite, and nitrosatable nitrogen compounds. These sites include saliva, the hypochorhydric stomach, the small bowel, infected urinary bladder, the *colon,* and the vagina of women infected with *Trichomonas vaginalis.*

Most body secretions contain nitrate, which must be converted to nitrite, the latter being involved in N-nitrosation. This conversion requires the presence of the enzyme *nitrate reductase,* and the only unambiguous source for this enzyme is in the bacterial flora, where it is widely distributed.

As to *nitrosatable amino compounds,* these occur within the body and may consist of alkylureas, *secondary amines,* and amides. Such secondary amines as *dimethylamine, piperidine,* and pyrrolidine result from *bacterial action in the colon.* From here, they are absorbed and transferred to body secretions such as saliva and gastric juices, to be eventually excreted via urine. The secondary amine named dimethylamine is also produced from *lecithin,* which is first hydrolyzed by the enzyme lecithinase C to form *choline,* which on dealkalation becomes dimethylamine. The secondary amine *piperidine* has *lysine* as a source, which is first decarboxylated to yield a diamine. This, in turn, is deaminated to form an amino aldehyde and ultimately is hydrogenated to piperidine. The secondary amine piperidine, by a similar sequence of reactions, is formed from ornithine. *Considerable amounts of dimethylamine, and lesser amounts of piperidine and pyrrolidine, are synthesized in the large bowel of humans* and finally end up in the urine.

Bile Acids

The liver synthesizes the bile acids, which are the taurine and glycine conjugates (linked together) of cholic and chenodeoxycholic acids (Hill, in *Role of the Gut Flora*, p. 470). More specifically, these acids are respectively known as 3,7,12-trihydroxycholanic acid and 3,7-dihydroxycholanic acid. Gut bacteria metabolize these acids by means of several enzymes in a complicated reaction sequence. Thus, cholanoylamide hydrolase releases the free bile acids from their conjugates. Hydroxysteroid dehydrogenase is active at the 3,7, an 12 sites, above, converting the hydroxyl groups to oxo groups and even hydroxyl groups. The enzyme 7a-dehydroxylase removes the 7a-hydroxyl group from both cholic acid and chenodeoxycholic acid to yield respectively deoxycholic acid and lithocholic acid. Further dehydrogenation reactions occur yielding unsaturated bile acids, and involve the enzymes 4-dehydrogenase and aromatase.

The carcinogenicity or mutagenicity of bile-derived acids is backed by a large body of evidence. There is no evidence, however, showing that the primary bile acids, as produced in the liver, are carcinogenic or mutagenic.

Cholesterol

Gut bacterial flora metabolize ubiquitous cholesterol ($C_{27}H_{45}OH$), the reactions occurring at two positions in the molecule (Hill, in *Role of the Gut Flora*, p. 472). That is, the 5-6 double bond is hydrogenated, and the 3-hydroxyl group may either be oxidized or inverted. The main metabolic product or metabolite formed is coprostanol, with sometimes significant amounts of coprostanone.

The verdict about the carcinogenicity of cholesterol is mixed, however. On the one hand, subcutaneous injections were found to increase the occurrence of tumors in rats—possibly caused by the crystals of cholesterol formed. On the other hand, if it is carcinogenic, then bacterial metabolism could be a protective process, since the coprostanol formed is insoluble and is removed from solution.

6.5.2 STUDIES ON LABORATORY ANIMALS

Studies on the role of gut flora in laboratory animals use germ-free animals as the basis of comparison (Hill, in *Role of the Gut Flora*, p. 473). These animals have been treated with antibiotics to free their systems of bacteria.

In studies on liver tumors in mice that were treated with the carcinogenic agent *dimethylbenzanthracene (DMBA)*, the normal animals developed hepatic tumors in a ratio of 17 of 21, and 10 of the 21 subsequently developed lung tumors. *For the germ-free animals the ratio for liver tumors was only 3 out of 23, and 1 of 23 for lung tumors.*

In the untreated animals used as controls, 7 of 21 of the normal mice developed hepatic tumors, but only 1 of 16 of the germ-free mice developed hepatic tumors. However, neither the normal mice nor the germ-free mice developed lung tumors.

In other experiments involving the introduction of bacterial mixtures back into germ-free mice, 39 percent developed hepatomas as compared to 82 percent in normal mice.

With respect to the injection of specific bacteria species, it was found that *Bacteroides multiacidus* produced hepatomas in 100 percent of the mice. *Clostridium indolis* produced 74 percent, and *Bif. infantis* produced 79 percent, whereas *Bif. adolescens* produced 69 percent. *Strep faecalis* produced 67 percent. *E. coli* combined with other specified bacteria produced up to 95 percent. However, when *Lactobacillus acidophilus* was added, the hepatoma rate fell dramatically to 46 percent.*

It was also noted that *the rate of hepatic tumor formation increased with increased dietary protein intake,* possibly due to the formation of volatile *phenols* produced by the gut flora.

With regard to intestinal tumors, it has been reported that *cycasin is carcinogenic in normal rodents but has no effect in germ-free rodents,* in that bacterial β-glucosidase is not formed. It is further mentioned that there are no other cases in which a specific bacterial enzyme has been traced unequivocally to the formation of any sort of tumors.

There is an effect of the gut bacterial flora, however, when various intestinal carcinogens are used to produce tumors. Thus, in using dimethylhydrazine (DMH) as the tumor agent, the rate is much higher in normal rats than in germ-free rats, where the rate was zero for carcinomas and only slight for benign adenomas. *Not only were the germ-free rats protected from cancer of the colon, but also of the ear duct, kidney, and small intestine.* On the other hand, *when N-methyl-N-nitro-N-nitrosoguanidine (MNNG) was used to produce tumors, the rate was as high in the germ-free rats as in the normal rats.* And in using azoxymethane (AOM), the cancer rate was higher in the germ-free rats than in the normal rats, for all sites except the kidney.

---

* The contrary argument surfaces that *Lactobacillus* bacteria produce the enzyme lactate dehydrogenase, involved in sustaining cancer cell metabolism. It can also be argued that some other things are going on.

In further studies involving DMH carcinogenesis, it was found that an antibiotic cocktail would suppress tumor formation. Another study showed that DMH carcinogenesis was suppressed by dietary *Lactobacillus acidophilus*. This also caused a decreased activity in several fecal enzymes, notably β-glucuronidase, azoreductase, and nitroreductase.

It was also found that beef, which increased the fecal enzyme activity, resulted in increased colonic tumors and small bowel tumors. In using supplemental *Lactobacillus acidophilus*, the rate of tumor formation was decreased, but not the final number of tumors.

Further studies on the effects of AOM have proven inconsistent. Whereas it had previously been shown that germ-free status had no effect on the tumors formed by AOM, it was subsequently shown that diversion of the fecal stream reduced the tumors formed in the defunctionalized colon. It was concluded that the fecal stream has more to it than simply bacteria, and that something else is going on. The rate of tumor formation could be restored in part by using diluted feces to irrigate the colonic remnant.

6.5.3 STUDIES ON HUMANS

The role of the gut flora has also been studied for human cancers of the stomach, colon, urinary bladder, and breast. It is observed that, whereas *stomach cancer* is very common in East Asia and the Andean countries of Central and South America, it is comparatively rare in North America and Australasia (Hill, in *Role of the Gut Flora*, p. 478). It varies in Europe, being higher in the south and east and lower in the north and west. Moreover, the incidence seems to be decreasing in all these locales.

Studies on migrants from Japan to the U.S., or from Eastern Europe to the U.S. or Australia, indicate that environmental factors during the formative years of life (up to 15 years) play an important part. The risk varies inversely with socio-economic status, of which diet may be the most significant factor—although no specific dietary component has been indicated in controlled studies. Based on recall only, there is a strong indication that *a mixed western diet that includes milk and other dairy products, along with meat, correlates with a low incidence of gastric cancer*. On the other hand, *a diet mainly of root vegetables and cereals correlates with a high risk*. There is also an apparent correlation with salt and nitrate intake. Moreover, there seem to be two main types of gastric cancer, with one associated with environmental factors (intestinal type) and the other with genetic factors (diffuse type).

With regard to the intestinal-type gastric cancer, among the theories proposed, a resident bacterial flora may play a part. Called the *Correa hypothesis,* the gut flora reduce nitrate to nitrite and then catalyze the formation of N-nitroso compounds, which are the carcinogenic agents proper. The reference weighs the evidence.

In turn, the formation of N-nitroso compounds can cause cancer at other sites with resident bacterial flora (Hill, *Role of the Gut Flora*, p. 483). These sites include a chronically infected urinary bladder, infected vagina, chronic small bowel overgrowth, and the colon of patients with ureterocolic anastomosis.

Human colorectal cancer has been shown to be related to colonic flora (Hill, in *Role of the Gut Flora*, p. 488). While colorectal cancer is more common in northern and western Europe, North America, and Australia, it is less common in Africa, Asia, and the Andean countries of Central and South America (the inverse of the occurrence of gastric cancer). A further breakdown shows a higher risk in northern and western Europe than in the south and east, and in Britain it is more common in Scotland and Ireland than in southeastern England. *Colorectal cancer is more prevalent in urban than rural areas, and in the higher socio-economic class than in the poorer.*

More specific studies show a *strong correlation with diets high in fat and meat. A high dietary fiber intake offsets this higher risk.* With populations having a low-fat/meat diet, the fiber intake is irrelevant (a low-fat/meat diet may indicate a high -fiber diet, anyway).

Studies about the causes and initiation of colorectal cancer are necessarily after the fact, there being a long incubation period, and circumstances (and diet) may have changed. *This indefiniteness has caused almost any and every dietary item to be implicated, either as a cause or as a treatment or cure.* Probably the most important study has been that of some 250,000 Japanese, which indicates *a causal relationship with fats and meat, and a protective relationship with green and yellow vegetables.*

In the search for a mechanism or theory, dietary carcinogens are placed foremost. That is, the human diet contains an array of carcinogens per se, mutagens, and tumor promoters. Some occur naturally (e.g., cycasin in cycad seeds and alkylhydrazine in mushrooms); others are present in food additives (nitrates to nitrites to N-nitroso compounds, food colors, and so on). Still others are formed during cooking (the polycyclic aromatic hydrocarbons and the wide range of pyrolysis products from fried or grilled foods). And others may result from food spoilage (aflatoxin or other mycotoxins). In spite of this presence, *none of the dietary carcinogens seems to correlate with the incidence of colorectal cancer.*

As an alternative cause, it has been proposed that *colorectal cancer may be the end result of a metabolite produced in the colon by bacterial action on an otherwise benign substance or substrate.* These possibilities encompass a wide variety of carcinogens/promoters/mutagens produced in the human colon, some of which have already been mentioned. Evaluation has been from two standpoints, namely the nature of the substrate or reacting substances and the bacteriological aspects.

As to the bacteriological aspects, the makeup of the fecal bacterial flora, which was first studied, was eventually abandoned. For one thing, there was no significant variation in the fecal bacteria counts for the six population groups studied, although there was a wide variation in the incidence of colorectal cancer. A tabulation is furnished in the reference.

For another thing, it was concluded that the fecal bacterial mixture is too complex for correlation. Moreover, whereas the site of bacterial metabolism is in the proximal colon, the fecal bacteria flora per se differ from the caecal flora. Furthermore, *the formation of a particular metabolite may be due to the action of enzymes rather than due to compositional changes in the flora.* Accordingly, the emphasis was then placed on the study of enzyme activity.

The particular enzymes selected for study included nitro reductase, β-glucosidase, β-glucuronidase, and 7-cholanoyldehydroxylase, referred to as "sentinel enzymes," since *in vitro* investigations indicated their involvement in the formation or release of carcinogens or mutagens. The studies here were also discounted, however, since there was no evidence to indicate that the activity of fecal enzymes is the same as in the caecum. That is, the bacterial flora are different, but not necessarily the enzymes, in comparing one part of the colon to another.

Since there is a strong relationship between bile acids and colorectal cancer, the enzymes involved in bile acid metabolism were studied next. The two enzymes receiving the most attention were 7α-dehydroxylase and 3-oxo-steroid 4-dehydrogenase. The former converts cholic acid (CA) to lithocholic acid (LA) and converts deoxycholic acid (DCA) to chenodeoxycholic acid (CDCA). These two products are noted to be carcinogenic to the rodent colon, whereas the reactants (or substrates) are not. It was found that the *fecal bile acids are considerably more dehydroxylated* (due to the action of the enzyme) *in populations at high risk of colorectal cancer.* In a comparison of cases to controls, the activity of the enzyme proved much higher for the cases than for the controls.

The latter enzyme, cited above, converts 3-oxo-5α reactants (or substrates) to steroids with a 3-oxo-4-en structure, in the chemical shorthand used. These products may in turn be reduced under intestinal conditions, to form the original reactant or substrate, or else to form steroids with a 3-oxo-5" configuration (called the allo bile acids). The allo bile acids have been observed to have mutagenic activity. *The particular enzyme is noted to be present in the feces of populations of high colorectal cancer risk, as compared to populations of low risk.* As a further note, it is stated that *colorectal cancers originate from preexisting adenomas,* with the possibility increasing with the adenoma size, villousness (the villi are finger-like projections), and the severity of dysplasia or abnormal tissue growth. (Adenomas are benign tumors, here presumably the *polyps* that may occur inside the colon.)

A tabulation is listed in the reference showing the production of the two enzymes by various gut bacteria. For the enzyme 7α-dehydroxylase, the most productive bacteria were *Bacteroides* spp., followed by *Clostridium* spp. and *Bifidobacterium* spp. Lesser amounts were produced by fecal streptococci and *Veillonella* spp.

For the enzyme 3-oxo-steroid 4-dehydrogenase, by far the most productive bacteria were *Clostridium paraputrificum* and *Cl. tertium.* Lesser amounts were produced by *Cl. indolus* and by *Clostridium* spp. as a whole.

Although the best evidence points toward bile acid metabolites and the enzyme 3-oxo-steroid 4-dehydrogenase as causing colorectal cancer, these agents are not implicated in the causation of the adenoma to start with, nor its subsequent displasia, although they may be correlated to adenoma size and the severity of displasia.

It has been stated that *breast cancer is highly correlatable with colorectal cancer,* both in individuals and in populations (Hill, in *Role of the Gut Flora,* p. 495). *Both cancers are at high risk in North America, western Europe, and Australasia,* but at low risk in Africa, Asia, and the Andean countries of Central and South America. *Both cancers are more prevalent among the more affluent.* Furthermore, *women who have been treated for breast cancer are at greater risk for subsequent colon cancer. Both cancers show a higher risk for dietary fat and meat.*

Since there is mounting evidence that bacteria may be involved in colorectal cancer, there may be a bacterial role also in breast cancer, a subject for further investigation. Thus there may be a connection between and among gut flora, estrogen circulation, and breast cancer. There may also be a connection between bacteria, bile acids, and breast cancer.

It is mentioned that a large body of evidence exists *implicating estrogens in human breast cancer.* This evidence arises from investigations on animal models for breast cancer, from the effects of surgery (as in ovariectomies, adrenalectomies, and so on) on slowing tumor growth, and from the effects of long-term estrogen therapy (for example, as pertains to the use of contraceptive pills).

With regard to steroid estrogens, observations on both animals and humans indicate that the processes are complex. For example, while there is evidence that estradiol causes tumors, there is also evidence that it inhibits tumor growth. The reference enumerates the various reaction or metabolic sequences which involve the steroid estrogens, and their retention and excretion. *It is noted in particular that antibiotic therapy affecting the gut flora also has a profound effect on estrogen activity.* For instance, women taking antibiotics while on contraceptive pills may experience failures. *Dietary changes may also have an effect on estrogen activity,* and this could lead to consequences on the rate of growth of breast tumors.

In comparing vegetarian and non-vegetarian women, the former had much higher estrogen excretion (and a lower incidence of breast cancer). Furthermore, the levels of blood plasma estrogens decreased as the levels increased in fecal excretion. Additionally, in the vegetarians the β-glucuronidase activity showed a decrease.

There is also an apparent correlation with bile acids and bile acid metabolites (and bacterial flora). In a study of women with breast cancer, much higher fecal bile acid concentrations occurred in post-menopausal cases than in the controls. However, there were no differences between premenopausal cases and the controls. A further conclusion reached was that fecal secondary bile acids, rather than primary bile acids, may play a significant role as tumor promoters in breast carcinogenesis.

6.5.4 ENZYME INHIBITORS

Inhibitors for the particular enzymes involved in producing carcinogenic metabolites may be presumed to exist, if not known. Referral is made to the particular enzymes selected in the previous subsection titled Studies on Humans. For the record, no inhibitors for cholanoyl 7α-dehydroxylase (or 7-cholanoyl-dehydroxylase) and 3-oxo-steroid 4-dehydrogenase could be found in either Jain or Zollner. Jain listed nitrofurantoin as an inhibitor for nitro reductase. Both Jain and Zollner listed inhibitors for various glucosidases and for β-glucuronidase. (Jain uses the symbol B for β.)

Thus for β-**glucosidase**, Jain lists arabino-1 5-lactone, conduritol-B-epoxide, 6-bromo-6-deox con-duritol, D-fucono-1 5-lactone, galactosylamine, glucono-1 4-lactone, gluconolactone, **D-glucose**, gluc-osylamine, N-(N-hexyl)-O-glucosylsphingosine, **nojirimycin**, glucosyl-sphingosine, 4-methyllumbel-liferyl xylopyranoside.

For β-**glucosidase**, Zollner lists **Ag⁺**, conduritol, conduritol epoxide, **Cu²⁺**, N-ethylmaleimide, **Fe³⁺**, fuconolactone, gluconolactone, glycosylmethyl-p-nitrophenyltriazene derivatives, **Hg²⁺**, phosphatidyl-choline, phosphatydylinositol, phosphatidylserine.

For β-**glucuronidase**, Jain lists **carotene, cholesterol**, D-glucaro-D-lactam, glucaro-1 4-lactone, D-glucaro-1 4-lactone, glucuronic acid, glucuronidase inhibitor, methayl-α-glucuronide, 2-diarylmethyl-1,3-ondanedione, poly-methacrylic acid, **peroxides**, phenolphthalein glucuronide, phenylbutazone, **ret-inol**, saccharo-1 4-lactone.

For β-**glucuronidase**, Zollner lists **ascorbate, Cu²⁺**, galacturonic acid, D-glucaro-1,4-lactone, glucu-ronic acid, **Hg²⁺, Ni²⁺**, saccharo 1,4-lactone.

Items of more than casual interest are highlighted above. It is informative to note that such substances as glucose, the antibiotic nojirimycin, carotene, cholesterol, peroxides, retinol, and ascorbate appear variously as inhibitors. Furthermore, that ions of silver (Ag), copper (Cu), iron (Fe), nickel (Ni), and even mercury (Hg) make an appearance. *Some of these substances—even some of the metals or their compounds—surface in medical folklore as anticancer agents.*

6.5.5 ENDOCRINE-DISRUPTING CHEMICALS

Among the latest developments is the argument that pesticides and other chemicals disrupt the endocrine systems of both wildlife and humans. This viewpoint has been set forth in a book by Theo. Colborn,

Dianne Dumanoski, and John P. Myers, titled *Our Stolen Future: Are We Threatening Our Fertility, Intelligence, and Survival?—A Scientific Detective Story*, with a foreword by Al Gore. The subject is referred to by the acronym EDCs. The suspect list looks like a "who's who" of hazardous chemicals, including such common names as PCBs, DDT, lead, cadmium, and various phthalates or phthalic acid derivatives, and even styrene. The initial listing comprises about 50 chemicals, but it is said that there may be hundreds more—even thousands.

Whether this kind of disruption of the endocrine system can also lead to cancer remains to be seen, although many such chemicals have been found to be carcinogens. It may be reasonably assumed that the endocrine-disrupting action will also involve enzyme inhibition, or at least "endocrine inhibition."

6.5.6 MUTAGENS AND BOWEL CANCER

In a chapter by S. Venitt, titled "Mutagens in Human Feces and Cancer of the Large Bowel," cancer of the large bowel is described as the second most common malignancy in the rich, industrialized countries (Venitt, in *Role of the Gut Flora*, p. 399). However, the quotation is qualified by a prominent group of fecal genotoxicologists who state, "All theories regarding the cause of colon cancer suffer from the lack of solid proof." The role of dietary factors and fecal mutagens are further examined by Venitt, as follows.

Mutagenic fecal activity has been known since 1977. And although the usual platitudes may apply about high-fat, high-meat diets versus high-vegetable, high-fiber diets, there appear to be exceptions, e.g., in studies of the Maori and non-Maori New Zealanders. *The study of carcinogenicity in fecal matter is mostly impractical* for laboratory rodents, for various reasons, and even more so for humans. Accordingly, *there is an emphasis instead on detecting biological indicators that are associated with carcinogenicity.* These biological indicators include *DNA-damaging activity, mutagenicity,* and *clastogenicity* (structural origins).

6.5.7 SHORT-TERM TESTS

Cancer development evidently occurs in two steps: initiation and promotion (Venitt, in *Role of the Gut Flora*, p. 401). Initiation is short lived and irreversible and involves DNA damage and mutagenic events such as chromosomal damage. "Tumor promotion is a longer-term process which may be reversible." Tumor promotion and the later stages of carcinogenesis are insufficiently understood, but if mutation occurs, it is probably not a factor here.

Accordingly, *short-term tests will only detect agents that have initiating activity.* This, moreover, is the role of the Ames test, or *Salmonella* test. However, *there is little evidence supplying a quantitative relationship between bacterial mutagenicity and carcinogenicity.* A weak mutagen does not necessarily correlate with a weak carcinogen, nor does a strong mutagen necessarily correlate with a strong carcinogen.

The reference furnishes a table listing summaries of studies of mutagenic activity in human feces, and further describes the Ames or *Salmonella* test, and test results (Venitt, in *Role of the Gut Flora*, p. 403ff).

6.5.8 DIET

Although diet is generally considered a prominent factor in carcinogenesis of the large bowel, studies involving the variables of high meat, high fat, and low fiber have not proven conclusive (Venitt, in *Role of the Gut Flora*, p. 419). In fact, the existence of fecal N-nitrosamines has been challenged. This challenge has in turn been challenged, in studies showing that a high-fat, high-meat diet yielded feces with nitrosamine levels 5 to 10 times higher than a typical Japanese diet of rice, fish, and vegetables. The argument remains unresolved, in part due to the difficulty in assaying fecal nitrosamines.

On the other hand, in its position report "Guidelines on Diet Nutrition, and Cancer Prevention: Reducing the Risk of Cancer with Healthy Food Choices and Physical Activity," issued in 1996, the American Cancer Society has gone on record, along with many others, about the importance of diet as a means for the chemoprevention of cancer. There is the promotion of fruits and vegetables for both main meals and snacks, and of other foods from plant sources, such as breads, cereals, grain products, rice, pasta, and beans. Whole grains are preferred, and beans furnish an alternative to meat. The notation is that there is particularly strong evidence that increasing the consumption of fruits and vegetables will reduce the risk of colon cancer. *It may be concluded that the ACS guidelines evidently favor both bulk and phytochemicals.*

In an Associated Press article by Paul Recer, dated on or about January 10, 1997, the findings of John Pezzuto and coworkers of the University of Illinois at Chicago were described, which were concerned with an *anticancer substance found in grapes.** The Associated Press article indicated that Pezzuto was the senior author of an article to appear in the journal *Science*, a publication of the American Association for the Advancement of Science, or AAAS.

The substance, called *resveratrol*, was found to help prevent cells from turning malignant and also to inhibit the spread of cells that were already malignant. It was indicated that this substance is the best chemopreventive for cancer yet studied, and there is the suggestion that even more potent anticancer agents may exist in other natural foods. (It can be wondered if resveratrol serves as an enzyme inhibitor for cancer cell metabolism and, if so, for which enzyme—say for instance lactate dehydrogenase?)

The aforementioned studies of grapes is a reminder that there is a book by Johanna Brandt titled *The Grape Cure*. The emphasis is on grapes as a cure for cancer. Apparently, it was originally published in 1927/1928; it has been republished in many editions by several different publishers and is still in print (Benedict Lust, Santa Barbara CA, 1971). A computer search of the information retrieval system called FirstSearch OCLC—which includes WorldCat, a data base of all books published—provides a listing of the many editions as well as peripheral books, mainly in substantiation. Johanna Brandt was born in 1876, and one entry listed suggests a publication date as early as 1900, although this could be in error.

In any event, the use of grapes against cancer is at least embedded in medical folklore, and the plant family *Vitaceae* is prominently represented in Hartwell's *Plants Used Against Cancer*, in particular the genus *Vitis*, and the species *Vitis vinifera*. Some of the citations provided by Hartwell go all the way back to the 9th and 10th centuries, even back to the Roman scholar known as Pliny the Elder (A.D. 62–113).

Just what kinds of compounds might be responsible has heretofore not been definitely known, but there has been the supposition at least that *flavonoids* or *bioflavonoids* may be involved (Moss, *Cancer Therapy*, p. 63). (The designator "bioflavonoids" is used to designate the more biologically active of the flavonoids.) The reference notes that some of the best known are *citrin, hesperidin,* and *rutin*, which occur abundantly in the *white pulp of citrus fruits*. (Oranges, notably, are presently being promoted as a cancer preventive. Hesperidin, for instance, may act against angiogenesis via inhibiting histamine release, as indicated in John Boik's *Cancer & Natural Medicine*.) Additional sources listed are grapes, plums, black currants, apricots, buckwheat, cherries, blackberries, and rose hips. They may be said to act as *chelating agents, removing toxic copper from the body, for instance,* thus protecting vitamin C from the adverse action of certain copper-containing enzymes. Believed to be nontoxic in reasonable amounts, there is the speculation that bioflavonoids assist in the anticancer effects of Vitamin C.

Speaking of chelating with copper and other toxic metals such as iron, the commonly mentioned compound *EDTA*, or ethylenediamine tetraacetic acid, is said to be this sort of a chelating agent (Walters, *Options*, pp. 254–259 and in particular p. 256). Ordinarily used as a chelating agent for treating cardiovascular disease by removing plaque deposits from the inside walls of the circulatory system, EDTA has also been tried as an anticancer agent but with conflicting reports. It is said to serve as a free radical inhibitor by removing such free-radical generators as copper and iron (or their compounds) from the body. The free radicals are thought to damage the DNA in cells, leading to a cancerous condition.

Vitamin C is also said to react with copper in the blood, and *high intravenous injections of vitamin C* (like 20 to 100 grams) have been given by metabolic practitioners with the additional idea that, in reacting with copper, the compound *hydrogen peroxide* is formed, which destroys tumors by oxidation. Without taking sides, it may be observed that *EDTA itself is an inhibitor for many enzymes*. Jain provides four listings for inhibition by EDTA, including collagenase, enzymes for DNA synthesis, and enzymes for prostaglandin synthesis. Zollner has an astounding 77 listings. In other words, there is a lot going on besides, say, copper chelation. A similar listing can be made for vitamin C or ascorbic acid (or ascorbate) as an enzyme inhibitor. Jain, for instance, has 13 listings, and Zollner has 6. *Very seldom is a single inhibitor found for a single enzyme—and even a reported one-to-one correspondence can be regarded as open to question and an error of omission. For chemical substances acting as enzyme inhibitors by and large are nonselective, which intensifies the difficulty in treatment, often expressed as producing adverse side effects.*

---

* This is the same John M. Pezzuto of the team Suffness and Pezzuto, cited extensively in Part 2, in the section on Cancer and Anticancer Agents. Mathew Suffness, who was with the National Cancer Institute, is deceased. Their joint contribution appeared in Volume 6 of the series, *Methods in Plant Biochemistry*, with the series edited by P.M. Dey and J.B. Harborne, and published by Academic Press, London, in 1990–1991. Specifically, Volume 6 was titled *Assays for Bioactivity*, edited by K. Hostettmann, with a 1991 publication date.

Inasmuch as the War on Cancer has been going on since 1971, one may well ask why proper investigations into grapes as a source of anticancer agents were not instituted much sooner. One may suspect that there is a prejudice against things natural, as spelled out by Jim Duke in the foreword to Hartwell's book, whereby on October 2, 1981, the Board of Scientific Counselors, Division of Cancer Treatment, National Cancer Institute, voted to abolish the NCI research contract program for developing antitumor agents from plants. The research, such as it might prove to be, was apparently left to the pharmaceutical firms, but firms "who have shown relative disinterest in plant products." (It may be presumed that there are no big profits in natural products, or at least not as much as in producing and marketing synthetic drugs where a patent position may be obtained.) The game now is one of catch-up in the arena of naturally derived pharmaceutical substances.

6.5.9 VITAMINS

There have been claims that diet supplementation with ascorbate (vitamin C) and alpha-tocopherol (vitamin E) reduces fecal mutagens (Venitt, in *Role of the Gut Flora*, pp. 420–421). This has been both challenged and affirmed.

For instance, in subjects who took vitamin capsules, the level of fecal mutagenicity fell to 21 percent of the control value. *"The changes in fecal mutagenicity seen in some of the donors are dramatic, and as yet not easily explainable in terms of a direct antioxidant effect, bearing in mind the anaerobic environment of the colon."* (The colon also displays a reducing condition.)

6.5.10 FRIED MEAT AND MUTAGENIC PYROLYSATES

There is a apparently a consensus that the processes of cooking produce mutagenic activity in foods, especially high-protein foods (Venitt, in *Role of the Gut Flora*, p. 421). The results of controlled tests described in the reference were mixed, however, with the qualification that the fecal mutagenic activity is transient, requiring sophisticated methods to separate and detect the mutagenic constituents.

If the evidence remains inconclusive about fecal mutagens and fried meat, on the other hand, it is observed that *raised levels of urinary mutagens can be found within a few hours after the ingestion of fried meat.*

In response to the question, "Are active carcinogens swallowed or are they formed in the colon?", a quoted response is as follows:

> The mucosal surface of the small intestine is over 100 times as great as that of the colon, yet *both benign and malignant tumours are over 100 times as frequent in the large as in the small bowel;* thus tumour risk relative to mucosal area is more than 10,000 times greater in the large than in the small bowel. Allowing for the fact that large-bowel mucosa appears more likely to undergo neoplastic change, this observation must suggest that the agents responsible for colon cancer are either formed or activated in the gut rather than being consumed in food in an active form and traversing the small intestine without modifying it.

6.5.11 FECAPENTAENES

A novel class of elusive mutagens called the *fecapentaenes* (or fecapentanes) occurs in the human colon (Venitt, in *Role of the Gut Flora*, p. 425). The reference provides examples of the chemical formulas, which are of the general type $R-O-CH_2-CHOH-CH_2OH$, where R is a partly unsaturated hydrocarbon chain.

It is noted that *fecapentaenes and other mutagens are the products of bacterial metabolism in the human colon, which increases with anaerobic incubation,* but is offset by antimicrobial agents. Furthermore, *bile and bile acids stimulate mutagen production,* but only at elevated bile levels.

Of the anaerobic bacteria species tested, five of the genus *Bacteroides* were particularly active: *B. thetaiotaomicron, B. fragilis, B. ovatus, B. uniformis,* and *Bacteroides* group 3452A. All are commonly present in human intestinal microflora.

Fecapentaenes appear active at very low doses, possibly forming a carbonium ion (or carbocation), and an increase in the hydrocarbon chain length increases mutagenicity. Synthetic fecapentaenes have assisted further studies, in which some of these substances appear to be 900 times more mutagenic than the potent mutagenic alkylating agent N-methyl-N-nitrosurea.

6.5.12 THE FLUCTUATION TEST

Inconsistencies with the Ames or Salmonella test results have led to the use of an alternative called the *fluctuation test* (Venitt, in *Role of the Gut Flora*, p. 432). The test involves the use of cultures of a small quantity of an amino acid in what is called an *amino-acid auxotroph* (growth culture). On standing overnight, the bacteria undergo cell division until the amino acid is exhausted. On the addition of a further amino-acid–free medium, only the revertent or prototrophic bacteria will be able to grow and divide. ("Prototrophic" signals that these are the bacteria that do not require the amino acid to proliferate.) A change in the pH of the mixture indicates the degree of growth. The degree of growth is an indication of the degree of mutation. The chemical or substance to be tested is added just prior to the period of auxotrophic growth.

In utilizing this test on population groups, giving the mutants per microliter of fecal extract, the following mean values were obtained: strict vegetarians, 0.66; ovo-lacto-vegetarians, 0.93; nonvegetarians, 0.92. The values ranged widely, and in fact the most mutagenic samples were found in the vegetarian groups.

Further tests are set forth in the reference, and it is noted in particular that *the addition of fiber to the diet significantly lowered mutagenicity* (Venitt, in *Role of the Gut Flora*, p. 438).

6.5.13 AEROBIC VS. ANAEROBIC TESTS

In the fluctuation test results so far indicated, the mutation assays were performed under aerobic conditions, and no special care was taken to exclude air (Venitt, in *Role of the Gut Flora*, p. 439) It was then found that even a brief exposure of an anaerobic sample to air would produce a positive result for mutagenicity, whereas an aerobic sample assayed negative when tested anaerobically.

A tentative conclusion reached is that feces may contain substances that fortuitously remain dormant and nonmutagenic under the anaerobic (and highly reducing) conditions of the bowel.

6.5.14 DNA-REPAIR TESTS

Due to the inherent problems in using either the Salmonella test or the fluctuation test in assaying fecal extracts, DNA repair can be used as the measure rather than revertent mutation. Moreover, indirect methods can be used to facilitate the assaying for this manifestation of genotoxic activity.

Strains of bacteria are available which are more susceptible to the lethal effects of DNA damage. The diameter of an incubated bacterial culture on a test plate can be used as an indication of the mutagenicity of an added agent or substance.

In testing fecal samples from several population groups, ranging from lactovegetarians to omnivores, the results were inconclusive.

Another test employed is called the SOS chromotest, the "SOS" system consisting of a set of genes promoting DNA repair. Without going into further details, this test also proved inconclusive.

Other studies used chromosomal nuclear damage as the criteria, again with inconclusive results.

6.5.15 GENOTOXICITY OF BILE ACIDS?

Further studies on the genotoxicity of bile acids yield some mixed results (Venitt, in *Role of the Gut Flora*, p. 447). Whereas it has been advanced that bile acids are not responsible, it has nevertheless been suggested that water-soluble fecal mutagens are composed principally of bile acids, and that these in turn may be a primary cause of colon cancer. The aforementioned investigation was supported by experiments, and given a statistical analysis (always a questionable procedure). The reference concludes that the premise was not sustained.

6.5.16 OTHER CONSIDERATIONS

Among the other considerations are factors affecting gut microflora, and the bacterial metabolism of proteins, fats, carbohydrates, nitro compounds, and nitrate, nitrite, and N-nitroso compounds, as well as toxic metals. Also of consideration are dietary fiber, lignans and phyto-oestrogens, intense sweeteners, and the hydrolysis of glycosides and esters. These are variously covered in chapters in the *Role of the Gut Flora in Toxicity and Cancer* and are briefly discussed in the following text.

6.5.17 FACTORS AFFECTING GUT MICROFLORA

It has been found that antibiotic drugs often suppress some, but not necessarily all, of the normal gut microflora (A.K. Mallett and I.R. Rowland, in *Role of the Gut Flora*, p. 347ff). This disturbs the microbial community of the gut in its prevention of disease by potentially pathogenic exogenous organisms. Moreover, there will be the development of antibiotic-resistant organisms.

Other drugs have an effect as well, notably the hydrogen-blocking agents such as cimetidine and ranitidine, as occur in *gastric secretions.* This may also be accompanied by increased nitrite and nitrosamine concentrations.

Certain diseases result in a bacterial colonization of the stomach and duodenum, which are normally sterile to these bacteria. And whereas the mammalian gut is sterile at birth, it is rapidly colonized. In most animals, the initial colonization is by lactic acid bacteria such as *Lactobacillus* spp. and *Bifodobacterium* spp. Next enter facultative anaerobes such as *Streptococcus* spp. and *E. coli*, which, as the descriptor "facultative" implies, can exist under differing conditions. With the ingestion of solid food, however, strict anaerobes such as *Bacteroides* gain ascendency at the expense of the facultative organisms and then become the defining flora.

Dietary processes involve the transformation of chemical structures by intestinal bacterial enzymes to yield end products that may have toxicological and pharmaceutical properties (Mallett and Rowland, in *Role of the Gut Flora*, p. 352). Indigestible plant cell-wall materials play a part, which may explain the protective role of fiber in offsetting toxicity. On the other hand, *the effect of pectins present may be otherwise.** Thus, *certain pectins may enhance nitrate reductase activity for converting nitrate to nitrite.* Furthermore, *pectins may affect the activity of nitro reductase,* involved in converting nitro compounds to amines that possess toxic, mutagenic, or carcinogenic properties.

The reference in fact carries a multipage table listing the effects of various dietary components on digestive enzymes (Mallett and Rowland, in *Role of the Gut Flora*, pp. 354–362). The dietary components include the following:

- **Non-starch polysaccharides** (pure form) designated as various celluloses, and various *pectins,* including citrus pectin and apple pectin, plus various *guar gums,* carrageenan, agar-agar, gum acacia in combination with locust bean gum and carboxymethyl cellulose, hemicellulose
- **Non-starch polysaccharides** (plant cell-wall products, mixtures) designated as wheat bran, maize bran in combination with soya (soy) bean bran and wheat bran, carrot fiber, and carrot fiber in combination with cabbage fiber
- **Carbohydrates** designated as lactose, rice starch, amylomaize starch, potato starch
- **Protein** designated as lactalbumin
- **Fat** variously designated as corn oil, lard, animal fat, and beef fat, cocoa butter, olive oil, safflower oil in combination
- **Meat** variously designated as beef, pork, lamb, and chicken in combination, beef (autoclaved), red meat

The *enzymes, enzymatic actions,* or *agents* variously involved in the above-mentioned tabulation include azoreductase (AR), cholesterol dehydrogenase (CDH), 7αdehydrogenase (7αDH), ammonia production from endogenous substrates, β-glucuronidase (GN), β-glucosidase (GS), nitro reductase or nitroreductase (NR), nitrate reductase (NT), urease (U), mucinase (MU), conventional flora (CV). Sometimes a single enzyme would be the case, but most usually a combination was involved.

Further brief remarks about some of these or other enzymes are as follows, and the effect of pectin or dietary fibers—as noted mainly in rodents (rats). For starters, and generally speaking, *pectin increases bacterially mediated toxicity,* at least *in vivo,* as indicated by a table supplied in the reference (Mallett and Rowland, in *Role of the Gut Flora*, pp. 353, 365). This is no doubt contrary to expectations, in that pectin is an ubiquitous form of dietary fiber.

Pectin affects enzyme activity. Thus, *nitrate reductase activity,* for the conversion of nitrate to nitrite, *is significantly increased by high-methoxyl pectin.* This is evidenced, for example, as a marked increase in blood methaemoglobin and a condition of nitrate-induced maethaemoglobinaemia. (Methaemoglobin, or methemoglobin, is the substance formed by the oxidation of blood hemoglobin or by drugs.) There is, in turn, the formation of genotoxic N-nitroso compounds, which is catalyzed by the enzymes from several common gut microorganisms. It is concluded that the formation of N-nitroso compounds may be increased manyfold by a pectin-containing diet.

---

* For the record, pectins are described as being structurally based on a polymer of galacturonic acid residues containing rhamnose and arabinose substituents, and having a variable proportion of uronic carboxyl groups esterified with methanol.

Nitro reductase activity, for the reduction of aromatic and heterocyclic nitrocompounds to carcino-genic, mutagenic, or toxic amines, *is increased by pectin ingestion.* Thus diet-related alterations in bacterial metabolism may increase the hepatotoxicity of agents such as 2,6-dinitroluene. Pectin was found to increase the degree of methaemoglobinaemia caused by nitrobenzene.

β-*Glucuronidase activity is increased by pectin* and other fermentable fibers. One consequence is the retention of toxic agents within the body. This may also play a role in the metabolism and tumorigenicity of carcinogens in the liver.

Azoreductase activity is increased in pectin-fed animals. This can result in carcinogenic or other adverse effects.* On the other hand, the enzyme methylmercury dimethylase serves to demethylate toxic methylmercury, lowering the body burden and tissue levels of mercury. And various *dietary fibers* have been found to enhance the activity of this enzyme, resulting in an increase in mercury excretion from the body.

Flavonoids are polyphenolic compounds that are common in plant materials and are conjugated with or linked to such sugars as L-rhamnose, D-glucose, glucorhamnose, galactose, or aribinose to form the corresponding *glycoside or glycosidic derivative* (Mallett and Rowland, in *Role of the Gut Flora*, p. 366). Whereas, by their hydrophilic nature and high molecular weight, they are poorly absorbed in the small intestine, these structures are readily *hydrolyzed by bacterial enzymes in the large intestine. The resulting aglycones may undergo further reactions and degradations.*

Flavones, a flavonoid subgroup, are common in vegetable matter, and about thirty flavones have been found to be *mutagenic.* For instance, *fecal microorganisms* in the presence of rutin or the compound known as quercitrin will form the *genotoxic* aglycone *quercetin.* (The preceding is an interesting statement, in that *quercetin is also considered to be an anticancer agent.*)

As a further statement, it is noted that flavonoid aglycones (such as quercetin) may either induce or inhibit the metabolic activity of certain mammalian enzymes. In short, flavonoid aglycones, in addition to being genotoxic, may also act as enzyme inhibitors (or promoters).

The nonnutritive sweeteners cyclamate and saccharin are suspect with regard to the causation of bladder cancer and may affect the gut flora in the process.

In a section on "Diet and Gut Flora Interaction in Cancer," the aforecited reference notes that the presence or absence of intestinal flora influences the development of liver cancer, being much higher in normal mice than in germ-free mice. Feeding the mice konjac mannan, however, significantly decreased the hepatic tumor incidence. (Konjac mannan is a glucomannan derived from the tubers of *Amorphallus konjac* or *Amorphophallus konjac* or *Conophallus konjac* of the plant family Araceae. This species or another is listed as an anticancer agent in Hartwell's *Plants Used Against Cancer*—as pertaining to India and China.)

It is also observed that the liver tumor promoting effect of a mixture of the intestinal bacteria *E. coli, Streptococcus longum,* and *Clostridium paraputrificum* was suppressed by *Bifodobacterium longum.*

As to intestinal tumors, the reference notes that the effect of dietary components—e.g., fat versus fiber—seems to be inconsistent. There is an effect of the kind of dietary fiber, however, and it is noted that both lignin and pectin are regarded as dietary fibers (Mallett and Rowland, in *Role of the Gut Flora*, p. 372).

Another consequence of a high-fiber diet is a lower pH in the colon (indicating a more acidic condition). The bacterial fermentation of dietary fiber and the poor absorption of carbohydrates, e.g., lactulose (not lactose) and short chain fatty acids (SCFA), may be responsible for lowering the pH. Some short chain fatty acids, and in particular butyric acid, suppress tumors cells *in vivo*, which may explain their action against colon cancer (Mallett and Rowland, in *Role of the Gut Flora*, p. 373).†

Ammonia occupies a prominent position in nitrogen metabolism as occurs in the large intestine. On the one hand it functions as an end product for the microbial degradation of endogenous and exogenous nitrogen compounds such as amino acids and urea. (Urea, incidentally, is viewed in some quarters as

---

* The prefix "-azo" signifies nitrogen, and more specifically refers to chemical compounds containing two joined nitrogen atoms, –N:N–, attached on either side to carbon, as in azo-benzene, H_5C_6–N:N–C_6H_5. Expectedly, the reduction of an azo-compound by hydrogen or its equivalent—as catalyzed, for instance, by the enzyme azoreducatase—would first yield amines and eventually ammonia, NH_3. Thus, for example, H_5C_6–N:N–C_6H_5 + 2 H_2 → 2 H_5C_6–NH_2, which may also be written as 2 C_6H_5–NH_2. In turn, 2 C_6H_5–NH_2 + 2 H_2 → 2 C_6H_6 + 2 NH_3. *Amines,* signified by the group –NH_2, are noted to be *carcinogenic.* At higher intestinal levels, *ammonia or NH_3 may be associated with gut cancers,* a matter to be mentioned subsequently.

an anticancer agent.) On the other hand, ammonia also serves as the starting point for the bacterial synthesis of cell constituents. Its existence in high concentrations may indicate cell proliferation, and it has been suggested that ammonia may be associated with cancer formation in the gut.

Ammonia concentrations increase with high protein levels but fall in the presence of fermentable carbohydrates. Thus, the addition of monosaccharides and disaccharides such as glucose, lactose, and lactulose inhibits ammonia production in human fecal suspensions, as do sugars such as sorbitol and mannitol. Human fecal ammonia concentrations also decrease with the intestinal ammonia concentrations.

More information about ammonia and other nitrogenous compounds is presented in the following section and subsection.

6.6   DIGESTIVE METABOLISM

Various foodstuffs and other ingested materials undergo many and various biochemical reactions, depending on their makeup and chemical content. Chief among these are, of course, proteins and their nitrogen content, fats and oils and associated compounds, and carbohydrates of many kinds. Also of consideration are inorganic nitrogen compounds and toxic metals. Dietary fiber also plays a role. The reactions involved are in the main catalyzed by bacterially produced enzymes and such other enzymes as may be ingested or formed.

6.6.1   BACTERIAL METABOLISM OF PROTEIN AND ENDOGENOUS NITROGEN COMPOUNDS

In a chapter with the foregoing title, clinical physiologist O.M. Wrong discusses more fully the bacterial metabolism of nitrogenous compounds. Wrong leads off with the statement, previously mentioned, that research on alimentary flora has concentrated on the large intestine, and that there has been an emphasis on bacteria to the exclusion of fungal and protozoal denizens (Wrong, in *Role of the Gut Flora*, p. 228).

As to the metabolism of nitrogenous substances, the most important aspect is the breakdown of proteins by the processes of *proteolytic digestion*. This is followed by the deamination and decarboxylation of the amino acids so formed, accompanied by the bacterial generation and metabolism of ammonia. In terms of amounts, the nitrogenous substances are less than the carbohydrates processed. Nor are nitrogenous substances an important source of energy; rather, their importance is in other types of metabolic reactions and as a potential source for systemic toxins. The bound nitrogen that reaches the large intestine is still mainly in the form of protein, and perhaps 60 percent of the fecal nitrogen leaving the large intestine is in the form of bound nitrogen of bacterial bodies.

Mucins make up an important substrate for large bowel bacteria (Wrong, in *Role of the Gut Flora*, p. 231). These are described as complex high-molecular-weight molecules with *protein cores* and *extensive polysaccharide side chains*, which in turn contain significant compositional units of N-acetyl glucosamine, galactose, sialic acid, fucose, phosphate, and sulfate. Certain fecal bacteria such as *Bifidobacteria* digest mucin to yield various other compounds. Short chain fatty acids (SCFAs) also occur, chiefly of acetate, propionate, and butyrate.

Ammonia is not only an end product of bacterial metabolism, it is utilized by bacteria in their own protein synthesis. Ammonia absorbed into the portal blood is converted to urea in the liver.

Urea, an endogenous nitrogen compound in relatively large amounts, is in turn degraded by bacteria in the intestinal tract to yield ammonia, a part of the nitrogen cycle (Wrong, in *Role of the Gut Flora*, p. 247). Urea, as a rule, is absent in the feces of normal subjects; *the administration of antibiotics, however, will raise urea concentrations to blood levels.*

The degradation or hydrolysis of urea to ammonia and water is accomplished by *urases*, which are the selective enzymes produced by both aerobic and anaerobic bacteria, particularly the latter. Renal or

---

† The anticancer effect of butyric acid is noted elsewhere, as supplied in the reference by John Boik (Boik, *Cancer & Natural Medicine*, pp. 10, 13, 248). It has also been commented that cytotoxic cancer drugs in high doses cause cell death directly by necrosis, whereas in low doses they induce apostosis or cell death by "suicide" (Boik, *Cancer & Natural Medicine*, p. 13). This is in line with the advocacy of the famous English physician Denis Burkitt, discoverer of Burkitt's lymphoma, of using chemotherapy drugs only in small doses.

kidney failure affects urea degradation, leading to uraemic (or uremic) poisoning, but the processes are complicated and unresolved.

Other nitrogen compounds discussed include *creatinine* and uric acid (Wrong, in *Role of the Gut Flora*, p. 250). It is noted that *creatinine is not degraded in mammalian tissues, but rather in the large bowel by bacterial activity. The products identified include creatine, considered in some quarters as an anticancer agent, as is urea.* Uric acid is evidently degraded by intestinal bacteria. (Both *creatine* and *urea* are cited as anticancer agents in Moss's *Cancer Therapy*.)

6.6.2 METABOLISM OF FATS, BILE ACIDS, AND STEROIDS

In a chapter of this title, H. Eyssen and Ph. Caenepeel take up the subject. As to fat absorption, it is noted that the effect of microflora is controversial and, in any event, is apparently small. Both natural and synthetic steroids are transformed by sulphatases and glucuronidases of bacterial origin to yield a variety of metabolites. The synthesis and catabolism of the sterol called *cholesterol* is markedly accelerated by intestinal bacteria, which also interfere with cholesterol absorption.

In rats, cholesterol has been noted to intensify the effect of the carcinogen dimethylhydrazine. On the other hand, plant sterols have a protective effect against the colon tumor carcinogen N-methyl-N-nitrosourea.

The epoxide of cholesterol has *in vitro* cell transforming activity and in animals has proven tumorigenic. Since hydrolysis of the epoxide will yield certain compounds found in human feces, the implication is that the epoxide exists in the large intestine.

The reference reexamines the role of bile acids in colorectal cancer (Eyssen and Caenepeel, in *Role of the Gut Flora*, p. 276). Apart from the usual arguments about high fat versus low fat and high fiber versus low fiber, it is noted that low fiber intake and low fecal bulk both increase the intestinal transit time. This contributes to an increase in the concentrations of the microbially formed metabolites such as bile acids, whereas a high fiber intake shortens the transit time. Thus, it can be inferred that intestinal transit time may be as much a factor in carcinogenesis as the nature of the metabolites.

The particular subject of *trans*-fatty acids (TFAs) as occur in hydrogenated vegetable oils is not mentioned in the foregoing reference. Nevertheless, we hereby address the subject.* Now referred to as shortening or hydrogenated vegetable oils, these *trans*-fatty acids are ubiquitous in baked goods, for instance—notably in pastries. At least some individuals believe that TFAs throw a monkey wrench into the complex cell machinery of the body. An advocate of this conclusion is Walter C. Willett, MD and PhD, who is chairman of the department of nutrition at the Harvard School of Public Health, and professor of epidemiology at the Harvard Medical School. May we add cancer to the list of potential consequences?

6.6.3 METABOLISM OF CARBOHYDRATES

The subject is presented in a chapter of the same title (Marie E. Coates, in *Role of the Gut Flora*, p. 287ff). It is noted that carbohydrates can be classified as "available," being readily digested and utilized as an energy source. This is as distinguished from "nonavailable," indicating those sources that are resistant to mammalian digestion and that may contribute little or nothing, nutritionally speaking. The principal concerns involve starches, lactose, lactulose, and polyols.

The hydrolysis of starches occurs mostly by the action of the pancreatic enzyme amylase. There is little or no microbial digestion occurring in the upper part of the intestinal tract. However, some starches escape undigested to the large intestine and are subject to fermentation by microflora, and in humans it is in fact estimated that perhaps 20 percent of the starch content reaches the colon. At the same time, this starch provides a substrate for the growth of bacterial flora—with the starch and proliferating bacteria contributing to fecal bulk. This is presumably the case for some Asian and African populations on a low-fiber diet.

Some of the starch reaching the lower gut cannot be broken down by amylase, and is termed "resistant starch." Dietary starches for the most part consist of about 20 percent amylose and 80 percent amylopectin,

---

* In most natural unsaturated fats, the molecules are arranged in what is called the *cis* position, in which kinks occur in the molecule such that the carbon atoms are opposite one another. After processing or hydrogenation, the molecules become rearranged so that the carbon atoms exist in line, called the *trans* position. As a result, the entirety of the molecules can be viewed as more packed together, whereby what was liquid before hydrogenation then becomes semi-solid or solid.

and during the course of storage, baking, or freezing, the amylose fraction will become highly resistant to hydrolysis by the enzyme. This resistant starch can be broken down by colonic bacteria, however.

There is, on the other hand, a high-amylose maize starch (amylomaize) that is resistant even to bacterial action. *Amylomaize has the interesting capacity to reduce cholesterol concentrations in the liver.* Moreover, it causes an increase in bile acid concentrations in the lower gut, interfering with bacterial transformations of both cholesterol and bile acids. Any effects on carcinogenesis were not noted.

The disaccharide *lactose* is decomposed by the enzyme lactase to yield glucose and galactose, both monosaccharides. Lactose or milk sugar, as the name implies, is found in milk. In individuals who are lactase deficient, the accumulation of lactose causes diarrhea, and the further microbial fermentation of lactose produces bloat, flatulence, and abdominal cramps. The use of yogurt in lactase-deficient subjects has been advanced, due to the presence of the enzyme bacterial β-galactosidase, which may aid in digestion, but apparently this is not the case. *Yogurt in the diet, however, may raise the activity of the enzyme β-glucuronidase in patients with large bowel cancer.*

Fermentation of lactose in the lower gut lowers the pH value, that is, increases the acidity, which may disturb the normal microbial equilibrium and may affect the activities of the microbial enzymes azoreductase, β-glucosidase, β-glucuronidase, nitroreductase, and urease. Although left unsaid, this may have bearing on carcinogenesis.

The action of lime water on lactose can be used to yield lactulose, otherwise known as 4-*O*-β-D-galactopyranosyl-D-fructofuranose. Although resistant to the enzymes that are disaccharidases, a degree of digestion nevertheless occurs, presumably by microbial fermentation. Not present in raw milk, lactulose is formed when the milk is heated. This is of concern in the use of heat-sterilized milk formulas for feeding infants. There are changes in the colonic bacterial population that may or may not be beneficial, a point of argument.

Lactulose is used as a laxative and for the treatment of portal systemic encephalopathy, where its benefits may be partially due to a lowering of the colonic pH. The disease called *portal systemic encephalopathy*, associated with severe hepatic cirrhosis, is described as a disorder of the central nervous system (CNS), *whereby an impaired liver permits the ammonia concentration to increase in systemic blood. This results in toxicity to the brain.*

The sequence includes the formation of ammonia in the colon by bacteria acting on amino acids. Although it would be expected that the acidic condition of the colon would neutralize the ammonia, apparently no such action occurs. There is an accompanying decrease in urea levels. In net sum, there is a general reduction in bacterial metabolism, including that for ammonia-forming bacteria. This could be beneficial against carcinogenesis per se but, of course, may have undesirable side effects.

What are called lactitol and maltitol are examples of *polyols*, which are chemical forms of sorbitol. They are used in the food industry as sweeteners and are noted for having low carcinogenicity. (The possibility of anticarcinogenicity was not taken up.)

Lactitol is not absorbed in the small intestine, nor is it hydrolyzed by mammalian enzymes. Metabolism instead occurs by the action of colonic bacteria. Maltitol, on the other hand, is hydrolyzed by the intestinal enzyme maltase to yield glucose and sorbitol, which may be further degraded by microorganisms. Maltitol is also absorbed and hydrolyzed by host tissues.

6.6.4 METABOLISM OF NITRO COMPOUNDS

The nitroaromatic chemicals are ubiquitous and include, for instance, antibiotic, antiparasitic, and radiosensitizing drugs as well as environmental contaminants from the (incomplete) combustion of fossil fuels (Douglas E. Rickert, in *Role of the Gut Flora*, p. 145ff). The manufacture of several thousand consumer products requires their use, estimated at ten percent of chemical industry sales.

The nitro group itself is reduced by mammalian and bacterial enzymes, and some of the reduction products are readily oxidized by molecular oxygen. The compounds of most interest here are nitrobenzenes, nitrotoluenes, and nitropyrenes.

The reduction of *nitrobenzene* by intestinal microorganisms results in such compounds as nitrosobenzene, phenylhydroxylamine, and aniline, each toxic or genotoxic in its own right.

Used in the manufacture of dyes and plastics, for example, the *nitrotoluenes* and their metabolic products are genotoxic.

The environmental pollutants known as *nitropyrenes,* as resulting from (incomplete) combustion, are very potent mutagens in the Ames *Salmonella* test. Moreover, *this mutagenicity depends on (bacterial) reduction.* Among the more active anaerobic bacteria that have been tested are *Bacteroides thetaiotaomicron, Clostridium perfringens, Peptococcus anaerobus, Clostridium* spp., and *Peptostreptococcus productus.* Less active were *Bifidobacterium infantis* and *Citrobacter* spp. Still less active were *Lactobacillus acidophilus, E. coli,* and three strains of *Salmonella typhimurium.*

6.6.5 NITRATE, NITRITE, AND N-NITROSO COMPOUNDS

Nitrate is widely distributed in the environment, and nitrite, its reduction product, is noted for being toxic (A.K. Mallett, in *Role of the Gut Flora,* p. 153ff). Intestinal bacteria produce this reduction, in turn inducing methaemoglobinaemia (anemia) or else forming genotoxic N-nitroso compounds.

Ingested nitrates have sources in most water supplies and in plants. Nitrate is the predominant form of the inorganic nitrogen oxides, although the nitrite form is also widely distributed but at much lower levels. Although nitrate occurs as a consequence of the oxidation of organic nitrogen by soil bacteria, most enters the environment from the leaching of natural mineral deposits and inorganic fertilizers.

It has been found that *there is more nitrate occurring in the body than can be accounted for from outside nitrate sources.* This endogenous nitrate evidently occurs via synthesis from *ammonia* (Mallett, in *Role of the Gut Flora,* p. 155). (It may be presumed that the *ammonia precursors include protein and amino acids in the diet.*) The conversion of ammonia to nitrate may be influenced by activation of the reticuloendothelial system with such agents as *E. coli* endotoxin. (The term *reticular* pertains to a meshwork. Endothelium is the tissue that lines the internal cavities of the body. The reticuloendothelial system helps promote the immune system.) There are additional mechanisms for endogenous nitrate formation, as set forth in the reference. In sum total, the *endogenous synthesis of nitrate each day equals that ingested in the diet, "with attendant toxicological risks for the host,"* as noted in the reference.*

Nitrate per se (that is, unreacted nitrate) is absorbed from the proximal small intestine to become part of the total body water, and is eventually excreted in the urine. Otherwise, nitrate is reduced by bacterial metabolism and may also be converted or metabolized by certain as yet ill-defined metabolic pathways, the latter as detected in experiments on germ-free animals (Mallett, in *Role of the Gut Flora,* pp. 158–159).

Nitrate reduction to nitrite results in the condition known as methaemoglobinaemia (or anemia, as previously mentioned) and in the eventual formation of N-nitroso compounds.

Nitrite undergoes a chemical co-oxidation with the respiratory pigment oxyhaemoglobin of the blood, resulting in the regeneration of nitrate and the formation of methaemoglobin. The conversion occurs at levels beyond the capacity of the host enzymes to restore the function of the oxyhaemoglobin. (On combining with oxygen, hemoglobin or haemoglobin becomes oxyhemoglobin or oxyhaemoglobin.) Infants are particularly at risk.

Nitrite, which exists in acidic aqueous solution as nitrous acid, can itself cause genotoxic changes in mammals and microbes. *Nitrate is considered not a particularly strong carcinogen,* although it may induce lymphomas in rats.

However, the *nitrite can react with certain amino groups* to yield *N-nitroso compounds that act as carcinogens or mutagens.* "*Various chemicals, including thiocyanate and ascorbate, are reported to catalyze or inhibit this process.*"†

In addition to being involved in the formation of nitrite, bacteria may promote nitrosation by nonenzymatic methods. More significantly, however, microbial enzymes are directly involved in the formation of N-nitroso compounds (Mallett, in *Role of the Gut Flora,* p. 161). Among the microbes involved is the well known species *Escherichia coli* as well as other intestinal bacteria. Inhibitors noted are cysteine and sodium tungstate.

Nitrosamine formation in the stomach is catalyzed by gastric acid in the presence of nitrite produced by oral microflora. It may also occur in individuals with pernicious anemia, caused by the lack of an intrinsic factor for the uptake of vitamin B12. In both cases, there is an increased risk for stomach cancer.

---

* One may therefore again speculate on the advantages of a low-protein diet, that is, upon vegetarianism—although vegetables and fruits contain amino acid-nitrogen as well, albeit at reduced levels.

† Once again, we possibly encounter the cyanic effects of Laetrile or amygdalin, if indirectly, and vitamin C as well. And note that N-nitroso compounds may be merely referred to as nitroso compounds, or nitrosamines.

There is apparently an increased risk of stomach cancer where the drinking water is high in nitrates. There may be an additional association of stomach cancer with a high carbohydrate intake, which may enhance bacteria activity and numbers. Nitroso compounds, incidentally, also occur in saliva.

An infected urinary bladder is a prime site for nitrosation, with bacteria and nitrate and amines all readily available.

Apparently, N-nitroso compounds are at low levels in the large bowel, or at least in the feces, and their role in cancer of the large bowel, or colon cancer, remains unsubstantiated.

6.6.6 METABOLISM OF TOXIC METALS

Toxic metals and metalloids include mercury, lead, cadmium, and arsenic, selenium, and tin, though the chemical form can be the determining factor in absorption and excretion, and on the distribution and accumulation in the tissues (I.R. Rowland, in *Role of the Gut Flora*, p. 207ff). More than this, these metals or their compounds may undergo biological transformations via the gut flora in mammals, including man. Mercury, notably, has been detailed with regard to biological transformations.

Mercury may exist in the metallic state or as the monovalent or mercurous form, or as the divalent of mercuric form. The mercuric salts are the more toxicologically important, entering the food chain via food and beverages, albeit in extremely small concentrations. Methyl mercury, MeHg, is particularly toxic, affecting the brain and central nervous system, with (oceanic) fish being a principal source.

It has been observed that *mercuric chloride can be converted to MeHg by intestinal flora*, both *in vitro* and *in vivo*. Whereas mercuric salts are poorly absorbed in the gut, *the methyl form is nearly completely absorbed*. Further reactions may occur in the gut due, for instance, to the presence of *hydrogen sulfide*.

Conversely, gut flora (or caecal flora) may demethylate MeHg to produce mercuric mercury (Rowland, in *Role of the Gut Flora*, p. 211). And while bacteria in general would be suspected of being susceptible to mercury poisoning, *some genera, species, or strains of bacteria are resistant not only to mercury but to other toxic metals* (Rowland, in *Role of the Gut Flora*, p. 216). Examples of mercury-resistant bacterial genera include *Escherichia*, *Proteus*, *Klebsiella*, *Staphyloccus*, and *Pseudomonas*.

Arsenic occurs in the environment and in food in a number of forms. These forms include such inorganic salts as the arsenate and arsenite, and such organo-arsenicals as, for example, monomethyl-arsenic acid (MMA) and dimethylarsenic acid (DMA).

Arsenic occurs mostly in the inorganic form as arsenate and arsenite in such sources as drinking water and wine (Rowland, in *Role of the Gut Flora*, p. 218). *Skin cancer, for instance, has been blamed on arsenic in the drinking water, and occupational exposure has been associated with lung cancer.*

Arsenic is observed to be metabolized by gut flora both *in vitro* and *in vivo*. Thus, sodium arsenate was found to be reduced to arsenite and, in turn, methylated to form MMA followed by DMA. The presence of bile acids accelerates the reduction. The presence of hydrogen sulfide further accelerates the reduction and also enhances methylation. Such reducing agents as cysteine and thioglycollate reduce arsenic. Generally speaking, the reducing conditions generated by gut flora favor the chemical reduction of arsenate.

While arsenic reduction and methylation also occurs *in vivo* in humans and experimental animals, the evidence is that this occurs by routes other than by the action of gut flora. For one thing, there is a rapid absorption of arsenate and arsenite in the mammalian gut, limiting the opportunity for the microflora to act. Furthermore, the rate of reduction and methylation of inorganic arsenic is extremely rapid—much more rapid than occurs *in vitro*.

The mechanisms for *in vivo* arsenate reduction and methylation were not supplied, although methylation apparently occurs in the liver. It was stated, moreover, that since MMA and DMA are much less toxic than arsenite, *the biomethylation of arsenic can be regarded as a detoxification process.*

6.6.7 DIETARY FIBER AND COLON MICROFLORA

Resident bacteria serve to digest dietary fiber in the colon (Robert L. McCarthy and Abigail A. Salyers, in *Role of the Gut Flora*, p. 295ff). Studies in the main have been directed at the taxonomic aspects, that is, the kinds and concentrations of bacteria present, and on digestibility experiments involving the incubation of fiber with fecal bacteria specimens. The statement is made that "the normal human colon is one of the most complex microbial ecosystems known." Furthermore, the occurrence of fungi and protozoa is very low. Although most of the predominant bacteria have been isolated and studied, there may remain unknown species.

All of the predominant colonic bacteria are designated as obligate (limited to a single condition) anaerobes, which produce the *anaerobic fermentation of carbohydrates* and yield short chain fatty acids (such as acetate, propionate, and butyrate), and also lactate and succinate, plus gases, notably carbon dioxide, hydrogen, and methane. (*Butyric acid,* for instance, is considered to be an anticancer agent as noted elsewhere, e.g., Boik, *Cancer & Natural Medicine*, pp. 10, 13, 248).

A table of the main genera of colon anaerobes is provided in the reference, consisting of *Bacteroides*, *Fusobacterium*, *Eubacterium*, *Bifidobacterium*, and *Peptostreptococcus*. These genera comprise about 60 percent of all colon bacteria. The genus *Bacteroides* has been studied the most extensively, and there are at least five species that occur in the colon.

There is some variation in the bacterial makeup among persons, with some people harboring higher concentrations of methane-producing bacteria and others having low concentrations of bacteria able to utilize microcrystalline cellulose. Bacteria that have long generation times, e.g., methanogenic and cellulolytic bacteria, may be vulnerable to diets that lower the transit time in the colon. Increasing the dietary fiber increases the number of colonic bacteria.

The reference provides a diagram for the utilization of carbohydrates in the colon. Polysaccharide-fermenting bacteria act on undigested polysaccharides to yield lactate and succinate and also to yield acetate, propionate, butyrate, and gaseous CO_2 and H_2 directly, as well as by the further bacterial conversion of lactate and succinate.

If bacterial methanogens exist, the CO_2 and H_2 are converted to methane. (In inorganic catalysis, CO_2 and H_2 will convert to methane in the presence of activated nickel oxide catalysts at elevated temperatures, the process called methanation.) The main methanogen is *Methanobrevibacter smithii*. Another methanogen, *Methanosphera stadtmaniae*, converts methanol and hydrogen to methane. (Methanol can be produced in the colon by the demethoxylation of pectin by pectinolytic bacteria.) An acetogenic bacterium named *Eubacterium limosum* converts CO_2 and H_2 to acetate. Still other bacteria with still other functions may be present but have not yet been identified in these very complex microbial and biochemical systems located in the colon.

None of the major colonic bacteria species is proteolytic in that these species cannot utilize protein as a sole source for carbon and energy. There is the possibility, nevertheless, that some of the carbohydrate-fermenting species can utilize protein providing a carbohydrate energy source is available. Thus, another process or two that may be going on is the incorporation of amino acids directly into cellular protein and/or the removal of amino groups to serve as a source of nitrogen. For example, *Bacteroides* will introduce exogenous amino acids such as leucine and isoleucine into cellular protein. On the other hand, *Bacteroides* has also been found to incorporate deaminated amino acid carbon skeletons into phospholipids (phosphorus-containing fats).

It is noted that *dietary fiber is not digested by the enzymes in the small intestine, but awaits the colon or large intestine* (McCarthy and Salyers, in *Role of the Gut Flora*, p. 303). A definition used is that *dietary fiber is the sum of cellulose and hemicellulose* (the latter consisting of polysaccharides less complex than cellulose and which are readily hydrolyzable to simple sugars), *with pectin and soluble gums sometimes included for good measure.*

Some colonic bacteria are not able to utilize cellulose, hemicellulose, or pectins but grow readily on monosaccharides and disaccharides. Another source is starch ("resistant starch") that is not digested by amylases. This leads to another definition for dietary fiber, as polysaccharides that are not digested in the small intestine, and that produce a physiological effect on account of bacterial fermentation in the colon.

It has been found that hydrogen in the breath correlates with the degree of microbial fermentation in the colon. Breath hydrogen also parallels blood acetate levels. Carbohydrate breakdown can be monitored by the level of breath hydrogen.

Other processes involving colonic bacteria and their metabolism include the modification of bile acids, sterols, and steroids (McCarthy and Salyers, in *Role of the Gut Flora*, p. 307). Fecal pentaenes are also produced, as previously indicted, and are mutagenic, but the correlation to cancer incidence has not yet been established. Neither is it known why some people excrete mutagens and other don't, whereas high concentrations of the mutagen-producing *Bacteroides* species occur in everyone's colon.

The control of bacterial growth in the colon may be mostly due to competition all up and down the bacterial food chain, since the degradation products of one group of organisms are the food source for another. Toxic metabolites may also have an effect, in particular hydrogen sulfide, which is known to inhibit the growth of some colonic microorganisms. *Short chain fatty acids or bile salts may delay the multiplication of an invading bacterium until it is excreted.* (Of note once more is butyric acid, regarded as an anticancer agent, e.g., in Boik's *Cancer & Natural Medicine*, pp. 10, 13, 248.)

What particular roles all the foregoing may play in carcinogenesis has not yet been spelled out. *However, there is the conjecture that such easily measurable quantities as breath levels of hydrogen or other gases may be an indicator or marker for the progression or diminution of cancer.*

6.7 LIGNANS AND PHYTO-OESTROGENS

It is stated that the Western-type diet, which is high in fat and protein but low in complex carbohydrates and fiber, is associated with many diseases, from coronary heart disease to cancer (K.D.R. Setchell and H. Adlercreutz, in *Role of the Gut Flora*, p. 315ff.) Among cancers, colon cancer is singled out, as well as hormone-dependent cancers such as mammary, endometrium (the mucous membrane lining the uterus), and prostate cancers. The bacterial metabolism of macro- and micro-nutrients and xenobiotics (foreign biotics) as found in food plays an important role. Endogenous substances such as bile acids and oestrogens (estrogens) also are involved. Moreover, bacterial metabolism may act either positively or negatively in the development of disease.

In identifying unusual compounds appearing in urinary steroid profiles (as analyzed by gas/liquid chromatography), a class was encountered and identified as *lignans*. These are compounds having a 2,4-dibenzylbutane structure. They exist as minor constituents of many plants. (*We distinguish lignans from lignin,* the latter being the essential part of woody plant tissue and a precursor for the eonic formation of coal.) For the record, the major urinary lignan identified has the structure written as (α)*trans*-2,3-bis-(3-hydroxybenzyl)-(-butyrolactone), designated HBBL, and called enterolactone for short. Others have used the same name enterolactone for a similar compound. Still other lignans have been uncovered, such as what is referred to as enterodiol. (The prefix "entero-" signifies the intestines.)

Compounds having oestrogenic (or estrogenic) activity are ubiquitous in plants. Notable among these compounds are isoflavones and coumestans, called phyto-oestrogens or plant estrogens, of which isoflavones have been the most studied. The phyto-oestrogens are heterocyclic phenols resembling oestrogenic steroids. Phyto-oestrogens were found to cause *infertility* in sheep in Western Australia, a condition traceable to a species of clover, *Trifolium subterraneum,* and called *Clover Disease.*

The most abundant plant isoflavones are called formononetin, daidzein, and genistein. A bacterially modification is called *isoflavan,* an example of which is called *equol,* the agent responsible for the trouble with the sheep. *Not only present in animals, it has been identified in human urine.*

The human diet, particularly as containing grains and other fiber-rich foods, is also noted to contain lignans (Setchell and Adlercreutz, in *Role of the Gut Flora*, p. 322). *These lignans function as precursors for the bacterial synthesis of enterolactone and enterodiol in the digestive tract.* Flaxseeds are especially rich in lignans and produce a corresponding high level in excretion. (Flaxseed or linseed, or flaxseed oil or linseed oil, incidentally, is a *folkloric anticancer agent.*) Lignans, as well as isoflavones, are hormonally active, with further details supplied in the reference.

More than this, *"Many plant lignans exhibit antimitotic activity and have been shown to be effective in vitro and in vivo against animal tumors,"* and *"Other dietary phenolic compounds inhibit neoplasia"* (Setchell and Adlercreutz, in *Role of the Gut Flora*, p. 328). Enterolactone has in fact shown a cytotoxic effect against breast cancer cells but not against normal cells. On the other hand, enterolactone has been observed to stimulate the growth of breast cancer cells. The evidence is conflicting and may be complicated by whether oestradiol is present.

Being diphenols, the lignan compounds maybe considered weak oxidants (or autroxidants) and possibly beneficial as inhibitors for carcinogenesis (Setchell and Adelcreutz, in *Role of the Gut Flora*, p. 329). As a matter of fact, *the plant lignan that is named norhdihydroguaiaretic acid (NDGA) was once used by the food industry as an effective antioxidant but was discontinued because it showed liver toxicity in rats.* That is, there is a bacterial conversion to an *o*-quinone in the intestines, which in turn leads to cystic nephropathy. (NDGA, which is found in *creosote bush* or *chaparral,* is sometimes regarded as an anticancer agent, or at least is listed as an enzyme inhbitor for a step in glycolysis—as is the creosote bush itself, for that matter.)

Other tests have shown mammalian lignans not to be carcinogenic although, in general, phenolic compounds are regarded as carcinogenic. Similarly, phyto-oestrogens have neither tumor-promoting nor

-inhibiting effects. However, more recent studies have indicated that enterolactone inhibits placental aromatase and passes freely into the cells of human choriocarcinoma (a chorion is a membrane enveloping the fetus of mammals). Enterolactone acts as an enzyme inhibitor for the enzyme designated P-450.

Although the results of *in vitro* studies are conflicting, studies on animals show that *the ingestion of phyto-oestrogens produces definite physiological and pathophysiological responses* (Setchell and Adlercreutz, in *Role of the Gut Flora*, p. 330). An example already cited was that of reproductive failure for sheep grazing on a certain clover species high in phyto-oestrogens.

Soybean products, notably, contain relatively high levels of the phyto-oestrogens daidzein and genistein. Uterotrophic effects occur in laboratory animals, and soy protein may turn out to be an efficient growth promoter comparable to the synthetic oestrogen (estrogen) known as diethylstilbestrol or DES. On the other hand, *there may be a connection between phyto-oestrogen intake and liver disease and infertility,* as observed in captive cheetahs, whereas there is no such evidence for wild cheetahs. In fact, liver disease is a major cause of death for captive cheetahs, a roadblock for the survival of this endangered species. *When the diet of captive cheetahs was changed to eliminate soy protein products, a marked improvement occurred, both in the elimination of liver lesions and in promoting fertility.*

Another interesting circumstance occurs with California quail. *In a dry year, the quail eat the leaves of stunted desert plants that are rich in phyto-oestrogens, and their reproduction is limited, therefore not compromising the limited food supply.* In a good year, meaning a wet year, the opposite occurs.

As to humans, there have been studies on the potentially beneficial role of lignans and phyto-oestrogens in common diseases such as colon cancer (Setchell and Adlercreutz, in *Role of the Gut Flora*, p. 333ff). Groups of women labeled as omnivores, lactovegetarians, and macrobiotics (vegetarians) have been compared as to the urinary secretions of various lignans and isoflavonic phyto-oestrogens, namely enterolactone (a lignan), enterodiol (a lignan), daidzen (an isoflavone), equol (an isoflavone), and *o*-desmethylangolensin (an isoflavone). *The highest urinary excretion rates were for the group of macrobiotics,* followed by lactovegetarians. *Omnivores came in last. Antibiotics reduced the excretion of lignans* by destroying the microflora responsible.

There is epidemiological evidence, at least, that women with much higher levels of enterolactone excretion have much lower risks of breast cancer. For women already with breast cancer, the level of excretion is nearly identical to that of the omnivores.

It is further mentioned that *nonhuman primates are highly resistant to the carcinogenic effects of oestrogens,* even when combined with another carcinogen. Thus, for chimpanzees, both lignan and isoflavone excretion is high—approximately the same as for human macrobiotics.

The inference above is that high excretion rates imply high concentrations in the gut, which in turn translates to protection against cancer.

It was noted that *there is a close correlation between breast cancer and colon cancer* (Setchell and Adlercreutz, in *Role of the Gut Flora*, p. 337). Thus, the frequency of adenomas or polyps and the incidence of colon cancer have both been found to be high following primary cancer of the breast.

6.8 INTENSE SWEETENERS

The intense sweeteners on the world market can be divided into organic acids and peptides (A.G. Renwick, in *Role of the Gut Flora*, p. 175ff). The latter category, consisting of aspartame and thaumatin, digest in the upper intestine and for the most part do not interact with gut microflora. Of primary interest here, therefore, are the organic acids, known as saccharin, cyclamate, and acesulfame-K. (Stevioside, obtained from leaves of the Paraguayan and Brazilian shrub *Stevia rebaudiana* of the plant family Compositae, can be regarded as a glycoside, a different category to be discussed subsequently.) These three organic acid sweeteners are incompletely absorbed from the gut, and there results an interaction with the gut microflora. Either the sweeteners affect the microflora, or the microflora affect the sweeteners.

In establishing the acceptable daily intake (ADI) for the ingestion of foods such as intense sweeteners, high-dose animal toxicity studies are used as the basis. The dosage levels can be as high as 10 percent by weight of the total dietary intake. As may be expected, at these levels, some drastic changes occur in the homeostatic balance, including changes in the metabolic activity of the gut microflora.

High dosages of saccharin produce changes in protein and carbohydrate digestion, and in the catabolism of intestinal microbes. The accompanying effect on tumor development is unclear, however. There are major differences between test animals and control animals, and both the interpretation and the extrapolation to humans is complicated and argumentative. The debate over saccharin continues, based on findings that three percent w/w sodium saccharin in the diet of succeeding generations of rats produces bladder cancer in the second generation. Single-generation studies, however, show no increased incidence of bladder tumors. The reference further discusses changes in carbohydrate and protein metabolism and changes in saccharin metabolism.

The subject of saccharin further introduces that of protein digestion, to the effect that *there may be a link between bladder cancer and protein, tryptophan, and other amino acids.* Thus, *the incidence of bladder tumors in rats follows a high protein diet.* Furthermore, *the protease inhibitor leupeptin promotes bladder cancer in rats. High dietary levels of the amino acids leucine and isoleucine promote bladder cancer in rats. A large increase in dietary tryptophan produced a hyperplasia in the epithelium of dogs.*

Finally, *microbial metabolites of aromatic amino acids may promote carcinogenesis.* Thus, *the metabolite indole is a more active promoter for bladder cancer than is the parent amino acid tryptophan.*

And *simple phenols such as cresol, which are microbial metabolites of tyrosine, are cancer promoters.*

As to *cyclamate,* it was banned in the U.S. and U.K. in 1969 based on experiments showing an increased incidence of bladder tumors in rats (Renwick, in *Role of the Gut Flora,* p. 185ff). The rats were fed a diet of cyclamate, saccharin, and cyclohexamine, the latter being a microbial metabolite of cyclamate. *The decision, however, was contingent on a single bladder tumor found in a group of rats given cyclohexamine alone. Duplication of the test results have been unsuccessful, and a consensus has been reached among interested parties that neither cyclamate nor cyclohexamine is carcinogenic. Cyclamate is used as a sweetener in other countries around the world, including Germany, Switzerland, and Australia.* Cyclohexamine has been found to be more toxic than cyclamate, and cyclamate intake levels are set by the degree of toxicity of this metabolite.

The reference furnishes additional information about the metabolism of cyclamate and the bacteria species responsible. An inspection of a table presented in the reference lists the following bacteria genera or species: *Clostridium* spp., including *C. perfingens* and *C. sordelli, Pseudomonas* spp., *Corynebacterium* spp., *Campylobacter* spp., *Propionibacterium acnes* and *P. acidipropionici, Enterobacterium* spp., *E. coli, Streptococcus faecalis, Bacillus* spp., and *Enterococci* spp. These bacteria were found variously in the feces, caecal contents, and gut contents of rats, guinea pigs, rabbits, dogs, and man. *Only the last-mentioned bacteria species showed up in man.*

It was further noted in the reference that evidently the enzyme involved in converting cyclamate to cyclohexamine is cyclate sulphomatase (Renwick, in *Role of the Gut Flora,* p. 195).

Acesulfame-K is described as a cyclic sulfonic acid derivative that is extremely water soluble. It is not metabolized *in vivo* and does not show antibacterial properties. It causes diarrhea and caecal enlargement in rats at very high doses, which may be related to an altered carbohydrate metabolism.

Stevioside, to be further described in a subsequent section, is a glycoside that occurs in the leaves of the Brazilian and Paraguayan plant *Stevia rebaudiana.* Stevioside is the most abundant of the several glycosides occurring in the plant. Other minor constituents, such as rebaudioside, probably contribute to the sweetness. *High dosage levels are nontoxic.* There is a report that, although stevioside and the leaf extracts are not mutagenic, *the pure aglycone (steviol) becomes a bacterial mutagen when activated.* The incubation of stevioside with rat caecal bacteria yields a stoichiometric conversion to steviol.

On account of the varying interpretations of toxicological data, the use of *Stevia* preparations has heretofore been confined to Japan, Paraguay, South Korea, and the People's Republic of China—although it can no doubt be obtained in the U.S. as well, if only under the counter.

6.9 HYDROLYSIS AND OTHER INTERACTIONS BETWEEN INTESTINAL FLORA AND CHEMICALS

Intestinal microflora play a significant role in the hydrolysis of glycosides and esters, and in other biochemical reactions, a role that has toxicological consequences (Joseph P. Brown, in *Role of the Gut Flora,* p. 109ff). Glycosides are first mentioned in the reference in describing the role of intestinal microbial glycosidases (or glucosidases). The action of these enzymes results, for instance, in both mucin degradation and laminarin degradation. Mucin can be regarded as a muco-protein originating from mucous membranes or the like; laminarin is defined as a type of glucan (a polymer of glucose) similar to that found in plant and fungal walls.

6.9.1 GLYCOSIDES

The numerous plant glycosides in the human diet include such classifications and compounds as the flavonoids, cyanogenic glycosides, amygdalin, cycasin, esculin, and so on. These glycosides are hydrolyzed by the intestinal flora (e.g., flora-produced enzymes) to yield various aglycones. (An aglycone is defined as a noncarbohydrate group, usually an alcohol or a phenol, which is combined with a carbohydrate or sugar to form a glycoside or glucoside). In turn, the aglycones released may produce significant physiological or toxicological effects.

Hydrolysis is accomplished by the enzyme β-glucosidase. Chief among the β-glucosidase-producing bacteria are the lactobacilli, the bacteroides, and the bifidobacteria. Others include the species *E. coli,* and the enterococci and the clostridia.

In a further paraphrasing, explanation, and distinction of terms (e.g., Peter A. Mayes, in *Harper's Biochemistry*, pp. 139–140), glycosides are formed from a condensation reaction between the hydroxyl group (–OH) of the "anomeric" carbon of a monosaccharide or monosaccharide residue and a group occurring in a second compound that may or may not be (as in the case of an aglycone) another monosaccharide. If the reacting group of the second compound is also a hydroxyl group, the glycosidic bond consists of an acetyl link denoted by –O–. The prevailing example for the second compound is a generalized alcohol, meaning it contains an –OH group (Voet and Voet, *Biochemistry*, p. 256). To continue, if the second compound is glucose, the resulting compound is a *glucoside;* if galactose, the resulting compound is a galactoside; and so forth. If the second group is an amine, the result is an N-glycoside. In general, especially if the second group is not a saccharide, we are speaking of *glycosides*—but herein the terms *glycoside* and *glucoside* may be used interchangeably. The prefix α or β denotes on which side of the anomeric carbon atom the reactant group is located, as in β-glycosides versus α-glycosides. The one position is the opposite of the other.

The subject of *cycasin* and related *azoxyglycosides* is also taken up by the reference. Cycasin is derived from cycads, plants of the tropics and subtropics, which comprise about 100 species in nine genera and are of the plant family Cycadiaceae. (As previously noted, this plant family does not appear in Hartwell's *Plants Used Against Cancer.*) Ingestion of the plants or plant parts (seeds or nuts) results in gastrointestinal and neurological effects of a severe nature, although the normal methods of preparation (washing) removes the toxic components.

A number of toxic constituents have been identified through the years, and the potential carcinogenicity is due to azoxyglycosides, producing tumors in the liver and/or kidney. The carcinogenic principle was identified as the *aglycone* called *methylazoxymethanol (MAM).*

Of particular note are *cyanogenic glycosides* such as amygdalin and prunasin. These compounds are found in many plants, notably of the family Rosaceae, which in particular contains the genus *Prunus.* Dietary cyanide can result in acute poisoning or chronic neurological disease. An example of the cassava root is provided, which contains cyanic glycosides and yet is used as a food source in many tropical countries. It is rendered safe by the food preparation methods of soaking and washing, roasting, and sun drying, which eliminate or decompose the cyanide.

If eaten without prior preparation, cyanide detoxification can be accomplished by an enzymatic conversion to thiocyanate, *a conversion that depends on the presence of sulfur-containing amino acids.* A deficiency of these amino acids compounds the toxic effects of dietary cyanide intake, producing neuropathies such as spastic paraparesis (partial paralysis of the lower limbs).

It turns out that the intestinal metabolism of cyanogenic glycosides is not quite like that of the azoxyglycosides. The enzymes responsible are apparently in the small intestine and in the intestinal contents and kidneys, at least in rats.

Apart from Laetrile or amygdalin being considered a (controversial and ineffective) treatment for cancer, it is pointed out that mandelonitrile, the aglycone of amygdalin and prunasin, displays mutagenic activity by the *Salmonella* test. In fact, amygdalin itself displays mutagenicity by the same test. (For more on Laetrile, or laetrile, consult Part 8 within the section "Phytochemicals That May Act Against Cancer," in the subsection titled "Laetrile Again?")

6.9.2 QUINONES

The quinones consist of such compounds as benzoquinones and naphthaquinones and are widely distributed in plants in the form of certain hydroxybenzoquinones—in particular, in the plant family Myrsinaceae (which, incidentally, has a couple of specie entries in Hartwell's *Plants Used Against*

Cancer). These quinones are found to have both antihelminthic (acts against intestinal worms) and purgative properties. Although not described as existing in the glycoside form, some have displayed similar mutagenic properties.*

The most widely distributed of the naturally occurring quinones are the 9,10-anthraquinones (AQs). *The majority that occur in the fungi and higher plants are phenolic.* Both natural and synthetic have been used as colorants and for other purposes. Those from the genera *Cassia* (from the family Legumi- nosae), *Rhamnus* (from the family Rhamnaceae), and *Rheum* (of the family Polygonaceae) have been used in purgative preparations. (All these families and genera are represented in Hartwell's *Plants Used Against Cancer*.)

What are called the *hydroxy anthraquinones* occur in fungi and higher plants. Most of these plants are considered nonedible with the exception of *Rheum palmitum* (rhubarb) and possibly *Cassia* (senna).

In addition to cathartic effects, some of the AQs exhibit hepatotoxicity, and a high percentage of the hydroxy AQs show mutagenicity (Brown, in *Role of the Gut Flora*, pp. 122–123). Whether natural or synthetic, occurring as food contaminants or constituents, or used as drugs or medicinal preparations, hydroxyanthraquinones demonstrate complex interactions between intestinal microflora and host metab- olism.

6.9.3 FLAVONOIDS

What are classed as flavonoids or flavonoid compounds have the basic structural feature of the 2- phenylbenzo[α]pyrane nucleus, or what is more readily called the *flavane nucleus* (Brown, in *Role of the Gut Flora*, p. 123). This nucleus consists of two benzene rings, denoted as A and B, which are linked through what is described as a heterocyclic pyrane C ring. There is a widespread natural occurrence in human foods and a further use in drugs and nutritional supplements. This emphasizes the interest in their potential mutagenic and carcinogenic properties.†

About 2,000 different flavonoids have been identified, and flavonoids are ubiquitous among vascular plants. *Quercetin* (as distinguished from, say, quercitrin) is the most common flavonol, existing in more than 70 glycosidic combinations, and what are called *kaempferol* and *myricetin* exist in nearly as many. All told, the separate compounds total some 400 in number.

Although there are claims for a *vitamin-like activity* in certain groups of food flavonoids, the matter remains unresolved. *Antioxidant properties are due to their phenolic nature.* And *antimicrobial activity is pronounced* against bacteria such as staphylocci, *E. coli*, and salmonellae, and against viruses and fungi. This antimicrobial activity is most evident for the methylated, lipophilic flavones such as nobiletin, tangeretin, and sinensetin.

Likewise, *certain methylated flavones and flavonoids exhibit cytotoxic effects against human cancer cells.* Otherwise, the therapeutic action pertains to some physiological and biochemical effects such as smooth muscle relaxation and anti-inflammation as well as diuretic effects and decreases in capillary fragility. The supportive mechanisms are mostly unknown but may involve *enzyme inhibition* and *copper chelation.*

Ingested *flavonoic glucosides are poorly absorbed* in the small intestine, and since they are largely β-glycosides, they are *poorly hydrolyzed by mammalian digestive enzymes* and pass mostly unaltered into the large bowel. A number of experiments are described in the reference about the metabolic fate of flavonoids, with the general conclusion that there is little evidence that aglycones persist after the ingestion of food flavonoids.

Food flavonoids are regarded as virtually nontoxic, and there have been conflicting reports about carcinogenicity, especially for quercetin (Brown, in *Role of the Gut Flora*, pp. 128–129). On the other hand, *flavonoids exhibit genetic toxicity, or mutagenesis,* including quercetin.

---

* The compound quinone, or benzoquinone, is an unsaturated six-carbon benzene-ring structure with two oxygens attached, and it has the stoichiometric formula $C_6H_4O_2$. Generalized, quinones are compounds based on, or involving, this sort of structure. Naphthoquinones are made up of two benzene rings joined side by side, with two oxygens attached. Anthraquinones involve three benzene rings joined side by side, again with two oxygens attached. Hydroxy quinones will have an –OH group or groups attached, and so on.

† The reference supplies a figure with an example of a flavonoid as well as other types of compounds mentioned. What are termed *flavones* and *flavanones* have a ketone linkage or linkages involving oxygen as –O–. What are termed *flavonols* involve the –OH group. It may be added that there is considerable mixing up of the prefixes "flava-" and "flavo-".

It is noted in the reference that *flavonol glycosides, notably of quercetin and kaempferol, are found in the edible parts of most food plants* (Brown, in the *Role of the Gut Flora*, p. 130). These sources include citrus and other fruits and berries, leafy vegetables, roots, tubers and bulbs, herbs and spices, legumes, cereal grains, and tea and cocoa. In fact, it is stated that about 25 percent of the flavonol dietary intake is from tea, coffee, cocoa, fruit jams, red wine, beer, and vinegar. Of the total intake of flavonols, about five percent can be regarded as mutagenic. *Caution is advocated about consuming excess flavonols or their glycosides, say in the form of rutin, in nutritional supplements.*

6.9.4 GLYCOSIDE SWEETENERS

The *ent*-kaurene glycosides are examples of diterpenoids and include substances such as stevioside, previously discussed, plus steviolbioside and rebaudioside (Brown, in *Role of the Gut Flora*, p. 131). These substances are included among the eight sweet *ent*-kaurene glycosides that occur in the leaves of the Paraguayan and Brazilian shrub *Stevia rebaudiana* of the plant family Compositae. These substances occur in the extracts from the leaves, and in totality are generically called stevia. The extracts of the plant and stevioside, the major sweetener component, are used as commercial sweeteners in Japan for confectioneries and soft drinks. For the record, stevioside has the complicated chemical name 19-*O*-β-glucopyranosyl-13-*O*-[β-glucopyranosyl (1-2)]-β-glucopyranosyl-13-hydroxykaur-16-en-19-oic acid.*

A study of the metabolic fate of stevioside and rebaudioside A indicated that they were both completely hydrolyzed to steviol by anaerobic whole-cell suspensions of rat caecal bacteria *in vitro*. In turn, the steviol was almost completely absorbed by the intestinal tract. A similar metabolic sequence for the *ent*-kaurene glycosides was predicted in humans.

The mutagenicity for steviol and steviol glycosides has been determined using a *Salmonella* test. It was found that six glycosides were nonmutagenic, being stevioside, steviolbioside, dulcoside A, and rebaudiosides A, B, and C. The metabolic product steviol, on the other hand, showed considerable induced mutagenic activity.

6.9.5 ROLE IN DRUG ADMINISTRATION

As previously presented, there is a colon-specific delivery of bioactive compounds involving the release of aglycones from the ingestion of poorly absorbed plant glycosides (Brown, in *Role of the Gut Flora*, p. 132). This release is mediated by the action of enzymes, the glycosidases produced by various colonic bacteria. Another bacterial enzyme, *azoreductase,* has been used as the means for activating therapeutic agents in the lower bowel. Thus, sulphasalazine and a polymer-based producing system both convert—upon reduction of their azo bonds—to 5-aminosalicylate in the colon. In these and other examples, the use of *prodrug glycosides* exploits intestinal microbial glycosidases to produce a site-specific therapy.

Glucosides and galactosides of various *steroids* can be slowly hydrolyzed by the action of intestinal bacterial enzymes, as can cellobiosides. This provides a method to introduce steroid prodrugs in the mammalian system, particularly for larger, more lipophilic drug molecules that cannot be introduced in any other way.

6.9.6 MISCELLANEOUS GLYCOSIDES

There are a number of miscellaneous glycosides which are involved in synthetic or natural toxicants (Brown, in *Role of the Gut Flora*, p. 133). Thus, certain *insecticides* such as cypermethrin, deltamethrin, and fenvalerate may show up as residues in plants in the form of glycoside conjugates 3-phenoxybenzyl alcohol (PB alc) and 3-phenoxybenzoic acid (PB acid). The metabolic fate is complicated, and no inferences were made about metabolite toxicity or carcinogenicity.

Another type of compound discussed in the reference is the insecticide *carbofuran,* which is partically oxidized to 3-hydroxycarbofuran (3–OH–C) in both animals and plants. In animals, 3–OH–C is degraded and excreted. In plants, however, the 3–O-glucoside of hydroxycarbofuran (3–OH–C-gluc) is formed as

---

* The famous South American explorer Colonel P.H. Fawcett, in traversing the Brazil–Paraguay border in his explorations during 1906–1909, noted a plant about 18 in. high with small aromatic leaves, *several times sweeter than ordinary sugar,* and which was called *Caa-he-eh* (Fawcett, *Lost Trails, Lost Cities*, p. 122). (Another small plant, called *Ibira-gjukych,* had leaves that tasted *salty*.) As of today, there are about 150 known plant species in the genus *Stevia*, but the genus is not represented in *Hartwell's Plants Used Against Cancer*, although there are many entries for the family Compositae.

a major residue and is considered equally toxic. On ingestion, microbial *hydrolysis* occurs in the intestines, and it can be inferred that exposure to the *toxic aglycone* will result.

A compound named *miserotoxin,* a glucoside, is internally synthesized by the plant species of the genus *Astragalus* of the family Leguminosae. (The genus *Astragalus* includes the poisonous *milkvetches* of the American West, which pick up selenium from the soil and serve as selenium indicators—and can cause selenium poisoning. The glucosides in milkvetches cause respiratory problems and paralysis in the hind legs of livestock, noted in *Weeds of the West*.) After ingestion by sheep and cattle, the *glucoside is hydrolyzed by ruminal organisms to release the aglycone,* which is 3-nitropropanol (NPOH). Miserotoxin is less toxic to rats, for instance, since there is a lower degree of microbial hydrolysis. What hydrolysis does occur in mammals evidently results in nitropropionic acid (NPA). This latter toxic compound is found in certain legume forages but does not occur simultaneously with NPOH. The compound NPA, however, is more toxic to monogastric animals as compared to ruminants, which rapidly detoxify the substance. It is stated that NPA toxicity apparently occurs by the inhibition of mitochondrial respiratory enzymes. No statements, pro or con, were made about mutagenicity or carcinogenicity, albeit several *Astragalus* species from different parts of the world are entered in Hartwell's *Plants Used Against Cancer,* notably as the Asian species called *gum tragacanth,* or tragacanth. This yields the gummy substance of the same name, which swells up in water and introduces firmness, and is used in the arts and in pharmacy.

6.9.7 ESTERS

Ester is the generic name for compounds between what are perceived as alcohols (RCH_2OH) and organic acids ($HOCOR'$) to eliminate HOH—that is, H_2O or water—by the condensation reaction

$$RCH_2O\text{–}H + HO\text{–}COR' \rightarrow RCH_2OCOR' + HOH$$

That is, esters may be regarded as acylated alcohols in which the hydroxyl hydrogen of the alcohol is replaced by the acyl group ($-COR'$ or $R'CO-$) as furnished by the acid. Alternatively, the acid hydrogen may be viewed as being replaced by an alkyl group (RCH_2-) furnished by the alcohol:

$$RCH_2\text{–}OH + H\text{–}OCOR' \rightarrow RCH_2OCOR' + HOH$$

The reference is concerned with the esterification of bile acids and sterols and with ester hydrolysis (Brown, in *Role of the Gut Flora*, pp. 135–136).

Human fecal bacteria were found to have cholate transforming abilities, including the formation of the ester called methyl deoxycholate. This particular metabolite was formed by most *Bacteroides* spp. and by a few strains of *Eubacterium* and *Lactobacillus*. Such bile acid esters are less soluble and exhibit less bacterial action than normal, and conceivably esterification could serve as a detoxification mechanism for the bacteria. That is, in some instances at least, esterification could preserve the bacterial flora.

When humans (and animals) consume a high-beef-fat diet, the feces contain an important bile acid, named lithocholic acid, which is associated with a high incidence of large bowel cancer. A study of lithocholic acid anaerobic metabolism by rat intestinal flora found a number of esters produced, notably ethyl esters of lithocholic acid or its isomer, isolithocholic acid. The animals were fed a high-meat diet for six months prior to the test. The toxicological properties of these esters have not yet been investigated, nor have they been found in human feces.

The pyrethroid insecticides *fluvalinate* and *fenvalerate* yield acid metabolites, which in turn form novel conjugates involving what is referred to as 3-hydroxyl esterification. There may be further ramifications in the cause of granulomatous changes in the brain, kidney, and spleen of animals, notably of rodents, dogs, and rhesus monkeys. (A granuloma is a tumor or growth of granulated or grain-like tissue.)

The hydrolysis of xenobiotic esters (of foreign biological origin, from outside the system) is generally thought to be by the action of mammalian intestinal or hepatic enzymes known as *carboxylesterases*. These enzymes are capable of hydrolyzing not only carboxyl esters, but thiol esters and aromatic amides. Furthermore, intestinal microflora are also involved—presumably in the production of the necessary enzymes. As an example, mixed rat caecal bacteria caused the hydrolysis of methyl gallate to gallic acid, pyrogallol, and resorcinol.

In other experiments, *Escherichia coli* were found to hydrolyze a series of *trans*-cinnamyl esters. It is noted that trans-cinnamyl acetate for instance is found in *cassia oil* derived from the plant species

Cinnamomum sieboldii of the family Lauraceae. (The genus *Cinnamomum* is well represented in Hartwell's *Plants Used Against Cancer*, although the aforementioned species is not listed. Generically speaking, we are talking about the spice known as *cinnamon*. The genus *Cassia*, on the other hand, belongs to the family Leguminosae and is also listed in Hartwell. Its product is better known as the laxative *senna*.) The derived spice, here called cassia oil, is noted to be used as a food flavoring. Of the several esters tested, only *trans*-cinnamyl formate was hydrolyzed to any significant degree.

The chemical di-(2-ethylhexyl)phthalate (DEHP) is commonly used as a plasticizer and, as a consequence, has become an environmental contaminant. Employed in the manufacture of polyvinyl chloride, it can be surmised that human exposure will accompany the use of such items as blood bags and food wrappers. Although the acute toxicity of DEHP is low, chronic toxicity surfaces in the form of several diseases, notably testicular atrophy and *liver carcinogenicity*, at least in rodents. The intestinal metabolism of DEHP has been shown to be alleviated by the use of antibiotics. This metabolism involves hydrolysis to yield the monoester (MEHP), which is equally toxic and moreover tends to promote intestinal absorption. Fortunately, there is a threshold below which DEHP does not reach the liver but is largely excreted in the liver and the feces.

All the foregoing illustrates the complexity of the interactions between chemicals and bacterial flora and whether the results are to a degree toxic, mutagenic, or carcinogenic.

6.10 ALL-MEAT AND ALL-VEGETARIAN DIETS

Vilhjalmur Stefansson, the famous explorer of the Canadian Arctic, has written two books extolling an all-meat diet, high in fat, as once practiced by the Eskimos. His experiences and observations commenced in 1906, when the more remote Eskimos still embraced a stone-age, nonwestern culture.

In *The Fat of the Land*, originally published in 1946 as *Not by Bread Alone*, it is noted that such an all-meat diet is sufficient in itself, *if enough fat is present*. But a diet on lean meat alone, such as rabbit, will leave the eater permanently unsatisfied, with still other unwelcome symptoms—which can be corrected easily enough by taking in fat (Stefansson, *Fat*, p. 31). Furthermore, the intestinal flora accommodate to this type of meat/fat diet (Stefansson, *Fat*, p. 56). Similarly, *an all-vegetarian diet will also be accommodated*. The bacteria flora that are not needed cease to exist. *It is when an omnivorous diet is adopted, with both meat and fruits and vegetables, that the problems commence.* This kind of diet is, of course, characteristic of Western Civilization.

It can be argued that Eskimos also take on fresh berries in the summer months (Stefansson, *Fat*, p. 94). There is the possibility as well that, like the plains Indians, they may add berries to pounded meat and fat to make (berry) pemmican, as distinguished from all-meat and fat (plain) pemmican. It is stressed, however, that the berry content is not essential to good health, that fresh meat with adequate fat suffices.

In chapters on scurvy or blackleg, from the documentation, it appears that the causes of scurvy can be traced to the use of salted or preserved meats rather than fresh meats, and/or a lack of fresh vegetables and fruits. *Even the rations of lime juice supplied to sailors were insufficiently effective. As to salt itself, the Eskimos called it evil tasting, disliking it even more than the partly herbivorous Indians* (Stefansson, *Fat*, p. 50). Stefansson himself kicked the salt habit.

Stefansson, as have many others, takes special note of the dramatic increase in sugar consumption, his figures showing a per capita increase from 7.5 pounds in 1791 to 114.1 pounds in 1941 (Stefansson, *Fat*, p. 118). Even higher at present, *at approximately 150 pounds per person*, the inference, of course, is that *sugar (e.g., sucrose) will cause an extra degree of intestinal putrefaction, releasing still other potentially carcinogenic compounds*. Stefansson follows this by some good words about whale blubber and adds the old saying that a person likes eating what he is used to eating (Stefansson, *Fat*, 124).

In *Cancer: Disease of Civilization?*, *Stefansson states that he initially did not encounter any sign of cancer in the more primitive or stone-age Eskimos—nor any tooth decay*. The same kind of observations have been made about cultures or societies on an all-vegetarian diet, e.g., the Hunzas of Asia. Again, it is civilization that intrudes.

An interesting comment supplied by elusive French personage M. Tanchou was that, circa 1840, Paris had four times the cancer incidence of London (Stefansson, *Cancer*, p. 28). No answers were provided other than to suggest that Paris was maybe four times more civilized than London. The doctrine that cancer is a disease of civilization was evidently first pronounced by this same M. Tanchou, and Stefansson describes the unsuccessful searches for further information about Tanchou and the comparative data on which his doctrine was based. Now, of course, there are all sorts of statistics as to the present state of affairs, but little is known about the incidence of cancer in Tanchou's time and before. Tanchou's pronouncements were perhaps most avidly promoted by John Le Conte, an American physician who practiced in the mid to late 1800s (Stefansson, *Cancer*, p. 27), and additional investigations were made by American cancer specialist Dr. Philip R. White in the 1950s. These latter investigations were inconclusive, however, and the status of cancer incidence in "precivilized" times remains an enigma.

In the annals of Africa, Dr. Albert Schweitzer, the famous missionary surgeon and founder of the hospital at Lambaréné, did not encounter any cancer when he first arrived at Gabon in 1913 (Stefansson, *Cancer*, p. 37). He viewed this absence as due to the differences in nutrition for the natives as compared to Europe.*

In Chapter 2, Stefansson describes the search for cancer among the Eskimos as conducted by Captain George B. Leavitt and others. Leavitt was commander of the steam whaler *Narwhal*. Leavitt arrived in the Canadian Arctic in 1906, the same time as Stefansson. The results can be summed up by the conclusion that no cases of cancer were found. Raold Amundsen, who explored these regions and noted the corrupting and death-dealing effects of civilization on other tribes, wrote that "My sincerest wish for our friends the Eskimos is, that civilization *never* reaches them."

In succeeding chapters, Stefansson describes further searches for cancer in the Canadian North, e.g., in Labrador, along the Anderson River, located to the east of the Mackenzie River and still farther east from Alaska, and among the woodland or forest Indians of northern Canada. *Initially, the results were nil, then cancer incidences began to occur.*

In a chapter titled "The Twentieth Century Forgets the Nineteenth," Stefansson provides some extensive quotations from *Cancer: Civilization and Degeneration,* by John Cope, published in London in 1932, of which one paragraph is as follows, and which still seems apropos (Stefansson, *Cancer*, pp. 130–133).

> Experimental cancer research has, in short, become so isolated and so entrenched that, without being aware of it, the researcher now almost instinctively regards those who criticize his opinion, question his authority, or adopt other methods of working, not as fellow workers, but as amateurs, as "outsiders," or even as positive enemies....

Stefansson also provides some prophetic statements by Sir Charles Dodds, who was professor of biochemistry at the University of London and a famous authority on malignant diseases. In an article titled "The Problem of Cancer," published in the *London Science News* for October 1949, Dodds reviews the success of certain synthetic chemotherapeutic drugs against bacteria, as in the case of salvarsan against syphilis. Other examples are the sulphonomides and the antimalarial drugs. (We could since add antibiotics.) Sir Charles goes on,

> It is only natural that attempts should have been made to apply the same general principles to cancer...[but] *the would-be chemotherapist is on very uncertain grounds, since he does not know the nature of the process he is attempting to reverse.* The only knowledge he has got is that the cancer cells grow in an unrestrained and disorganized manner as compared with normal cells...."

Parenthetically, it may be commented that German biochemist and Nobel Prize-winner Otto Warburg had discovered the fundamental difference between the metabolism of cancer cells and normal cells back in 1926.

In the succeeding chapter, "The Twentieth Century Rediscovers the Nineteenth," Stefansson recounts the parallel trend emerging toward looking at demographic differences, age differences, diet differences, cooking differences, chemical contamination, and so on, which is still underway. He concludes the chapter with a statement about the meat eaters versus the vegetarians being both right and both wrong. They are each right in praising their own diet but wrong in condemning the other.

---

* In a chapter on lung cancer in *Hypothyroidism*, by Barnes and Galton and published in 1976, it was stated that *150 years ago tumors were relatively infrequent* but were noted as becoming more prevalent in the late 1800s, notably in England. In 1898, a Dr. Roger Williams reported in the British medical journal *Lancet* that *during the 50-year period from 1840 to 1890, there was a five-fold increase,* from 17 deaths per 100,000 to 88, whereas circa 1976 the rate was 150 deaths. Today, this figure in the U.S. is more like 200 per 100,000—or about a *twelve-fold increase.*

Stefansson wraps things up with a chapter titled "A 'Cancer-Free' People of Asia," about the long-lived Hunzas, who are lacto-vegetarians, and a chapter on prevention. According to Sir Robert McCarrison, who served in northern India and investigated the Hunzas during the period 1904–1911, cancer-resistant health can be attained in three key ways. The first key is that, in the few months before birth, there be a healthy mother eating healthy foods. The second is protracted breast feeding. The third is the preponderant use of fresh and raw foods, with a minimum of processing. (More on the Hunzas is presented in Part 8, within the section "Phytochemicals That May Act Against Cancer," in the subsection "Laetrile Again?".)

Maladies that are rarely found when cancer is also rare were listed by Stefansson as appendicitis, constipation, and corpulence. Other difficulties that are rarely found include arthritis, asthma, beriberi, dental cavities, colitis, diabetes, duodenal ulcers, epilepsy, gallstones, gastric ulcers, hypertension, night blindness, pellagra, rickets, and scurvy.

Called the frontier doctor's prescription, the above thoughts correlate with an absence of cancer.

REFERENCES

"American Cancer Society Guidelines on Diet, Nutrition, and Cancer Prevention: Reducing the Risk of Cancer with Healthy Food Choices and Physical Activity," prepared by the American Cancer Society 1996 Advisory Committee on Diet, Nutrition, and Cancer Prevention, *CA—A Cancer Journal for Clinicians*, 46(6), 325–341 (November/December, 1996)

Atlas, Ronald M., *Microbiology: Fundamentals and Applications*, 2d ed., Macmillan, New York, 1984, 1988.

Barker, Rodney, *And the Waters Turned to Blood: The Ultimate Biological Threat*, Simon & Schuster, New York 1997.

Barnes, Broda O. and Lawrence Galton, *Hypothyroidism: The Unsuspected Illness*, Crowell, New York, 1976.

Boik, John C., *Cancer and Natural Medicine: A Textbook of Basic Science and Clinical Research*, Oregon Medical Press, Princeton MN, 1995.

Brandt, Johanna, *The Grape Cure*, Benedict Lust, Santa Barbara CA, 1971.

Brock, Thomas D. and Michael T. Madigan, *Biology of Microrganisms*, 6th ed., Prentice Hall, Englewood Cliffs NJ, 1970, 1974, 1979, 1984, 1988, 1991.

Colborn, Theo., Dianne Dumanoski and John Peterson Myers, *Our Stolen Future: Are We Threatening Our Fertility, Intelligence, and Survival?—A Scientific Detective Story*, Dutton, New York, 1996. Little, Brown, Boston, 1996. Dutton, New York, 1997. Penguin, New York, 1997. Foreword by Al Gore.

CRC Handbook of Microbiology, 2nd ed., in seven volumes, Allen T. Laskin and Hubert A. Lechevalier Eds., CRC Press, Cleveland OH, Boca Raton FL, 1977–. Vol. I. Bacteria. Vol. II. Fungi, Algae, Protozoa, and Viruses. Vol. III. Microbial Composition: Amino Acids, Proteins, and Nucleic Acids. Vol. IV. Microbial Composition: Carbohydrates, Lipids, and Minerals. Vol. V. Microbial Products. Vol. VI. Growth and Metabolism. Vol. VII. Microbial Transformation.

Cutaneous Melanoma: Status of Knowledge and Future Perspective, U. Veronesi, N. Cascinelli and M. Santinami Eds., Academic Press, London, 1987.

Fawcett, Col. P.H., *Lost Trails, Lost Cities*, Funk & Wagnalls, New York, 1953.

"Guidelines on Diet, Nutrition, and Cancer Prevention: Reducing the Risk of Cancer with Healthy Food Choices and Physical Activity," prepared by the American Cancer Society 1996 Advisory Committee on Diet, Nutrition, and Cancer Prevention, *CA—A Cancer Journal for Clinicians*, 46(6), 325–341 (November/December, 1996)

Handbook of Microbiology, see *CRC Handbook of Microbiology*.

Harper's Biochemistry, see Murray, Robert K. et al.

Hartwell, Jonathan L., *Plants Used Against Cancer*, Quarterman Publications, Lawrence MA, 1982. Foreword by Jim Duke.

Hasselberger, Francis X., *Uses of Enzymes and Mobilized Enzymes*, Nelson-Hall, Chicago, 1978.

Jain, Mahenda Kumar, *Handbook of Enzyme Inhibitors (1965–1977)*, Wiley, New York, 1982.

Mallis, Arnold, with contributing editors, *Handbook of Pest Control: The Behavior, Life History, and Control of Household Pests*, Franzak & Foster, Cleveland OH, in seven editions, 1945–1990, e.g., the 6th ed., 1982.

Methods in Plant Biochemistry, P.M. Dey and J.B. Harborne Series Eds., Academic Press, London, 1990–1991. Vol. 1. *Plant Phenolics*, J.B. Harborne Ed., 1991. Vol. 2. *Carbohydrates*, P.M. Dey Ed., 1990. Vol. 3. *Enzymes of Primary Metabolism*, P.J. Lea Ed., 1990. Vol. 4. *Lipids, Membranes and Aspects of Photobiology*, J.L. Harwood and J.R. Bowyer Eds., 1990. Vol. 5. *Amino Acids, Proteins and Nucleic Acids*, L.J. Rogers Ed., 1991. Vol. 6. *Assays for Bioactivity*, K. Hostettmann Ed., 1991.

Moss, Ralph W., *Cancer Therapy: The Independent Consumer's Guide To Non-Toxic Treatment & Prevention*, Equinox Press, New York, 1992.

Murray, Robert K., Daryl K. Granner, Peter A. Mayes and Victor W. Rodwell, *Harper's Biochemistry*, 24th ed., Appleton & Lange, Stamford CT, 1990, 1993, 1996. Lange Medical Publications, 1988.

Rifkin, Jeremy, *Beyond Beef: The Rise and Fall of the Cattle Culture*, Dutton, New York, 1992.

Role of the Gut Flora in Toxicity and Cancer, I.R. Rowland Ed., Academic Press, London, 1988.

Sidransky, David, "Nucleic Acid-Based Methods for the Detection of Cancer," *Science*, 278, 1054–1058 (November 7, 1997).

Sigma Chemical Company Catalog, *Biochemicals, Organic Compounds, and Diagnostic Reagents*, St. Louis MO, 1996–.

Stefansson, Valhjalmur, *Cancer: Disease of Civilization?: An Anthropological and Historical Study*, Hill and Wang, New York, 1960. Introduction by René Dubos.

Stefansson, Valhjalmur, *The Fat of the Land*, Macmillan, New York, 1956. With Comment by Frederick J. Stare, M.D., and Paul Dudley White, M.D. Originally published as *Not by Bread Alone*, Macmillan, New York, 1946.

Stress Proteins in Biology and Medicine, Richard I. Morimoto, Alfred Tissiéres and Costa Georgopoulos Eds., Cold Spring Harbor Laboratory Press, Plainview NY, 1990.

Taguchi, H. and M. Yoshida, "Chaperonin from *Thermus thermophilus* Can Protect Several Enzymes from Irreversible Heat Denaturation by Capturing Denaturation Intermediate," *J. Biol. Chem.*, *268*(8), 5371–5375 (March 15, 1993).

Vaccination Strategies of Tropical Diseases, F.Y. Liew Ed., CRC Press, Boca Raton FL, 1989.

Voet, Donald and Judith G. Voet, *Biochemistry*, 2d ed., Wiley, New York, 1995.

Walters, Richard, *Options: The Alternative Cancer Therapy Book*, Avery Publishing Group, Garden City Park NY, 1993.

Weeds of the West. Tom D. Whitson, Editor. Authors: Larry C. Burrill, Steven A. Dewey, David W. Cudney, B.E. Nelson, Richard D. Lee, Robert Parker. With a list of Contributors. Published by the Western Society of Weed Science in cooperation with the Western United States Land Grant Universities Cooperative Extension Services, College of Agriculture, University of Wyoming, Laramie, January, 1991.

Zollner, Helmward, *Handbook of Enzyme Inhibitors*, VCH Verlagsgellschaft mbH. Weinheim, FRG, 1989. VCH Publishers, New York.

Zollner, Helmward, *Handbook of Enzyme Inhibitors*, 2d ed., revised and enlarged, in two volumes, VCH Verlagsgellschaft mbH. Weinheim, FRG, 1993. VCH Publishers, New York.

Viruses and Cancer

Part 7

Viruses and Cancer

Increasingly, there seems to be a connection between viruses and cancer, seen in the further establishment of a biological mechanism whereby viruses invade a cancer cell to create cancer-forming oncogenes. This is as distinguished from the usual role of viruses to invade a cell and destroy the cell, at the same time proliferating.

Additionally, viruses may be the (so far) unsuspected causes involved in other strange illnesses, and the subviral particles known as prions have entered the scene. Genetic alterations that may be induced by viruses are, of course, a concern—for instance, with the onset of German measles or rubella during early pregnancy, caused by what is known as a *togavirus*. In fact, viruses may conceivably explain the mutations occurring in different species of frogs worldwide. These minute bits of molecular matter called viruses are indeed of consequence, not only with regard to cancer but with other phenomena as well.

7.1 MORE ABOUT VIRUSES AND OTHER PATHOGENS

A definition of viruses that has been supplied is as follows (Voet and Voet, *Biochemistry*, p. 1074):

> Viruses are parasitic entities, consisting of nucleic acid molecules with protective coats which are replicated by the enzymatic machinery of suitable host cells.

Furthermore, lacking metabolic machinery, technically, viruses are not alive. The intact virus particle, or virion, is composed of a nucleic acid molecule encased by a protein capsid. The capsid is said to be constructed of one or several protein subunits that are juxtaposed in a symmetrical or nearly symmetrical fashion. The two possibilities found are helical viruses in which the protein subunits form helical tubes, and spherical viruses in which the coat proteins aggregate in closed polyhedral shells. (The arrangements can be considered as the natural state.)

In instances, the nature of the proteins has been identified (Voet and Voet, *Biochemistry*, p. 1076ff). Perhaps the most studied is the *tobacco mosaic virus* or *TMV*. Its protein subunits each consist of 158 amino acid residues, arranged in a helix, with a single RNA strand composed of approximately 6400 nucleotides. In the reference, the structure of TMV protein includes polypeptide chains as ribbons.

Suffice it to say, we are also speaking of *proteins* and *peptides* when we are speaking of viruses. The inference, therefore, is that *heat shock proteins (hsp)* or *molecular chaperones* are also involved in the transmission of viruses to and from the host cell. In turn, the viruses expectedly affect the metabolic machinery of the host cell and, depending on the virus, there is the latent possibility for the creation of a cancerous condition in the cell as well as causing other diseases specific to the particular virus or viruses. *The usual action of a disease-causing virus is to invade a cell, where it replicates, but which results in the dissolution and death of the cell. In mammals, some viruses will invade the cells of the nervous system,* producing brain encephalitis for instance, as in case of the rabies virus. *Some viruses infect bacteria* and are called *bacterial viruses* or *bacteriophages* ("phage" meaning to eat—to "eat" the bacteria, in this case) and may sometimes be designated by letter, as by the Greek letter λ. Viruses may be further classed as *virulent*, in which they "lyse" cells in a process called lysogeny, or classed as *temperate*, in which they do not always kill the host cell.

A virus such as the rabies virus can be classed as virulent and, in this case, is always or nearly always fatal to humans unless remedial action is taken by the Pasteur treatment. Pretreatment by immunization can also be induced, both to humans and animals, and is a means for the control of rabies in animal populations. The subject will be further discussed in a subsequent section on rhabdoviruses.

The use of the term *lysogeny* also occurs in a broader sense, as explained in a following section titled "Lysogeny, Viruses, and Cancer." That is, viruses may invade a cell and combine with the chromosomal genes to become what are called *proviruses*, which in turn result in the formation of *oncogenes*—that is, tumor-inducing genes. Thus, not only may oncogenes be *inherited*, or otherwise occur, but they may be virus induced. In consequence, *viruses must remain suspect as a principal cause of cancer,* directly or indirectly. Exactly which viruses are involved seems not yet to be spelled out in full, although *papovaviruses*, for instance, are candidates.

In fact, in *Infectious Cancers of Animals and Man*, by Richard N. T-W-Fiennes, the potential carriers of cancer-causing viruses have been listed (in 1982) as the herpesvirus group, the oncornovirus group, the papilloma virus group (part of the papovaviruses), and the adenovirus group (T-W-Fiennes, *Infectious Cancers*, pp. 103–104). It may be expected that the range of cancer-causing virus families is considerably larger than this, especially since the classification of cancer families is to some extent arbitrary. It may be noted, moreover, that the oncornoviruses (oncogenic RNA viruses) include the retroviruses, which are increasingly indicted, a subject to be further considered.

Beyond their involvement with cancer and their causation of known diseases, viruses are increasingly found to be the unsuspected causes of diseases both common and rare. Thus, *virus-caused illnesses are turning out to be much more ubiquitous than formerly thought*—above and beyond what is already known, which is considerable. The tantalizing prospect is always immunization by vaccines.

In further explanation, many of the common infectious diseases are caused by viruses (such as polio, mumps, measles, influenza, hepatitis, herpes simplex, smallpox, chickenpox), and conventional vaccines have been developed in a considerable number of cases, although there remain many other diseases for which a vaccine is not available (F.Y. Lieu, in *Vaccination Strategies*, p. 4ff.; Martin J. Carrier, in *Vaccination Strategies*, p. 12ff). *With conventional vaccines, moreover, there is the risk for virulence or contamination, and effectiveness.* *

Accordingly, as described in the aforecited references, there is much interest in developing synthetic vaccines by genetic engineering via recombinant DNA (rDNA) techniques using such organisms as vaccinia virus and salmonella mutants as carriers. *The end products are peptides or proteins, which to a degree provide protective immunity,* whether a given antigen provokes a B cell or a T cell response. Such synthetic vaccines may be called *subunit vaccines* and are further described in the references. In addition to *viral* subunit vaccines or possibilities for hepatitis, influenza, herpes simplex, foot-and-mouth disease, and hopefully AIDS, there are *bacterial* subunit vaccines, such as for tetanus toxin, diphtheria toxin, bacterial toxins in general, pertussis or whooping cough, and mycobacteria. (These would conceivably replace or augment the vaccine series for diphtheria, pertussis, and tetanus—better known as DPT—and presumably could be extended to typhoid.) Beyond this is the potential for *parasite* subunit vaccines. (No possibilities are indicated for a *synthetic cancer vaccine*.)

Another possibility in the development of vaccines is the utilization of *vaccinia virus,* the source for smallpox vaccine (Geoffrey L. Smith, in *Vaccination Strategies*, p. 32ff). The vaccinia virus is closely related to the cowpox virus, both being orthopoxviruses which interact, and vaccinia may serve as a carrier for vaccine antigens. The genome is described as a double-stranded DNA (dsDNA) molecule, and the poxviruses are unusual in that they replicate in the cytoplasm. There are very few complications in the use of vaccinia virus, noted in the reference, and there is the potential of constructing polyvalent vaccines that act against a number of diseases—including malaria. (And maybe against cancer-inducing viruses.)

---

* A concomitant problem with such diseases as measles and mumps is that encephalitis or brain inflammation may develop not only from the disease itself but from the vaccine (Moses Grossman, in *Vaccination Strategies*, pp. 589–591, 577). Varicella zoster or chickenpox and herpes zoster are other sources for the problem. The old rabies vaccine, vaccinia vaccine for smallpox, and pertussis or whooping cough vaccine have been implicated. The symptoms of encephalitis are fever, chills, malaise, and headache, which may be followed by lethargy, somnolence, vomiting, coma, and convulsions. In general, we are talking of infections of the central nervous system (CNS) caused by such varied agents as pyogenic (pus-forming) bacteria, mycobacteria, parasites, fungi, yeasts, and viruses, and which can result in encephalitis, meningitis, meningoencephalitis, or brain abscesses. There may be an accompanying disruption of the absorption of cerebrospinal fluid (CSF). *Any suspected infection of the CNS represents a medical emergency.*

In discussing recombinant vaccinia viruses as vaccines, the above reference includes the subject of inducing antibodies to internal antigens. (The adjective *recombinant* signifies a hybrid form or crossover; that is, a "recombined" form.) These antibodies are mostly *immunoglobulin G* (IgG), but local secretory IgA is also produced using vaccinia virus. The generalization is literally to scores of different vaccinia antigens. It is also mentioned that live vaccines will usually evoke good cell-mediated immune responses as well as antibody responses. Furthermore, the following statement was made:

A human vaccinated with a recombinant vaccinia virus expressing the human immunodeficiency virus (HIV) gp160 envelope protein also developed a T cell response to this protein.

Similar kinds of results were obtained with influenza virus HA. (As previously noted, to the extent that cancerous cells may be virus-induced, these findings are of concerted significance.)

The action of viruses as cell destroyers is as distinguished from the action of bacteria, which produce toxins (exotoxins and enterotoxins). These toxins or poisons are proteins or proteinaceous compounds such as lipoproteinsaccharides, which in effect act as enzyme inhibitors for one or another of the body functions, some of which may be vital, with a fatal outcome. (This is also why, in fact, that there is an occasional interest in bacteria of one kind or another as anticancer agents. *Presumably the toxin produced could be specific against cancer cells.*) An example of a serious disease caused by bacteria is typhus or typhus fever. Epidemic typhus is caused by *Rickettsia prowazekii*, a bacterium carried by the body louse *Pediculus humanus corporis*. In general, these bacteria are of the family designated Rickettsiae and are called coccabacillary organisms, as found in arthropod insect hosts such as lice and fleas. Moreover, these microorganisms are *pleomorphic* or may otherwise occur in several distinct forms (*Encyclopedia Americana*, under Typhus Fever). The consequences are vascular and neurological disorders, which can lead to death. *Antibiotics act against typhus, and a vaccine is available.*

Another serious bacterial disease is the plague or black death, in particular bubonic plague, which may end up as pneumonic plague or in another form called septicemic plague. It is caused by the bacillum *Yersinia pestis,* which produces toxins affecting the normal functioning of the circulatory system. The disease, fortunately, responds to antibiotics. The bacterium may be carried by the oriental rat flea *Xenopsylla cheopis* or by other fleas. The reservoirs for the fleas are rodents, notably the common black house rat *Rattus rattus*—but various other rodents may also serve, such as gophers, chipmunks, jack-rabbits, and prairie dogs as found in the American West. There are other kinds of plague, caused by other bacteria of the same genus, that may be carried by other kinds of fleas or arthropods and involve other reservoirs such as the Norway rat or the house mouse. Bubonic plague may very well have had its origins in the Central Asia or Eurasia, from which it spread to other parts of the world, but its evolution evidently remains a mystery.

The origins not only of bacteria but of viruses can, in fact, be of great concern. Among other things, this will shed light on how the disease may erupt and can be countered or contained. For example, certain viruses interact with both plants and insects, and others interact with both insects and mammals or humans—not to mention that viruses interact among humans and other animals or mammals. Thus, knowing the sources for mysterious and newly emerging viruses such as the Marburg and Ebola viruses would be of inestimable value in the fight against these disease-causing microorganisms.

The two principal virus structures are the rod and the icosahedron, although bacterial viruses or bacteriophages have completely different structures of their own, indicating a separateness in origins. A classification of the kinds of viruses will include such names as adenoviruses, herpesviruses, myxoviruses (e.g., which cause influenza), paramyxoviruses, picornaviruses, poxviruses, reoviroses, rhabdoviruses (e.g., species of which cause rabies), and togaviruses (e.g., which cause German measles or rubella), some of which will be further discussed. A brief rundown of virus families is provided in Table 7.1 based on information in the *Encyclopedia Britannica*, 15th ed., as published in 1995. Some of the viruses will be further elaborated upon. Furthermore, the emphasis henceforth will in the main be on cancer-causing aspects.

In an article by Bernard Le Guenno, published in the October, 1995 issue of the *Scientific American*, it is stated that the Ebola virus is a hemorrhagic fever virus and is among the most dangerous biological agents yet known. *New ones are discovered yearly, and their spread is triggered by natural and artificial environmental changes—including the destruction of tropical rain forests.*

Le Guenno explains that the speedy evolution found among hemorrhagic fever viruses is due to the nature of their genetic makeup. Instead of being composed of DNA, as with most living things, the

Table 7.1 Classification of Virus Families

DNA Viruses

Adenoviridae (dimension, about 80 nm). Genome consists of linear dsDNA. The subgroup Mastadenoviruses infect mammals, and Aviadenoviruses infect birds. These viruses cause respiratory and gastrointestinal disorders in humans, and some types may produce **malignant transformations** in culture cells and animals.

Herpesviridae (dimension, about 105 nm). Genome consists of linear dsDNA. The subfamily Alphaherpesvirinae is comprised of human **herpes simplex** viruses types 1 and 2, bovine mamillitis virus, SA 8 virus and monkey B virus, pseudorabies virus, equine herpesvirus, and **varicella-zoster** virus. Betaherpesvirinae is composed of various cytomegaloviruses. Gammaherpesvirinae is composed of **Epstein-Barr** virus, baboon herpesvirus, chimpanzee herpesvirus, Marek's disease virus of chickens, turkey herpesvirus, herpesvirus saimiri, and herpesvirus ateles.

Iridoviridae (dimension, 130–300 nm). The virions or virus particles contain linear dsDNA. The genera include iridovirus and chloridirovirus, known to infect insects. Other genera comprise African swine fever virus and lymphocystic disease virus.

Papovaviridae (dimension, 45–55 nm). Virions contain covalently linked circular DNA. The genus comprising polyomaviruses consists of SV40 and polyoma viruses, and cause **malignant transformations** in infected cells. The genus comprising papillomaviruses (which, incidentally, do not grow in cell cultures) usually produces warts and benign papillomas.

Parvoviridae (dimension, 18–26 nm). Virions contain ssDNA. Infect both vertebrates and insects. The vertebrate viruses may be divided into those which replicate unaided, and those which replicate with the assistance of adenoviruses or herpesviruses, and which are also called adenoassociated viruses (AAV) or dependoviruses.

Poxviridae (dimensions, 400 × 200 nm, large with complex structures). Genome consists of linear dsDNA. The subfamily Chordopoxvirinae infects vertebrates. The subfamily Entomopoxvirinae infects arthropods. The former includes groups called orthopoxviruses, parapoxviruses, and avipoxeviruses which variously infect rabbits, sheep, swine, and birds.

RNA Viruses

Arenaviridae (dimension, 100–200 nm). Virions contain 2 segments of minus-strand RNA and small amounts of ribosomal RNA. The family is divided into 4 genera, with the viruses widely distributed in animals. The viruses are transmitted by insects, and cause serious diseases.

Bunyviridae (dimension, about 95 nm). Virions contain single-strand RNA of negative sense. The four genera are bunyvirus, phlebovirus, nairovirus, and uukuvirus. It is noted that many viruses occur in this family.

Caliciviridae (dimension, about 38 nm). Genome consists of single plus-strand RNA. The prototype virus is known as the vesicular exanthema of swine virus.

Coronaviridae (dimension, 60–22 nm). Genome contains single plus-strand RNA. Club-shaped glycoprotein spikes in capsid envelope resemble a crown or corona. The viruses produce gastrointestinal disease in humans, bovines, and poultry.

Filoviradae or Filaviridae (among the largest viruses, circa 850–950 nm × 20–30 nm). This is a new classification for the **Marburg and Ebola viruses**, both causing viral hemorrhagic fevers, and not yet listed in the *Encyclopedia Britannica* as of 1995 (e.g., Joseph B. McCormick and Susan Fischer-Hoch, in *Tropical and Geographical Medicine*, p. 713ff.; Scott B. Halstead, in *Tropical Medicine and Parasitology*, p. 20).

Flaviviridae (a newly designated family, described as enveloped and spherical in shape). Genome consists of nonsegmented single plus-strand RNA. Transmitted either by insects or arachnids (spiders). The viruses cause such severe diseases as **yellow fever, dengue**, tick-borne encephalitis, and Japans B encephalitis.

Orthomyxoviridae (dimension, about 100 nm). Virions contain eight segments of negative-strand RNA and endogenous RNA polymerase. The viruses of this family consist only of **influenza** viruses of the three antigenic types A, B, and C.

Paramyxoviridae (dimension, 150–300 nm). Virions contain a single negative-strand nonsegmented RNA and an endogenous RNA polymerase. The lipoprotein envelope has two glycoprotein spikes designated as hemagglutinin-neurominidase (HN), apparently an enzyme, and fusion factor (F). The principal genus of the family is denoted as paramyxovirus, and consists of human parainfluenza viruses and **mumps** virus, and also the **Newcastle disease** virus found in poultry. The genus called morbillivirus includes viruses responsible for **measles** in humans, **distemper** in dogs and cats, and **rinderpest** in cattle. Another genus, known as pneumovirus, is responsible for what is called **respiratory syncytial virus disease**, a serious disease occurring in human infants.

Table 7.1 Classification of Virus Families *(continued)*

Picornaviridae (dimension, 27–30 nm). Virions contain nonsegmented ss, plus-strand RNA. There are four known genera. The enteroviruses consist of **polioviruses, Coxsackie viruses**, and **echoviruses**. The cardioviruses are not further described. The rhinoviruses consist of the **common cold** viruses. The aphthoviruses include the **foot-and-mouth disease** virus of cattle.

Reoviridae (dimension, 60–80 nm). Virions contain dsRNA in 10–12 segments. The viruses are known to infect many plant and animal species. There are four genera, called orthoreoviruses, orbiviruses, rotaviruses, and cypovirus. The orbiviruses occur widely in insects and vertebrates, an example being the bluetongue virus disease of sheep. Rotaviruses are the widespread agents causing gastroenteritis in mammals, e.g., in humans. The cypovirus prototype produces the insect disease named cytoplasmic polyhedrosis.

Retroviridae (dimension, about 90 nm). Nondefective virions contain two identical copies of single plus-strand RNA and the enzyme reverse transcriptase. The latter, the enzyme also known as RNA-dependent DNA polymerase, catalyzes the synthesis of dsDNA from the viral RNA template. A feature of the RNA templates is what are called long terminal repeat (LTR) nucleotide sequences. **This feature serves to integrate DNA into the chromosomes of the host cell.** Retroviridae are known to cause **cancers** in many species of animals, notably humans. This consequence very likely originates from normal cell nucleotide sequences known as **proto-oncogenes**.

Rhabdoviridae (dimensions 180–300 × 65 nm, bullet-shaped). Virions contain single minus-strand RNA and endogenous RNA polymerase. The lipoprotein envelope contains a single glycoprotein, the type-specific antigen. The viruses infect a wide variety of both plants and animals, ranging from insects to humans. There are two genera that, in particular, infect animal. The one genus is known as vesicular virus, causing vesicular stomatitis in swine, cattle, and equines. The other genus is called lyssavirus, which includes the **rabies** virus.

Togaviridae (dimension, about 30 nm). Genome consists of single plus-strand RNA. Of the three recognized genera, one is transmitted by arthropods, namely mosquitoes. Called alphaviruses, the members of this genus are the prototype examples for the Sindbis virus, and eastern and western encephalitis viruses. The other two genera are not arthropod-borne, and consist of rubivirus, which causes **German measles**, and pestivirus, which comprises such mucosal disease viruses as bovine virus (or diarrhea virus) and **hog cholera** virus.

Source: Data from the *Encyclopedia Britannica*, 15th ed., 1995, pp. 510–511; also 15th ed., 1997.

Note: The symbol "nm" stands for nanometers, a nanometer being one-billionth of a meter, or one millionth of a millimeter, or one thousandth of a micron. By comparison, an angstrom is one tenth of one billionth of a meter, so that 10 Å equal 1 nm. The symbol "ds" stands for double-stranded, whereas "ss" stands for single-stranded.

genes of these viruses consist of RNA and must be converted by an enzyme called RNA polymerase (in this case, RNA-directed DNA polymerase or reverse transcriptase), which leads to frequent errors in the conversion process. The result is an accumulation of mutations. This conversion or reversion is connoted by the commonly used name "retrovirus."

It may be added that these successive mutations work against ever developing a successful vaccine.

7.1.1 SOME OBSERVATIONS ON VIRUSES AND CANCER

A paper presented by G.J. Todaro at the seventh Cold Spring Harbor Conference on Cell Proliferation was titled, "Summary: Tumor Virus Genes in the 'Real World'—Current Status," and appears as the concluding chapter in *Viruses in Naturally Occurring Cancers*, Book B, edited by Myron Essex, George Todaro, and Harald zur Hausen, published in 1980. The thrust of the conference was that viruses cause naturally occurring cancers and sometimes should be taken seriously as risk factors in human cancers. It was noted, however, that although viruses are risk factors, it is doubtful that they are, by themselves, "necessary and sufficient to produce the disease."

Furthermore, *finding a virus in a tumor cell does not necessarily mean that viral infection contributed to the development of the tumor.* But the converse is also not true, namely that "not finding a virus in tumors in no way can be taken that viruses were not involved." A mere portion of the virus—the transforming region—may be all it takes. It is stated that viral proteins needn't be gene-expressed, and the cancer-inducing mechanism may involve host cell gene-activation. This pertains especially to large DNA-continuing viruses. That is, since the DNA is so complex, only a small part of the total genome (complement of genetic information) is required. Efforts that try to find the entire genome may be misleading. And the effects of viral infection may be more indirect and be secondary to cell necrosis and regeneration. Such may not necessitate the continued presence of the virus.*

Todaro, writing in *Viruses in Naturally Occurring Cancers*, affirms that the three main viruses for which there is considerable evidence for causing human cancer are the *Epstein-Barr virus (EBV)*, the *hepatitis B virus,* and the group of *papilloma viruses.*

Thus, it is becoming increasingly evident that the Epstein-Barr virus is a major risk factor for Burkitt's lymphoma (BL) and for nasopharangeal carcinoma (NPC). Moreover, the virus acts with other factors such as immune depression, genetic factors, and maybe even malarial infection.

The hepatitis B virus appears to be the major risk factor in one of the most common tumors in the world, hepatocellular carcinoma (liver cell cancer), and vaccines are a possibility. Papilloma viruses, also called papovaviruses, cause benign cell proliferation in the epidermis and in mucosal surfaces, but which can lead to malignancies. (Human papillomavirus or HPV is a very common type of virus, with more than 75 different strains now identified, that are numbered. Some cause ordinary warts on the hands, arms, or legs. Cervical cancer is directly linked to HPV, with most related to numbers 16 and 18.) Squamous-cell carcinomas may develop at sites exposed to light. (The descriptor "squamous" means scale-like or covered with scales, but in anatomy pertains to the anterior upper portion of the temporal bone, the sides of the skull which are designated the temples.) A particularly intriguing fact observed by Todaro is that *"Although papilloma virus particles can be seen in the papillomas, they can no longer be found in the carcinomas."*†

Todaro goes on to supply sections dealing with oncogenic DNA viruses, herpes viruses of animals and man, hepatitis B virus, infectious type-C viruses, endogenous retroviruses, transmission of retroviruses and oncogenes, and retroviruses in human tumors. Although published in 1980, the material seemingly remains up to date, and beyond that, is uncommonly readable. Information items gleaned from the various sections are as follows.

The oncogenic DNA viruses include hepatitis B, probably the most important DNA tumor virus in man. The papilloma viruses or papovaviruses are classed within this group, and include Simian virus 40 (SV40) DNA, which was a contaminant in some early polio vaccine stocks, but the recipients have shown no excessive cancer risk. The human viruses called BK and JC are widely distributed, with the former infecting 86 percent of the human population before age five. These viruses have been found to cause a wide variety of tumors in hamsters, including abdominal tumors. The JC virus has caused brain tumors in owl monkeys. Evidence for an extrapolation to humans is not compelling. Back to SV40, closely related if not identical strains have been reported from melanoma patients and from human tissues, and also from the glioblastoma multiforme cell line (glioblastoma is a kind of brain tumor). It is noted that the papovavirus T antigen is a potent immunigen and may provide cellular immunity to tumors (as a potential vaccine).

The African green monkey lymphotropic papovavirus (AGM-LP) indicates an entire new class of viruses (the implication is to AIDS and to the Marburg and Ebola viruses). The papilloma virus HPV-5 can be detected in patients with epidermodysplasia, with malignant conversion occurring in 20 to 30 percent of the cases. A synergistic connection has been found between papilloma virus infections and environmental carcinogens, e.g., the malignant conversion of esophageal papillomas to cancers associated with the consumption of *bracken fern,* which contains a strong chemical carcinogen.

Kansas cottontail rabbits have been studied for the progression of naturally occurring virus-induced cancers. *The natural regression that occurs in many tumors may be connected to substances released*

---

* It is of interest to compare the above with the results of Naessen and others as mentioned by Moss and by Walters. Naessen, for instance, advanced the idea, if not the irrefutable evidence, of particles smaller than viruses. Enter the finding of subviral pathogens, as introduced in Part 1 and elsewhere—e.g., prions (Voet and Voet, *Biochemistry*, p. 1113ff). We may in fact be talking of a whole spectrum of particles and particle sizes, ranging from remnants or pieces to aggregates or agglomerates, or polymers. It may, in large part, be a problem in semantics; that is, just what is to be called a virus?

† It can be asked, *are papilloma viruses involved in the formation of intestinal polyps on the intestine inner surfaces? These polyps are considered to be the source for colon cancer—which, it may be added, all too readily metastasizes to the liver and other parts of the body such as the lungs.* A keyword search of MEDLINE over the five-period 1992–1996 did not turn up any connection. But, then, maybe the subject has never been investigated from this standpoint.

by the lymphocytes. It was also found that the DNA extracted from the papillomas or from carcinomas would produce tumors when inoculated into the skin of other rabbits, indicating that the viruses have transforming genes. Among the human DNA-containing viruses, adenoviruses ("adeno-" signifying gland or glandular) are said to be the least likely candidates for causing human cancers.

The herpes viruses of animals and man have a large complicated genome (the complement of genetic information) by comparison with other tumor viruses, although cell transformation can be made from only small fragments of the genome. *The Epstein-Barr virus (EBV) is the clear cause of mononucleosis but is also a major risk factor candidate for Burkitt's lymphoma (BL) and for nasopharyngeal carcinoma (NPC).* Improvements in sanitary conditions reduce the risk of BL, and *the association between EBV and undifferentiated carcinomas of the nasopharynx is observably "high, consistent, and specific the world over."* Early detection is possible in terms of IgA (immunoglobulin A) titrations to EBV viral capsid antigens. (The capsid is the protective protein coat of the virus.) The herpesvirus papio (HVP) produces lymphomas in baboons and is a close relative of EBV. The herpes simplex virus type 2 (HSV-2) has been implicated as the necessary cause of some cervical cancers. Furthermore, HSV-2 can produce morphological transformations in hamster, mouse, and rat cells, and the cells become *tumorigenic.**

The hepatitis B virus shares a similarity with a virus isolated from the Eastern woodchuck. This latter virus is associated with the occurrence of hepatomas (liver cancers) in woodchucks, which is fairly common. Human hepatitis B itself has been related to hepatocellular carcinoma, or liver cancer, one of the most common cancers in the world, with at least 100,000 new cases every year. At the time of publication of the reference, it was noted that vaccine trials had begun in parts of Asia. The polypeptide surface antigen of hepatitis B may prove to be the best source of vaccine. It had not yet been proven that hepatitis B is a full-fledged tumor virus in that it has so far failed to produce specific transforming genes.

We further distinguish between *hepatitis A* and *hepatitis B,* collectively known as *viral hepatitis* (Richard A. Weisiger, in *Tropical Medicine,* p. 47ff.; Ian D. Gust, in *Tropical and Geographical Medicine,* p. 586ff.) There is also a third kind, known as *non-A, non-B.* Hepatitis A can also be described as infectious hepatitis (IH), epidemic hepatitis, or short incubation period hepatitis. Hepatitis B can be called serum hepatitis (SH), homologous serum jaundice, or long-incubation-period hepatitis. Still another kind is delta hepatitis, also called L-hepatitis or hepatitis D.

Hepatitis A is caused by a virus designated HAV. The virus particle is small, circa 27 nm, characterized as an unenveloped RNA virus of the family of enteroviruses. The disease is described as ancient and ubiquitous in humans. Although it can be transmitted to primates, it evidently doesn't occur naturally in the wild. Most people have been infected without clinical signs, and the symptoms are mild or not noticed. There is no specific treatment save rest, but recovery is complete. Occasionally gamma globulin may be employed.

Hepatitis B is caused by an enveloped virus designated HBV. As distinguished from HAV, it contains an unusual partially double-stranded DNA genome. The double-shelled virus particle or virion is circa 42 nm in diameter with an inner core circa 28 nm containing DNA, hepatitis B core antigen (HBcAg), and the enzyme DNA polymerase. (It may be commented that there are a number of known enzyme inhibitors for DNA polymerase, as listed in Appendix E.) Similarly to hepatitis A, hepatitis B has been found to be an ancient and ubiquitous disease in humans and is common and widespread. Again, although transmission to primates can occur, there appears to be no animal reservoir.

Formerly, hepatitis A or infectious hepatitis was thought to occur mainly from injections or by way of the mouth (e.g., from fecal contamination), whereas hepatitis B or serum hepatitis was thought to

---

* Incidentally, there is the possibility of a vaccine for Burkitt's lymphoma (Charles L.M. Olweny, in *Tropical and Geographical Medicine,* p. 53). The vaccine would utilize the high-molecular weight glycoprotein component found in the membrane antigen of the Epstein-Barr virus. *This possibility indicates a hope for vaccines against other cancer types, perhaps all cancers.* It may be added that experimental animals have been immunized against the Friends leukemia virus and against erythroleukemia, with the possibility of utilizing vaccinia recombinant vaccines (e.g., cowpox- or smallpox-type vaccines) against virus-induced cancers (Geoffrey L. Smith, in *Vaccination Strategies,* p. 38). These experimental vaccinia recombinants expressed polyoma large or middle T antigens, either before exposure or after the tumors had developed. In further explanation, vaccine proteins can be produced by the techniques of recombinant DNA technology (genetic engineering), which involve the *in vitro* manipulation of foreign DNA into a suitable host cell or organism (Martin J. Carrier, in *Vaccination Strategies,* pp. 12–14). Among the host cells that have been used are *E. coli, Bacillus subtilis, Saccharomyces cerevisiae,* or mammalian cells in culture.

occur mainly from blood transfusions. The sources are now considered more general, and the viruses or strains may coexist in the same source. The most obvious symptom of both is the sometimes yellowing of the skin called *jaundice,* although, on other occasions, the victim will hardly be aware. Still other cases are life threatening. The liver is the principal organ affected. Albeit having either form of the disease results in an immunity to that type, *the development of immunity for the one does not confer immunity for the other.*

Hepatitis B can be a much more serious disease than hepatitis A. For what is designated as acute hepatitis, the symptoms can vary from mild (usually in children) to extremely severe, resulting in fulminate (meaning explosive or sudden) hepatitis in a few percentages of cases, with fatal consequences. Thus, the outcome may range from complete resolution with attendant immunity to massive necrosis and death. Otherwise, a chronic infection may ensue, first evident as persistent hepatitis which, if not resolved, will transit into chronic active hepatitis.

Beyond these stages, *primary hepatocellular carcinoma* may be incurred. This is the most prevalent cause of cancer deaths in parts of tropical Africa, Southeast Asia, Japan, and other countries, as noted elsewhere.

Treatment is essentially the same for hepatitis B as for hepatitis A, which fundamentally means no treatment, with the disease running its course. Passive immunization has recently become commercially available using a recombinant subunit vaccine, as mentioned elsewhere (Martin J. Carrier, in *Vaccination Strategies,* p. 23). Treatment for the other forms of viral hepatitis is the same, which means no overt drug therapy.

An interesting aside about the herbal treatment of hepatitis is found in Harold Stephens and Albert Podell's *"Who Needs a Road?",* the story of the Trans World Record Expedition which, starting in the Winter of early 1966, circled the globe via Toyota Land Cruiser and Jeep—more than 40,000 land miles on the original tires. In his Chapter 17, titled "Remove Blanket for Access to MLG Torque Shaft," Stephens describes a bout with hepatitis. Marooned in and about Dacca in East Pakistan, Stephens came down with the usual symptoms, including intense jaundice, possibly from the water or from an unsterilized cholera shot in Afghanistan. The attending doctor prescribed two months in bed followed by another four months of convalescing. As an expediency, Stephens went to a Chinese herb doctor, who administered a routine based on some 2,500 years of Chinese herbal experience. Besides receiving acupuncture treatments, five times each day Stephens "swallowed two dozen green objects that looked like slugs." And three times a day took on a dozen large red-colored pills which he though might be vitamins. Plus, twice a day, he chewed-up a handful of sawdust-looking stuff. Meals consisted of bitter berries and high-protein mixtures remindful of shark's eyes and toad bellies. The most important feature was a two-gallon bucket of foul-smelling liquid. But Stephens got better each day, and after 10 days was up on his feet and ready to proceed on to Bangkok.

What are called the *infectious type-C viruses* include viruses that are the major causes of leukemias and lymphomas in chickens, mice, cats, cows, and a primate, the gibbon ape. In a section on endogenous retroviruses, the Todaro reference indicates that *RNA tumor virus genes are contained in chromosomal DNA of most vertebrates.* (We distinguish endogenous or internally generated from exogenous or externally generated, which may also be referred to as infectious.) Furthermore, there may be a vertical transmission from parents to progeny, and a horizontal transmission as infectious particles. Thus, the type-C viruses live and replicate as part of the cellular genetic machinery or may escape from the host's cell genome. *After escaping, they are able to reinsert themselves in other parts of the same cellular DNA, not only in other cells of the body, but in other animals of the same species, or even in other species.*

It is mentioned that *increasing numbers of retroviruses (both endogenous and infectious) are being found in tissues and cell lines of primates, that is, from several species of Old and New World monkeys*—e.g., woolly monkeys, baboons, langmuirs, and gibbon apes. *(The premonition, of course, is of HIV and AIDS, and maybe the Marburg virus and the Ebola virus or other newly emerging viruses.)*

Endogenous retroviruses can be viewed as cellular genes that can cause infectious and potentially pathogenic viral particles. (In so many words, *there is a connection between retroviruses and oncogenes,* which may be partly a game of semantics, but which is further explored in the section on "Lysogeny, Viruses, and Cancer.") Animals raised from birth in complete isolation show a greatly reduced incidence of tumors, although the answer is different for certain strains of inbred mice that are cancer prone. The latter develop leukemias or breast cancers because they contain virogenes or proviruses that, when activated, lead to cancer. *In studying relatives of the laboratory mouse, new families of retroviruses were discovered. It seems that much of the cellular genomes of vertebrate species is occupied by retroviral genetic material.*

The transmission of retroviruses and oncogenes is an important aspect of the overall tumor virus picture, for it is stated that *retroviruses clearly have the potential to pick up, recombine with, and transport genes to different sites. This may involve cells of the same tissue, or other tissues from the same animal or from animals of the same species, or even cells of tissues from other species.* Primates contain a number of different endogenous retroviruses, several of which exist in the cellular DNA as multigene families. In some species, activation may be easy, in others not so much so, and in still others not at all. As an example, among the infectious viruses, *the family of gibbon leukemia viruses transmit readily from primate to primate. Bovine leukemia virus (BLV), originally discovered in Europe, now has almost worldwide distribution and has also appeared in sheep. With regard to human cancers, there is as yet a lack of epidemiological (read statistical) evidence that horizontally transmitted retroviruses are a risk factor in human cancers.* (We exclude HIV.) However, *there is at least isolated empirical or experimental evidence linking transmissible agents to nasopharyngeal carcinoma, hepatocellular carcinoma, and cervical carcinoma.*

Speaking further of AIDS, it has evidently reached epidemic proportions in parts of Africa, however transmitted. Thus, Tudor Parfitt, in *Journey to the Vanished City*, published in 1992, about his search for a lost tribe of Israel in Africa, had some telling information at the start of his Chapter 28. In visiting with an Israeli doctor on a flight between points over eastern Africa, the doctor mentioned the extreme seriousness of AIDS in Malawi, in particular. In a survey of Malawi children who were under 12 years of age, it was found that *50 percent* were sero-positive. And, regarding child mortality, even before the advent of AIDS, only three countries had a higher infant mortality rate, these other countries being Borkina Faso (or Burkina Faso, formerly known as Upper Volta, located in West Africa south of Mali and north of Ghana), Yemen, and Afghanistan.

Now, with the onset of AIDS, the doctor thought the infant death rate must be incredible. "But the government does all it can to conceal the statistics." Malaria, for instance, is given a higher priority. The doctor added, "I think that AIDS can destroy Africa." He further mentioned that the so-called confrontation states are fighting political battles when the real enemy is AIDS. (In comment, this reinforces the need for general antiviral agents or viricides to act against such elusive and ever-changing or ever-mutating viral diseases. Some of these agents may potentially be derived from plant or herbal sources, as set forth in Part 2 and Appendix J. And it is not beyond conjecture that there may be a common link with cancer, not only the disease but the cure.)

As to *retroviruses in human tumors,* although there are potential pitfalls in linking retroviruses to human cancers, the same as in trying to associate papovaviruses or papilloma viruses with specific human cancers, there are nevertheless some reports deserving serious consideration. For instance, *substantial evidence is accumulating that both the papilloma virus group and the hepatitis virus group are major contributors to the etiology or causes of important human cancers.* There are in fact striking features in common, notably the very narrow tissue specificity and the difficulty of *in vitro* propagation. Thus, a rare cell type (a diffuse histiolytic lymphoma), when cultivated, released a type-C virus. Viral proteins cross-react with analogous proteins from other primate viruses. Type-C virions (virus particles) are found in cultures of both human teratocarcinoma cells ("terato-" denotes monster or monstrous) and testicular tumor cells. Cultures of fresh human lymphocytes derived from patients with cutaneous T-cell lymphomas contain novel type-C viral particles. A human breast cancer cell line contained an antigen with properties related to mouse mammary tumor virus (MMTV). The search was to continue for the *protein* responsible for the antigenic reaction.

Todaro concludes that *viruses are examples of what may be called environmental carcinogens* and that health and sanitary measures have eradicated certain once-common cancers in the U.S. and Europe, although they are still common in other parts of the world. He observes that, with the exception of smoking-related cancers, the major risk factors appear to be biologic agents, especially viruses, as well as microorganisms such as the aflatoxin-producing *Aspergillus flavus.*

In further comment, it can be judged that *viruses provide but one more way to cause aberrations—read genetic aberrations—in cells, along with radiation and chemicals.* If, as the latest point of view has it, cancers are caused by oncogenes and only oncogenes, then wherefrom the oncogenes? In fact, what exactly is to be meant by an oncogene? Are we merely dealing with tautologies, redundancies, or circularities? If we say that oncogenes cause cancer, is not this merely a different way of saying that cancer is caused by oncogenes? The one means the other; that is, the one is tautological with the other, and vice versa.

And are these genes merely inherited, to become "activated" during the course of time, or are other factors at work such as viruses, radiation, and/or chemicals? In fact, all possibilities seem valid and interconnected, and such differences as there appear to be, may only be another case of the blind men and the elephant. There seems to be a semantics problem imposed on the technical problems.

Which gets back around to such other matters as, for instance, how do such causal agents as viruses and chemicals enter cells and micelles in the first place, there to result in diseases such as cancer? And how may antidisease or anticancer agents such as enzyme inhibitors thereby penetrate into the cells? The answers, very possibly, may lie in stress proteins or heat shock proteins, or molecular chaperones, which may prove either beneficial or not so beneficial, depending on whether we are talking about cures or causes.

The descriptor "stress" seems especially appropriate, since medical folklore itself indicts stress as a major underlying cause of illness. There we supposedly have it.

Or we can attribute everything to viruses, even the effects of chemicals and radiation. Thus, in a chapter on the role of viruses, in particular retroviruses, the authors mention that endogenous proviruses can be induced to replicate by a variety of chemicals, e.g., halogenated pyrimidines and protein synthesis inhibitors (Duplan, Guillemain, and Astier, in *Radiation Carcinogenesis*, p. 74ff.) The same reference indicates that retroviruses can also be the causative agent in radiation carcinogenesis, that is, there is proviral activation by the radiation. (As to be further explained, a provirus is a virus that has been integrated into the cell chromosome.) Otherwise, the radiation is said to damage DNA structures, altering many sites in the purine and pyramidine rings, destroying ribose residues, breaking one or both strands of DNA, and producing DNA-protein crosslinks (James E. Cleaver, in *Radiation Carcinogenesis*, pp. 45–46.) Another reference, for instance, speaks in terms of radiation-induced chromosomal rearrangements and interactions or interchanges (C.R. Geard, in *Cell Transformation and Radiation-Induced Cancer*, p. 163ff). Chemical carcinogenesis, on the other hand, may be attributed to the chemical reactions or interactions with the four bases in DNA, notably with nitrogen or oxygen, as well as with the sugar residues and phosphates of the DNA backbone (Bernard Weinstein, in *Mechanisms of Chemical Carcinogensis*, p. 109). These various contributing effects are in part countered by the processes of DNA repair.

For the record, we repeat that *immunity is conferred by the type of white blood cells called lymphocytes* (Voet and Voet, *Biochemistry*, p. 1207). *Whereas, cellular immunity guards against virally infected cells, fungi, parasites, and foreign tissue, and is mediated by T cells originating in the thymus, humoral (body fluid) immunity acts against bacterial infections and extracellular viral infections, and is mediated by proteins known as antibodies or immunoglobulins produced by B lymphocytes or B cells, originating in the bone marrow. The immune response per se is triggered by the presence of foreign macromolecules, which are normally proteins, carbohydrates, and nucleic acids, collectively known as antigens.*

While bacterial infections are certainly included above, viruses and viral infections are the more pervasive, both within cells and outside of cells, that is, in body fluids.

And as to viruses and viral infections, cancer may be included as a consequence, whether expressed in terms of oncogenes, inherited or induced, or in terms of the genetics of viruses.It has now been found that *both cellular and humoral immunity are under genetic control,* albeit this is a truism, since every body component is affected by genes (Lucio Luzzatto, in *Tropical and Geographical Medicine*, p. 89). *This is contrary to the former viewpoint, where it was assumed that the immune response signified an acquired resistance to infectious agents rather than an innate resistance.* Thus, genetic variability turns out to be an important consideration. Moreover, there are considerations of *genetic polymorphism* (where allelic or contrasting genes occur at frequencies higher than would be expected for mutations), and there are different consequences in what are called *families* versus *populations*. (The subject is further represented in the reference in such rarefied terms as linkage disequilibrium, *major histocompatability complexes or MHCs,* and histocompatability loci antigens or HLAs. Suffice to say, the subject becomes increasingly complex, and the knowledge so far is said to be very limited.)

In a review paper by P.J. Fischinger, in a publication from the National Cancer Institute, published in 1992, it is remarked that over the last 25 years *there has been a major effort to identify human viruses that can cause human cancers either directly or indirectly.* By the latter qualification is meant that viruses can at least be considered significant cofactors or promoters of cancer. It is further stated that the prevailing view is that *tumor-associated viruses are necessary but not sufficient to cause tumors.* Moreover, there is a long latent period between the initial infection and the appearance of cancer, and the virus so implicated becomes part of the cellular DNA. *The virus types identified include both DNA- and RNA-containing viral agents from the hepadnavirus, herpesvirus, papovavirus, picornavirus, and lentivirus groups* (which is a somewhat longer listing than generally supplied). It is noted that these viral agents are not near as prevalent in the developed world, but *worldwide hundreds of millions of people are infected, and about one million of these develop virus-associated tumors each year.* It is further noted that nonviral cofactors are either suspected or have been identified in the formation of many virus-associated cancers. Fischinger concludes by calling for a major global approach to develop anticancer vaccines against the initial viral infections. He observes that such a human vaccine already exists in one case, and there is the promise that other candidate vaccines will soon be available. (This, of course, remains to be seen.)

7.1.2 ANTIVIRAL AND OTHER AGENTS

There are a number of antiviral, antibacterial, antifungal, antiparasitical, and other antidisease agents listed in Part 2 and in Appendices I, J, K, and L, and which are for the most part of plant origins. Such substances as vitamin C (ascorbic acid) are a possibility, perhaps, as is of a certainty the role of fever in combating disease, in particular infectious diseases. Even the cancer patient may note the onset of fever and an increased heart rate as the body attempts to throw off the cancer.* Whether these antidisease substances or phenomena may act as critical enzyme inhibitors is not fully explained in the literature.

Vitamin C, or ascorbic acid, in particular is a known inhibitor for a number of enzymes, as has been mentioned elsewhere. Thus, as listed in Jain's *Handbook*, the enzymes which are inhibited include adenylate cyclase, Na, K-ATPase, catalase, catechol o-methyltransferase, ferredoxin-NADP reductase (as derived say from spinach leaves), glucose-6-P dehydrogenase, lipase, fatty acid oxygenase, peroxidase, cAMP phosphodiesterase, tyrosinase, and what are referred to as *urea levels.* Jain also observes that vitamin C dehydroascorbate (an ascorbic acid conversion product) also acts as an inhibitor for Na, K-ATPase. [Dehydroascorbic acid is an oxidation product of ascorbic acid and further degrades to oxalic acid (Aree Valyasevi and Hamish N. Munro, in *Tropical and Geographical Medicine*, p. 1054). Oxalic acid is in itself an inhibitor for various enzymes.] Furthermore, it is indicated in Jain that the ascorbic acid inhibition of glucose-6-P dehydrogenase is associated with the presence of butanol (butyl alcohol) and is, in turn, due to hydrogen peroxide, and so on.†

As listed in Zollner's *Handbook*, the enzymes inhibited by ascorbate (i.e., ascorbic acid) are o-aminophenol oxidase, catalase, J-glucuronidase, GTP (guanosine triphosphate) cyclohydrolase I, hydroxymethylglutaryl-CoA reductase, lactoylglutathione lyase.

In further comment *ascorbic acid is related to the production or stabilization of collagen* (Voet and Voet, *Biochemistry*, p. 156). Collagen is a protein that is the main constituent of the fibrils of connective tissue and bones. An enzyme named prolyl hydroxylase is involved in its biosynthesis. Thus, if collagen is formed under conditions that inactivate prolyl hydroxylase, the collagen will denature, that is, lose its normal conformation (technically, denatured collagen is called *gelatin*). Ascorbic acid or vitamin C is necessary to maintain or promote the activity of prolyl hydroxylase, whereas without ascorbic acid the collagen will not form fibers in a proper manner, resulting in the disease known as *scurvy*.

Another consideration is the relation between *nutrition and infection,* and *nutrition and the immune function* (Leonardo Mata, in *Tropical and Geographical Medicine*, pp. 174-177; Gerald T. Keusch, in *Tropical and Geographical Medicine*, pp. 178-184). These twin topics, perforce, collide headlong with the controversies about the role of vitamins and minerals in combating disease and maintaining health. If vitamin and mineral deficiencies are indeed a part of the problem, especially in the Third World, then

---

* The pulse rate increases about 15 beats per minute for each 1° C rise in body temperature; the patterns of fever may be affected by modern chemotherapeutic agents and by the use of often irrational self-medication, and chronic fever of more than two weeks duration is usually due to infections or *malignancies* but is rarely caused by connective tissue diseases (Herbert M. Gilles and David A. Warrell, in *Tropical and Geographical Medicine*, pp. 4–6).

† It may be added that hydrogen peroxide has been prominently mentioned, albeit controversially, as an anticancer agent (Walters, *Options*, pp. 234-238). It may also be noted that butyric acid (in the form of its sodium or potassium salt) is said to be an agent for cellular apostosis, or selective cell death (Boik, *Cancer & Natural Medicine*, p. 13). And butanol is a reduction product of butyric acid.

consider the statement by Keusch that "the frequency of infectious diseases among the people in the developing world is astounding." Furthermore, a common sign of infection is fever, which places extra energy demands on the victim's body.

The reference further comments that infection alters the metabolism of the host, as if no food will be forthcoming, and loss of appetite, or anorexia, is an early sign of infection (Keusch, in *Tropical and Geographical Medicine*, pp. 178–179). It is noted that glucose is then supplied from endogenous sources, and that body protein is degraded to yield amino acids, the source for new protein synthesis. All in all, there is an efficient mobilization of the body's resources. *The proteolysis of muscle tissue, for example, produces amino acids that the liver then converts to glucose by the processes of gluconeogenesis.* Other of the amino acids so produced are deployed to synthesize proteins involved in the inflammatory response. The latter proteins formed are called acute phase reactants (or substrates), and include what are called complement components—that is, they backup or complete, or complement, the immune response. These proteins also form enzyme inhibitors and serve as transport or binding proteins for a few necessary minerals that are involved in the host responses to infection. Notable among these minerals are iron, zinc, and copper. (These also surface in the literature as anticancer agents.)

Along with other signals, fever ensues, which increases energy demands, that are partially compensated by the tendency to rest or sleep and conserve energy. Muscle metabolism, instead of relying on glycolysis, converts over to the *in situ* oxidation of branched-chain amino acids that are released during proteolysis. This so-called *functional insulin resistance* reduces glucose demands in muscle tissue. The synthesis of less-critical proteins such as albumin or transferrin is shut down. The resulting lack is designated as *hypoalbumenia* or *hypotransferrinemia*, signifying that infection has occurred. (There is the latent possibility that this condition can be also be interpreted as a potential indicator for monitoring the progression or regression of cancer.)

The foregoing infection-related phenomena are regulated by the small peptides called *cytokines*, which are released from infected macrophages or other cells. In addition to regulating metabolism, these cytokines regulate the immune response. These regulator proteins or cytokines include *interleukin 1 (IL-1)* and *interleukin 6 (IL-6)*, plus what is referred to as *cachectin/tumor necrosis factor (C/TNF)*, to be further described subsequently. IL-1 is said to be the principal endogenous pyrogen that produces fever. It is also a key regulator for T lymphocytes or T cells in that it induces the synthesis of interleukin 2 (IL-2), which is recognized as the T-cell growth factor.

What are called the *interferons* can also be considered to be *cytokines* and more specifically are *glycoproteins* (Voet and Voet, *Biochemistry*, p. 1005). Interferons are secreted by virus-infected vertebrate cells and were discovered from the fact that virus-infected persons will be resistant to a second type of virus. Interferons bind to the surface receptors of other cells, converting them to an antiviral state, a condition that acts against the replication of various DNA and RNA viruses.

The Voet and Voet reference further specifies three families of interferons. The first is type alpha or leukocyte interferon (the leukocytes or leucocytes being white blood cells). The second is type beta or fibroblast interferon (fibroblasts being the cells of connective tissue). The third is type gamma or lymphocyte interferon (lymphocytes being cells of the immune system).

Interferons are said to be potent antiviral agents, even at very low concentrations, and have been clinically used against cancers caused by viruses. (However, for cancers in general, the results have been disappointing.)

In a chapter on "Cancer, Cancer Genes, & Growth Factors," Robert K. Murray mentions and tabulates polypeptide growth factors, which include IL-1 and IL-2 among others (Murray, in *Harper's Biochemistry*, pp. 766–768). As the growth factor descriptor implies, they are mitogenic, that is, assist in cell division. While some growth factors interact with oncogenes and are involved in cancer cell proliferation, others may act as inhibitors, that is, act in a negative fashion. In the case of IL-2, it stimulates the growth of T cells, and this production is further stimulated or enhanced by Il-1. Thus these interleukins assist in the immune response. (The immune response is by and large ineffective against cancer cells, however, since the T-cells do not usually recognize cancer cells. The subject is further discussed in a subsequent section on immunity.)

For the record, the Sigma catalog lists interferons and several interleukins under the category "Alphabetical List of Compounds." Further listings of interleukins and other growth factors are presented under the category *immunochemicals*, in a section on "Growth Factors, Cytokines and Antibody Reagents." Growth factors include stem cell factors, transforming growth factors, and tumor necrosis factors.

(Various growth factors may also be called *cytokines*, e.g, in *Harper's Biochemistry*, p. 716.) If these listings are any indication, numerous substances have been tried against cancer outside of the realm of plant chemicals.

It is further stated in the foregoing Keusch reference that IL-1 induces the synthesis of other cytokines. The include, notably, IL-2, previously mentioned, which serves to activate the T-cell responses. Also mentioned is that IL-1 activates B cells for antibody production, namely by the induction of other cytokines such as IL-3 and IL-6, which in turn act on the B cell. Noted as well is that IL-6 stimulates what is called the *hepatic acute protein response* and may actually regulate some of the processes laid to IL-1.

Among the many other biochemical changes or processes is the depletion of lipid or fat stores which is regulated by a substance first named *cachectin* and later found to be identical to the *tumor necrosis factor,* or *TNF*—and henceforth designated as *C/TNF* (Keusch, in *Tropical and Geographical Medicine*, pp. 179–180). Another example of a metabolic change is the rapid uptake of iron and zinc by liver cells and mononuclear cells, accompanied by the release of copper-ceruloplasmin. [Cachectin or TNF is described as a 15,000-dalton protein produced from macrophages in response to various stimuli—such as the presence of malarial and trypanosome (e.g., sleeping sickness-causing) protozoan organisms (James H. McKerrow, in *Tropical Medicine and Parasitology*, p. 9).]*

It is stated by Keusch that *the most common nutritional problem in the world is protein-energy malnutrition, or PEM*. It is noted, furthermore, that PEM alters cell-mediated immunity. Among the biochemical changes are alterations in the circulating populations of T-lymphocytes. Also mentioned is a depression in the proliferative response to mitogenic lectins such as phytohemagglutinin (PHA).

The Keusch reference further outlines the action of some specific nutrients on T lymphocytes. Thus, *zinc deficiency may mimic the effects of PEM on the thymus*. The explanation provided is that many of the enzymes needed for the immune response are zinc-containing metallopeptides. The listing includes thymidine kinase, DNA polymerase, and DNA-dependent RNA polymerase (but evidently not RNA-dependent DNA polymerase, or reverse transcriptase, as occurs in retroviruses). Other zinc-containing enzymes are thymic hormone factors and terminal deoxynucleotidyl transferase.†

A figure is also provided in the reference that diagrams the effect of nutrients on the immunological network. Iron deficiency is noted to affect peripheral blood T lymphocytes.‡ Other deficiencies affecting the immunological network occur for such substances as pyridoxine (vitamin B6), vitamin A, copper, selenium (?), vitamin C, magnesium, and vitamin E. (Most or all of these various substances have found their way into medical folklore as anticancer agents. As to minerals, selenium and magnesium, for instance, rate chapters in Moss, and copper is mentioned frequently in both Moss and Walters.) Also shown in the aforecited diagram are the several immunoglobulins.

The Keusch reference concludes with a discussion of phagocytic cells. It is believed that bacterial infections in malnourished subjects could result from an acquired phagocytic (eating or destroying) cell dysfunction and/or defects in the complement system.

Whereas antibodies only function to identify foreign antigens, the complement system in turn inacti-vates and disposes of the invaders (Voet and Voet, *Biochemistry*, p. 1230ff). The complement system is made up of a complex set of 20 interacting plasma proteins. Its functions are to kill foreign cells by binding to and lysing the cell membranes; to stimulate the phagocytosis of the foreign particles; and to trigger local acute inflammatory reactions which seal off the area and attract more phagocytic cells. Voet and Voet further diagram the pathways and provide a tabulation for the various components of the

---

* There is the inference here that blood levels of TNF, iron, zinc, and/or copper could potentially be correlated to the progression or regression of cancer.

† Apparently, the folkloric remedy for taking zinc supplements against colds and the flu has a basis in scientific fact. The projection can be made to other infectious diseases, maybe even to cancer. There is a chapter on zinc and numerous other references in Ralph Moss's *Cancer Therapy*. There are citations also in Richard Walter's *Options*, e.g., in a chapter on the therapy of Hans Nieper, M.D. Thus, it is remarked that Dr. Nieper utilizes zinc and dry beta-carotene, with the comment that *zinc assists the lymphocytes or white blood cells to attack and destroy cancer cells,* activating the enzymes within the lymphocytes, which in turn digest the cancer cells. "Cancer patients nearly always show a deficit of zinc in their total blood."

‡ It has been noted that iron-deficient anemia generally accompanies cancer, but an excess of iron can be toxic (Walters, *Options*, pp. 178, 256). Moreover, chelation therapy can remove zinc and iron and other necessary minerals, adversely affecting immunity.

complement system. A further complexity is the alternate pathways by which certain proteins of the complement system target invading microorganisms and their pathway activators (Voet and Voet, *Biochemistry*, p. 1231). An example of the activators are polymers of microbial origin, for example, lipopolysaccharides of Gram-negative bacteria, called *endotoxins,* and what are called *cell wall teichoic acids* from Gram-positive bacteria. Other activators include certain bacteria, fungi, and virus-infected cells. The reference further notes, in this very complicated picture, that persons deficient genetically in certain components of the complement system will be highly susceptible to infection. We may ask if these infections extend to the causes of cancer?

It has been reported that *the bactericidal activity of polymorphonuclear leukocytes is diminished by an iron deficiency* (Keusch, in *Tropical and Geographical Medicine*, p. 182). This effect is probably due to a reduced MPO (myeloperoxidase) activity. On the other hand, the oral or intramuscular injection may increase the virulence of some microorganisms, since the excess iron is available for bacterial metabolism. It is noted that a zinc deficiency impairs chemotactic (directed toward—or away—from a chemical substance) activity of polymorphonuclear leukocytes or PMLs, which corrects itself on the administration of zinc. Contrarily, *an excess of zinc inhibits phagocytosis and the microbial activity of both PMLs and macrophages.*

A table is provided in the reference summarizing the effects of PEM on the immune system components. The division is by T lymphocytes, phagocytic cells, B lymphocytes, and the complement system.

A chapter on "Zinc and Other Trace Metals" by Noel W. Solomons and Manuel Ruz is presented in *Tropical and Geographical Medicine*, pp. 1083–1094. (The chapter following this particular chapter deals with "Iodine, Endemic Goiter, and Endemic Cretinism.") Trace elements are defined as those elements that make up approximately 0.01 percent of total body mass. An enumeration includes a number of elements proven to be of nutritional importance to mammalian species, and assumably to humans: iron, zinc, copper, manganese, chromium, selenium, molybdenum, cobalt, iodine, fluorine, nickel, vanadium (and limited others, such as the rare earth metals). The aforementioned chapter confines the discussion to zinc, copper, selenium, and chromium.

It is stated that the main role of zinc in mammalian metabolism is as a component of metalloenzymes. Examples are alkaline phosphatase, carbonic anhydrase, carboxypeptidase, and Zn-Cu superoxide dismutase. There are in fact many zinc-containing or zinc-activated enzymes involved in nuclear regulation and cell proliferation. Thus in cellular protein synthesis, zinc serves as a stabilizer for polyribosomes, and RNA polymerases contain zinc. It is further mentioned that the stabilizing membranes of circulating cellular elements involve zinc. Such cellular elements are red blood cells, macrophages, and platelets. The important immune-regulating, circulating thymus-derived hormones thymulin and thymosin contain zinc. Furthermore, zinc interacts with other nutrients, serving for instance in the transport of vitamin A from the liver and the conversion of retinol (vitamin A) to the aldehyde form (retinal), to be further converted to the pigment for night vision. *High levels of dietary zinc are noted to reduce the absorption of copper.* There is conceivably an interaction between zinc and essential fatty acids in humans, not yet defined.

Copper is efficiently absorbed from the diet, to be transported via the portal blood stream to the liver, with albumin as the carrier. There, the copper is either stored, to be distributed to the tissues via the hepatic protein ceruloplasmin, or else recycled to the gut via biliary secretions. The pancreatic secretion may regulate copper absorption. Copper is a component of several *cuproenzymes,* which are all involved in oxidation-reduction reactions. These cuproenzymes include lysyl oxidase, cytochrome c oxidase, *tyrosinase,* and Zn-Cu superoxide dismutase. Ceruloplasmin is noted to have enzymatic activity in the form ferroxidase I. *Copper is involved in a wide range of physiological functions:* erythropoiesis, lekopoiesis, *skeletal mineralization, connective tissue synthesis,* myelin formation, melanin pigment synthesis, catecholamine metabolism, *oxidative phosphorylation, thermal regulation, antioxidant protection, immune function, cardiac function,* and *glucose regulation. Ascorbic acid reduces the absorption of copper. Excess copper is pathogenic, and can result in hepatic cirrhosis.*

Selenium is obtained from normal dietary components, although milk is a poor source. Dietary levels from, say, cereal grains will depend on the selenium content of the soil. Nutritional yeasts are ordinarily low in selenium, but can be enhanced by the growth medium used. The major role is as a constituent of the enzyme glutathione oxidase. In this capacity, selenium provides antioxidant protection for the cytosolic milieu of the cell. Selenium is apparently involved in the hepatic detoxification of drugs by the cytochrome. *Selenium interacts with tocopherol (vitamin E),* providing a stabilizing effect, one to the other, to prevent liver necrosis and muscle disease. (Apparently of benefit in cardiac problems, given the publicity about vitamin E.) *Selenium absorption is favored by vitamin C.* Selenium evidently acts against mercury toxicity, e.g., from methylmercury. Selenium deficiency appears to be connected with what is called Keshan's disease, e.g., in China, which is a progressive myocardiopathy in children. It may also be related to PEM, or protein-energy malnutrition.

Inorganic *chromium* is absorbed inefficiently, although organic complexes in food are absorbed much more readily. The active form of chromium has in fact been found to be an organic complex of the trivalent chromic ion, Cr(III), with nicotinic acid (e.g., niacin) and glutathione, or at least with the latter's amino acid makeup. *Involved in the metabolism of glucose, this complex has been referred to as the "glucose tolerance factor."* There is an involvement, apparently poorly understood, with the functions of *insulin.* Chromium may also be connected with nucleic acid metabolism, leading to the inference that it plays a part in gene regulation.

One may choose to speculate, therefore, that the foregoing trace elements, and others, may be involved in many ways with cancer cell formation and metabolism, as well as with normal cells. The problem is that these ways are not sufficiently known.

With further regard to *fever*, it is a universal indicator for an infection and with some diseases is of a prominence to be used in the naming of the disease, e.g., dengue fever, and so on. Fever, however, is a more universal phenomenon. Thus, the *Encyclopedia Britannica*, 15th ed., 1997, mentions that, though fever is ordinarily associated with infections, it may be observed with "*cancer,* coronary artery occlusion, and disorders of the blood," and may follow from physiological stresses such as produced by "exercise or ovulation." Similarly, the *Encyclopedia Americana*, 1995, states that fever can accompany body tissue injuries, and occurs with many types of *tumors.* The latter include, particularly, "*lymphomas and certain cancers, such as of the lung, kidney, stomach, or pancreas."* Fever may follow a stroke or an immune system malfunction as with collagen diseases. Such metabolic disorders as gout may induce a fever. Fever resulting from a heart attack may be due to heart muscle injury. Brain injuries may affect the temperature-regulating centers, as may hyperthyroidism or other diseases affecting body heat production. Drugs may cause an increase in the rate of metabolism, or there may be a fever of unknown origin, or FUO. Heat stroke is perhaps the most severe example, producing temperatures of 110 to 112° F, or 43.3 to 44.4° C, versus a normal temperature of approximately 98.6° F or 37° C.

As to the causes of fever, the maintenance of a balanced body temperature can be disrupted in a number of ways, the prime example being the appearance of a fever, as noted, such as happens from a bacterial infection, or other such cause. Thus, bacterial toxins affect the sensitivity of hypothalamic cells, which then act to conserve heat and cause the body temperature to rise by one or another of several ways. (The hypothalamus, a part of the brain located below the thalamus, regulates many bodily functions including body temperature, and the secretions of the pituitary gland. It is associated with several other names, e.g., diencephalon, forebrain, and so on.)*

Fevers have been broken down into a number of classifications (Gilles and Warrell, in *Tropical and Geographical Medicine*, pp. 4–7). The reference states that fevers result from thermoregulatory disturbances, e.g., the action of endogenous pyrogens such as interleukin-1. (A *pyrogen* is merely another name for a fever-producing substance.) These pyrogens are released from macrophages due to a number of causes or stimuli, which include bacterial endotoxins or other microbial constituents, and immune complexes. That is, the immune system will also produce fever. The reference further states that "fever is associated with an array of metabolic changes, immunological responses, and inflammatory reactions involving humoral mediator systems." Of clinical significance is that there is an increased hepatic synthesis of certain proteins, notably fibrinogen and C-reactive protein. The fibrinogen is said to cause an increase in erythrocyte sedimentation rates.

In further explanation, *fibrinogen* is a soluble protein that occurs in the blood and other body fluids, which is converted to insoluble fibrin by the action of the blood enzyme thrombin. The end result is coagulation. An *erythrocyte* is a red blood corpuscle. The term *C-reactive* may pertain to reaction with the C-terminus of a protein or polypeptide—that is, with a carbon atom—or, more likely, it pertains to

---

* It may be mentioned in passing that there is a theory that solar radiation may stimulate the hypothalamus and in turn promote general health and well-being (Moss, *Cancer Therapy*, p. 70). And speaking of radiation, there is the conjecture at least that radio frequency radiation may adversely affect the growth of tumor cells, as advanced by Rife and others (Walters, *Options*, pp. 268–272).

what is called the C-protein, a protein associated with a particular muscular filament structure (Voet and Voet, *Biochemistry*, pp. 108, 1236, 1243).

Left mostly unsaid is that, very possibly, these interrelated immune-system processes may be accelerated by an increase in temperature, since it is a well enough known fact that chemical reaction rates increase with temperature. Moreover, there may be a threshold temperature for some of the immune-system phenomena to respond or kick in. (On the other hand, too high a body temperature will result in deadly side effects or end effects, as is all too well known. As with so many things, including medicinal agents, there is apparently an optimum range or window of effectiveness. It may be added that this upper body-temperature limit is well below the usual temperature levels for the sterilization of most microorganisms, e.g., see the section dealing with viruses in animal or meat products.) In further comment, however, the *Encyclopedia Britannica*, 15th ed., 1997, furnishes the statement that *higher-than-normal body temperatures serve to stimulate the motion, activity, and multiplication of white blood cells, at the same time enhancing the formation of antibodies.* It is also mentioned, moreover, that these *elevated temperature levels may kill or inhibit certain bacteria or viruses which are especially heat sensitive.*

Of further interest is the use of externally induced hyperthermia against cancer and other diseases (e.g., Walters, *Options*, pp. 240–247). Since, as indicated above, the body's internal initiation of a fever is a greatly complicated process and involves among other things the action of the immune system, there is a good deal more going on than would be represented by a mere application of external heat. In other words, a fever indicates that the immune system is working, or trying to work, in ways not fully understood. Contrarily, however, the application of heat from an external source does not necessarily signify that the immune system will be so stimulated. Nor, very possibly, will other external agents necessarily stimulate the immune system in desirable directions.*

In final analysis, the action if any may be regarded as occurring at the molecular level, in the parlance of enzyme inhibitors. Thus, with bacteria or other cellular forms, the antidisease agent may act as an inhibitor for the formation of toxins, say, or for the metabolism of the cell itself. In the case of viruses, the agent may act as an inhibitor for the functions of the virus-infected cell or for the vital functions of the virus particle itself. Viruses also operate and replicate via enzymes—e.g., the various DNA and RNA polymerases and, in the case of retroviruses, the enzyme known as reverse transcriptase or RNA-directed DNA polymerase. Clearly, further investigation is in order, directed at the role of particular enzyme inhibitors in acting against diseases—up to and including cancer.

7.1.3 REFERENCES ON SPECIFIC MICROORGANISMS

For more about specific viruses, several references may be consulted. For instance, there is the *CRC Handbook of Microbiology*, 2nd ed., in seven volumes, edited by Allen T. Laskin and Hubert A. Lechevalier and published in 1977–. These volumes take up not only viruses, but bacteria, fungi, algae, protozoa, and a number of other topics.

Roger Hull, Fred Brown, and Chris Payne compiled *Virology: Directory and Dictionary of Animal, Bacterial, and Plant Viruses*, published in 1989. The *Encyclopedia of Microbiology*, in three volumes, was edited by Joshua Lederberg and published in 1992.

Additionally, there is the continuing series *Advances in Virus Research*, published by Academic Press. The first volume was published in 1973, and Volume 46 was published in 1996. The name of the journal *Virology Abstracts* was change to *Virology and AIDS Abstracts*. These listings are aside from the many other books and publications extant about virology or viruses. A popularization by Ann Giudici Fettner is titled *Viruses: Agents of Change*, published in 1990.

As to bacteria per se, there is *The Prokaryotes: A Handbook on Habitats, Isolation, and Identification of Bacteria*, in two volumes, edited by Mortimer P. Starr et al., and published in 1981. Robert C. King served as editor for the *Handbook of Genetics*, in five volumes, published in 1974–1976, which includes the subjects of bacteria, bacteriophages, and fungi; plants, plant viruses, and protists (unicellular organisms); as well as a volume on invertebrates of general interest and another on molecular genetics.

A standard reference work is *Bergey's Manual of Systematic Bacteriology*, published in four volumes. A companion volume is *Bergey's Manual of Determinative Bacteriology*. The former contains a wealth

---

* All of which may suggest why *hypothermia may not be a conclusive remedy* for cancer, for example, or for other diseases—nor are all substances classed as immunostimulants. Things are a great deal more complex.

of detailed information about members of the different genera and species. The latter volume is directed more at identification, but summarizes considerable information. Moreover, as the editors state, it contains information about only a small fraction of the total bacteria found in nature. So far, in the latter regard, about 2,000 or so bacteria species have been identified and classified. Although in sheer individual-specimen numbers, bacteria may be the most numerous of all living creatures, as to the number of different species, the insects no doubt are runaway winners. As to the naming of most bacteria species, there is the *Index Bergeyana: An Annotated Alphabetical Listing of Names of the Taxa of the Bacteria*, published in 1966, and its *Supplement*, published in 1981. The taxonomy or classification of bacteria is arbitrary to a great extent, the same as with viruses, since there is not the diversity of characteristics as with higher animals and plants.

At the outset, *Bergey's Manual of Determinative Bacteriology* distinguishes a bacterium or prokaryote (or procaryote) from a microscopic eukaryote (or eucaryote), examples of the latter being molds, yeasts, algae, or protozoans. Bacteria are further categorized or divided into Gram-negative eubacteria with cell walls, Gram-positive eubacteria with cell walls, eubacteria without cell walls (commonly called *myco-plasmas*), and archaeobacteria (or archeobacteria). The prefix of the last-mentioned division signifies a more primitive or ancient form. (The prefix "eu-" ordinarily signifies *good* or *advantageous*. Here, *eubacteria* denotes those prokaryotic organisms exclusive of archaeobacteria.)

Further technical information is provided in *Bergey's Manual of Determinative Bacteriology*, for instance, for distinguishing prokaryotes, and about each of the four categories. (The comment is supplied that the varies divisions and subdivisions, or categories and subcategories, do not necessarily correspond with the species classifications.) *The main distinguishing feature is that prokaryotes do not have a nuclear membrane as do eukaryotes.*

Mycoplasmas are singled-out as being highly pleomorphic and may be saprophytic, parasitic, or pathogenic, causing diseases in animals, plants, and tissue cultures.

As to *archaeobacteria*, a most unusual category, they are both terrestrial and aquatic, occurring in anaerobic or hypersaline environments and in hydrothermally or geothermally heated environments. Some also act as symbionts (living in close conjunction with dissimilar organisms) in the digestive tract of animals. They comprise both aerobes and anaerobes, and facultative anaerobes (able to live under widely varying conditions), and may be mesophiles or thermophiles (living under both ordinary and higher temperatures). Some are able to exist and grow at boiling-water temperatures, even above 100° C. Some other unique properties are listed in that these microorganisms may be methanogenic (methane-producing), sulfate reducers, halophilic (able to survive in saline environments), without cells, and thermophilic sulfur metabolizers.

An ubiquitous bacterial grouping of interest comprises the *methanogens*, which may fall across several of the four categories or divisions previously set forth. By definition, all methanogens are microbes that yield methane as a major catabolic product. All other organisms are excluded.

Of note is the genus *Methanobacterium* of the family Methanobacteriaceae, found in flooded soils, sediments, or other anoxic (oxygen-deficient) environments. Energy metabolism requires the reduction of carbon dioxide to methane. (Interestingly, the final product gases will be about one-half methane and one-half carbon dioxide. In other words, the carbon dioxide is formed first, and then in part reacts with water or hydrogen, or with other reducing agents such as formate or carbon monoxide, and so on, to form methane. In the reduction of carbon dioxide, it may be presumed that oxygen is produced as an intermediate—the reverse of oxidation—to further react with something else. The processes are very involved, to say the least.) The conversion needs a nitrogen source (as ammonia) and a sulfur source, a necessity found for other of the methanogenic bacteria. These gaseous products may emanate from ponds, for instance, where in former times the natives would collect the gas in bags to be burned as fuel.

Another methanogenic genus of interest, from the same family, is *Methanobrevibacter*. In addition to nitrogen and sulfur, one or more B vitamins are required for metabolism. These bacteria are found in the gastrointestinal tract of animals and humans, in anaerobic digestors, or in other anaerobic environments. In animals and humans, they are a source for intestinal gas. Of the several other methanogens, another genus, *Methanococcus* of the family Methanoccaceae, is found in anoxic salt marshes and in marine or estuarine environments. The genus *Methanosphaera* is also found in the gastrointestinal tract. The list could go on.

Of more concern as a pathogen is the genus *Bacteroides*, of the family Bacteroidaceae, previously encountered in Part 6 within the section on "Intestinal Flora and Cancer." As further set forth in *Bergey's*

Manual of Determinative Bacteriology, the genus is found in a wide range of anaerobic habitats (for example, in gingival [gum] crevices, the intestinal tract, and sewage sludge) and occurs under infective and purulent conditions in both humans and animals. Gram-negative and anaerobic, many of the species are *pleomorphic* and may be either motile or nonmotile—generally the latter. Metabolism involves carbohydrates, peptones, or other metabolic intermediates. Species that are strongly saccharolytic (utilize or catabolize sugars as the source for metabolism) will yield fermentation products such as acetate, succinate, lactate, formate, or propionate. *Butyrate* may also be formed (*butyric acid is said to induce apoptosis in cancer cells,* ref. Boik, *Cancer & Natural Medicine*, p. 13). In many species, there will be high levels of branched-chain fatty acids. It is further noted that vitamin K and hemin act as stimulants for the growth of many species.

One may also consult other microbiology or biochemistry references about such subjects as bacterial genetics, bacteriophages, and viral genetics (e.g., Voet and Voet, *Biochemistry*, p. 838ff). As noted elsewhere, a *bacteriophage*, as its name implies, is a bacteria-destroying agent and may be called a *bacterial virus*. (It may be mentioned in passing that the Sigma catalog provides a listing by subject and title of some 300 technical books in a section on "Techware.")

7.2 LYSOGENY, VIRUSES, AND CANCER

There is a section on "Tumour-Producing Viruses" under the entry "Virus in the Macropaedia" of the *Encyclopedia Britannica*. The 15th edition, as published in 1974, will first be reviewed. Although dated, it may still be assumed to have bearing, although there is an increased interest and concern with such other matters as oncogenic behavior, or oncogenes. A later edition will be subsequently consulted.

Thus, according to the above-cited article, the first indication that tumors can be caused by a viral infection occurred in 1908, when investigators were able to transmit leukemia from one chicken to another, and in 1911 it was found that a solid tumor could be transmitted between chickens. Biologists were for many years reluctant to admit that viruses could produce cancer, but now the evidence is regarded as incontrovertible, since *tumors of many kinds can be caused by viral infections in almost all kinds of experimental animals.* Moreover, *many virus-like particles with the morphology of tumor-producing viruses have been found in human tumor tissues.* There has heretofore been a difficulty in directly demonstrating viral carcinogenicity in humans due to ethical considerations, although comparative biological studies indicate that this must be the case.

The problem of infective transmission of viruses between humans is explained away by the assumption that cancer is not especially contagious—at least for humans. Moreover, the available evidence is said to be such that oncogenic or tumor-producing viruses are not readily transmitted between individual animals.*

It has been found that cells in cultures will respond to tumor-producing viruses by either dying or by a *transformation*. The latter involves changes in the cell morphology and surface properties. Additionally, *following transformation, the cells divide rapidly and do not exhibit normal growth inhibition or contact inhibition under crowded cell culture conditions.* Moreover, *such transformed cells will cause a tumor when injected into an animal.* The analogy is made that the tumor-producing viruses will cause cancer in an animal, starting from scratch.

It is further noted that, *in many cases, the infecting virus cannot be recovered from the transformed cell.* This is due to the fact that *the virus now exists as a provirus, that is to say, it has been integrated into the chromosomes of the host cell.* The sequence is described as similar to that of the *lysogeny* of bacteria by *lysogenic* bacteriophages. (The term *lysogeny* pertains to a virus infecting its DNA into the chromosome of a host cell.) It is also noted that *genes of the oncogenic provirus continue to be expressed, thus maintaining the transformed or malignant state.* Therefore, as indicated, the transformation of animal cells by oncogenic viruses can be judged similar to the conversion produced by lysogenic bacteriophages.

---

* It can be added that the activity of the immune system of the second party may be such that, in this case, it works against an outside infective virus or viruses. At the least, the immune system of the second party will destroy cancer cells injected from the first party. A corollary is the difficulty in transplanting cells or organs form one individual to another. The body of the second party will likely reject the transplant unless the immune system is suppressed—something about the immune response recognizing differences in the cellular makeup.

The section in the *Encyclopedia Britannica* concludes by stating that, just as a bacterial prophage can be induced by various treatments, the evidence indicates that *oncogenic viruses can exist in a latent form, to be induced to multiply and infect other cells, resulting in tumors.* Moreover, *X-rays have been found to induce mouse leukemia, which in turn is transmissible by a virus occurring in the leukemic cells.* The article further states that *it is suspected that chemical carcinogens may produce cancers by activating a latent virus.* (Such may conceivably occur in the gut and may occur inversely. That is, *bacteria and viruses in the colon, particularly, may produce chemical carcinogens that are absorbed and enter the bloodstream, to produce mutagenesis or carcinogenesis by altering the cellular machinery,* almost at random. See, for instance, the section in Part 6 on "Intestinal Flora and Cancer.") According to the article, the mechanisms by which oncogenic viruses alter the biochemistry of a cell, changing it to a malignant cell, were still under consideration at the time of publication.*

A detailed explanation of *lysogenic* behavior requires a consideration of two alternatives, or alternative lifestyles (Voet and Voet, *Biochemistry,* pp. 1090–1091). In the one, the virus or phage or bacteriophage (bacterial virus) follows the familiar lytic mode in which the phage or virus is replicated by the host or host cell such that the host *lyses* (self-destructs) to release numerous progeny phages or viruses. (This is the usual course of events for a viral infection, where the virus is replicated in the cell to produce more virus particles, destroying the cell in the process.)

In the other, the phage or virus may proceed by the so-called *lysogenic life cycle* whereby its DNA is inserted at a specific site in the host chromosome. Here, the phage DNA is said to passively replicate with the host DNA. (It is further added that, even after many bacterial generations, the phage DNA may eventually be excised from the host DNA to initiate a lytic cycle.) Another technical term used is prophage (or provirus), indicating phage DNA that follows a lysogenic life cycle. In turn, the host cell is called a *lysogen.*

Furthermore, lysogens have the intriguing property that they cannot be reinfected by phages of the type with which they are lysogenized. That is, they are *immune* to superinfection or superimposed infection. A bacteriophage, for instance, that can follow either a lytic or lysogenic life style is called a *temperate* phage, but those having only a lytic mode are called *virulent* and are said to be engaged in vegetative growth. (*A cancer-causing virus would therefore be temperate as distinguished from virulent.*) Interestingly, *over 90 percent of the thousands of known types of phages or viruses can be classified as temperate*—that is, can engage in either lysis or lysogeny Whereas, *most bacteria in nature are lysogens,* that is, are hosts for invading bacteriophages or viruses. Moreover, the presence of prophages or proviruses goes mostly unnoticed, since they seem to have little apparent effect.

The Voet and Voet reference further observes that the advantage of lysogeny lies in the fact that a parasite can form a stable association with its host, ensuring a *long-time survival.* (*Which may be projected to the survival of cancer-causing viruses and cancers.*) On the other hand, a virulent phage proceeds to destroy its host or host colony, albeit it multiplies prodigiously in the process. After the host is wiped out, however, the progeny may not encounter another suitable host. By contrast, *a prophage will multiply with its host indefinitely as long as the host remains viable.* (The resemblance to the behavior of cancer is uncanny.)

If the host is fatally injured or undergoes trauma, such as the exposure to agents that damage the host DNA or disrupt its replication, there is a shift to the lytic phase, called the *lifeboat* response. The prophage escapes via the formation of infectious viral particles having at least some chance for repli-cation. (*This may have bearing on cancer metastasis that sometimes accompanies the treatment of cancer with various agents such as used in chemotherapy or radiation, or even surgery.*)

It is further mentioned that *lysogeny is triggered by poor nutritional conditions for the host,* since phages or viruses can only lytically replicate in an actively growing host (the alternative being lysogeny for an unhealthy host cell). Otherwise, lysogeny is triggered by a large number of phages infecting each host cell, which signals that the phages are on the verge of destroying the host and need to go to the lysogenic mode. (*Again, the behavior to cancer is uncanny, in that poor nutrition favors or*

---

* It can alternately be speculated that the chemical or biochemical carcinogens produced in the gut, or ingested, or otherwise entering the bloodstream, or absorbed through the skin or acquired during respiration, in one way or another reach and enter body cells and may in turn alter the cellular genetic code. *This alteration very possibly may proceed by affecting or inhibiting the particular enzymes responsible for normal cell replication and metabolism.* In a way, this gets to be an exercise in semantics. A similar analysis may be made for the effects of radiation.

triggers a cancerous or lysogenic condition, and infections may also trigger a cancerous or lysogenic condition.)

In the Macropaedia of the *Encyclopedia Britannica*, 15th edition, as published in 1995, there is an update under the heading *Viruses*. Within this, under "Viral DNA Integration," there is section titled "Lysogeny," followed by another titled "Malignant Transformation." The thrust of the presentation by and large agrees with the Voet and Voet reference as presented above (Voet and Voet, *Biochemistry*, pp. 1090–1091).

It is mentioned first in the section on *Lysogeny* that many bacterial and animal viruses may lie dormant in an infected cell, and at the same time their DNA may be integrated into the chromosome of the host cell. Furthermore, as the cell genome replicates, so do the integrated DNAs of the virus. On cell division, the integrated viral DNA is copied and ordinarily is distributed evenly between the two resulting cells.

With regard to bacteria that carry the noninfective precursor phage, called the *prophage*, these bacteria will remain healthy and continue to grow until stimulated and disturbed by some extraneous factor. *Ultraviolet light* is an example of such a factor. *This causes the prophage DNA to be excised from the bacterial chromosome* and is followed by replication of the phage, resulting in many progeny phages. *At the same time, the host bacterial cell is lysed or destroyed.* It is added that this sequence was first discovered in 1950 as occurring in temperate bacteriophages and is known as *lysogeny*, as previously described.

An example furnished for a temperate bacteriophage involves the lambda (λ) virus, which readily induces lysogeny in several variants of the bacterium species *Escherichia coli* or *E. coli*. Thus, the DNA of the lambda bacteriophage integrates into the DNA of the *E. coli* host chromosome. This occurs at specific regions, referred to as *attachment sites*.

The integrated phage DNA, or prophage DNA, signals the inherited, noninfectious form of the virus. A gene present in the prophage acts to suppress the lytic functions of the phage and thus guarantees that the host cell will continue to replicate both the phage DNA and its own. Furthermore, the host cell *will not be destroyed by the virus*.

On the other hand, *the action of ultraviolet light or other stimulating factors is to markedly increase the replication of DNA in the host cell*. In the process, the enzyme recA protease is formed, which serves to break apart the lambda phage repressor. At the same time, lambda phage replication is induced, leading to the destruction of the (oncogenic) host cell.

Other ramifications ensue. An excision of the prophage DNA from the DNA of the host cell chromosome becomes the initial step for the synthesis of an *infective lytic virus*. The excision also may be accompanied by the removal of part of the host cell DNA. This removed portion becomes packaged into bacteriophages, which then become defective. In turn, part of the bacteriophage DNA is excised, to become positioned at the other end of a gene of the host bacterium. The gene can be said to be captured by the lambda phage DNA, and the resulting virus particle is called a *transducing phage*. When this transducing phage infects a bacterial cell, it transmits the gene into the infected cell. Thus, *transduction by bacteriophages provides a method to transfer genetic information from one bacterial cell to yet another.*

There is more. The example lambda bacteriophage and similar phages are regarded as specialized transducing phages since the only genes transmitted are those next to the lambda prophage attachment site whereas, in other cases, the prophages can integrate almost anyplace on the chromosomes of the host cell. On account of this randomness, the term generalized transducing phages is used. Furthermore, *this random transduction becomes a means to create bacteria with new gene functions, or to replace those that have been lost by mutations.*

The foregoing means for transferring genetic information is called *lysogenic conversion* and is a way to impart genes with special functions to bacterial cells lacking these functions. The phenomenon is common in nature. A consequence is that a bacteriophage released from one cell can infect another cell, imparting new genetic information in the process. As an example, consider the bacterium species *Corynebacterium diphthereiae*, the causative agent for the disease known as *diphtheria*. To be activated, however, it must contain the prophage of the bacteriophage designated beta (β), which codes for the *toxin* actually responsible for the disease. Other examples of lysogenic conversion by bacteriophages include those that code for, or induce, bacterial toxins such as occur with the *streptococci*. Thus, what are called group A streptococci contain a prophage that codes for the toxin responsible for *scarlet fever*.

It may be concluded that the foregoing is an important aspect of epidemiology—the study of the incidence, distribution, and control of infectious diseases. In other words, the mere presence of a certain bacterium does not necessarily indicate the corresponding disease, because the bacterium must first be "activated" by a bacteriophage (bacterial virus), in turn producing the toxin that is the actual cause of the disease.

In the section on "Malignant Transformation," the subject becomes that of *animal* cells infected with certain viruses. The phenomenon may be viewed as analogous to bacterial cell lysogeny. It is noted that animal viruses do not at first necessarily cause disease, at least for certain animal cells. Rather, animal cells have a *persistent* infection with such viruses. That is, the DNA of these viruses (which now may be called *proviruses*) remains integrated into the chromosomal DNA of the host cell.

> In general, cells with integrated proviral DNA are converted into cancer cells, a phenomenon known as malignant transformation.

The animal cell so transformed will have no infectious virus, which is similar to the case for bacterial prophages as already discussed. It will have only the integrated provirus DNA, which replicates in concert with the chromosomes of the dividing cells. Subsequent to the preliminaries of cell division, called *mitosis*, each new cell formed is furnished a copy of the proviral DNA. A property of these transformed animal cells is that of uncontrolled growth. Furthermore, this growth is not inhibited by being in contact with other cells, and there is a loss of the ability to remain stuck to certain kinds of surfaces. (In other words, the latter effect is related to why cancerous cells metastasize, migrating and adhering to other sites.)

The article cites several different animal virus families or viruses that produce malignant transformations. As to DNA viruses, those of the family Papovaviridae were among the first found to produce malignancies, resulting in illness or death in animals. Of these, polyoma virus is common to mice and also other rodents and can induce tumors in infected animals in general. Another virus from the same family, known as simian virus 40 (SV40), was first found in the African green monkey. Here it shows rapid growth, at the same time killing the cells. When rodent or human cells are infected, however, the infection is aborted. This is said to be on account of an incompatibility between the virus and the host cell. Nevertheless, an occasional malignancy results, of the sarcoma or lymphoma type. There are, moreover, viruses related to both the polyoma virus and the SV40 virus that have been found in humans. One of these, called the *JC virus*, is associated with progressive multifocal leukoencephalopathy, a fatal neurological disease. For the most part, however, human papovaviruses are not viewed as being associated with diseases (other than tumors or cancer).

The family Papovaviridae also includes the papilloma viruses, which are implicated in the formation of usually benign tumors on human skin surfaces, and they are referred to as papillomas or polyps, an example being warts.

The foregoing statement brings up a question to be asked. Could these viruses be associated with polyps in the colon? These polyps are commonly regarded as the source for colon cancer. In this regard, on p. 47 of a chapter by J.P. Sundberg in *Papilloma Viruses and Human Disease*, it is noted that polyps have been experimentally induced in the urinary bladders of calves. The particular volume also has several chapters that deal with the human papilloma virus or HPV and its connection with tumors or cancers in various parts of the body, e.g., the concluding chapter by K.J. Syrjänen.

The Adenoviridae contain certain viruses implicated in the malignant transformations of certain cells. These viruses were first noticed in human tonsils and adenoids, hence their name. Although widely studied, the evidence indicates that the more common adenoviruses do not produce human cancers.

The family Herpesviridae, on the other hand, has been implicated. Thus, the common herpes simplex viruses—which cause cold sores, for instance—are also suspect in cancer formation. These viruses produce malignant transformations in the same fashion as adenoviruses. In fact, the Epstein-Barr virus, a herpesvirus, produces Burkitt's lymphoma, an often fatal childhood cancer. Another herpesvirus results in chicken pox, or varicella, and the virus will lie dormant in the body tissues, maybe for years, finally to be resuscitated so as to cause shingles, the very painful neurological and skin disease also known as herpes zoster. Still other herpesviruses are the sources for diseases in animals, such as Merek's disease in chickens, and there are herpesviruses in monkeys and even in frogs.

As to RNA viruses, the Retroviridae constitute the most widespread group of the transforming viruses, infecting eukaryotic cells in nonbacterial species ranging from yeasts to humans. Early on, there was the suspicion that viruses cause lymphomas and leukemias in birds and, as early as 1911, a virus was found to produce sarcomas in chickens.

A feature of retroviruses is that the virions or virus particles can be described as spheres or polygons enclosed by a lipid (fat-like) membrane that contains a glycoprotein. The glycoprotein serves to recognize and bind to cell receptors of a particular species; these are further denoted as type-specific glycoproteins. It is in turn stated that the retrovirus genomes are made up of two identical RNA molecules, each having from 7,000 to 10,000 nucleotides.*

The enzyme called *RNA-dependent DNA polymerase,* or *reverse transcriptase,* is associated with virion RNA. Using the virion RNA as a template (or model), this particular enzyme catalyzes the formation of a linear DNA molecule, which can be regarded as complementary to the virion RNA. In turn, with the linear DNA molecule so formed serving as the template, the same enzyme catalyzes the formation of a second or anticomplementary DNA molecule. The end result is *double-stranded DNA,* or *dsDNA.*

Further stated in the article is that, for fully infected bird retroviruses that can replicate autonomously, there are four genes whose essential functions are to code sequentially for group-specific antigens, the enzyme reverse transcriptase, the envelope glycoprotein, and the sarcoma-transforming protein. The genome contains still other nucleotide sequences, called *long terminal repeats* or LTRs, which function to integrate proviral DNA into the recognized and receptive DNA sequences of the host cell chromosome.

This highly complicated procedure is annotated with the observation that *many retroviruses are defective* and cannot replicate in cells unless assisted by other, nondefective *helper retroviruses.* These helper retroviruses are most usually involved in transforming fibroblastic cells (cells that contribute to the formation of connective tissue). The result is *malignant sarcomas.* Otherwise, without helper retroviruses, the defective retroviruses transform blood-cell precursors, with the end-result being leukemias (or blood-related cancers). *The foregoing establishes the difference between the formation of sarcomas and leukemias.*

The article goes on to say that many different retroviruses have been found to act as agents for producing cancers in birds, rodents (notably mice), domestic cats, and monkeys. The list has been recently extended to humans. It is further noted that the human T-cell leukemia virus (HTLV) causes certain lymphatic leukemias in humans. As is well known, the retrovirus named human immunodeficiency virus (HIV) is the source for the *acquired immune deficiency syndrome (AIDS).*

The observation is made that the origins of retroviruses are from the genes of many species of animals, and even from lower life-forms. There is the qualification, however, that *retroviruses do not ordinarily cross species barriers* and are therefore limited in their range of hosts. Thus, the origins for every retrovirus studied so far can be tied to the genes normally found in animals (including humans). That is, there is an analogy between the genes found in a particular retrovirus and the genes found in the correspondingly virus-infected animal. The retroviruses can almost—*but not quite*—be said to be animal-specific. These genes are called *proto-oncogenes* and have the potential to transform into cancer-causing genes.

Proto-oncogenes are further described as having deoxynucleotide sequences that are closely, *but not entirely,* homologous to the nucleotide sequences of a corresponding viral cancer-causing gene, called simply an *oncogene.*

Although the integration of retrovirus DNA into cell chromosomes will result in cancer, such is not the case for proto-oncogenes, as *proto-oncogenes do not become cancer-causing until triggered by another event.* A circumstance is provided in terms of the action of *chemical or physical carcinogens,*

---

* Again, for the record, a nucleotide is a chemical compound called an *ester,* formed by the interaction or reaction of phosphoric acid with a nucleoside. And, according to a dictionary definition, a nucleoside is any of a class of compounds consisting essentially of ribose or deoxyribose combined with the nucleic acid bases adenine, guanine, cytosine, uracil, or thiamine. (For instance, see Part 1, or see Voet and Voet, *Biochemistry,* p. 796.) Interestingly, adenine, for example, can be considered an alkaloid, as can the other nucleic acid bases, in a manner of looking at it. Adenine, by the way, may itself be involved in the biosynthesis of the alkaloids caffeine, theobromine, or theophylline (Cordell, *Alkaloids,* p. 958). Furthermore, the adenine in tRNA, or transfer RNA, likely takes part. There are some strange and mysterious biochemical interactions of which the kind of nitrogen-containing ring structure occurring in alkaloids is apparently involved, in one way or another.

which may produce alterations in the proto-oncogene sequences, resulting in a conversion to oncogenes. A specific example furnished is that of DNA tumor viruses such as SV40 or adenoviruses, which may induce a malignant transformation if their DNA is integrated next to the site of a proto-oncogene.

The foregoing can be judged as an extremely sophisticated way to explain why viruses may or may not cause cancer, directly or indirectly, and that a given retrovirus, at least, may or may not cross species lines. That this sometimes happens is of course noted in tracking influenza virus and is suspected for HIV as well, and it may yet prove to be the case for such newly emerging viruses as the Marburg and Ebola viruses.

A later word is that the agent triggering the transformation or mutation of a normal cell to become a cancerous cell is an obscure *protein* called *beta-caterin*. The fact that viruses may also be looked upon as proteins makes one wonder about what is what. Given that some sort of proteinaceous agent can induce normal cells to become cancerous cells, what enzyme or enzymes are involved, if any, and what inhibitors will serve? More than this, if cancerous growth ensues, what enzymes are critical, and how may these be blocked?

7.3 RETROVIRUSES AND ONCOGENES

The statement has been made that contemporary research on oncogenes traces its roots to work on several lines of tumor viruses (Robert A. Weinberg, in *Oncogenes*, p. 1). Work on the papovaviruses, namely polyoma and SV40, and also on the Rous sarcoma virus, led to the finding that cultured cells which were infected with these viruses would acquire many of the phenotypes (characteristics) of cancer cells, including tumorigenicity. "The importance of these observations is hard to overestimate." It permitted the study of cancer genesis in cultures rather than in living tissues. The processes of malignant transformation were demystified.

Not only this, but it permitted insights at a molecular level for the cellular transformations. For instance, the genomes for the viruses were only a minute part of the total DNA content of the cell, and it could be concluded that this very small amount of genetic information was sufficient to orchestrate malignant transformations. Only a small number of regulators within the cell controlled growth. Among the developments was the discovery that the viral oncogene associated with the Rous sarcoma virus genome was itself derived from a normal cellular gene. The generalization was then made that the cellular genome has genes that can be converted into oncogenes by specific types of genetic change, aside from infecting tumor viruses. These conversions in human tumor genomes involve what are called *point mutation, chromosomal translocation, gene truncation,* and *amplification.* Central to this conclusion is that the cell genome carries among its various genes the seeds for cancer formation and for the organism's own destruction. In other words, the human animal carries the seeds for its own destruction.*

The now generally accepted principles of oncogenetics may be listed as follows (Harold Varmus, in *Oncogenes*, p. 4ff.):

1. Eukaryotic (or nonbacterial) cell genomes have probably from 50 to 100 genes that may participate in neoplasia or cancer cell formation, the consequence of mutations.

2. Most of these genes, called *proto-oncogenes* ("proto-" meaning first), can be divided into gene families according to sequence or function, or both.

3. The mutations converting proto-oncogenes into active oncogenes may involve changes in sequence (e.g., single-nucleotide substitutions) or may involve extensive rearrangements (e.g., insertions, deletions, gene amplifications, or chromosomal translocations), which may be induced by chemical, physical, or viral presences.

4. Some cancer-inducing mutations may deactivate other genes, called *tumor-suppressive* genes.

5. Many viruses contain one to several genes that can induce neoplastic change, but retroviral oncogenes are derived directly from cellular proto-oncogenes.

6. Combinations of oncogenes are necessary for the conversion of a normal cell to a tumor cell.

---

* In comment, the search for cause and effect is open ended, for one may ask, if point mutation, chromosomal translocation, gene truncation, and amplification are the causes of genetic transformations, then what are the causes for these causes, now regarded as effects? And so on, ad infinitum.

With respect to viruses per se, DNA viruses, as the name implies, contain DNA. Examples include polyomavirus and simian virus 40 (SV40) as well as the adenoviruses, the papilloma viruses, and a few of the herpes viruses, notably the Epstein-Barr virus or EBV (Varma, in *Oncogenes*, pp. 10–11).

Retroviruses were formerly called RNA tumor viruses but are now known simply as retroviruses, and they include Rous sarcoma virus and the papovaviruses (Varmus, in *Oncogenes*, p. 11ff). Retroviruses are the source of many oncogenes and, for the record, retroviral genomes are composed of two identical strands of RNA, capable of encoding 1-10 polypeptides.

In fact, there is a volume titled *RNA Tumor Viruses*, published by the internationally recognized Cold Spring Harbor Laboratory, in the series *Molecular Biology of Tumor Viruses*. The volume has several chapters and contributors dealing with retroviruses. A previous volume in the series was titled *DNA Tumor Viruses*. These terms are also used, for instance, in *Viral Oncology*, which under "RNA Tumor Viruses" has sections or chapters dealing with Oncornaviruses of various sorts. (That is, as noted previously, the term *oncornaviruses* is short for the expression "oncogenic RNA viruses," with retroviruses a special case.) Thus, other terms supplied include *oncogenic DNA viruses* and *oncogenic RNA viruses*, as per the divisions in *Viruses Associated with Human Cancer*. These works are but several in a flurry of technical monographs published in the early 1980s whose findings have since been sifted and have entered the general literature. (The proliferation continues, whereby a word search of MEDLINE will find approximately 15,000 to 20,000 publications each year about cancer, mostly technical articles or papers.)

We repeat that the retroviruses are RNA-containing eukaryotic viruses, which include certain tumor viruses and others such as the human immunodeficiency virus (Voet and Voet, *Biochemistry*, p. 1041.) These viruses contain an enzyme called *RNA-directed DNA polymerase* (or *reverse transcriptase*). The enzyme can be viewed as synthesizing DNA from RNA.

The particular circumstances involving HIV are further set forth in a chapter "Retroviruses and the Human Immunodeficiency Syndrome" by Robert Colebunders and Thomas C. Quinn, in *Tropical and Geographical Medicine*. We defer to the reference.

In the same volume, published in 1990, relative to successes in the development of new or improved killed rabies, polio, and hepatitis B vaccines, the remark is made that "the celebratory note of the past decade has been shattered by the emergence of viruses which are simultaneously invisible and lethal to the human immune system" (Scott B. Halstead, in *Tropical and Geographical Medicine*, p. 558). "HIV-1 and its virological cousins are the all-too-real Andromeda strain." Originally centered around Africa's Lake Victoria, the virus has since been seeded worldwide.

Although retroviruses show some similarity with SV40 and other DNA viruses as experimental carcinogens, they have several other distinguishing characteristics, as follows. Whereas most DNA viruses only transform foreign host cells, which are cells in which they fail to grow, *retroviruses can transform their natural host cells*. The oncogenes of DNA tumor viruses are required for both replication and transformation, whereas retroviral genes are required only for transformation. The origins of the DNA virus oncogenes are unknown, but retrovirus oncogenes are derived from normal cellular genes, for example, from proto-oncogenes. Although many retroviruses do not carry viral oncogenes and will not transform cells in culture, *they will nonetheless cause tumors in animals*, albeit after a lengthy latent period. The small DNA tumor viruses and many retroviruses generally cause only sarcomas (a relatively rare form of human cancer), whereas the retroviruses for the most part cause various leukemias and carcinomas. ("Sarco-" means flesh, but in the usage here, *sarcomas* are designated as occurring in nonepithelial tissue such as connective tissue, lymphoid tissue, cartilage, and bone. "Carcinoma" itself means cancer, but in the specialized usage, carcinomas occur only in epithelial tissue, that is, in the layered, cellular, membrane-like tissue covering a surface or lining a cavity.)

Cellular genes have also been discovered that contribute to oncogenesis (Varma, in *Oncogenes*, p. 19). This line of investigation was pursued after observing that *retroviruses that lack their own oncogenes can nevertheless induce tumors*. In another development, *genes have been isolated that normally suppress tumorigenesis* (Varma, in *Oncogenes*, p. 25).

Oncogenes and proto-oncogenes produce protein products, or *oncoproteins*, in small amounts relative to other cell proteins, and they are therefore difficult to identify and characterize (Varma, in *Oncogenes*, p. 28ff). It has been possible to generate antibodies, however, that act against these oncoproteins, thus identifying them in the process. (Which calls to mind that it is conceivable to develop anticancer serums or sera, or anticancer vaccines, in similar fashion.)

The biochemical properties of oncoproteins, the proteins encoded by oncogenes and proto-oncogenes, have been used to group these proteins into functional families. Thus there are the protein kinases, the growth factors, the signal transducers, and the transcription factors. (Incidentally, the terms oncoprotein and oncogene seem to be used synonymously in the reference.) There is evidence that oncoproteins, read oncogenes, meddle in growth control and either alter the level of activity in one or more of the metabolic pathways implicated in growth control, or else replace pathway regulation, with the consequences of uncontrolled growth. Among the possible pathways, the reference lists tyrosine phosphorylation, phosphatidylinositol metabolism, and cAMP-dependent pathway. (No mention is made of anaerobic glycolysis.)

As to growth factors (GFs), they generally pertain to the tissue of origin or to function but may share common characteristics (Weinberg, in *Oncogenes*, p. 46ff). *Oncogenes may induce the release of growth factors* and, in instances at least, *oncogenes are activated by viruses*, e.g., by the mouse mammary tumor virus or MMTV (Weinberg, in *Oncogenes*, pp. 55, 57). [No details were supplied in the reference as to the chemical makeup of growth factors, although growth hormones per se are polypeptides (Voet and Voet, *Biochemistry*, p. 845).]

Protein kinase is noted to be an oncogene product in the cell cytoplasm (Tony Hunter, in *Oncogenes*, p. 147ff.) Protein kinase is the enzyme that can transfer phosphate from ATP (adenosine triphosphate) to protein, the process of *protein phosphorylation*, which changes the protein activity. The protein kinases include both protein tyrosine kinases and protein serine kinases. There are cellular versions and oncogenic versions of each. The reference provides schematic structures in terms of the number of amino acids.

The oncogenic protein kinases have their origins in normal cellular enzymes that do not have transforming properties, and the differences between oncogenic and normal protein kinases require explanation (Hunter, in *Oncogenes*, pp. 153–155). In other words, what gives oncogenic protein kinases their oncogenic potential? It is mentioned in the reference that the mutations that change normal protein kinase genes into transforming genes also abolish regulatory domains, thus turning normal protein kinase into a nonregulated protein kinase, which may then catalyze phosphorylation.

The reference states that more than half of the approximately 30 known oncoproteins that act *outside* the nucleus have proved to be protein kinases. Most are protein tyrosine kinases, but three oncogenes encode protein serine kinases.

It may be mentioned in passing that *the nucleus, the eukaryotic cell's most conspicuous organelle, contains its genetic information* (encoded in the base sequences of DNA molecules that form the discrete number of chromosomes that characterize each species) that exists in the cell nucleus rather than in the cytoplasm (Voet and Voet, *Biochemistry*, p. 8). The cytoplasm is *not* the repository of genetic information, hence it may be assumed that if the oncogene resides in the nucleus, *the protein products, the oncoproteins, diffuse from the nucleus to the cytoplasm.*

It may be mentioned, furthermore, that the DNA encoded information is transcribed into molecules of RNA in the nucleus, which are then transported to the cytoplasm, where they direct the synthesis of protein at the sites called ribosomes or ribosmal structures or particles (Voet and Voet, *Biochemistry*, p. 8). These sites occur in the cytosol, which is the part of the cytoplasm exclusive of its membrane-bound organelles. The cytoplasm also contains numerous enzymes, both in the cytosol and in the organelles. The nucleus is enclosed by a double-membrane envelope whose numerous pores permit and regulate the flow of components between the nucleus and cytoplasm. In turn, the plasma membrane or cell membrane controls the passage of molecules in and out of the cell.

In the above regard, the heat shock proteins or molecular chaperones presumably play an instrumental role in the passage of molecular components between and among the various cellular compartments—the nucleus, the cytoplasm, and its cytosol and organelles, and in and out of the cell proper. To the list of molecular components may be added enzymes and enzyme inhibitors.

With regard to the preceding paragraphs, there are therefore oncogenes in the cell nucleus, although the work on retroviral oncogenes indicated that the oncoprotein action was largely confined to the cytoplasm and the plasma membrane (Robert N. Eisenman, in *Oncogenes*, p. 176ff). It is noted, furthermore, that these proteins now appear to interact with DNA elements that stimulate or repress transcription. In short, they serve as gene regulatory proteins.

The *myc* family of nuclear oncogenes has been studied the most extensively. (The designator is for myelocytomatosis, a kind of tumor which occurs in chickens.) *These oncogenes have been shown to be associated with neoplasms (tumors or cancers) in a wide variety of species.* Presumably of a regulatory nature, *its alteration may very well underlie the genesis of neoplasia in many different cell types.* It has also been discovered to be a retroviral transforming gene, whose action directly affects cell proliferation (Eisenman, in *Oncogenes*, p. 179). Further details are provided in the reference for these and other similar oncogenes, as well as oncogenic hormone receptors.

A chapter in *Oncogenes* is devoted to the oncogenes in DNA tumor viruses, namely the papovaviruses (Walter Eckhart, *Oncogenes*, p. 223ff.) As previously indicated, the papovavirus family includes the polyomaviruses, notably polyoma and SV40, and the papillomaviruses. The polyoma virus has been found to cause a wide variety of tumors. The SV40 virus was found as a contaminant in cultures of rhesus monkey cells, the common source for polio vaccines. (*Note:* Some attribute this contaminant or other contaminants to producing the lethargic so-called "hippy generation.") Papillomas or warts occur in many species, and a variety of papillomaviruses have been isolated, with some implicated in the progression of benign warts to malignant tumors. Further details are furnished in the reference, with an emphasis on the role of papillomaviruses in human cancer.

Three basic types of warts are induced in humans by papillomaviruses (Eckhart, in *Oncogenes*, p. 235). These types are common warts, flat warts, and genital warts, and unlike polyoma and SV40, papillomaviruses are involved in human tumors, both benign and malignant. Beginning as benign lesions, warts may progress to malignancies, although rarely.

Papillomaviruses, however, are also associated with squamous cell cancers, which include cervical and anogenital carcinomas, laryngeal oral carcinomas, and cutaneous carcinomas. The extension is particularly apt for persons with epidermodysplasia verruciformis or EV, which is characterized by disseminated skin lesions that resemble flat warts. (It has already been asked whether intestinal polyps are a variant caused by papillomaviruses.) It is noted that EV is influenced by environmental as well as genetic factors, and *sunlight* may play an important role, since tumors tend to develop in areas exposed to the sun.

The aforecited reference work *Oncogenes* has another chapter on oncogenesis by DNA viruses that is devoted to the adenovirus (Thomas Shenk, in *Oncogenes*, p. 239ff.), and still another devoted to herpesviruses (Elliott Kleff and David Liebowitz, in *Oncogenes*, p. 259ff).

A chapter on heritable cancer and suppressor genes provides some interesting insights (Eric J. Stanbridge and Webster K. Cavenee, in *Oncogenes*, p. 281ff). It is emphasized that *two or more cooperating oncogenes are required for neoplastic transformations,* at least in normal rodent cells, and other as yet unidentified genetic changes are also required.

Somatic cell fusions between a normal cell and a malignant cell have shown that malignancy is suppressed in the resulting hybrid. (Somatic cells pertain to the body wall, as distinguished from the viscera or inner body parts.) The results can be explained in terms of chromosomes.

Renal-cell carcinomas and small-cell lung carcinomas have been examined in terms of genetic abnormalities, as have colorectal carcinomas. With regard to the last-mentioned, there are consistent rearrangements of chromosome 17, including deletions. Still other kinds of tumors have been examined in terms of chromosomal changes, and the results are tabulated in the reference. Past and ongoing work is described for finding tumor suppressor genes, which are variously called *tumor suppressors, growth suppressors, emerogenes,* or *anti-oncogenes* (Stanbridge and Caveanee, in *Oncogenes*, p. 298). Among the latest are the *p53* gene and the *erbA* gene. Generally speaking, however, the functions of most of the candidate tumor suppressor genes remain unknown.

The final chapter of *Oncogenes* is devoted to oncogenes and clinical cancer (J. Michael Bishop, in *Oncogenes*, p. 327ff). Emphasized is the discovery of the proto-oncogenes from which retroviral oncogenes arise in birds and animals and make the leap to oncogenesis in humans. The provisional answers sustain the conviction that genetic damage is an important vehicle for tumorigenesis.

In the next to last section of the reference, there is a brief discussion about the foundations for cancer therapy (Bishop, in *Oncogenes*, p. 348). There is a statement about the desire for a more rational treatment of cancer, which is followed by the statement that this may be in terms of malfunctioning genes. "The prospects still seem real but distant." However, it is indicated that analyses of the oncogenes may soon influence therapy choices for at least a few kinds of tumors.

A possibility mentioned is the repair or removal of damaged proto-oncogenes, but the likelihood seems small. Published in 1989, it is concluded, "Effective therapy against cancer founded on our knowledge of oncogenes will probably be slow to come."

An unsuspected adjunct to retroviruses is that there are what are called *Ty* elements in the yeast species *Saccharomyces cerevisiae* (bakers yeast), related structurally to retroviruses (Jef D. Boeke and David J. Garfinkel, in *Viruses of Fungi and Simple Eukaryotes*, p. 41ff). In further explanation, *Ty* elements stand for "transposable genetic elements," which have in fact been identified in almost every organism so far studied at the molecular genetic level (Fred Winston, in *Viruses of Fungi and Simple Eukaryotes*, p. 41ff). Studied in the most detail for prokaryotes, the common characteristic observed is the ability of this genetic element to transpose to different positions in the host genome, with the likelihood of encoding a reverse transcriptase enzyme. The inference therefore is that there are other, long-range avenues for oncogenic cellular activity, with the immediate prospect of mutations in yeast cells proper. Additional chapters in the same volume are concerned with yeast killer systems.

7.4   VIRUSES AND DEGENERATIVE DISEASES

Viruses are also the suspected agents in other intractable diseases. These include such demyelinating diseases as multiple sclerosis or MS. (MS involves myelin, the soft, white, fatty substance that forms a protective sheath around nerve fibers.) Thus, R.T. Johnson notes that infectious agents have been postulated for over a century as the cause of MS. This is supported by data that:

1. Childhood exposure to viral infections is involved.
2. Infections can cause diseases with long incubation periods, accompanied by periods of remission followed by relapsation and, in this case, by demyelination.
3. MS patients have abnormal immune responses to viruses.

Three other demyelinating diseases are also discussed in terms of viral causation. Thus, in progressive multifocal leukoencephalopathy, a papovavirus is the causative agent. In postmeasles encephalomyelitis, the virus disrupts immune regulation, but is not evident as an infection of the central nervous system or CNS. In human immunodeficiency virus-caused encephalopathy and myelopathy, there is viral evidence in macrophages, for instance, and the myelin abnormalities may be caused by such factors as viral proteins, cytokines, or neurotoxins.*

A research paper by Orefice et al. presents evidence that papova-like viral particles have been detected in the cerebrospinal fluid of AIDS patients who have progressive multifocal leukoencephalopathy (PML). This disease is characterized as a neurological opportunistic viral infection. The authors hypothesize that the severe cell-mediated immunodeficiency reactivates the papovavirus from a latent state in the brain, which leads to PML.

It has been observed elsewhere that the subviral pathogens called *prions*, or prion proteins, may be responsible for diseases affecting the mammalian central nervous system (e.g., Voet and Voet, *Biochemistry*, p. 1116). These diseases, under the umbrella of *spongiform encephalopathies*, include the animal disease called *scrapie*, the human disease called *Creutzfeldt-Jakob disease*, and *kuru*, a disease similar to Creutzfeldt-Jakob, if not the same. Prions are distinguished from the subviral particles known as viroids, in that *prions apparently are only protein molecules*, whereas *viroids are small, single-stranded RNA molecules* (Voet and Voet, *Biochemistry*, pp. 1114-1119).

A book going into the facts of the matter is Richard Rhodes' *Deadly Feasts: Tracking the Secrets of a Terrifying New Plague*. (Rhodes received the Pulitzer Prize and a National Book Award for an earlier book titled *The Making of the Atomic Bomb*, published in 1988.) The title pertains to the cannibalistic New Guinea ritual of consuming the brains of the enemy, whereby the disease *kuru* is spread. Cessation of this ceremonial practice seems to be effective in stopping the disease. *Mad cow disease, or bovine spongiform encephalopathy (BSE)*, as found in England and which is similar to scrapie, seems to be on the wane since the abandonment of the cannibalistic practice of using brain material as animal feed. A similar sort of disease has been observed in wild game animals in Colorado and Wyoming, especially in animals that may have been penned-up for various purposes. Called *chronic wasting disease*, no spread

---

* By way of further explanation, the suffix "-pathy" refers to a disease of a specific designated type, as does the suffix "-itis." The prefix "leuko-" or "leuco-" denotes white, as in leukocytes or leucocytes for example, which are white or colorless blood cells or corpuscles. In turn, "-encephalo-" pertains to the brain. The suffix "-myelitis," as used above, indicates a diseased condition for the myelin, here the sheath protecting the brain, whereas the term *encephalitis* denotes inflammation of the brain itself.

to humans has been noted, or to domestic animals, though Richard Rhodes indicates that, in certain cases at least, *spongiform encephalopathies may have crossed the animal/human boundary*. In fact, the term *transmissible spongiform encephalopathy* or TSE is now being used.

Another book on the subject is *Mad Cow USA: Could the Nightmare Happen Here?*, by Sheldon Rampton and John Stauber. The authors claim that, despite assurances, the practice of animal cannibalism has been allowed to continue in the U.S. and is more extensive than anywhere else in the world. (The authors are associated with an organization called the Center for Media and Democracy, Madison WI, which publishes an investigative quarterly called *PR Watch*.)

An article by Ellen Ruppel Shell about TSE or transmissible spongiform encephalopathy appeared in the September, 1998 issue of the *Atlantic Monthly*. In particular, there was cited the rendering of farm animals to provide animal protein for cattle feed. (Game farm animals are also fed animal protein.) There is the possibility, therefore, that by these means mad cow disease or an equivalent form such as Creutzfeldt-Jakob Disease or CJD could be spread, not only between animals but to humans. It may be further noted that there is no antibody reaction, for the body's immune system does not recognize prions—and such diseases as CJD and kuru are at present incurable.

There is the speculation also that Alzheimer's disease may be caused by prions or viroids. Thus, in Part 8 for example, in a section titled "A Review of Anaerobic Glycolysis," there is mention of slow virus diseases, and prions and viroids, and it is suggested that there may be a causal link for Alzheimer's disease, Parkinson's disease, and Lou Gehrig's disease (Tortora et al., *Microbiology*, pp. 15, 370–371, 567–569). The reference further describes a causal link between a virus and cancer (Tortora et al., *Microbiology*, p. 367).

And if peptides are sometimes viewed as anticancer agents, can they also be the causes as well—and if not only of cancer, then of other diseases? Thus, in Table 8.6 in Part 8, it is commented that peptide fragments have been found in the brains of Alzheimer's disease patients (Sigma catalog, p. 1130). The particular peptide fragment was an amyloid J-protein fragment, designated Fragment 1-40. A peptide, moreover, can be viewed as merely a short protein molecule. So are these peptide fragments what we call prions, or what?

In summation, it has been commented that there are many human chronic degenerative diseases whose causes remain unknown (Voet and Voet, *Biochemistry*, p. 1118). The causes may very well be viruses of one kind or another, in one form or another, and in one molecular size or another.

7.4.1 RHABDOVIRUSES, E.G., RABIES VIRUS

The rhabdoviruses or Rhabdoviridae are characterized by the rod-like shape of the member viruses, of which the most notorious is the rabies virus in its several forms or strains. A succinct but comprehensive overview of the disease and its aspects is provided in the monograph *Rabies: The Facts* by Colin Kaplan, G.S. Turner, and D.A. Warrell. Although there is a similarity in the bullet-like or rod-like morphology of the Rhabdoviridae, apparently there is no genetic relationship between the several rabies subgroups and the more than 80 other viruses that have been placed in the same virus family (Kaplan et al., *Rabies*, p. 2). However, in addition to a similarity in shape, the rhabdoviruses all have similar protein and nucleic acid structures. The entirety occurs variously in diverse plants and invertebrate and vertebrate hosts.

For the purposes here, a discussion of perhaps among the most deadly of all viruses, the rabies virus, may have bearing on manifesting a resistance to cancer, either natural or induced by the action of vaccines or serums.

The aforecited reference observes that the infectivity of rabies virus is destroyed by a number of agents, including most organic solvents, oxidizing agents, and surface-active agents. The last-mentioned category includes soaps, detergents, and quaternary ammonium compounds. *Treating the virus with proteolytic enzymes and with ultraviolet radiation or X-rays will also destroy the virus, as will exposure to markedly acidic and alkaline conditions.* Its survival rate depends in large part on the temperature. When freeze dried or kept at −70° C, it will survive indefinitely; at approximately 0° C, it survives for several days, and in saliva at room temperature, it survives for about 1 day. At 40° C (104° F), its half-life is 4 hr, but at 60° C (140° F) only 30 s.

Rabies virus particles are noted to enter cells by engulfment or else by a fusion between the viral envelope and the cell membrane, with replication occurring in the cytoplasm of the infected cells (Kaplan et al., *Rabies*, p. 3). It can be wondered if this invasion is not assisted by stress proteins or molecular chaperones. Viral synthesis involves the formation of an excess of ribonucleoproteins (RNP) which constitutes the matrix of cellular inclusions known as *Negri bodies,* whose presence is used to diagnose rabies.

It is further noted that what is called *L protein* is associated with the activity of the enzyme transcriptase, which is necessary for replication (either a DNA-dependent DNA polymerase, also simply called DNA polymerase, or else DNA-dependent RNA polymerase, also called RNA polymerase), and what is called *glycoprotein G* is associated with the attachment of the virus to cell surfaces, and is related to virulence (Kaplan et al., *Rabies,* p. 4). Furthermore, glycoprotein G apparently will function as an antigen for the rabies virus, and this immunological activity may ultimately prove of great importance in developing other kinds of rabies vaccines.*

Whereas rabies virus was heretofore regarded as unique, there have been rabies-like or rabies-related viruses isolated from some highly disparate hosts (Kaplan et al., *Rabies,* p. 5). It is noted that, although these viruses appear morphologically and immunologically similar to rabies virus, vaccination against rabies does not necessarily provide immunity to infection by rabies-like viruses. So far, these *rabies-like viruses have been found for sure only in Africa,* although there was an occurrence in two bats found near Hamburg, Germany; they were presumed to have been carried on a ship from Africa.†

A further potential complication is that *antibodies display antigenic behavior according to geographical area.* While standard vaccine strains so far appear to give the necessary protection worldwide, at some future date it may be necessary to tailor vaccines and antiserums according to geographical area.

Also mentioned is that rabies infections, in common with other viral infections, induce the infected cells to produce the particular protein known as *interferon,* which then interferes with virus growth (Kaplan et al., *Rabies,* p. 7). *In the case of rabies, however, this natural interferon induction does not happen soon enough to inactivate the virus.* It has been noted, on the other hand, that *the prompt administration of interferon protects experimental animals from rabies.* (The administration of interferon evidently does not provide protection against cancer, however, or at least does not provide a cure, in spite of some high hopes.)

While recovery from the attack of an infectious disease usually makes the patient immune to subsequent attacks of the same disease, *recovery is so rare in humans that this immunizing effect has not been observed* (Kaplan et al., *Rabies,* p. 8). However, *infection and recovery have sometimes been observed in wildlife reservoirs and, less frequently, in dogs.*

The foremost problem with rabies in humans and animals is lack of an immune response until late in the cycle, as indicated above. *"In common with many other diseases, the initial infecting dose of rabies virus is unlikely to be sufficient to provoke an immune response by itself."* The spread and proliferation of the virus occurs within the nervous tissue, apart from the immune system. Only after the virus multiplies in the brain is an immune response produced, which by then is too late.

Several types of rabies vaccines have been developed over time (Kaplan et al., *Rabies,* pp. 11–14). The original rabies vaccines were derived from suspensions of infected rabbit spinal cord, which had been dried for various intervals of time. The shorter the drying period, the more live virus remained, and the more infective the suspension. Resistance is built up by the daily injection of successively more active suspensions. The potential hazards of using even attenuated live vaccines caused the procedure to be modified, killing the virus with carbolic acid, called Semple's method. Duck-embryo vaccines were next developed, a much safer vaccine that avoided the possibility neurological accidents. This, in turn, has been succeeded by cell-culture vaccines. A further development in the last-mentioned approach

---

* The enzyme called RNA-dependent RNA polymerase or RNA-directed RNA polymerase (according to the index in Voet and Voet, this is DNA-directed RNA polymerase or simply RNA polymerase) catalyzes the transcription step (Noel Tordo and Olivier Poch, in *Rabies,* p. 30). It may be concluded therefore that *the rabies virus is not a retrovirus.* That is, a retrovirus utilizes the enzyme called RNA-directed DNA polymerase (or reverse transcriptase).

† While rabies virus is the prototype, both rabies virus and rabies-related viruses belong to the genus *Lyssavirus* (Tordo and Poch, in *Rabies,* p. 25). And whereas rabies-related viruses were formerly thought to be confined to Africa, they have more recently been found in European countries, as indicated above. The reference further states that rabies virus has an unsegmented negative strand RNA genome, a structure common to two viral families, the Paramyxoviridae and the Rhabdoviridae. The host range of the Rhabdoviridae is especially wide, ranging from insects to fishes and mammals. The two main genera are *Vesiculovirus* and *Lyssavirus.* The former consists primarily of vesicular stomatitis virus or VSV and its subtypes and related viruses. As noted, rabies virus is the prototype or original form for *Lyssavirus.*

is the use of a vaccine prepared in cultures of special human cells, designated as human diploid cell strains (HDCS). The search continues for even better (and cheaper) vaccines for humans.

As to vaccinating cats and dogs, it is said that *if more than 70 percent of the canine population is immunized, this is said to break the chain of transmission and extinguish the disease* (Kaplan et al., *Rabies*, p. 14). Live virus vaccines heretofore have been used for domestic animals but have subsequently been questioned, so now there is a choice of many potent inactivated veterinary vaccines. As to wildlife, it has been shown that attenuated live virus, administered by mouth, will produce an immune response in foxes, and its use is expected to spread by the use of baits containing the virus.

Current practice for widespread rabies control is to impregnate feed pellets or biscuits with serum, to be spread widely over the landscape, for instance from airplanes. This was used successfully, for instance, to contain a rabies outbreak in southwestern Texas and has also been used in Australia. A widespread rabies outbreak is of great concern in the Serengetti Plains region of East Africa. It is of the canine strain and spreads to wildlife, apparently by domestic dogs. Steps are being taken to immunize village dogs as a means of control. Although rabies has been minimized in the United States, the human death estimates in Africa range up to 25,000 per year, mostly children. Many who are bitten cannot afford the Pasteur treatment, or it is not easily available. All of this makes an inexpensive prophylactic or after-the-fact oral antivirus/antirabies agent—such as a plant substance—even more desirable. That there may be an anticancer activity connected with antiviral activity is a possibility, since viruses have been associated with at least some kinds of cancer.

Modern immunological practice indicates that rabies vaccine dosage levels could be drastically reduced, as practiced in other countries, although the fatal nature of the disease makes one want to be on the safe side (Kaplan et al., *Rabies*, pp. 15–17). And whereas pre-exposure vaccination has proven highly effective, it is difficult to judge the effectiveness of post-exposure vaccination.

> Many subjects receiving treatment may not be infected, for—despite popular mythology—man is relatively resistant to rabies and natural infection is therefore uncertain.*

The reference continues,

> It is, of course, ethically impossible to withhold treatment, and so controlled studies cannot be made.†

> None of the animal models, including those in Pasteur's original experiments, convincingly demonstrated a protective effect of vaccine administration after infection. The retrospective examination of more than a million cases of post-exposure treatment in the 1940s also proved inconclusive. The most credible evidence of value in man comes from a 20-year survey in India where 56 per cent of untreated exposed subjects died of rabies, whereas only 7 per cent died after post-exposure treatment.

Part of the difficulty probably lies in the antigenic inadequacy of early vaccines. However, in controlled tests on animals, it has been demonstrated without a doubt that potent cell-culture vaccines successfully protect animals after experimental infection, and sometimes with only a single dose.

It was stated that the experience of the Pasteur Institute of Southern India during the period 1907 to 1923 found that 35 percent of the people bitten by known infective animals died if not vaccinated (Kaplan et al., *Rabies*, p. 26). Similar results were reported in 1887, before the advent of Pasteur's original vaccine.

---

* It may be mentioned, in passing, of the instance in the frontier army where two soldiers were bitten by the same rabid animal. One died and one survived. There may, of course, have been differences in the activities of their immune systems, and differences in the presence or absence of stress proteins or molecular chaperones that assist viruses in crossing cell barriers. Or the bite may have been more severe for the one than the other, that is to say, more of the rabies virus was transmitted for the one than the other. Three cases are provided in the reference (Kaplan et al., *Rabies*, pp. 56–57). And as will subsequently be noted, *in a study of the many cases of rabies-exposed victims in India, nearly 50 percent survived without treatment.* Still another reference cites recovery, albeit rarely (K.M. Charlton, in *Rabies*, p. 136).

† This matter of ethics gives pause for concern about double-blind tests, say, for, judging the effectiveness of cancer treatments.

Being a communicable disease, the spread of rabies corresponds to the same patterns as other communicable diseases (Kaplan et al., *Rabies*, p. 94). In a way of speaking, subjects that have immunity to a given agent will withstand infection by it, and those that don't, won't. And recovered subjects will be immune to reinfection by rabies. Furthermore, part of those infected may never show any signs of the disease and will develop immunity. Also noted is that, during an epidemic, the number of susceptible subjects will progressively diminish. A point will be reached at which there are too few susceptible subjects to transmit the disease, ending the epidemic. The causative agent will not reestablish itself until the number of susceptible targets again increases, by immigration or by birth.

Among the ways for the body to provide specific protective immunity is by the formation of soluble substances involving the serum proteins of the blood (Kaplan et al., *Rabies*, p. 17). These substance may be referred to as *circulating* or humoral antibodies. Another way is by a response connected directly with cellular activity. This latter response is called *cell-mediated* immunity. These are subjects still under investigation in the development of a serum. Cell-mediated immunity can be induced by rabies antigens in both humans and animals, but the cytotoxic reactions produced can be either protective or pathogenic.

On the other hand, the serum antibodies neutralize rabies virus, and the effects can be estimated with some degree of accuracy. However, administration of the serum can sometimes cause the *early death phenomenon*—at least in animals that had previously been vaccinated. Thus, *the anti-rabies serum may ether protect or may accelerate death from the disease.* In any event, in all severe exposures, the early administration of both anti-rabies serum and vaccine was recommended, before the virus has reached the central nervous system.*

For various reasons—including the sometimes long incubation period—the incidence of rabies is viewed as under-reported (Kaplan et al., *Rabies*, p. 21ff). *England, however, is said to have remained free from rabies since 1903, although there are a few instances of the return and treatment of victims who were infected abroad.* (Australia may also be rabies-free.)

The severity of the rabid animal bite will have an effect on the time for the symptoms of rabies encephalitis to make an appearance, with bites around the face, neck, and hands being the most serious, the location accelerating the transmission of the virus to the central nervous system (Kaplan et al., *Rabies*, p. 26). In an early study reported in 1887, previously cited, *the mortality rate was 21 percent from leg bites, ranging up to 88 percent for facial bites.*

As to the incubation period, the symptoms of rabies encephalitis may show up in as little as four days after exposure, or may not show up for years (Kaplan et al., *Rabies*, pp. 27–28). In a study of rabies victims in Thailand, *the incubation time was a minimum of four days and a maximum of four years.* Reports of 19-year-incubation times, or more, have been reported in the scientific literature, but these may be due to a second exposure. Alternatively, *the rabies virus may lie dormant until activated by another infection, or even stress.* It is noted that *herpes viruses act in the same way.* Thus, the childhood chickenpox virus can be reactivated in later life to cause shingles. Cold sores caused by the herpes simplex virus are another example. The virus stays latent until activated by a fever such as may occur with the common cold.

Although generally the result of a bite, *airborne rabies may be transmitted by inhalation.* In 1956, two men died from rabies after exploring caves in Uvalde County, Texas. These caves are resident to millions of insectivorous Mexican free-tailed bats. In another case, during early investigations of rabies in bats roosting in caves, a worker—who was not bitten—came down with rabies and died (Kaplan et al., *Rabies*, p. 89). The vectors were considered to be either insects or the aerial route. Subsequently, animals were caged in insect- and bat-proof cages and put around the caves inhabited by colonies of bats. One by one the animals—ranging from mice to foxes—contracted rabies and died. The dust on the cave floor was found to be heavily contaminated with rabies virus, left there by the saliva and urine of the bats roosting above. The virus could very well be transmitted among the bats during quarrels or fights in the roosts, and by breathing the contaminated dust (or air), then transmitted to terrestrial animals when they entered the cave.†

The two clinical forms of rabies are (1) *furious*, or *agitated*, or *excited* (or *virulent*) rabies and (2) the rarer *paralytic* or *dumb* rabies (Kaplan et al., *Rabies*, p. 34ff). Both are the result of an acute inflammatory reaction in the central nervous system (CNS), which accompanies the invasion and multiplication of the

---

* The use of serum is sometimes called "passive" immunization, whereas the use of vaccine is sometimes called "active" immunization. Serum is obtained from an immunized donor, human or animal.

virus in the cells of the nervous system. In the former, the brain is primarily affected. In the latter, it is the spinal cord. Moreover, there is the indication that the two forms may be caused by different strains of rabies virus. Not only are rabies viruses not all of one type, but there are distinct strains varying with geographical area and with the species of animal serving as the vector. Strictly speaking, hydrophobia—the fear of water—while sometimes used as a synonym for the rabies disease, pertains to this dreaded and unexplainable symptom, which occurs in about 80 percent of the victims of furious rabies. A similar uncontrollable symptom is aerophobia—dread of air—such as produced by a draft of air on the face.

No mention is made in the reference of the effect of plants or plant substances such as rue and elecampane as folkloric rabies cures, as mentioned in the section "Antibacterial and Antiviral Agents" in Part 2, and again in the section "Alkaloids and Anticancer Agents" in Part 4. *Attempts to cure rabies by intensive care have largely failed, although it may prolong life* (Kaplan et al., *Rabies*, p. 57). On the other hand, *there is a commercially available antiviral agent called ribavirin or "Virazole" which shows activity against RNA viruses,* although its use against rabies virus is uncertain. Interferon has proved unsuccessful. Whereas some mammalian species such as dogs can recover from rabies, and this recovery can be further promoted by various immunological manipulations, it has not been projected to humans.

Nevertheless, for the record, Parts 2 and 4 as previously indicated, and also Appendix J, mention or list various plants that are cited as antiviral agents according to medical folklore, with the possibility that some of these might also act as anticancer agents.

As a further comment, *there is the sometimes rumor that a few rabies victims who have received the vaccine may die of mysterious causes at a future date.* In the past, this may have been due to an allergic reaction produced from the duck-embryo proteins that occur in the vaccine. (This is, in fact, why the vaccine was formerly administered successively in the stomach area—to spread out and slow down any allergic reactions that might occur, which, such as there were, would be expected to happen during or shortly after the vaccination sequence.) Mitigation is not necessary with the modern vaccines developed from human diploid* cell lines, there being few allergic reactions. As an additional note, with the modern vaccine, pre-exposure vaccinations are given epidermally, whereas post-exposure vaccinations are given intramuscularly.

Rabies or hydrophobia was an intermittent but serious concern on America's western frontier. Bernard DeVoto, in *Across the Wide Missouri*, describes an incident and the consequences of a nocturnal visit by a rabid wolf to a camp of the Rocky Mountain Fur Company (DeVoto, *Across the Wide Missouri*, pp. 104–106). The incident occurred in late July, 1833, when everyone was sleeping in the open, as was reported by Charles Larpenteur, a fur trader on the Upper Missouri (Larpenteur, *Forty Years a Fur Trader*, pp. 30–34). The wolf bit three men at the RMF Company camp and nine more at another camp located four or five miles away. An Indian was also bitten, as well as one of the bulls that were being driven to a new outpost. Several victims went into paroxysms and died before camp was broken up. Some were later stricken on the trail and wandered off to their deaths, and the bull also died. DeVoto adds that several inexplicable deaths in the next two years were attributed to this visit by the wolf. DeVoto repeats Larpenteur's description of the way one of the bitten men went mad, developing a phobia against water, and who had to be covered with a blanket to get him across small streams. Abandoned by the party, when searchers were sent back, they found that the man had removed all his clothes and wandered off, never to be found.

---

† Another speleological hazard in exploring caves is *histoplasmosis*, a fungal infection produced by the inhalation of dust containing *Histoplasma capsulatum*. This is a soil fungus that grows on decaying vegetation. According to the article in the *Encyclopedia Americana*, the infection usually occurs only in the lungs but may at times spread to other parts of the body via the bloodstream. Pneumonia is the primary acute result but may be followed by infection in the liver and adrenal glands and, lastly, by chronic cavitary pulmonary disease. The treatment of choice is the antifungal agent amphotericin B. Other references speak of histoplasmosis as a disease of the reticuloendothelial system, whose proper function is to maintain immunity. (The term "reticular" means mesh-like, and the endothelium pertains to a layer of cells lining the heart, blood vessels, lymphatics, and serous cavities—"serous" in turn implying serum-containing, serum being a body fluid of a watery consistency.) The usual, more noticeable signs of the disease are fever, anemia, and emaciation. The spread of the fungus is evidently through the excretions of bird life, notably, and even mites may be involved. Examples of carriers include chickens, pigeons, starlings, and even the oil birds of South American caves. Very likely, bats can be added to the list.

* Diploid, meaning having double the basic or haploid number of chromosomes.

Robert M. Wright, a frontiersman and founder of Dodge City, Kansas, mentions problems with mad wolves and skunks (Wright, *Dodge City*, pp. 70, 72). This was in the 1870s and earlier. The rabid animals would invade the early-day forts and camps, and in one incident at Fort Larned, northeast of Fort Dodge and present-day Dodge City, a wolf bit several of the men, including a Lt. Thompson. The others all died, but Thompson was able to go east for treatments. Wright indicated that Thompson was never the same, however, and didn't know whether this was from the treatment or from the continual dread of coming down with the disease.

Wright also mentioned that, in the early days, skunks were numerous around Dodge City. Inasmuch as their bite was nearly always fatal, it was supposed that they were rabid. The first year of Dodge City's existence (founded in 1872), there were 8 or 10 persons who died from skunk bites. The custom was to sleep outdoors, and the skunks would climb right into bed and bite the person, usually on the face, hands, or feet.

Col. Richard Irving Dodge, commander at Fort Dodge and a cofounder of Dodge City (after whom Dodge City is said to have been named), wrote that rabies was not a Plains malady, and that he personally never knew of a single case on the Plains save for white men bitten by a skunk (Dodge, *Our Wild Indians*, pp. 320–321). Indians, on the other hand, say they are troubled by mad wolves that usually make their appearance in February and March. They will enter an Indian village and attack everybody in sight until killed or disabled. The result from even a scratch is, in every case, death by hydrophobia. At the first sign of paroxysms, the victim goes off alone to await death or commit suicide.*

Col. R.I. Dodge added that *Indians were not affected by the bite of a skunk,* which is so very fatal to white men. The Indians seem to suffer no injurious effect whatsoever, other than the pain of the bite. Either the Indian is genetically different and therefore is immune to the particular rabies strain of the skunk (if there is one), or else the Indians knows something about a cure that the white man doesn't.†

The foregoing leads to the subject of antiviral agents and, in particular, to potential antirabies agents, as previously described in Part 2 within the section "Antibacterial and Antiviral Agents." Thus, Carl Lumholtz, who explored the American Southwest and Northwest Mexico in the early 1900s, pinpointed rue as a native cure for rabies (Lumholtz, *Unknown Mexico*, II, p. 347). In a later book, he mentioned that the Papago Indians of the region had a secret, undisclosed cure for rabies (Lumholtz, *New Trails*, pp. 184–185). Furthermore, in an article appearing in the August, 1961 issue of *Arizona Highways*, Dr. Joseph G. Lee emphasizes rue as a Navajo remedy for rabies. (Albeit, without a doubt, we would prefer the latest Pasteur treatment.) Not to be overlooked, the herb known as rue (*Ruta graveolens* of the family Rutaceae) contains many alkaloids, and can therefore be considered hazardous to take, if not downright toxic.

John Heinerman's book, *Healing Animals with Herb,* contains several references to plants that act against rabies, in instances going all the way back to pioneering English herbalist Gervase Markham's *Cheape and Good Husbandry,* first published in London in 1614. Although rue (*Ruta graveolens* of the family Rutaceae) and yarrow (*Achillea millefolium* of the family Compositae) are mentioned, the most space is given to elecampane (*Inula helenium* of the family Compositae). Incidentally, these three plant species are also listed in Hartwell's *Plants Used Against Cancer.*

---

* There is a point of confusion between two different and unrelated Dodges. There was also a Gen. Grenville M. Dodge, prominent during the Civil War, and before and afterward, as a railroad construction engineer. (Not to mention a Gen. Henry Dodge, also famous on the frontier.) Grenville M. Dodge may or may not have been the namesake for Fort Dodge, located just east of what became Dodge City. General G.M. Dodge became chief engineer for building the Union Pacific Railroad westward to Promontory Point, Utah Territory, to meet up with the Central Pacific, the historical event of May 10, 1869.

† Speaking of genetic differences, there is case of the Navajo Indians, mentioned in John Heinerman's *Spiritual Wisdom of the Native Americans,* who have such a low natural cancer incidence but who also do not eat poultry products and boil their mutton for a long time—presumably avoiding or killing viruses present. (The Indians are also supposed to know about such plants as chaparral, a folklore agent against cancer.) It can be wondered, in turn, if the low cancer rate is genetic or if the Navajo cancer rate has increased upon adopting the usual American diet, as found in Japan for instance. Another presumed genetic difference for the Indians is their superb sense of balance, as evidenced by the Mohawk steelworkers who walk the girders of skyscrapers and high bridges with aplomb. This, however, may be attributed to the way they walk, one foot directly in front of another, similar to a tightrope walker, as noted by Alex Shoumatoff in *The Rivers Amazon.* The Indians of Amazonia walk in this way, making a path only a few inches wide, and display extraordinary balance (Shoumatoff, *The Rivers Amazon,* p. 166).

Alma R. Hutchens' *Indian Herbalogy of North America* also lists a number of herbs that, according to medical folklore, act against hydrophobia or rabies.

It may be commented that, if these plants contain substances that in fact act against rabies virus, then there very likely are other plant substances that act against still other viruses. Whether this action is as an enzyme inhibitor for certain critical biochemical pathways is yet to be spelled out—but this sort of action may be suspected, either in the replication of the virus per se or in the host cell.

Lastly, there is the interesting conjecture that rabies-bearing bats inhabit caves, and there is the suspicion that the *Ebola virus,* for instance, may have had its origins or presence in a cave or caves of equatorial Africa. What kind of mutations or crossovers could conceivably have occurred or evolved is an item for intense speculation, inasmuch as the *Ebola virus is a retrovirus.* Although rabies virus per se is not regarded as a retrovirus, and presumably is always a *stable entity—evidenced by the fact that vaccines can be prepared and effectively used—*there may still be the possibility of mutations or crossovers with other kinds of viruses.

Influenza virus in its various strains is such an example (e.g., Voet and Voet, *Biochemistry,* pp. 1105–1113). Migratory birds are in fact regarded as the major worldwide vector (Voet and Voet, *Biochemistry,* p. 1109)—though bats are not mentioned. (Interestingly, glycoproteins are involved in the influenza virus structure.) There are, of course, different types and strains of rabies virus, which can lead to aberrations in treatment. And if rabies virus is excluded, there are still other kinds of viruses that potentially may interact, and that may involve such life forms as other mammals, birds, reptiles, insects, plants, fungi, bacteria, and protozoa.

It may be further added that with the decimation of tropical rain forests, notably in Amazonia, *there is talk of the emergence of strange viruses from the soil itself.* What eventual impact this may have remains to be seen. *Inasmuch as rain forests have also been destroyed in equatorial Africa, this may have also played a part in the emergence, say, of the Marburg and Ebola viruses or viruses yet to be discovered.*

Speaking of the potentially enormous number of different virus species that may occur from all sources, it will subsequently be noted that *some 100 different enteric (intestinal) viruses have been found in humans* (Kilgren and Cole, in *Microbiology of Marine Products,* pp. 197–209). Furthermore, of the picornaviruses or Picornaviridae, so far the largest virus family yet known, *there are approximately 200 species that are specific merely to humans, of which 69 are enteroviruses found in the intestinal tract.*

7.4.2 REOVIRUSES

Reoviruses, of the family Reoviridae, constitute a commonly found family of viruses, with the acronym "reo" standing in for *r*espiratory *e*nteric *o*rphan viruses. (The designator *enteric* signifies that the viruses pass through the stomach unaffected and proceed on to the intestines proper to disintegrate, be expelled, be absorbed, or otherwise act in ways that are not always known. "Orphan" viruses are those that have not yet been classified as specifically causing a disease.) Reoviruses are associated with respiratory infections of vague causation, with intestinal infections such as may be called the *intestinal flu,* and with more unusual diseases such as encephalitis and phlebotomus fever. That which is called a *human virus* is said to be a reovirus.*

Reoviruses are found in certain animal and human tumors.

More generally speaking, from further information supplied from various scientific dictionaries, reoviruses occur in a wide variety of hosts, including vertebrates, insects, and plants. The virus particles are said to be unenveloped and isochedral. The virus is further described as an echovirus. (ECHOviruses, or echoviruses, comprise a genus of entero viruses of the family Picornaviridae. The acronym stands for *e*nteric *c*ytopathic *h*uman *o*rphan viruses. These viruses replicate in the intestinal tract, some apparently being harmless, but others associated with such disorders as aseptic meningitiis.) Also, the Reoviridae are referred to as a group of ribonucleic acid-containing viruses, indicating that they can be called

---

* What is known as the *rhinovirus* is blamed for the human cold, "rhino-" meaning nose. It, along with the poliovirus, are examples of *picornaviruses* ("pico" plus RNA), which is a very large family of very small, RNA-containing animal viruses, and which also includes the viral agents that cause hepatitis A in humans and foot-and-mouth disease in cattle, sheep, and swine (Voet and Voet, *Biochemistry,* p. 1086).

RNA viruses, utilizing the enzyme sometimes called simply *transcriptase* (DNA-directed RNA polymerase).

The penetration of reovirions (reovirus particles) into the host cell has been said to be accomplished "by an active yet nonspecific process of phagocytosis, termed viropexis" (Helmut Zarbl and Stewart Millward in *The Reoviridae,* p. 113). Presumably, this process may be viewed as assisted by means of molecular chaperones, previously described. It is further mentioned in the reference that the penetration of reoviruses can be inhibited by cationic polymers such as diethylaminoethyl [DEAE]-dextran. The mechanism of inhibition is not understood.

The virions end up in the interior of the cell and fuse with lysosomes, the membrane-bound organelles containing hydrolytic enzymes. Within the lysosomes, the virus particles are uncoated by hydrolytic enzymes, as further described below.

The same reference speaks of intermediate subviral particles (ISVPs) that enter the host cell by direct penetration (Zarbl and Millward, *The Reoviridae,* p. 114). Furthermore, it has been observed that the ISVPs can be produced *in vitro* by digestion using the enzyme chymotrypsin in the presence of sodium ions. The action is to remove part of the coat of the virions. In other words the virions lose essentially all the outer capsid proteins. These ISVP particles are resistant to proteolysis, but on exposure to potassium ions (K^+), there is a further uncoating, and the enzyme *transcriptase* is reactivated. This has been observed both *in vitro* and *in vivo.* Thus, when cells are infected with ISVPs where the particles penetrate the cell membrane, followed by exposure to K^+ in the cytoplasm, this produces particles with an active RNA transcriptase. The end result is that the ISVPs become infectious agents.

Whereas most animal viruses are destroyed by lysosomal hydrolases, this will defend the cell against viral infections (Zarbl and Millward, in *The Reoviridae,* p. 119). Reoviruses are the exception, however, since they utilize this same defense mechanism against the host cell. In turn, there is a slow escape of the uncoated particles or virions, called parental SVPs (subviral particles), which is an essential step in the infectious cycle (Zarbl and Millward, in *The Reoviridae,* p. 120).

It is set forth in the reference that an infection with reoviruses does not shut down host cellular protein synthesis at first, but synthesis is slowly diminished so that, after about 10 hours, viral proteins predominate (Zeebl and Millward, in *The Reoviridae,* p. 162).

In a discussion of plant Reoviridae and plant-virus relationships, it is stated that *all plant-infecting Reoviridae* are transmitted only by *insect* vectors (R.I.B. Francki and Guido Boccardo, in *The Reoviridae,* p. 533)—a vector, of course, being a carrier or agent of transmission. Among the plant reoviruses or phytoreoviruses studied are rice dwarf virus (RDV) and Fiji disease virus (FDV). Another discovered is wound tumor virus (WTV). The last is of particular interest due to its tumor-inducing properties. It is further noted that *WTV infects only dicotyledonous plants to produce neoplastic growths,* whereas RDV infects only Gramineae (or Poaceae) and produces no neoplasia. Another example is rice gall dwarf virus (RGDV), which infects only rice, inducing neoplastic growths.*

It has been observed that the reoviruses transmitted by their (insect) vectors multiply in these same vectors (Francki and Boccardo, in *The Reoviridae,* p. 544). *"Although the viruses multiply in their vectors, no neoplastic growths like those in plants are produced."* This is, in turn, qualified as to other effects in that *"cytopathological effects similar to those induced in plant cells have been observed in all the organs of the various vectors"*—the exception being the testes. Further statements are made to the effect that phytoreoviruses (plant-reoviruses) have been studied in intact insects as well as in vecto-cell monolayers, with WTV the most extensive virus studied. (WTV for instance is transmitted by an insect or insects called the *planthoppers.* Another insect vector mentioned is the leafhopper.)

It is further stated that, of the six Reoviridae genera, four genera include viruses that multiply in insects (Francki and Boccardo, in *The Reoviridae,* p. 551). *There is only a single genus pathogenic to insects alone,* having no alternative plant or vertebrate hosts, this being the genus *Cypovirus.* The other three genera of insect-infecting viruses also have either plant hosts or vertebrate hosts. Thus the two insect-infecting genera that also have plant hosts are *Phytovirus* and *Fujivirus.* The single insect-infecting genus which has vertebrate hosts is *Orbivirus.* These species of the former genera are referred to as plant viruses; the species of the latter genus are referred to as vertebrate viruses.†

---

* If insects act as vectors, presumably the possibilities can be generalized to include other invertebrates, or the term "insect" can be used to denote invertebrates in general.

It is commented in the reference that the ability of these reoviruses to replicate in insect hosts without any indication of disease may signify that *both the vertebrate reoviruses and plant reoviruses may have evolved from common insect-infecting ancestors.*

Thus, in a roundabout way, one may conclude that there are viruses that will not only infect plants but also will infect insects. In turn, there are viruses that will not only infect insects but will also infect vertebrates. But the statement is not made that some viruses will make the leap from plants to humans, or vice versa.

A special case to consider is that of the arborviruses, denoting arthropod-borne viruses that are transmitted by the phylum of invertebrates known as arthropods, which includes insects, arachnids or spiders, and crustaceans. *Arborviruses cause such human diseases as yellow fever and dengue fever, with the viruses transmitted by mosquitoes. Furthermore, by definition, the arthropod or insect is merely a vector or carrier—the agent of transmission between an animal or human host, or victim, and another. It may be asked in this case, however, can the virus actually infect the arthropod or insect vector, and thus be called an arthropod virus or insect virus? Evidently not, for these particular viruses—at least according to conventional wisdom. But if otherwise, then there is a potential relationship not only to insects as an infectious agent as well as a vector, but to plant viruses as well and also to humans. The question has bearing on whether there are some unsuspected sources in unexpected places for emerging viruses, say the Ebola virus.

To continue, the above-cited genus *Orbivirus* encompasses a number of arthropod-borne viruses that have certain unique and distinct morphological and physicochemical criteria (Barry M. Gormon, Jill Taylor, and Peter J. Walker, in *The Reoviridae*, p. 287). They may, in turn, infect mammals, notably humans—e.g., Colorado tick fever.†

Colorado tick fever, for instance, was first recognized in 1930 as an acute febrile (fever) illness in humans, and it was later shown to be tick-borne (Gorman et al., in *The Reoviridae*, p. 300). The major vector is the tick *Dermacentor andersoni*, found in the mountainous regions of the northwestern U.S. and Canada. Vertebrate reservoirs for the virus include rodents, ground squirrels, pine squirrels, chipmunks, meadow voles, and porcupines.

We may also choose to include bacterial or prokaryotic viruses (bacteriophages), which widens the scope of possibilities even further. That is, conceivably, not only could bacteria act as vectors for viral diseases, but they could be the infected repository for viruses affecting not only bacteria per se but also humans, insects, and plants—not to mention that bacteria are in themselves disease-causing agents.

7.5 PLANT AND INSECT VIRUSES

The conventional wisdom is that plant viruses do not and cannot infect animals or humans, nor can they mutate with animal or human viruses—albeit certain insect or insect-borne viruses can infect animals or humans. (Human and other viruses may interact or mutate, however, being the source, for example, of various newly encountered influenza strains. In particular, this is a property of retroviruses.) Nevertheless, with such new-found viruses as the Marburg and Ebola viruses, perhaps there is good and sufficient reason to wonder about plant viruses making the leap to humans. There are insect viruses, of

---

† For the record, let it be said that *vertebrates* comprise a subphylum of animals that have a segmented backbone or spinal column and may include a few more primitive forms having a backbone represented by a notochord—an elastic rod such as occurs in lampreys. Humans, of course, are vertebrates, as are all mammals as well as birds, reptiles, amphibians, and fishes. By exclusion, vertebrates are not invertebrates, the latter represented by insects, arachnids, and crustaceans.

* More specifically, arthropods constitute the phylum Arthropoda, which consists of animals with articulated bodies and limbs. Examples, as previously indicated, are insects, arachnids, and crustaceans.

† Colorado tick fever is as distinguished from Rocky Mountain spotted fever. The latter, as its name implies, was first discovered in the Rocky Mountain region but has since been found to be much more widespread. Rather than by a virus, it is caused by a bacteria-like microorganism called *Rickettsia*, more specifically the species *Rickettsia rickettsii*. (It may be noted that the genus *Rickettsia* also pertains to the microorganism that causes typhus fever.) Colorado tick fever is identical with the disease called São Paulo fever in Brazil and with the spotted fever of Colombia. The microorganism for RM spotted fever is parasitic on arthropods, namely on ticks (the means by which it is spread) and is pathogenic to animals and humans. It is spread by the same tick that carries the virus for Colorado tick fever and also by the common dog tick *Dermacentor variabilis*, and by yet other tick species in other locales. The disease can be treated by antibiotics, and immunization is routinely available for workers who expect to encounter the disease.

course, that are already capable of making the leap. Add to this the possibility that bacterial viruses may somehow enter the loop, and the picture becomes increasingly complex.

Moreover, in the destruction of the tropical rain forests and the attendant disturbance of the soils, the thought is sometimes expressed about the emergence of other still-unknown and potentially lethal viruses. The question can be asked, are these emerging microorganisms plant viruses, insect viruses, bacterial viruses, or what? And are these viruses in themselves a threat to humans, and/or will they mutate or interact with human and other animal viruses?

There is no shortage of books about plant viruses. In fact, the tobacco mosaic virus (TMV) has probably been studied more than any other, and studies on plant viruses have formed the basis for fundamental studies on human and animal viruses. One of the more extensive works is that of R.E.F. Matthews, titled *Plant Virology*, now in its third edition. In a chapter on variability, Matthews takes up the subject of "The Molecular Basis of Variation" (Matthews, *Plant Virology*, p. 474ff). It is noted that *mutations or nucleotide changes can occur due to a number of causes, denoted as chemical mutagens, irradiation, elevated temperature, and those that are natural mutations.*[*]

Aside from the technical descriptions, it is set forth that chemical mutagens will also inactivate viruses. Nitrous acid is mentioned in particular as a mutagen used for *in vitro* studies. However, the commonly used cytotoxic chemotherapy agent 5-fluorouracil is also mentioned as a mutagenic agent. It is said to replace the uracil residues occurring in RNA. The changes are denoted as uracil6 cytosine and as adenine6 guanine. If these things occur in plant viruses, the questions can be asked, what goes on in viruses affecting humans, and what in turn may be going on in human cells?

Ionizing radiation and UV radiation are observed to inactivate viruses and to produce mutations in those viruses. Elevated temperatures induce variant strains but may also favor the invasion and multiplication of other strains. As to natural mutations, there may be involved only a single-amino acid substitution in the viral protein. For example, in 16 spontaneous mutants observed for the tobacco mosaic virus, six had one amino acid exchange in the coat protein, another had two exchanges, and one had three such exchanges. It was surmised that most of the mutants were the result of copying errors made by the enzyme *RNA-dependent RNA polymerases* during viral RNA duplication. The distinguishing phrase here is "RNA-dependent RNA polymerases"—whereas if it had been "RNA-dependent *DNA* polymerases" or RNA-directed *DNA* polymerases," or *reverse transcriptase,* then we would be talking *retroviruses.* In any event, *mutations in virus populations are apparently common enough, at least in plants,* and if this degree of mutagenicity can be projected to viruses in humans, then we may be speaking of all kinds of infectious agents, for various cancers and for many other disease variations. These agents, being mutations, are both similar and different at the same time.

In another chapter dealing with nomenclature and classification, Matthews speculates on origins and evolution (Matthews, *Plant Virology*, p. 650ff). He considers several possibilities for viral origins—as descendants of primitive precellular life forms, by development from the normal constituents of cells and by degeneration from cells. In the course of describing these possibilities, Matthews regards viruses as highly developed obligate (limited to a single-life condition) parasites that use the same genetic code as cellular organisms but are dependent on the host cell for protein synthesis on ribosomes, tRNAs, and associated enzymes. It is observed that *amino acids occur in viral proteins in the same frequency as in the globular proteins of other organisms.* Although viral particles are relatively simple in structure, they seem to be no more primitive, from an evolutionary standpoint, than do cellular organisms.

There is reason to believe that viruses may develop from an escaped cell constituent and are outside the cell-regulating machinery. Or *a normal cell component from one organism may act as a virus when introduced into the cells of another.* Thus, *a possibility is that certain plant viruses, for instance, may have come from the cellular components of the insects that feed on the particular plants.* (Here, we would have an interaction between viral plant and animal life, or at least insect life.)

In support of statements in the preceding paragraph, *there is relationship between certain genetic elements in bacteria and bacterial viruses.* Thus, *plasmids* can be regarded as autonomous extrachromo-

---

[*] It may be mentioned that *viral infections have been used for centuries in plant breeding to change the coloration of tulips.* Probably the most commonly used agent for producing plant mutations is the alkaloid *colchicine.* The foregoing serves to emphasize that a number of different kinds of agents, both organic and inorganic, will affect the DNA or nucleotide chemistry of organisms. In the case of viral agents, the process may be referred to as *lysogeny,* and has been previously discussed.

somal genetic elements found naturally in many types of bacteria. (A *plasmid* can be designated as a DNA molecule that is distinct from the bacterial chromosome replicated by the cell. Furthermore, plasmids can integrate into the bacterial chromosome to be replicated along with the chromosomal DNA.) In a sense, therefore, *a plasmid can be perceived as an additional smaller host chromosome. It has been found possible to convert some viruses into plasmid-like entities by a deletion of some of the genes. On the other hand, by adding the appropriate viral genes, it may be possible to change a plasmid into a virus-like entity.* *

The very fact that the DNA of some viruses will integrate into a host cell genome supports the theory that these viruses could have originated there (Matthews, *Plant Virology*, p. 652).†

The RNA tumor virus family, which may also be called the Retroviridae and which infect eukaryotic cells, are of special interest as to viral origins. The genome consists of a form of RNA, ssRNA, but upon infection, this is copied by means of a viral-coded enzyme, *reverse transcriptase* (also called RNA-directed DNA polymerase) to be integrate into the host cell genome.

Assorted "proviruses" or "protoviruses" have also been proposed wherein viral genes are regarded as normal but "repressed" components of the genome of the cell. On "de-repression" by some form of stress such as radiation or chemical carcinogens, there is a production of the infectious virus.

Carried farther, this line of theorizing indicates that *new viruses are constantly being created due to degenerative processes occurring in cells*. Thus, it has been proposed that some RNA animal viruses, and even small DNA-containing viruses, have originated from retroviruses. On the other hand, there is the possibility that viral-related genetic sequences as found in normal individuals may be the remnants of a viral integration in the distant past.

If there is a complete *integration* of the viral genome into the host genome without damage to the host, this should permit the survival and dissemination of the virus through many generations of the host. Such an integration would provide an ideal scenario for survival of the virus. If viruses did indeed originate in this way, however, the reference then asks, "Why is it so few established virus families and groups appear to have retained this survival mechanism?" Fortunately for the human species, and all species, these few exceptions predominate.

The reference asks if there is a fundamental distinction between viruses that infect prokaryotes or bacterial cells, and those that infect eukaryotes—that is, between the viruses (bacteriophages) infecting bacteria cells and those infecting nonbacterial cells, in this case, namely plant cells (Matthews, *Plant Virology*, p. 666). This is answered by the statement that *"There is no authenticated example of a virus of one sort completing its life cycle successfully in cells of the other type."* (Apparently, the evolutionary origins are simply different, although the option is left open for a common ancestor.) *There are, however, a few instances of a short-sequence similarity between the two types of viruses.* (It should again be emphasized that *the eukaryotes pertain here only to plant cells.*)

The extrapolation to prokaryotic (bacterial) viruses versus animal or mammalian eukaryotic viruses was not made. There is the inference that bacterial viruses (bacteriophages) are dissimilar to other kinds of viruses in almost every way (e.g., Voet and Voet, *Biochemistry*, pp. 841-843, p. 1089ff).

The foregoing, of course, bypasses the question of whether there is a distinction between viruses infecting plants and viruses infecting vertebrates, e.g., mammals or humans. That is, as stated in the opening paragraph of this subsection, *the conventional wisdom is that plant viruses and vertebrate viruses do not cross over.*‡ As to plant viruses versus vertebrate viruses, however, the final word may not yet be apparent.

---

* Here again, we encounter microorganism transformations which are in some respects alike to the previously noted phenomena of *pleomorphism*, as advanced by such investigators as Rife, Livingston, and Naessens, and as set forth by Moss and by Walters.

† Again, for the record, a *genome* can be perceived as the totality of DNA sequences in an organelle of a cell or in an organism as a whole, as the case may be, and it represents the genetic endowment of a species. On a microscopic scale, the term applies to the complete chromosomal gene complement of an organism contained in a single set of chromosomes (for the eukaryotes or eukaryotic cells of non-bacteria), in a single chromosome (for the prokaryotes or prokaryotic cells of bacteria), or in a DNA or RNA molecule (for viruses). For a human individual, there may be 50,00 to 100,000 in a single haploid set of chromosomes. More encompassingly, the term genome can also be used to denote the entirety of the genes in an individual specimen. For a human individual, this totality may amount to perhaps 10 million genes.

‡ On the other hand, there are some vertebrate viruses—namely *retroviruses*—that occasionally mutate or crossover. Possibly this interaction can be extended to a degree to vertebrate viruses in general.

The reference also mentions the reoviruses, or Reoviridae, in discussing viral evolution (Matthews, *Plant Virology*, p. 669). It is affirmed that the family Reoviridae *"has members that infect both vertebrates and invertebrates, and others that infect both invertebrates and plants."* It is further commented that the more ancient invertebrates could have been the original source for this particular virus family, the Reoviridae.

Similarly mentioned is the fact that members of the virus family Rhabdoviridae also have a particle morphology and genome strategy such that vertebrates and invertebrates can both be infected, or that invertebrates and plants can both be infected. A common evolutionary origin from their insect vectors is indicated.

The reference provides other examples of invertebrate origins, stressing a common taxonomy (Matthews, *Plant Virology*, p. 670). More than this, there is the comment that *"Another feature favoring an ancient origin for present-day viruses is the geographical distribution of some groups"* (Matthews, *Plant Virology*, p. 672). This, in turn, is related to the geographical distribution of the particular plants they infect. As an example, the potato is considered, of the *Solanum* species, which probably had its origins in the Andean regains of Peru and Bolivia. "This diversity of virus strain, climatic adaptation, and geographical restriction of some strains to parts of the region support the idea that the section of the genus *Solanum* comprising the potatoes and the major viruses of potatoes have coevolved and are still coevolving in the Andean region."

Similar speculations about origins can be made regarding such new-found viruses as the Marburg virus and the Ebola virus, both originating from parts of Africa. It is less obvious for the older-found viruses, which have had time to spread around the world. Nevertheless, there is the possibility that one or another could be traced back to its ancient origins. And, in turn, these origins conceivably may be of a plant, bacterial, invertebrate, or vertebrate source, in a particular geographical region.

7.5.1 MORE ON INSECT VIRUSES AND OTHER ASPECTS

In a communication from Hans A. Nieper, M.D., of Hannover, Germany, which appeared in the November, 1997 issue of the *Townsend Letter for Doctors & Patients*, the subject of insect viruses is discussed, along with other subject areas. To wit:

After first mentioning *calcium diglucarate* as a breast cancer preventive, Dr. Nieper indicated that he had used *calcium-1-dl-aspartate* to suppress pain in the fibrocystic tissue of the female breast, and *in a follow-up of the 78 patients so treated, only one malignancy occurred*, which was successfully removed. (This is significantly less than the normal incidence.) It is his thought that the calcium-dl-aspartate *blocks* the transfer of DNA information from the mitochondria into the nuclear genomes. In a way of speaking, the substance may act as an enzyme inhibitor.

Comments were next made by Dr. Nieper about flies and insects in general, and the fact that *insects such as ants can carry enormous loads of viruses within themselves*. Furthermore, the insects do not get sick, although they do not have a vertebrate-like immunosystem. It is further stated that *ants are rendered disease-resistant* due to the presence of a substance Nieper calls *Iridodial*, an activatable dialdehyde referred to as an ant enzyme.

In treating advanced cancer patients with very limited dosages of Iridodial (which is itself available only in very limited quantities), it was observed that *even advanced malignancies will "suffocate" from the effects of ant-derived Iridodial*.

Another pointed observation by Dr. Nieper is that *for every malignancy, the levels of herpes 2, Cytomegaly, or EB-IGG-CBR titers were elevated*. (Cytomegaly pertains to a viral infection in newborn infants that produces liver enlargement, fever, and retardation.) There is the thought by Dr. Nieper, therefore, that offshooting *herpes group virus genomes perform an essential part in causing long-lasting oncogenesis*. He further asks the question of whether Iriodial acts by pulling the viral "key" out of the malignancy.

On the other hand, insect bites have been implicated in melanoma, at least in terms of anecdotal evidence that melanomas occurred at the sites of bee stings. Whether this was due to viral causes or toxins in the bee venom is a subject for further speculation. Interestingly, ant bites and bee stings are a folkloric remedy for relieving the pains of arthritis, as noted for instance in George St. George's *Soviet Deserts and Mountain*, not to mention that the dangerously toxic root of the genus *Aconitum* or monkshood, properly used, is claimed to be a "true miracle drug for arthritis" (St. George, *Soviet Deserts*, pp. 110, 167). For more information about the toxins present in ant venom and bee venom, consult the section on "Enzyme Inhibitors for Melanoma" in Part 8.

The therapy of Hans Nieper, MD is the subject of Chapter 19 in Richard Walters' *Options*. Generally speaking, Walters describes Nieper's *eumetabolic* therapy as a complex, multifaceted, metabolic-nutritional therapy involving the correction of mineral imbalances in the body, the use of "deshielding" enzymes for dissolving the mucous layer that may surround tumor cells, and the deployment of what are said to be natural "gene-repair" substances to reprogram incorrect genetic information in cancerous cells. (As previously noted, the prefix "eu-" connotes *good* or *advantageous*.)

Good words are said for *shark-liver oil*, whose active anticancer ingredient is *squalene*, but which must be accompanied by equal doses of vitamin C to be effective against cancer. Observing that sharks rarely have cancer, although other fish do, Nieper hypothesizes that this may be in part due to the elimination of excess sodium by the action of the compounds taurine and isaethionic acid, which are produced in the shark's liver. It may be commented that any parallels with shark cartilage therapy may be only coincidental.

Nieper uses laetrile only when the body's natural defenses are working, but he calls the banning of laetrile in the U.S. "the greatest and most depressing tragic comedy of modern medicine." He is in favor of beta-carotene, and his patients drink beta-carotene-rich carrot juice, mixed with cream or butter for better intestinal absorption.

Along the way, the formation of oncogenes is dealt with. *Some scientists believe that oncogenes are pieces of genetic material from infectious viruses, but others believe these pieces may be inherited from an ancestor first infected with a virus.* Examples furnished of such viruses are HIV, Epstein-Barr, and hepatitis B. Other factors listed are *stress*, radiation, carcinogenic chemicals, and *strong electromagnetic fields*.

A substance that, according to Nieper, *cancels the genetic information in cancer cells is the steroid tumerosterone*, which is marketed in Germany as *Resistocell* and *Ney-Tumorine*. Another substance is an organic compound called *didrovaltrate*, derived from Himalayan valerian plants (genus *Valeriana* of the family Valerianaceae or Valerian family).

It is noted that *such insects as cockroaches, beetles, and ants may carry all kinds of viruses and infect humans with them.* However, the insects do not get sick, although they have no immune system, and Nieper traces this fact to the presence of *iridodials*, which repair the body system and/or destroy virus genomes. *The claim is made that these substances act against cancer and cancer viruses, including herpes virus, and may possibly act against AIDS.* It is noted that *squalene, found in shark-liver oil, is a chemical precursor to iridodials.*

The use of *Carnivora*®, derived from the Venus flytrap, is also discussed. (The insectivorous Venus flytrap—the lone member of its genus—is the species *Dionaea muscipula* of the Sundew family, or family Droseraceae, of the order Sarraceniales, and which is native to the bogs of North and South Carolina. It is not listed either in Hartwell's *Plants Used Against Cancer* or in Cordell's *Alkaloids*, although other members of Droseraceae appear in Hartwell, all of the genus *Drosera*.) Available commercially in Germany, and noted to have been developed by Helmut Keller, M.D. of Bad Steben, Germany, *it is said to slow tumor growth and stimulate the T-cells of the immune system.* Acting against cancer and other immunosuppressive diseases, *it is also reported to work against AIDS.*

7.5.2 ISOPRENOIDS AND TERPENES

The substance named *squalene*, mentioned above as part of the Nieper therapy, and also called *spinacene*, is an oily unsaturated hydrocarbon involving ring structures, with the stoichiometric formula $C_{30}H_{50}$. It is found in fatty tissue, including that of humans, and is a chemical intermediate in the synthesis of cholesterol.

In further explanation, squalene belongs to the class of organic compounds called *isoprenoids*, found in both plants and animals, and which are named after isoprene. Isoprene has the stoichiometric formula C_5H_8, but more exactly is named 1,3-butadiene, 2-methyl- or 2-methyl-1,3-butadiene, with the structural formula $CH_2:CHC(CH_3):CH_2$ where the symbol ":" or "=" is used to represents an unsaturated double bond. The substances named *terpenes* or *terpenoids*, derived from terpentine, are mixtures of isoprenoids. Isoprenoids occur in the essential oils and gummy exudates of plants, as substances affecting growth, and as red, yellow, and orange pigments—e.g., *carotenoids*. Chlorophyll is part isoprenoids, as are some alkaloids. In animals, isoprenoids are found in fish-liver oils and wool wax, and they occur as the *yellow pigments in egg yolks, butterfat,* and even in feathers and fish scales.

Isoprenoids are vitally involved in animal metabolic processes, and *vitamins A, E, and K are wholly or in part isoprenoids*, as are the ubiquinones (*coenzymes Q*). *Steroids are derived directly from isoprenoids.*

Other chemical groups or radicals may be attached to the structure such as the hydroxyl group (alcohols), the carbonyl group (aldehydes and ketones), and the carboxyl group (organic acids). *Menthol* is an example of an isoprenoid alcohol. The halides for instance may be attached, forming the corresponding chlorinated isoprenoid, and so forth.

Isoprenoids are built up in myriad ways from the basic isoprene structure, the examples ranging from volatile oils with the stoichiometric formula $C_{10}H_{16}$ to the giant molecules of *natural rubber* containing circa 4,000 isoprene units. (Synthetic rubbers, which are polymers say of isoprene or butadiene, involve the same general sort of molecular structure.)

In general, there are the classes denoted as monoterpenes ($C_{10}H_{16}$), sesquiterpenes ($C_{15}H_{24}$), diterpenes ($C_{20}H_{32}$), triterpenes ($C_{30}H_{48}$), tetraterpenes ($C_{40}H_{64}$), and polyterpenes designated as (C_5H_8)$_n$. There may be subclasses, depending on structural and other variations. For example, *beta-myrcene* is an acyclic monoterpene, *limonene* is a monocyclic monoterpene, *alpha-pinene* is a bicyclic monoterpene, and *vitamin A* is an oxygenated monocyclic diterpene.

The essential oils as obtained from odiferous plants are usually monoterpene or sesquiterpene hydrocarbons or their oxygenated derivatives, e.g., alcohols, aldehydes, or ketones, and *menthol, citral, camphor, limonene,* and *alpha-pinene* are specific examples. The nonvolatiles present in resins from the pine family contain diterpene carboxylic acids. The lattice structure of a few plants contain the polyterpene hydrocarbons known as rubber or gutta-percha.

It is informative to note that these kinds of compounds are in the main *bioactive* and some have been used against cancer. For additional information about isoprenoids, consult for instance the *Encyclopedia Britannica*.

7.5.3 CROSSOVERS AND VACCINE CONTAMINATION

The reoccurring question, of course, is, can knowing the origins assist in containing and conquering the diseases caused by these plant and insect viruses, potentially including cancer? More than this, what arrays of virus mutations or crossovers are potentially possible, and may these be indicted in many diseases, known or yet unknown, including cancer? More importantly, given these facts, how can these diseases be cured or at least controlled? Which, of course, gets around full circle to the role of enzyme inhibitors in modern medicine.

A controversy renewed is in regard to the origins and spread of the AIDS virus or HIV—which also has inferences for the Marburg and Ebola viruses. In *Emerging Viruses: AIDS and Ebola—Nature, Accident or Intentional?*, author Leonard Horowitz explores the possibility of contaminated vaccines. That is, *the problem is that of crossovers or mutations between specie viruses in preparing and utilizing the vaccines.* Dr. Horowitz, described as a Harvard graduate, independent investigator, and internationally known public health authority, speaks to the *origins of AIDS*. Among other things, documentation is provided—including National Cancer Institute reports—that contracts were entered into for the purposes of developing and testing *immune system-destroying viruses* on *both monkeys and humans*. Horowitz implicates the Centers for Disease Control (CDC), the Federal Drug Administration (FDA), and Merck & Company as being involved in developing 200,000 doses of a *contaminated experimental hepatitis B vaccine.**

Horowitz charges that, back in 1974, this vaccine was given to thousands of Central Africans, to gay men in New York City, and to mentally retarded children on Staten Island, prior to the 1978 outbreak of AIDS cases in these areas. Horowitz states that the CDC and the pharmaceutical company experts "don't really know whether they are harming or killing more people than they are helping or saving." A moratorium on vaccines is being considered until the issues can be resolved.

Furthermore, it would be of extreme importance to have more specifics about the exact origins of such immune system-destroying viruses, and of whether they are crossovers from the animal, plant, or insect world, or what. In other words, is the viral system stable, or is it undergoing continual change or mutation, as is charged with the AIDS virus, therefore precluding a successful vaccine.

---

* The possibility of a link between the AIDS epidemic and hepatitis B vaccine was noted in 1984, and was investigated by the CDC and Merck.

7.6 FUNGAL VIRUSES

There are also viruses that invade fungi and that may be referred to as *mycoviruses*, with the subject called *fungal virology*. In a way of speaking, if a fungus is regarded as a plant, then fungal viruses could be considered a special case of plant viruses. On the other hand, if the fungi or Mycota are sometimes regarded as allied with bacteria, we may be speaking also of bacteriophages or bacterial viruses. Not to mention that protozoa may be viewed as bacteria with a cell nucleus, and protozoan viruses and bacterial viruses may share a relationship of sorts and merge with fungal viruses. Or they may not. (As explained earlier in Part 5, bacteria, fungi, and protozoa have each been assigned their own designated kingdom.)

Howsoever, fungal virology has its own specialized body of literature. Among the more ready references are *Fungal Virology,* edited by Kenneth William Buck; *Fungal Viruses,* edited by H.P. Molitoris, M. Hollings, and H.A. Wood; *Viruses and Plasmids in Fungi,* edited by Paul A. Lemke; and *Viruses of Fungi and Simple Eukarotes,* edited by Yigal Koltin and Michael J. Leibowitz.

A fungus, for the record, may be defined as any of a group of thallophytic plants devoid of chlorophyll and that reproduce by asexual spores. Examples include molds, mildews, rusts, smuts, mushrooms, and so on. As noted in Part 5, the fungi or Mycota range from unicellular forms to the higher forms such as mushrooms, where the plant body is a thallus, showing no demarcation into roots, stems, and leaves. In general, thallophytes (of the phylum Thallophyta) can be said to include algae, bacteria, fungi, and lichens, and there is the sometimes problem of whether we are speaking of plant life, animal life, or what. Further information is furnished in Part 5.

We are therefore interested in whether some forms of fungi are somehow involved in cancer formation. And if so, we are also concerned about what means might be available for counteracting this carcinogenic action. Fungicides are, of course, the most noticeable possibility, but there are fungal viruses, and if bacteria are in some way involved, there are bacterial viruses, more usually called bacteriophages. We therefore first take up the subjects of *mycoplasmas* and *mycobacteria*, which by their prefix signal a relationship to fungi and which may have further consequences.

7.6.1 "MYCO-" MICROORGANISMS AND PLEOMORPHISM

The prefix "myco-", denoting fungus, appears in such names as mycoplasma and mycobacteria, indicating a connection of sorts. The subject gets back to the question of whether a fungus is a plant, an animal, or a bacterium, or maybe even sort of virus-like, or what. In fact, as previously noted, the fungi or Mycota have been classed as a separate kingdom independent from plants or animals. It may be further observed, however, that fungi are considered to be composed of eukaryotic cells, as are animals or non-bacteria, as distinguished from the prokaryotic cells of bacteria proper. What are called slime molds (or slime-molds), for instance, have been particularly troublesome as to whether to consider them plant-like or animal-like, or both, calling for their own kingdom. There are other distinctions, such as obligate fungi that cannot grow apart from the host, and, otherwise, there are the facultative fungi, which can grow most anywhere, under varying conditions. For example, some of the former are called *rusts,* whereas the latter are called *smuts.* Some further considerations are as follows.

The pathogenic *mycoplasmas* constitute the sole genus *Mycoplasma* of the family Mycoplasmataceae. And, according to *Webster's Third New International Dictionary,* the family Mycoplasmataceae (coextensive with the order Mycoplasmatales) are minute *pleomorphic* Gram-negative microorganisms that in some respects are *intermediate between viruses and bacteria.* Mostly parasitic in animals, they are nonmotic (non-mobile) and have complex life cycles.*

The *Encyclopedia Britannica,* 15th edition, 1995, notes that mycoplasmas are among the very smallest of bacterial microorganisms, ranging from 300 to 800 nm in a spherical or pear shape, to perhaps

---

* The designator *Gram-negative* or *Gram-positive* depends on whether the microorganisms take up *Gram stain* (Voet and Voet, *Biochemistry,* p. 5). This test was devised by Christian Gram in 1884. Heat-fixed cells are first treated with crystal violet dye, or gentian dye, and then with iodine, followed by destaining with the solvent acetone or ethanol. The *Gram-negative* microorganisms do not retain the stain and will be found to have *two structurally distinct layers in the cell wall.* They include the cyanobacteria or blue-green algae, some of which are able to fix nitrogen, that is, to convert atmospheric nitrogen to organic nitrogen compounds, as happens with legumes. The *Gram-positive* microorganisms, which retain the stain, will have only a *monolayered cell wall.* Although the designators are usually applied to bacteria, microplasmas are *not* considered bacteria in the strict sense of the word, as noted above.

150,000 nm (150 μm) for a branched filament. However, they are described as mostly facultative or mobile, as distinguished from nonmotic or nonmobile as indicated above, and are further described as *anaerobic*. Significantly, *Mycoplasma* species do not have cell walls, which distinguishes them from bacteria, and which is in line with the property of being *pleomorphic*. They are parasitic in the *joints* and in the mucous membranes, notably as line the respiratory, genital, and digestive tracts variously of ruminants, carnivores, rodents, and humans, and yield toxic by-products that invade the host's tissues. *Virus pneumonia,* produced by *Mycoplasma pneumoniae*, is widespread but seldom lethal, although mycoplasma infections can also cause a *severe immune reaction.*

The *Encyclopedia Americana*, 1994, states that mycoplasmas are intermediate in size between viruses and bacteria, and refers to them as *pleuropneumonialike organisms*, abbreviated as PPLO. However, *unlike viruses, they don't require a host cell in order to replicate*. And some microbiologists have placed mycoplasmas in a new bacteria class named *Mollicutes*. In addition to causing virus pneumonia, they are also noted to be associated with *arthritis*. (*There is even talk of viruses being associated with obesity.* Also unexpectedly, bacteria are now regarded as a cause of stomach ulcers, and ulcers are so treated, using antibiotics.) It is noted in the reference that, in addition to not having a cell wall, and having only a thin cell membrane instead, *there are forms of mycoplasmas so small that they pass through filters used to retain and separate bacteria from viruses and rickettsia*. In size, mycoplasmas are said to range from 125 to 250 nm in diameter, and they may require steroids such as cholesterol for growth. (*This is within the size range of viruses.*)

It may be observed in passing that *plants contain little cholesterol,* and the most common sterol components of their membranes are *stigmasterol* and β-*sitosterol* (Voet and Voet, *Biochemistry*, p. 284). Interestingly, *both the latter have been found to be anticancer agents,* and especially β-sitosterol, as noted in Part 4 in the section "Common Garden Vegetables and Alkaloids," e.g., Table 4.6.

It is further observed in the above-cited *Encyclopedia Americana* article that under certain environmental conditions true bacteria (e.g., *Proteus* and *Salmonella*) can change into stages lacking a cell wall and resemble mycoplasmas in this respect. These forms are denoted as *L forms*. The loss of the cell wall can be induced by an antibiotic such as penicillin or by a toxic substance such as lithium chloride. Furthermore, some types of L forms, designated *L phase* cells, may revert to the original bacterial form. No disease has yet been attributed to the L forms.

More and more, the *viral/bacterial pleomorphism* described by Livingston, Rife, and Naessens, and further described by Moss in *Cancer Therapy* and by Walters in *Options*, seems to be a fact of life.*

There is in addition the classification *Mycobacterium*, denoting a genus of nonmotive acid-fast *aerobic* rod-shaped *bacteria* of the family Mycobacteriaceae (of the order Actinimycetales), which are difficult to stain for the purposes of determining if the microorganism is Gram-positive or Gram-negative (e.g., *Webster's Third* and the *Encyclopedia Britannica*, 1995). The species *Mycobacterium tuberculosis* is the source for *tuberculosis*, transmitted between humans, and the species *M. leprae* causes *leprosy*. While some mycobacteria are obligate parasites, others are saphrophytes, living on decaying organic matter, plant or animal. They may occur in soils and in water as free-living forms or may be found in diseased tissue. *Fortunately, some of the antibiotics can be used successfully to treat the resulting infections.*

Another source for tuberculosis is *M. bovis,* transmitted from cattle to humans (Reynard J. McDonald and Lee B. Reichman, in *Tropical Medicine and Parasitology*, p. 133). Still another source is named *M. africanum*. With tuberculosis, referred to as a granulomatous infection, *not only does the infection affect*

---

* *Rickettsia* may be described as small Gram-negative microorganisms that are different from other bacteria due to their obligate intracellular parasitism, and that vary in size from 1000 to 2000 nm by 300 nm (Theodore E. Woodward and Joseph V. Osterman, in *Tropical and Geographic Medicine*, p. 920). *Pleomorphism* is common. The morphology of *Rickettsia prowazecki* (the cause of epidemic typhus fever) is affected by its intracellular growth. Moreover, *Coxiella burnetti* (the cause of Q fever) is an *extremely pleomorphic* Gram-variable microorganism, with dimensions of 100 to 300 nm by 100 to 2000 nm. (These numbers are also on the order of virus dimensions.) Other references confirm the *pleomorphism of rickettsia* (e.g., Rudolf Brezina and Jan Kazár, in *Tropical Medicine and Parasitology*, p. 64). Rickettsia are further described in the particular reference as short, Gram-negative, rod-shaped microorganisms, approximately 200 to 500 nm in diameter by 800 to 2000 nm long. It is noted that these obligate intracellular parasites cannot be grown on artificial media, with the exception of *Rochalimaea quintana*, the source of trench fever in humans, transmitted by infected lice whose feces are deposited into broken skin. In addition to noting *several forms of typhus fever as rickettsial diseases,* the reference also cites various spotted fevers, including Rocky Mountain spotted fever, transmitted mainly by the bite of ticks, and whose reservoirs are mostly rodents and dogs.

the respiratory system primarily, but it may affect any organ. The disease occurs worldwide and results in more than 130,000 deaths annually in developing countries. It is noted that a small proportion of primary infections may ultimately disseminate hematogenously to produce miliary (skin eruptive), meningeal (brain and spinal cord), or other extrapulmonary lesions. (That is, the disease may be spread via the blood to cause tubercles or spots in other organs and in the membranes surrounding the brain or spinal cord, or in still other regions outside the lungs.)

A further breakdown of extrapulmonary tuberculosis includes what are called *tuberculous pleuritis,* laryngeal tuberculosis, genitourinary tuberculosis, bone and joint tuberculosis, tuberculosis of the lymph glands, gastrointestinal tuberculosis, meningeal tuberculosis, tuberculous pericarditis (meaning near the heart, or enclosing the heart, e.g., as spread from the lungs), and still other forms involving the adrenals, ears, skin, and spleen (McDonald and Reichman, in *Tropical Medicine and Parasitology,* pp. 136-137). *The most common final cause of death for all forms is either meningitis or miliary tuberculosis.* (It may be commented that *these locations are also sites for cancer occurrence.*)

Drugs of choice in the treatment of tuberculosis are presented in the reference, with side effects, including hepatotoxicity and nerve damage (McDonald and Reichman, in *Tropical Medicine and Parasitology,* pp. 140-141). Several antibiotics are listed, and their side effects make one hesitant about their routine use. (At the same time, if there should be some sort of a connection between tuberculosis and cancer, could some of these drugs serve as anticancer agents, that is, as selective enzyme inhibitors for the processes involved?)*

Leprosy or Hansen's disease, a chronic infectious disease caused by *mycobacterium leprae,* varies between the *lepromatous* type and the *tuberculoid* type (Robert H. Gelbert, in *Tropical Medicine and Parasitology,* p. 143). In the former type, there is extensive multiplication and dissemination of the mycobacteria with no protective cell-mediated immunity. In the latter, there are relatively few microorganisms with intact cell-mediated immunity. Skin manifestations range from nodular lesions in the former, to pigmented anesthetic macules (spots on the skin) in the latter. It is noted that leprosy is the only bacterial disease that infects the peripheral nerves, resulting in a loss of sensation. The parasite is obligate and intracellular but is not easily identified, since it does not grow *in vitro.* It is an acid-fast and alcohol-fast, Gram-positive, rod-shaped mycobacterium about 500 nm in diameter and 6,000 to 8,000 nm long (Richard A. Miller and Thomas M. Buchanan, in *Tropical and Geographical Medicine,* p. 851). The mode of transmission is not precisely known, sometimes taking years, and since the microorganisms do not grow *in vitro,* this complicates the study of the disease. However, infections can be established in mouse footpads and the congenitally athymic nude mouse, in the nine-banded *armadillo,* and in various nonhuman primates including the mangahey monkey. Chemotherapeutic drugs used in treatment include *rifampin, dapsone,* and *clofazimine.* These have side effects such as hepatotoxicity.†

Whether any of these drugs might be used as an anticancer agent is apparently unknown. For one thing, there is the question of whether the action of the drugs is solely as enzyme inhibitors for the bacterial processes versus, say, cancer cell metabolism.

Work continues on developing a vaccine for leprosy (M.J. Colston, in *Vaccination Strategies,* p. 166ff). A vaccine tried is *BCG* (Bacillus Calmette-Guérin vaccine), which has produced widely varying results. More favorable results have been obtained using killed *M. leprae. Armadillos were used to grow the bacteria,* since the bacteria cannot be grown *in vitro.* It is noted that the development of a leprosy vaccine raises more questions than it answers. *Still not known is why some individuals are resistant to the microorganism, but others are not.* Nor are the dynamics of transmission known, establishment of which may take many years. Furthermore, no methods exist for measuring the levels of transmission

---

* The afore-used adjective "granulomatous" pertains to *granuloma,* an inflammatory growth or tumor composed of granulation tissue. The latter term, in turn, refers to tissue formed in ulcers and in early wound-healing and repair. It consists of newly growing capillaries and is named for the irregular wound surface. *The potential similarity to cancerous tissue and angiogenesis is striking* and brings up the possibility at least *that bacterial infections can conceivably result in cancer, as can viral infections.* The connection of carcinogenesis with the factors relating to blood clotting and wound healing has previously been noted (e.g., Boik, *Cancer & Natural Medicine,* p. 15ff). However, no apparent epidemiological correlation between tuberculosis, say, and cancer has surfaced.

† Chaulmoogra oil was once employed against leprosy and other skin diseases. The oil is derived from the seeds of the East Indian tree *Taraktogenos kurzii* or *Hydrocarpus kurzii* of the family Flacourtiaceae, and is listed in Hartwell's *Plants Used Against Cancer.* It is an acrid, clear oil containing unique fatty acids with a cyclic or cyclopentenyl structure.

other than the incidence of occurrence. All these factors interfere with evaluating the efficacy of a vaccine. (As with cancer, what is needed is a near-instantaneous test that indicates whether the disease is progressing or regressing, from which the efficacy of treatment can be evaluated—and the treatment changed if so required.)

Additionally, *there are other nontubercular or atypical mycobacteria*, which include *M. Kansasii, M. marinum, M. scrofulaceum, M. gordonae, M. intracellulare, M. avium, M. fortuitum, M. chelonei* (McDonald and Reichman, in *Tropical Medicine and Parasitology*, p. 152). Interestingly, *M. avium* and *M. intracellulare* have been associated with AIDS. In turn, the acquired immunodeficiency syndrome is associated with certain kinds of cancer. Prominently cited is *Kaposi's sarcoma*, described as an angio-proliferative disorder of endothelial origin (e.g., Robert Colebunders and Thomas C. Quinn, in *Tropical and Geographical Medicine*, pp. 735–736).

It may be added that vaccines are under continued investigation for such mycobacterial diseases as tuberculosis and leprosy, as well as for other diseases (Martin J. Carrier, in *Vaccination Strategies*, p. 26; Marilyn J. Moore and Juraj Ivanyi, in *Vaccination Strategies*, p. 80ff).

7.6.2 MYCORRHIZA

In passing, another variation employing the prefix "myco-" may be mentioned. This is the term mycorrhiza or mycorhiza, which connotes the association between a fungus and the roots of a higher plant. The hyphae, the branched tubular filaments of the fungus, establish a symbiosis with the plant roots, contributing to the nutritional support of both the symbiont and the host. It is further stated in the *Encyclopedia Americana*, 1994, that such beneficial combinations of a fungus (myco) and the root system (rhiza) of a higher plant involve many tree species, and also members of the orchid and heath families. It is observed that trees requiring this association will grow poorly in soils lacking the proper fungi, an example being pine trees planted in Australia and in Puerto Rico, which remained stunted until fungi-containing soils were introduced. Orchids are said to be unable to survive without the correct fungi at their roots. Mycorrhizal fungi are for the most part from the family Basidiomycetes, commonly known as club fungi, and oftentimes a particular fungus species may be associated with only a single species of woody plant (or, at the most, only a few). Thus, *Amanita muscaria* or fly agaric will be located under birch and pine, whereas truffles are found under oaks and beeches. The complex mycorrhizal relationship is accented if the soil is mineral deficient, a common situation in the tropics. The fungi can obtain these minerals from the forest litter, trading the minerals for sugars and growth hormones from the plant. There is also saprophytic behavior among some of the higher plants, which depend entirely on fungi for food. An example is the rhododendron relative known as the Indian pipe, which lacks chlorophyll and depends on a fungus for food. A further comment is that mycorrhizal plants do not ordinarily have root hairs, their mineral- and moisture-absorbing function being performed instead by the fungi.

Expectedly, there will be viruses that attack mycorrhizal systems.

7.6.3 PLASMIDS

Another term encountered in discussing viruses is that of a plasmid. A plasmid has been defined as a small circular DNA molecule that replicates independently of the DNA in the host cell, and that contains the nucleotide sequence necessary for self-replication (Edward Glassman, in *Textbook of Biochemistry*, p. 987). It can be perceived as a virus or virus-like particle, but it does not utilize cellular DNA. As an additional note, plasmids and bacteriophages, as well as yeast artificial chromosomes, have been used as cloning vectors in genetic engineering (Voet and Voet, *Biochemistry*, p. 897).

Thus, a common strategy used by viruses is to act so that the host cell survives unharmed (Jeremy Bruenn, in *Fungal Virology*, p. 86). Some bacteriophages, for example, may act as though they were plasmids. Other strategies are noted to vary from the nonlethal infection of DNA bacteriophages to the more complex pathways of the retroviruses. There may result, at least among prokaryotes or bacterial cells, an immunity to infection. In fungi, which are simple eukaryotes, plasmids or viruses may confer a selective advantage for the host cell.

7.6.4 KILLER SYSTEMS

In yeast cells (fungus cells) with a certain double-stranded RNA (dsRNA) virus, or with a linear double-stranded DNA (dsDNA) plasmid, a toxin is synthesized and secreted that kills cells of the same (and, in some cases, different) species that lack the virus-like particle or plasmid. These actions comprise the so-called killer systems found in at least eight yeast genera and first observed in the species *Saccharomyces cervisiae*. The inference is that there may be ways to produce killer-system toxins that are selective toward destroying cancer cells but not normal cells.

It may be further noted that *Saccharomyces cervisiae* of the family Saccharomycetaceae is listed in Hartwell's *Plants Used Against Cancer* in the section on Fungi at the end of Hartwell's book. Whether these toxins act as enzyme inhibitors was not stated in the reference, nor was the chemical formula of the toxin identified.

Apparently, there is an inhibiting action, however, as evidenced by studies on a standard Petri-plate assay (M.H. Vodkin and G.A. Alianell, in *Fungal Viruses*, p. 109). There may be mutant killer strains—even superkillers. Toxin activity is normally greatest at 23° C (73.4° F), falling off as the temperature is decreased or increased. Superkiller strains have been shown to remain active over a wider temperature range, from 20° C (68° F) to 30° C (86° F). The latter temperature is approaching normal body temperature 37° C (98.6° F).

It is commented that different strains such as brewer's yeast, sake yeast, and other nonlaboratory strains will yield different types of toxins and patterns of resistance (Vodkin and Alianell, in *Fungal Viruses*, p. 116).

The killer system or killer phenomena—or killer factors or killer substances or killer strains, also called killer proteins—so far remain unidentified (Y. Koltin and R. Levine, in *Fungal Viruses*, p. 120ff). In common with other mycotoxins, they are proteins. Furthermore, they may interact to regulate the formation of secondary metabolites, or reaction products, for example as in the production of antibiotics such as penicillin or toxins such as aflatoxin, depending on the organism (R.W. Detroy and K.A. Worden, in *Fungal Viruses*, pp. 94-95). In other words, viruses may interact with the fungi and therefore are involved in the production of metabolites such as antibiotics or toxins.

Thus, there may be a connection with cancer treatment in that some antibiotics are known to act as anticancer agents. That is, the antibiotic per se can be regarded as a toxin. Not only are antibiotics toxic to prokaryotic or bacterial cells, acting as enzyme inhibitors that interfere with bacterial metabolism or other functions, but they can also act against eukaryotic cells. These eukaryotic cells may be cancer cells but, unfortunately, may also be normal cells, judging from the toxicity or side reactions of some of the more dangerous antibiotics. Some of these matters were discussed in Parts 1 and 5.

Additional work on killer strains has been based on physicochemical differences (E. Alan Bevin and Diane J. Mitchell, in *Viruses and Plasmids in Fungi*, pp. 188–194). The different strains were labeled TOX1, TOX2, TOX3, and TOX4. It was further noted that the killer system in yeast exhibits many similarities with the colicinogenic system of *Escherichia coli*. Purification experiments on the TOX1 group isolated a protein with an estimated molecular weight of 10,000 daltons, which was assumed to be the actual toxin, and which has most of the initial toxin activity.

Subsequent work on the killer toxin indicates a protein molecule consisting of a disulfide-linked dimer (Howard Bussey et al. and Thierry Vernet et al., in *Viruses of Fungi and Simple Eukaryotes*, p. 170). The dimers, in turn, can form a ladder of multimers ranging up to octamers. Whether the multimers are necessary for toxic action was yet to be determined.

Given all the above, fungal viruses may play a varied role, because there is at least the latent possibility that certain viruses may not only act against fungi but against fungus-related or fungus-type organisms or microorganisms, notably those prefixed with "myco-", and may also act against toxins produced. That is to say, viruses may not only cause disease but potentially may cure disease.

7.7 BACTERIAL AND PROTOZOAN VIRUSES

Whereas a bacterium consists of a single cell without a nucleus, a protozoan (or protozoon) is a single cell that has a nucleus. (The preferred plural form is protozoa rather than protozoans or protozoons. To further confuse the variations, either protozoan or protozoic serves as the adjective form.) A bacterium is a prokaryote, a classification which pertains to bacteria alone. On the other hand, a protozoan is an *eukaryote,* the same cellular classification as for multicellular organisms, plant or animal. And whether a protozoan is considered plant or animal depends on one's viewpoint (a problem that may also arise with bacteria, but which has been resolved by assigning each its own kingdom).

An *amoeba* (of the rhizopodon order Amoebida) is for example a (unicellular) protozoan and is *animal-like*, as are many other microorganisms, some of which are infectious or pathogenic. Amoebae or amoebas range from the common species *Amoeba proteus* found in the decaying vegetation at the bottom of streams and ponds to those that produce such illnesses as *amoebic dysentery*, as caused by the species *Endamoeba histolytica*. In comparison, *algae* (the singular is alga), for instance, are primitive *plant-like* organisms that may vary from a single cell to such complex structures as seaweed.

Bacteria and protozoa (or protozoans or protozoons) also differ in size and are conveniently measured in microns. Thus, a bacterium may have a linear dimension on the order of one micrometer (micron), a millionth of a meter. A protozoan may have a dimension of 10 to 100 μm and a corresponding volume of 1000 to 1,000,000 times that of a bacterium. By comparison, a virus has a dimension measured in nanometers—e.g., 50 nm or only 0.05 μm, where a nanometer is 1/1000 μm.

A more general classification sometimes used is that of the *protists*, or *protista*, where protist denotes the singular. The classification pertains to both unicellular and acellular organisms (the latter term signifying that the organism is not made up of a cell or cells). This classification comprises bacteria, protozoa, many algae and fungi, and sometimes viruses. The classification can be viewed as constituting a kingdom or other division of living organisms or beings distinct from multicellular plants and animals. A further distinction can be made by dividing the classification into such as Animalia, Plantae, and Protozoae (for instance, consult Part 5).

Another distinction that has been made is for the animal kingdom to be broken down into two sub-kingdoms or phyla, called the Protozoa and the Metazoa. The Metazoa, by difference and definition, consists of all animals except the Protozoa. This distinction, in turn, can compromise both the animal and plant kingdoms if some at least of the Protozoa are to be admitted into the latter. Thus, there is the class called Mycetozoa or Myxomycetes, or plant-animals, notably the slime molds, which defy a rigid classification as plant or animal. Still other divisions or nuances can be made in this sometimes inexact science of classification, as per the arrangements of Part 5.

Inasmuch as bacterial viruses or bacteriophages have been previously mentioned from time to time, the emphasis here will be on the viruses of protozoa as such.

There is not as yet very much appearing in the literature specifically about the viruses of protozoa, an exception being a paper by A.L. Wang and C.C. Wang titled "Viruses of the Protozoa," published in 1991 in the *Annual Review of Microbiology*. References related to their investigation are cited. Of particular note is that all viruses of protozoa are RNA viruses, and furthermore, most if not all are double-stranded RNA (dsRNA) viruses. This configuration occurs in certain yeast fungi as set forth in the previous subsection on Fungal Viruses, and are associated with so-called killer systems where a toxin is produced.

The enzyme involved is RNA-dependent RNA polymerase (which may also be called *transriptase*, as is the enzyme DNA-dependent RNA polymerase), the same as for say rabies virus, which indicates that *protozoa viruses also are not retroviruses*. *Retroviruses*, as noted elsewhere, are distinguished by the enzyme RNA-dependent DNA polymerase, also called RNA-directed DNA polymerase (or *reverse transcriptase*).

The early reports of *virus-like particles (VLPs)* in protozoa relied on electron micrographs of thin cell sections. Indications were observed in species of the protozoa genera *Plasmodium*, *Naegleria*, *Leishmania*, and *Entamoeba*. However, with the possible exception of *Entamoeba*, exact differentiation could not be made from prokaryotic inclusions within the eukaryotic cell. (That is, virus-like particles could not be definitively distinguished from bacterial or prokaryotic cells occurring within the protozoan or eukaryotic cell.) In the case of the protozoan species *Entamoeba histolytica*, however, three distinct types of VLPs were found, reported in the year 1976. The linear dimensions were observed to be 75–80, 7, and 17 nm. In micrometers, these dimensions would be, respectively, 0.075, 0.007, and 0.017 μm. At about the same time, VLPs were found in several strains of *Leishmania hertigi*, a *kineoplastid* that infects porcupines. (A *plastid* has been defined as a minute body of protoplasm occurring in the cytoplasm of some cells, including plant cells and certain protozoans. As used here, it has the connotations of a protozoan itself. In the reference, the VLPs were said to be cytoplasmic, that is, occurred in the cell cytoplasm.) A diameter of 55 to 60 nm was reported. Subsequent work identified VLPs in still other species of protozoa genera such as *Eimeria* and *Babesia*. All the foregoing protozoa were described as obligatory parasites (requiring a host), as distinguished from free-living protozoa.

Additional work was carried out by the authors on the prototozoan *Trichomonas vaginalis* which identified the *T. vaginalis* virus (TVV) as composed of double-stranded RNA (dsRNA). Subsequently, the protozoan *Giardiavirus lamblia* was also studied, and the *G. lamblia* virus (GLV) was also identified as composed of double-stranded RNA.

It is further mentioned that TVV and GLV are distinct viruses which don't cross-hybridize. Neither do their capsid polypeptides cross-react immunologically with each other or with mycoviruses such as ScV, which designates the yeast killer virus (Wang and Wang, p. 258). (This yeast killer virus is *Saccharomyces cervisiae* of the family Saccharomycetaceae, previously mentioned in the section "Fungal Viruses," and which is listed in Hartwell's *Plants Used Against Cancer.*)

The reference continues, "Nevertheless, many of the physical and biological characteristics of TVV and GLV are quite similar to those of the killer yeast virus or *Ustilago maydis* virus (UmV)."

It was further noted that the above three viruses overproduce single-stranded RNA (ssRNA) in the infected cell that could serve as a viral message and replicative intermediate. Accordingly, a decision was made in 1990 by the International Committee on the Taxonomy of Viruses *"to recognize and accept GLV as the first fully identified virus of protozoa."* GLV was therefore classified within the family Totiviridae, which includes such nonsegmented dsRNA viruses as the mycoviruses, and was given the genus name *Giardiavirus.**

A candidate RNA virus, designated LR-1, was identified in 1988 (Wang and Wang, p. 259). It was found to be present in the promastigotes (flagella or fibrils) of the protozoan species *Leishmania braziliensis guyanensis*, designated CUMC1-1A, but was not found in a subspecies nor in 10 other *Leishmania* species. It was found, however, that LR-1 did not cross-hybridize with genomic DNA of the infected cells. *This indicates that LR-1 is not copied into the cellular genome, and rules out the possibility that LR-1 is a retrovirus.*

The reference provides some additional examples of other newly discovered virus-like particles of protozoa, for instance in the sporozites of the protozoan species *Eimeria stiedae*. It was found, furthermore, that the RNA associated with the virus-like particle of *E. stiedae* cross-hybridizes strongly to the giardiavirus RNA but not to that of TVV. There is thus a strong possibility of similarity, if not of identity, between the virus-like particles of the two species. (*On the other hand, we may be on occasion talking of retroviruses after all*—and all that may imply.)

Going back in time, there was a series of books by J. Jackson Clarke, the last of which was published in 1922 as *Protists and Disease*. Clarke was senior surgeon to the Hampstead and North-West London Hospital and surgeon to the Royal National Orthopaedic Hospital. He was particularly interested in cancer. In a chapter on *Cancer-Bodies*, protozoa are described as appearing in cancers, although protozoa are said not to be peculiar to cancer (Clarke, *Protists and Disease*, p. 92). *Clarke further speaks of parasites found in the examination of pathological cancer sections* (Clarke, *Protists and Disease*, p. 183ff).

Clarke earlier had mentioned protozoa as a cause of cancer in a previous series of books (Clarke, *Protozoa and Disease*, Part III, p. 66, 1912). In any event, it is evidently a direction that modern medical research has not pursued.

The foregoing brings to mind the book by Hulda Regehr Clark titled *The Cure for All Cancers*. Clark is or was adamant that an intestinal fluke parasite is the cause of cancer. (The fluke singled out by Clark is the species *Fasciolopsis buskii*, studied at least since 1925.) Furthermore, the growth of flukes is said to be accelerated by the presence of propyl alcohol (propanol) in the body. A deworming or anthelminthic procedure was recommended using, notably, small amounts or extracts of the plant known as *wormwood*, also called *absinthe* (*Artemisia absinthium* of the family Compositae)—a substance that has its own built-in toxic hazards.† It is listed in Hartwell's *Plants Used Against Cancer*, however, and is well known in medical folklore as a deworming agent, hence the common name. In further comment, according to microbiologists, the above-cited fluke species is but rarely found in humans. Moreover, what Clark classifies as "cancer" is not necessarily cancer in the conventional sense.

---

* It may be mentioned that *Giardia* is a genus of *flagellate protozoans* of the order Diplomonadida, which are parasitic in the intestines of vertebrates. The accompanying disease in humans is called *giardiasis*, most often caused by drinking water contaminated with animal feces, such as may sometimes happen in the streams of the Rocky Mountain West. The genus *Trichomonas* of the order Trichomonadida pertains to flagellate protozoa called trichomonads, which are found in the digestive tract of many animals. The resulting disease is called *trichomoniasis—as distinguished from trichinosis*, the latter an infestation of the roundworm *Trichinella spiralis*, usually caused by eating undercooked pork. There are three species of Trichomonas that occur in humans, e.g., the species *T. hominis* affects the intestines.

In further explanation, a fluke is defined as a flattened, parasitic, trematode worm, of the order Digenetica and class Trematoda, the most common of which are the liver flukes, notably the sheep fluke, *Fasciola hepatica*, found in the livers of cattle, sheep, swine, and humans—who may become infected by eating raw, uncooked vegetables.* There is also the *Chinese liver fluke Optisthorchis sinensis* or *Chlonorchis sinensis*, and the *cat liver fluke Opisthorchis felineus*, both of which require fish as an intermediate host and which may infect humans. The species *C. sinensis*, for example, may enter the human system by eating raw or partially cooked fish. *Blood flukes* make up the genus *Schistosoma*, three species of which can infect humans, producing the tropical disease called *bilharzia* or *schistosomiasis*.

The most notorious example of a parasitic fluke or trematode is the schistosome. Schistosomes are of the genus *Schistosoma*, and the cause of the disease *schistosomiasis*, more commonly known as *bilharziasis* or *bilharzia*, as previously mentioned. There are three main forms of the disease, depending on the particular fluke species. The East and Southeast Asia variety of the disease is caused by *S. japonicum*. Another kind, called intestinal or Manson's schistosomiasis, occurs in a region extending from the Mideast, across Africa, to the West Indies and northern South America. It is caused by *S. mansoni*. Vesical or urinary schistosomiasis occurs throughout Africa and into the Mideast, even into Portugal, and is caused by *S. haematobium*. In the first two types, the female fluke, which may range from 10 to 25 mm (0.4 to 1 in.) long, releases eggs that find their way into the veins of the small and large intestines.

In the third and more serious type, the cycle can be said to start when fluke eggs are laid in the veins of the bladder and pelvic regions and then are eventually evacuated in the urine and feces. The eggs hatch on contact with fresh water, producing larvae that find a snail host and further grow into fork-tailed larvae called *cercariae*. After emerging from the snail, they may contact the skin of a mammal, whereby the larvae drop their tails and penetrate the skin into the tissues, ending up in the bloodstream to feed, grow and mature, and complete the cycle by laying more eggs. The first symptoms are allergic reactions, followed by the impacting of eggs into all parts of the body, interfering with body functions. Autopsies have shown fluke eggs in almost all parts of the body. *There is the saying that the parasitic larvae penetrate the soles of the feet and eventually end up in the brain.* Estimates by the World Health Organization indicate that *more than 200 million people may be infected, with the numbers increasing, and second only to malaria.*

Chemotherapy is the prescribed treatment for the disease, aimed at killing the adult flukes. *Antimony compounds* have been used, no doubt serving as enzyme inhibitors for the vital functions of the flukes. The disease is most usually contracted by being in water containing snails that carry the flukes or flatworms, and *a means of control is to use molluscides such as copper sulfate or other molluscidal compounds.*

Malaria, the number one tropical disease, *is a protozoan disease* caused by several species called blood Sporozoa, which are of the single genus *Plasmodium*. The disease was common enough in the Old World, being known to the ancients, but was evidently introduced to the New World, possibly via Columbus's voyages. *The first severe epidemics were in fact observed in 1493.* In some parts of the

---

† The stems and leaves of the wormwood plant provide the source. Presumably, the active ingredient in wormwood is not an alkaloid—or at least *Artemesia* is not mentioned in Cordell's *Introduction to Alkaloids: A Biogenetic Approach.* Instead, the active ingredients in this herb include *absinthin* and *anabsinthin*, which have the characterisiic "-in" ending of glycosides and which, in this case, are glucosides. These compounds give the bitter taste. A mixture of I- and J-thujone, a ketone, constitutes the major toxic element, which can produce profound physical and mental changes in the user. Wormwood is a component of the alcoholic drink called absinthe, which is presumed to have caused artist and addict Vincent van Gogh to cut off his ear and mail it to a lady friend. More information is found in Varro E. Tyler's *The Honest Herbal.* Other sources of miscellaneous chemical information include such standard reference publications as the *Biochemists' Handbook* and the *Dictionary of Organic Compounds* and its supplements. The question, of course, can then be asked, whatever the active components, do these not then act as enzyme inhibitors for the metabolism of the internal parasites? And possibly even for cancer cells? And at the same time, unfortunately, act against other vital body functions, being the so-called side reactions? These particular questions, however, avoid the other question of whether the parasites are the cause of the cancer in the first place.

* Apropos of Hulda Regehr Clark's book, cited above, the following quote was obtained from the 15th edition of the *Encyclopedia Britannica* under the category Liver, Human. *"Of the instances of primary cancer of the liver observed in Hong Kong, about one case in six occurs after infestation with liver flukes."* The question, of course, next can be asked, what proportion of the general Hong Kong population was infected with flukes in the first place—was it about one out of six?

world, almost the entire population is infected at any given time and, for instance, in the mid-twentieth century, the death rate was as high as 1,000,000 persons per year in India alone. Although the main vector is the anopheline or anopheles mosquito, it can also be transmitted from person to person by drug needles and by blood transfusions. Some persons may have a natural or acquired immunity.

The progression of malaria is marked by chills and fever, anemia, enlargement of the spleen, and in some cases the disease may move to the brain with quickly fatal consequences. The course of the disease will depend on which form of malaria is contracted, that is, on which species of *Plasmodium* is involved—and sometimes more than one species may be involved. The control of mosquito populations is one factor in controlling the disease, and the former widespread use of DDT has been compromised by its adverse effects on still other populations. A means of immunization by vaccination would be most welcome, if possible.

The use of the alkaloids from the stems and bark of the genus *Cinchona* date back to 1633, when first used by a Jesuit priest (Cordell, *Alkaloids*, p. 707). The name was given by Linnaeus in 1742, after a former consort of the Spanish Viceroy of Peru. (The genus *Cinchona* of the family Rubiaceae also appears in Hartwell's *Plants Used Against Cancer.*) There are eight alkaloids, the principal one being quinine. Quinine is toxic to many bacteria and unicellular organisms, e.g., protozoa (Cordell, *Alkaloids*, p. 720). May we assume this action is as an enzyme inhibitor for critical functions in these microorganisms? It also serves as a local anesthetic and is effective for a considerable period of time. The reference states that 1.5 million people worldwide died of malaria in 1976, and that malaria is again on the increase as a major health threat to humankind. This is in large part due to the fact that malaria strains are becoming resistant to the synthetic antimalarial drugs now used.

Another tropical scourge is the protozoan disease known as *sleeping sickness,* also called African sleeping sickness or African *trypanosomiasis.* Generally fatal, it is caused by the protozoan *Trypanosoma gambien* or the closely related *T. rhodesiense.* Transmission is by one or another of the 21 species of the *tsetse fly,* which is of the genus *Glossina*—e.g., *Glossina palpalis*—of the family Muscidae in the order Diptera. (This protozoan disease is as distinguished from the viral disease also called sleeping sickness, but more properly is epidemic or lethargic encephalitis, which affects the brain. There is also a version of the latter sometimes called *equine sleeping sickness* or *equine encephalitis.*) The progress of the disease is characterized by fever, inflammation of the lymph nodes, and involvement of the brain and spinal cord. Early treatment with the arsenic compound *tryparsamide* has proved successful ("tryp-" for the disease, "-ars-" for arsenic), but there may be side effects such as a loss of vision. May it be assumed that enzyme inhibition is involved? Control has sometimes required moving entire villages from the tree/brush regions favored by the flies, for instance in West Africa, to disease-free zones, and the extermination of domestic or wild game reservoirs of the disease.

Hookworm or hookworm disease is caused by various bloodsucking nematode worms, such as *Ancylostoma duodenale* or *Necator americanus,* which are parasitic in the intestines of animals—notably dogs and cats—and humans. (A nematode is a roundworm, having a long cylindrical shape, and is of the class Nematoda and phylum Aschelminthes). The major symptom is severe anemia. The length of *N. americanus* is approximately 5 to 11 mm (0.2 to 0.4 in.), and this species causes perhaps 90 percent of the infections that occur in the world's tropical and subtropical regions. The species *A. duodenale* is somewhat larger at 8 to 13 mm and is found mostly in warm regions. Another species, named *A. braziliense,* is parasitic mainly in dogs and cats but sometimes infects humans in Asia, South America, and the southern U.S. The eggs are laid in the host's intestines and are discharged in fecal matter to hatch and become larvae. On contact, a larva penetrates the skin of another host and, burrowing-in, it enters the bloodstream and locates in the lungs. From there it migrates to the mouth and is swallowed, winding up in the intestines, where it grows and mates, to start the cycle over. (Infants exposed to dog-scat may short-circuit the process.) Living for up to seven years in the host, large infestations will suck the host's blood in sufficient quantities to produce bowel inflammation and anemia. The eradication of hookworm was once a top priority in the southern United States and Africa. Such measures as ingesting *carbon tetrachloride* were once used—no doubt with untold side effects.

Heartworm, a parasitic disease of more recent prominence among veterinarians and pet owners, is caused by *Dirofilaria immitis,* a parasite which lives in the right ventricle and pulmonary artery of dogs.

These few examples serve notice that the field of *parasitology* is a large and complicated one. It may be assumed that these various eukaryotic parasites—single-cell protozoa or multicellular trematodes and nematodes, or whatever—will have their own array of viruses.

Whether protozoan viruses, say, are also involved in cancer in one way or another, positively or negatively, is a question apparently not yet asked. But given the action of fungal viruses on yeast fungi to produce killer systems involving the formation of toxins (which may potentially act as anticancer agents), there is much left to be considered. And at the lower end of the complexity spectrum, fungi in the limit merge into the unicellular domain of protozoa and bacteria. Obviously, there is much left to be uncovered, and there may be yet unsuspected applications for the control or cure of cancer.

Beyond this, we mention again the possibility that different kinds of viruses can mutate or cross over, resulting in forms deadly to humans. (The example of most concern is of course that of the *retroviruses*, which involve the enzyme called RNA-directed DNA polymerase, also called *reverse transcriptase*.) Remote as this may be in most or nearly all instances involving widely disparate kinds of viruses (say, plant viruses versus animal viruses or fungal or protozoan viruses versus animal viruses), it is nevertheless a possibility that should be considered. The phenomena involved potentially may be related to the emergence of such strange tropical viruses as the Ebola virus, with their origins in unexpected places such as caves and forests, and which may variously involve mammalian life (such as bats), bird life, reptilian life, insect life, plant life, and fungal, bacterial, or protozoan life.

7.8   VIRUSES IN ANIMAL PRODUCTS

In the previous section titled "Viruses and Degenerative Diseases," and in the subsection on Rhabdoviruses, a footnote mentions that the Navajo of the American Southwest do not eat poultry products, neither chicken nor eggs, and boil their mutton for a long time. The inference was that chickens and eggs may contain some weird viruses to be avoided, as does meat—especially the feedlot variety. The apparent clincher was that Navajos have a very low cancer incidence from natural causes. (The effect of radiation from working in the uranium mines was excluded.) There is evidently a similar low incidence among other native peoples who do not follow a "civilized diet" and instead emphasize a vegetarian diet.

Inasmuch as the presence of viruses in animal products may therefore be of concern, a closer look will be taken at this particular subject.

Most textbooks or references on meat hygiene, or on related subjects, do not take up the matter of viruses that may be present (e.g., *Meat Microbiology*, edited by M.H. Brown). The emphasis is rather on bacterial microorganisms and fungi such as molds and yeasts. The topic of viruses is instead usually confined to texts on the microbiology of various animal products, notably meat and milk. A number of references have been consulted, and the findings are reviewed as follows.

If subviral pathogens are included, the list of possibilities may be extended, as previously indicated in Part 6 within the section on "Cancer Initiation, Enzymes, and Enzyme Inhibitors." In brief review, subviral pathogens include what are labeled viroids and prions (Voet and Voet, *Biochemistry*, p. 1113ff). The former are small single-stranded RNA (ssRNA) molecules; the latter are evidently only protein molecules (the word "prion" stands for *pro*teinaceous *in*fectious particle). Somehow, prions are able to replicate, and the reference lists three scenarios, the most plausible of which is thought to be that the susceptible host cells may carry a genetic code which is activated by the prion infection.

Animal diseases that are considered to be caused by prions include the neurological disease called *scrapie,* mentioned previously also in the section on "Viruses and Degenerative Diseases." Originally found only in sheep (causing them to scrape off their wool), it is apparently now found also in cattle—and called *bovine spongiform encephalopathy or BSE,* better known as *mad cow disease.* The speculation is that the disease was passed on to cattle by utilizing cattle feed containing sheep brains. A similar disease called *chronic wasting disease* has been noted in deer and elk, particularly in Colorado and Wyoming, but the word so far is that there is no danger of transmission to humans.

As also previously noted, there may be a close relationship with the cerebellar disorder found in humans that is known as *Creutzfeldt-Jakob disease,* which is said to be similar or identical to *kuru,* a degenerative brain disease transmitted via ritual cannibalism in Papua New Guinea. Other possibilities in humans are Alzheimer's disease and what is called the Gerstmann-Straussler syndrome (Atlas, *Microbiology,* pp. 237, 244).

7.8.1   VIRUSES IN MEAT AND POULTRY

Food-borne viral diseases have not had much study and are considered only a small part of the totality of food-borne diseases (Constantin Genegeorgis, in *Elimination of Pathogenic Organisms*, p. 134).

Statistically, during the period 1977 to 1981, viral illnesses were said to make up only 3.5 percent of the food-borne outbreaks in the U.S., and 2.6 percent of the totality of illnesses where the etiologies (causes) were determined. Nevertheless, the numbers can still be regarded as significant.

The reference observes that a variety of viruses can be found in the animal at the time of slaughter and are noted to be responsible for animal infections. In fact, fresh meat and meat products are sources for spreading a number of animal viruses, including those causing foot-and-mouth disease, hog cholera, African swine fever, and Newcastle disease. (Foot-and-mouth disease, an acute disease such as occurs in cattle, sheep, and swine, is characterized by blisters and ulcers in the mouth and around the hooves. Hog cholera, often fatal, is characterized by fever, diarrhea, and hemorrhaging in the liver and kidneys. African swine fever, for instance, is a variant of hog cholera. Newcastle disease is a viral disease of birds and domestic fowl, resulting in the loss of egg production by the latter and causing paralysis in chicks.)

Human cholera, denoting a wide variety of diarrheal diseases with various names, is generally caused by bacteria. The notable example is the bacterium species *Vibrio cholerae,* which produces a toxin (e.g., Voet and Voet, *Biochemistry,* p. 1278). The resulting disease in this instance is called Asiatic cholera and in the past has risen to epidemic levels in parts of Southeast Asia, particularly. The toxin is said to block the sodium pump in the small intestine that normally serves to absorb sodium chloride (salt) into the body. The excess which is unabsorbed then acts as a severe saline cathartic.

In animals, in addition to hog cholera, noted above, there are other forms of the viral disease called fowl cholera and sheep cholera. Presumably these and other animal viral infections can be controlled by vaccination—e.g., foot-and-mouth disease—although the more usual means is to destroy infected animals and, better yet, not let the infection get started in the first place. In practice, the latter route will involve restrictions on the importation of animals or meat from countries or areas that have infected animals.

The Genegeorgis reference further states that, fortunately, the above-cited animal viruses are not transmitted to man, nor are animal leukemia viruses, rotaviruses, and enteroviruses. (It is not explicitly stated, however, that these viruses will not mutate or cross with human viruses, as would retroviruses. And as will be subsequently noted, foot-and-mouth disease is occasionally transmitted to humans.) Only the human hepatitis A viral infection has been associated with meats. There is the suspicion, however, that human viral gastroenteritis (caused by a rotavirus) can be transmitted by meat, as can the Norwalk viruses. Infected animals discharge these viruses in large numbers in the feces.*

It is further mentioned that the survival of viruses in meat products takes on new dimensions, since imported raw or processed meats potentially may contain exotic animal diseases. However, perishable canned meats such as partly cooked hams have been found safe if heated to an internal temperature of 69° C (156° F). This degree of heating will destroy swine vesicular disease virus, foot-and-mouth disease, hog cholera virus, and African swine fever virus. On the other hand, fermentation processes have only a small effect on eliminating echovirus, poliovirus, and swine vesicular virus. And curing salts at legal levels, with sodium chloride up to 20 percent, do not kill the foot-and-mouth disease virus. For the latter reason, no cured or dried products are allowed entry into the U.S. from countries where foot-and-mouth disease occurs. The exception is made if the product is to be processed further by heating to an internal temperature of 74.4° C (165.9° F).†

7.8.2 VIRUSES IN MILK

Although cows themselves usually are not seriously affected, the cowpox virus produces blisters or postules on the udder, and the virus can be transmitted to the hands of milkers (A. Gilmour and M.T.

---

* The Norwalk virus, or Norwalk agent, resembles human caliciviruses and is so classified in this virus family by some scientists (Marilyn B. Kilgen and Mary T. Cole, in *Microbiology of Marine Food Products,* pp. 197, 204). It produces viral gastroenteritis and is transmitted from waters and food contaminated with human fecal matter from various sources. More than 100 enteric or intestinal viruses occur in human feces and belong variously to the picornaviruses, reoviruses, adenoviruses, caliciviruses, astroviruses, and unclassified viruses. The unclassified viruses include Norwalk and Norwalk-like viruses, what is called the Snow Mountain agent, small round viruses, and non-A-non-B-hepatitis virus (NANB).

† Foot-and-mouth disease may occur in humans, although rarely—e.g., as noted in the *Encyclopedia Britannica.* It is transmitted to humans by contact with, or ingestion of, infected animal products. The disease in humans shows up first as a high fever, followed by the formation of blisters or vesicles in the mouth and pharynx, and also on the palms of the hand and soles of the feet. Although no treatment is available for affected humans, the disease seems to heal itself after a few weeks. An immunization vaccination is available for animals.

Rowe, in *Dairy Microbiology*, 1, pp. 71–75). Lesions subsequently occur on the back of the hands, on the forearms, and on the face. The virus itself appears oval, with no true envelope and only a multilayer covering, and contains double-stranded DNA, or dsDNA.*

In instances, both raw and pasteurized milk have been shown to be vehicles of infection for poliomyelitis. The polio virus may be spread by inhalation or by the ingestion of foodstuffs that have been contaminated with fecal material from a carrier or infected person. Usually, the only sign of the disease will be fever, headache, and vomiting. But in an infrequent number of cases, the virus will become localized in the central nervous system, which produces paralysis.

The polio virus is described as having an icosahedral shape, with a diameter of 27 nm, which encloses a core of ssRNA with no envelope. It has a narrow host range, that of primates, and displays a strong affinity for nervous tissue. Temperatures of 74–76° C (165–169° F) will destroy the virus at lower concentrations.

A viral disease called *Central European tick-borne fever* may be transmitted by the ingestion of raw goat's milk. The vectors are two species of ticks of the same genus, *Ixodes ricinus* and *Ixodes persulcatus*. The virus is described as spherical, with a 20–50 nm diameter. The core is ssRNA with an envelope. Heating for 10 min. at 60° C (140° F) will kill the virus.

What is called *hepatitis* in humans can be caused by a number of agents. Sometimes defined as inflammation of the liver, the causes are varied. Among the causative agents are a variety of viruses such as rubella and adenovirus, and also nonviral organisms such as *Coxiella burnetii* and *Toxoplasma* (Gilmour and Rowe, in *Dairy Microbiology*, 1, pp. 73–74). In temperate regions, the principal causative agents are hepatitis A virus (producing *infective* hepatitis) and/or hepatitis B virus (producing *serum* hepatitis). The latter is distinct from the former, being found in the serum or blood of victims and carriers, and is spread by tissue penetration with insufficient *asepsis*. (That is to say, in a roundabout way, *asepsis* denotes a state or condition where the system is not sufficiently aseptic or antiseptic, that is, free of pathogens—and such may inadvertently occur during blood transfusions and in kidney dialysis units. The system may therefore be described as septic, involving a condition or state of sepsis, where pathogens are present.)

As to infective hepatitis, the hepatitis A virus may be found in food processing operations if polluted water is used, or may be introduced via fecally contaminated insects and rodents. Infected workers may also transmit the disease via handling prepared foods that are not further cooked. Symptoms generally occur within 15 to 50 days, and most commonly within 28 to 30 days after ingestion. The systems usually include fever, nausea, vomiting, and stomach ache, which precede the enlargement of the liver. A yellowing of the skin, called jaundice, may ensue, depending on how the virus affects the liver.

The hepatitis A virus is said to be 12–18 nm in size and encloses RNA. Since it can survive for 30 min. at 50° C (122° F), somewhat higher temperatures are required to kill the virus.† The hepatitis A virus is a picornavirus, as are the polio virus as well as the foot-and-mouth disease virus and the rhinovirus, the latter the cause of the common cold (Voet and Voet, *Biochemistry*, pp. 1086–1088). They are among the smallest of the RNA-containing animal viruses.

The aforementioned RNA viruses—the polio virus, that of Central European tick fever, and the hepatitis A virus—leave the possibility open that they may in instances behave as retroviruses, interacting with still other viruses, if the necessary enzyme, reverse transcriptase or RNA-directed DNA polymerase, is somehow present. The same may be conjectured for the foot-and-mouth disease virus and other picornaviruses.

To continue, the fate of human pathogenic viruses in cheese has not been studied to any significant degree (Helen R. Chapman and M. Elisabeth Sharpe, in *Dairy Microbiology*, 2, p. 286). However, experimental studies on milk infected with polio virus, certain enteric viruses, and the influenza virus indicate that such viruses are destroyed or are to a large extent inactivated by pasteurization. Cheesemaking, on the other hand, uses unheated milk but nevertheless has been found to reduce virus levels, although the surviving viruses may be around for a long time. Thus, polio virus has been found to last seven months in cheddar cheese and five to six weeks in cottage cheese.

---

* As was to become well known, *people who have had cowpox are made immune to smallpox*. This was the basis for the inoculation against smallpox first developed by the great English physician Edward Jenner in 1796.

† In the U.K. at least, milk pasteurization conditions were originally 30 min. at 64° C (147.2° F), but these have been replaced by the high-temperature, short-time (HTST) method of 15 s or more at 74° C (164.2° F) (W. Banks and D.G. Dalgiesh, in *Dairy Microbiology*, p. 20).

The same reference notes that whenever bovine tuberculosis is endemic in raw milk, there is the possibility that the bacterium *Mycobacterium tuberculosis* may show up in cheeses. Although killed by pasteurization, the bacterium is resistant to acidic conditions, which will relate to the type of cheese. Thus, the survival time in cheddar is approximately 220 days, in tilsit 300 days, in camembert 90 days, and in Edam 60 days or longer.

Other viruses present in milk or milk products are the bacteriophages (bacterial viruses) of lactic acid bacteria, which are noted as a cause for the slow growth of starter cultures (Gilmour and Rowe, *Dairy Microbiology*, 1, p. 74). Worthy of further mention is that it is not always possible to distinguish between virulent phages and temperate phages. The bacterial phages described in the reference include the following:

- Phages of mesophilic lactococci, which include *Lactococcus lactis* and various of its subspecies
- Phages of thermophilic *Streptococci*
- Phages of *Lactobacilli*
- Phages of *Leuconostoc* spp.

These phages are said to belong variously to what are called Bradley's group A or B. The last three genera or species mentioned, especially, produce the enzymes involved in the conversion of carbohydrates or sugars (e.g., milk sugar or lactose, or glucose) to lactic acid or lactate. In particular, the enzyme lactate dehydrogenase is produced, which catalyzes the last step in the formation of lactic acid or lactate.

Accordingly, the several bacteriophages can in this instance be considered as enzyme inhibitors. That is to say, the bacteriophages which may infect *Streptococci*, *Lactobacilli*, and *Leuconostoc* will block or interfere with the production of the necessary enzymes for producing lactic acid or lactate. In this respect, therefore, these bacteriophages are potential anticancer agents. The reference did not provide ways for producing or growing these particular bacteriophages.

7.8.3 VIRUSES IN SEAFOODS

It has been previously noted in the subsection on "Viruses in Meat and Poultry" that more than 100 different enteric (intestinal) viruses can be found in human feces (Kilgren and Cole, in *Microbiology of Marine Food Products*, pp. 197–209). Furthermore, as previously indicated, these viral pathogens are picornaviruses, reoviruses, adenoviruses, caliciviruses, astroviruses, and as yet unclassified viruses. As also previously indicated, the unclassified viruses included the Norwalk virus and Norwalk-like viruses, Snow Mountain agent, small round viruses, and, by exclusion, the non-A-non-B hepatitis virus (NANB). Hepatitis A and B viruses belong to the family of picornaviruses.

Of the above-cited enteric viruses, most have been documented as causing seafood-related illnesses. These are the hepatitis A virus (HAV), the Norwalk virus, the Snow Mountain agent, caliciviruses, astroviruses, the NANB virus, and other unspecified hepatitis viruses. Excluding HAV contamination from infected food handlers, the sources of seafood-related viral infections are raw or improperly cooked molluscan shellfish.

It is mentioned, furthermore, that human enteric viruses remain inert in food but are activated inside the host, as are all viruses. Not only this, but the viruses are species specific and may be receptor specific for certain kinds of cells. Transmission is most often by the feces-oral route and may involve contamination by human sewage, as in the fouling of marine waters. The water conditions in turn determine the survival and persistence of the viruses, salinity and (ultraviolet) sunlight being two factors. Lower water temperatures, less than 10° C (50° F), favor survival as does protection from the organic material in the water. Aside from these factors, food handling may also introduce viruses, notably hepatitis virus A, as previously mentioned.

The picornavirus family constitutes the largest of all viral families, and approximately 200 specific picornaviruses have been identified in man. Furthermore, 69 different enteroviruses from the picornavirus family have been found in the intestinal tract. These enteroviruses are described as having a naked icosahedral capsid which is 25 to 30 nm across and appear in outline as being smooth and round. They are built up from 60 protomers, and replication takes place in the cytoplasm. [Proteins with identical subunits are called *oligomers*, and the protomers are the identical subunits that make up the oligomer (Voet and Voet, *Biochemistry*, p. 181).] Each protomer consists of a single molecule composed of four polypeptides, designated as VP 1, VP 2, VP 3, and VP 4, or correspondingly as 1D, 1B, 1C, and 1A. The genome is a single-stranded RNA (ssRNA) molecule.

It is stated that the enteroviruses are resistant to the acidic conditions and the proteolytic enzymes and bile salts in the gut. The hepatitis type A virus or HAV (also designated enterovirus Type 72) is less acid stable than other enteroviruses but, on the other hand, is more heat stable. It can survive temperatures of 60° C (140° F) for up to four hours.

These *enteroviruses* may in turn be divided into the species groups that are *polioviruses* (PV), *Coxsackieviruses, echoviruses,* and *enteroviruses* as such. (*The Coxsackie virus is similar to the polio virus* and causes the infectious diseases called *herpangia* and *epidemic pleurodynia.* The former affects children especially, producing fever, appetite loss, and throat ulcerations. The latter produces sudden chest or side pains, accompanied by a mild fever and a third-day recurrence. (The Coxsackie virus was named after the town of Coxsackie NY, located in the southeast part of the state, where it was first discovered. Incidentally, regarding the Norwalk virus, there is a town by that name in southwest Connecticut and another in southwest California. As to the Snow Mountain agent, there must be many sites by that name.) The clinical features, and the epidemiology and control, can be classified by syndromes, save for the poliovirus and HAV. (A *syndrome* can be characterized as a group of signs and symptoms that occur simultaneously, as distinguished, say, from a single definitive symptom.)

As to poliovirus, the three wild types are designated PV1, PV2, and PV3. No longer endemic in the U.S., the reference further states that "no cases of seafood-associated polio have been reported in this country." Furthermore, it is added that "there is virtually no risk of infection with wild-type PV from fecally contaminated seafood, or from seafood processing and handling." The wild types are to be distinguished from the vaccine strains of poliovirus, which have evolved during the course of widespread polio vaccination programs.*

The reference further observed that "vaccine strains of PV are generally the most common enteroviruses found in estuarine waters and molluscan shellfish." It goes on to mention that PV infections were relatively minor, even before the advent of the Salk inactivated polio vaccine (IPV) and the Sabin oral polio vaccine (OPV). Epidemiological studies indicate that the odds are 1 in 100 that persons infected with PV will develop clinical symptoms. Spread mainly by the fecal-oral route or by direct contact, in this country food-borne polio had been spread mainly by raw milk, which was eliminated by pasteurization. Underdeveloped countries, however, still may have epidemics caused by contaminated water and food supplies. Further information about symptoms and control are provided in the reference. The few reported polio cases in the U.S. are said to be due to the failure of OPV, manifested as an inadequate reduction of virulence or as immunosuppression in the recipient of the vaccine.

Hepatitis A virus or HAV (also designated as enterovirus Type 72) is also spread by the fecal-oral route. Countries that are overcrowded, with inadequate sanitation and poor hygiene, are rife with the disease. Usually, in these undeveloped countries, the infections occur during childhood and are called subclinical, meaning that at this early age the disease is not as virulent. (That is, the victim is not entirely sick, but is sick enough.) In developed countries, the disease occurs most often in those between 15 and 30 years of age.

Contaminated food and water, along with person-to-person contact, remain the principal sources for hepatitis or HAV disease, and the Centers for Disease Control (CDC) still report 20,000 to 30,000 cases each year in the U.S. The first case to be documented of shellfish-related HAV was reported in Sweden in the 1950s, followed by the U.S. in the 1960s. Between 1961 and 1984, there was a report of approximately 1,400 cases of HAV from molluscan shellfish. Between 1973 and 1987, the CDC reported 437 cases of seafood-associated HAV from 11 outbreaks. The incidence is decreasing, however. A tabulation by year between 1973 and 1987 is provided in the reference. Interestingly, finfish show relatively few outbreaks and cases. The main exception, which occurred in 1982, was from a contaminated food handler. As to other sources, the finfish record is zero. As to unknown etiologies, which are probably not all microbiological pathogens, the shellfish total was 3,524 cases as compared to 482 cases for finfish.

---

* As an aside, a news release from the Centers for Disease Control in Atlanta, on or about January 30, 1997, stated that almost every polio case in the United States between 1980 and 1994 was caused by the vaccine itself. Out of 133 cases contracted, some 125 were attributed directly or indirectly to the oral vaccine, which contains a weakened but live virus. As a precaution, young persons will now receive a killed-virus vaccine first, to build up resistance, before the oral live-virus vaccine is administered.

Another tabulation by specific viruses or pathogens in shellfish, for cases reported between 1973 and 1987, shows the following total cases: HAV, 356; Norwalk, 11; Snow Mountain, 71; NANB, 1, unspecified hepatitis, 4479; unknown etiologies, 5342.

Since *HAV infection results in permanent immunity,* a vaccine could be developed to eradicate the disease. A trial live vaccine was noted to be undergoing tests by the U.S. Army, although no licensed vaccine is available to the public (as of the 1990 date of publication for the reference). *Control is obtained, nevertheless, by passive immunization with gamma-globulin following exposure.*

The other enteroviruses considered in the reference are the Coxsackie, echo, and enteroviruses proper. Even if usually subclinical as such, these viruses can produce syndromes of neurological disease, cardial and muscular disease, enanthems and exanthems (eruptions inside and outside the skin), respiratory disease, ocular disease, and abdominal disease. (No mention is made of cancer.) The main points of growth for the viruses are the throat and intestinal tract, both part of the gut or alimentary canal. The viruses are discharged in the feces and in respiratory secretions, the former over a longer period of time than the latter, and move via the bloodstream to target organs. On a positive note, none of these other enteroviruses has ever been shown to be seafood related.

The family of reoviruses includes the rotaviruses. And the rotaviruses are the most significant source, worldwide, for infantile gastroenteritis, resulting in many deaths in underdeveloped countries. Feces are mainly responsible for the spread of the virus, accented by poor hygiene. In the U.S., there have been no documented cases of rotavirus infections from seafood sources. No human vaccine is available (as of 1990), although research is underway to develop a live oral vaccine.

Adenoviruses were originally found in human adenoids, hence the name. They have also been found to be connected with gastroenteritis. Being enteroviruses, they are shed in human feces, to be spread by the fecal-oral route, which involves direct contact, contaminated food and water, and contaminated swimming or bathing waters. As with rotaviruses, however, no documented cases of adenovirus infections have been traced to seafood. No vaccine is available.

Human caliciviruses are another source of gastroenteritis, and the Norwalk virus resembles the caliciviruses, although it may be considered an unclassified virus. Transmission for both the caliciviruses and the Norwalk virus are essentially the same as for the other enteric viruses. Although not confirmed, *caliciviruses have been reported to be involved in shellfish-related outbreaks.* Slightly larger than picornaviruses, with an icosahedral capsid containing only one polypeptide and having 32 cup-shaped depressions or calices, caliciviruses are resistant to both heat and acids.

Astroviruses are found in the feces of infants by means of immune electron microscopy, or IEM. Having a dimension of approximately 28 nm, they are named after their star-shaped centers. Again, good sanitation is the most effective means for control.

The unclassified viruses include the nonspecific agents for gastroenteritis, notably the Norwalk virus or agent and Norwalk-like agents, the Snow Mountain agent, and the small round viruses or SRVs. Also unclassified is the non-A-non-B (NANB) enteral hepatitis virus.

Viral gastroenteritis from the Norwalk agent is from the usual contaminated sources, including the consumption of undercooked shellfish from estuaries containing human fecal matter. The first documented shellfish-related outbreak of the Norwalk virus occurred in Australia in 1979, followed by many more in the U.S. It continues to be a problem and is on the increase, with the possibility that there are more infections than reported.

The diameter of the Norwalk virus is circa 25–32 nm, and that of the SRVs is approximately the same, or approximately 27–40 nm. As has been the case for the astroviruses, the SRVs have been found in the feces of infants suffering from diarrhea using immune electron microscopy, or IEM.

The disease called *enteral NANB hepatitis* is transmitted in the usual ways from the usual sources, and is endemic in the Mideast and Africa. It is also found in India and Soviet bloc countries, as well as in Mexico, and no doubt occurs in the U.S. Shellfish are suspect. Enteral NANB can be more severe than HAV and is usually accompanied by cholestasis (bile inactivity). It is further commented that, in general, unspecified hepatitis is a clinical syndrome that can be caused by a number of unknown viral agents or bacterial infections, as well as by hepatitis A virus, hepatitis B virus, and NANB viruses. (Hepatitis or inflammation of the liver is also a catch-all term for liver problems that may be caused by still other agents, such as drugs and even folk medicines, read anticancer agents.)

Further information is analyzed in the reference about hepatitis A virus and its occurrence and frequency from seafood-related sources. Data from the CDC and the New England Technical Services

Unit (NETSU) of the U.S. Food and Drug Administration was used as the basis. Other enteric viruses from seafood were discounted.

As has been previously indicated, the possibility of cancer-causing viruses was not mentioned. However, there is a bacterium named *Listeria monocytogenes* that produces a disease called *listeriosis*, which is of concern for cancer patients and others taking immunosuppressive chemotherapy (John E. Kvenberg, in *Microbiology of Marine Food Products*, p. 273). The disease can also affect pregnant women, diabetics, cirrhotics, and the elderly, and even normal healthy individuals. The consequences are septicemia (blood poisoning), meningitis, and encephalitis, as well as enteritis. A milk-related outbreak in New England was reported to have a 29 percent mortality rate. No cases in the U.S. have been traced to seafood, although the *Listeria* genus is widely distributed in the environment.

Other observations on viruses, particularly as related to seafood, are as follows. In research on enteric viral diseases such as may be attributed to shellfish, it has been proposed that enteroviruses such as poliovirus be used as indicators for the diseases (Howard Kator and Martha W. Rhodes, in *Microbiology of Marine Food Products*, p. 175). As an alternative, bacteriophages or bacterial viruses have also been proposed. They are noted to have a resistance to disinfection, that is, have a resistance to being disinfected or rendered inert.

Bacterial and viral microbes enter shellfish mainly via the feeding route (Gary P. Richards, in *Microbiology of Marine Food Products*, p. 400ff). Mucus is secreted by the shellfish, whereby strands of mucous entrap food and contaminants, in turn to be swept into the mouth by the action of cilia. Bacteria and viruses not only appear in the feces but accumulate in molluscan shellfish tissues. Most microbes accumulate in the digestive gland/hepatopancreas. At the same time, there are not only mechanisms for carrying nutrients to the tissues, but mechanisms for inactivating or dispelling the contaminants. Thus, hemocytes (blood cells) isolate foreign materials by phagocytosis, pinocytosis, or encapsulation. (That is, the blood cells eat and digest, immobilize, or surround the contaminants.) Nevertheless, the accumulation of viruses in shellfish of special concern, in particular with regard to hepatitis A virus (Robert M. Grodner and Linda S. Andrews, in *Microbiology of Marine Food Products*, p. 437).

It is noted in the reference that the effects of irradiation on viruses is not encouraging.

7.8.4 EFFECT OF TEMPERATURE

Natural ice cut or sawed from frozen ponds, lakes, or rivers was once commonly used as a refrigerant. It is a potential source of pathogens. It has been noted that virus infections from natural ice have had very little study but, in the meantime, natural ice contaminated by domestic sewage obviously should not be harvested for potable or edible purposes (Jensen, *Microbiology of Meats*, p. 218).*

It is further noted in the reference (last published in 1954) that extreme cold has a preservative effect on both bacteria and viruses. In fact, virus-containing tissues that are frozen and stored at −76° C (−104.8° F) show no viral deterioration.

The above findings about low temperatures having no effect on viruses is contrary to other information. Thus, it has since been stated that viruses such as the foot-and-mouth disease virus cannot survive freezing, nor can nematodes (roundworms) such as Trichinella, nor protozoa (Daniel Y.C. Fung, in *The Microbiology of Poultry Meat Products*, p. 22).

As to fishery products, the statement has been made that the purpose of freezing is not to kill bacteria, but to stop metabolism and growth, which would produce spoilage (David W. Cook, in *Microbiology of Marine Food Products*, p. 32). There is, however, an initial reduction in the bacterial count, followed by a further decline during storage. It has also been found, moreover, that the ideal freezing procedure of a fast freeze and the subsequent maintenance of a constant low temperature is also most protective to bacteria (Russell J. Meget, in *Microbiology of Marine Food Products*, p. 78).

---

* The reference mentions the different kinds or phases of crystalline ice that can occur, depending on the temperature and pressure, and interestingly mentions noncrystalline or vitreous ice (Jensen, *Microbiology of Meats*, p. 212). Vitreous ice can be formed by quickly chilling water droplets to a temperature considerably below freezing, namely to -12° C (or 10.4° F). The resulting vitreous ice is very transparent, with no microcrystalline structure. Two types are said to exist, one more like a true glass and the other like a supercooled liquid. (Very possibly, the foregoing distinction is signaled by the so-called "glass point," whereby the heating or cooling curve will show a distinct change in slope, denoting a slight change in physical properties for the amorphous or glassy state.)

Microbial activities, being related to chemical and enzymatic reactions, are affected by the well known temperature analogy that each 10° C rise doubles the reaction rate, and each 10° C lowering halves the reaction rate (Daniel Y.C. Fung, in *The Microbiology of Poultry Meat Products*, pp. 21–22). As a rule, slow freezing is more likely to act against microbes due to the formation of large extracellular ice crystals that damage the cell membranes as well as removing cell components by osmosis. In quick freezing, small intracellular crystals form, doing less damage to the cells.

Although freezing temperatures will kill some microbes, the more common bacteria tend to be preserved and will grow again at warmer temperatures. And *some bacteria, called psychotrophs, can grow at chilling and refrigeration temperatures.*

Freeze drying (also called *lyophilization*) involves first freezing the food and then applying a vacuum. At the lower pressure, the phase behavior of the system is such that the ice content sublimes; that is, it is converted directly to water vapor. In the absence of water, the bacteria naturally present cannot grow, so that the material need not be refrigerated. Once water is added, however, spoilage may occur, the same as before freeze drying. Albeit some microorganisms are killed off during freeze drying, for most, it is the most effective way to preserve bacterial cultures.

7.8.5 DRYING

As to simple drying, by controlled dehydration or by the sun, this is perhaps the most common means of food preservation whereby cereals, meat, fish, and fruit can be preserved for lengthy times (Fung, in *The Microbiology of Poultry Meat Products*, p. 20). By removing water, the microorganisms present cannot grow, and enzymatic activity ceases, but the food is not sterilized. Plus, the spores of bacteria and mold survive such that, on rehydration, spoilage may ensue.

An option, akin to drying, is *smoking* (D.M. Janky, J.L. Oblinger and J.A. Koburger, in *The Microbiology of Poultry Meat Products*, p. 350). In "hot-smoke" processing, a degree of cooking occurs, as distinguished from "cold-smoke" processing at relatively low temperatures (less than 40° C, or 104° F). Although the former will have a lower yield of product, the reference indicates that the resulting microbiological profiles will be the same after cooking the final products. However, increasing the surface temperature during smoking will increase the deposition of phenolic and formaldehyde compounds, which have a bacteriostatic and bactericidal effect on the smoked product. Furthermore, Gram-positive organisms are more heat resistant, whereas Gram-negative organisms are less heat resistant.

Inasmuch as most smoked products are precured with a brining step, the topic of *salting* is also of interest (Janky et al., in *The Microbiology of Poultry Meat Products*, pp. 348–349). The curing solution may not only contain common salt but sugar, nitrates, and nitrites as well. The last-mentioned produce the "cured" color of the product, may contribute to flavor, and have a bacteriostatic effect, especially on the bacterium *Clostridium botulinum*. (Nitrates and nitrites are also ultimately carcinogenic by microbial actions that take place in the gut, as set forth in Part 6 on "Intestinal Flora and Cancer.")

The reference notes that raw poultry contains a broad spectrum of microorganisms. The most prominent spoilage bacteria are of the genera *Pseudomonas* and *Acienetobacter*. These are both aerobic and psychrotrophic (will grow at low temperatures). Pathogenic genera include *Salmonella* and *Campylobacter*. Additionally, handling the raw product may introduce *Staphylococcus aureus*. Representative coliform counts are cited as are yeast and mold counts. (Coliform bacteria occur in the large intestines of man and animals and are principally of the genera *Escherichia*—e.g., the ubiquitous species *E. coli*—and *Aerobacter*. Their presence in water is an indication of fecal pollution.) Specific viruses were not cited.

Brine treatment may or may not reduce the microbial load on raw carcasses and is probably dependent on the brine concentration and temperature. Dry massaging with salt, or dry salt packing, may adversely affect certain microorganisms, although other organisms may develop a tolerance. Whereas dry salt-cured hams have a relatively long shelf life at room temperatures, poultry is seldom treated this way.

7.8.6 EFFECT OF HIGH TEMPERATURES

Elevated temperatures kill microorganisms by the denaturing (changing the nature) of protein and by inactivating enzymes (Fung, in *The Microbiology of Poultry Meat Products*, p. 22). Pasteurization generally means treatment for 30 min. at 63° C (145° F) or for 15 s at 72° C (161° F). Most vegetative (fertile) cells are destroyed at these conditions, notably *Mycobacterium tuberculosis* and *Coxiella burnetti* such as in milk. Organisms described as thermoduric will survive pasteurization unless the pasteurized food is refrigerated.

Higher temperatures are used in what are called very high temperature (VHT) or ultra high temperature (UHT) treatments. Conditions are for one second or more at temperatures of 130° C or higher. Flavor, however, can be affected. Commercial canning achieves sterilization temperatures by cooking under pressure in sealed containers—a practice also of home-canning procedures, when conducted properly. The time and temperature are to be such that *Clostridium botulinum* spores are destroyed. Whereas commercial canning has a good record, such is not always the case for home canning.

7.8.7 EFFECT OF IRRADIATION

Two types of radiation may be distinguished: ionizing and nonionizing (Fung, in *The Microbiology of Poultry Meat Products*, p. 23). The former has the energy to ionize compounds to create reactive free radicals. The latter does not have sufficient energy to produce ionization but can stimulate molecular vibration and generate heat.

The forms of radiation called alpha and beta particles, and gamma rays and X-rays, will destroy microorganisms. Since alpha and beta particles can be stopped by paper and aluminum, this poor penetrating power negates their use for food preservation. Both gamma rays and X-rays have the necessary penetrating power—being stopped only by lead—and have been tried for preserving foods.

The preserving effect of radiation is apparently due to the breaking of the chemical bonds or structures of essential macromolecules such as the DNA of the microorganisms, and/or to the formation of highly reactive free radicals from the water or moisture present. These free radicals (such as HO^- and H_2O^-) disrupt the carbon-carbon bonds in the macromolecules of the microorganisms. No heat is generated in the process of radiation sterilization, or irradiation, which is known as *cold sterilization*. In less than lethal doses, however, ionizing radiation can produce mutations in the microorganisms.

Regarding nonionizing radiation, ultraviolet radiation or ultraviolet light (UV) for instance, will sterilize only the surface of foods. The most effective wavelength is said to be 2600 Å, which has an affect on nucleic acids and proteins. Incidentally, nonionizing UV can also produce mutations in organisms as well as their destruction.

Microwaves are another form of nonionizing radiation. Most often at a frequency of approximately 2540 megahertz (MHz), these waves induce a vibration in asymmetric, dielectric molecules such as of water, in turn generating heat. (A hertz is a frequency unit of one cycle per second. A megahertz is a unit of 1,000,000 Hz.) Along with cooking the food, the heat is said to be most responsible for destroying microorganisms present. Interestingly, microwaves heat from the inside of the food outward, the reverse of normal cooking.

It has been observed that the effect of radiation, at least on viruses in shellfish, and in particular on hepatitis A virus, has been relatively ineffective (Robert M. Grodner and Linda S. Andrews, in *Microbiology of Marine Food Products*, p. 437).

7.8.8 EFFECT OF CHEMICALS AND DEPURATION

Chemicals that kill microorganisms are called *bacteriocidal* or *bactericidal*, whereas those that merely prevent the microorganisms from growing are called *bacteriostatic* (Fung, in *Microbiology of Poultry Meat Products*, p. 24). These chemicals may be injected or otherwise introduced into the live host or into the meat products. Antibiotics, for instance, are used in this way against infective bacteria. The processes of curing also touch on the subject. Sometimes an internal gut cleansing of the live host will serve, if maintained over a sufficient time interval. That is, so to speak, the animal is exposed to clean food and water. This is the objective for the depuration of fish, and especially shellfish.

In the case of shellfish, therefore, merely a simple cleansing with clean seawater may suffice. The process is called *depuration* (Richards, in *Microbiology of Marine Food Products*, p. 395ff). Also called *controlled purification,* the stock is held in tanks of clean seawater for a necessary and sufficient length of time. The water cleanses both externally and internally. The process may sometimes be accelerated by using chlorinated water or ultraviolet light if no adverse effects occur.

Ordinarily of most concern are bacteria, and moderately contaminated shellfish can be depurated in approximately 72 hours (Richards, in *Microbiology of Marine Food Products*, pp. 397–398). An exception is that of indigenous marine bacteria of the genus *Vibrio*, which persist for extended periods and may require as many as 16 days for depuration, though ozone can be used to accelerate the process.

The family Vibrionaceae includes the genus *Vibrio* among others (Gary E. Rodrick, in *Microbiology of Marine Food Products*, p. 285ff). The genus *Vibrio* contains more than 50 bacteria species, at least

11 of which are known pathogens. *The diseases that are caused include gastroenteritis, wound infections, ear infections, and primary and secondary septicemia (blood poisoning).* The reference further discusses several of the species, of which *Vibrio cholerae* is of the most concern. As its name indicates, its *toxigenic strains* (as distinguished from nontoxigenic strains) are capable of producing a *cholera toxin,* or a toxin that is very similar. Pandemics that began in Hong King and Macao have spread to Russia, Africa, the Mideast, Europe, and the U.S. Although the U.S. has not had a serious outbreak since 1911, there were sporadic clusters of cases in the 1970s occurring on the Gulf Coast in Texas, southwestern Louisiana, and in Florida. *Vibrio cholerae* is widely distributed, moreover, occurring even where there is no pollution. Perhaps 95 percent of the strains are nontoxigenic, but even these can cause gastrointestinal illness.

Although studies on the depuration of viruses are not entirely conclusive, in at least one investigation it was found that moderate levels of poliovirus could be depurated in 3 days (Richards, in *Microbiology of Marine Food Products*, pp. 398–399). Hepatitis A virus, however, is especially resistant to depuration. Bacterial viruses or bacteriophages such as coliphage-13 were also found to be resistant to depuration.

It has also been found that toxins, heavy metals, petroleum hydrocarbons, and radionucleotides are extremely resistant to depuration, requiring extended periods if successful at all, and become uneconomical (Richards, in *Microbiology of Marine Food Products*, p. 399).

Ultraviolet light has been used for the depuration of seawater used in shellfish processing and is noted to reduce the content of both bacteria and viruses (Richards, in *Microbiology of Marine Food Products*, p. 410).

Ozone is a chemical agent that can be used for the disinfection of waters used in depuration (Richards, in *Microbiology of Marine Food Products*, pp. 410–411). While it destroys bacteria and viruses, it is also toxic to shellfish. As a special case, activated oxygen has been tried. Known also as *UV-generated ozone,* or known commercially as *Photozone* (developed by Water Management Inc. of Englewood, Colorado), tests have indicated that it is not toxic to fish. The reference supplies other parameters relating to the effectiveness of depuration, including the water temperature maintained.

Whereas chlorine is used effectively against bacterial contamination (that is, for depuration), no mention of its effectiveness against viruses is made, e.g., in *Microbiology of Marine Food Products*. Similarly, no mention of the effect of chlorine on viruses occurs in *Elimination of Pathogenic Organisms from Meat and Poultry*, although its effect on bacteria is described. That is, chlorine-water sprays are used to reduce the bacteria content on the surface of the carcasses, although they are not consistently effective (Anthony W. Kotula, in *Elimination of Pathogenic Organisms*, pp. 188–190). The maximum chlorine concentration allowed by the USDA is 200 ppm, which is below the threshold for many bacteria, according to a table furnished in the reference.*

Chlorine in chilled water has been found to extend the shelf life of poultry carcasses (J.S. Bailey et al., in *Microbiology of Poultry Meat Products*, p. 202). This may be attributed to the effect on bacteria. A general statement is that where there are bacteria, there are also viruses—and, furthermore, shellfish-associated enteric viral illnesses are on the increase, whereas bacterial illnesses are decreasing (John R. Chipley, in *Microbiology of Poultry Meat Products*, p. 96).

Moreover, regarding bacteria or microbes, chlorine/hypochlorite disinfection in depuration waters is marginal in processing shellfish on account of its extreme toxicity to shellfish (Richards, in *Microbiology of Marine Food Products*, p. 409). The use of *iodophors* (for instance, *iodoform* or *triiodomethane*, CHI_3, is a well-known antiseptic) seems to be successful, however. (It may be commented that iodine and bromine, as well as chlorine and hypochlorite, have been used to treat swimming pool water.) Other chemical decontaminants tried or proposed for microbes include the following (Peter S. Elias, in *Elimination of Pathogenic Organisms from Meat and Poultry*, p. 349ff.): acetic acid and its potassium and sodium salts; propionic acid and its calcium, potassium and sodium salts; *lactic acid and its ammonium, calcium, potassium, sodium, and magnesium salts;* formic acid.

---

* The reference also discusses airborne contamination, antibiotic and pesticide residues, and *Trichinella spiralis*, the larvae of which occur in pork and lead to the disease called *trichinosis* (Kotula, in *Elimination of Pathogenic Organisms*, pp. 190–194). The detection of the larvae using the trichinoscope, which is only 63 percent effective, is of first concern, followed by ways to treat pork to kill the larvae. Extended freezing is effective at –30° C (–22° F), and extended cooking with heat above 55° C (131° F) is effective, but microwave cooking is unreliable.

7.9   THE TROPICAL CONNECTION

As has been noted in Parts 2 and 3, the tropics, and especially the neotropics, are the source places for the preponderance of bioactive plants and the most debilitating diseases. Here grow the great tropical rain forests with their myriad plant species, many yet to be cataloged, and many more yet to be assayed for bioactivity. And here occur such strange disease-causing agents as the Marburg and Ebola viruses, and viruses yet to be known, to which can be added fungal-related diseases, and in particular protozoan-caused diseases.

7.9.1   SOME INFORMATION SOURCES ABOUT BIOACTIVE PLANTS IN NEOTROPICA

Starting with the common disease hepatitis in one form or another, we reintroduce the subject of bioactive plants and viruses, or viral diseases. Plants have been used to treat this virus-caused illness (Franklin Ayala Flores, in *Ethnobotany in the Neotropics*, p. 6). Thus, the Achual Indians employ the young root of the plant species *Iriartea exorrhiza*, pounding the root, adding water, and boiling the mixture to markedly reduce the volume. The dose is drunk before breakfast. Also, the flower of the cotton plant *Gossypium barbadense* is prepared in similar fashion. (This latter species is of the family Malvaceae and is listed in Hartwell's *Plants Used Against Cancer*.) The root of *Physalis angualata* is used to make a tea. (This species, of the family Solanaceae, is also listed in Hartwell. Interestingly, common names used for the genus *Physalis* in Hartwell include strychnos and winter-cherry, an indication that toxic alkaloids are present.) The Iquitos Indians utilize the rhizome of *Calathea* spp., drinking the juice extract once per day or soaking the pounded rhizome in water to make an infusion.

The Flores reference also lists and describes plants that contain *alkaloid hypotensive drugs* and also *alkaloid relaxants* for the smooth or skeletal muscles. There are *anti-rheumatic* plants and plants used against snakebites, plus plants used to treat diabetes, and anti-inflammatory plants, not to mention plants used in folk *odontology*, including the *latex* from *Chlorophora tinctoria*. The latter, when placed in a cavity, will cause the tooth to disintegrate. On the other hand, the pounded leaf bud or young leaf of *Couroupita guianensis*, when placed in the cavity, will relieve toothache. (The genus *Chlorophora* of the family Moraceae is listed in Hartwell's *Plants Used Against Cancer*.) There are plants used in ophthalmology, antimalarial plants, antihelminthic plants, antidiarrhetic plants and, to round things out, plain poisonous plants.

For the record, some of this information is presented in Table 7.2, according to plant family, genera, and species, and compared with Hartwell's compendium. It may be assumed that the plants listed in the tabulation contain substances that act as enzyme inhibitors or promoters for critical enzymatic reactions that are variously involved in the several categories, or may even supply enzymes.

Another author in the volume cited is Michael J. Balick, who contributes a chapter on "Ethnobotany of the Palms in the Neotropics." Rosita Arvigo and Balick later wrote *Rainforest Remedies: One Hundred Healing Herbs of Belize*. This latter work is cited in Part 2 under the section "Antibacterial and Antiviral Agents," and in Part 3, within the section "Investigations in Other Countries," in the subsection on "Neo Tropica," and also in Appendix J, notably, which pertains to antiviral plants.

In *The Rivers Amazon*, published in 1978 by Sierra Club Books, Alex Shoumatoff commented on the immense biodiversity of Amazonia (Shoumatoff, *Rivers*, pp. 74–76). He notes that some of the more bioactive plants which he collected in Amazonia belonged to the families *Menispermaceae, Bignoniaceae,* and *Apocynaceae*. (All are represented in Hartwell.) Shoumatoff further quotes Dr. Richard Evans Schultes of Harvard, described as the dean of Amazonian ethnobotany:

Of all the known plant species of the Amazon valley, "Only a mere fraction have even *superficially* been looked at chemically.* While there is certainly no reason to presume that people in primitive cultures possess any particular insight into the discovery of biodynamic plants, it is true that they do live in a much more intimate relationship with their ambient vegetation than do those of urbanized, advanced civilizations. *Trial and error and the experience of centuries have built up a rich store of folklore. It is, therefore, a shortcut, as it were, for us today to use to our advantage....*" (italics added) (Schultes is featured in Wade Davis' *One River*.)

---

* Some estimates indicate that perhaps 90 percent of all living species worldwide are still yet to be discovered.

Table 7.2   Medicinal Plants of the Neotropics

Acanthaceae	*Mendoncia** spp. **Poisonous.** Used as fish poison. Active ingredient unidentified.
Anacardiaceae	*Anacardium occidentale*: cashú, marañón. **Antidiarrhetic.** Bark boiled and liquid drunk for bacterial diarrhea.
Anacardiaceae	*Spondias* mombin*: ubos. **Antidiarrhetic.** Bark boiled and liquid drunk for bacterial diarrhea. Also used as disinfectant.
Apocynaceae	*Ambelania* lopezii*. **Ophthalmology. Poisonous.** Leaves mixed with bark of *Martinella* and bark of *Districtella racemosa* for **arrow poison.**
Apocynaceae	*Rauvolfia* serpentina*. **Hypotensive alkaloids.** This species is not native to Peru. It contains more than 50 alkaloids, of which reserpine and rescinamine are the most important. The latter is also found in other species of the genus. In addition to being hypotensive, rescinamine acts as a tranquilizer.
Apocynaceae	*Rauvolfia* sprucei*: huevo de gato (Shipibos, Yaguas, and Achuals). **Hypotensive alkaloids. Poisonous.** Contains reserpine, tetraphylline, tetraphyllicine.
Apocynaceae	*Rauvolfia* tetraphylla*: misho runto (Shipibos, Yaguas, and Achuals of Amazonian Peru). **Hypotensive Alkaloids. Poisonous.** Root contains reserpine, tetraphylline, tetraphyllicine. Used primarily as an **arrow poison**, but has also been used for treating nervous disorders.
Aracaceae	*Anthurium** spp.: jergón quiro (Achuals of the Rio Tigre). **Snakebite.** Pounded corn put on snakebite.
Aracaceae	*Iriartea* exorrhiza*: cashapona (Achuals). **Hepatitis.** Pounded root with water.
Bignoniaceae	*Crescentia cujete*: huingo (Achuals). **Anti-inflammatory.** Fruit used for cough medicine in form of macerated mesocarps.
Bignoniaceae	*Distictella* racemosa*. **Poisonous.** Bark mixed with bark of *Martinella* and leaves of *Ambelania lopezii* to make arrow poison.
Bignoniaceae	*Mansoa* alliacea*: ajo sacha (Achuals). **Antirheumatic.** Root contains dimethyl sulfide, divinyl sulfide, diallyl sulfide, propylallyl sulfide, alline, allicine, disulfoxide allyl. This array of compounds evidently indicates a kinship with garlic (*Allium sativum* of the family Lilicaceae).
Bignoniaceae	*Martinella* obovata*: remio (Candoshi-Shapras of Rio Pastaza, natives of Colombia and other parts of Amazonia). **Ophthalmology. Poisonous.** A few drops of the juice of the root for conjunctivitis. However, the Barasnas of Colombia use the bark plus the leaves of *Distictella racemosa* of the family Bignoniaceae to make **arrow poison**. An infusion of the bark of *Martinella* is a dangerous but effective febrifuge (reduces fever).
Bignoniaceae	*Spathicalyx* xanthophylla* (Tikunas of Colombia). **Ophthalmology.** Infusion of the yellow leaves for severe conjunctivitis.
Caricaceae	*Carica papaya*: papaya. **Anthelmintic.** Seeds and latex of young fruit contain the digestive enzyme papain, and are also used as a vermifuge or anthelmintic.
Caryocaraceae*	*Caryocar* glabrum*: almendra. **Poisonous.** Pounded mesocarp and endocarp are mixed with water and used as fish poison. Contain saponins.
Celastraceae	*Maytenus ebenfolia**: chuchuhuasi (used in Amazonian Peru). **Antirheumatic.**
Chenopodiacea	*Chenopodium ambrosioides* var. *anthelminticum**: paico (folk medicine). **Anthelmintic.** Specific against roundworms, namely the species *Ascaris lumbricoides* and *Oxyurus vermicularis*. Contains ascaridol
Compositae	*Clibadium* asperum*: huaca. **Poisonous.** Pulverized leaves mixed with ashes is a fish poison. May be stored in leaves of *Helicona* spp. for future use.
Cucurbitaceae	*Momordica charantia**: papailla (Indians of Iquitos, Peru). Diabetes. Infusion from leaves.
Cyclanthaceae*	*Asplundia** spp.: calzón panga (Achuals of Rio Corrientes). **Snakebite.** Chew young petiole.
Cyperaceae	*Cyperus* spp.: vibora piripiri (Achuals). **Snakebite.** Pounded rhizome put on snakebite.

Table 7.2 Medicinal Plants of the Neotropics *(continued)*

Euphorbiaceae	*Alchornea* * *castaneifolia*: ipurosa, ipururo, ipururu (Candoshi-Shapras, Shipibos). **Antirheumatic**.
Euphorbiaceae	*Hura* * *crepitans*: catahua. **Poisonous**. Cream-colored latex is very caustic and poisonous, and can injure the eyes of axmen. Tree-trunk taps yield the latex which is used as a fish poison and to kill anacondas.
Euphorbiaceae	*Nealchornea* * spp. **Poisonous**. Used as fish poison. Active ingredient unidentified.
Euphorbiaceae	*Phyllanthus acuminatus* *. **Poisonous**. Used as fish poison. Active ingredient unidentified.
Gramineae	*Paspalum conjugatum*: torurco (Achuals of Rio Tigre). **Ophthalmology**. **Anti-inflammatory**. A few drops of the stem sap for conjunctivitis. Also a good anti-inflammatory.
Gramineae	*Paspalum conjugatum*: torurco (Achuals of Rio Tigre). **Anti-inflammatory**.
Helicontiaceae*	*Heliconia* * spp.: bijao, situlli. **Poisonous** adjunct. Leaves used to store *Clibadium asperum*, to be used as fish poison.
Icacinaceae*	*Calatola* * *costaricense*: piu, pio (Candoshi-Shapras from the Morona and Pastaza Rivers). **Odontology**. Chew leaves against cavities, which stains teeth black.
Iridaceae	*Eleutherine* * *bulbosa*: yaguar piripiri (Indians of Iquitos, Peru). **Antidiarrhetic**. Wine-red bulb is boiled and the extract drunk to treat diarrhea and colic resulting from bacteria or amoebas such as the species *Entamoeba hystolitica*.
Lecythidaceae	*Couroupita* * *guianensis*: ayahuma (Indians of Rio Tigre). **Odontology**. Pounded leaf bud or young leaf will relieve toothache when placed in cavity.
Leguminosae	*Campsiandra* * *angustifolia*: huacapurana (used in Amazonian Peru). **Antirheumatic**.
Leguminosae	*Cassia reticulata* *: retama (Achuals, medicine men of Iquitos, Peru; Boras of Brillo Nuevo). **Anti-inflammatory**. **Poisonous**. Contains antibiotics in the perianth and leaves in the form of rhein (cassic acid). Contains copaiba balsam that is rich in the anthraquinone called emodine, having a strong purgative action. Used against renal and hepatic diseases, and venereal and skin diseases.
Leguminosae	*Inga* * *coriacea*: bushilla (Achuals of Nuevo Canaan and Intuto on Rio Tigre). **Antimalarial**. Pounded bark seeped in water, strained, and consumed as tea ("agua de tiempo").
Leguminosae	*Lonchocarpus nicou* *: barbasco, cozapi, cube, huasca, pacai. **Poisonous**. Pounded root used as a fish poison. Contains rotenone. Also of great value as a commercial **insecticide**.
Leguminosae	*Pithecolobrium laetum* *: remo caspi (Achuals of Nuevo Canaan and Intuto on Rio Tigre, "campesinos" near Iquitos, Peru). **Antimalarial**. Pounded bark, steeped in water, drained, and consumed as tea.
Leguminosae	*Tephrosia sinapou*: barbasco, cube, muyuy, tingui, tirana. **Poisonous**. Pounded roots used as fish poison.
Loganiaceae	*Potalia* * *amara*: curarina, sacha curarina (Boras, Huitotos, Ocainas, Yaguas). **Snakebite**. Root contains squalene and fatty acid methyl esters. Used orally and topically.
Malvaceae	*Gossypium barbadense* or *G. vitifolium*: algod\n, algod\n silvestre (Achuals). **Hepatitis**. Pounded flower with wtaer.
Marantaceae	*Calathea* * spp.: guisador (Indians of Iquitos). **Hepatitis**. Juice from rhizome.
Menispermaceae	*Abuta imene* *. **Poisonous**. **Alkaloid Relaxant**. Contains the active curare principle. See *Chondrodendron tomentosum*.
Menispermaceae	*Abuta rufescens* *. **Alkaloid relaxant**. **Poisonous**. Contains the active curare principle. See *Chondrodendron tomentosum*. Contains the oxoaporphines imenine, homomoschatoline, and imerubine, and the azafluoroanthenes imeluteine, rufescine, and norrufescine.
Menispermaceae	*Chondrodendron* * *limacifolium*. **Alkaloid relaxant**. **Poisonous**. Contains the active curare principle. See *Chondrodendron tomentosum*.

Table 7.2 Medicinal Plants of the Neotropics *(continued)*

Menispermaceae	*Chondrodendron* tomentosum*: amphiuasca curare (indigenous peoples of Peru). **Alkaloid relaxant. Poisonous.** Contains D-tubocurarine, the active curare principle, an alkaloid of the bisbenzylquinoline group. Natives macerate the bark of root and stem and use extract as arrow poison. Western medicine uses it as a muscle relaxant.
Menispermaceae	*Curarea* toxicofera*. **Alkaloid relaxant. Poisonous.** Contains the active curare principle. See *Chondrodendron tomentosum*. Contains the alkaloids curine, isochondodendrine (of the benzylquinoline group), toxicoferine.
Menispermaceae	*Telitoxicum* minuteflorum*. **Alkaloid relaxant. Poisonous.** Contains the active curare principle. See *Chondrodendron tomentosum.*
Menispermaceae	*Telitoxicum* peruvianum*. **Alkaloid relaxant. Poisonous.** Contains the active curare principle. See *Chondrodendron tomentosum*. Contains the alkaloids norufescine, lysicamine, subsesseline, telitoxine, peruvianine, telazoline.
Moraceae	*Chlorophora tinctoria**: insira ("campesinos" from Marañón River). **Odontology.** Drops of latex in tooth cavity will disintegrate tooth. Also has a diuretic and antivenereal action due to presence of the benzyl amine called moringin, an antiseptic for the urinary tract and the eyelids. The antiseptic compound phloroglucine and the astringent compound gallic acid are also present.
Moraceae	*Ficus insipida** or *F. anthelmintica**: oje. **Anthelmintic.** White latex used as vermifuge or anthelmintic. Contains phylloxanthine, B-amyrine or lupeol, lavandulol, phyllanthol, eloxanthine. The last-mentioned produces the vermifuge action, being toxic to parasites.
Musaceae	*Musa paradisiaca*: banana. **Antidiarrhetic.** Unripe fruit boiled and liquid drunk for bacterial diarrhea.
Myrtaceae	*Psidium* guajava*: guyaba. Shoots are boiled and the liquid drunk for bacterial diarrhea.
Nyctaginaceae	*Neea parviflora**: piosha, yanamuco (Candoshi-Shapras in Tintiyaca, near Andoas, Peru). **Odontology.** Chew leaves against cavities, which stains teeth black.
Piperaceae	*Piper* spp.: cordoncillo (Yaguas of Itaya River, Indians of Amazonian Peru). **Odontology.** Chew leaves against cavities, which stains teeth black.
Polygonaceae	*Triplaris surinamensis*: tangarana (curanderos in area of Iquitos, Peru). **Antimalarial.** Prepared from bark.
Rubiaceae	*Calycophyllum* spruceanum*: capirona colorada (Indians of Iquitos, Peru). **Diabetes.** Boil stembark.
Rubiaceae	*Genipa americana*: huito (Achuals and "campasenos" near Iquitos, Peru). **Anti-inflammatory.** Fruit and seeds are boiled to heal ulcerations. Contains genepine, mannitol, tannins, methyleter, caffeine, hydantoin, tannic acid. Also used as cough medicine and for anti-inflammatory effect on membranes.
Rubiaceae	*Manettia* divaricata*: yumanasa (Candoshi-Shapras). **Odontology.** Chew seeds against cavities, which stains teeth black.
Rubiaceae	*Simira* rubescens*: pucaquiro caspi (Achuals of Rio Tigre). **Odontology.** Chew bark against cavities, which stains the teeth pink or red.
Solanaceae	*Brunfelsia* grandiflora*: chiric sangango (Achuals). **Antirheumatic.**
Solanaceae	*Physalis angulata*: bolsa mullaca (Achuals). **Hepatitis.** Roots used to make a tea.
Solanaceae	*Solanum mammosum**: veneno, tintoma, reconilla dulce. **Poisonous.** Fruit used against rats.
Thymelaeaceae	*Schoenobiblus* peruvianus*: barbasco caspi. **Poisonous.** Triturated root mixed with water used as fish poison.
Verbenaceae	*Stachytarpheta cayennensis*: sacha verbena, verbena regional (Indians of Iquitos, Peru). **Diabetes.** Extract of stem and leaves. Seeds and pericarp contain a saponic glycoside which yields a cucurbitin called elatrin. Also contain alkaloids. Side effects are vomiting and diarrhea.

Source: Data from *Ethnobotany in the Neotropics*, edited by G.T. Prance and J.A. Kallunki, The New York Botanical Garden, Bronx, New York, 1984.

Note: Indian names are supplied where known, and parentheses indicate Indian tribes who use the plant. Plant families, genera, and species that do **not** appear in Hartwell's *Plants Used Against Cancer* are denoted by an asterisk.

Shoumatoff adds that maybe 10 percent of the Amazonian flora has been analyzed chemically, and there remain many blanks to be filled in. For example, the antibiotic compounds in the fungi have not been studied, nor have the lichens been investigated for bacteria-inhibiting compounds and chemovars (chemical variations or variants). The ferns and their allies have not been studied for the presence of, for instance, sesquiterpenoid lactones, ecdysones, alkaloids, and cyanogenic glycosides. (Laetrile and amygdalin are cyanogenic glycosides.) Although the angiosperms may be better known, there are still numerous genera that have not been analyzed for phytochemicals.

As to the high country west of Amazonia, in the Andes Mountains of Peru, called *Quechualand*, the most common plant families are *Compositae, Umbelliferae,* and *Cactaceae* (Shoumatoff, *Rivers*, p. 211). These are also families that comprise the most common wildflowers of other alpine zones, well-represented in Hartwell. Lupines, clovers, and other members of the *Leguminosae*, the nitrogen-fixers, are also present.

Also mentioned by Shoumatoff is Dr. João Mirá Pires of Belém, who at the time estimated that *at least 25,000 plants had been identified in Amazonia, with about that many more remaining to be discovered—which is somewhat at odds with Dr. Schultes, who estimated 62,000 known species from the Amazon valley with another 20 to 25 percent to be discovered* (Shoumatoff, *Rivers*, p. 76, 111). Dr. Pires added that only the margins of the rivers had been studied. In short, Shoumatoff states, "No one knows how many species there are in the Amazon." In any event, the last word has yet to be said, updating matters even unto today.

Another authority mentioned is Dr. Ghillean Prance, who was curator of Amazonian botany at the New York Botanical Garden (Shoumatoff, *Rivers*, pp. 75, 111–115.) (The work of the New York Botanical Garden is prominent, not only in the tropics as per the several volumes cited elsewhere, but world-wide—as per Thomas H. Everett's *The New York Botanical Garden Encyclopedia of Horticulture*, in 10 volumes.)

Still another noted authority on South American plant species is Alwyn H. Gentry, author of *A Field Guide to the Families and Genera of Woody Plants of Northwest South America (Colombia, Ecuador, Peru)* and editor of *Four Neotropical Rainforests*. Gentry also contributed a monograph (no. 31) on Bignoniaceae in *Flora Neotropica*. The subject of neotropical plants has been further discussed, notably in Part 3.

It may be mentioned in passing that Karl Friedrich Philipp von Martius compiled the two-volume set *Flora Brasiliensis,* from forays during 1817 to 1820 and published in 1833, followed by the 15-volumes in a set of 40 with the same leadoff title *Flora Brasiliensis*, published during the period 1840–1906.

In the former, Maximilian, Prinz von Wied is prominently mentioned, and he contributed his own *Beitrag zur Flora Brasiliens*, published in 1825, based on a trip to the tropical jungles of Brazil during 1815–1816. This same Maximilian, Prince of Wied-Neuwied (or Weid-Neuweid), a small royal house of Rhenish Prussia, later led an expedition up the Missouri River of North American in 1833, resulting in his account titled *Travels in the Interior of North America*. He was accompanied by the Swiss artist Karl Bodmer, whose portraits of Indians and other features of the Upper Missouri became world famous and are exhibited at such notable places as the Thomas Gilcrease Institute of American History & Art in Tulsa OK. Maximilian is commemorated by the Maximilian sunflower, *Helianthus maximiliani* of the family Compositae, a sunflower of the North American Plains. (This particular species does not make Hartwell's *Plants Used Against Cancer*, though the common or Kansas sunflower *H. annuus* is listed—as used in Venezuela.)

7.9.2 DISEASES OF THE TROPICS

Amazonia, as with some other parts of the tropical world, in addition to common diseases, has some strange and not so strange tropical diseases for which the native folkloric agents have not been very successful. At the top of the list is malaria, with tuberculosis, hepatitis A and B, typhoid, and venereal diseases as additional hazards (Shoumatoff, *Rivers*, pp. 16–18). Introduced diseases include pneumonia, measles, and influenza. Yellow fever can still be contracted in the jungle, but smallpox has largely been wiped out. There may be occasional outbreaks of diphtheria and bubonic plague, but beriberi, a malnutrition problem during the rubber-boom days, is no longer widespread. Schistosomiasis is common in northeastern Brazil, but there are only two other river locations in Amazonia at which the disease occurs. Intestinal worms are widespread, and the resulting diseases include trichocephaliasis, ancilostomiasis, strongiloidiasis, and belhausis. Various protozoa parasitize the intestines, the most common being the amoeba acquired from consuming feces-contaminated water or vegetables. While some amoeba are benign, others enter the liver, and still other protozoa inhabit the bloodstream.

An example of the last of these is *Trypanosoma crusii*, the cause of Chagas' disease, which Darwin contracted during his brief stopover in central Brazil. *This unusual disease is transmitted in the feces of the hissing beetle, which bites its sleeping victims on the face and defecates by the bite. When the victim unconsciously scratches the bite, the dung is rubbed into the wound, transmitting the protozoa to the bloodstream. The symptoms may not appear until 20 years later, in the form of cardiac and digestive dysfunctions.* It is said, however, that the disease is now under control in most of Amazonia. In fact, there was the Evandro Chagas Institute located at the edge of Belém, a tropical research center under the direction of a lady doctor, a Dr. Gilberto (Shoumatoff, *Rivers*, p. 15).

Worms called microfilia are also found in the bloodstream, and one in particular results in onchocerciasis, also called *African River blindness*. The disease, like elephantiasis, is carried by the *black fly*. Some of the injected microfilia travel to the eye, dying there and producing blindness. *It is estimated that two-thirds of the Yanomamo nation have the disease—the Yanomamo being the largest group of Indians in Amazonia, and who occupy the Venezuela border.*

Ectoparasites may become attached as a person walks through the jungle. These include various ticks and chiggers, and the scabies mite, presumably *Sarcoptes scabiei*, the source for the itch or mange. Another problem is called *bichus de pe*, comprising gravid (pregnant) female insects of the species *Tunga penetrans*, which bore through the skin to lay their eggs. The botfly *Dermatobia hominus* lays its eggs on the proboscis of a different insect known as the *mutuca*, which in turn feeds on humans and passes the eggs along. *The larvae grow into inch-long maggots,* finally breaking the skin after about 40 days. The botfly itself causes the disease known as *miiasis*. All the ectoparasites can cause secondary infections, aside from the bites of various mosquitoes and sandflies, that also serve as vectors for such *arboviruses* as may cause *equine encephalitis*.

As has been previously mentioned, the acronym *arbor* stands for *ar*thropod-*bor*ne; that is, the virus carriers are such arthropods as mosquitoes and ticks or other insects. Although some or many arboviruses are benign, others are not. The more dangerous viral diseases transmitted, in addition to equine encephalitis, include *yellow fever, dengue fever,* and *louping ill*. The last-mentioned is an acute, viral, infectious disease that affects sheep, and it is transmitted by the bites of a tick known as the castor-bean tick, *Ixodes ricinus*, which also may attack humans. It causes encephalomyelitis (inflammation of the brain and spinal cord) and is so named because the sick sheep, as were found in northern England and Scotland, were ill and would leap or "loup" about.

In general, arthropods belong to the phylum Arthropoda and consist of animals with an articulated body and limbs—in other words, invertebrates. The notable classes within the Arthropoda are the insects, arachnids, and crustaceans.

Of further mention by Shoumatoff are other assorted fevers such as *Oripush fever,* which is transmitted by the *acuticordes* mosquito. Occurring in seven-year cycles, the victim is laid up for about three days each time. The infamous jungle sickness called *blackwater fever,* or *febre negra de Lábrea,* is still under study, its etiology apparently unknown. An outbreak of another mysterious fever, or *febre,* which occurred in the northeastern Brazilian state of Pará previous to Shoumatoff's book, *resulted in 71 deaths—which included the people on the research team trying to identify the disease. The area was closed off until the disease died out of its own accord, a period taking several weeks. (The course of events has a similarity with the Ebola virus outbreak in Africa.)*

Shoumatoff provides the observation that *most of these diseases could be treated with pills or injections, save for those diseases that did not appear until years afterward. (Elephantiasis or filariasis* is an example of such a treatable disease. It is a disease in which the skin becomes hardened and fissured like an elephant's hide, and the affected body part becomes enormously enlarged due to inflammation and obstruction of the lymphatics. The most severe form is caused by an infestation of the parasitic worm or nematode, *Wucheraria bancrofti,* of the superfamily Filarioidea, and is transmitted by mosquitoes such as *Culex fatigans*. The disease is endemic to the tropics and subtropics, but effective therapy exists in the form of the drugs *diethylcarbamazine* and *sodium caparsolate,* which kill adult worms and microfilariae. Interestingly, *when the victim reaches northern climes, the infestation dies out*. Still other forms and carriers of the disease exist in many parts of the tropical world, for example in the Far East, Guatemala and Mexico, and West and Central Africa.

Leprosy is observed to be active in western Amazonia, notably in the state called Acre, with slightly more than 10 persons per thousand being infected (Shoumatoff, *Rivers*, pp. 16, 107–108). There are two basic kinds, with one kind chronic and the other of shorter duration and more amenable to treatment by sulfa drugs. Some persons may be more genetically susceptible than others, but *the exact means of transmission remain a mystery, although skin contact and contact with shared objects are no doubt involved. Tuberculoid leprosy yields to a few years of treatment with sulfone drugs, but the lepromatous kind is only arrested and may return without warning.* (There are also two intermediate kinds.) The microbe *Mycobacterium leprae* is reiterated as the source and thrives in the colder extremities, namely the fingers, toes, nose, ears, and cheekbones, deadening the nerve endings.

A disease named *leishmaniasis* is caused by a protozoan, which is said to be transmitted by a mosquito whose habits and life cycle are not yet completely understood (Shoumatoff, *Rivers*, pp. 16, 104–105). Other experts blame it on sandflies. The results can be grotesque in the extreme, for in the advanced stages both the palate and nose disintegrate. Shoumatoff comments that five new cases per day enter the Hospital for Tropical Diseases at Manaus, Brazil, and the treatment utilizes chemicals whose effects are as debilitating as the disease. (Manaus has its share of vendors for herbs, potions, and amulets, as reported on p. 109 of Shoumatoff's book, and a few Quechuan remedies are also indicated on p. 209.) During the mid-rainy season, the peak for leishmaniasis transmission, military groups entering the jungle will have up to 80 percent casualties. By invading the lymphatic system, the protozoa can cause extensive muco-cutaneous damage, first signaled by open sores on the arms or legs, and eventually eating away the nose and palate in from 2 to 20 years. Treatment involves 30 injections of pentavalent antimony over a 50- to 140-day period. Unfortunately, there are severe side effects—e.g., cardiac involvement and swelling of the joints. For this reason, the antibiotic Rifampicin is sometimes used, stretched over a 5-month period.

As to the febrile disease called *malaria*—caused by the protozoan known as the *malaria parasite* of the genus *Plasmodium* and transmitted by the *Anopheles* mosquito, the drug *chloroquine* is good only for *Vivax* malaria, whereas the sulfa-based drug called Fansidar worked for *Falciparum* malaria, and one can hope that the malaria was not one of the resistant strains, which, as indicated by the foregoing remarks about various diseases, may prove rapidly fatal (Shoumatoff, *Rivers*, p. 105).

Other tropical travelers remind us from time to time of the medical possibilities of Amazonia—for instance, Mark Jenkins' sketch in the October, 1997 issue of *Men's Health*. Thus, there is mention of *cat's-claw* or *uña de gato* (*Pithecolobium Unguis-cati*) as an antitumor agent. The record hardly bears this out. In fact, the comments previously indicated are pertinent, in that the native shamans cannot for the most part cure their own serious tropical diseases, a couple of examples being malaria and bilharziasis or schistosomiasis. Still....

It would seem that Amazonia itself should provide a fertile place to try out the plants and phytochemicals derived from the tropical rainforest. It may be commented, however, that *the white man's treatments or cures seem, so far, to be the best answer for most tropical diseases*. Nevertheless, there is an occasional instance when a native remedy is reported to cure the white man, as reported for example by Michael Swan in *The Marches of El Dorado: Brtish Guiana, Brazil, Venezuela*, published in 1958. An early-day white settler of British Guiana contracted a fever that was cured by an infusion of bark (Swan, *Marches*, p. 125). In common with so many other such reports, the plant species was not stated.

Swan has many other interesting information items to report in his book. For instance, he describes the *Ité palm* (*Mauritia flexuosa* of the family Marantaceae), also called the *Arbol de la Vida* or *Tree of Life,* and *the source for the nutritional starch called arrowroot* (Swan, *Marches*, p. 36). This species may or may not be distinguishable from the Biblical version, but it certainly differs from the several species known as arbor vitae, which are of the genus *Thuja* of the family Pinaceae. (Although Marantaceae is represented by a single species in Hartwell's *Plants Used Against Cancer*, this species is not of the genus *Mauritia* but is the Brazilian species *Thalia geniculata*, also called *Cortosa arundinacea* or *Maranta geniculata*. The species *Thuja occidentalis* has many entries under Pinaceae.) Also mentioned is a device for squeezing the hydrocyanic acid from cassava, with the acid extract further processed into a treacle-like substance called *casareep*, which acts to preserve meat. It is kept in a "pepper-pot," to which meat is added as needed (Swan, *Marches*, p. 87). Furthermore, the Indian tribes of the tropical forests are sustained by a cassava culture, whereas the Mayas of Central America had a maize culture (Swan, *Marches*, p. 90). Then as now, fires were set by the Indians (and settlers), who believed that soil productivity was enhanced by this practice (Swan, *Marches*, p. 143).

Erythroxylum coca and *cocaine* are briefly mentioned, and a longer description of urari or *curare* is provided, which specifies the alkaloid component *curarine* as the active ingredient, which causes paralysis, in turn blocking respiration and causing death by asphyxiation (Swan, *Marches*, pp. 145–148). As previously indicated, ordinary salt tends to counter the effects, and the drug prostigmin is said to be an effective neutralizer for curare (Price, *Amazing Amazon*, pp. 169, 174). As further noted, Willard Price has listed many more herbs and oils, including *mandrake against cancer*, and supplies a noteworthy compendium of medicinal plants from Amazonia (Price, *Amazing Amazon*, pp. 175–179, 283).]

Another strange disease is caused by the bite of a sandfly called the *Verruga*, as noted in Christopher Isherwood's *The Condor and the Cows*, published in 1948. A fever and warts (verrugas) are produced, with the warts ulcerating, and the end result may be fatal (Isherwood, *The Condor*, p. 132). *Sandfly attacks occur at night in what is called the Verruga belt*, e.g., in the subtropical regions of eastern Peru, and it was formerly thought that the sandfly injected a toxin, possibly from plants on which the flies settled. Later investigations showed, however, that the illness is caused by a bacterium named *Bartonella bacilliformis,* and the disease is called *bartonellosis* (Hugo Lumbreras and Humberto Vuerra, in *Tropical Medicine and Parasitology*, pp. 172–174). The anemic stage is called *Oroya fever,* and the eruptive state is called *verruga peruana* (or peruviana). Transmission is by the sandfly *Lutzomyia verrucarum*, and infected persons are the hosts. Native children are generally resistant due to neonatal exposure, but outsiders develop severe, sometimes fatal, symptoms. Most newcomers to certain Andean valleys located in Peru, Ecuador, and Colombia, at elevations between 1000 and 2000 m, are affected within months. Antibiotics successfully treat the disease, however.

Another comment by Ishelwood, perhaps worth mentioning, is to the effect that visitors to, say, Lima, Peru should take extra vitamins, since there aren't enough vitamins inherent in the local vegetables due to the cloudy weather (Ishelwood, *The Condor*, p. 126)

Tabulations of arborvirus families and species that cause various diseases consist of some 10 different virus families and 35 different virus species (Scott B. Halstead, in *Tropical Medicine and Parasitology*, pp. 19–22). The Marburg and Ebola viruses have been classified as *Filaviridae*, and what are called the *Bangui* and *Quaranfil* viruses remain unclassified. The major arborviral and related viral diseases are divided as occurring in the following regions: the Americas; Africa and the Middle East; Asia, India, and Southeast Asia; and Australasia and the Pacific. The arthropod fever-causing vectors include the mosquito, the phlebotomine fly, the tick, and the culicoides. The reference provides further details.

The statement has been made that there are more than *400 known arthropod-borne viruses in vertebrates* (Robert B. Tesh, in *Tropical and Geographical Medicine*, p. 73). Add to this all the other known virus species (such as enteroviruses), and the potential for invasion is indeed great, which translates to the potential for inducing cancer cell formation.

Another microorganism classification of interest consists of the parasitic bacterial family *Chlamydiaceae* (Julius Schachter, in *Tropical Medicine and Parasitology*, p. 82ff). These are characterized as *obligate intracellular parasites*, approximately 300–400 nm in diameter, and are closely related to Gram-negative bacteria. (The descriptor *obligate* indicates that the organism is restricted to a particular condition of life. This is as distinguished from *facultative*, indicating that an organism can live under more than one set of environmental conditions, e.g., can live either a parasitic or nonparasitic existence.) Among the chlamydial diseases is *psittacosis,* also called *ornithosis* or *parrot fever.* It is caused by *Chlamydia osittaci* and is manifested as an acute febrile infection. It can lead to pneumonia and potentially fatal results if untreated. Occupational exposure occurs *in the poultry industry,* although human-to-human transmission is rare.

A chapter on "Malignant Diseases," by Alexander C. Templeton, is contained in the volume *Tropical Medicine and Parasitology*. In the leadoff paragraphs, the statement is made that

> in the industrial countries, about 50 percent or half the population will develop a malignant tumor during the course of their lifetimes, and about 20 percent will die as the result. In the tropics however, the corresponding figures are much lower, about 10 and 5 percent. These differences are in large part attributed to the age distribution of the populations.

In industrialized countries, there is a low infant mortality rate, followed by a minimal loss of life until the sixth decade, when vascular disease and cancer become pronounced. In tropical countries, there is a high infant mortality rate, followed by a significant adult mortality rate due in considerable part to infectious diseases, leaving a relatively small old-age population to be affected by vascular disease and cancer.

A table is provided in the reference showing the regional variations for various tumors in the tropics. Among the observations is that, *in Bombay, tumors of the mouth comprise about 50 percent of the tumors found in males,* whereas the rest of the world averages about *2 percent.* The cause is the interminable chewing of a quid of tobacco and betel nut, with or without the addition of lye. Bile duct cancers are common wherever *Clonorchis sinensis* infection is endemic. Large intestinal neoplasm or colon cancer, in contrast with affluent meat-eating populations, is relatively unusual throughout the tropics where meat products are a dietary rarity.

In a chapter on "Neoplasms and Malignancies," by Charles L.M. Olweny in *Tropical and Geographical Medicine,* a number of epidemiological facts about cancer are presented. Worldwide, there are an estimated *4.3 million deaths per year* from cancer, with death rates increasing in developing countries. It is further stated, for instance, that hepatocellular carcinoma (HCC) accounts for over 90 percent of primary liver cancers. High incidences occur in sub-Saharan Africa, southeast Asia, and in western Pacific countries. It is the commonest form of cancer in tropical Africa, particularly in Mozambique, and is rapidly increasing in China. Furthermore, *about 80 percent of HCC cases can be traced to hepatitis B virus (HBV) infection. Aflatoxin is also a causative agent—e.g., from molded peanuts or grains.* The comment is furnished that *hepatitis B* may be the *initiating* factor, and such other factors as *aflatoxin* may be *promoting* factors.

7.10 IMMUNITY

Resistance or immunity to disease may be natural or induced, the latter introducing the continuing subject of vaccines. Vaccines have been successfully developed and applied for a number of infectious diseases, viral and otherwise, some of which have already been mentioned. Newer developments in the subject include what may be called synthetic vaccines, and information is presented for instance in *Vaccination Strategies of Tropical Diseases,* edited by F. Y. Lieu and published in 1989. Some of the topics taken up are recombinant DNA technology, vaccinia virus (cowpox- or smallpox-type viruses) as a carrier of antigens, salmonella vaccines as carriers of antigens, and peptide vaccines.

Vaccinia vaccines, for example, have been successfully used on experimental animals against such diseases as hepatitis B (HBV), influenza, herpes simplex virus (HSV), vesicular stomatitis (VSV), respiratory synctial (RSV), and rabies (Geoffrey L. Smith, in *Vaccination Strategies,* p. 38). Additionally, vaccinia vaccines have also been used successfully against *polyoma virus-induced tumors* and against *Friends murine (mouse) leukemia virus* (Fm-LV).

The immunization techniques and principles applied to the prevention or cure for many pathogenic diseases are to some degree applicable to cancer, or at least to certain types of cancer. Further particulars are as follows, both with regard to the development and administration of vaccines, and to the immune system or immune response per se.

7.10.1 VACCINES

It may be noted that work continues on vaccines for such mycobacterial diseases as tuberculosis and leprosy, as well as for other diseases (Martin J. Carrier, in *Vaccination Strategies,* p. 26; Marilyn J. Moore and Juraj Ivanyi, in *Vaccination Strategies,* p. 80ff). Whereas conventional vaccines consist of live attenuated or killed organisms, there are other possibilities. Such approaches as manipulation of the idiotype network are a possibility.*

What is known as BCG, for Bacillus Calmette-Guérin vaccine, has been tried, with a degree of success. Synthetic peptides are also a possibility (e.g., Fred Brown, in *Vaccination Strategies,* pp. 66, 68). Inasmuch as peptides may sometimes be viewed as anticancer agents, the connection with the immune system is obvious. On the other hand, there may be other considerations to take into account, such as the vaccine functioning as an enzyme inhibitor (or inhibitors) for critical metabolic processes, both in mycobacterial cells say and in cancer cells.

---

* Idiotypes, or Ids, are designated as antigenic determinants associated with various regions of the antibody molecules. Another term employed on p. 81 of the latter reference, above, is "paratope," designated as the antigen-combining site. Still another terms used is "epitope," which may be defined as an antigenic site (Voet and Voet, *Biochemistry,* p. 1216).

Speaking further of vaccines, the conventional technologies may be placed in the major categories of whole organisms and semipurified subcellular components (Carrier, in *Vaccination Strategies*, p. 22). The whole organisms can be subdivided into attenuated strains such as for *Salmonella* bacterial vaccines, and the virus vaccines for measles and mumps, or killed viral strains as for rabies. The subcellular components can be divided into inactive toxins, notably the toxoids of tetanus and diphtheria, and into protective nontoxic components. An example of the latter is the human plasma-derived particles of hepatitis B in the 22-nm size range. Although acknowledged to be generally effective, nevertheless a table is provided in the reference of some of the drawbacks. The listing includes killed whole cells for the bacterial diseases of typhoid, whooping cough or pertussis, and cholera. The toxoid is used against tetanus, also a bacterial disease (the toxoid is produced by the microorganism *Clostridium tetani*). Killed whole viruses are used against the viral diseases influenza and hepatitis.

It may be further mentioned that whole cell techniques have been used in the attempt to develop cancer vaccines. In other words, the antigen is the cancer cell itself, generally taken from the individual patient, to serve potentially as the vaccine to produce the antibodies for immunization. Considering that this route has not been demonstrated to be entirely successful in every case, the above-cited reference furnishes the following remark.

> ...the very nature of utilizing whole organisms and cellular cocktails means that potentially large numbers of components in the vaccine either are not required or are harmful to some degree.

An illustrative example is that of tetanus toxoid preparation, where 30 to 50 percent of the vaccine is the toxoid, and the rest consists of other components of *C. tetani*.*

The reference, in turn, puts in a good word for the development of new kinds of vaccines from modern biotechnology. The techniques variously utilized include recombinant DNA technology, peptide synthesis, monoclonal antibodies, and sophisticated immunological analysis. From these techniques, it is possible to determine the antigens leading to protection, and to clone and express these antigens in an appropriate host. It is added that many pathogenic antigens have been identified, cloned, expressed, and sequenced, although not all of these subunit antigens are protective. Where this might lead in developing cancer vaccines was not identified.

As indicated elsewhere, vaccines—particularly live attenuated vaccines—may need to be stabilized by what are called *adjuvants* (Robert Bomford, in *Vaccination Strategies*, p. 94ff). While alum has been used for this purpose in the past, and mineral gels such as of aluminum hydroxide are now used, other substances are under investigation. Notable among these are the triterpene glycosides occurring in plants, called *saponin* or *saponins*, which may be even more active in the form of ISCOMS or "immunostimulatory complexes." The subject is further mentioned in that *saponins* are recognized *medicinal agents* of one kind or another, and are potential *anticancer agents*.

7.10.2 THE IMMUNE SYSTEM

The subject of vaccines and immunization further brings up the matter of globulins and gamma globulins, and of immunoglobulins. For the purposes here, dictionaries, encyclopedias, reference books, and textbooks will be relied upon to review the appropriate definitions. What are called the *gamma globulins* or *gammaglobulins* constitute a protein-containing blood fraction that contains antibodies effective against certain diseases such as measles, rubella, infectious hepatitis, and poliomyelitis. (It can be seen why gamma globulin administration is sort of a catch-all treatment, or immediacy, for a variety of circumstances.)

The more encompassing term is *globulin*, indicating proteins that are insoluble in water and that may be precipitated, for example, by salts such as ammonium sulfate. Examples of the latter include serum globulin found in blood serum, J-lactoglobulin found in milk, and ovoglobulin found in egg whites. It is indicated that most of the proteins in plant seeds have the properties of globulins, for example, *edestin* from hemp seeds, another called *amandin* from almond seeds, and *canavalin* from jack beans. *Legumin*

---

* In the case of cancer-cell proliferation, the disease may already be too advanced for any kind of vaccine treatment. In other words, vaccines are directed at immunization prior to the onset of the disease. An exception, maybe, is rabies vaccine, but even here, there is ordinarily only a brief respite period after infection in which the vaccine is effective. After this, it is too late.

occurs in peas and lentils, while *excelsin* is found in Brazil nuts. (The inference could be that these globulins may have an adverse effect on cancer cells, in that these plants and/or seeds are entered in medical folklore as anticancer agents.)

The proteins of the immune system are referred to as *immunoglobulins* (Voet and Voet, *Biochemistry*, p. 105). They may also be called *antibodies*. In further comment, it has been stated that "antibody molecules are immunoglobulins produced by an organism in response to the invasion of foreign compounds, such as proteins, carbohydrates, and nucleic acid polymers" (Richard M. Schultz, in *Textbook of Biochemistry*, p.105). It is further stated that the antibody associates noncovalently with the foreign substance, to start a process in which the foreign substance is eliminated from the body. Furthermore, the materials or substances that stimulate antibody production are known as *antigens*. (The foregoing interpretation would assume that microorganisms produce, or consist of, chemical compounds that stimulate an immune response.)

The immune system, in turn, can be described as an elaborate protective array of functions that act against disease-causing microorganisms or pathogens, including bacteria and viruses (Voet and Voet, *Biochemistry*, p. 1207ff). This action constitutes the immune response and is conferred by certain kinds of white blood cells known as *lymphocytes*. These arise from precursor cells, or stem cells, in the bone marrow. In addition to patrolling the blood vessels, lymphocytes can leave the blood vessels to enter the intercellular spaces, also to act against foreign invaders (antigens). Eventually returning to the blood by way of the lymphatic vessels, along the way they interact with lymphoid tissues such as the thymus, the lymph nodes, and the spleen. Much of the immune response happens in these tissues.

The reference distinguishes two types of immunity, called cellular immunity and humoral immunity. *Cellular immunity* responds against virus-infected cells, fungi, parasites, and foreign tissue, and is mediated or carried out by T lymphocytes or T cells, whose development occurs in the thymus. On the other hand, *humoral immunity* (signifying "fluid") acts predominantly against bacterial infections and viral infections outside the cells. It is mediated by an extensive and diverse collection of proteins related to one another. These proteins are called *antibodies* or *immunoglobulins*, as previously noted, and are produced by B lymphocytes or *B cells* that mature in the bone marrow.*

There are five different classes of the immunoglobulins, or Igs (Voet and Voet, *Biochemistry*, pp. 1211–1214). Technically speaking, the structures consist of subunits designated as light chains (L) and heavy chains (H), which are associated by disulfide bonds and by noncovalent interactions, resulting in a Y-shaped dimer representable as $(L-H)_2$. The "Y" may be divided into fragments, with the upper, identical branches each designated fragment "ab" or Fab, and the lower stem designated fragment "c" or Fc.

Furthermore, immunoglobulins are *glycoproteins* whereby each heavy chain has an N-linked oligosaccharide. (The emphasis on the use of glycoproteins as a curative measure is seen in the foregoing fact.)

An enumeration is provided in the reference of the secreted immunoglobulins in humans. These are denoted as immunoglobulin A or IgA, and in the same fashion as IgD, IgE, IgG, and IgM. They differ in their corresponding types of heavy chains, which are respectively designated I, L, M, K, and T. It is noted that these various classes of secreted immunoglobulins have different physiological functions.

Thus, *IgM* works best against invading microorganisms. Mostly confined to the blood, it is the first antibody secreted in response to an antigen, usually 2 to 3 days after the infection.

The most common immunoglobulin is *IgG*, which is evenly distributed between the blood and interstitial fluids. It is able to cross the placenta and furnish the fetus with immunity, and production ensues 2 to 3 days after IgM appears.

The immunoglobulin *IgA* is found, for the most part, in the intestinal track and in saliva, sweat, tears, and other such secretions. Its action is to bind to the antigenic sites of pathogens, thus blocking their attachment to epithelial (outer) surfaces. It is mentioned that IgA is the major antibody of first-milk or colostrum and of ensuing milk, and it serves to protect nursing infants from pathogens in the intestinal tract.

Immunoglobulin E or *IgE*—present in the blood in dilute concentrations—acts against parasites and, in addition, may be involved in allergic reactions.

---

* Inasmuch as peptides are involved in synthetic vaccines, even as anticancer agents, the connection to immunity is obvious; peptides are merely shorter-chain proteins formed from various combinations of amino acids. Or proteins can be viewed as long-chain peptides.

Lastly, and occurring in the blood in minute amounts, the functions of *IgD* were said to be as yet unknown.

It may be further commented that all the foregoing immunoglobulins are variously cited in *Vaccination Strategies* except IgD.

For example, the immune response to the number one tropical scourge, malaria, may be referenced to immunity and IgG, with respect to the development of a vaccine (Michael J. Lockyer and Anthony A. Holder, in *Vaccination Strategies*, pp. 129–135). Thus, the reference observes that, in endemic areas, the persons most at risk to the parasite are children between 1 and 5 years of age. Children who survive this window of susceptibility will slowly acquire an immunity with increasing age. Although parasites can be found intermittently in the blood of so-called *immune* individuals, along with antibodies, the infected parties seem to reach a stage of equilibrium. Moreover, it seems that a continued exposure to malarial infection is required to sustain immunity. This presumably has bearing on the development of a successful malarial vaccine, with boosting by natural infections or multiple immunizations.

Various species of the parasitic genus *Plasmodium* have in fact been considered in the development of a vaccine, and notably against *P. falciparum* sporozoites.*

In brief summary, it has been found that the surface of infective, mature sporozoites is covered with a stage-specific protein, or circumsporozoite (CS) protein, characterized as immunodominant. Monoclonal antibodies (Mabs) will act against the CS protein, abolishing their infectivity. Recombinant proteins or synthetic peptides were used in a vaccine, with positive results, although relatively high doses were required to cause IgG responses (Lockyer and Holder, *Vaccination Strategies*, pp. 134–135). The work continues and illustrates the fact that IgG antibody response is a measure of the effectiveness of a malaria vaccine or other parasitic vaccines.†

An even more down-to-earth picture of the effect of devastating diseases can be described in the following terms. Thus, malaria and its causative agent *Plasmodium*, transmitted via the *Anopheles* mosquito and thought to have been exported from the Old World to the New, post-Columbus world, is perhaps less contagious than some other diseases. As to the latter category, it has been noted that some of the South American native tribes had a horror of highly contagious epidemics and would resort to extreme measures for containment—torching hut and victim, killing and burying victims, or even burying them alive (Price, *Amazing Amazon*, p. 165). The search for vaccines for these dreaded diseases—whatever the cause—is of the highest priority.

The action of the cellular immune response can be described in terms of the destruction of the offending cells (Voet and Voet, *Biochemistry*, p. 1208). A macrophage, a type of white blood cell, will engulf and partially digest a foreign antigen. (This digestion is said to proceed "lysosomally"—lysosomes being membrane-bounded organelles or "bags" within the cell, and which contain hydrolytic *enzymes*, whose function is to digest ingested materials.) The macrophage then displaces the antigenic fragments so formed on its surface, which are then thought to bind to cell-surface proteins known as major histocompatability complex (MHC) proteins. It is found that the MHC is *polymorphic*, changing into numerous genetic forms or alleles. Furthermore, any two unrelated individual specimens of the same species are highly unlikely to have the exact same set of MHC proteins, which are therefore referred to as "markers of individuality."

On consulting the *Encyclopedia Britannica* under "Allergy and Anaphylactic Shock," tumor cells are said to be different antigenetically from normal cells. *Either the tumor cells have fewer or no histocompatability antigens, or they have new and different antigens.* In the introductory section of the article, it is emphasized that two successive contacts with an allergen or antigen—which is a proteinaceous substance—are required to induce an allergic reaction, the first contact developing sensitization for the second. The substances formed during sensitization are called antibodies. In comment, however, there may be cases in which no prior contact could have existed, as with newly prescribed drugs, so it can be speculated that some other agent or agents may have induced sensitization. *In any case, there is the*

---

* Sporozoites are the minute, active bodies formed from the division of spores, which in turn develop into adult spores—the latter being designated the primitive reproductive bodies, usually unicellular but also multicellular, and which are produced by lower plants and some protozoa. Examples of spore-producing organisms include algae, fungi, ferns, liverworts, and mosses, all of which yield spores analogous to the seeds of flowering plants and develop directly into the mature organism.

† For the further purposes here, if somehow cancer is related to parasitic agents, as advanced in the book by Hulda Regehr Clark, then there may be an additional avenue open for cancer vaccines.

hazard that in using any biochemical substance or drug, a severe allergic reaction may ensue within a given individual, another example of biochemical individuality. In fact, it sometimes becomes difficult to say whether the individual was "poisoned" by the substance or suffered a severe allergic reaction, that is, anaphylactic shock. Thus, the venom say from sting of a bee or even the bite of a rattler may cause little reaction in some individuals, while others may rapidly go into death-threatening anaphylactic shock. Reason enough, obviously, for carrying such emergency histamine-countering drugs as *Benadryl*® or *epinephrine* (adrenalin), otherwise known as antihistamines. A *histamine*, by the way, is a definite chemical compound, being an amine with the stoichiometric formula $C_5H_9N_3$, and which is naturally present in the human body and in plants. Its normal functions are stated to include capillary dilation, smooth muscle tissue contraction, enhancement of gastric secretions, and the stimulation of heart rate. Excess histamine, however, is released from the tissues during conditions of allergic reaction, inflammation, and stress. If too much is released, for example from the lung mast cells, causing contraction of the smooth muscle cells, then asphyxiation can result. Classed as *autocoids*, other compounds or groups similar to histamine include serotonin, polypeptides, adenyl compounds, and prostaglandins. Interestingly, such kinds of compounds are mentioned from time to time in discussing the many aspects of cancer, suggesting a web or network of some sort—and potential indicators for the progression or regression of cancer. Antihistamines provide countering effects by competing at the sites of histamine action. (Further details are furnished for instance in the *Encyclopedia Britannica* in the section on "Histamine and Antihistamines.")

What are called Class I MHC proteins are found on the surface of vertebrate cells and are recognized by other proteins known as T cell receptors, existing on the surfaces of cytotoxic T cells. Macrophages having antigenic fragments that are linked to what are called Class II MHC proteins, which are bound to helper T cells, having a cognate receptor protein. The one recognizes the other, and both are necessary and serve to concentrate the action of the immune system on diseased cells.

A complicated series of processes follow in turn, involving the so-called cytotoxic T cells, or killer T cells, which bind to antigen-bearing host cells. At the site of contact, these T cells release a 70-kD protein called *perforin*, which lyses or destroys the targeted cells by creating pores in the plasma membranes of the diseased cells.

The cellular immune system will in finality kill virus-infected host cells, thus in the main serving to prevent the spread of *viral infections*. It also acts against *fungal infections, parasites,* and certain types of *cancers*. (Hence, all the talk about stimulating the immune system for protection against cancer—even curing cancer.) May we also say that the immune system acts against *bacteria*, that is, bacterial cells—in turn obviating their products, namely *bacterial toxins*?*

The surfaces of the B cells of the humoral immune system have both immunoglobulins and Class II MHC proteins. Encountering a surface-binding antigen, the B cell proceeds to surround and partially digest the antigen, displaying the fragments on the surface in a complex formed with the Class II MHC protein. Helper T cells in turn bind to the B cell, releasing interleukins that cause the B cells to proliferate. There is thus an as-needed stimulating and proliferating effect not only for B cells but for T cells.

An ancillary effect in this complicated chain of events is that an animal is rarely infected twice by the same kind of pathogen. In other words, recovery from a pathogenic infection generally makes an animal immune. Called a *secondary immune response,* it is promulgated by what are known as long-lived memory T cells and memory B cells. It is mentioned that the Greek historian Thucydides observed this phenomenon over 2400 years ago, in that the sick and recovered could care for the sick.

Exactly what enzymes and inhibitors might be involved in these immune response was not spelled out in the reference. In other words, do T cells and B cells in a way of speaking inhibit the metabolism of diseased cells? More specifically, can we include cancer cells?

Furthermore, the immune system ideally is described as self-tolerant (Voet and Voet, *Biochemistry*, pp. 1210–1211). And since nearly all biological macromolecules are antigenic, to suppress self-destruction, the immune system must distinguish between self-antigens and foreign antigens. As the reference states, this process has to be "exquisitely selective," since a vertebrate for example has macromolecules

---

* It is observed in the reference that HIV attacks helper T cells. Moreover, it causes problems incurred by modern medicine that do not otherwise occur in nature. These include tissue and organ grafts, which will be rejected unless immunosupressants are used—drugs that suppress the immune response, but hopefully will not leave the body completely defenseless against pathogens.

numbering in the tens of thousands, each molecule with many different antigen sites. It is noted that the immune system of mammals is activated at about the time of birth. However, if a foreign antigen is implanted in the embryo before birth, the birthed animal cannot mount an attack against that particular antigen. The T and B cells that should recognize the antigen are apparently eliminated. New cells are created, however, and these are cells having receptors with no affinity for self-antigens, but instead bind to what are called MHC (major histocompatability complex) proteins, to be discussed subsequently. On rare occasions, however, the immune system becomes intolerant to some of the self-antigens, resulting in an *autoimmune disease*. Examples of such autoimmune diseases include *myasthenia gravis*, where a person produces antibodies that act against the acetylcholine receptors of the skeletal muscles. Another example is *temphidus vulgaris*, which produces oral and body sores, lesions, or blisters. Other examples are *rheumatoid arthritis, insulin-dependent diabetes mellitus*, and *multiple sclerosis*. (The term "mellitus" pertains to honey.)

The study of antibodies or immunoglobulins and their structures and binding sites has been based on the cells of an *immune system cancer* named *myeloma* (Voet and Voet, *Biochemistry*, pp. 74, 1214–1215). For instance, by fusing a desired antibody-producing cell with a myeloma cell, the hybridoma cell that results has an infinite capacity to reproduce. Whereas ordinarily antibody cells die off after a few divisions, by means of this fusion with myeloma cells, extensive cultures of monoclonal (cloned) antibodies can be made available for study. ("Myeloma" pertaining to marrow.)

A further consideration involves what are called *myeloma proteins*, which are generated by cancer cells that originally proliferated for causes known or unknown, very possibly on account of antigens. Interestingly, this antigenic effect can be produced by small organic groups called *haptens*. An example is the 2,4-dinitrophenyl (DNP) group, which covalently attaches to a carrier protein, for example bovine serum albumin. When, in this instance, the combination or complex is injected into an animal, antibodies are produced that bind to the hapten in the absence of the protein carrier.

In turn, X-ray studies of hapten-myeloma protein complexes have pinpointed the immunoglobulin's antigen-binding sites. Follow-up studies utilizing hen egg white (HEW) lysozymes (cell wall-destroying enzymes) indicate more extensive areas of binding sites. Further generalizations, moreover, suggest that "a protein's entire accessible surface is potentially antigenic."

For the purposes here, these few things are mentioned in that they may somehow relate to cancer, both to the initiation and proliferation of cancer cells and to potential means of control or immolation.

In discussing MHC proteins, or major histocompatability proteins, their highly *polymorphic* nature has been stressed (Voet and Voet, *Biochemistry*, p. 1224). What are called Class I and Class II MHC genes are regarded the most highly polymorphic genes found in higher vertebrates. The consequence is that two unrelated individuals are extremely unlikely to have the same set of MHC genes. However, the statement is made that "epidemiological studies indicate that certain polymorphs of MHC genes are associated with increased susceptibilities to particular infections and/or autoimmune diseases." This is a basis, no doubt, for the ongoing work linking certain kinds of cancer to certain genes.

The reference asks the question, however, "what is the function of MHC protein polymorphism?" That is, if all members of a particular vertebrate species had an identical set of MHC proteins, and a pathogen occurred whose epitopes (antigenic determinants) interacted but poorly with these proteins, then the outcome could be disastrous. It would be possible for a pathogen to obliterate a species. With polymorphism, there is such a large variety of MHC proteins within a species population that the species should survive. (Which brings up the obvious question, could we also speak of the extinction of a species that does not maintain the requisite MHC protein polymorphism?)

Along the way, it is mentioned that T cell receptors do not recognize antigens unless they are presented together with MHC proteins. This, possibly, indicates a way for MHC proteins to act as anticancer agents.

7.10.3 IMMUNIZATION AGAINST CANCER

A major objective of modern medicine has been, and remains, the development of a vaccine that will act against cancer cells. The search is severely complicated by the fact that the body's immune system does not normally recognize its own cancerous cells as antigens. In other words, cancer cells mimic normal cells, at least as far as the immune system is concerned, which does not recognize the cancerous cells as invaders.

This does not pertain to cancerous cells from a different individual. As is well known, if cancer cells from another individual are injected into a subject, the subject's immune system will make short work of the imposters. The same sort of phenomenon arises in organ transplants, where the body will reject the transplant unless the immune system can be compromised.

The objective in the case of cancer, therefore, is to cause the immune system to act against the body's own cancer cells. Ordinarily, it seems that, no matter how powerful the body's immune system is, it does not recognize and destroy the body's own cancer cells. The infrequent exception is called a *spontaneous remission,* by causes seemingly unknown. (That a mystical element can be involved is described by Lewis Mehl-Madrona, MD, in Coyote Medicine.) Enter the suject of the immune system and anticancer vaccines, which would act selectively against the body's own cancer cells. In other words, it is believed that cancerous cells may display antigens on the cell surfaces that may invoke an immune response.

Some of the latest developments are explored by Stephen S. Hall in an article called "Vaccinating Against Cancer," which appeared in the April 1997 issue of the *Atlantic Monthly.* (Hall, an editor for *The New York Times Magazine,* has also written a book about immunology, titled *A Commotion in the Blood: Life, Death, and the Immune System.*) Hall's lengthy article may be paraphrased as follows.

Emphasized are the pioneering studies of German physician Alexander Knuth and Flemish-born and American-trained molecular geneticist Thierry Boon. Their work, which essentially began in 1982, was directed at understanding the connection between cancer cells and the immune system, the ways the immune system can distinguish a cancer cell from a normal cell, and how the immune system can attack the cancerous cell. Central to the studies was the case of a German lady known as Frau H., who lived in a small town southwest of Frankfurt. She was afflicted with a rapidly growing form of skin cancer, normally fatal. In the course of events, however, Knuth found that Frau H's white blood cells—that is to say, her immune system—could somehow recognize her cancer cells with "exquisite specificity." This led to exciting developments, to be further described by Hall.

Along the way, Hall notes that immunological approaches so far have not been successful, nor have other forms of treatment save maybe surgery, at least in some cases. Of about 1.4 million new cases of cancer each year in Americans, nearly half are incurable, in part because the cancer has already spread. The further statistic is supplied by George Canellos, a professor of medicine at Harvard Medical School, that, although about half the patients with cancer survive for five years (the threshold for being cured), the vast majority of these are treated by surgery, with about 10 percent cured by radiation alone, and 5 percent by a combination of radiation and chemotherapy. It is added that chemotherapy alone rarely yields a five-year remission except for childhood cancers and a few adult malignancies (which assumably are blood-related cancers, e.g., leukemias).*

In the case of Frau H., the cancerous condition started in a pigmented cell, or melanocyte, to cause the deadly skin cancer known as melanoma, which in turn had spread to an ovary and to the adrenals, and then to a lymphnode below the armpit. Both surgery and chemotherapy had proven ineffective.

The patient had been referred to Knuth, who had previously worked on an experimental melanoma vaccine at Sloan-Kettering in New York City. In a particular instance, a patient had been injected with cells from his own aggressive melanoma, and in this "rare and remarkable" instance the patient's immune system had responded, with the patient still alive today.

Repeating the same strategy, melanoma cells from Frau H's excised tumor were cultured, to create a cell line called MZ2, to become an important tool in cancer research, and was used to establish a relationship between "cell-killing" or cytolytic T lymphocytes of the immune response and the melanoma cells. Although T lymphocytes are efficient killers, retaining a memory for viral and bacterial antigens, even identifying virus- or cancer-containing cells, they do not ordinarily recognize the body's own cancer cells. In the case of Frau H's cancerous system, however, her cytolytic T lymphocytes not only recognized the melanoma cells but proceeded to kill them in a test tube.

To reinforce this kind of immune response, Knuth proposed that a cancer vaccine be developed, which would involve altering or mutagenizing Frau H's melanoma cells. Whereupon it was suggested that Knuth communicate with Thierry Boon (pronounced "Bone"), providing him with some of the cells.

---

* The statistics can be summarized by saying that the total number of cancer cases can be roughly divided into 50 percent incurable and 50 percent curable, with the interpretation that 10 percent of the total are cured by radiation, 5 percent cured by a combination of radiation and chemotherapy, and the remaining 35 percent presumably by surgery. The basis for cure is a five-year remission. On the other hand, the numbers above may be meant to imply that 10 percent of the 50 percent cured are cured by radiation and 5 percent by radiation and chemotherapy, leaving 85 percent cured by surgery. Whichever, the overall record is dismal—with the figure supplied elsewhere that nearly 600,000 people per year die from cancer.

Boon was already aware that certain chemicals would produce mutations, and that with the injection of mutated cancer cells into the body, the unmutated cancerous cells sometimes become "visible" and are then attacked and destroyed by T lymphocytes or T cells. Although demonstrated with mice, the extrapolation had never been made to humans. Accordingly, after further conventional treatments of Frau H's condition failed, vaccination was commenced using approximately 100 million cancer cells from the tumor, which had been chemically mutated and then killed by irradiation. Injection intervals were four to six weeks, from February until September 1984. The remaining cancerous mass proceeded to diminish during the course of injections, to disappear and never to return.

The case results have never been published in the medical literature on account of an agonizing decision that was made: not to make a biopsy on the shrinking cancerous mass to determine if it was a recurrence of the original cancer. Knuth knew that such a biopsy would wrap up a convincing case for the vaccine, but there was another consideration.

He also knew that in snipping away even a small piece of malignant tissue they might endanger Frau H. by accidentally disseminating tumor cells, promoting the spread of what had already proved to be a highly malignant cancer.

Thus, they were left with but an anecdote rather than definitive proof that their vaccine had made a difference.

The foregoing emphasizes that taking a biopsy on a cancerous mass may in itself cause the cancer to spread. There is already folklore that surgery can cause cancer to spread, presumably by inadvertently unleashing cancerous cells into the bloodstream, an excuse for using follow-up chemotherapy. One gets the sinking feeling that biopsies may be but more business for the medical business.

A spin-off discovery by Boon, Knuth, and their colleagues was that of the first known T-cell-specific tumor antigen in humans. Reported in 1991 in the journal *Science*, research into tumor immunology has been invigorated, and several highly specific cancer vaccines are being tried on patients who are deemed most likely to respond, but with as yet no guarantees for success.

Hall's article continues by describing the career and work of Thierry Boon, characterized as an "accidental immunologist," who first studied medicine and then came under the influence of molecular biology, but kept his own counsel, "getting advice from first-rate people and never following it." Among his earlier investigations was one on tetracarcinoma in mice, which is manifested as grotesque aberrations during embryonic development, resulting usually in spontaneous abortions—not only in mice but in other animals, including humans. The genetic pathways are somehow short-circuited, producing a repetition of specialized tissues such as teeth, hair, bone, muscle, and so on.

Boon and a colleague, Odile Kellermann, used a chemical agent to form mutations in tetracarcinoma cells and injected these cells into mice. To their surprise, the mutated cells never took hold in about 30 percent of the mice, whereas unmutated cells would almost always take hold in mice. Although no cancer expert, Boon figured that the genes of the cancer cells had been changed such that the cells were no longer cancerous. This change was found to be not an alteration of the cancer's malignancy but of marking the cells such that they were visible to the immune system. In net sum, Boon and Kellerman had produced man-made tumor antigens. Although tumor immunology had fallen into disrepute in the 1970s, Boon had rocked the boat.

These findings were reinforced by the discovery in 1969, by the French hematologist Georges Mathé, that injections of an attenuated live bacterium known as Baccillus Calmette-Guérin (BCG) would produce a prolonged remission in childhood leukemia. Known to stimulate the immune system, BCG has by now been used successfully on more than two billion people as a vaccine against tuberculosis. Tried on cancer, BCG vaccine was an almost total failure.

In addition to the BCG failure, there had been other exhaustive experiments that seemed to confirm that tumors do not excite an immune response. Conducted over a 20-year period in England, with the results first published in 1976 in the *British Journal of Cancer*, these experiments seemed to forever refute the idea that cancers could cause an immune response. The traditional line of investigation had heretofore been only with animal tumors in which the cancerous condition had been caused by viruses or by chemical carcinogens. (An example cited of the latter was painting animals with methylcholanthrene, an ingredient of coal tar.) In many cases, these experimental or "man-made" cancers could be detected by the immune system, and animals vaccinated with these cancer cells did not develop cancer.

However, a researcher named Harold B. Hewitt and his coworkers pointed out that such man-made cancers were not representative. Rather, human cancers more usually arrived spontaneously, probably on account of a sequence of genetic mistakes. Hewitt's team studied 27 different kinds of spontaneous cancers via some 20,000 transplants in mice. Not a single one of these "natural" tumors could be influenced by an immune-system attack.

Despite this contrary evidence, Boon as before injected mice with mutated cancer cells—which tended not to produce cancer—then injected the same mice with unmutated cancer cells. It was found that three-fourths of these mice had rejected the tumor cells, whereas all the control animals ended up with cancer.

The conclusion reached was that the mouse immune system had a memory. Once the immune system had recognized and acted against a mutated cancer cell, it would then have the ability to "see" the formerly invisible parent unmutated cancer cell.

Boon and his chief collaborator, Aline Van Pel, proceeded to work over most of the next ten years to detect changes in the antigens of the mutated tumor cells. (As Hall notes, it was a lengthy process not conducive to support from say the National Institutes of Health, for which progress must be shown every three years in order for the grant to be renewed.) The work proved nearly interminable, but they were able to isolate and clone populations of mouse T cells that had the ability to recognize specific antigens, and in turn were able to pinpoint the gene responsible for the antigen.

As part of the investigation, Aline Van Pel repeated Hewlitt's experiments with spontaneous or "natural" tumors, but this time around the results were different: it was demonstrated that mice vaccinated with mutated versions of the cancer cells would then reject the unmutated cancers. The next step was to try it in humans, and fortuitously the cancer cells of Frau H. arrived at Boon's laboratory in Brussels.

Hall next turns to a philosophical sort of question, of self versus nonself. For the immune system is designed for violent attack against pathogens such as viruses or bacteria that are foreign to the body, and T cells will also rapaciously attack transplanted organs unless mitigated in some way. It is observed, however, that cancer cells can be regarded as intermediate between self and nonself, occupying a kind of no-man's land. This is described by Hall as breaching normal cell behavior in terms of relentless cycles of replication and the sabotaging of normal internal check points, and as the cells grow, there is an apparent reactivation of the genes deployed even for fetal development. The immune system, however, remains mostly "tolerant," not distinguishing the slight differences in cancer cells from normal cells, and not recognizing any antigens that might exist.

Boon's group further intersected with the immunological discoveries made by Rolf Zinkernagel and Peter Doherty in the 1970s. The work of the latter investigators had shown that T cells are able to recognize antigens only in a very special way. This has to do with the molecule known as the "major histocompatibility complex" or MHC, previously discussed. This work, for which they were eventually awarded a Nobel Prize, delineated that MHC "cradled" antigens so as to furnish a "necessary intimacy of contact" with T cells.

Subsequent to this previous discovery about MHC, another team, immunologist Alain Townsend and associates, found that a similar mechanism occurs in normal cells. That is, each cell cannibalizes every different type of protein made inside it and permits the immune system to "sample" a bit to determine whether the protein is of itself or nonself. The agents of surveillance are the lymphocytes, that is, the cytolytic T lymphocytes.

In further explanation, there are millions of different T lymphocytes, with each preprogrammed to recognize a specific antigen. If the corresponding antigen is encountered, the particular T lymphocyte will replicate explosively, literally into tens of millions of new cells in a week or so. This selective programming occurs in the thymus early in our life. Only T cells that distinguish nonself proteins are programmed. Any T cells that recognize self proteins are ablated or destroyed.*

Another aspect is that the T cells have a memory. Once an antigen has been detected, this antigen will be attacked more swiftly the next time around. (One can wonder as well to what degree the selective natal or prenatal programming that occurs in the thymus is an inherited characteristic from the parents, sort of an acquired immunity—maybe reinforced via mother's milk. Thus, some populations, for instance, are more resistant to certain diseases than others, malaria being an example.)

---

* Hall notes that breakdowns in selectivity can happen, as there are T cells that attack our own tissues, manifested in such autoimmune diseases as lupus and some forms of diabetes. The previously mentioned disease called *temphidus vulgaris*—or vulgar blisters—is another.

The cannibalization of proteins in the cell interior results in the subunits known as peptides. These are loaded into the grooves of the MHC molecules, and shipped to the cell surface, so to speak. Here, the MHC molecules display their "wares" so that the T cells are able to examine the peptide fragments.

The complexity and incredible precision of this examination is illustrated by the fact that each peptide fragment or snippet may be composed of from one to twenty different amino acids—the fundamental twenty. An antigen is said to constitute a chain of nine amino acids, and if so, the reference states that a simple probability-type calculation indicates that there are 9 raised to the twentieth power possible combinations. A T cell is said to be able to differentiate between self and nonself on the basis of a change in merely one amino acid in a single peptide.

The quantity "9" raised to the 20th power is equal to about 1.2 times the quantity 10 raised to the 19th power, or is equal to about 12 billion × 1 billion. As to other means of looking at the problem, consider the combination and permutation calculations as follows. (This determination will be re-emphasized in a discussion about the number of peptides as potential inhibitors, in the section titled "Enzyme Inhibitors for Anaerobic Glycolysis," in Part 8.) For a nine-member chain made up from the 20 fundamental amino acids, if no distinction is made between amino acids, then the number of combinations or ways for expressing a sample size r out of a total of n items is given by

$$\frac{n!}{r!(n-r)!} = \frac{20!}{9!\,11!} = 167,960$$

where the factorials are represented by, say, $9! = 9 \times 8 \times 7 \times 6 \times 5 \times 4 \times 3 \times 2 \times 1 = 362,880$. And so on. If each amino acid has a label on it, that is, if the 20 amino acids are each different and distinct and may be ordered, then the total number of possible permutations is given by the formula

$$\frac{n!}{(n-r)!} = \frac{20!}{11!} = 60.0949324 \text{ billion}$$

That is, the result is 60 billion, as compared to the previously stated number of 12 billion × 1 billion. Whichever, the number of possibilities is almost beyond belief for attempting to determine just what particular peptide chains could serve as antigens for stimulating the immune system. The work by Boon and Knuth and the other investigators is monumental.

Parenthetically, it may be remarked that the foregoing astronomical calculations further confirm the premise of biochemical individuality, whereby an individual's cellular makeup in terms of combinations and permutations of amino acids, peptides or polypeptides, and proteins will be unique—even absolutely unique. This is in fact seen in the uniqueness of the DNA imprint, anticipated in biochemist Roger Williams' *Free and Unequal: The Biological Basis of Individual Liberty*. And it may mean that the cards are stacked against using the immune system against the body's own cancerous cells, indicating that *selective* biochemical agents will have to suffice. Nevertheless, read on.

As an example of how the foregoing system is supposed to work, T cells will ignore a normally constituted protein, but if, let's say, a flu virus has invaded the cell, some of the viral protein will be fragmented and transferred to the cell surface, along with normal peptide fragments. The antigen-specific T cells acknowledge this foreign presence by perforating the wall of the marked cell with tiny pores. The alarm is sounded, and still other T cells transmit the alarm by producing molecules called *cytokines*, some of which serve to recruit reinforcements of T cells to the site, while others cause the particular antigen-specific T cells to multiply.

Examples of cytokine molecules include interferon and interleukin-2. These are noted for being highly active, even in small amounts. In fact, such flu-like symptoms as fever, aches and pains, and malaise are caused by the action of the cytokines rather than by the flu virus per se. These symptoms signal an aroused and active immune system, trying to do its work. It is further remarked in the reference that after an infective agent is identified, there is a period of seven to ten days before the T-cell response reaches its maximum.

Acknowledging that there must be genes that carry instructions for making cancer-specific antigens, Boon, Knuth, and colleagues searched in both mice and humans for such a gene, and in particular examined the cancer cells in Frau H's blood sample for recognition by her T cells. This required making cuttings at the cancer cell surface and trying to identify a single protein as uniquely antigenic.

(There is now an improved technology for doing this, courtesy of Donald Hunt and colleagues at the University of Virginia.) Boon's group had previously located a tumor-specific antigen in mice, which was named PIA. Using the same Frau H's DNA, it was subjected to the same procedures, made all but insurmountable by the fact that a human cell may contain approximately 100,000 genes, with each gene containing DNA-coded instructions for synthesizing a particular protein. Each such protein can be regarded as a three-dimensional chain containing a multitude of amino acids, from dozens up to hundreds.*

Inasmuch as T cells only notice what fits onto an MHC molecule, the peptide fragments that can be recognized by the immune system are limited to about nine amino acids. These peptide fragments are the result of the cannibalization of the larger globular proteins but serve as a sample for the protein. Therefore, a human antigen would constitute a 27-letter portion of a gene that could have up to, say, 2 million DNA code letters. (The comparison is made that finding this antigen is like finding a 5-word sentence in a 300,000-word book, buried in a 3 billion-letter text of fine print.)

Boon's Brussels lab proceeded to chop up the DNA of Frau H's melanoma cells, amounting to about 100,000 genes, with 3 billion base pairs. The chopped-up DNA was divided into approximately 700,000 "cosmids"—sort of a subdirectory of the entire DNA complement. Each so-called cosmid was inserted into a special recipient cell. Each recipient cell was from one from many distinct cell colonies, and the recipient cells within the colony would manufacture the encoded proteins that would appear at the cell surfaces, to be scanned by Frau H's T cells.

Out of a group of 29,000 colonies tested, only 5 contained the gene encoding of the antigen recognized by the T cells. In another set of experiments, out of 13,000 colonies, 2 more colonies tested positive.

The concluding result was a tiny molecular bump on the cell surfaces, of an active colony, arching outward and having exactly nine amino acids. Utilizing known recombinant DNA techniques, the cell was entered and the gene was identified and further produced in its complete sequence. The gene was supplied with the acronym MAGE, after "melanoma antigen," and in late 1991 the findings were published in the journal *Science*. The scientific study of human tumor immunology was given new life.

In a following section on Altered Selves, Hall comments that the discovery of a new gene is only the beginning, for the protein that the gene makes must be determined and understood, and its subsequent role in the biochemistry of the body must be spelled out. It turned out that MAGE was a small part of the X chromosome and remained silent in normal cells. At times, however, it became active—or was "expressed"—for instance in about 30 percent of melanoma cases, and less frequently in other tumor cases such as breast cancer and lung cancer. In turn, it was found that there were many similar related genes, so that MAGE became MAGE-1, and so on. All were previously unknown and normally silent. The gene designated MAGE-3 was subsequently found on the surface of many tumors, as were two others in the MAGE family, and genes called BAGE and GAGE were also identified, both of which encode tumor antigens. All were discovered using Frau H's T cells.

These normally silent genes may have other purposes. Thus, Boon reasons that they may have functions in the earliest embryonic or placental development, enabling cellular movement or metastasization. Subsequently, these genes lay dormant. However, a cell that becomes cancerous (say by chemical carcinogens or genetic predisposition) can resurrect or activate these genes, which then allow it to move around or metastasize.

In a continuation of the work, it has been found that a gene may produce more than one antigen, which may associate with more than one MHC molecule. And in some melanoma patients, the T cells recognize antigens in normal proteins, sort of an autoimmune response. One of these antigens is called Melan-A; another is *tyrosinase*, interestingly an enzyme. Other antigens under study include the unusual protein known as *mucin*, found in certain breast, colon, and stomach cancers. A better known protein found is *CEA*, for "carcinoembryonic antigen," occurring in breast, colon, and lung cancers. Still others have been reported, and there is the possibility that literally hundreds of antigens may be uncovered, inaugurating a new era in cancer treatment. (There is the unstated possibility: can these antigens in themselves, if administered to the patient, institute an anticancer action?)

---

* As an example, at the higher end of the scale, the large gene for producing the complex muscle-tissue protein called dystrophin—which has been linked to muscular dystrophy—has about 2 million base pairs or letters of DNA. At the other end of the scale, the code for the hormone known as insulin contains less than 2,000 letters, producing a protein of only 51 amino acids.

There are, however, obstacles to further progress, as Hall explains in a section titled "The Houdini Phenomenon." That is to say, tumor cells have ways to protect themselves, to fool the T cells, hence the titled used for the section. Hall supplies a remark attributed to Joost Oppenheim, a researcher at the National Cancer Institute, that "viruses know a lot more about the immune system than immunologists do, and the same could be said of tumors." For instance, if T cells recognize an antigen, the tumor cell may mutate to turn off the gene that encodes the antigen. Furthermore, this mutated cell will be favored by survival and replication, also known as "survival of the fittest." Other tricks include the chemical jamming of the immune system, turning out genes that produce molecules signaling the immune system to cease and desist, and deleting the production of genes that produce molecules carrying signals between T cells. The tumor may even act to shut down the genes making the MHC molecules. Collectively, these tumor protective tactics are termed "tumor escape mechanisms."

It is emphasized that tumors play the same game as antibiotic-resistant bacteria, where the most malignant of the cells are the ones that survive and reproduce. More than this, Boon made the discovery that melanomas being able to remain invisible to the immune system has as much to do with the genes of the patient as with tumor characteristics. In other words, there may be an enormous variation in the MHC system between one human and another. This variation can be explained in terms of the MHC transport molecules, denoted as HLA markers, of literally hundreds of subtypes such as HLA-A1, HLA A-2, HLA B-24, and so forth. Only certain antigens will fit into a particular subtype. A person not only must have a tumor that displays the antigen but must have inherited the corresponding MHC molecule. If there's no fit, the T cells will never see the antigen.

It so turns out that the blood of Frau H. showed that the antigen from gene MAGE-1 will fit only into MHC molecule or marker HLA A-1. Moreover, it was found that about 26 percent of Caucasians carry the A-1 marker, including Frau H. This translates to mean that heredity will determine whether a melanoma is immunogenic, that is, whether the immune system will respond to the melanoma. The example is supplied that if 30 percent of melanoma victims produce MAGE-1 antigens, and if 26 percent of Caucasians carry the HLA A-1 protein molecule, then the probability of Caucasians having the correct combination is $(0.30) \times (0.26) =$ about 0.08 or 8 percent. If this probability sounds low, the odds are improved by the presence of still other antigens. Thus, the antigen from gene MAGE-3, which fits A-1 and A-2 markers or molecules, appears in 70 percent of metastatic melanomas, as well as in many lung tumors, bladder tumors, and head-and-neck squamous-cell carcinomas. The conclusion furnished by Boon is that there is the possibility of preselecting candidates most likely to benefit from immunization.

It may be added that, rather than working through the correct combination of genes, antigens, and MHC molecules to make the cancer cell visible to the immune system, why not just destroy the cancer cell by negating its metabolism? This is, of course, the purpose of using enzyme inhibitors for cancer cell metabolism, in particular inhibitors for lactate dehydrogenase in one or another—or all—of its several forms.

In a section headed "Experiments With Vaccines," Hall reaffirms the long-held objective of a cancer vaccine, an idea that has waxed and waned through the years. Probably the first primitive vaccine was developed in 1893 by William B. Coley, M.D. of the Memorial Hospital in New York City.*

As to melanoma vaccines, several first-generation vaccines were tested, starting in the 1970s. These used the traditional method of grinding up or irradiating tumor cells, which were injected into the patient—as Knuth and Boon had tried with Frau H. Although the experimenters did not have exact knowledge of all the mechanisms involved, there were some successes. In fact, the indication is that 10 to 20 percent of the patients responded, as did Frau H. What had been heretofore lacking was an explanation for what is going on, an explanation provided by Boon and Knuth at the molecular level.

The comment is further provided that a physician may now be able to predict which patients will respond, merely from a blood sample and an analysis of the tumor. The application has proceeded, with

---

* Coley's mixed bacterial toxins are described in Ralph Moss's *Cancer Therapy* and Richard Walters' *Options*. The toxins are a by-product of the two common bacteria *Streptococcus pyrogenes* and *Serratia marcescens*, and the bioactive constituent was found to be lipopolysaccharide or LPS, also called *endotoxin*. This agent was previously discussed in the section "More about Viruses and Other Pathogens," in the subsection "Antiviral and Other Agents."

laboratories in both Europe and the United States performing the tests, and patients are being administered experimental tumor vaccines.

It is stressed that each antigen will connote a *different* cancer vaccine. A very large number of vaccines are being tried, for the most part to test safety, but some are also showing promise. For example, in 1993, Boon's team, in conjunction with Knuth in Germany and doctors variously in Italy, France, Belgium, and the Netherlands, tried out a simple, all-purpose vaccine utilizing a small immunogenic fragment, the MAGE-3 peptide. The objective was to determine if there was a pronounced rise in T cells in genetically compatible patients, indicating an immune response.

There were some dramatic remissions in several of the patients—all of whom had rapidly advancing cancers—which are detailed by Hall. Overall, of 16 melanoma patients who took the full treatment, there were 5 who had significant responses.

The vaccination strategies continue, e.g., by Steven Rosenberg at the National Cancer Institute, who so far has treated 141 patients. His work includes inserting genes encoding tumor antigens into several common viruses, notably adenovirus and vaccinia virus, and using these treated viruses as vaccines. Additionally, a dose of the cytokine interleukin-2 is sometimes used. The results are characterized as "sporadic."

At the University of Virginia, a team directed by Craig Slinguff and Victor Engelhard have commenced testing a melanoma vaccine based on the gp100 antigen, accompanied by one or two adjuvants of oil, water, and other ingredients that seem to enhance the immune response.

At Stanford University, Ronald Levy and colleagues are investigating a vaccine against non-Hodgkin's lymphoma. Isolating an antigen specific to each patient and inserting it into the immune cells called dendritic cells, a notably vigorous T-cell reaction ensues. A small number of patients have shown encouraging responses.

At the University of Pittsburgh, Walter Storkus and associates are trying a dendritic-cell vaccine, in this instance against melanoma.

At Johns Hopkins, Drew Pardoll's group is using a vaccine against advanced kidney cancer. In this case, a desirable gene is inserted into the patient's cells, a process called gene therapy. A fuller description of the gene is that of a cytokine or signaling molecule, called GM-CSF, the acronym for "granulocyte macrophage colony stimulating factor."

Also, at the University of Pittsburgh, Michael Lotze and Hideaki Tahara are using gene therapy with the cytokine interleukin-12, and so far there have been "interesting" responses in 5 out of 26 patients.

At Fordham University, a group led by Pramod Srivastava has found *heat shock proteins* inside cells, and which collect peptides. The claim is made that, on isolating these heat shock proteins, the entire antigenic complement of the tumor is also captured and can be administered as a vaccine. An initial trial has been concluded in Germany, and a further trial is scheduled in the U.S.

Further work by Alex Knuth in Frankfurt, however, sounds a cautionary note. In safety studies conducted injecting GM-CSF followed by vaccination with peptides from several different antigens, in addition to favorable responses, there was also evidence of the "Houdini phenomenon." Some tumors simply stop expressing the targeted antigen.

Nevertheless, there is reason for optimism, with the odds shifting toward the patient, although Hall states in his wrap-up that the value of a cancer treatment takes five years for assessment. Accordingly, the word "cure" is avoided, and instead the phrase "complete durable remission" is preferred.

As a final comment, we may again observe that it would be most opportune if a simple and non-invasive test were forthcoming that would indicate whether the cancerous condition is in progression or in remission. In other words, the efficacy of treatment—e.g. of administering an anticancer agent or vaccine—could be determined almost immediately. Either the treatment could be continued, or something else could be tried, if so indicated.

REFERENCES

Arvigo, Rosita and Michael Balick, *Rainforest Remedies: One Hundred Healing Herbs of Belize*, Lotus Press, Twin Lakes WI, 1993.

Atlas, Ronald M., *Microbiology: Fundamentals and Applications*, 2nd ed., Macmillan, New York, 1984, 1988.

Bergey, D.H., *Bergey's Manual of Determinative Bacteriology*, 9th ed., John G. Holt, Noel R. Krieg, Peter H.A. Sneath, James T. Staley and Stanley T. Williams Eds., Williams & Wilkins, Baltimore, 1994.

Bergey, D.H., *Bergey's Manual of Systematic Bacteriology*, John G. Holt, Ed., Williams & Wilkins, Baltimore, 1984. Vol. 1 edited by Noel R. Krieg. Vol. 2 edited by Peter H.A. Sneath. Vol. 3 edited by James T. Staley. Vol. 4 edited by Stanley T. Williams.

Bergey, D.H., also see *Index Bergeyana*.

The Biology of Heat Shock Proteins and Molecular Chaperones, Richard I. Morimoto, Alfred Tissiéres, and Costa Georgopoulos Eds., Cold Spring Harbor Laboratory Press, Plainview NY, 1994.

Boik, John C., *Cancer and Natural Medicine: A Textbook of Basic Science and Clinical Research*, Oregon Medical Press, Princeton MN, 1995.

Cell Transformation and Radiation Induced Cancer, K.H. Chadwick, C. Seymour and B. Barnhart Eds., A. Hilger, Bristol, New York, 1989.

Clark, Hulda Regehr, *The Cure for All Cancers*, ProMotion Publishing, 10387 Friars Road, Suite 231, San Diego CA 92120, (800) 231-1776, 1993.

Clarke, J. Jackson, *Protists and Disease: Vegetable Protists; Algae and Fungi, including Chytridiineae; Various Plassomyxineae; the Causes of Molluscum Contagiosum, Smallpox, Syphilis, Cancer, and Hydrophobia; Together with the Mycetoza and Allied Groups*, Baillière, Tindall and Cox, London, 1922.

Clarke, J. Jackson, *Protozoa and Disease*, in four parts, Baillière, Tindall and Cox, London, 1902, 1908. Part I. No title, 1903. Part II. Sections on the Causation of Smallpox, Syphilis, and Cancer, 1908. Part III. The Cause of Cancer, 1912. Part IV. Rhizoid Protozoa: The Cause of Cancer and Other Diseases, 1915.

CRC Handbook of Microbiology, 2nd ed., in seven volumes, Allen T. Laskin and Hubert A. Lechevalier Eds., CRC Press, Boca Raton FL, 1977–.

Dairy Microbiology, 2nd ed., R.K. Robinson Ed., Elsevier, London, 1981, 1990. Vol. 1. The Microbiology of Milk. Vol. 2. The Microbiology of Milk Products.

Davis, Wade, *One River: Explorations & Discoveries in the Amazon Rain Forest*, Simon & Schuster, New York, 1996, 1997.

DeVoto, Bernard, *Across the Wide Missouri*, Houghton Mifflin, Boston, 1947, pp. 104–106.

Dodge, Colonel Richard Irving, *Our Wild Indians: Thirty-Three Years' Personal Experience among the Red Men of the West. A Popular Account of Their Social Life, Religion, Habits, Traits, Customs, Exploits, etc. with Thrilling Adventures and Experiences on the Great Plains and the Mountains of Our Wide Frontier*, Archer House, New York, 1959. Introduction by General Sherman. Originally published in 1882.

Elimination of Pathogenic Organisms from Meat and Poultry, F.J.M. Smulders Ed., Elsevier, Amsterdam, 1987.

Encyclopedia of Microbiology, in three volumes, Joshua Lederberg Ed., Academic Press, San Diego, 1992.

Ethnobotany in the Neotropics, G.T. Prance and J.A. Kallunki Eds., The New York Botanical Garden, Bronx, New York, 1984. Proceedings of the Ethnobotany in the Neotropics Symposium, Society for Economic Botany, Oxford OH, 13–14 June, 1983.

Everett, Thomas H., *The New York Botanical Garden Illustrated Encyclopedia of Horticulture*, in 10 volumes, Garland Publishing Co., New York and London, 1980.

Cordell, Geoffrey A., *Introduction to Alkaloids: A Biogenetic Approach*, Wiley, New York, 1981.

DNA Tumor Viruses, John Tooze Ed., Cold Spring Harbor Laboratory, Cold Spring Harbor NY, 1980, 1981.

Fettner, Ann Giudici, *Viruses: Agents of Change*, McGraw-Hill, New York, 1990.

Fiennes, see T-W-Fiennes.

Fischinger, P.J., "Prospects for Reducing Virus-Associated Human Cancers by Antiviral Vaccines," *Monogr. Natl. Cancer Inst.*, *12*, 109–114 (1992).

Flora Neotropica. Published for the Organization for Flora Neotropica by the New York Botanical Garden, New York, 1968. As of 1994 there were 65 monographs, namely by plant families.

Four Neotropical Rainforests, Yale University Press, New Haven CT, 1990. Edited by Alwyn H. Gentry with the editorial assistance of Myra Guzman-Teare, and coordination of avian and herpetological chapters by James R. Karr and William E. Duellman.

Fungal Virology, Kenneth William Buck Ed., CRC Press, Boca Raton FL, 1986.

Fungal Viruses, H.P. Molitoris, M. Hollings and H.A. Wood Eds., Springer-Verlag, Berlin, 1979. From XIIth International Congress of Microbiology, Mycology Section, Munich, 3–8 September, 1978.

Gentry, Alwyn H., *A Field Guide to the Families and Genera of Woody Plants of Northwest South America (Colombia, Ecuador, Peru), with Supplementary Notes on Herbaceous Taxa*, Conservation International, Washington DC, 1993. Illustrations by Rodolfo Vasquez.

Gentry, Alwyn H., also see *Four Neotropical Rainforests*.

Hall, Stephen S., *A Commotion in the Blood: Life, Death, and the Immune System*, Holt, New York, 1997.

Hall, Stephen S., "Vaccinating Against Cancer," *Atlantic Monthly*, *279*(4), 66–84 (April, 1997).

Handbook of Genetics, in five volumes, Robert C. King Ed., Plenum Press, New York, 1974–1976. Vol. 1. Bacteria, Bacteriophages, and Fungi. Vol. 2. Plants, Plant Viruses, and Protists. Vol 3. Invertebrates of Genetic Interest. Vol. 5. Molecular Genetics.

Harper's Biochemistry, see Murray, Robert K. et al.

Hartwell, Jonathan L., *Plants Used Against Cancer*, Quarterman Publications, Lawrence MA, 1982. Foreword by Jim Duke.

Heinerman, John, *Healing Animals with Herbs*, BiWorld, Provo UT, 1977, pp. 55, 61–65.

Heinerman, John, *Spiritual Wisdom of the Native Americans*, Cassandra Press, San Rafael CA, 1989, pp. 133–135.

Horowitz, Leonard, *Viruses: AIDS and Ebola—Nature, Accident or International?*, Tetrahedron Publishing Group, Rockport MA, 1997.

Hull, Roger, Fred Brown and Chris Payne, *Virology: Directory and Dictionary of Animal, Bacterial, and Plant Viruses*, Stockton Press, Macmillan Publishers, New York, 1989.

Hutchens, Alma R., *Indian Herbalogy of North America*, Shambhala, Boston, 1969, 1991. Peter Smith, Magnolia MA, 1992. MERCO, Windsor, Ontario, 1969, 1970, 1973.

Index Bergeyana: An Annotated Alphabetic Listing of Names of the Taxa of the Bacteria, Robert E. Buchanan, John G. Holt and Erwin F. Lessell, Jr. Eds., Williams & Wilkins, Baltimore, 1966. *Supplement to Index Bergeyana*, Norman E. Gibbons, Kathleen B. Pattee and John G. Holt Eds., Williams and Wilkins, Baltimore, 1981.

Isherwood, Christopher, *The Condor and the Cows: A South American Travel Diary*, Random House, New York, 1948, 1949.

Jain, Mahenda Kumar, *Handbook of Enzyme Inhibitors (1965–1977)*, Wiley, New York, 1982.

Jenkins, Mark, "The Secret Garden," *Men's Health*, *12*(8), 143–149 (October, 1997).

Jensen, Lloyd B., *Microbiology of Meats*, Third Edition, Garrard Press, Champaign IL, 1942, 1945, 1954.

Johnson, R.T., "The Virology of Demyelinating Diseases," *Ann. Neurol.*, 36 Suppl., S54–S60 (1994).

Kaplan, Colin, G.S. Turner and D.A. Warrell, *Rabies: The Facts*, 2nd ed., Oxford University Press, New York, 1986.

Larpenteur, Charles, *Forty Years a Fur Trader on the Upper Missouri: The Personal Narrative of Charles Larpenteur, 1833–1872*, The Lakeside Press, R.R. Donnelley & Sons Co., Chicago, 1933, pp. 30–34. Historical Introduction by Milo Milton Quaife.

Le Guenno, Bernard, "Emerging Viruses," *Scientific American*, *273*(4), 56–64 (October, 1995).

Lee, Dr. Joseph G., "Navajo Medicine Man," *Arizona Highways*, *XXXVII*(8), 2–7 (August, 1961).

Lumholtz, Carl, *Unknown Mexico: A Record of Five Years' Exploration among the Tribes of the Western Sierra Madre; in the Tierra Caliente of Tepic and Jalisco; and among the Tarascos of Michoacan*, in two volumes (1902). Reproduced by the Rio Grande Press, Glorieta NM, 1973.

Lumholtz, Carl, *New Trails in Mexico: An Account of One Year's Exploration in North-Western Sonora, Mexico, and South-Western Arizona 1909–1910* (1912). Reproduced by the Rio Grande Press, Glorieta NM, 1971.

Matthews, R.E.F., *Plant Virology*, Third Edition, Academic Press, San Diego CA, 1970, 1981, 1991.

Meat Microbiology, M.H. Brown Ed., Applied Science Publishers, London, 1982.

Mechanisms of Chemical Carcinogenesis, Curtis C. Harris and Peter A. Cerutti Eds., Alan R. Liss, New York, 1982.

Mehl-Madrona, Lewis, *Coyote Medicine: Lessons from Native American Healing*, A Fireside Book, Simon & Schuster, New York, 1997, 1998.

The Microbiology of Marine Food Products, Donn R. Ward and Cameron Hackney Eds., Van Nostrand Reinhold, New York, 1991.

Microbiology of Meats, see Jensen, Lloyd B.

The Microbiology of Poultry Meat Products, F.E. Cunningham and N.A. Cox Eds., Academic Press, Orlando FL, 1987.

Moss, Ralph W., *Cancer Therapy: The Independent Consumer's Guide To Non-Toxic Treatment & Prevention*, Equinox Press, New York, 1992.

Murray, Robert K., Daryl K. Granner, Peter A. Mayes and Victor W. Rodwell, *Harper's Biochemistry*, 24th ed., Appleton & Lange, Stamford CT, 1990, 1993, 1996. Lange Medical Publications, 1988.

Oncogenes and the Molecular Origins of Cancer, Robert A. Weinberg Ed., Cold Spring Laboratory Press, Plainview NY, 1989.

Orefice, G., G. Campanella, S. Cicciarello, A. Chirianni, G. Borgia, S. Rubino, M. Mainolfi, M. Coppola and M. Piazza, "Presence of Papova-like Viral Particles in Cerebrospinal Fluid of AIDS Patients with Progressive Multifocal Leukoencephalopathy. An Additional Test for 'in vivo' Diagnosis," *Acta. Neurol. Napoli.*, *15*(5), 328–332 (October, 1993).

Papillomaviruses and Human Disease, K. Syrjänen, L. Gissmann and L.G. Koss Eds., Springer-Verlag, Berlin, 1987.

Parfitt, Tudor, *Journey to the Vanished City: The Search for a Lost Tribe of Israel*, St. Martin's, New York, 1992, pp. 221–222.

Price, Willard, *The Amazing Amazon*, John Day, New York, 1952.

The Prokaryotes: A Handbook on Habitats, Isolation, and Identification of Bacteria, in two volumes, Mortimer P. Starr, H. Stolp, H.G. Troper, A. Balows and H.G. Schlegel, Eds., Springer-Verlag, Berlin, 1981.

Rabies, James B. Campbell and K.M. Charlton Eds., Kluwer Academic Publishers, Boston, 1988. No. 7 in the series *Developments in Veterinary Virology*.

Radiation Carcinogenesis, Arthur C. Upton, Roy E. Albert, Frederic J. Burns and Roy E. Shore Eds., Elsevier, New York, 1986.

Rampton, Sheldon and John Stauber, *Mad Cow USA: Could the Nightmare Happen Here?*, Common Courage Press, Monroe ME, 1997.

The Reoviridae, Wolfgang K. Koklik Ed., Plenum Press, New York, 1983.

Rhodes, Richard, *Deadly Feasts: Tracking the Secrets of a Terrifying New Plague*, Simon & Schuster, New York, 1997.

RNA Tumor Viruses, Robin Weiss, Natalie Teich, Harold Varmus and John Coffin Eds., Cold Springs Harbor Laboratory, Cold Springs Harbor NY, 1982.

Shell, Ellen Ruppel, "Could Mad-Cow Disease Happen Here?," *Atlantic Monthly,* 282(3), 92–106 (September 1998).

Shoumatoff, Alex, *The Rivers Amazon*, Sierra Club Books, San Francisco, 1978.

Sigma Chemical Company Catalog, *Biochemicals, Organic Compounds, and Diagnostic Reagents*, St. Louis MO, 1996.

St. George, George and the Editors of Time-Life Books, *Soviet Deserts and Mountains*, Time-Life Books, Amsterdam, 1974, pp. 110–111. With photographs by Lev Ustinov of the Novostic Press Agency, Moscow.

Stephens, Harold and Albert Podell, *Who needs a road?: The Story of the Trans World Expedition*, Bobbs-Merrill, Indianapolis IN, 1967. pp. 254–256.

Swan, Michael, *The Marches of El Dorado: British Guiana, Brazil, Venezuela*, Beacon Press, Beacon Hill, Boston, 1958.

Textbook of Biochemistry with Clinical Correlations, Thomas M. Devlin Ed., Wiley, New York, 1982.

Tortora, Gerard J., Berdell R. Funke and Christine L. Case, *Microbiology: An Introduction*, 2nd ed., Benjamin/Cummings, Menlo Park CA, 1982, 1986.

T-W-Fiennes, Richard N., *Infectious Cancers of Animals and Man*, Academic Press, London, 1982.

Tropical and Geograpical Medicine, 2nd ed., Kenneth S. Warren and Adel A.F. Mahmoud Eds., McGraw-Hill, New York, 1984, 1990. Associate Editors: David A. Warrell, Louis H. Miller, Adel A.F. Mahmoud, Scott B. Halstead, Charles C. Carpenter, John E. Bennett, Gerald T. Keusch.

Tropical and Geographical Medicine: Companion Handbook, 2nd ed., Adel A.F. Mahmoud Ed., McGraw-Hill, New York, 1993.

Tropical Medicine and Parasitology, Robert A. Goldsmith and Donald Heyneman Eds., Appleton & Lange Eds., Norwalk CT, 1989.

Tyler, Varro E., *The Honest Herbal: A Sensible Guide to the Use of Herbs and Related Remedies*, 3rd ed., Pharmaceutical Products Press, New York, 1992. Haworth Pess, Binghamton NY, 1993. Revised edition of *The New Honest Herbal*.

Vaccination Strategies of Tropical Diseases, F.Y. Liew Ed., CRC Press, Boca Raton FL, 1989.

Viral Oncology, George Klein Ed., Raven Press, New York, 1980.

Viruses Associated with Human Cancer, Leo A. Phillips Ed., Marcel Dekker, New York, 1983.

Viruses and Plasmids in Fungi, Paul A. Lemke Ed., Marcel Dekker, New York, 1979. Volume 1 in *Series on Mycology*.

Viruses in Naturally Occurring Cancers, Book B, Myron Essex, George Todaro and Harald zur Hausen, Eds., Cold Spring Laboratory Press, Plainview NY, 1980. Volume 7 in the series Cold Spring Harbor Conferences on Cell Proliferation.

Viruses of Fungi and Simple Eukaryotes, Yigal Koltin and Michael J. Leibowitz, Marcel Dekker, New York, 1988. Volume 7 in *Series on Mycology*.

Voet, Donald and Judith G. Voet, *Biochemistry*, 2nd ed., Wiley, New York, 1995.

Walters, Richard, *Options: The Alternative Cancer Therapy Book*, Avery Publishing Group, Garden City Park NY, 1993.

Wang, A.L. and C.C. Wang, "Viruses of the Protozoa," *Annu. Rev. Microbiol.*, 45, 251–263 (1991).

Williams, Roger, *Free and Unequal: The Biological Basis of Individual Liberty*, University of Texas Press, Austin, 1953.

Wright, Robert M. (Marr), Plainsman, Explorer, Scout, Pioneer, Trader and Settler, *Dodge City: The Cowboy Capital and the Great Southwest: In, the Days of: The Wild Indian, the Buffalo, the Cowboy, Dance Halls, Gambling Halls and Bad Men*, Wichita Eagle, Wichita KS, 1913, pp. 70–72. Reprinted by Ayer Company Publishers, New Salem NH, 1975.

Zollner, Helmward, *Handbook of Enzyme Inhibitors*, 2nd ed. revised and enlarged, in two volumes, VCH Verlagsgellschaft mbH. Weinheim, FRG, 1993. VCH Publishers, New York.

Anticancer Agents as Enzyme Inhibitors
and Other Issues

Part 8

Anticancer Agents as Enzyme Inhibitors and Other Issues

8.1 BIOACTIVE PLANTS AS ENZYME INHIBITORS

The plants or plant substances (or still other substances) that are of most interest are what may be labeled *bioactive* or *biodynamic*, a descriptor that encompasses medicinal plants. With regard to bioactive plants per se, these plants are at the same time, by and large, toxic or poisonous, but this is a matter of degree or dosage. The bioactivity is produced by plant substances that are composed of compounds belonging to different chemical classifications such as alkaloids, glycosides, and so forth, and that are known to display biological/physiological activity. The compounds may be known or yet unknown, as may the full array of chemical classifications. In lieu of the plant itself, these compounds may be regarded as the bioactive source.

Inasmuch as modern drug practice is for the most part based on the use of medicines that serve as enzyme inhibitors, it is of vital concern that these plants or plant substances, or other substances, be investigated for their specific functions as enzyme inhibitors (or, sometimes, as promoters or activators). In particular, the chemical classes and compounds themselves should be identified and further studied as to their particular role as enzyme inhibitors. While many plant chemical classes and compounds have been so identified, their further role as enzyme inhibitors is known only in a relatively few instances.

Beyond this, of course, is the use of other chemicals or chemical substances that are not identified with or derived from plants. Inasmuch as the use of such chemicals may be arbitrary for the most part, it is no doubt preferable to emphasize plants or plant substances that have some sort of positive track record, say from medical folklore.

Furthermore, the relatively few enzyme inhibitors that have been used against cancer have mainly involved cytotoxic activity. That is, the compounds destroy both cancerous cells and normal cells by disrupting the sequence of DNA/RNA/protein synthesis. This nonselective cell toxicity may be incurred with both synthetic and naturally derived drugs. The outstanding beneficial example, of course, is that of antibiotics that selectively destroy prokaryotic cells that include bacteria but do not harm the mammalian eukaryotic cells that constitute the human body.

The action of antibiotics includes that of inhibiting bacterial DNA replication (as by novobiocin), transcription (as by rifamycin B), and bacterial wall synthesis (as by penicillin)—but most antibiotics block translation (Voet and Voet, *Biochemistry*, p. 1002). An example provided by the reference is streptomycin, which acts against prokaryotic ribosomes,* causing a misreading of messenger RNA or mRNA, and at higher concentrations blocks proper chain initiation, producing cell death. Another example provided is chloramphenicol, which inhibits peptidyl transferase activity in prokaryotic ribosomes.

On the other hand, there are examples of antibiotics that will destroy cancer cells but are too toxic to use—that is, they are cytotoxic to all cells and destroy normal and cancerous eukaryotic cells as well as prokaryotic cells.

Conventional chemotherapy drugs work in similar fashion against cancer cells, as set forth in Part 1. The problem is, the chemotherapy drugs used are nonselectively cytotoxic, destroying all body cells—normal cells as well as cancer cells.

___

* Ribosomes are the cellular sites for protein synthesis, and consist of particles made up of both RNA and protein (Voet and Voet, *Biochemistry*, p. 981). Ribosomal protein or polypeptide synthesis involves three separate phases, namely chain initiation, chain elongation, and chain termination.

Accordingly, it would be most desirable if plant substances or compounds could be found that act in other ways, namely as enzyme inhibitors for other cellular processes involved in diseases. Specifically, in the case of cancer as indicated in Part 1, it may be possible to negate the anaerobic glycolysis displayed by cancer cells—or at least slow it down. At the same time, the object would be not to disrupt normal cell aerobic glycolysis and other vital cell functions. This would amount to selectively "starving" cancer cells. An encapsulation of this approach is presented in an article titled "Enzyme Inhibitors for Cancer Cell Metabolism" by E.J. Hoffman, published in the May, 1997 issue of the *Townsend Letter for Doctors & Patients*. Other and similar aspects of this approach were examined by Anthony G. Payne in "Achieving Oncolysis by Compromising Tumor Cell Metabolic Processes," which appeared in the December 1996 issue of the *Townsend Letter*.

There are no doubt many other diseases that could be attacked by use of the appropriate enzyme inhibitors, most appropriately as derived from bioactive plants. These diseases may include not only bacterial, but viral and fungal diseases as well. The vast array of possibilities in attempting to match-up diseases with plant substances or compounds requires some sort of preliminary screening, which is where folklore, anecdote, and hearsay come into play. Beyond this, theories would be most welcome that relate the type of compound to the particular disease.

Another facet that should be kept in mind is diet and nutrition. The foods we eat contain many bioactive substances, known or unknown. Moreover, these substances are in minute concentrations so as to not be life-threatening, which often enough can be questioned for other plant or herbal sources. What we recognize as foodstuffs are those that can be readily consumed in quantity without undesirable side effects, which is definitely not the case for what we refer to as medicinal and poisonous plants. The winnowing process has already occurred, and each kind of foodstuff evidently has its place.

Such bioactive ingredients are in addition to, or are above and beyond, what we ordinarily classify as vitamins. Such ingredients can be more properly classified as medicinal substances.

Furthermore, the argument can be made that these kinds of bioactive substances occur most usually in raw vegetables and fruits and thereby retain their bioactivity. This is as distinguished from cooked or processed foods. Moreover, there is the argument that "junk food" foodstuffs that are essentially protein, carbohydrate, and/or fat do not contain these bioactive constituents to a sufficient degree—the familiar refrain of "empty" calories. The answer, of course, is to emphasize the more complex (carbohydrate) food sources, notably uncooked vegetables and fruits.

At the same time, the array of folkloric herbal remedies remains a potential source for more scientific studies—e.g., as to their role as enzyme inhibitors. In the New World, not only is Amazonia to be reckoned with, but the southwestern deserts of North America are of continued interest. Thus, Sam Hicks' *Desert Plants and People*, with a foreword by Erle Stanley Gardner, revived some of these possibilities. The toxic herb rue or *ruda* is mentioned, along with *gobernadora* or creosote bush—although nothing is specified with regard to cancer. Farther north, however, retired University of Wyoming chemistry professor Owen Asplund's work on yucca and alpine sunflower extracts as anti-melanoma agents is bearing fruit, but not in the U.S. Although not approved for use in the United States, the word is that the product is in routine use in Switzerland as a successful treatment for melanoma. (U.S. drug companies are currently working on a vaccine for melanoma. The FDA reluctance toward approving a competitive herbal cure seems predictable.) The injections are made in the stomach area, whereby the substance is more slowly absorbed into the body system, a procedure also used for more toxic-like substances such as the old rabies vaccine.

It turns out that the extract from the alpine sunflower did not pass the toxicity test. The alpine sunflower, incidentally, is of the genus *Hymenoxis*, with the most representative species being *H. grandiflora*, more commonly called the "old man of the mountains."

The extract from the yucca flower passed the toxicity test, however, and is being used in Switzerland against melanoma, as previously noted. Specifically, it is the species *Yucca glauca*, found in Wyoming and Colorado. Albeit banned in the U.S., it is nevertheless not approved. It may be added that the yucca plant contains saponins, evidenced by its soap-like qualities. (By the way, neither *Hymenoxys* nor *Yucca* is listed in Hartwell's *Plants Used Against Cancer*.)

Present-day toxicity tests utilize human tissue rather than mouse tissue. All kinds have been used, both from normal tissue and cancerous tissue, as well as from other pathological tissues. It would be interesting to know what cytotoxic chemotherapy agents pass the modern toxicity tests—for, after all, cytotoxic indicates cell-destroying properties. Perhaps there is a "grandfather" clause. And maybe it is more a matter of the concentrations used, exposure times, and other variables or parameters. And there is always a fine line between toxicity and effectiveness in the performance of bioactive substances. It may be added, furthermore, that cancer tissue toxicity is the measure of effectiveness for a chemotherapy agent. The objective of course is to destroy cancerous tissue *selectively* without adversely affecting normal tissues.*

The yucca flower extract treatment is specific for melanoma and does not affect other kinds of cancer, indicating that melanoma is unique. In other words, melanoma, like blood-related cancers, can be viewed as markedly different from what are ordinarily called solid tumors or cancers and should be distinguished by its own special category. The subject will be further discussed in the section on "Enzyme Inhibitors for Melanoma."

8.2 A REVIEW OF ANAEROBIC GLYCOLYSIS

The above things said, we wish to pursue a more specific tack, namely the role of enzyme inhibitors for anaerobic glycolysis, which—according to the Warburg theory, as set forth in Part 1—is the main metabolic sequence for cancer cells. In other words, the idea is to block anaerobic glycolysis, thereby selectively "starving" cancer cells, so to speak. This is as distinguished from the usual cytotoxic action of conventional chemotherapy drugs, in which *all* cells are adversely affected, normal cells as well as cancer cells.

As per Figure 1.1 in Part 1, the enzymes for the controlling reactions in the glycolysis sequence to produce pyruvic acid or pyruvate are hexokinase, 6-phosphofructokinase, and pyruvate kinase. (A controlling reaction is generally one-way, as distinguished from reversible or two-way reactions, and will often [but not always] be the slowest reaction in a sequence. In another way of saying it, reversible reactions are more likely to have reached an equilibrium condition.) In anaerobic glycolysis, the pyruvic acid or pyruvate is further converted to lactic acid or lactate, a reaction catalyzed by the enzyme lactate dehydrogenase as indicated in Figure 1.2 in Part 1. Some inhibitors for these several enzymes have been set forth in Appendix A. These inhibitors are taken from the compilations of M.K. Jain's *Handbook of Enzyme Inhibitors* and from H. Zollner's compilation of the same title.

We will hereby be interested in additional enzyme inhibitors for anaerobic glycolysis—in particular as exist in the form of *nontoxic* plants or plant substances, or the pure compounds.

To continue, we are most interested in anaerobic glycolysis to produce lactic acid or lactate, called *lactic acid fermentation*. There are three important genera of lactic acid bacteria that accomplish this conversion, which are described as homofermentative or homolactic bacteria since only lactic acid is produced. These genera are *Streptococcus*, *Lactobacillus*, and *Leuconostoc*. (The name *Streptococcus* has been changed to *Lactococcus* to be rid of the disease-bearing connotations associated with the former name.) Among the several monographs that discuss this conversion is *Microbiology: An Introduction*, by Gerard J. Tortora, Berdell R. Funke, and Christine L. Case. A simplified diagram is supplied in the reference (Tortora et al., *Microbiology*, p. 138), which is utilized here as the basis for Figure 8.1. (Figure 8.1 encapsulates the steps shown in Figures 1.1 and 1.2.)†

It is noted that, if alcoholic fermentation should occur instead, ethanol or ethyl alcohol is produced. Alcoholic fermentation is enzymatically catalyzed by a type of fungus, namely a yeast of the genus *Saccharomyces*. Still other microorganisms will produce both lactic acid and ethanol or ethyl alcohol, as well as other acids and alcohols, even acetone. These organisms are described as *heterofermentative*

---

* The fact that there are now techniques to grow all sorts of human tissue, and notably cancerous tissue, indicates that these can also be tested for substances that may act as growth inhibitors and that may be toxic to cancerous cells but not normal cells. This direction of investigation has, of course, been pursued with various standardized cancer cell lines but in the main can be said not to project to successful clinical use. There is the problem, no doubt, addressed elsewhere, that cells are unique to each individual, whether cancerous or normal. What are needed, therefore, are substances that *selectively* act against all cancerous cells, independent of the particular individual.

† *Note:* The reference also mentions *slow virus* diseases, and *prions* and *viroids*, and there is the speculation that there is a causal link for *Alzheimer's disease, Parkinson's disease,* and *Lou Gehrig's disease* (Tortora et al., *Microbiology*, p. 15, 370–371, 567–569). It in turn describes a *causal link between a virus and cancer* (Tortora et al., *Microbiology*, p. 367).

Glucose

$C_6H_{12}O_6$

$2\ ADP \rightarrow 2\ ATP \downarrow$

2 Pyruvic acid

$CH_2COCOOH$

$2\ NADH_2 \rightarrow NAD \downarrow$ (or) $\downarrow\ \rightarrow 2\ CO_2$

2 Lactic acid   2 Acetaldehyde

$CH_3CHOHCOOH$ CH_3CHO

$\downarrow 2\ NADH2 \rightarrow 2NAD$

2 Ethanol

CH_3CH_2OH

Figure 8.1 Anaerobic glycolysis or fermentation to produce either lactic acid or lactate, or ethanol or ethyl alcohol. Observe that the NADH + H⁺ NAD⁺ → + 2[H] reaction is represented somewhat differently from that of Figure 1.1, whereby the hydrogen delivered is used to form the product, in this case lactic acid. (Based on information from Tortora, Funke, and case, *Microbiology: An Introduction*, p. 138.)

or *heterolactic*. The comment is made that the production of ethanol is a low-energy process, slightly less so even than for the production of lactic acid, in that most of the energy of the glucose remains in the ethanol product. (The heat of combustion of glucose is 673 kcal per gram-mole, and each gram-mole of glucose yields two gram-moles of either ethanol or lactic acid. The heat of combustion of ethanol is 326.8 kcal per gram-mole, and the heat of combustion of lactic acid is 325.8—which for two moles of product is 653.6 and 651.6, respectively, for a net of 19.4 and 21.4 kcal per gram-mole of glucose converted) By contrast, the aerobic conversion of glucose to carbon dioxide and water is a high-energy process, giving off by far the most energy (that is, the conversion has a high exothermic heat of reaction or heat of combustion, being 673 kcal per gram mole, as originally stated).

Ronald M. Atlas's *Microbiology: Fundamentals and Applications* also provides a diagram for the lactic acid fermentation pathway and notes that *Lactobacillus delbrueckii* is commonly used for the production of lactic acid (Atlas, *Microbiology*, pp. 132, 515). A representative medium is 10 to 15 percent glucose or other fermentables, plus 10 percent calcium carbonate to neutralize the lactic acid formed (which helps drive the conversion). Corn sugar, sugar beet molasses, potato starch, and whey are typical carbohydrate sources. Conversion temperatures are 45–50° C (113–122° F) at a pH of 5.5–6.5, which is a slightly acid condition.

In the *Biology of Microorganisms*, by Thomas D. Brock and Michael T. Madigan, the particular enzymes involved are spelled out, along with the fermentation pathway. The enzyme *aldolase* is noted as a key enzyme, determining whether homofermentation or heterofermentation takes place (Brock and Madigan, *Microorganisms*, pp. 102–104, 772–773). It is mentioned in passing that the conversion of glucose to pyruvic acid or pyruvate is called the Embden-Meyerhof pathway (or Embden-Myerhof-Parnas pathway, with the alternate spelling "Myerhoff"). *The presence of aldolase assures that pyruvic acid or pyruvate will be converted to lactic acid or lactate rather than to ethanol or other products.* This is informative, since *aldolase is also the enzyme for the (reversible) conversion of fructose-1,6-bisphosphate to glyceraldehyde-3-phosphate, which is Step (4) in Figure 1.1 in Part 1.* Ordinarily, this is not a rate-controlling step. No particular mention is made of the enzyme lactate dehydrogenase, which is responsible for lactic acid or lactate formation from pyruvic acid or pyruvate. Evidently, aldolase is produced by the homofermentative bacteria, along with the other necessary enzymes for glycolysis, plus lactate dehydrogenase for the final step.

The reference work *Microbial Physiology*, by Albert G. Moat and John W. Foster, takes into account that quite a number of enzymes are indeed involved. "The complete sequence of reactions in glucose fermentation via the Embden-Meyerhof pathway involves at least 10 steps, each catalyzed by a different enzyme." (Moat and Foster, *Microbial Physiology*, pp. 24–25) Subsequently, the entire sequence (sometimes also called the Embden-Meyerhof-Parnas pathway or EMP, as previously noted) is diagrammed with all the enzymes shown, including lactate dehydrogenase for the formation of lactic acid or lactate (Moat and Foster, *Microbial Physiology*, p. 120). The enzymes involved are exactly the same enzymes as in the sequence or pathway presented in Figure 1.1 in Part 1.

Thus, we can assume that the formation or production of lactic acid or lactate from glucose or glycogen is the same whether *in vitro* or *in vivo*, or *in the human body*.

Expectedly, the array of biochemical reactions involved will be more complicated than appears at first glance. As indicated in Part 1, aerobic glycolysis will also occur to a limited extent, and glutaminolysis may be involved, as well as the conversion of still other amino acids. Moreover, the conversion of fructose 6-phosphate to fructose 1-6-bisphosphate may be especially important (Atlas, *Microbiology*, p. 122). This is Step (3) of Figure 1.1, illustrating the glycolysis sequence or pathway. The enzyme-catalyst is phosphofructokinase (PFK). The reference notes that this is a significant regulatory step in the glycolysis pathway. The supporting reaction that occurs simultaneously is the conversions of ATP to ADP (adenosine triphosphate to adenosine diphosphate). However, the presence of ATP also inhibits the activity of the enzyme phosphofructokinase. (ATP is described as an allosteric inhibitor, meaning that it binds near to active sites on the enzyme, thereby affecting enzyme activity.) Thus, if the cell is sufficiently supplied with ATP, the glycolytic pathway is blocked near the beginning, which in turn will prevent the production or recycle of ATP further along the pathway via Step (7) and Step (10) of Figure 1.1. As the ATP is depleted, the remaining ADP tends to be hydrolyzed to AMP (adenosine monophosphate). AMP, however, is an allosteric activator or promoter for the enzyme phosphofructokinase. This will then have the effect of restoring glycolysis and stimulating the production of ATP by Steps (7) and (10).

The overall process, above, may be described as the *allosteric control* or *regulation* of phosphofructokinase activity. *It is observed that in the presence of oxygen, less carbohydrate reacts, paradoxically, and some microorganisms will grow more slowly than in the absence of oxygen.* Called the *Pasteur effect,* and previously touched upon in Part 1, this difference will occur because during aerobic respiration, an accumulation of ATP can occur that reduces phosphofructokinase activity, and this greatly slows the rate of carbohydrate conversion or aerobic glycolysis.

On the other hand, in the absence of oxygen, where fermentative metabolism or anaerobic glycolysis is proceeding, it is said that less ATP is produced, and the glycolysis sequence is not inhibited. The reference concludes with a statement about the importance of regulating phosphofructokinase activity.

> The allosteric regulation of phophofructokinase activity is the key to controlling the flow of carbon through the metabolic pathways of a cell, directing the cell toward ATP-generating or ATP-utilizing pathways.

Inasmuch as cancer cells are found to undergo anaerobic glycolysis at rates up to 20 times that of normal aerobic glycolysis, *the regulation of phosphofructokinase activity may be a deciding factor in controlling cancer growth.* The question is, however, should the phosphofructokinase activity be *enhanced* or *inhibited,* and by what means? Furthermore, should ATP be added or ADP (or AMP) be added, or whatever other inhibitors or promoters? And how can the differentiation be made between the glycolytic effects or metabolism in cancer cells as compared to normal cells?

Based on the preceding statements, it would seem that adding ATP or another specific phosphofructokinase enzyme inhibitor could be used to (partially) deactivate phosphofructokinase and slow down glycolysis, that is, slow down aerobic glycolysis for normal cells and anaerobic glycolysis for cancer cells. Strictly speaking, we are talking of the glycolysis sequence per se, which produces pyruvic acid or pyruvate. In the presence of oxygen, the pyruvic acid, say, is converted to carbon dioxide and water. In the absence of oxygen, it is converted to lactic acid or lactate. Fundamentally, therefore, for the glycolysis sequence or pathway proper, the pathway is the same for the production of pyruvic acid or pyruvate under either aerobic or anaerobic conditions. The only difference is that in aerobic glycolysis, there is an accumulation of ATP that inhibits phosphofructokinase, and hence glycolysis is also inhibited. In anaerobic glycolysis, there is less ATP produced, so the phosphofructokinase is not inhibited, and glycolysis is not inhibited.

On the other hand, by adding ADP or AMP, or adding another specific phosphofructokinase activator or promoter, glycolysis will be enhanced for producing pyruvic acid or pyruvate, apparently under both aerobic and anaerobic conditions.

The above may be further qualified in that, although oxygen is available to both normal cells and cancerous cells, the cancer cells apparently operate more in the fermentative mode so as to produce lactic acid or lactate. And if so, the lactate dehydrogenase enzyme must be present to convert pyruvic acid to lactic acid.

From the foregoing, we may draw some inferences, if not conclusions, about *cancer cell metabolism.* For one thing, the cancer cell surface may be so altered that oxygen does not penetrate into the cell.* Or if it does, the oxygen may not be able to penetrate the mitochondrion, the organelle where respiration can take place. Or else the mitochondrions are defective (or nonexistent, so to speak). But even if oxygen can make its way into the mitochondrions, there may not be sufficient specific and active enzymes present or manufactured to consummate the tricarboxylic acid cycle to produce carbon dioxide and water, as in normal cells. And/or there may be a sufficient preponderance of the active enzyme lactate dehydrogenase to preferentially convert the pyruvic acid or pyruvate to lactic acid or lactate.

Considering all this, *the inhibition, say, of phosphofructokinase may be only a partial solution.* Perhaps a more decisive solution would be to introduce an inhibitor or inhibitors for *lactate dehydrogenase,* with the acknowledgment that this conversion is also supported by the reaction $NADH + H^+ \rightarrow NAD^+ + 2[H]$, as shown in Figure 1.2. Thus, inhibition of this latter reaction may be another possibility. The reverse of this latter reaction occurs during the glycolysis pathway, namely Step (6) of Figure 1.1 for the conversion of glyceraldehyde 3-phosphate to 1,3 bisphosphoglycerate using glyceraldehyde 3-phosphate dehydrogenase as the specific enzyme. The reverse also occurs in several steps of the tricarboxylic acid cycle as shown in Figure 1.4.

The exothermic heat of reaction in the anaerobic conversion of glucose to lactic acid is small compared to that for the aerobic conversion of glucose to carbon dioxide and water, so that it takes a lot more glucose converted to yield the same amount of metabolic energy. This is manifested as a higher glycolytic rate for cancer cells as compared to the aerobic glycolysis rate for normal cells.

Since lactic acid is the final product of cancer cell metabolism, its *concentration in the blood could conceivably be used to indicate and monitor the progression of cancer.* Other things being equal, increasing concentrations could indicate cancer growth, decreasing concentrations could indicate cancer regression, and near-zero concentrations could indicate the absence or complete remission of cancer. Moreover, instead of taking blood samples, it might be possible to use other more indirect measurements, such as the presence and concentration of lactic acid or lactate in the breath or saliva or urine. (There is an analogy with testing for diabetes by the presence of waste products from incomplete metabolism—e.g., acetic acid, and so on.) Ideally, it might be possible to use an electronic device on the body surfaces to monitor lactic acid concentrations within the body by measuring some such physical property as conductivity and calibrating against lactic acid content.

Presumably, the buildup of lactic acid/lactate would be in small, minute, or trace concentrations, since lactic acid is converted in the liver back to glucose or glycogen. Incidentally, this latter conversion is an endothermic reaction, requiring energy in the exact same theoretical amount as produced by the exothermic conversion of glucose to lactic acid. *There is therefore no overall net production of energy in cancer metabolism.* This fact can be construed as a further reason for cancer victims losing weight.

Another observation: The lactic acid-forming bacteria are ubiquitous in our surroundings and can sometimes be deadly in their own right, e.g., members of the genus *Streptococcus.* Furthermore, if described in terms of *infective bacteria* rather than beneficial ones, their production of enzymes supporting anaerobic glycolysis may conceivably be tied in with cancer cell metabolism. *In other words, the question can be asked, "does the presence of the lactic-acid forming bacterial genus Streptococcus within the human body further support cancer cell growth and proliferation?"* Viewed from this perspective, maybe the big surprise is not that there are so many cases of cancer but that there are not even more.

Lactic acid fermentations are not only involved in producing milk products such as buttermilk, sour cream, yogurt, and cheese, but in producing other sorts of products. Ronald M. Atlas, for instance, has a section on the "Microbiological Production of Food" (Atlas, *Microbiology,* p. 478ff). Thus, there are *fermented meats* and *fermented vegetables.* Of the latter, the production of sauerkraut from cabbage, pickles from cucumbers, and green olives from harvested olives are notable. There is generally a succession of bacteria involved, which often occur naturally in the raw material itself, topped off by a fermentation to yield *lactic acid,* which imparts a *sour taste* and acts as a *preservative.*

---

* *Cancer cells are noted to have altered surface properties* (Atlas, *Microbiology,* p. 257), an item to be further discussed.

All in all, the situation can be much more complicated than it first appears, and the final resolution may lie in actually trying different bioactive *nontoxic* substances, say, as enzyme inhibitors (or promoters) for lactic-acid producing bacterial cultures. A first screening could be *in vitro* utilizing either a test tube, culture or Petri dish, or watch glass—and presumably under air-free or anaerobic conditions, which would favor the use stoppered test tubes—and with the admonition that *in vitro* results do not necessarily project to *in vivo* or clinical results. For one thing, substances digested may be altered or inactivated, suggesting intravenous application, if possible. For another thing, there is the matter of dosage levels or concentrations, and of activity or purity.

Some representative sources for cultures, enzymes, and inhibitors will be introduced next.

8.3 ENZYMES AND INHIBITORS FOR ANAEROBIC GLYCOLYSIS

As has been noted, above, a complete listing of enzymes variously involved in glycolysis and associated reactions has been presented in Part 1, notably in the sequences displayed in Figures 1.1 through 1.4, with various enzyme inhibitors listed in Appendix A. The enzymes of most interest here are those involved in anaerobic glycolysis, the conversion of glucose to produce, ultimately, lactic acid or lactate. These enzymes named in the order of usage are

1. **hexokinase**
2. hexose phosphateisomerase
3. **phosphofructokinase**
4. aldolase
5. trios phosphate isomerase
6. glyceraldehyde 3-phosphate dehydrogenase
7. phosphoglycerate kinase
8. phosphoglyceromutase
9. enolase
10. **pyuvate kinase**, and last but not least,
11. **lactate dehydrogenase**

The controlling enzymes are highlighted in boldface.

In addition to the previous citations for enzyme inhibitors as found in Jain's *Handbook of Enzyme Inhibitors* and Zollner's *Handbook of Enzyme Inhibitors*, used as the basis for Appendix A, other information can be found by a search of the comprehensive and continuing multivolume series, *Methods in Enzymology*, edited by Sidney P. Colwick and Nathan O. Kaplan et al. and published by the Academic Press. For the purposes here, however, a briefer volume will first be examined, *The Regulation of Carbohydrate Formation and Utilization in Mammals*, edited by Carlo M. Veneziale.

With regard to the enzyme hexokinase, glucose 6-P (that is, the compound designated glucose 6-phosphate) has long been known as an *inhibitor* (Herbert J. Fromm, in *The Regulation of Carbohydrate Formation and Utilization*, pp. 45–68). The inhibiting effect is offset by the presence of P_i (orthophosphate ion), which tends to *promote* the activity of hexokinase. Inasmuch as glucose 6-P is the product of the glucose conversion catalyzed by hexokinase, it would naturally be expected that a buildup or increase in glucose 6-P would tend to suppress the conversion.

The action of the enzyme *phosphofructokinase* (PFK) is counteracted by the presence of the antagonistic enzyme D-fructose bisphosphatase (FBPase), which reverses the reaction, and PFK is itself inhibited by α-D-fructose 6-P (Younathan, Voll, and Koerner, in *The Regulation of Carbohydrate Formation and Utilization*, pp. 70, 89). FBPase, incidentally, is allosterically activated by β-D-fructose-6-P, whereas PFK is allosterically activated by α-D-fructose-1,6-P_2.

The enzyme *pyruvate kinase* is regulated by the action of the pancreatic hormones glucagon and insulin (James B. Blair, in *The Regulation of Carbohydrate Formation and Utilization*, pp. 135–136). The *glucagon acts as an inhibitor,* whereas *insulin reverses the inhibition and produces hypoglycemia. Incidentally, alanine, a nonessential amino acid, has been found to enhance the inhibition of pyruvate kinase by glucagon.* Other findings about alanine are as below.

The more usual functions of glucagon and insulin are in opposition as well. That is, glucagon stimulates glucose release through glycogenolysis and stimulates lipolysis, whereas insulin stimulates glucose uptake through glucogenesis, protein synthesis, and lipogenesis (Voet and Voet, *Biochemistry,*

p. 1263). Inasmuch as cancer cell metabolism can be construed as involving pyruvate kinase, as can normal cell metabolism, one can infer that *there may be a connection between the production and functioning of these hormones and cancer,* and *an imbalance may conceivably lead to a cancerous condition.*

A search of MEDLINE for the period 1992–1996, under the word combination "anaerobic glycolysis," reveals that, according to a paper by Guerra et al., *alanine is a marker for anaerobic glycolysis.* The cited study was directed at the buildup of amino acids in neuronal injury caused by CNS (central nervous system) insults due to ischemia (deficiency in oxygenation), trauma, hypoglycemia, epilepsy, and in particular by bacterial (pneumococcal) meningitis. Significant increases were found for the cerebrospinal fluid concentrations of glutamate, aspartate, glycine, taurine, and *alanine. Glutamate concentrations* in fact increased by 470 percent. Whether this is somehow connected to cancer per se was not an object of the investigation.

The aforementioned volume, *The Regulation of Carbohydrate Formation and Utilization,* has considerably more information about the regulation of carbohydrate metabolism, most of it of a highly technical nature. Another reference dealing with the subject is *Regulation of Carbohydrate Metabolism,* in two volumes, edited by Rivka Beitner and published in 1985. In particular, note Volume I. In Volume II, a chapter by Eigenbrodt et al., is of particular interest, titled "New Perspectives on Carbohydrate Metabolism in Tumor Cells," and which is cited elsewhere. We next turn to biologically oriented possibilities.

In a chapter on "Microbial Technology," authors Brock and Madigan list a number of sources for *culture collections of microorganisms* (Brock and Madigan, *Microorganisms,* p. 349). They provide the comment that the ultimate source for all microorganisms is the natural environment, but through the years there have been improvements, yielding strains of commercial importance that have been deposited in culture collections. Thus, whenever an industrial process is patented, the patent application must include a deposit of a microbial strain that is capable of reproducing the process as stated in the application. It is further noted that there are generally further improvements in a given strain, which are not deposited in the repositories. Examples for culture collections of industrial microorganisms are furnished in Table 8.1, with the annotation that many universities and research organizations keep special collections of specific microbial groups.

Table 8.1 Microorganism Culture Collections and Locations

Canada	Ottawa	Canadian Department of Agriculture (CDDA)
Czechoslovakia	J.E. Purkyne Univ, Brno	Czechoslovak Collection of Microorganisms (CDDA)
France	Paris	Collection of the Institut Pasteur (CIP)
FRG	Göttingen	Deutsche Sammlung von Mikrooranismen (DSM)
Japan	Tokyo University of Tokyo	Faculty of Agriculture, Tokyo University (FAT) Institute of Applied Microbiology (IAM)
The Netherlands	Baarn	Centraalbureau voor Schimmelcultur (CBS)
Scotland	Aberdeen	National Collection of Industrial Bacteria (NCIB)
U.K.	Kew London	Commonwealth Mycological Institute (CMI) National Collection of Type Cultures (NCTC)
U.S.	Peoria IL Rockville MD	Northern Regional Research Laboratory (NRRL) American Type Culture Collection (ATCC)

A representative commercial source for cultures is Rhône-Poulenc of Madison WI. Its Marschall Products division produces *bacterial cultures for converting sugars to lactic acid,* e.g., for the dairy industry. These cultures contain the complete array of enzymes for the anaerobic glycolysis sequence, with the exact same enzymes produced by the bacteria culture as by humans. As a specific example, Rhône-Poulenc Dairy Ingredients has a yogurt culture consisting of a blend of specially selected freeze-dried strains of *Streptococcus thermophilus, Lactobacillus delbrueckii* var. *bulgaricus, Lactobacillus acidophilis,* and *Bifidobacterium longum.* It can be added that the genera *Lactobacillus* and *Bifidobacterium* are increasingly mentioned as agents for promoting good health. They are thought to enhance bowel health by producing organic acids and other *inhibitory* metabolites, which suppress the growth of undesirable pathogens in the intestinal tract.*

To continue, a culture of *Lactobacillus delbrueckii* or some other lactic acid-producing culture could be used in testing (nontoxic) bioactive plants or plant extracts and compounds as enzyme inhibitors for lactic acid formation. Possibilities include plants or plant extracts containing various alkaloids, notably, or containing various glycosides and cyanoglycosides, saponins, flavonoids, etc., in progressively minute concentrations. Alternatively, the particular known pure alkaloid, glycoside, saponin, flavonoid, and so on, can itself be tested. (There is, of course, the qualification that concentration also determines the dividing line between toxicity or nontoxicity.)

The tests could be conducted *in vitro* in a test tube, Petri dish, or watch glass, preferably under anaerobic conditions. If the mixture grows cloudy, it is a sign that the culture is multiplying or reproducing, and the substance or compound added is ineffective as an inhibitor. On the other hand, if the culture remains clear, then the substance is effective as an inhibitor.

Whereas the main interest has been in what part a few particular bacteria genera and species play in producing the enzymes for anaerobic glycolysis, there are the many, many other genera and species of bacteria, some of which are beneficial and some of which are pathogenic. Just what enzymes or enzyme inhibitors these many other genera and species might generate is a topic unto itself, but there is always the prospect that some few might act against cancer. The argument can even be extended to fungi and viruses—although some viruses are thought to be cancer causing, a thought that can be generalized also to bacteria and other microorganisms.

Contrarily, some of the antibacterial agents that have so far been found very possibly might serve as anticancer agents. (For instance, a certain few antibiotics will act against cancer, although they are usually too toxic to use.) Similarly with antiviral, antifungal, and other miscellaneous agents. Listings of some of these agents have been provided in Appendices I, J, K, and L. In turn, interestingly, some of these same agents have been listed in Hartwell's *Plants Used Against Cancer* and are so noted in the respective appendices.

It may be added that the search for these kinds of natural agents is apparently intensifying, in particular for antiviral agents, and one of the investigators is former University of Wyoming pharmacy professor Steve Gillespie, now of the Mayo Clinic, who has been checking out Wyoming plants for medicinal properties. As a specific instance, several Wyoming species of the plant called *osha* or *lovage* have been found to have antibacterial, antiviral, antifungal, and antispasmodic properties and were used by American Indians variously for colds and sore throats, stomach aches, and even wounds. These several native species are *Ligusticum porteri, L. filicinum,* and *L. tenuifolium* of the family Ammiaceae or Apiaceae, or Carrot family, of which celery is also a member, and they have their counterpart species and uses in the Old World. For the record, these plants have relatively high levels of the chemical compounds known as *ligustilides* and also the compound *butylidenephthalide.* The first-named plant species, above, generally preferred by native Americans, has the highest levels of ligustilides, and it may be further noted that a specific ligustilide is being mentioned in Japan as a treatment for *Alzheimer's disease*. Of further interest would be the question of if and how these compounds act as enzyme inhibitors.

There are, of course, many organic and inorganic chemical compounds that could be tested and that may be judged as nontoxic in the amounts or concentrations to be used. Thus, it may be noted in passing that such substances as sodium fluoride and iodo-acetic acid are general enzyme inhibitors and will kill off these particular lactic acid-forming bacteria cultures. In fact, it is said that fluorides kill off the bacteria in the mouth (around the teeth) by blocking bacterial enzymes. This is a reason why fluoridation reduces cavities. (The usual reason assigned is that fluoride replaces the calcium compounds in the tooth surfaces or enamel, a condition more resistant to decay.) Of course, one can wonder what fluorides do in the rest of the body. There are other known agents that will readily kill off these kinds of bacteria, but they are too toxic for human use.

The potential problem of fluoride toxicity as may be encountered in municipal water supplies has been a common enough topic and has been given added emphasis in a book titled, *Our Stolen Future*,

---

* There is of course the inference that there may be an inhibition of cancer-causing pathogens.

by T. Colborn, D. Dumanoski, and J.P.Myers. Additionally, the adverse effects of DES or diethylstilbestrol are also discussed. Among other things, a lowering of children's IQs is suspected.

These matters are reviewed by Richard G. Foulkes, MD, in an article titled, "The Fluoride Connection," in the April, 1998 issue of the *Townsend Letter for Doctors & Patients*. The leadoff caption on the cover is, "Is Fluoride Making Us Act Like Devils?"

We may also mention peptides or polypeptides, which are short-chain proteins—that is, relatively short as compared to other proteins. The presence or use of these sorts of compounds is a feature of both shark cartilage therapy and the *Burzynski therapy*, e.g., as mentioned in Richard Walters' *Options*. According to Burzynski, polypeptides act as enzyme inhibitors—although for what particular enzyme or enzymes seems not to have been made clear. (For a source of bioactive peptides, see Tables 8.5 and 8.6.)

Interestingly, *peptides are also known to provide an immune response* and are under study in the preparation of *synthetic vaccines* (F.Y. Liew, in *Vaccination Strategies*, p. 6; Fred Brown, in *Vaccination Strategies*, p. 65ff). *Polysaccharides* are a possibility (and which are sometimes considered as *anticancer agents*, as indicated, for example, in John Boik's *Cancer & Natural Medicine*). For another instance, it is known that a *peptide* chain of as few as six amino acids will elicit *virus-neutralizing antibodies* (Brown, in *Vaccination Strategies*, p. 68). The connection to developing a cancer vaccine was not specifically mentioned in the reference.

In work described by Stephen S. Hall, in an article "Vaccinating Against Cancer," published in the April 1997 issue of the *Atlantic Monthly*, based on the research by physician Alexander Knuth and molecular geneticist Thierry Boon and coworkers, it is noted that *a peptide chain of nine amino acids will act as an antigen, stimulating the immune response*, at least in the case of melanoma. Further details have been provided in Part 7 under the section "Immunity" in the subsection titled "Immunization Against Cancer."

As to the odds for determining and identifying the particular amino acids making up a nine-member chain out of the 20 fundamental amino acids, consider the question of combinations versus permutations. If no distinction is made between amino acids, then the *number of combinations* or ways for expressing a sample size r out of a total of n items is, for the case at hand,

$$\frac{n!}{r!(n-r)!} = \frac{20!}{9!\,11!} = 167,960$$

where, say, $9! = 9 \times 8 \times 7 \times 6 \times 5 \times 4 \times 3 \times 2 \times 1 = 362,880$. And so on. If each amino acid has a label on it, that is, if the 20 amino acids are each different, then the total number of possible permutations is given by

$$\frac{n!}{(n-r)!} = \frac{20!}{11!} = 60.0949324 \text{ billion}$$

Clearly, there can be a gargantuan number of possibilities for ascertaining just what particular peptide chains could serve as antigens for stimulating the immune system, which serves to illustrate the enormity of the work by Boon and Knuth and other investigators. More than this, however, there are involved such things as *major histocompatibility complex* (MHC) molecules, which are required to transport an antigen from the cell interior to the cell surface, there to activate or signal the roaming T cells or T lymphocytes. They then proceed to perforate and destroy the cell. This complicated sequence was further described in Part 7, in the section and subsection on dealing with immunity and immunization.

Whether the administration of an antigen or peptide could serve the same sort of function is apparently not known. That is, if, for example, an antigen or peptide enters the bloodstream, would it become selectively attached to the diseased cell surface and there activate the T cells to destroy the cell? Or can the antigen or peptide be introduced into the cell, say by a virus? In this regard, there are ongoing studies to utilize viruses against cancer, as indicated in the following footnote. *Adenoviruses* in particular are a candidate vaccine component.*

There is the further possibility of using *adjuvants* to activate the vaccine, *the function of immunological adjuvants being to stimulate the vaccine's specific immune response to the antigens* (Robert Bomford, in *Vaccination Strategies*, p. 94). That is, in the case of vaccines that utilize purified proteins or synthetic peptides, an adjuvant is required to sustain vaccine activity. (There are problems also with *live attenuated vaccines,* especially in the tropics, for there may be a *reversion to virulence.* The vaccines are unstable and must be stored at low temperatures.) Mineral gels such as of aluminum hydroxide or phosphate have been used as adjuvants. Newer possibilities enumerated in the reference include muramyl dipeptide, pluronic purols, liposomes, *saponin,* and *ISCOMS.*

Saponin or *saponins* are already widely used as an adjuvant in veterinary vaccines, notably against foot-and-mouth disease (Brown, in *Vaccination Strategies,* p. 99). Saponins are classified as *triterpene glycosides of plant origin,* and those used as adjuvants are specifically derived from the South American tree *Quillaia saponaria* of the family Rosaceae. (The triterpene ring structure is said to be lipophilic, with the attached sugars hydrophilic, such that the molecule is surface active. Accordingly, *the soft drink industry uses saponins as a foaming agent.* Quillaia or quillaia bark in fact is commonly known as soapbark.) Saponins have been previously discussed as a major classification of plant chemicals or phytochemicals, as are, say, alkaloids. Furthermore, some saponin-containing plants are known *anticancer agents.*

Quillaia is not listed in Hartwell's *Plants Used Against Cancer,* although the family Rosaceae is well represented. Speaking further in these directions, the family Sapindaceae is represented in Hartwell but does not include the genus *Sapindus,* the soapberry of North America. The species *Sapindus drummondi,* for instance, occurs in western Oklahoma, and the berries were used by the Plains Indians for soap. Another species, *S. saponaria,* is found in Florida and ranges on down through the West Indies into Venezuela and Ecuador. The genus and these and other species are detailed in Sargent's *Manual of the Trees of North America.* Whether there is a kinship between the genera is not readily discernible, other than that they both contain saponins of one kind or another. Another plant with soap-like qualities is, of course, the yucca, of the genus *Yucca* of the family Liliaceae or Lily family. The genus *Yucca* is not listed in Hartwell, albeit the family Liliaceae is well cataloged. The genus *Aloe* is also prominent in the Liliaceae, with many entries in Hartwell, as are garlic and onions (and wild iris, for good measure, which produces a stomach ache—and which is an indication of some kind of bioactivity).

ISCOMS are particles called immunostimulatory complexes, resulting from the discovery that saponins will bind directly to proteins that have been removed from cell membranes or viral envelopes. These complexes can be separated from the free saponin left over and are found to be more immunogenic than simple micelles of the cell-surface antigen.

> ISCOMS prepared from the surface antigen of feline leukemia virus were protective in cats, a result with an obvious implication for other retroviral diseases such as AIDS.

In that some cancers, at least, may be caused by viruses or retroviruses, the extrapolation is also obvious.

In general, therefore, we may also speak of what are called immunostimulants, to further activate the immune system. (For a source of immunochemicals, also see Table 8.7.)

With further regard to viruses, it is known that some viruses, such as the influenza virus, undergo *antigenic shifts,* requiring the regular production of new vaccines (Marilyn J. Moore and Juraj Ivanyi, in *Vaccination Strategies,* p. 80). In further comment, this is the sort of problem encountered with retroviruses—e.g., with HIV in AIDS—that are constantly changing or mutating into something else.

The influenza virus, or viruses, is an RNA virus but *not* a retrovirus, and it is described as *antigenic*—that is, related to antigens, but here meaning that there is an antigenic variation such that immunological resistance is lowered against new infections.

The influenza virus family is the Orthomyxoviridae, which includes what are called the influenza types A, B, and C, as per Table 7.1 in Part 7. Its most distinct property is the ability of the type A virus to infect animals as well as humans, with the ability to cross over and form new strains against which there is little human resistance.

---

* Thus, in a parallel line of investigation, it has been announced, in fact, that a *special strain of adenovirus* is being tried. Ordinarily, when adenoviruses infect a cell, they yield a protein that disarms what is called the *p53* tumor suppressor gene, and the adenovirus will proliferate and destroy a normal cell. A special strain of adenovirus has been developed, however, that has lost the ability to disarm the p53 tumor suppressor gene. Hence, the virus will not affect normal cells in which the tumor suppressor gene is functioning. However, in cancerous cells, the tumor suppressor gene is likely to have been damaged, and the virus is free to proliferate and destroy the cell.

A similar line of investigation to that of Knuth and Boon and coworkers is being conducted by physician and researcher Steven A. Rosenberg, MD, PhD, and associates, who are connected with the National Cancer Institute of the National Institutes of Health at Bethesda MD. Dr. Rosenberg's work against melanoma was featured in a presentation by The Learning Channel, or TLC, on or about March 6, 1998. A peptide immunization vaccine is utilized, which is enhanced using interleukin 2, or IL-2 (which is not active in itself). *The peptide vaccine has no side effects,* albeit this is not the case for IL-2. Furthermore, IL-2 is not tolerated by smokers, so an alternative enhancer is used, evidently designated as GNCSF. The results so far are mixed, with a 42 percent response reported versus a baseline 18 percent response.

The vaccine is supplied by a drug company, and Dr. Rosenberg made the interesting comment that it has been required that some of his findings be kept confidential and not shared to protect the investment of the drug company. The FDA initially proved clinical tests on only 50 patients, but presumably these efforts will be expanded as more vaccine becomes available. The hotline for the NCI is 1-800-4CANCER or 1-800-422-6237.

It may be further mentioned that Steven A. Rosenberg and John M. Barry are authors of *The Transformed Cell: Unlocking the Mysteries of Cancer*, first published in 1992. Rosenberg is also an editor of *Cancer: Principles and Practices of Oncology*, published in five editions, the latest in 1997. The work of S.A. Rosenberg and associates is more than amply documented on MEDLINE, with numerous citations.

For the pure enzymes per se, a representative source is the Sigma Chemical Company of St. Louis MO. Stated again, the controlling enzymes involved are evidently hexokinase, 6-phosphofructokinase, pyruvate kinase, and in particular *lactate dehydrogenase.* The Sigma catalog is available also on a CD or on diskettes, and can be searched by computer, not only for reactants and enzymes, but for potential inhibitors and other information. Reactants and enzymes involved in (anaerobic) glycolysis are shown in Table 8.2 as obtained from the Sigma catalog. The controlling enzymes are highlighted. The catalog also lists reaction rates and enzyme sources.

The testing of reacting systems—that is, of reactants (or substrates), enzymes, and inhibitors—for activity is a standardized clinical procedure, and routine in its application, with some equipment capable of running as many as 24 tests at a time. In some instances, the diagnostic kits are available, as indicated in the previously mentioned table, Table 8.2. In particular, *a kit is available for testing lactate dehydrogenase.*

In principle, a spectroscope is used, set for a specified wave length or wavelengths of light. In other words, the reacting system of substrate, enzyme, and/or inhibitor is tested for its transmission of light. A decrease in the degree or rate of light transmission indicates a reduction in activity, as caused, for example, by the addition of an inhibiting substance. An increase, on the other hand, would indicate that the added substance functioned as a promoter instead of an inhibitor.

With regard to all the above, we are most interested in which *foods, vitamins,* or *minerals* contain, or are, enzyme inhibitors—and specifically, for what enzymes or enzyme-catalyzed reactions. It is especially so for controlling, regulating, or modulating the enzymes for anaerobic glycolysis, namely the controlling enzymes hexokinase, 6-phosphofructokinase, pyruvate kinase, and lactate dehydrogenase, as has been noted previously. In a way of speaking, we are talking of *nutritional immunology,* a term coming into favor. If not this, then we can fall back on the term *nutritional therapy.*

More than this, we are also interested in whatever bioactive plants or plant substances, or herbs, might serve as enzyme inhibitors for anaerobic glycolysis—*with the condition that these substances be nontoxic to other body processes or functions, and not be cytotoxic to normal cells.* Ordinarily, we think of what we call herbs as being fairly benign, although curative, but this is not necessarily the case. Efficacy versus toxicity will in large part depend on *dosage levels,* as is well recognized in homeopathic medicine—and trace dosage is indeed an underlying feature.

An inspection of the small but comprehensive volume titled *Pocket Manual of Homœopathic Materia Medica: Comprising the Characteristic and Guiding Symptoms of All Remedies [Clinical and Pathogenetic]* will substantiate this dichotomy. Written by William Boericke, MD, and first published in 1901, it continues today in the form of its ninth edition, published in 1927, as revised and enlarged with a repertory by Oscar E. Boericke, MD. Many of the most common herbs or herbal medicines are entered along with riveting descriptions of their toxic effects—which are often numerous and severe indeed. But presumably, these toxic effects are caused by large dosage levels. And, according to the principles of

Table 8.2 Commercially Available Reactants and Individual Enzymes for (Anaerobic) Glycolysis

Production of Pyruvic Acid or Pyruvate

Glucose [D-(+)-glucose, also known as dextrose or corn sugar]

    (1) **Hexokinase** (known also as ATP: D-hexose-6-phosphotransferase). Obtained variously from **bakers yeast**, bovine heart, and from beaded agarose in bakers yeast. (Agarose is a linear polymer of alternating D-galactose and 3,6-anhydro-L-galactose structures, e.g., as obtained from red algae.) Reaction rate and impurities are listed. Diagnostic kit is available.

Glucose 6-phosphate [D-(+)-glucopyranose 6-phosphate]

    (2) Hexose phosphateisomerase (listed as phosphoglucose isomerase, known also as D-glucose-6-phosphate ketol-isomerase). Obtained variously from *Bacillus stearothermophilus*, **bakers yeast**, rabbit muscle, lyophilized yeast (dispersed in water), and beaded agarose from bakers yeast. Reaction rate and impurities are listed. Diagnostic kit is available (phosphohexose isomerase or PHI).

Fructose 6-phosphate

    (3) **Phosphofructokinase** (listed as fructose 6-phosphate kinase; known also as 6-phosphofructokinase or ATP: D-fructose 6-phosphate 1-phosphotransferase). Obtained variously from rabbit muscle, rabbit liver, and from *Bacillus stearothermophilus*. Reaction rate and impurities are listed.

Fructose 1,6-bisphosphate (see D-fructose 1,6 diphosphate)

    (4) Aldolase (known also as D-fructose-1,6-bisphosphate-D-glyceraldehyde-3- phosphate-lyase). Obtained from rabbit muscle, trout muscle, **spinach**, *Staphylococcus aureus*, and **bakers yeast**. Reaction rate and impurities are listed. Diagnostic kit is available.

Glyceraldehyde 3-phosphate

    (5) Trios phosphate isomerase or triose phosphate isomerase (known also as TPI or as D-glyceraldehyde-3-phosphate ketol-isomerase). Obtained variously from **bakers yeast**, rabbit muscle, dog muscle, and porcine muscle. Reaction rate and impurities are listed.

    (6) Glyceraldehyde 3-phosphate dehydrogenase (known also as GAPDH or as D-glyceraldehyde 3-phosphate:NAD$^+$ oxidoreductase [phosphorylating]). Obtained variously from human erythrocytes (red blood corpuscles), *Baccillus stearothermophilus*, chicken muscle, porcine muscle, rabbit muscle, **bakers yeast**, and beaded agarose in bakers yeast. Reaction rate and impurities are listed.

1,3 Bisphosphoglycerate (lists only 2,3-diphospho-D-glyceric acid, as sodium salt, etc.).

    (7) Phosphoglycerate kinase (listed as 3-phosphoglyceric phosphokinase, p. 838; known also as ATP:3-phospho-D-glycerate 1-phosphotransferase). Obtained variously from *Bacillus stearithermophilus*, rabbit muscle, and **bakers yeast**. Reaction rate and impurites are listed.

3-Phosphoglycerate [D(–)3-phosphoglyceric acid, as calcium, sodium salts, etc.]

    (8) Phosphoglyceromutase (listed as phosphoglycerate mutase, known also as 2,3-diphospho-D-glycerate: 2-phospho-D-glycerate phosphotransferase). Obtained from rabbit muscle. Reaction rate and impurities are listed.

2-Phosphoglycerate [D(+)2-phosphoglyceric acid, as sodium salt]

    (9) Enolase (known also as phosphopyruvate hydratase or 2-phospho-D-glycerate hydro-lyase). Obtained variously from **bakers yeast** and rabbit muscle. Reaction rate and impurities are listed.

Phosphoenolpyruvate (2-[phosphonooxyl]-2-propionic acid, as sodium salt, etc.).

Table 8.2 Commercially Available Reactants and Individual Enzymes for (Anaerobic) Glycolysis *(continued)*

---

(10) **Pyruvate kinase** (known also as PK or as ATP:pyruvate 2-O- phosphotransferase). Obtained variously from rabbit muscle, dog muscle, rabbit liver, *Bacillus stearothermophilus*, porcine heart, chicken muscle, and polyacrylamide in rabbit muscle. Reaction rate and impurites are listed. Diagnostic kit is available.

Production of Lactic Acid or Lactate from Pyruvic Acid or Pyruvate

Pyruvate (α-ketopropionic acid or 2-oxopropanoic acid, as acid or sodium salt)

(11) **Lactate dehydrogenase** (listed as D-lactic dehydrogenase, known also as [R]-lactate: NAD⁺ oxidoreductase). From *Lactobacillus leichmanii*, *Leuconostoc mesenteroides*, *Staphylococcus epidermidis*. Reaction rate and impurities are listed.

Lactate dehydrogenase (listed as L-lactic dehydrogenase, known as L-LDH, LAD, or LD, or as [S]lactate: NAD⁺ oxidoreductase). From rabbit muscle and heart, pigeon breast muscle, bovine adrenal glands, heart, and muscle, porcine heart and muscle, chicken heart, liver, and muscle, human erythrocytes and placenta, lobster tail, dog muscle, trout muscle, *Bacillus stearothermophilus*, human liver, bovine semen. Reaction rate and impurities are listed. Diagnostic kits are available.

Source: Taken from the catalog *Biochemicals, Organic Compounds, and Diagnostic Reagents*, Sigma Chemical Company, St. Louis MO, 1996-, in a section on Compounds and another section on Diagnostic Kits.

Note: Reactants and the numbering of enzymes for the glycolysis sequence or pathway corresponds to Figure 1.1 in Part 1. Reactants are shown in **boldface** as are the enzymes for the controlling reaction steps, as well as other information items of potential interest. The further enzyme-catalyzed anaerobic conversion of pyruvic acid or pyruvate to lactic acid or lactate corresponds to Figure 1.2 in Part 1. Catalog pages listing the enzymes are entered in parens, along with alternative names for the enzymes. The various sources for the enzymes are set out in separate paragraphs, including bacterial sources. Reaction rate and impurities are supplied in the catalog citations for each enzyme-catalyzed conversion. In a few instances, notably for lactate dehydrogenase, the respective diagnostic kits for the reactants or enzymes listed are available from the Sigma catalog in the section titled Diagnostic Kits and Reagents. Spectroscopic equipment for use with the diagnostic kits are available from such laboratory and chemical supply houses as Van Waters and Rogers, or Fisher, etc.

Homeopathy (take it or leave it), these same (toxic) herbal drugs administered in minute or trace amounts will tend to cure or offset the very symptoms caused by large amounts.

The same dichotomy, however, is encountered time and again in chronicling cancer treatments. An anticancer agent used in small amounts may act curatively, whereas in large amounts it will be known to cause cancer.

We may continue this line of discussion in terms of some of the most toxic bioactive substances known: aconite or aconitine, ricin, and abrin. All three substances are listed in the Sigma catalog (the first under "Compounds," and the later two under "Lectins"). All three of the plant sources are entered in Hartwell's *Plants Used Against Cancer*.

Aconitine is an alkaloid, whereas ricin and abrin are listed in the Sigma catalog under *lectins*, which are described as *proteins or glycoproteins* of nonimmune origin that agglutinate cells and/or precipitate complex carbohydrates. This agglutinating (adhesive) property is noted to be *inhibited by monosaccharides or di- or tri-saccharides, or by polysaccharides.*

Interestingly, as set forth in Part 6, in the section on "Metastasis and Glyoproteins," migrating or metastasizing cancer cells have a stickiness that causes them to adhere at other places in the body. Thus, with regard polysaccharides acting as inhibitors for cell adhesion, it may be emphasized that polysaccharides are considered to be anticancer agents, as indicated in Part 3 in the section on "Other Information about Chinese Anticancer Agents." Not only are polysaccharides found in higher plants, but they also occur in fungi.

On the other hand, cancer cells tend to break away from the cancerous mass, losing cohesion and thus metastasizing. It can therefore be asked whether polysaccharides inhibit cohesion and thus accelerate metastasis. The distinction may be crucial.

Aconite or *aconitine* is derived from the genus *Aconitum* (of the family Ranunculaceae) and is more commonly known as monkshood or wolfsbane. (The wild species with dark blue flowers found in the

Rocky Mountains is *A. columbianum*, and a similar species with light-colored flowers is called *A columbianum* var. *ochroleucum*, whereas *A. napellus* is regarded as the domesticated or cultivated species. As mentioned in the footnote, the species *A. sibiricum* grows wild in Asia, e.g., in the Tien Shan Range.) Prepared from the root, the substance is so toxic that only a drop to a few drops of the alcoholic extract may be tried, as indicated in Part 4 in the section on "Toxicity versus Medical Benefits," where Alexander Solzhenitsyn described its apparent use in his book *Cancer Ward*.*

Ricin is derived from the *castor bean plant, Ricinus communis* (of the family Euphorbiaceae or Spurge family). *Abrin* is derived from the *jequirity bean,* also called Indian licorice, as found in India and other parts of the tropics. The scarlet and black seeds have served for beads and necklaces and, because of their uniform size, have even been used for standard weights. Further information is presented in Part 4 in the section on "Toxicity versus Medical Benefits."†

Of main interest here is whether any of these substances have been found to be enzyme inhibitors. Furthermore, do they or their derivatives possess any inhibiting action toward cancer cell metabolism, or are their effects mainly life threatening due to other inhibiting actions? The results of an inspection of Jain's *Handbook* and Zollner's *Handbook* are both conclusive and inconclusive.

For the record, Jain's *Handbook* lists aconitine as an inhibitor for binding to the "sodium channel." Aconitic acid acts as an inhibitor for glutamate decarboxylase. Trans-aconitic acid acts as an inhibitor for aconitase and fumarase. Zollner's *Handbook* lists trans-aconitate as an inhibitor for fumarate hydratase—which presumably is the same as fumarase.

Glutaminase, if it is the same or approximately the same as glutamate decarboxylase, is an enzyme involved in glutaminolysis, as per Figure 1.3 in Part 1. The inhibition of this enzyme can be viewed as not particularly life-threatening.

Aconitase is the enzyme for step 2 in the tricarboxylic acid cycle, as per Figure 1.4 in Part 1. Fumarase is the enzyme for step 7 in the tricarboxylic acid cycle. *The conclusion is that aconite or aconitine or its derivatives block or interfere with respiration, a serious circumstance indeed, and one not likely to be offset by any beneficial effects.*

Nevertheless, there is always the long-shot possibility that, in trace amounts, aconitine or its derivatives might not unduly interfere with respiration yet might act against cancer cell metabolism by interfering with one or another of the enzymes involved in anaerobic glycolysis (read, cancer cell metabolism). This would be the thin line between toxicity and beneficence as is so often encountered with other drugs—e.g., digitalis—where the dosage is the poison. (And there is the further fact that the enzyme called *aconitase* is itself necessary for respiration to take place—indicating an association of sorts.)

Jain's *Handbook* lists ricin as an inhibitor for the binding of EF-2 (elongation factor 2), and for GTPase and ribosome-dependent GTPase, and for protein synthesis. (Protein synthesis is inhibited because ricin inhibits the binding of EF-2 and of ADPR-E2 to ribosomes, the last-mentioned category consisting of particles of RNA and protein that occur in the cell cytoplasm, the part exclusive of the nucleus). Presumably, ricin is severely cytotoxic to all cells.

Jain's *Handbook* lists abrin also as an inhibitor for the binding of EF-2 and as an inhibitor for protein synthesis. Presumably, abrin is also severely cytotoxic.

No mention could be found for one or another of these three substances blocking or inhibiting any of the enzymes involved in cancer cell metabolism, namely in anaerobic glycolysis. Either they have not been so tested, or they were found to be inactive toward the particular enzymes. Evidently, they have at some time been tried against cancer, however, for they are listed in Hartwell's compendium. If in any

---

* The subject of *aconite* is mentioned in George St. George's Time-Life book titled *Soviet Deserts and Mountains*, in which he sought the elusive species *Aconitium sibiricum*, the Siberian species similar to *Aconitum columbianum*, the wild monkshood found in the Rocky Mountains (St. George, *Soviet Deserts*, p. 167). He stated that "the aconite root, properly used for medicinal purposes, is claimed as a true miracle drug for arthritis." Referred to as the "Issyk-Kul root," by St. George, and described as a terrible plant, it was said to grow in the vicinity of Lake Issyk-Kul in the great Tien Shan Range, which separates southwestern Siberia from western China. St. George didn't locate any that day.

† The plant source for abrin is *Abrus precatorius*, of the family Leguminosae. It is to be distinguished from another "Indian" licorice, or wild licorice, the North American species *Glycyrrhiza lepidota*, also of the family Leguminosae. The common licorice used to flavor candy is *G. glabra*, found in Europe and Asia, although the root of wild licorice is equally sweet and was an important food source for American Indians. Although *G. glabra* is listed in Hartwell, *G. lepidota* is not, albeit there is a general listing for *Glycyrrhiza* spp.

way effective, their use would seem more like a game of Russian roulette. Presumably, less dangerous anticancer agents exist.

Not to be overlooked are *electromagnetic effects,* and in particular, *radiation.* Most generally, what is called electromagnetic radiation is described in terms of either *wavelength* or *frequency,* the one being inversely proportional to the other. Thus, electromagnetic radiation may vary in wavelength or frequency, and may range from, say, the low end of radio-transmission waves on up to X-rays, gamma rays, and cosmic rays. Thus, radio waves are of longer wavelength and lower frequencies, whereas X-rays are of ultra-short wavelength and ultra-high frequencies. Otherwise and in between are microwaves and short-wave radio signals, visible light, and so on. In addition to the measure of wavelength or frequency is the *intensity* of radiation.

It would be of interest to determine what effect the various electromagnetic radiation frequencies and intensities will have on the enzymes of anaerobic glycolysis—not to mention other enzymes. In other words, can electromagnetic radiation serve as an enzyme inhibitor or regulator? And if so, at what frequencies and intensities? The work of Rife on radio frequency (RF) radiation, described in Richard Walters' *Options,* is indicative that there may well be such an effect, to be further studied and substantiated. Enter the subject of *electronic medicine.*

Radiation or radiant energy and its transmission can be described in terms of either wave theories or "corpuscular" theories, the latter category having been favored by Isaac Newton, for instance. A purpose of what is called quantum mechanics or quantum theory is to reconcile the two interpretations by mathematically describing radiant energy as a function of both—a matter of "duality."

In terms of decreasing wavelength or increasing frequency, radiation varies from radio waves and then to microwaves, into the infrared region, through the visible light spectrum, to the ultraviolet region, and thence to X-rays and gamma rays. Long-wave radio and AM radio waves start out at about 10^5 or 10^6 cycles per second or cps, whereas gamma rays are approximately 10^{22} cps (10 multiplied by itself 21 times). By comparison, ordinary household electrical current is 60 cycles per second, or of the order of 10^2 cps second.

As the wavelength decreases and the frequency increases, radiation becomes increasingly photon-like—manifested in the terms of so-called "packets" or quanta of radiant energy. Radiation from nuclear sources includes not only gamma but particle radiation—e.g., alpha particles, beta particles, and various other particles and radioactive particle fragments. Cosmic rays consist of gamma rays plus protons, neutrons, and heavier nuclei or particle fragments, and mesons and other strange particles or elementary particles, and so on—not to mention electrons.* We may also speak of sound radiation or ultrasonics, for instance, but this is a different proposition from electromagnetic radiation.

Very possibly, there can be enzyme-inhibiting effects with electric fields or with magnetic fields. There are indications at least that magnetic fields, for instance, may have such an effect. (For example, what is called *magnetic field therapy* is regarded as a facet of alternative medicine.) Further independent and impartial substantiation is needed. And what better and easier way to perform the initial, necessary tests than on the critical or controlling enzymes themselves?

The use of *oscillating electric currents* is again being explored. Once a tool of the chiropractic, there is now considerable research into what is called *cranial electrostimulation* or *CES.* Two electrodes are placed at opposing positions on the head, and an electric potential of from a few volts to maybe line voltage is applied, at frequencies of from perhaps one hertz to several hundred, a hertz being one cycle per second. (Information about ongoing CES research has been compiled by Tools for Exploration, 4460 Redwood Highway, Ste. 2, San Rafael CA 94903, 415-499-9050.) Cranial electrostimulation has been variously used against drug addiction, anxiety and depression, insomnia, and cognitive dysfunction. (The treatment, reportedly first used by Russian scientists for insomnia, has been termed *electrosleep.*) Successes have been reported for the various applications.

No mention is made of CES for cancer treatment; however, as complex as is the human body, almost anything remains a possibility. And who knows? Maybe an oscillating electric current applied across a cancerous location can have beneficial effects—with the optimum voltage and frequency to be determined. At the very least, it could be tried as an inhibitor or regulator for one or another of the enzymes controlling anaerobic glycolysis.

---

* For more, consult for example the section on "Electromagnetic Radiation" in the *McGraw-Hill Encyclopedia of Science and Technology.*

Also making the news is what is called *transcranial magnetic stimulation* or *TMS*. In the presence of strong magnetic fields, the brain does some peculiar things, with unexpected consequences, particularly on the nervous system. It can be assumed that TMS is related to magnetic field therapy, and magnetic effects on other parts of the body remain to be confirmed decisively—in particular, as pertains to cancer treatment. In other words, mainstream medicine will have to be convinced of the benefits, if any.

Another prospect remains that of using *antibiotics* of one sort or another. Thus, for instance, if anaerobic glycolysis is induced by the presence of lactic acid-producing organisms in the body system, perhaps an antibiotic is indicated that will destroy these particular bacteria (by blocking critical bacterial enzymes). The indication so far, however, is that the use of antibiotics is not a systematic therapy for cancer, although some antibiotics are noted to act as anticancer agents but are generally too toxic to be used. Other assorted antibacterial, antiviral, antifungal, and antidisease agents may also have a beneficial effect against cancer, yet to be determined.

Still another possibility is the use of such biochemical compounds or agents as cAMP, ADP, and ATP, which are involved in glycolysis and other vital biochemical reactions. In this regard, the Sigma Chemical Company catalog lists many of these particular compounds, some with radioactive tags. Additional information is provided in Table 8.3. Furthermore, there are sections in the Sigma catalog for bioactive peptides and for immunochemicals, which may also have potential as anticancer agents, and which are also noted in Tables 8.4 through 8.7. *Of paramount interest is the potential for synthesizing peptides (or peptide chains of amino acids) that would be active as enzyme inhibitors against the controlling enzymes of anaerobic glycolysis.* This, of course, ties in with the work of Burzynski, previously mentioned, and with the use of shark cartilage against cancer, also mentioned.

Table 8.3   Some Biochemicals Involved in Cell Metabolism

Adenosine 5´-monophosphate—AMP
Adinosine 5´-diphosphate—ADP
Adinosine 5´-triphosphate—ATP
Adinosine 3´,5´-cyclic monophosphate—cAMP
Cyclic nucleotides index
β-Nicotinamide adenine dinucleotide, oxidized form—NAD+
β-Nicotinamide adenine dinucleotide, reduced form—NADH
β-Nicotinamide adenine dinucleotide phosphate, oxidized form—NADP+
β-Nicotinamide adenine dinucleotide phosphate, reduced form—NADPH
Nucleosides and nucleotides (in a section on Standards and Controls)
Bioactive Peptides (in a section on Bioactive Peptides)
Immunochemicals (in a section on Immunochemicals)

Source: Data from the catalog *Biochemicals, Organic Compounds, and Diagnostic Reagents*, Sigma Chemical Company, St. Louis MO, 1996–, in a section on Compounds. 1996 edition consulted.

Note in particular, with regard to Table 8.6, about three-fourths of the way through, that *platelet factor 4 fragment 58-70* acts as an *angiogenesis inhibitor*. Thus, conceivably, it could act against the formation of the vascular system of blood vessels within solid cancers.

In speaking further of chemical substances or compounds, above, there is a question of *purity*. It should be kept in mind that purification processes become increasingly involved and expensive as more stringent purification levels are reached. Thus, for chemicals as such, particularly inorganics, there are generally several grades, starting notably with the commercial grade or grades and progressing upward to the USP or pharmaceutical grade, suitable for human use, and finally to the analytical grade, the most nearly pure of all. Thus, in testing "pure" substances, there is the likelihood that contaminants may be present in varying degree, and the contaminants may be the more active constituents for the purposes at hand. (Pharmaceuticals also come in a grade or quality for animal or veterinary use—although there are some who contend that it all comes out of the same vat, and any differences may be in the degree of sterility maintained in bottling or packaging.)

The alternative is to use the naturally occurring or naturally derived substances, mostly "as is." And although, in some instances at least, it may be theoretically possible to analyze for the array of compounds

Table 8.4   Categories of Bioactive Peptides

Adrenocorticotropic Hormones (ACTH) and Fragments. Regulate adrenal cortex. Affect motivation, learning, and behavior.

Angiotensin and Related Peptides. Comprise enzyme substrates and inhibitors for renin-angiotensin system of renal hypertension.

Atrial Natriuretic Peptides (ANP). Have natriutetic (sodium- or salt-related), diuretic, and vasorelaxant effects, and affect blood volume and blood pressure hemeostasis.

Bradykinin and Related Peptides. Regulate fluid and electrolyte balance, smooth muscle contraction, vasodilation, and capillary permeability.

Chemotactic Peptides. Reported to be leukcyte chemoattractants that direct cell migration.

Dynorphin and Related Peptides. Family of endogenous opioid peptides having affinity for the kappa receptor.

Endorphins and β-Lipotropin Fragments. Affect analgesia, behavioral changes, and growth hormone release.

Enkephalin and Related Peptides. Include leucine enkophalin and methionine enkophalin that interact with opioid receptors.

Enzyme Inhibitors. Most are isolated from microbial sources. For further information, see Table 8.2

Fibronectin Fragments and Related Peptides. Large glycoproteins that favor cell-to-cell adhesion, cell-to-basement-membrane attachment, and clot stabilization.

Gastrointestinal Peptides. Found in the endocrine and nervous systems., these peptides are involved in functions of the gastrointestinal tract, pancreas, respiratory tract, and central nervous system.

Growth Hormone Releasing Peptides. Growth Hormone Releasing Factor (GRF) causes the release of the pituitary growth hormone (GH). Certain other short peptides are also noted to cause the release of the growth hormone.

Luteinizing Hormone Releasing Hormone (LH-RH) and Related Peptides. Also called the gonadotropin releasing hormone (GnRH), it is the principal mediator in the neuroregulation of the release of gonadtropins, and of the luteinizing hormone (LH) and the follicle stimulating hormone (FSH).

Melanocyte Stimulating Hormone (MSH) and Related Peptides. May play important part in the control of vertebrate pigment cell melanogenesis, neural functioning involving learning and behavior, and fetal development.

Neurotensin and Related Peptides. Involved in many pharmacological activities, e.g., hypertension, hyperglycemia, gut contraction, enhanced vascular permeability, the increased secretion of growth hormone, and hypothermic effects.

Opioid Peptides. Miscellaneous opioid peptides other than dynorphins, endorphins, and enkaphalins, and that elicit miscellaneous biological responses.

Oxytocin, Vasopressin, Vasotocin and Related Peptides. Peptide hormones with a wide spectrum of biological properties. Oxytocin for instance is involved in lactation and other female functions. Vasopressin causes antidiuresis and raises blood pressure. Both play a role in regulating the central nervous system.

Parathyroid Hormone (PTH) and Related Peptides. Modulates serum calcium concentration, thus affecting mineral and bone metabolism.

Protein Kinase Related Peptides. Act on target proteins by phosphorylating specific serine, threonine, and tyrosine residues. This is crucial to regulating many cellular processes.

Somatostatin and Related Peptides. Modulates physiological functions at such sites as the pituitary, pancreas, gut, and brain. Also inhibits the release of growth hormone, insulin, and glucagon.

Substance P and Related Peptides. Proposed as a neuromodulator connected with the transmission of pain. Also affects the contraction of smooth muscle, the reduction of blood pressure, and the stimulation of secretory tissue.

Miscellaneous Peptides. Some of the more interesting are listed in Table 8.6.

Source: Data from the catalog *Biochemicals, Organic Compounds, and Diagnostic Reagents*, Sigma Chemical Company, St. Louis MO, 1996–, in a section on Bioactive Peptides. 1996 edition consulted.

Table 8.5 A Listing of Bioactive Peptides that Act Specifically as Enzyme Inhibitors

n-Acetyl-LEU-LEU-methioninal. Calpain Inhibitor II.

n-Acetyl-LEU-LEU-norleucinal. Calpain Inhibitor II.

Acetyl pepstatin. Inhibitor for HIV-1 proteinase and HIV-2 proteinase.

Amastatin. (Zollner: inhibits aminopeptidase A; cytosol aminopeptidase)

(2S,3R)-3-Amino-2-hydroxy-4-(4-nitrophenyl)-butanoyl-L-leucine (hydrochloride). Analog of bestatin with five times the inhibitory activity.

Antipain (hydrochloride). Protease inhibitor.

Bestatin (hydrochloride). (Jain: inhibits aminopeptidase B)

Nα-t-BOC-deacetylleupeptin. Protease inhibitor.

Chymostatin. (Jain: inhibits chymotrypsin; protease, acid)

Conduritol B epoxide. Glucosidase inhibitor.

Elastatinal. (Jain: elastatinol inhibits elastase; Zollner: elastatinal inhibits leucocyte elastase)

Epiamastatin (hydrochloride). See Amastatin.

Epibestatin (hydrochloride). See Bestatin.

Foroxymithine. Angiotensin-converting enzyme inhibitor.

Histatin 5. Human salivary peptide that serves as an inhibitor for the protease of *Bacteroides gingivalis*, and of clostripain.

Leupeptin. Protease inhibitor.

Propionyl-Leupeptin (hemisulfate). Protease inhibitor.

NLE-STA-ALA-STA. Pepstatin analog, for inhibiting renin activity.

Pepsinostrepin. Complexes with pepsin and inhibits its activity.

Pepstatin A. Effective inhibitor for acid proteases, e.g., pepsin, renin, and cathepsin D.

N-(αRhamnopyranosyloxyhydroxyphosphinyl)-LEU-TRP.

Source: Data from the catalog *Biochemicals, Organic Compounds, and Diagnostic Reagents*, Sigma Chemical Company, St. Louis MO, 1996-, in a section on Bioactive Peptides and subsection on Enzyme Inhibitors. Abbreviations stand for amino acids. 1996 edition consulted.

---

present in a plant, which may already be known to some extent, the plant or plant substances is taken at "face value." The situation is complicated by the fact, moreover, that the plant compounds present may vary with geographic location and with the season, even with the soil—not to mention variations within the plant species itself.

If it is preferred instead to use a pure compound or compounds, however, the synthesis of the pure compound or compounds of interest may range from the difficult to the impossible, at least on a production basis. This can be further complicated by the problems of separation. Thus, it may sometimes be far simpler and far less costly to use the plant or plant substance, or extract.

As to just which plants or plant substances to test against the controlling enzymes in anaerobic glycolysis (read, lactic acid or lactate formation), there have been presentations of many potential anticancer possibilities in Parts 2 through 5, and in one way or another, in Appendices H through W, and also in Appendices X and Z. In many cases, these listings include the chemicals or compounds obtained by actual chemical analysis. There is the admonition of toxicity, however, and the fact that the

Table 8.6   Some Miscellaneous Bioactive Peptides that Act as Enzyme Inhibitors (or Activators) or Serve Other Purposes or Functions

[Ala^5-β-Ala^8]-α-Neurokinin fragment 4-10 (**anti-ulcer**)

[cys(bzl)]^{84}-fragment 81-92 (inhibits **HIV-1** induced cell fusion and infection)

adenylate cyclase activating polypeptide fragment 6-27 amide (inhibitor of PACAP-27)

adenylate cyclase activating polypeptide-38 (stimulates adenylate cyclase)

ALA-LYS-PRO-SER-TYR-HYP-HYP-THR-TYR-LYS (bioadhesive peptide)

amyloid β-protein fragment 1-40 (peptide that deposits in the brain of **Alzheimer's disease** patients)

C-reactive protein fragment 174-185 (enhances **tumoricidal** activity of human monocytes and alveolar macrophages)

calpain inhibitor peptide, carbomethoxycarbonyl-D-PRO-D-PHE benzyl ester (inhibits binding of protein of the **HIV-1 virus**)

carcinoembryonic antigen fragment 101-115 (possibly involved in **hepatic metastasis**)

CD4 fragments (cell surface glycoprotein receptor for **HIV** or **AIDS** virus)

cecropins (**antibacterial** peptides)

conotoxin M1 (blocks acetylcholine receptor)

CYS-ASP-PRO-GLY-TYR-ILE-GLY-SER-ARG amide (experimentally **inhibits metastasis**)

D-ALA-SER-THR-THR-ASN-TYR-THR amide (**HIV** inhibitor)

dermaseptin (**antifungal**)

exendin-4 (from venom, stimulates **cAMP increase** in pancreatic acini)

GLN-ARG-ARG-GLN-ARG-LYS-SER-ARG-ARG-THR-ILE (C-terminal sequence for human **interleukin-2** receptor)

GLY-GLY-HIS (**copper binding** peptide)

GLY-GLY-TYR-ARG (**papain** inhibitor)

GLY-PRO-GLY-GLY (inhibits dipeptidyk peptidase IV and inhibits entry of **HIV-1** or **HIV-2** into cell lines)

his-ASP-MET-ASN--LYS-VAL-LEU-ASP-LEU (**anti-inflammatory peptide** 2, inhibits phospholipase A$_2$)

HIS-PRO-PHE-HIS-LEU-D-LEU-VAL-TYR (**renin** inhibitor)

HIV envelope protein (gp 120) fragment 315-329 (causes production of **HIV-specific cytotoxic T lymphocytes**)

HIV-related peptide (list provided)

hypercalcemia of malignancy factor (a parathyroid hormone fragment)

indolicidin (**antibacterial and antifungal**)

interleukin-1β fragment 163-171 (**T cell activator** without inflammatory properties of interleukin-1)

LEU-LEU-methyl ester hydrobromide (toxic to natural killer cells)

MET-GLN-MET-LYS-LYS-VAL-LEU-ASP-SER (**anti-inflammatory** peptide 1)

N-acetyl-LEU-VAL-phenylalaninal (potent **HIV** protease inhibitor)

N-acetyl-THR-ILE-NLE-R-[CH2NH]-NLE-GLN-ARG amide (**HIV-1** protease inhibitor)

N-pro-Calcitonin (potent **bone-cell mitogen**)

Table 8.6 Some Miscellaneous Bioactive Peptides that Act as Enzyme Inhibitors (or Activators) or Serve Other Purposes or Functions *(continued)*

platelet factor 4 fragment 58-70 (**angiogenesis inhibitor**)

PRO-HIS-PRO-PHE-HIS-PHE-PHE-VAL-TYR-LYS (human renin inhibitor)

PRO-LEU-GLY amide (inhibits melanocyte-stimulating hormone)

PRO-THR-PRO-SER amide (IgA1 **proteinase** inhibitor)

pseudostellarin G (inhibits tyrosinase and melanin formation)

ranalexin (amphibian **antimicrobial** peptide)

sauvagine (releases ACTH and endorphins)

sendai virus nucleoprotein fragment 321-336 (peptide recognized by cytotoxic T lymphocytes and provides immunization in mice against lethal virus infections)

SER-GLN-ASN-PHE-R(CH2N)-PRO-ILE-VAL-GLN (**HIV-1** protease inhibitor)

THR-CYS-GLY (hemastopoietic cell adhesion peptide).

THR-VAL-LEU (**schizophrenia**- related peptide)

tuftsin fragment 1-3 (macrophage inhibitory peptide)

tumor necrosis factor-α

VAL-GLU-PRO-ILE-PRO-TYR (**immunostimulating peptide**)

VAL-PRO-ASP-PRO-ARG (**appetite suppressant**)

Source: Data from the catalog *Biochemicals, Organic Compounds, and Diagnostic Reagents,* Sigma Chemical Company, St. Louis MO, 1996-, in a section on Bioactive Peptides and subsection on Miscellaneous Peptides. 1996 ed.

Note: In many instances the amino acid sequences are denoted by three-letter capitalized groupings, e.g., SER-ARG-LEU-MET-PHE-..., etc., or by Ser-Arg-Leu-Met-Phe-..., etc. Fragments may be specified by a numbered interval. An inspection of the various peptide sources reveals that not only are bacterial sources represented, but insects, snails or mollusks, reptiles, and higher animals. Plant sources seem to be conspicuously absent. For further detailed information, the Sigma catalog may be consulted. A running account is provided rather than an itemization, with some of the potentially more interesting aspects highlighted in **boldface**. The main interest, of course, is whether one or another of these or other peptides could be used against cancer.

dosage level determines toxicity. Furthermore, there is the warning that plant substances or compounds that in any way act against respiration, and the central and autonomous nervous systems should be avoided. This includes cardiac arrest. Less deadly are those substances that are cytotoxic or cell-toxic, but here as well the word is avoidance. In other words, the search is for substances and compounds that act selectively against cancer cells—more specifically, substances that selectively block the enzymes of cancer cell metabolism, but not normal cell metabolism.

The presentations mentioned above are in the main by plant family, which is about as far as systemization can be carried out at this date. In other words, some plant families contain more bioactive genera and species than others, and some are more likely to contain say alkaloids of a particular class, alkaloids being the most bioactive plant substances of all.

This great degree of *bioactivity for alkaloids* may in large part be attributed to the *special nitrogen-containing ring structure* found in alkaloids, which indeed is for the most part the distinguishing feature defining the classification. This particular chemical structure may be presumed to enable these compounds to act as enzyme inhibitors in one way or another, such as by attachment to an active site on the enzyme molecule, which interferes with the functioning of the enzyme. In other words, alkaloids may block the biochemical purposes of enzymes and, in the broader sense, act as enzyme-catalyst poisons. Furthermore, a particular alkaloid may specifically affect a particular enzyme or group of enzymes, and this effect

Table 8.7   Assorted Antibodies and Immunochemicals

Monoclonal Antibodies to Human IgG Subclasses. Antibodies for Human IgG1 through IgG4.

Monoclonal Antibodies to Human Immunoglobulins. Include antibodies to Human IgA. IgA1, IgD, IgE, EgG. IgM, Kappa Light Chains, Lambda Light Chains, Human Secretory Component.

Monoclonal Antibodies to Human Antigens. Include antibodies to Human glycoprotein, serum albumin, alkaline phosphatase, serum amyloid P component, antithrombin III, C-reactive protein (CRP), epithelial specific antigen (ESA), factors V-X, fibrinogin, macrophages, neutrophils, proteins C and S, thyroglobulin, etc. Notable among the listing are antibodies to **Human carcinoembryonic antigen or CEA.** (An antigen or foreign body acts as a toxin, normally stimulating the formation of antibodies—or "anti-antigens.") The antibody or **anti**human carcinoembryonic antigen is produced using CEA isolated from a human colon adenocarcinoma cell line as an immunogen. **The antibody acts specifically against human CEA from several types of malignant tissues including colorectal, lung, and breast tumors. The product reacts strongly with the cell surface and cytoplasm of malignant glands in colorectal adenocarcinomas.** Weak reactivity occurs with normal colon mucosa and occasionally with bile canilacular and pancreatic acinar cells.

Monoclonal Antibodies to Human Red Cell Antigens. Comprise antibodies to Band 3, glycophorin A (α), glycophorin A, B (α,δ), glycophorin C (β), and red cell Wrb antigen.

Species Specific Monoclonal Antibodies to Animal Immunoglobulins. Include Bovine IgG, Cat IgG, Chicken IgG, Dog IgG, Goat/Sheep IgG, Guinea Pig IgG, Hamster IgG, Mouse Kappa and Lambda Light Chains, Rabbit IgG, Rat IgA -IgM, Rat Kappa and Lambda Light Chains, etc.

Monoclonal Antibodies to Hormones and Drugs. Include antibodies to digoxin, folic acid, human growth hormone, insulin, progesterone, vitamin B12.

Monoclonal Antibodies to Enzymes. Include antibodies to alkaline phosphatase, ATpase, carboxypeptidase, CNPase, β-galactosidase, glucose oxidase, glutathione-S-transferase, peroxidase, prostatic acid phosphatase, terminal deoxynucleotidyl transferase, tyrosine hydroxylase, urease. No antibodies are listed for any of the enzymes involved in (anaerobic) glycolysis.

Miscellaneous Monoclonal Antibodies. Include antibodies to bovine serum albumin, chicken egg albumin, hemocyanin, phycoerythrin, mouse ascites fluid.

Other immunochemicals of cancer-related interest include the following entries from the same Sigma catalog section, with acronyms supplied.

Hepatocyte Growth Factor (HGF). Stimulates growth of hepatocytes. **Inhibits mouse melanoma cells, human squamous carcinoma cells, and human hepatoma cells.**

Interferons (IFN). Of the several interferons, interferon-γ is said to have antitumor effects. It is produced by activated T cells and natural killer cells that are stimulated by alloantigens, tumors, and mitogens. It is noted to activate macrophages, boost the cytoxicity of natural killer cells, and stimulate T cell cytoxicity.

Interleukins (IL). Interleukins 1α and 1β on through 12. Variously activate T cells, and have other effects and side effects.

Leukemia Inhibitory Factor (LIF). Suppresses the proliferation of the murine (rodent, e.g., mouse or rat) M1 myeloid leukemia cell line, and inhibits the differentiation of other cells.

Stem Cell Factor (SCF). A potent stimulator for human and murine bone marrow cells.

Transforming Growth Factor-β (TGF-β). Inhibits growth of hepatocytes, epithelial cells, T and B lymphocytes.

Tumor Necrosis Factors (TNF). Both TNF-α and TNF-β exhibit antitumor activity, and TNF-α is undergoing clinical testing for the treatment of certain cancers.

Source: Data from the catalog *Biochemicals, Organic Compounds, and Diagnostic Reagents,* Sigma Chemical Company, St. Louis MO, 1996-, in a section on Immunochemicals. 1996 edition consulted.

Note: According to the Sigma catalog, monoclonal antibodies are produced from hybridomas generated from the fusion of spleen cells of immunized mice with myeloma cells. After cloning, the hybridomas are used to produce antibodies in cell cultures or ascites fluid. Other immunochemicals are produced in other ways. For additional information, consult the Sigma catalog. The main interest here, of course, is whether such antibodies could be formed that would act against cancer cells.

may be moderated or enhanced by still other features of the chemistry and structure of the particular alkaloid. Thus, different alkaloids will behave differently in their role as enzyme inhibitors. That is to say, some are poisonous in the extreme, adversely affecting some vital body function or functions in one way or another, but others are much less so.

As to a cancer cure, the objective is to find, say, an alkaloid or alkaloidal substance that would interfere with cancer cell metabolism *only* and would not noticeably interfere with normal cell metabolism, in particular as pertains to the functions of such vital organs as the heart and lungs, and the liver and kidneys.

The best of all worlds, of course, would be to find foods or food substances that act as enzyme inhibitors for cancer cell metabolism. And this may involve, in particular, determining enzyme inhibitors for anaerobic glycolysis. Of a certainty, *vitamins and minerals* may be included under the category of food substances, either in the foods or as the chemical compounds per se, better known as nutritional supplements. Vitamins and minerals are bioactive substances, some of which have been noted to have some sort of a beneficial effect in cancer treatment. To what extent seems largely unresolved. To name two examples, there are ongoing studies on folic acid and on vitamin A, with the possibility that still others may yet prove demonstrably effective. The same goes for minerals or mineral compounds, such as selenium and germanium, as discussed in Moss's *Cancer Therapy* and Walters' *Options*. Some exist in plants, usually in trace amounts, and are derived from the soil.*

The more common mineral or metallic compounds such as of sodium, potassium, calcium, magnesium, iron ... may play roles in cancer cell inhibition yet to be determined. Dosage levels will no doubt play a part, inasmuch as some (or all) of these mineral compounds can be toxic—depending on the concentration.

Studies at the University of Wisconsin Comprehensive Cancer Center (UWCCC) indicate that the *oil from lavender flowers has anticancer activity.* The work, by scientist Michael Gould, first focused on a family of natural substances called *monoterpenes* that *shrink tumors in laboratory animals.* The investigation was subsequently extended to humans, using perillyl alcohol as found in the oil from lavender flowers. It is noted that *monoterpenes apparently exhibit anticancer activity against breast, prostate, ovarian, liver, and pancreatic tumors, and against leukemias. Not only do they act as cancer-prevention agents but as therapeutic agents against existing tumors.* Whether this anticancer action is as an enzyme inhibitor was not specified. (It may be added that Hartwell's *Plants Used Against Cancer* lists several species of *lavender*, which are of the genus *Lavandula* of the family Labiatae.)

Even such bland and apparently innocuous foods as the common *banana, Musa sapientum* of the family Musaceae, may have phytochemicals of some sort that interfere with cancer cell metabolism—or at least it is listed in Hartwell's *Plants Used Against Cancer.* (Maybe the purported extra-high potassium content has something to do with it.)

Incidentally, although Hartwell indicates it has been used (or tried) against cancer in the South American countries of Brazil and Venezuela (not to mention England as well), it said that edible bananas are not native to South America (Shoumatoff, *The Rivers Amazon*, p. 80). It is thought that the banana came originally from the Burma-Thailand area of southwestern Asia (Shoumatoff cites T.W. Purseglove's three-volume *Tropical Crops*). From there it was taken to Africa by the Portuguese, then to the Canary Islands, and finally to the New World. Now, every tropical forest tribe in South America has access to bananas, for reasons yet to be explained. The movement of other plant families and species is attributed to continental drift and other geologic upheavals, or to still other phenomena (Shoumatoff, *The Rivers Amazon*, pp. 111–113). Thus, for example, Central America is presumed to have risen from the sea and formed a land bridge for the movement of species both north and south, and both plant and animal. While firs, alders, sweetgums, beeches, walnuts, and elms went south, the South American creosote bush for instance—native to the drylands of Argentina—headed north to become a folkloric remedy in Mexico and the American Southwest.

---

* The more active metals are rarely found uncombined and usually exist as an oxide, sulfide, or chloride, and so forth. In the raw form, these substances occur in varying concentrations with major nonmetallic impurities, mostly earthen compounds of silica and aluminum in the form of silicates or aluminates, or some chemical combination of the two, and the bulk mixtures are then referred to as *ores*. For maximum absorptivity in the human body system, minerals may be chemically combined with organic structures, a process also called *chelation*, which enhances solubility and uptake by the body.

Figs, of the genus *Ficus* (of the Mulburry family or family Moraceae), appear in medical folklore as anticancer agents, as per Hartwell's compilation. In William Langewiesche's *Sahara Unveiled,* published in 1996, it is mentioned that *dates,* the fruit of the date palm (species *Phoenix dactylifera* of the family Palmae or Arecaceae), are under investigation as anticancer agents (Langewiesche, *Sahara,* p. 119).*

The family Erythroxylaceae makes Hartwell in several species designated as of the genus *Erythroxylum.* This is the genus otherwise known as *Erythroxylon,* of which *E. coca* or *E. truxillense* furnishes the familiar *coca leaf,* the source of the concentrated alkaloid *cocaine* for the drug traffic (Cordell, *Introduction to Alkaloids,* p. 102). The word supplied is that merely chewing the leaf is only mildly problematical and that, in addition, the leaf furnishes many nutrients. The leaf called khat or kat (or qat), the favorite chew of the Mideast and East Africa, does not make Hartwell, however. Known and used for perhaps 3000 years, the leaf is of the species *Catha edulis* of the family Celastraceae, and contains several alkaloids, notably *d*-norpseudoephedrine (Cordell, *Introduction to Alkaloids,* p. 287).

In his book *The Rivers Amazon,* published by the Sierra Club in 1978, Alex Shoumatoff mentioned that *the Coca-Cola Company imports 500 tons of coca annually* (Shoumatoff, *Rivers,* p. 227). It may be reliably assumed that this is used for *flavoring only,* and that *all of the cocaine content has been extracted and immolated.*

In Michael Swan's *The Marches of El Dorado: British Guiana, Brazil, Venezuela,* published in 1958, another commercial product is mentioned, namely *Flit®,* which once contained a chemical substance derived from a bush-rope evidently called Ishal and used by the natives as a fish poison (Swan, *Marches,* p. 169). Swan was traveling through the savannahs of southern British Guiana, now Guyana, in the country generally of tribes of a branch of the West Indian Carib Indians, once known for cannibalism or anthropophagy. (Appendix B of Swan's book is devoted to the Caribs.) This substance is very likely *rotenone,* or similar to it, a poisonous crystalline ketone with the stoichiometric formula $C_{23}H_{22}O_6$, used as both a fish poison and an insecticide. (Rotenone proper is obtained from the roots of East Indian plants of the genus *Derris,* and from neotropical plants of the genus *Lonchocarpus,* both being of the family Leguminosae. A species of the latter genus is listed in Hartwell's *Plants Used Against Cancer.*) On the next page of his book, Swan has a few things to say about the modus operandi of tribal medicine men.

> They have their sessions in their hut at night in the dark, and they're wonderful ventriloquists. They can fill a hut with strange noises that they say are the spirits. They're terrible frauds.

As to North America, the Plains Indians used the crushed roots of *Tephrosia virginiana* (of the family Leguminosae) as a fish poison. A common name is goat's rue (although it is not of the Rue family or family Rutaceae), an dit is also the common name for the European plant Galega officinalis. Other names are cat gut, turkey pea, rabbit pea, and devil's shoestring. Found in dry areas, the flowers are spectacular, combining yellow and purple, and are remindful of the sweetpea *Lathyrus odoratus,* itself of the family Leguminosae, and it also displays toxicity. Certain species of milkweed have also been known to be used as native fish poisons.

It goes almost without saying that clinical testing and clinical therapy should start out with extremely small amounts of any therapeutic agent tried and proceed from there. *Of particular interest, therefore, is the point-wise or near-instantaneous measurement of efficacy.* In other words, at any particular moment, is the agent doing its job? And without toxic side effects, which also need to be monitored. If not, adjustments (or substitutions) need to be made, immediately. It is analogous to the well known *feedback* loop as used in industrial processes, whereby the measurement of a process variable (or variables) is used to control the process. The same biofeedback can be applied to cancer treatment if the necessary measurements or indications can be obtained expeditiously, on the spot or nearly so.

---

* Other interesting information is supplied, such that date palms can utilize water 10 times more salty than humans can consume; that dates have an arresting vitamin and mineral content, with dried dates consisting of half sugar; and furthermore that the deep water found under the Sahara is "old" water from confined aquifers, that is, so-called geopressured or abnormally pressured reservoirs or formations, sealed off from their surroundings (namely the natural aquifer), and which when drilled into may flow as artesian wells and may even have to be capped to prevent flooding (Langewiesche, *Sahara,* pp. 116, 118, 120).

As indicated previously, this measurement might be made indirectly, for instance in terms of the buildup of lactic acid or lactate from anaerobic glycolysis, or of the enzyme lactate dehydrogenase, or of the amino acid alanine, said to be a marker for anaerobic glycolysis as per the work of Guerra et al.

The Sigma catalog contains additional information that may be of potential interest and relevance, as follows: Venoms (under "Compounds"); a section titled "Molecular Biology Products," regarding DNA/RNA studies and nucleic acids; a section titled "Tissue Culture Media and Reagents" with subsections variously dealing with Sera, Antiboiotics, Growth Factors, Hormones, Lectins, and Lipopolysaccharides, and so forth.

8.4 ENZYME INHIBITORS FOR MELANOMA

The metabolic processes for melanoma are different from those for solid tumors (and both are different from processes for blood-related tumors). In specialized cells called melanocytes, there is the conversion of *tyrosine* to *levodopa*, which is in turn converted to the pigment *melanin*. The tyrosine conversion requires the action of the enzyme known as *tyrosinase*. If there is an excess of tyrosinase, melanoma may develop. Accordingly, there is an interest in enzyme inhibitors for tyrosinase, and this very possibly may be the role played by the yucca/arctic sunflower extract mentioned previously, the result of the work by retired University of Wyoming chemistry professor Owen Asplund, noted elsewhere.*

For the record, a listing of tyrosinase inhibitors is provided in Table 8.8, as obtained from Jain's *Handbook*. Zollner's *Handbook* has listings for tyrosine aminotransferase, tyrosine 3-monooxygenase, tyrosine phenol-lyase, and tyrosine-tRNA ligase, with their corresponding code numbers as found in the reference volume *Enzyme Nomenclature*. (Jain lists some of these inhibitors as well.) The Sigma catalog lists the enzyme tyrosinase.

The compounds of most interest as tyrosinase inhibitors are highlighted. Thus, *ascorbic acid* or *vitamin C* appears prominently. Also the several *halide ions. Butyric acid,* a butter constituent, is a presumed cancer inhibitor. *Lactic acid,* the final product of anaerobic glycolysis and cancer-cell metabolism, is on the list. (It is also a component of sour milk or buttermilk.) *Oxalic acid* is an inhibitor for one or more of the steps in glycolysis. *Formic acid* is an active agent in ant stings—and bee stings are cited elsewhere as a potential cause for melanoma. Other components in ant stings include toxins that contain large amounts of fatty acids rather than short-chain protein molecules (or peptides). Histamines and hemolytic factors are present as well as formic acid, and fire ants have venom that contains unique alkaloids. (Andrew Mallis, *Handbook of Pest Control*, sixth edition, p. 428). *Tyrosine,* interestingly, is listed as an inhibitor (ordinarily tyrosine, the reactant, would favor the conversion to the levodopa product). And not to be overlooked is *cyanide ion,* as per Laetrile or amygdalin.

8.5 PHYTOCHEMICALS THAT MAY ACT AGAINST CANCER

There are a very few sources for plant chemicals or phytochemicals per se that may act against cancer. A principal source is by James A. Duke, titled *Handbook of Biologically Active Phytochemicals and Their Activities*. It is a companion book to Duke's *Handbook of Phytochemical Constituents of GRAS Herbs and Other Economic Plants*, which has been cited for instance in Part 3. Another potential source is *Hager's Handbuch der Pharmazeutischen Praxis*, also previously cited.

There is a computer-generated database of this sort of information on phytochemicals available from Dr. James A. Duke via the World Wide Web at the following Internet address:

http://www.ars-grin.gov./~ngrlsb/

Further information may be obtained from the Herbal Vineyard, Inc., 8210 Murphy Road, Fulton MD 20759. It may be noted in passing that Duke is also the author of *The Green Pharmacy*, a popularized book about herbal remedies, which contains a chapter or section on cancer prevention that emphasizes a vegetarian-type diet—but avoids any specifics about a cancer cure.

---

* What are called *freckles* are the result of the pigment cells responding unevenly to sunlight. The melanin pigment is laid down irregularly, appearing as benign freckles. These are as distinguished from birthmarks or *nevi*, which can occasionally become cancerous.

Table 8.8   Enzyme Inhibitors for Tyrosinase

Acetic acid, phenyl-	Anisic acid
Ascorbic acid	Benzamide
Benzoic acid	Benzoic acid, 4-hydroxy-
Bromide ion	**Butyric acid**
Carbamate, diethyldithio-	**Chloride ion**
Cyanide ion	Cyclohexane carboxylic acid
Diethylcarbamate	**Fluoride ion**
Formic acid	Fusaric acid
Indole derivatives	Indole-3-acetic acid, 5-hydroxy-
Indole, 5-hydroxy-	**Iodide ion**
Lactic acid	Minosine, L-
Oxalic acid	Phenylzine
Phenylalanine, L-	Phenylalanine, p-fluoro-DL-
Phthalic acid	Phthalic acid, ter-
Pyruvic acid, phenyl-	Thio reactants
Thiourea	Tryptophan, 5-hydroxy-DL-
Tyrosinase inhibitor	**Tyrosine**
Tyrosine, M-Fluro-DL	Tyrosine, N-acetyl-L-
Tyrosine, N-formyl-L-	Tyrosine, 3-Amino-L
Tyrosine, 3-Fluoro-L	Veratric acid

Source: Data from *Handbook of Enzyme Inhibitors*, 1965–1977 by M.K. Jain, Wiley, New York, 1982.

Another herbal information source is from Michael Moore, whose several books have been cited elsewhere. There is, in this regard, an Internet address, as follows:

http//chili.rt66.com/hrbmoore/HOMEPAGE

The business name and new mailing address are: Southwest School of Botanical Medicine, P.O. Box 4565, Bisbee AZ 85603. As part of the information supplied, the chemical constituents or phytochemicals in some 250 different medicinal plant species are listed.

With further regard to herbs per se, other organizational names include the Herb Research Foundation at Boulder CO, which operates in conjunction with the American Botanical Center in Austin TX. They jointly publish an HerbalGram. There is also the American Herbalists Guild.

A selection of phytochemicals that may act against cancer has been made from the first-mentioned reference work by James A. Duke, above, and is presented in Appendix W. One or another of these chemicals could conceivably be tried against a lactic acid-producing culture to see if anaerobic glycolysis could be stopped. Presumably the tests should be made in an inert or oxygen-free atmosphere.

Another qualification would be to try to select phytochemicals known to be *nontoxic* at the dosage levels used or anticipated. That is, no adverse side effects are admissible.

As a means of further introducing the subject, Table 8.9 contains a miscellany of phytochemicals or other plant substances selected from Appendix W and from Part 4, notably the bioactive constituents of common garden vegetables and fruits. For the most part, these compounds are alkaloids, but there are exceptions. For instance, Laetrile or amygdalin is mentioned, about which more can be said, and that serves to distinguish the points of view.

The substances listed in Table 8.9 are commercially available, e.g., from the Sigma Chemical Company, St. Louis MO, and/or from the Aldrich Chemical Company, Milwaukee WI and St. Louis MO.

One may observe that the alkaloids *vincristine* and *vinblastine*, used against blood-related cancers such as leukemia, are each classed as a **highly toxic teratogen**—that is, a substance that damages the fetus. (Apart from this, they are also cytotoxic—that is, are toxic to all cells.) Other compounds are variously listed as **toxic** or **highly toxic**.

And speaking of cytotoxic, the conventional chemotherapy drug 5-*fluorouracil* is described as **highly toxic**, whereas uracil has no such descriptor. The chemotherapy drug **methotrexate** (amethopterin hydrate) is described as a **highly toxic teratogen** that is a folic acid antagonist and a potent inhibitor of the enzyme dihydrofolate reductase.

Laetrile or *amygdalin* is listed as a matter of course. As noted, amygdalin has been given the chemical name D-mandelonitrile 6-O-β-d-glucosido-β-D-glucoside, or D-mandelonitrile β-gentiobioside (strictly speaking, the former is amygdalin, the latter is laetrile). Accordingly, *mandelonitrile* is also listed, along with some of its compounds.*

8.5.1 LAETRILE AGAIN?

Continuing on with the controversial subject of Laetrile or laetrile, Varro E. Tyler, in *The Honest Herbalist*, challenges Laetrile's proponents about the role of enzymes. Thus it is believed by Laetrile advocates that an enzyme called β-*glucosidase* exists in large amounts in tumorous tissue but not in the rest of the body (Tyler, *The Honest Herbalist*, p. 32). Moreover, it is said that this enzyme is capable of breaking down Laetrile to release toxic cyanide. And these proponents "further hypothesize that another enzyme, rhodanese [sic], which has the ability to detoxify cyanide, is present in normal tissues but deficient in cancer cells." Tyler concludes that no scientific proof for this proposed mechanism has ever been presented.†

Begging the latter point for the time being, the fact remains that these two enzymes are commercially available from the Sigma Chemical Company. The first-mentioned, β-*glucosidase*, is obtained from almonds (also a source for Laetrile) and is alternatively called β-D-glucoside glucohydrolase (Sigma catalog). Its activity is described as being such that one unit will liberate 1.0 μmole (micromole) of glucose from *salicin* per minute at pH 5.0 at 37° C, which is a slightly acidic condition, where a pH of 7.0 is neutral, and higher pH levels are alkaline or basic.‡

The second-mentioned, *rhodanese*, is obtained from bovine liver and is alternatively called thiosulfate sulfurtransferase or thiosulfate cyanide sulfurtransferase (Sigma catalog). Its activity is such that one unit will convert 1.0 μmole of *cyanide* **to** *thiocyanate* per minute at pH 8.6 at 25° C. It may be noted that the spelling "rhodanese" is used in the Sigma catalog, albeit Tyler questions this particular spelling (enzymes customarily should end in "-ase").

---

* In common with some other chemicals, the prefix "D-" signifies that the above compounds are optically active. In other words, they or their solutions will exhibit either *dextro* or *levo* rotary properties. That is, they will cause a polarized beam of light to rotate either to the right or to the left. These optical properties are further designated respectively by the prefixes D- or *d*- or (+) and by the prefixes L- or *l*- or (-), or by both—and are called a *racemic modification*, where the one cancels out the other.

† For more about the enzyme β-glucosidase, consult Part 6 within the section "Intestinal Flora and Cancer," in the subsection "Bacterial Metabolism and Carcinogens," which has entries for β-glucosidase and for enzyme inhibitors. Additional information is presented in Part 6 within the section "Hydrolysis and Other Interactions between Intestinal Flora and Ingested Chemical Types," in the subsection titled "Glycosides." The enzyme β-glucosidase is common enough and is involved in bacterial-related metabolism in the gut, serving as the catalyst for the hydrolysis of various glucosides, including cyanic glucosides, whereby the toxic cyanic aglycone results.

‡ *Salicin* is a glucopyranoside. Whether the particular enzyme will liberate cyanide from Laetrile or amygdalin is not stated. Suffice it to say, however, that Laetrile is a cyanoglycoside or cyanoglucoside, and very possibly, in liberating glucose, cyanide will also be liberated.

Table 8.9   Miscellaneous Compounds or Substances that May Act as Enzyme Inhibitors for Anaerobic Glycolysis or Cancer Cell Metabolism

Abrin, from *Abrus precatorius* or jequirity bean (Sigma). Listed under Lectins (proteins or glycoproteins of non-immune origin that agglomerate cells and/or precipitate complex carbohydrates). Contains two major toxic proteins, **highly toxic.**

Acetylcholine chloride (Aldrch), **irritant.**

Aconitine (Aldrich), **highly toxic.**

(+)-Amethopterin hydrate or L-Amethopterin hydrate (Aldrich, Sigma), **highly toxic teratogen.** Folic acid antagonist and potent inhibitor of dihydrofolate reductase.

(−)-Amethopterin hydrate or L-Amethopterin hydrate. Same as above.

(α)-Amethopterin hydrate or DL-Amethopterin hydrate. Same as above.

L-Amygdalin, from apricot kernels (Sigma). Also known as D-mandelonitrile 6-O-β-d-glucosido-β-D-glucoside; or D-mandelonitrile β-gentiobioside.

Betaine (Aldrich)

(+)-Borneol (Aldrich,), **flammable solid.**

[(1S)-endo]-(−)-Borneol (Aldrich), **flammable solid, toxic.**

Caffeine (Aldrich), **toxic.**

Campesterol (Aldrich), **flammable liquid, irritant.**

Camphor (Aldrich), **flammable solid, irritant.**

Camptothecin (Sigma)

Candelilla wax (Aldrich)

Capsaican (Aldrich). Also known as *trans*-8-methyl-N-vanillyl-6-nonenamide, **highly toxic irritant.**

Cartilage, bovine (Sigma)

Castor bean acetone powder (Sigma), **warning: extremely dangerous.**

Chrysophanic acid (Aldrich)

DL-Citrulline (Aldrich)

(α) Coniine (Sigma)

Ellipticine (Aldrich), **toxic.**

Emodin (Aldrich), **irritant.**

(1R,2S)-(−)-Ephedrine (Aldrich), **toxic irritant.**

Eugenol (Aldrich), **irritant.**

5-Fluorouracil (Aldrich), **highly toxic corrosive inhibitor of DNA synthesis.**

Folic acid dihydrate (Aldrich), **light sensitive.**

(+)-Glaucine (Sigma)

Gramine (Aldrich)

Harmaline (Aldrich)

Harmine (Aldrich)

Hordenine (Sigma)

Hyoscine, see Scopolamine

Hyoscyamine (Sigma)

Inulin, from chicory root (Aldrich)

Jojoba bean, meal, oil (Sigma,)

Juglone (Sigma)

Kaempferol (Sigma)

L-Citrulline (Aldrich)

L-Hyoscyamine (Sigma)

Laetrile, see Amygdalin

Linnalool (Aldrich)

(−)-Lobeline hydrochloride (Adrich), **toxic.**

Mandelonitrile or DL-Mandelonitrile (Aldrich; Sigma), **toxic.** See Amygdalin.

D-Mandelonitrile acetate (Sigma)

D-Mandelonitrile β-D-glucoside (Sigma)

Methotrexate, see Amethopterin

S-Methyl-L-cysteine (Aldrich)

Muscarine chloride (Sigma)

Table 8.9 Miscellaneous Compounds or Substances that May Act as Enzyme Inhibitors for Anaerobic Glycolysis or Cancer Cell Metabolism *(continued)*

(S)-(–)-Nicotine (Aldrich), **highly toxic irritant.**

NDGA, see Nordihydroguaiaretic acid

Nordihydroguaiaretic acid or NDGA (Aldrich; Sigma), **irritant.** From *Larrea divaricata* (creosote bush or chaparral).

Paclitaxel (Sigma Aldrich), **toxic irritant.**

Pilocarpine hydrochloride, nitrate (Sigma)

Piperidine (Aldrich)

Putrescine (Sigma)

Pyrrolidine (Aldrich)

Quercetin dihydrate (Aldrich; Sigma), **toxic, suspected cancer agent.**

Acts as enzyme inhibitor for mitochondrial ATPase and phosphodiesterase.

Quinidine (Aldrich)

Quinine (Aldrich), **toxic irritant.**

Rhein (Aldrich; Sigma), **irritant.** Oxidation product of aloe-emodin.

Ricin, from *Ricinus communis* or castor bean plant (Sigma). Listed under Lectins, **warning: extremely hazardous!** Be aware of the risks and familiar with safety procedures before using this product.

(+)-Rutin hydrate (Aldrich, p. 1305)

Sanguinarine chloride (Aldrich)

Saponins (Sigma)

Scopolamine hydrochloride (Sigma)

Shikimic acid (Aldrich)

β-Sitosterol (Aldrich)

Solanidine, from potato (Sigma)

α-Solanine, from potato sprouts (Sigma)

Solasodine (Sigma)

Solasodine (Sigma).

Spermidine (Aldrich), **corrosive.**

Spermine (Aldrich), **corrosive.**

Strychnine (Aldrich), **highly toxic.**

Tannic acid (Aldrich)

Tannin, see Tannic acid

Taxol, see Paclitaxel

Theobromine (Sigma)

Theophylline (Aldrich), **toxic.**

o-Toluidine (Aldrich), **highly toxic, suspected cancer agent.**

m-Toluidine (Aldrich), **highly toxic, suspected cancer agent.**

p-Toluidine (Aldrich), **highly toxic, suspected cancer agent.**

Tomatidine hydrochloride (Sigma). Contains up to 10% solasodine.

Tomatine (Sigma). Also called lycopersicin.

Tomato powder (Sigma)

Trigonelline (Sigma)

Tyramine (Aldrich), **irritant.**

Uracil (Aldrich)

Vinblastine sulfate (Aldrich), **highly toxic teratogen.** (Causes fetus deformation)

Vincamine (Aldrich)

Vincristine sulfate (Aldrich), **highly toxic teratogen.** (Causes fetus deformation).

Yohimbine (Aldrich), **highly toxic, light-sensitive.**

Yohimbine hydrochloride (Aldrich), **highly toxic, light-sensitive.**

Source: Data from the catalog *Biochemicals, Organic Compounds, and Diagnostic Reagents,* Sigma Chemical Company, St. Louis MO, 1996- and from the 1996–1997 *Catalog/Handbook of Fine Chemicals,* Aldrich Chemical Company, Milwaukee WI and St. Louis MO. *Note:* Descriptive comments are provided, where applicable. In some instances the entries occur in both sources.

Given the above information, it should be easy enough to test Laetrile using these enzymes. The question is, however, how do cancer cells react *in vitro* and *in vivo* vis à vis normal cells. Presumably this has been tested, but the results seem not to be readily available. And clinical results seem shrouded in mystery.

Further confusing the subject, there is an enzyme named *mandelonitrile lyase,* derived from almonds (Sigma catalog, Aldrich catalog). Its activity is such that one unit will form 1.0:mole of benzaldehyde and HCN from mandelonitrile per min. at pH 5.4 at 25° C. *Benzaldehyde, incidentally, is the characteristic odor of decomposed almonds* rather than hydrogen cyanide or HCN, which is odorless. The two go together, however.*

Compounding the problem, of course, is the fact that *HCN can act as an enzyme inhibitor for other vital body processes.* In particular, we are concerned about the carboxylic acid cycle of cell *respiration.* Besides this, there is the concern about cardiac arrest, caused for instance by what are called *cardiac glycosides* or *glucosides,* or by yet other substances.

Beyond this are problems that can be induced in the kidneys and liver, notably, categorized as nephrotoxicity and hepatotoxicity, not to mention other organs of the body, including the lungs and brain. In other words, the substances may conceivably act as enzyme inhibitors for vital body processes.

At the same time, *these kinds of adverse side effects can also be encountered with pharmaceutical drugs, as distinguished from plant or herbal substances.* It is, unfortunately, a feature of conventional cytotoxic or cell-toxic chemotherapy drugs as used against cancer that they act as well against all other cells in the body.

The objective, therefore, is to determine what substance or substances will act *selectively* against cancer cells without harming normal cells and their functions. Sometimes, as a last resort, it may be playing one thing against another, the trade-off of *benefits versus toxicity.* On the other hand, it may be not so much a question of the toxicity of the particular substance itself but of dosage levels and how it is administered. For there is a matter of degree whereby at one (lower) dosage level the substance may be beneficial, but at another (higher dosage) level may prove toxic and/or carcinogenic. And with some overtly toxic substances, the lower effective dosage level may be minute indeed, if it can be used at all.

Bitter almonds, for instance, have a much higher and more lethal amygdalin content than do confectionery or sweet almonds. According to the concluding chapter in Alan Schom's *Napoleon Bonaparte,* Napoleon met his final end from a dose of the oil of bitter almonds that had been put into a drink. Leading up to this, he had been systematically poisoned by arsenic added to his medicines.

8.5.2 THE HUNZAS AND APRICOT KERNELS

Albeit a few apricot or peach kernels are not considered harmful in some quarters, there are others who view the situation oppositely. However, in this regard, consider a book written by Ian Stephens and published in 1955 by the University of Indiana Press. Titled *Horned Moon: An Account of a Journey through Pakistan, Kashmir, and Afghanistan,* Stephens made a visit to the Hunzas (or Hunzakuts or Hanzawals) and their neighbors the Nagers (or Nagerwals), located on each side of the Hunza River in the canyons of the northwestern Himalayan massif, here named the Karakoram Range, one of the three great mountain ranges of the Himalayas, the other major ranges being the Everest Range and the Hindu Kush Range. Apricots were found to play a major role in the local economy—although apples, pears, peaches, cherries, and mulberries were also grown (Stephens, *Horned Moon,* pp. 169–170). In fact, apricot trees were planted with the ubiquity of potatoes.

The flesh of the ripe apricot fruit is eaten both fresh and dried, but the *kernel* is considered the more important, to be eaten as is, like a hard almond, or ground into flour or meal for bread and cakes. In turn the flour or meal is pressed to yield a valuable oil. In sum, the kernel has been judged as *exceptionally nutritious.* Stephens himself subsisted on apricot kernels in his travels, with a few raisins thrown in.

The vigorous health of these people was attributed to the dietary apricot factor, and maybe something in the water. An elderly man of confirmed age 97 looked and acted like 65. And the great stamina of

---

* While on the subject, the names amygdalin and Laetrile or laetrile are often used synonymously, although there is a slight difference in chemical makeup. Thus, the proper scientific name for amygdalin has been given as mandelonitrile β-gentiobioside, whereas the proper name for Laetrile or laetrile has been given as mendelonitrile β-glucoronide. The particulars, including the structural formula, are furnished in the *Dictionary of Plant Toxins,* edited by Jeffrey B. Harborne and Herbert Baxter. These chemical names are at variance with the versions appearing in the Sigma catalog.

the Hunzawals (and Nagerwals) on mountain expeditions was said by some to be even superior to that of the Sherpas of Nepal.

A subsequent book about the Hunzas, by Allen E. Banik and Renée Taylor, was published in 1960 as *Hunza Land: The Fabulous Health and Youth Wonderland of the World.* Directed more at nutritional aspects, there is a chapter on farming and food. The grains produced include wheat, barley, buckwheat, corn, millet, alfalfa, and rye. In addition to the fruits already named, watermelons and grapes are added—even a grape wine. Vegetables include potatoes, tomatoes, carrots, onions, garlic, peas, beans, and pulses. The nuts raised were restricted to walnuts. Goat milk was used for butter and cheese (with some cheeses extraordinarily well aged). Meat is scarce, confined mainly to mutton, and eggs are imported only for the wealthy and the royal family—with chickens suspect, due to their scratching up seeds and crops.*

Special attention is given to apricots as a staple, where the trees are allowed to grow for about 50 years, then cropped at about twenty feet from the ground, and afterward allowed to grow and produce for another 50 years or so—with prodigious yields. The huge trunks rival forest trees in size, and the apricot trees themselves are viewed as valuable property.

The apricot flesh is described as extra-sweet, but the seed kernels are considered the best part of the fruit. The kernels taste sweet and oily, a good deal like almonds. (The apricot is, of course, of the genus *Prunus* of the plant family Rosaceae, along with peaches and almonds.) The apricot oil looks a good deal like olive oil, and it was said that it could be taken a spoonful at a time as needed. Used also for deep frying, other uses are for external application, even for shining silverware.†

Apricots are also high in sulfur content, although perhaps having only one-fourth of the sulfur content of garlic, but ranking equally with onions and broccoli (Larry D. Lawson, in *Garlic*, p. 39). To which can be added that garlic, of the family Liliaceae, has long been cited as a folkloric anticancer agent, as are various of the cruciferous vegetables, so-named because their flowers are in the shape of a Greek cross—but which are of the family Cruciferae or Brassicaceae, or Mustard family.

An opposing viewpoint is expressed in John Clark's *Hunza: Lost Kingdom of the Himalayas*, published in 1956. Clark was a geologist who had taught at Princeton and elsewhere and had been in this part of the world before. His main purpose was not only to prospect and survey for minerals but to establish a school, and so on, and he took along supplies of medicines. As indicated in his preface, Clark spent 20 months among the Hunzas. They mostly re-educated him, but sometimes the reverse occurred.

From day one, Clark was involved in treating Hunza ailments, with a continuing parade of patients, e.g., some 62 on his fourth day (Clark, *Hunza*, p. 66). Sores were a big problem, along with other ailments, due to a lack of medical support over the previous years. Fortunately, antiseptics and antibiotics solved most of the cases (Clark, *Hunza*, p. 68). Clark notes treating 5,684 patients during his stay, mostly successfully, but with some deaths in spite of treatment, and some beyond hope.

Clark commented that the Hunza diet was lacking in oils and vitamin D, resulting in soft teeth, along with barrel chests and rheumatic knees, the signposts for subclinical rickets (Clark, *Hunza*, p. 205). This is viewed contrary to "Happy healthy Hunza, where everyone has just enough"! The long life spans attributed to the Hunzas are apparently not mentioned.

George B. Schaller's *Stones of Silence: Journeys in the Himalaya* was first published in 1979. In a chapter titled "Karakoram," Schaller described traveling over the new Karakoram Highway (or KKH), which runs into and through the Hunza country, up the Hunza River, and over Khunjerab Pass, there overlooking the Sinkiang or Sinkian (or Xinjiang) Province of China and following stretches of the old Silk Road. Describing the valley of the Hunzas as being scenically lovely, where Western visitors see it as a sort of Shangri-La, and where the people know the secrets of health and tranquillity and long life, Schaller instead viewed the people as no happier or sadder, or healthier or wealthier, than those in other valleys (Schaller, *Stones of Silence*, p. 87). Acknowledging that perhaps a disproportionate number of the Hunza people may become centenarians, he asked a local official about this, who scoffed at the

---

* With regard to raising garlic, above, the general region was very likely rife with its cousins, wild onions. This is mentioned by George St. George in his Time-Life book *Soviet Deserts and Mountains.* Thus, the Soviet explorer Peter Semyonov found the meadows within the Tien Shan Range to be covered with onions, a species subsequently named *Allium semenovi* (St. George, *Soviet Deserts*, p. 153). It was later learned that Chinese had given this part of the Tien Shan the Chinese name Tsun lin, or "onion mountains." Perhaps this onion species had something to do with Hunza health secrets.

† The above descriptions are in line with using apricot kernels in the raw state, without roasting.

idea. Schaller further indicated that no accurate records existed, and that there had never been an accurate comparison with other peoples in other valleys.

About apricots, Clark mentioned being served walnuts and apricot nuts (Clark, *Hunza*, p. 73). As to the inhospitable terrain, and the heroic attempts at cultivation, the Hunzas are called a "land-starved people," although visitors proclaim Hunza as the land where everybody has "just enough," and there are no poor (Clark, *Hunza*, p. 202). The climate, however, is judged ideal for apricots, mulberries, and grapes. Good horticulturists, the Hunzas have practiced grafting apricots trees for approximately 1600 years. It is noted that there were at least six local varieties, with some furnishing strong root systems on which to graft the more desirable cuttings (Clark, *Hunza*, p. 203). The children climb the trees and harvest the fruit—which becomes contaminated on the ground, a cause of dysentery.

In America, apricot trees are cut down when they become too high to pick the fruit from ladders, normally after about 35 years. As previously noted, however, the Hunza trees are cropped after 50 years and then grow for another 50 years, with enormous annual yields. The mature trees, as large as forest trees, yield a beautiful wood.

Apricot flesh is eaten both fresh and dried, and the seeds yield the almond-like kernels or nuts. The dried fruit being extra-sweet and soft, it barely lasts through the winter. Whereas *sweet* apricot kernels are eaten, the *bitter* apricot kernels are instead ground, to be squeezed to produce a *highly poisonous* apricot oil, for fuel in saucer-shaped lamps, using a cotton wick.

Evidently, there are *both sweet and bitter varieties of apricot kernels,* the same as with its close relative, the almond. Furthermore, maybe a spoonful of the oil once in awhile is nontoxic. As to its use for a cooking oil, it may be remarked that heat destroys the cyanic content—as it does for the cyanic content of beans.

At one point in his book, Clark mentions a rash of very sore stomachs among the Hunzas, but no accompanying side effects (Clark, *Hunza*, p. 181). It turned out that the Hunzas were flavoring their wine with the oil from bitter apricot nuts. Clark tried some of the wine himself and ended up with a terrific stomach ache. He concluded that those "who use prussic acid for bitters must expect a little gastric distress."

For more on the subject of apricot kernel toxicity, a computer search of the information base AGRICOLA turned up an article titled "Toxicological, nutritional and microbiological evaluation of tempe fermentation with *Rhizopus oligosporus* of bitter and sweet apricot seeds," by G. Tunáel, M.J.R. Nout, L. Brimer, and D. Göktan, variously of Ege University, Izmir, Turkey, the Agricultural University, Wageningen, The Netherlands, and the Royal Veterinary University, Frederiksberg, Denmark. What is called "tempe" is a food prepared from fermented soybeans, in this case fermented by the fungus *Rhizopus oligosporus*. It is noted that the apricot species *Prunus armeniaca* is a favorite fruit consumed during the summer season in Turkey—with a large amount of seeds left over after processing. The seeds can be used to produce both edible oils and bitter oil, depending upon the apricot variety, whether sweet or bitter. Further technical details are provided about leaching and fermentation and about amygdalin content and cyanic toxicity. The point is, that both sweet and bitter varieties exist, as in the case of almonds, and it has been previously noted that the Hunzas have some six different local varieties of apricots.

The reference books (e.g., *Hortus Third*) list the apricot as *Prunus Armeniaca* or *Prunus armeniaca* (as distinguished from a North American wild plum named *Prunus americana*). Native to Asia, the principal edible variety of apricot is denoted *Prunus Armeniaca* var. Armeniaca, and which has made its way to America—e.g., to California—to be raised commercially. There is, however, a variety that grows in Asia as far north as Siberia and produces small inedible fruit, with the scientific name *Prunus Armeniaca* var. sibirica (and that may or may not have toxic seed kernels). As previously indicated, the Hunzas apparently have many more varieties.

As to the almond, the species name as such is *Prunus dulcis*, with the bitter almond called *Prunus dulcis* var. amara, and the sweet or confectionery almond called *Prunus dulcis* var. dulcis. The references note slight differences in the appearance of the seeds or kernels.

An inspection of the sections on Peach and on Plum, Prune, and for the genus *Prunus* in the volume *Hortus Third* (initially published more or less as *The Standard Cyclopedia of Horticulture,* by L.H. Bailey, in three volumes) does not yield information about whether the seed kernels of the peach and/or the plum may sometimes also be toxic, although it makes the distinction definitely for almonds and leaves the door open for apricots. (Apple seeds, by the way, of the genus Malus of the family Malaceae or Apple family, are definitely said to contain toxic cyanogenic glycocides.) There are a number of species of peaches listed, the most common being *Prunus Persica* or *P. persica*—with the annotation that many cultivars exist—the varieties commonly cultivated. The species of what are called plums or prunes include *Prunus domesticus* or *P. domestica*, and *P. americana.*, plus *P. angustifolia*, here specifically referring to the wild plum or sand plum. Incidentally, the nectarine is listed as *Prunus Persica* var. nucipersica, and called a smooth-skinned peach. Folklore, on the other hand, sometimes considers the nectarine as a cross between a peach and a plum.

The expectations of Clark were that a growing Hunza population would outstrip its a resources, both for food and for fuel (Clark, *Hunza*, pp. 215, 204) Clark was wary of Western-style industrialization being a solution, with direct gifts definitely not (Clark, *Hunza*, p. 265ff).

His initial chapter goes back to WWII, when in 1944 Clark was a reconnaissance engineer on General Stillwell's staff, charged with surveying trails and roads in western China. At the time, the Chinese Nationalist government was relocating Chinese refugees and had plowed up the winter range of the native tribe, the Hazakh people—land unsuitable for any kind of crop. A Chinese Nationalist official, who was supervising the operation, admitted that the Chinese were out to "Sinify" the province—a term used for the genocide of a local native people, to be replaced with Chinese. A misguided missionary even called Clark's opposition unchristian. The result was warfare when the Hazakh came down from the hills in the autumn to reclaim their ancient pastures. The Chinese forces were assisted by U.S. equipment, and the people of Central Asia (including the Chinese refugees, who were helpless pawns in the game) came to hate America for this and overwhelmingly went Communist.

The Russians had previously established a presence in the area—since abandoned—that demonstrated how to make friends by working directly with the people rather than through the government or its political parties. The Russians built schools in every town, both to teach Russian political thought and to furnish a sound basic education. Poor students received free room and board. Local languages were always employed, even if extra teachers were necessary. Simple gravel roads and wooden bridges were built quickly. Small portable steam engines were furnished for power and electricity.

On the other hand, the horrible side of Russian colonization was also present. For instance, in one city, six square blocks were cordoned off, and every man and boy was killed to set an example for any opposition. The Russians viewed planned killing as part of the overall program, along with schools, roads, and little steam engines. As a Turki in Kashgar said, "The Chinese oppress us, kill our leaders, propagandize our children, and sell us no goods. The Russians oppress us, kill our leaders, propagandize our children, and do business with us. What does America expect of us, Effendi?"

A later book about the Hunzas or Hunzakuts, published in India in 1995, titled *Hunza: An Ethnographic Outline* by H. Sidky, gives considerable information about the history of these people and supplies numerous photographs. In his introduction, Sidky notes that the 1974 abolishment of Hunza's princely state by Pakistan, and the completion of the all-weather Karakoram Highway in the late 1970s, forever changed the Hunza's isolated way of life. The population of Hunza was estimated at about 32,300 and comprised 52 villages. The largest segment of the population, nearly 60 percent, consisted of the Hunzakuts, followed by the Shin and the Wakhi, each at about 20 percent, and the Bericho, only about 2 percent (Sidky, *Hunza*, p. 9). Many have Caucasoid features and fair skins, and a few even have blond hair and blue eyes, a fact noted by other travelers. Their physiognomy is remindful of the people of Iran and Afghanistan, evidenced in the many photos supplied.

Sidky goes on to say that there have been exaggerated accounts by 20th-century Western visitors about the outstanding health and longevity of the Hunzakut, with claims of life spans over 100 years. He notes that these claims originated with British medical officer Robert McCarran, who was stationed at the Gilkit Agency during the period 1904 to 1911. Sidky further mentions that the myth was sustained by the writings of E.O. Lorimer, who accompanied her husband David Lorimer into Hunza while he did field research there during 1934 to 1935. References are supplied. These claims, however, do not reconcile with the findings of medical practitioners and researchers, who observed that "the Hunzakut suffer from a host of diseases, such as rheumatism, intestinal worms, cataracts, goiter, trachoma, pneumonia, tuberculosis, dysentery, appendicitis, and heart disease." In a chapter on "Religion in Hunza," Sidky describes the role and functions of the Hunzakut shamans, called *bitans*, and notes that they also serve as healers, particularly when western medicine fails (Sidky, *Hunza*, p. 171).

Apricots are given prominent mention as a vital part of Hunza agriculture and diet (Sidky, *Hunza*, pp. 82, 87). Considered as a form of wealth, apricot trees are inherited from one generation to the next. Sidky describes the drying of the fruit on the roofs of the dwellings and the subsequent cracking of the apricot stones to get at the kernels, which are eaten raw or else dried and ground to become flour for bread. An alternate practice is also noted, that of pressing the kernels to recover the oil, which in turn is used variously for grooming, as a skin balm, and as fuel for lamps. However, no distinction is made by Sidky between sweet apricot kernels and bitter apricot kernels and their appropriate uses.

Another and later book about the Hunza by Sabine Felmy, published in 1996, is titled *The Voice of the Nightingale: A Personal Account of the Wakhi Culture in Hunza.* The Wakhan is described as a narrow valley in northeastern Afghanistan and is considered the origin for what are fundamentally called the Wakhani or Wakhi, the people of these high mountain valleys. Their flocks of sheep, goats, cattle, and yaks are considered their riches, and their principal vegetable crops are peas, beans, barley, and a little wheat, plus potatoes (Felmy, *Voice*, pp. 2, 46, 51). The apricot is still the main fruit crop—called the queen of fruits, with eight varieties acknowledged—and both sweet and bitter apricots are raised (Felmy, *Voice*, pp. 49, 50). Harvest time is in August, and the pulp or flesh is for the most part sun dried for future use. The sweet apricot kernels are still eaten, but the oil from the bitter apricot kernels is used for nonfood purposes (Felmy, *Voice*, p. 21). The excess or spoiled fruit is in turn used for livestock feed (Felmy, *Voice*, p. 53). Children falling out of trees and breaking bones during harvest time continues as a hazard (Felmy, *Voice*, p. 42), but no mention is made of long life spans for the elders.

8.5.3   OTHER BIOACTIVE SUBSTANCES AND MISCELLANEOUS AGENTS

While folic acid (as the dihydrate) is listed in Table 8.9, other vitamins are not, nor are minerals. It is assumed that these can be routinely obtained at the local health food store. Nevertheless, these substances should be tested, the same as phytochemicals. Moreover, most have the advantage of not being considered toxic, at least in recommended amounts—even in mega-amounts for most vitamins (save for vitamins A and D).

Vitamin C is no doubt an obvious possibility, as are *vitamins A and D,* maybe vitamin E, and one or more of the *B-vitamins,* and so on. In this regard, it has been found that *cancer patients characteristically have low vitamin C levels* (*Handbook of Vitamins,* second edition, p. 217). Whether increasing the levels of vitamin C will reverse the progress of cancer remains the debatable question. In an update, however, a survey of the scientific literature about vitamin C and the treatment of cancer has been conducted by Gary Null, Howard Robbins, Mark Tanenbaum, and Patrick Jennings. Their Part I labeled abstracts and commentary appears in the May, 1997 issue of the *Townsend Letter for Doctors & Patients,* with more to follow—but the final word is not yet evident. *Mineral compounds* of calcium, magnesium, and zinc are possibilities, as are traces of selenium and germanium compounds. Inorganic compounds such as *urea* crop up in listings of anticancer agents. In fact, all sorts of mineral compounds are potential possibilities, including those of iron and other Group VIII transitional elements of the periodic table, noted for their catalytic activity. (The metals in chemically similar chlorophyll and hemoglobin underscore their role in enzymatic activity.)

To the list may be added compounds of the platinum-group metals platinum, palladium, iridium, rhodium, osmium, and ruthenium, rarer still in the diet—not to mention the noble metal gold and its compatriots silver and copper—plus compounds of the rare-earth metals. Then enter metallo-compounds involving such elements as sulfur, phosphorus, arsenic, bismuth, antimony,..., intermediate in the periodic table, and some of which can be toxic in the extreme. The subject is in general that of trace elements, some of which are, or may be, vital to body processes. Not only this, but they may also play a role in normal cell metabolism, and conceivably may act against cancer cell metabolism.

In the parlance of catalysis—and in particular of heterogeneous catalysis, where two or more distinct phases or substances are involved—these enzyme inhibitors can be said to act as "poisons" to enzyme catalysts. This terminology is especially appropriate for the more overtly toxic substances such as arsenic, cyanide, and so on. The inhibitors or poisons in some way or another block the so-called active sites on the enzyme catalyst, as previously discussed in Part 1. There may be a structural or chemical resemblance, or reaction, with the inhibition mode classed either as competitive or uncompetitive (Voet and Voet, *Biochemistry,* p. 355ff).

Interestingly, on the same page, above, Voet and Voet describe cancer cells as "rapidly dividing cells" and therefore more susceptible to chemotherapy agents. Other authorities, however, regard cancer cells in the main as *slow growing. Fast-growing cells* comprise the immune system and blood cells, the gastrointestinal tract, and hair—all of which *are attacked first and more severely.* (Chemotherapy is relatively successful against blood-related cancers, however.) *Cytotoxic chemotherapy* drugs can therefore more accurately be described as *more selective against these normal cells* rather than against cancer cells, but in cold fact they serve to attack every type of cell in the body. The larger question becomes, if conventional chemotherapy (or surgery or radiation) doesn't work, then what does?

To continue, the myriad plants or herbs are notable possibilities as selective enzyme inhibitors, many of which are already recognized as anticancer agents, at least in medical folklore. *Pau d'arco* is an example, available from the local health food store, as is *condurango* or *condor vine,* which must be obtained more indirectly. The results evidently have not been favorable, however. Incidentally, pau d'arco (Spanish) or lepacho (Portuguese) is the only anticancer agent described in Andrew Chevallier's *The Encyclopedia of Medicinal Plants,* a colorful addition to the subject.

Among the more recent developments is the use of the *Venus flytrap, Dionaea muscipula* of the plant family Droseraceae or Sundew family, and called by Charles Darwin "the most wonderful plant in the world," as noted by Morton Walker in the November, 1997 issue of the *Townsend Letter for Doctors & Patients.* Walker describes its use against cancer and other diseases in the form of the registered trademark name Carnivora®. The product's discoverer is physician Helmut Keller, MD, of Bad Steben, Germany, and it is produced via a patented process by Carnivora Forschungs GmbH of Nordhalben Germany. A refined product of Venus-flytrap juice, the most active components are said to be *plumbagin* and *hydroplumbagin-glucoside.* The therapeutic effect is evidently via the action of the immune system. As part of the article, a tabulation is provided of some dozen immune system *biomarkers* for monitoring the patient's response.

Add to this list *bloodroot,* which contains the alkaloid *sanguinarine,* listed in Table 8.9, and a plant well embedded in medical folklore. Also on the list is *creosote bush* or *chaparral,* which contains NDGA and quercetin, both listed in Table 8.9—and it is a source for still other interesting substances such as 50-some volatile oils including vinyl and methyl ketones, camphor, and limonene, and the amber-like resin exuded contains not only these oils but flavonoids, lignins, saponins, and waxes (e.g., Gary Nabhan's *The Desert Smells Like Rain* and *Gathering the Desert*).

Unsuspectedly, *hyoscyamine*—the principal alkaloid found in *Jimsonweed* (or Jamestown weed or Jimtown weed), and an even more toxic chemical relative of atropine—can be induced to occur in tomato plants and tomatoes by grafting. Both Jimsonweed (*Datura stramonium*) and the tomato (*Lycopersicon esculentum*) are of the same plant family Solanaceae or Nightshade family, and it is possible to insert a tomato cutting into the cut stalk of a vigorous Jimsonweed plant, and thereby raise tomatoes. The phenomenon and consequences are described in a chapter titled "Something a Little Unusual," in Berton Roueché's *The Medical Detectives,* a collection of stories that originally appeared in *The New Yorker,* in his Annals of Medicine department. A family and friends who partook of the product, so raised, suffered *hallucinations and other classic symptoms,* some more severely than others, depending on the quantity eaten. Another experimenter who had previously raised tomatoes in this fashion suffered no symptoms from eating them. The difference turned out to be that the latter had taken off all the leaves from the Jimsonweed plant, and the leaves are the principal source for manufacturing hyosycamine.

Some of the aforesaid compounds or classes are considered as anticancer agents, although they may have some adverse side effects not yet fully documented. Plus, *Compound-X,* whatever it is, has been available by mail as indicated in an occasional advertisement. Naessen's *714X* is available by mail, and *Burzynski's polypeptides (or other agents)* may or may not be available—albeit *the Sigma Chemical Company is a source for a maze of bioactive peptides*—or fragments, or polypeptides, depending on how one views the circumstance.

The evidence for the efficacy for some of these therapies is controversial, to say the least. Thus, as an example, a critical view is provided by Cari Lynn, a former Burzynski patient, in the September, 1998 issue of *Health.*

Chaparral or creosote bush (*Larrea tridentata*) may or may not be an ingredient in the Indian remedy called Compound-X, cited above, as may bloodroot (*Sanguinaria canadensis*), which contains the alkaloid sanguinarine. Interestingly, this component has been found to be an anticavity agent and is used in toothpastes such as Vident®. Compound-X may also or instead contain redroot (*Lachnanthes tinctoria*). Redroot, however, is the colloquial name for still other species having red roots, such as alkanet, pigweed, and New Jersey tea. Thus, there may as well be confusion with bloodroot, a sometimes herbal remedy.

There is a story about pigweed, here of the genus *Amaranthus* of the family Amaranthaceae. (Pigweed is also the name used for members of the family Chenopodiaceae or Goosefoot family—e.g., the genus *Chenopodium.*) In Joseph J. Williams' *Voodoos and Obeahs: Phases of West Indian Witchcraft,* the observations of Edward Long are furnished (Williams, *Voodoos,* p. 180). Long's *History of Jamaica* was published in 1774. The term "Obeah" is more or less used to indicate witchcraft, and there was the observation than an Obeah man could return an apparently dead man to life.

> The method, by which this trick was carried on, was by a cold infusion of the herb branched calalue; which, after the agitation of dancing, through the party into a profound sleep. In this state, he continued, to all appearances lifeless, no pulse, nor motion of the heart, being perceptible; till on being rubbed with another infusion (as yet unknown to the whites), the effects of the calalue gradually went off, the body resumed its motions, and the party on whom the experiment had been tried, awoke as from a trance, entirely ignorant of anything that had passed since he left off dancing.

It so turns out that calalue is a species of pigweed, *Amaranthus spinosus*, also known as spiny Amaranthus or spiny pigweed. Among its ordinary effects are that of a laxative, of an antieczemic, and of an antirheumatic. A more common species in North America is *A. retroflexus* or redroot pigweed. In any event, there is again the caution that plant medicines can have untoward and unexpected side effects, sometimes dangerous in the extreme.

In addition to such naturally occurring hallucinogens as from the peyote cacti and certain mushrooms, there are other neuropharmacological plant and animal substances. A further example has been furnished by Harvard ethnobotanist Wade Davis regarding voodooism and zombiism, published in his *The Serpent and the Rainbow* and *Passage of Darkness*. The toxins of the puffer fish (family Tetraodontidae, and called *fugu* in Japan) have been implicated, e.g., tetraodontoxin.

For the record, the Sigma Chemical Company catalog organizes peptides as follows in a section on Bioactive Peptides: Adrenocorticotropic Hormone and Fragments; Anglotensin and Related Peptides; Atrial Natriuretic Peptides; Bradykinin and Related Peptides; Chemotactic Peptides; Chemotactic Peptides; Endorphins and β-Lipotropin Fragments; Enkephalin and Related Peptides; *Enzyme Inhibitors;* Fibronectin Fragments and Related Peptides; Gastrointestinal Peptides; *Growth Hormone Releasing Peptides;* Luteinizing Hormone Releasing Hormone and Related Peptides; Melanocyte Stimulating Hormone and Related Peptides; Neurotensin and Related Peptides; Opioid Peptides; Oxytocin, Vasopressin, Vasotocin and Related Peptides; Parathyroid Hormone and Fragments; Protein Kinase Related Peptides; Somatostatin and Related Peptides, Substance P and Related Peptides; Miscellaneous Bioactive Peptides. An index is also provided by peptide name. In the foregoing, a couple of categories are highlighted, notably *Enzyme Inhibitors*, but others are also of potential interest, such as *Somastatin*.

Immediately under the Sigma catalog heading *Enzyme Inhibitors,* as per the foregoing, the following statements are made.

> *Many of the following enzyme inhibitors were initially isolated from microbial sources.* They are useful tools in the analysis of homeostasis of living organisms and disease processes. *Many of these products have shown promise in cancer chemotherapy."* (*Homeostasis* is the tendency for an organism to regulate and maintain within itself a condition of *stability*.)

Shark cartilage or *bovine cartilage,* comprising its own category in the Sigma catalog, is said to contain *polypeptides.* It is routinely available at health food stores.

A sourcebook on the synthesis and physical data of peptides is, appropriately, *Peptides: Syntheses—Physical Data*, in six volumes, by Wolfgang Voelter and Erich Schmid-Siegmann, published in 1983.

Polysaccharides are another possibility, as indicated in Part 3 in the section "Other Information About Chinese Anticancer Agents," with a number of citations furnished in Table 3.13. Additional information appears in Part 5 in the section "Medicinal Fungi and Cancer." It may be noted in Table 5.1, which is comprised of fungal entries in Hartwell, that a fungus family is named Saccharomycetaceae. Further mention of polysaccharides appears in Part 5 within the section "Antibiotics," in the subsection "Anticancer Activity." A listing of polysaccharides is provided in Table 8.10.

There is some contradictory evidence, however. In the section on "Plant Carcinogens" in Part 2, the seaweed extract called *carrageenan* is described as a *sulfated polysaccharide extracted from seaweed,* and which contains ammonia, calcium, magnesium, and sodium salts of the sulfate esters of galactose and 3,6-anhydrogalactose copolymers. It was found to be *carcinogenic,* at least in the amounts used. However, Hartwell's *Plants Used Against Cancer* has several entries at the end of his book under the category Algae, which include the seaweed or kelp families Facaceae and Laminariaceae.

Table 8.10   Some Common Polysaccharides that May Have Possibilities as Enzyme Inhibitors or Anticancer Agents

Homopolysaccharides

Cellulose (Sigma; Aldrich). The sugar component is glucose, the function is structural, and it occurs throughout the plant kingdom.

Amylose (Sigma; Aldrich). The sugar component is glucose, the function is food storage, and it occurs in starches such as from corn and potatoes. Sources are corn and potatoes. IRRITANT. May contain up to 10% n-butanol

Chitin (Sigma; Aldrich). The sugar component is N-acetylglucosamine, the function is structural, and it occurs in insect and crustacean skeletons. Sources include crab shells, shrimp shells.

Inulin (Sigma; Aldrich). The sugar component is fructose, the function is food storage, and it occurs in such diverse plants as artichoke and chicory. Sources include chicory root, dahlia tubers, Jerusalem artichoke.

Xylan (Sigma; Aldrich). The sugar component is xylose, the function is structural, and it occurs in all land plants. Sources include birchwood, oat spelts. (The word "oat" may indicate the grain of *Avena sativa*, or the plant itself; "spelt" is a specific wheat named *Triticum spelta*).

Glycogen (Sigma; Aldrich). The sugar component is glucose, the function is food storage, and it occurs in the liver and muscle cells of all animals. Sources include mammalian livers: rabbit, bovine; other sources are oysters, mussels, slippery limpets (mollusks).

Dextran (Sigma). The sugar component is glucose, the function is unknown, and it occurs primarily in bacteria. Sources include *Leuconostoc mesenteroides*, Strain No. B-512.

Agar (Sigma; Aldrich). The sugar component is galactose, sometimes with sulfate groups, the function is structural, and it occurs in seaweeds.

Heteropolysaccharides

Hyaluronic acid (Sigma). The sugar components are D-glucuronic acid and N-acetyl-D-glucosamine; the functions are as lubricant, shock absorber, and for water binding; the distribution is in connective tissue and skin. Sources include bovine trachea, bovine vitreous humor, human umbilical cord, rooster comb, *Streptococcus zooepidemicus*.

Chondroitin-4-sulfate (Sigma). The sugar components are D-glucuronic acid and N-acetyl-D-glucosamine-4-O-sulfate; the functions are calcium accumulations, and cartilage and bone formation; the distribution is in cartilage. Linked to protein (about 10% protein). Sources include bovine trachea, porcine rib cartilage, bovine mucosa, porcine skin, porcine intestinal mucosa.

Heparin (Sigma). The sugar components are D-glucuronic acid, L-iduronic acid, and N-sulfo-D-glucosamine; the functions are as an anticoagulant; occurs in mast cells and blood. (Mast cells are certain cells that line the blood vessels.) Linked to protein. Sources include porcine intestinal mucosa, bovine intestinal mucosa, bovine lung, ovine (sheep) intestinal mucosa.

Gamma globulin, human blood (Sigma). The sugar components are N-acetyl-hexosamine, D-manose, and D-galactose; the function is as an antibody; distributed in blood. Linked to protein (better than 95% protein).

Blood group substance. The sugar components are D-glucosamine, D-galactosamine, L-fucose, and D-galactose; the function is blood group specificity; occurs in cell surfaces, especially red blood cells.

Source: Data from the catalog *Biochemicals, Organic Compounds, and Diagnostic Reagents*, Sigma Chemical Company, St. Louis MO, 1996–, and from the 1996–1997 *Catalog/Handbook of Fine Chemicals*, Aldrich Chemical Company, Milwaukee WI and St. Louis MO. Descriptive comments are provided where applicable. In some instances, the entries occur in both catalogs. Information source: *Encyclopedia Britannica.*, under "Carbohydrates."

In Part 3, however, in the section on "Other Information about Chinese Anticancer Agents," previously cited above, saccharides or polysaccharides are repeatedly mentioned (e.g., as an aloe component in the substance developed by Mannatech, Inc.) and are cited as components in a number of Chinese anticancer herbs. The latter, for the record, include the following plant families and genera:

- Actinidiaceae—*Actinidia*
- Araliaceae—*Acanthopanax*

- • Lilicaceae—*Aloe*
- • Polyporaceae—*Ganoderma*
- • Umbelliferae—*Angelica*

Polysaccharides also occur in fungi, as previously indicated relative to Part 5. The substances called glucans are polysaccharides. Furthermore, in Part 5 in the section on "Medicinal Fungi and Cancer," and the section on "Antibiotics" and subsection on "Anticancer Activity," it may be noted that *polysaccharides are sometimes classified as antibiotics.*

Continuing in a different direction, it may be added that electromagnetic radiation—e.g., radiofrequency waves—may possibly serve as an enzyme inhibitor for anaerobic glycolysis, that is, say for lactate dehydrogenase, as has been previously indicated. The connection is to, say, the Rife therapy, described by Walters in *Options* and also previously noted. The effectiveness, if any, would likely be a function of intensity and of frequency or wavelength.

In this latter regard, among the newer techniques proposed for cancer therapy is that of using an agent that is selectively absorbed by cancer cells then activating this agent by radiant energy (e.g., by light). The activated agent in turn destroys the cancer. Very possibly, a phytochemical or other substance could also be used to activate this agent.

The possibilities seem endless, especially when projecting from test tube or culture dish trials, to *in vitro* and *in vivo* tests on cancer cells, and finally to clinical trials involving either oral or intravenous administration—all this at varying concentrations and frequencies, with the optimum safe dosage to be established.

A potential food source that could be tested consists of the *edible oils*. These can be variously enumerated as sunflower oil (from *Helianthus annuus* of the family Compositae), safflower oil (from *Carthamus tinctorius* of the family Compositae), rapeseed oil or canola oil (from *Brassica napus* of the family Cruciferae), mustard seed oil (from *Brassica nigra* from the family Cruciferae), olive oil (*Olea europaea* of the family Oleaceae), corn oil (from *Zea mays* of the family Gramineae), wheat germ oil (from the genus *Triticum* of the family Gramineae), flaxseed or linseed oil (from the genus *Linum* of the family Linaceae), cottonseed oil (from *Gossypium herbaceum* of the family Malvaceae). There is peanut oil (from *Arachis hypogaea* of the family Leguminosae) and even an oil derived from sweet or confectionery almonds (*Prunus amygdalus* of the family Rosaceae). All the families and species are listed in Hartwell's *Plants Used Against Cancer.*

These oils, by their liquid or oily nature, connote the presence of unsaturated double chemical bonds that may pick up various chemicals such as hydrogen or oxygen. The use of hydrogenation is practiced to achieve solid-like status, for example as practiced with cottonseed oil to produce what are called hydrogenated vegetable oils. Some claim that *the hydrogenated product is not as satisfactory healthwise as is the oil itself.*

Most or all these oils have been promoted in one way or another as having beneficial health effects, e.g., as free-oxygen scavengers or as antioxidants. This, in turn, may be related to anticancer activity. This may be in part due to their unsaturated nature and their property of picking up oxygen. For this reason, some have long been used commercially for drying oils (e.g., linseed oil, rapeseed oil, mustard seed oil) whereby they oxidize into a solid-like substance or film. The use of linseed oil in paints is a notable example.

Flaxseed oil or *linseed oil* is still eaten in Europe and Asia, although it doesn't keep long due to its tendency to oxidize, and it appears in medical folklore as an *anticancer agent*. More than this, there have been some scientific studies backing this up (Moss, *Cancer Therapy*, pp. 241–246). The principal component is linoleic acid, but it is also noted to contain valuable vitamins and minerals. Flaxseed oil is marketed as an herbal remedy, generally in capsules.

This brings up the point that these oils may also contain other phytochemicals that may act as enzyme inhibitors, e.g., against cancer metabolism. These substance may be only in trace amounts, albeit they occur throughout the plant, but may be more concentrated in particular parts. It may be further emphasized that these oils are derived from the seeds or kernels, the most nutritionally active part of the plant.

In any event, some or all are worth further checking out as enzyme inhibitors. In this regard, *linoleic acid,* the principal component of flaxseed oil, is listed in Jain's *Handbook* as an enzyme inhibitor for elastase (the pancreatic enzyme for digesting fibrous and proteinaceous elastin), fatty acid synthesis, and phospholipase. (*Linolenic acid* is listed as an inhibitor for photosystem II. This effect, here and in other fatty acids, is noted to be *counteracted* by the manganate ion, Mn^{++}.) Zollner's *Handbook* lists linoleic acid as an inhibitor for arachidonate-CoA ligase and for 9-hydroxyprostaglandin dehydrogenase. These enzymes are not directly involved in anaerobic glycolysis, however.

Another unsaturated fatty acid of note is **oleic acid**. Jain lists it as an inhibitor for **ATP-P$_i$ exchange**, the binding of PGE1, chrymotrypsin, elastase, fatty acid synthesis, **glutamate dehydrogenase**, glycerol-3-P acyltransferase, **lipase**, PEP carboxykinase, **phosphofructokinase**, pyruvate carboxylase, **transphosphorylation**, **transport of adenine nucleotide**, transport of potassium, uptake of calcium. (*Lipase* is an enzyme that hydrolyzes fats to fatty acids.) Zollner lists oleic acid as an inhibitor for dolichol esterase. As the highlighted terms indicate, oleic acid is involved in anaerobic glycolysis and the tricarboxylic acid cycle, as well as other bioprocesses such as potassium transport and calcium uptake.

From the above paragraph, there is the suggestion that not only oleic acid but linoleic acid and other fatty acid components of vegetable oils may be similarly involved, and all may be involved to a greater degree than so far found. It is one more illustration of how complex and interrelated biochemical processes can be.

8.6 TESTING PROCEDURES

As to the initial testing or screening itself, the single biochemical reaction probably of most interest is the conversion of aqueous solutions of pyruvic acid or pyruvate to lactic acid or lactate, the principal distinguishing feature of anaerobic glycolysis as pertains to cancer cells. As has been noted, pyruvic acid or pyruvate (as the sodium salt) is available from both the previous cited sources (Sigma catalog, Aldrich catalog). The enzyme involved, lactate dehydrogenase, is also available (Sigma catalog). Expectedly, concentrations and pH will have to be adjusted to achieve the desired results. To the system can be added one or another of various substances as potential enzyme inhibitors. These potential enzyme inhibitors are to be nontoxic in the dosages used.* The criterion of effectiveness will be whether lactic acid or lactate makes an appearance, and to what degree. If no lactic acid or lactate forms, then the suspected inhibitor is probably effective. While various tests could be used for determining the lactic acid or lactate presence and concentration, perhaps the simplest would be to measure the change in the index of refraction of the mixture.

It would no doubt be better to add the proposed enzyme inhibitor to the pyruvic acid or pyruvate solution first, then add the enzyme itself—or at least add the inhibitor and the enzyme at the same time. This would prevent any unwarranted conversion to lactic acid or lactate. For a blank or reference, the conversion of pyruvic acid or pyruvate to lactic acid or lactate can be checked with only the enzyme added.

Even though the foregoing testing appears simple enough, it is probably better left to a professional. Moreover, there may be other mitigating factors involved that are not readily apparent to the untrained eye. Hence the need for medical/biochemical clinics, centers, or institutes specializing in the testing of bioactive substances as enzyme inhibitors for cancer cell metabolism.

At the same time, *it would be most opportune if a kit were made routinely available, with procedures spelled out, for testing the effectiveness of various suspected inhibitors.* If advisable, such could be used for the home screening of potential inhibitors.

In this connection it may be remarked that the Sigma catalog lists *diagnostic kits and reagents* for testing for lactate and for lactate deyhdrogenase and its isoenzymes or isozymes. The methods variously involve enzymatic, colorimetric, ultraviolet, kinetic, immunologic, and electrophoretic procedures.

This is only a start, however, for there is the problem of whether the substance would be effective in the body, and whether it should be administered orally or injected intramuscularly or intravenously. Furthermore, is the substance toxic to other body functions, and to what degree? That is, what are the side effects?

Therefore, what is to be the dosage level? (Minute, trace, infinitesimal, or what?) For these reasons, the care of a professional is generally advisable, at least until the methodology is proven to be both safe and effective, and probably afterward as well. The situation is entirely analogous to that of prescribing and using antibiotics.

---

* Laetrile or amygdalin, or it chemical equivalent, is of course a possibility although, according to the theory, it acts on an enzyme or enzymes completely differently from those involved in anaerobic glycolysis—where, as to the latter, lactate dehydrogenase is of particular interest. Furthermore, *cyanoglycosides* such as occur in Laetrile or amygdalin are suspect in cardiac arrest, and it is suspected that *free hydrocyanic acid or cyanide ion is a respiration inhibitor.*

At the same time, a *buildup of lactic acid or lactate* may in itself constitute an indication for the presence of cancer and could therefore be used to monitor the progress of cancer treatment. More than this, the presence and concentration of the enzyme *lactate dehydrogenase* might also be an indicator for cancer and could be used to monitor treatment. Any change in concentration of the enzyme from normal, up or down, may serve to indicate cancer and in turn the progress of treatment.

That is to say, an increase in enzyme concentration could mean that the enzyme reaction should be favored. On the other hand, an increase could mean that the enzyme is not being used, and so the reaction is disfavored. Or, a decrease in enzyme concentration could mean that the reaction is proceeding and the enzyme is being used up. Or, on the other hand, a decrease could mean that the reaction will not be favored. These speculations bring up the matter of whether enzyme catalysts are actually used up during the course of reaction and must therefore be replenished. This is contrary to the usual connotations for catalytic activity, however, whereby the catalyst is considered to remain unchanged. Nevertheless, *catalysts will ordinarily undergo a decrease in activity over the course of time and must be replaced or regenerated.*

An additional indicator or marker for anaerobic glycolysis is a buildup of the amino acid *alanine*, as has been previously indicated (ref. the work of Guerra et al.). (L-Alanine, incidentally, is an inhibitor for pyruvate kinase, as listed in Appendix A.)

In speaking of enzyme concentrations—minute though they may be—this introduces the question of how or by what pathways are enzymes manufactured in the body. In other words, are enzymes required to manufacture still other enzymes, and where does it all start? Any sort of resolution will, in turn, introduce other perplexities. This illustrates how complicated and interrelated body processes are, and it indicates the impossibility of a full understanding. Nonetheless, we will settle for a partial understanding as long as it leads to cures for disease, in this case cancer.

As to clinical tests, above, it would be most opportune if a ready indicator could be found that would function to monitor or measure the progression or remission of cancer, that is, whether the cancer or cancerous condition is increasing or decreasing. *Alanine*, mentioned above, is potentially such an indicator. Thus, possibly the concentration of alanine in the blood—that is, serum levels—might provide such an indication. Possibly, lactic acid concentrations could be used as a generalized measure. The presence or absence of cancer cells in the bloodstream might or might not be an indicator. Other proposed markers are Bence-Jones proteins, electroacupuncture, and various hormones, antigens, enzymes, and so on.

A newer development, applicable to detecting *lung cancer* early on, is an invasive test: the use of fluorescent light to indicate precancerous lung cells. The technique is called *fluorescent bronchoscopy* and is conducted similarly to conventional bronchoscopy. Instead of white light, however, fluorescence is used, which causes the precancerous tissue to appear dark red, whereas healthy tissue appears green. A positive test would be followed up by any one of several treatments. The possibilities include, say, inhaled gene therapy, the removal of cancerous tissue by laser, a vitamin A regimen, or photodynamic therapy by means of an endoscope. The procedure is being offered at several facilities in the U.S., including the Columbia Presbyterian-St. Luke's Medical Center at Denver, under the auspices of the University of Colorado Medical Center, in turn funded by a National Cancer Institute grant. Whatever, *the death rate from lung cancer is said to be about 85 percent,* and the rate hasn't changed much in the last 10 to 15 years.

In the case of *prostate cancer,* and prostate cancer only, an indicator routinely used is the PSA test, the acronym standing for prostate-specific antigen. Additional information on this particular test is available for instance in the current *Merck Manual* and in the volume *Current Medical Diagnosis and Treatment,* now in its 135th edition (Appleton & Lange, Stamford CT, 1996, p. 847). In further explanation, PSA is a *glycoprotein* produced only in the cytoplasm of *both benign and malignant* prostate cells. The test can be performed by radioimmunoassay methods. Another indicator is elevated *serum acid phosphatase* level, a test largely replaced by the PSA test—although the level of this enzyme is more predictive of metastatic diseases.*

In further comment, the progression and response to therapy involving elevated PSA levels are still being evaluated, particularly with regard to early detection and treatment. Roughly speaking, about 25

---

* Using levels of foregoing enzyme as an indictor suggests that other enzymes might serve for other cancers. A possibility, of course, is l*actate dehydrogenase,* the enzyme responsible for producing lactic acid or lactate, the principal end product of cancer cell metabolism. The subject of lactate dehydrogenase in its several forms will be subsequently discussed.

to 90 percent of patients with elevated PSA levels will have prostatic carcinoma, whereas maybe 30 to 50 percent of patients with elevated PSA levels will only have benign prostatic hypertrophy.

The above percentages outline the dilemma of the patient, regarding whether he has a malignant or benign condition—and may in considerable part explain the saying that many prostate cancer victims will outlive the cancer. That is to say, the condition may have been more benign than malignant, never mind the PSA levels—or maybe never mind even the biopsy.

The extended sequence of events that may ensue are illustrated by the experiences of a patient in Boulder CO. During approximately the 10 years preceding, the patient had undergone physical examinations indicating a swollen prostate with a lump in it. Since it wasn't causing any trouble, nothing was done. Finally, on consulting with experts in the field, even at the Fitzsimmons army hospital at Denver (the patient was a WWII veteran), there was a consensus of sorts that something ought to be done. The options seemed to be that of doing nothing or else undergoing surgery (the latter at appreciable cost, it may be added).

In the meantime, an article appeared in the *National Enquirer* about a procedure in which a needle or needles containing radioactive materials could be inserted in the lump, and done on an outpatient basis. The operation was said to be performed at hospitals in New York and Houston, and at the University of Washington Medical School at Seattle. A call to Seattle indicated that the operation seemed to be effective and reasonably simple. As to inquiring about a doctor in the Denver area who also performed the operation, the closest was apparently at Las Vegas NV. A trip to Las Vegas to see the doctor was positive, and an appointment was made to schedule the operation. In the meantime, the patient decided to check out things more closely in Denver, and after an unproductive lead or two, the Department of Urology at the University of Colorado Medical Center made a referral, which led to still another referral, and the last doctor said that the very same thing was being done at Boulder Community Hospital, which had a "radiation machine." The patient signed on with the appropriate doctor in Boulder, canceled the Las Vegas appointment, and had a series of treatments right there in his hometown of Boulder, and apparently remains cured to this day, with consistently low PSA levels.

The patient, however, thought that he had gotten the runaround in his initial inquiries. Either the doctors seen didn't seem to know about the new treatment, didn't care, or preferred the more expensive option—surgery. It was found out later that Fitzsimmons hospital in fact had a radiation unit, and there were doctors in Boulder who apparently didn't even seem to know about the treatment, much less that a radiation unit was right next door at the Boulder hospital.

This, then, is the sort of thing that cancer patients have to contend with. To put it charitably, as per the old saying, the right hand doesn't know what the left is doing.*

Another set of experiences is furnished by Elaine Nussbaum in *Recovery from Cancer: A Personal Story of Sickness and Health.* The list could go on, based on an underground of cancer patients willing to tell their story. Most such chronicles do not find their way into print, however.

8.7 ANTICANCER AGENTS AND ANGIOGENESIS

An ancillary question that can be asked is whether these or other bioactive substances may at the same time also act to prevent or reverse neovascularization or angiogenesis, the creation of the vast network of new blood vessels that are formed in cancerous growths. Or in another way of looking at it, is an anticancer agent also an antiangiogeneisis agent, or vice versa? Does not the one infer the other, somehow being the one and the same?

John Boik's *Cancer & Natural Medicine* has a chapter on angiogenesis, and it turns out that there are a number of plants or plant and other substances that may deter or otherwise affect angiogenesis, and these are listed in Appendix X.

These plants or substances serve to inhibit the formation of fibrin or stimulate fibrinolysis, the breakdown of fibrin, fibrin being a protein associated with blood coagulation, and is in fact the blood

---

* As to the insertion of radioactive needles into a tumor or cancerous tissue, this kind of operation was performed on Lee Atwater, who was the former chairman of the Republican Party and manager of George Bush's presidential campaign in 1988, as per John Brady's *Bad Boy: The Life and Politics of Lee Atwater.* Atwater had inoperable brain cancer. As a method of treatment, holes were drilled into his skull, and radioactive needles or rods were inserted into the tumor. The tumor was killed, but Atwater suffered disastrous side effects and subsequently died.

clot per se—albeit other factors enter, as set forth by Boik. For present purposes, these same kind of plant species are in many cases also known as anticancer agents and are referenced to Hartwell's baseline compilation *Plants Used Against Cancer.* It may be speculated, therefore, that at least some anticancer agents may act against angiogenesis. The one may go with the other.

Angiogenesis is found to variously involve blood coagulation, inflammation, and tissue repair (Boik, *Cancer & Natural Medicine*, p. 17). Among the angiogenic factors are those classed as angiogenic cytokines (cell-produced protein factors that regulate cellular growth and function), and noncytokine angiogenic factors. The former classification includes interleukins from the immune cells, basic fibroblast growth factor (bFGF), transforming growth factors (TGF-α,β), platelet-derived endothelial cell growth factor (PD-EGF), vascular permeability factor (VPF), platelet activating factor (PAF) from immune cells, tumor necrosis factor alpha (TNF-α, or cachectin). Undoubtedly, a lot is involved, with some things at cross purposes, and the use of the term "factor" indicates an element of ambiguity.

The noncytokine angiogenic factors include copper, fibrin degradation products, eicosanoids such as prostaglandins, lactic acid, kinins, heparin, insulin, nicotinamide (considered part of the B-complex), and thrombin. *Kinins* are described as highly bioactive *peptides* found in the pancreas and other tissues (Boik, *Cancer & Natural Medicine*, p. 23). *Heparin* is a *polysaccharide* whose primary function is to *inhibit coagulation* (Boik, *Cancer & Natural Medicine*, pp. 20–21). *Thrombin,* a blood serum component, reacts with fibrinogen (a protein) to form fibrin. Also involved is the biologically active amine compound *histamine,* $C_5H_9N_3$, whose action is evidently *inhibited by flavonoids,* which some authorities have divided into anthocyanins, anthochlors and aurones, plus minor flavonoids, flavones and flavonols, isoflavonoids, and tannins (Boik, *Cancer & Natural Medicine*, pp. 150–151). It is observed that low molecular weight flavonoids tend to give tartness or bitterness to fruits, whereas *high molecular weight flavonoids (tannins)* produce astringency.

The blood clotting pathway or cascade is spelled out in more detail in still other references (e.g., Voet and Voet, *Biochemistry*, p. 1197; York, in *Textbook of Biochemistry*, p. 212). It is noted, for instance, that *thrombin is an enzyme*—a *serine protease* comprising two disulfide-linked *polypeptide* chains (Voet and Voet, *Biochemistry*, p. 1201). *Vitamin K* enters the picture as an essential *cofactor*—but it may be inhibited by such agents as *dicoumarol* or *dicumarol* (found in spoiled sweet clover, and which causes *hemorrhaging* in cattle) and *warfarin* (a rat poison). Voet and Voet follow up their presentation with a section on immunity, but no mention is made of angiogenesis or vascularization, nor is mention made in the *Textbook of Biochemistry.* (The aforementioned substances or compounds are variously listed in the Sigma and Aldrich catalogs.)

Certain terms used in Appendix X or in the Boik reference require further clarification. Thus, *mast cells* are cells that line arterial walls, notably in the liver, and have intracellular granules (Voet and Voet, *Biochemistry*, p. 265). According to the *Academic Press Dictionary of Science and Technology, fibronectin* is "a protein that interacts with a variety of extracellular substances in plasma and tissues (such as collagen, fibrin, and heparin) to help cells, especially fibroblasts, bind to each other; aids in tissue repair." Fibroblasts, in turn, are cells that contribute to the formation of connective tissue fibers. The acronym PAF stands for platelet activating factor, and in the PCA test, PCA stands for passive cutaneous anaphylaxis (skin susceptibility or sensitivity).

The term *CAM,* as in the CAM assay, pertains to *Crassulacean acid metabolism* (Voet and Voet, *Biochemistry*, p. 658). It involves the storage of carbon dioxide by the synthesis of malate, which is an intermediate compound that occurs in the tricarboxylic acid cycle, as shown in Part 1 and diagrammed in Figure 1.4. The phenomenon was first observed in plants of the family Crassulaceae or Orpine family, which includes succulent herbs such as sedum or stonecrop. These plants store CO_2 in the cool of the night to avoid water losses by transpiration or evaporation that would occur in the daytime. The carbon dioxide is stored in *phosphophenolpyruvate* or phosphoenol pyruvate, called *PEP* (which is also the reaction intermediate that is converted to pyruvate in the last step or Step (10) of the glycolytic pathway, as diagrammed in Figure 1.1 in Part 1). That is, the PEP and carbon dioxide combine to form oxaloacetate that is further converted to malate, and then pyruvate, releasing the stored carbon dioxide in the process (Voet and Voet, *Biochemistry*, p. 658). There is then involved what is called the *Calvin cycle,* the usual nighttime process by which carbon dioxide is converted into carbohydrates, the category of *dark reactions* that occur in plants (Voet and Voet, *Biochemistry*, p. 649ff).

For the purposes here, a most interesting feature in Crassulacean acid metabolism or CAM is that pyruvate is created, which is converted back to phosphoenol pyruvate or PEP by the action of the enzyme pyruvate-phosphate dikinase, to complete the cycle. According to Boik, as set forth in Appendix X, *vitamin A analogs, for instance, not only inhibit cell growth but inhibit angiogenesis* in the CAM assay—maybe because *vitamin A inhibits collagen synthesis,* the protein that is the chief constituent of connective tissue (Boik, *Cancer & Natural Medicine*, p. 30). This correspondence may be an indicator for the fact that the concentration of pyruvate is affected, in turn affecting its further conversion to lactic acid in cancerous cells. Moreover, the concentration of carbon dioxide is affected, which relates to normal cell metabolism. The interactions are necessarily complicated. Suffice to say, something is going on.

The listing of *copper, lactic acid,* and *nicotinamide* as angiogenic factors is potentially enlightening (Boik, *Cancer & Natural Medicine*, p. 17). In fact, it is stated in the reference that *lactic acid is produced within tumors and may act to stimulate macrophages to secrete angiogenic factors.*

And we may again emphasize that lactic acid is the end product of anaerobic glycolysis, whereby pyruvic acid is converted to lactic acid by the enzyme lactate dehydrogenase.

It is interesting to note that shark cartilage is said to stop vascularization and contains *polypeptides*, that is, relatively short chain proteins or amino acid polymers. Similarly, the Burzynski antineoplastin therapy is said to contain *polypeptides*. Thus, again, we have the indication of *polypeptides as anticancer agents,* in one way or another. (Of course, most body components in some way or another are made up of peptides, read polypeptides, read proteins. The word is "ubiquitous.")

Very possibly, electromagnetic radiation—e.g., radiofrequency waves—could function as an *antiangiogenesis* agent, read anticancer agent, as previously indicated.

Among the newer agents that have shown promise against angiogenesis are *interleukin-12* and *angiostatin*. Several of the other interleukins have in fact been mentioned as antiangiogenesis agents (Boik, *Cancer & Natural Medicine*, p. 17), although *a general problem with interleukins is that of toxicity. Angiostatin* has been described as a 38 kDa (kilodalton) plasminogen fragment, plasminogen being a precursor to the plasmin as found in blood plasma and serum. (*Plasmin* is a proteolytic blood enzyme that dissolves the fibrin of blood clots.)

Angiostatin and a related substance called *endostatin* have in fact been publicized as *angiogenesis inhibitors*. Work has proceeded under the direction of Dr. Judah Folkman, who is a surgeon and biologist at Children's Hospital in Boston, and who is assisted by Dr. Michael O'Reilly. These angiogenesis inhibitors are further described as natural agents that act against blood capillary growth factors in tumors. Angiostatin, for instance, has been be collected from mouse urine in small concentrations and used against mouse tumors. Other angiogenesis inhibitors are in the offing from pharmaceutical companies, and which may act against human cancers. Evidently, angiogenesis inhibitors are not anticancer drugs per se but must be used along with conventional chemotherapy. An update was provided, for instance, on p. 82 of the December 9, 1996 issue of *U.S. News & World Report*, with the notation that these substances, even when made readily available, will require lengthy testing. Another update is provided by Keith I. Block, MD, in the September-October, 1998 issue of *Natural Health*, where it is noted as well that what works on mice does not necessarily work on humans. Block also lists 10 natural substances or combinations as anticancer agents:

1. soy genistein
2. bioflavonoids
3. omega-3 fatty acids
4. vitamins A and D
5. vitamin E
6. thiols (sulfur-containing compounds, e.g., from garlic and onions)
7. cartilage (e.g., shark and cow cartilage)
8. curcumin (a component of the spice tumeric)
9. anthocyanins and procanthocyanidins (the red, blue, and violet pigments found in vegetables and fruits)
10. bromelain, the protein-digesting enzyme from pineapple stems

The preceding subject continues to be of interest, as per a flurry of publicity circa May, 1998—but with the admonition that what works for mice doesn't necessarily work for humans. It also points to the need for cancer clinical research centers, or their equivalent, where promising therapies can be tried on advanced cancer patients, with their acquiescence, and under strict medical supervision in the event of any adverse or life-threatening side reactions, including anaphylactic shock—as discussed in Part 7 within the section on immunity, in the subsection titled "The Immune System."

A final comment:

Trying substances that affect blood coagulation can be very serious business indeed. It is no place for amateurs.

Inasmuch as we are also talking of cancer cell death, we may again turn to the subject of cell *necrosis* versus *apoptosis*. In necrosis, cell death is presumed caused by external factors, whereas apoptosis is produced internally (Boik, *Cancer & Natural Medicine*, p. 13). The latter may in fact be regarded as programmed into the cell.

Moreover, apoptosis occurs at random and does not cause inflammation or damage to adjacent cells. It can be viewed as a systematic way for the body to remove old or damaged cells that are no longer needed or wanted. *The failure of apoptosis to remove cells with damaged DNA has been advanced as a possible cause for cancer. It is also noted that cancer cells have lower apoptosis rates than do normal cells.*

Whereas higher doses of cytotoxic chemotherapy drugs produce necrosis, at lower doses these same drugs may produce apoptosis. Thus, there is in fact a reason for treating cancer with low levels of chemotherapy agents. This is a regimen advocated by English physician Dr. Denis Parsons Burkitt, discoverer of Burkitt's Lymphoma.

Among the agents observed to produce apoptosis in cancer cells *in vitro* are those shown in Table 8.11. Some of these same agents act against angiogenesis, as seen in Appendix X. Of particular note, *butyric acid* is an entry, which in the form of the glyceride is a significant component of *butter* or *butterfat.* May we therefore project that butter or butterfat acts as an anticancer agent—including cream, ice cream, and butter-rich desserts?

It is informative to note that *caffeine* also makes an appearance in Table 8.11, suggesting that there may be more than meets the eye in the fact that medical folklore includes caffeine as an anticancer agent. Moreover, as previously indicated, caffeine may be an enzyme inhibitor for one or another of the steps in anaerobic glycolysis. The question then arises, if this is so, *why do heavy coffee drinkers get cancer, the same as anybody else?*

8.8 PLANT OR HERBAL REMEDIES CHALLENGED

Varro E. Tyler, cited previously, is listed as the Lilly Distinguished Professor of Pharmacognosy at the Purdue University School of Pharmacy and Pharmacal Sciences and is the author of many other publications, including *The Honest Herbal,* and another book titled *Herbs of Choice: The Therapeutic Use of Phytomedicinals.* (It may be noted that Eli Lilly is a leading pharmaceutical company.) Tyler is both skeptical and wary of many herbs, undoubtedly with good enough reasons. That is, the herbal substance may be toxic or may be ineffective. But this is not the entire story, as previously indicated.

In his book, *The Alternative Medicine Sourcebook*, published in 1997, Fort Collins CO physician Steven Bratman, MD, takes on the pros and cons of using alternative medicines, e.g., in a chapter titled "Alternative Medicine: Myths and Realities." There is the problem of determining whether the treatments are actually effective, there being wide variation among individual patients. For one or a few, or for some, the treatment may work, for others it does not. Bratman also discusses such problems for cancer treatment but foregoes any specific recommendations (Bratman, *The Alternative Medicine Sourcebook*, pp. 233–235).

Other authors may mention some specific treatments, and one such is Melvyn Werbech, MD, in his *Healing Through Nutrition.* In his section on cancer, however, these treatments are more mentioned than recommended.*

It may be indicated concomitantly that there are some distinguished individuals or faculty members who have made extensive plant or herbal compilations, as noted and utilized in Part 3. (Although these compilations may be relegated to medical folklore, at the same time these listings furnish a place to start for developing alternative plant-derived treatments.) For example, there is Maurice M. Iwu, professor

Table 8.11   Agents Producing Cancer-Cell Apoptosis

Butyric acid	The sodium salt, sodium butyrate, produces apoptosis in colon cancer cells. This may be explained in part by the fact that intestinal bacteria act on fiber to yield butyric acid. Thus, the role of dietary fiber against colon cancer. Both the acid and the sodium salt are listed in the Sigma and Aldrich catalogs. Butyric acid is classed as a fatty acid. In the ester form, it is a component of animal fats and plant oils. As the ester of glycerol, called a glyceride, it constitutes 3 to 4% of butter or butterfat. It accounts for the disagreeable odor of rancid butter, whereby the glyceride hydrolyzes to yield butyric acid. (Can we therefore infer that butter or butterfat serves as an anticancer agent?)
Caffeine	Under certain conditions, caffeine can produce apoptosis and enhance the action of radiotherapy and of alkylating chemotherapy agents such as carboplatin, busulfan, and cyclophosphamide. With nonalkylating chemotherapy agents, however, caffeine may prevent apoptosis. Caffeine is listed in both the Sigma and Aldrich catalogs.
DMSO	Dimethylsulfoxide induced apoptosis in mice cancer cells. Mentioned by both Moss and Walters as an anticancer agent, it is listed in the Sigma and Aldrich catalogs.
Genistein	An isoflavone found in legumes, effective against some cell lines. It is listed in the Sigma catalog.
Quercetin	A flavonoid that induces apoptosis in leukemia cells and in Burkitt's lymphoma. Listed as the dihydrate in both the Sigma and Aldrich catalogs.
Retinoic acid	Promotes the enzymes called transglutaminases, which catalyze the cross linking of proteins. Affects blood clotting and macrophage functions, and is important in apoptosis. Also known as *vitamin A* acid, *all-trans*-retinoic acid is listed in both the Sigma and Aldrich catalogs and is described in the Aldrich catalog as an antitumor agent and an inducing factor in leukemia differentiation, with references cited. A form called 13-*cis*-retanoic acid is a *teratogen* (causes fetus abnormalities).
Umbelliferae	*Blupereum chinensis* (chai leu). Inhibited human hepatocellular carcinoma. The saponin constituent saikosaponin-α induced apoptosis in human hepatoma cells *in vitro*. The plant family and genus are listed in Hartwell's *Plants Used Against Cancer*, but not the particular species. The saponin constituent is not listed in either the Sigma or the Aldrich catalog.
Labiatae	*Scutellaria baicalensis* (huang qin). The flavonoid constituent baicalein completely inhibited cell growth. The flavonoid component baicalin inhibited human hepatoma cell growth. The plant family, genus, and species are listed in Hartwell's *Plants Used Against Cancer*. Baicalein is listed in the Sigma catalog; baicalein monohydrate is listed in the Aldrich catalog. Baicalin hydrate is also listed in the Aldrich catalog, with the spelling "Baicalin."

Source: Data from *Cancer & Natural Medicine* by John Boik, Oregon Medical Press, Princeton MN, 1995, pp. 13–14.

of pharmacognosy at the University of Nigeria, who wrote the *Handbook of African Medicinal Plants*. Nguyen Van Duong, formerly professor and chairman of the department of pharmacy at the University of Saigon, wrote the *Medicinal Plants of Vietnam, Cambodia and Laos*. Kee Chang Huang, professor of pharmacy at the University of Louisville, wrote *The Pharmacology of Chinese Herbs*. The subject of herbal use in turn rests on how plant chemicals may affect the body, for better or worse.

In an article by James Trefil in the December, 1995 issue of the *Smithsonian*, the subject is about how the body repairs itself from toxins, and in particular how DNA repairs itself utilizing enzymes. Interviewed along the way is Bruce Ames, who is a professor of molecular and cellular biology at the University of California, Berkeley, and the originator of the Ames test for cancer, a test based on cell mutagenicity. It is Ames' contention that the body is exposed to more toxic chemicals via those that exist naturally in the food we eat than occur from man-made chemicals. In fact, many plants produce

---

* As if in confirmation of the dilemmas encountered, the Home Box Office (HBO) TV channel presented a program on or about May 10, 1997, that encountered the world of alternative cancer therapies. The program was titled "Six Months to Live," and the particular cases investigated were not encouraging, either for alternative or conventional treatments. Both *Time* and *Newsweek*, in their respective issues dated May 18, 1998, reviewed what is going on in the unconventional world of conventional medicine—contrasting the hype and the hope.

toxins in self-defense. (Alkaloids are a prime example, as has previously been noted.) Furthermore, the body is able to repair itself against all this damaging bombardment. Among those agreeing with Bruce Ames is James Duke, cited elsewhere.

Of course, one can mention the now-ubiquitous halogenated organic compounds, notably of chlorine and fluorine, but also of phosphorus and sulfur—as in pesticides—that constitute a synthetic category far removed from nature. Maybe we're being bombarded from both directions. However, we're not in the habit of dining on hemlock, locoweeds, or Jimsonweed and their alkaloids—apparently there are enough alkaloids already in *Papaver somniforum, Erythroxylon coca, Cannabis sativa, Nicotiana tabacum, Coffea arabica,* and so on—not to mention the psychophysiological effects of ethanol.

In comment, sometimes the body is not able to defend itself, and cancer appears. It therefore can be wondered if some or many of these same plant-chemicals or phytochemicals—or call them poisons—cannot also assist the body's DNA in repairing itself. That is, potentially these phytochemicals may be either enzyme inhibitors or enzyme activators for DNA repair—not to mention inhibitors for cancer cell metabolism. (This same issue of the *Smithsonian* carries an article about garlic, but cancer is barely mentioned.) The possibilities seem nearly endless. Some authorities speak of *approximately 100,000 different chemical compounds that have already been found in plants.* Another item of information is that *perhaps 25 percent of all pharmaceuticals have plant origins.*

We continue. It is a given that many or most medicinal plants or herbs are poisonous to one degree or another. (If not, then by definition they are not medicinal plants or herbs.) The adjective "bioactive" in fact connotes this toxicity. For example, John K. Crellin and Jane Philpott, in the introduction to *Herbal Medicines Past and Present,* note that *hepatotoxic pyrrolizidine alkaloids are fairly common throughout the plant kingdom.* This may be for the worse or for the better, or both, depending on how much is consumed and whether the beneficial actions, if any, outweigh the toxic effects. (Unfortunately, as has been previously noted, in some countries the plants that contain these alkaloids are consumed as foods during drought times, in quantities sufficient to cause severe medical problems, even death.)

It can be added that *common garden vegetables and fruits contain bioactive substances or phytochemicals as well as vitamins and minerals, albeit in trace amounts.* These substances are evidently not toxic if foods are consumed in moderation—evidently the criterion to be classed as "foods"—and presumably may be beneficial read medicinal. Sometimes, in fact, there may be a fine line between what is beneficial and what is toxic.

The question becomes, can herbal or plant substances be used in trace amounts, or in the amounts necessary, to heal the body of disease without otherwise adversely affecting the body? That is, can these herbal or plant substances somehow be used to the benefit of body biochemistry by acting say as inhibitors for enzymes that are involved in disease-causing or disease-sustaining biochemical reactions? After all, it is said that modern medicine is based on enzyme inhibitors—antibiotics being the best known example.

Given the number and ranges of variables involved—the wide variation of active components and concentrations in plants or herbs—this is not an easy question to answer. In part, this may be central to the difficulty in accepting herbal remedies, which oftentimes appear as if at random, as if they were made up. Proffered in myriad array without an underlying scientific basis, these remedies do not have adequate substantiation and may lack even anecdotal evidence. There is often a vagueness using catchall explanations, such as volunteering that the substance stimulates the immune system—just whatever this is supposed to mean.

Nevertheless, something must be going on, and medical folklore may as often be right as wrong. It seems the proper function of science to try to ferret out what is correct from what isn't, rather than throwing out the baby with the bathwater. For "scientific" assessments can appear as random as remedies. In other words, what is the validity of the scientific assessment itself? Or, who's looking out for whom?

There is an informative article about cancer statistics versus cures in the June 1996 issue of the *Atlantic Monthly,* by David Plotkin, MD. Titled "Good News and Bad News About Breast Cancer," among the subjects discussed is longevity after diagnosis. It is often claimed that early diagnosis increases survival times. But this can be challenged in that early diagnosis only means that the patient knows about the cancer for a longer period of time. *Life spans are essentially the same whether the diagnosis is made earlier or later.* On the next to last page of his article, Dr. Plotkin also offers this remark about his experiences with conventional therapies: *"Cruelly, chemotherapy helps least those who need it most."*

About the new age of "pharmo-capitalism," Greg Critser has written "Oh, How Happy We Will Be: Pills, paradise, and the profits of the drug companies," which appeared in the June 1996 issue of

Harper's. If it seems that nutritional supplements are excessively promoted, then one ought to read Critser's article.

In another way of looking at it, not only are what we call vitamins and minerals apparently necessary to life, but other kinds of chemical compounds or phytochemicals may be equally necessary. For if not, all we would need in the way of nutrition is sugar water. Clearly, something is afoot, only we haven't found out the all of what it is.

Given the fact that this is not a subject for the pharmaceutical industry, since plants substances cannot be patented, then it becomes a function and responsibility for government. That is, government-supported research and development should fund projects that are in the public domain and in the public interest. Unfortunately, this conflicts with the purposes and profits of the private sector, and politics being politics.... Which may be one good reason that an absolute cure for cancer is still not in sight.

Perhaps as the last word, the German government has itself been involved in herbal remedies, as per the Commission E recommendations published by the German Federal Department of Health. This information has been translated, and the translation was published in 1998 by the American Botanical Council, Austin TX, as *The Complete German Commission E Monograph*. (The American Botanical Council, as part of its functions, publishes the newsletter *HerbalGram* and is affiliated with the Herb Research Foundation, Boulder CO.) The American Botanical Council has also issued a CD titled *Herbal Remedies*, prepared by T. Brendler, J. Gruenwald, and C. Jaenicke. This CD contains information about over 600 plants, including Chinese and Japanese traditional medicines and provides further information about dosages, side effects, interactions, contraindications, reference sources, and so on. German Commission E recommendations are included. See also the new *Physicians' Desk Reference for Herbs*.

8.9   AN UPDATE ON PLANT OR OTHER SUBSTANCES AS ENZYME INHIBITORS

The foregoing things said, we return once again to the subject of enzyme inhibitors for anaerobic glycolysis, that is, cancer cell primary metabolism. As noted, enzymes are the proteinaceous catalysts required for the many and varied biochemical reactions that sustain life. A comprehensive description of specific enzymes and their properties is contained in the multivolume *Enzyme Handbook*, edited by D. Schomburg and M. Salzmann.

Another source of information is *Enzyme Nomenclature 1978*, published in 1979, which comprises the recommendations of the International Union of Biochemistry on the nomenclature and classification of enzymes. The contents consist of the chapters designated "Historical Introduction," "The Classification and Nomenclature of Enzymes" (which includes a section on systematic and trivial, which do not necessarily correspond to the agreed upon method of classification), "Enzyme List," "References to the Enzyme List," "Index to the Enzyme List," plus an appendix dealing with the nomenclature of electron-transport proteins. The classification and numbering system assigns code numbers to the main divisions, subclasses, subsubclasses, and provides a serial number. The main divisions are: (1) Oxidoreductases, (2) Transferases, (3) Hydrolases, (4) Lyases, (5) Isomerases, (6) Ligases. As indicated, these formalized divisions do not necessarily correspond to the trivial or common names that have been used and that are still in use. This said, here we are most interested in enzyme inhibitors for the few controlling enzymes involved in cancer cell metabolism, which is referred to as *anaerobic glycolysis*.

In the enlarged and revised edition of H. Zollner's *Handbook of Enzyme Inhibitors*, published in 1993, a number of additional substances have been added to the listings of the original volume, published in 1989. The original listings were presented in Appendix A for the several controlling enzymes involved in anaerobic glycolysis, that is, the conversion of glucose to lactic acid or lactate, the primary sequence in cancer cell metabolism. Commentary was furnished in Part 1. The update is presented in Appendix Y, listing both the original substances that appeared in Appendix A and the additional substances.

The controlling enzymes have been perceived as *hexokinase* (HK), *phosphofructokinase* (PFK), *pyruvate kinase* (PK), and, perhaps most importantly, *lactate dehydrogenase* (LDH). Lactate dehydrogenase catalyzes the last step, the conversion of pyruvic acid or pyruvate to lactic acid or lactate, as shown in Figure 1.2. The preceding 10 steps for the formation of pyruvic acid from glucose are the same for aerobic glycolysis as for anaerobic glycolysis, as indicated in Figure 1.1. On the other hand, in aerobic glycolysis or normal cell metabolism, the pyruvic acid or pyruvate is converted to carbon dioxide and water via the tricarboxylic acid cycle, also called the Krebs cycle or citric acid cycle, as previously shown in Figure 1.4.

8.9.1 GARLIC AND ALLICIN

Among the several items of special interest are the chemical compounds shown in the previously mentioned Appendix Y. These may be natural or synthetic, and in some cases their sources may be indicated. The compounds or substances of most interest are shown in boldface in Appendix Y. Some of this information is supplied in the article "Enzyme Inhibitors for Cancer Cell Metabolism," by E.J. Hoffman and published in the May 1997 issue of the *Townsend Letter for Doctors & Patients*.

It may be noted in passing that, in Table Y.2 of Appendix Y, the compound *EDTA*, for ethylenediaminetetraacetic acid, is highlighted, it being the substance used in chelation therapy as a treatment for removing arterial plaque. It has also been tried against cancer, with inconclusive results, as described in Walters' *Options*. The substance called *disulfiram* (or Antabuse®) also appears in Table Y.2 as an inhibitor for L-lactate dehydrogenase but is listed in neither Moss nor Walters. Its chemical name is tetraethylthiuram disulfide or bis(diethylthiocarbamyl) disulfide, with the stoichiometric chemical formula $C_{10}H_{20}N_2S_4$, and it contains urea-type or carbamide structures as well as sulfur. It is listed in the Sigma catalog as possibly carcinogenic. Its principal use is in combating chronic alcoholism, causing unpleasant symptoms when alcohol is consumed. Another compound highlighted is *oxamic acid,* or monoamide oxalic acid, with the formula $HOOCCONH_2$, which bears a chemical resemblance to urea and hydrazine, both simple nitrogen-containing compounds. Oxamic acid or its compounds, similarly to the use of urea, has been proposed as a chemical fertilizer. Urea, an organic compound also known as carbamide or carbonyl diamide, has the chemical formula H_2NCONH_2. Hydrazine, which has the formula H_2NNH_2, is classed as an inorganic compound. Urea is described in Moss's *Cancer Therapy* as an anticancer agent, and hydrazine sulfate is described by both Moss and Walters as an anticancer agent.

Returning to garlic and its compounds, *allicin* is listed in Appendix Y as an *enzyme inhibitor* for both *hexokinase* and *L-lactate dehydrogenase.* It is a transitory sort of substance, derived from *raw garlic* via the conversion of the odorless and flavorless compound alliin by the enzyme alliinase (e.g., Heinerman, *The Healing Benefits of Garlic*, pp. 59-61). Heinerman states that, in the pure form, its half-life is less than three hours, indicating that the garlic source must be utilized fresh. Accordingly, allicin is not found in the chemical catalogs. And, it hardly needs to be said, garlic has been prominently mentioned in medical folklore as a treatment for cancer. (Increasingly, medical folklore cites garlic in some form or another as an anticancer agent, especially against colon cancer. We may wonder also about its cousin the onion.) For the record, there are a few commercial preparations that claim an allicin content, for example "Garlicin®," "Garlique®," and "Garlinase®." The allicin is formed after ingestion, however, from a powdered mix of alliin and allinase. Compressed into tablets, the active components make contact and form allicin by the time the mixture reaches the small intestine.

According to the handbooks, allicin may also be called S-oxodiallyl disulfide and is commonly given the stoichiometric formula $C_6H_{10}OS_2$. More precisely, the allyl group is $CH_2=CH-H_2-$ or simply C_3H_5- and the formula may be written as $C_3H_5S(:O)SC_3H_5$ or as $(CH_3H_5S)_2O$. It may be noted in passing that other garlic-derived compounds include diallyl sulfide or $C_6H_{10}S_2$, diallyl trisulfide or $C_6H_{10}S_3$, and allyl propyl disulfide or $C_6H_{12}S_2$. There is the possibility that one or another of these compounds may also act as an enzyme inhibitor or inhibitors.

The subject of garlic and garlic-derived agents is covered in a chapter titled "Chemoprevention of Gastrointestinal Cancer in Animals by Naturally Occurring Organosulfur Compounds in Allium Vegetables," written by Michael J. Wrgovich, Hiromichi Sumiyoshi, Allan Baer and Osamu Imada. It appears in the volume *Vitamins and Minerals in the Prevention and Treatment of Cancer*," edited by Maryce M. Jacobs. Of special note are the cancer-inhibiting effects of diallyl sulfide (DAS) and S-allyl-cysteine, and also garlic oil, although allicin as such was not mentioned. (It may be added that the *eye-watering property of onions* is said to be caused by a gaseous sulfur compound called *thiopropanal S-oxide*. This compound is formed when the cell structure is disturbed, which permits a certain enzyme to contact an existing sulfur compound, in turn producing and releasing thiopropanal S-oxide.)

The above-cited volume has other interesting information, e.g., a chapter by Carmia G. Borek on the antioxidant role of selenium and vitamin E, and vitamin C—an antioxidant role now apparently of common knowledge. The effect of folic acid deficiency is discussed in a chapter by Richard F. Branda, with mixed signals. *Lower than normal levels of folic acid are found in cancer patients, but increasing the folate intake may cause cancer to spread.* (Nevertheless, there is research ongoing directed at folic acid antagonists as chemo agents.) The relationship of potassium levels to cancer is the subject of a chapter by Maryce M. Jacobs and Roman J. Pienta. Epidemiological and other studies associate *increased potassium intake with a decreased cancer risk,* whereas an *increased sodium intake will increase cancer risk. Of even more significance is the potassium/sodium ratio, with higher values decreasing cancer risk.* As a general statement, potassium levels are higher in normal tissues, lower in cancerous tissues, except possibly for leukemic bone marrow. The authors conclude, however, that *a potassium-rich diet may or may not be of value in curing malignancies.*

Perhaps the authoritative reference on *garlic* to date is the volume *Garlic: The Science and Therapeutic Application of* Allium sativum *L. and Related Species,* second edition, edited by Heinrich P. Koch and Larry D. Lawson, and published in 1996. There is appended a list of 2580 references, 2240 of which are concerned with garlic. A chapter on "The Composition of Garlic Cloves and Processed Garlic," by Larry D. Lawson, contains tables listing the general breakdown for the composition of garlic cloves, and a bar chart showing that garlic has many times the sulfur content of other vegetables, including nearly four times that of onions, broccoli, and cauliflower. Interestingly, apricots have about as much sulfur as the latter three.

The reference gives the history behind the discovery of the chemistry of the sulfur compounds of garlic, notable of the allyl sulfides, of alliin and its conversion to allicin by the action of the enzyme alliinase, and of what are called the γ-glutamylcysteines. (Lawson, in *Garlic,* pp. 38–41). It was found early on, for instance, that *alliin itself had no antibiotic activity unless converted to allicin.* It is further noted that *allicin is the parent compound for the diallyl sulfides; the characteristic odor-producing compounds.*

A table is supplied listing the total known sulfur compounds in whole and crushed garlic. These compounds are divided into the four categories designated S-(+)-alk(en)yl-L-cysteine sulfoxides, g-L-glutamyl-S-alk(en)yl-L-cysteines, thiosulfinates, and others. The cysteine sulfoxides include alliin, methiin, and isoalliin. The thiosulfinates (THS) include allicin, and are products from the conversion of each of the first two categories, the cysteine sulfoxides being the primary source, the glutamylcysteines the secondary source. A figure is provided showing the steps and enzymes involved in the chemical conversion of both γ-glutamylcysteines and cysteine sulfoxides to thiosulfinates (THS). Information is also supplied about pathways for the biogenesis of garlic's sulfur compounds, starting initially with the sulfate ion (Lawson, in *Garlic,* pp. 72–75).

In addition to the cysteine sulfoxides, there are other parent compounds for alliin, which occurs abundantly in garlic cloves, as previously indicated. These and similar compounds constitute a reserve pool for the further production of alliin. These are called **γ-glutamylpeptides**, and occur in *onions* as well. Of the nine or so different compounds found, six contain the sulfur amino acid *cysteine,* and are therefore called γ-glutamylcysteines (Lawson, in *Garlic,* p. 41). Of the latter, the two of most significance are probably the γ-glutamyl-S-propenylcysteine and γ-glutamyl-S-*trans*-1-propenylcysteine. The amounts vary with storage. These two γ-glutamylcysteines may be the specific parent compounds for alliin (and isoalliin).

The reference specifically cites three S-alkylcysteine sulfoxides as the precursors for the thiosulfinates, and these particular sulfoxides are alliin, isoalliin, and methiin (Lawson, in *Garlic,* pp. 46-48). Alliin constitutes about 85 percent of the total, and a tabulation is provided of the allicin content from various strains of crushed garlic. A table is also provided for the distribution of cysteine sulfoxides and γ-glutamylcysteines in the several plant parts, where in mature plants the concentration is in the bulbs, but in premature plants most may be found in the leaves and stems. It is noted that the cysteine sulfoxides are rare in other plants outside the family Alliaceae or Liliaceae, e.g., the genus *Allium.* An exception is methylcysteine sulfoxide as found in the family Cruciferae or Brassicaceae.

The reference notes that dried garlic has a sulfur content of 1.0 percent of its dry weight, and the dried product is about 35 percent of its fresh weight (Lawson, in *Garlic,* p. 41). About 72 percent of the sulfur compounds consist of alliin, allicin, and two principal g-glutamylcysteines; there are 16 nonproteinaceous organosulfur compounds that have been identified in whole cloves, and 23 in crushed cloves. The totality of the sulfur compounds so far identified constitute about 86 percent of the sulfur content.

Of prime interest are the thiosulfinates, which include *allicin,* here given the formula (Lawson, in *Garlic,* pp. 40–42):

$$CH_2{=}CHCH_2\text{-}SS({=}O)\text{-}CH_2CH{=}CH_2$$

Its scientific or chemical name depends on the system of nomenclature used:

IUPAC name	allyl 2-propenethiosulfinate or 2-propenyl 2-propenethiosulfinate
Chemical Abstracts name	2-propene 1-1 sulfinothionic acid S-2 propenyl ester
Historically used name	allicin or diallyl thiosulfinate

The stability of allicin depends on the temperature and solvent (Lawson, in *Garlic*, pp. 57–68) and, in general, is longer than the half-life of a few hours stated by Heinerman, noted previously. At room temperature, pure allicin has a half-life of 16 hr, and in water a half-life of 30 to 40 days. At –70°C, allicin in water had no change in 2 years, but the pure compound had a half-life of only 25 days at the same temperature.

Of particular concern is the effect of cooking on garlic's sulfur compounds, since garlic is most often eaten cooked (Lawson, in *Garlic*, pp. 68–69). *Heat inactivates enzymes, and it has been found that alliinase becomes inactivated by cooking so as to prevent the formation of allicin and other thiosulfinates.* The information is supplied that boiling unpeeled whole garlic cloves for 15 min. completely inactivates alliinase, although there is a small amount of alliin conversion (about 0.5 to 1 percent) that may occur due to the cloves bumping into each during heating. The allicin, in turn, is converted to diallyl trisulfide for the most part, with smaller amounts of the di- and trisulfides also produced. Accordingly, even boiled cloves can produce garlic breath. Other reactions occurring include the hydrolysis of glutamylcysteines to still different forms.

The thiosulfinates (e.g., allicin) are very reactive and, in addition to reacting with reducing agents, undergo spontaneous reactions in various solvents and media (Lawson, in *Garlic*, pp. 59–65). The reaction products are more stable than the thiosulfinates but still contain the thioallyl groups (S-allyl) or thiomethyl groups, and are active components in garlic oils.

At room temperature, the thiosulfinates (e.g., allicin) in crushed garlic slowly convert to various diallyl and allyl sulfides, and so on, a conversion accelerated on heating, for instance, in steam distillations. *Pure allicin is an oily liquid, but is unstable,* and has been noted to disappear in less than 20 hr at room temperature (which corresponds to a half-life of a few hours, as reported by Heinerman). The decomposition products are said to be diallyl disulfide, diallyl sulfide, and diallyl trisulfide, but other products identified include the vinyldithiins and ajoene. In organic solvents, the conversion products are different than in water, and they include the vinyldithiins and ajoene. The thiosulfinates are relatively stable under acidic conditions, but under basic conditions undergo rapid hydrolysis to form disulfides. *Allicin has also been found to react rapidly with the amino acid cysteine to produce a mercaptocysteine.**

Allicin inhibits a large number of enzymes *in vitro* that contain cysteine at the active sites, but it inhibits very few otherwise (Lawson, in *Garlic*, p. 65). The same kind of inhibition reaction occurs with glycylcysteine, N-acetylcysteine, and protein-cysteine.

The reference further makes the following statement, that *"many of the explanations given for the biological effects of garlic focus on the ability of allicin to react with sulfhydryl enzymes."* Additionally, *"allicin reacts with the sulfhydril group of acetyl-CoASH, the building block of cholesterol and triglyceride synthesis."* (The compound acetyl-CoASH is also involved in the *tricarboxylic acid cycle,* as per Figure 1.4 in Part 1. Thus, presumably, there can also be some counter effects of allicin.)

In further comment, it is not known whether lactate dehydrogenase contains cysteine at the active cites. In any event, allicin functions as an inhibitor for this particular enzyme, as has been reported elsewhere (e.g., in Zollner's *Handbook*).

---

* The *vinyldithiins* occur as the isomeric forms 1,3-vinyldithiin and 1,2-vinyldithiin (Lawson, in *Garlic*, pp. 60–63). The respective chemical names given are 2-vinyl-4H-1,3 dithiin and 3-vinyl-4H-1,2 dithiin. The chemical formulas involve a sulfur-containing ring structure with the sulfurs at the 1,3- and 1,2-positions in the ring, and the vinyl group attached at the 2-position and 3-position, respectively. The overall conversion from allicin is as follows: allicin → H_2O + vinyldithiin. The compound designated *ajoene*—"ajo-" standing for garlic—comes in two isomeric forms, denoted as "E" and "Z." The chemical name given is E,Z-4,5,9-trithiadodeca-1,6,11-triene 9-oxide. The chemical formula may be designated

$$CH_2=CHCH_2-SS-CH_2=CH_2CH_2-S(=O)-CH_2CH=CH_2$$

Its chemical structure is somewhat similar to allicin and in fact is formed from allicin. The overall chemical conversion is as follows: 3 allicin → 2 ajoene + H_2O. Inasmuch as water is formed in both instances, the conversions can be viewed as condensation reactions.

In the aforecited volume on *Garlic*, in a chapter on "Therapeutic Effects and Applications of Garlic and Its Preparations," by Hans D. Reuter, Heinrich P. Koch, and Larry D. Lawson, sections are included on:

- Effects on the Heart and Circulatory System
- Antibiotic Effects
- Anticancer Effects
- Antioxidant Effects
- Immunomodulatory Effects
- Anti-inflammatory Effects
- Hypoglycemic Effects
- Hormone-Like Effects
- Enhancement of Thiamine Absorption
- Effects on Organic and Metabolic Disturbances
- Garlic in Homeopathy
- Dosing of Garlic and Its Preparations
- Deodorized Garlic Extracts
- Other Active Compounds in Garlic

Truly, garlic appears to be an all-purpose herb.

Regarding the section on "Anticancer Effects," the role of garlic in treating cancer is traced from ancient times, and more recent epidemiological studies indicate that there is a beneficial anticancer effect. Statistical studies in fact furnish evidence that cancer occurs least in countries where garlic and onions are a significant part of the diet. Examples include the French Province, Italy, the Netherlands, the Balkans, Egypt, India, and China. A specific citation (1936) refers to the connection between diet and cancer, whereby there is a cancer-inhibiting effect noted for leek or *Allium* plants, although the reasons were not known. Very possibly, the stimulation of gastric secretions and restoration of intestinal flora, along with the inhibition of gastrointestinal autointoxication, work against cancer formation. The notation is added that the use of black or green tea along with garlic can be correlated with the prevention of tumorigenesis.

As to clinical trials where garlic has been used against advanced cancer, only one study is known (Reuter, Koch, and Lawson, in *Garlic*, p. 176). In this one-and-only clinical investigation, conducted in Russia with the results published in 1962, a *garlic juice preparation* was introduced either intravenously or intramuscularly. The former was administered in 0.2 to 2 mL daily doses, the latter in 1 to 5 mL daily doses, over a period of 3 to 7 days. The 35 patients tested had cancers variously of the lung, cervix, stomach, lower lip, mammary gland, larynx, and also had leukemia. It is stated that 26 showed positive results in varying degree, but none experienced complete healing.

Another case cited, however, was of a man whose pituitary cancer shrunk by 50 percent over a 5-month period in which he ate 5 to 7 g of fresh garlic daily. This was noted to be the first case in which this particular kind of cancer regressed without the use of chemotherapy or surgery. The results were reported in 1993 in the journal *Neurochirurgia*.

In comment, the trials involving the intravenous or intramuscular dosage of garlic juice administered, above, were for only a very short period. If administered over a period of months, the results could have been dramatically more positive. Furthermore, no figures on allicin content were given. Presumably, allicin, the most active ingredient derived from garlic, would have been present if the juice was extracted by crushing the garlic. There is also the matter of freshness, in that allicin gradually decomposes, and rather rapidly under some conditions.

As to the man's daily consumption of fresh garlic, above, an amount of garlic weighing 5 to 7 g is relatively ordinary, being only about 0.2 to 0.3 oz, since there are 454 g or 16 oz to the pound. (*Fresh garlic weighs about one gram per clove,* so that 5 to 7 g amounts to about 5 to 7 cloves per day.) As a point of reference, a *garlic tablet* of one of the several brands that produce allicin from a powdered mixture of alliin and alliinase will yield an announced 5,000 µg of allicin, or 5 mg of allicin—albeit some may yield up to 14 mg/g (Lawson, in *Garlic*, p. 95). *Fresh crushed garlic will yield about 3 to 7 mg of allicin per gram of garlic,* depending on the variety and strain (Lawson, in *Garlic*, p. 46). Using an average of 5 mg/g for convenience, *in terms of allicin, one tablet would be equivalent to 1 g or one clove of fresh garlic.* Thus, 5 to 7 g per day of fresh garlic could be supplied by 5 to 7 tablets per day. The recommended dietary usage is ordinarily one tablet per day.

The reference further states that epidemiological studies support the fact that garlic consumption correlates with a reduced risk for cancer, especially of the gastrointestinal tract (Reuter, Koch, and Larson, in *Garlic*, pp. 176–178). In what was called the "Iowa Women's Health Study," which involved the intake of 127 different foods including 44 vegetables and fruits, it was found that *garlic was the only food that showed a significant statistical reduction in cancer risk*. While the foregoing study did not include onions, other studies have shown that *onions* and other *Allium* species correlate to a reduced gastrointestinal cancer risk. Another study conducted in the Netherlands showed *no correlation* between the consumption of garlic supplements (tablets) and a reduced risk for stomach, colon, rectum, lung, or breast cancers. The reference advises, however, that garlic supplements vary widely in composition according to type and brand.

Early *in vivo* experiments (1913) showed that garlic and its compounds, notably diallyl sulfide, inhibited tumors in mice, and similar results were subsequently obtained, both *in vivo* and *in vitro* (Reuter, Koch, and Lawson, in *Garlic*, pp. 178–186). For instance, for mice fed garlic or garlic juice, tumor growth could be inhibited. In experiments reported in 1949, *alliin freshly isolated from garlic bulbs was directly injected into rat sarcomas, resulting in reduction and dissipation. Parallel results were obtained by intramuscular injection*. On the other hand, *others subsequently could not find any alliin activity against transplanted and induced tumors*. Ehrlich ascites tumor cells were deactivated by fresh garlic extract containing allicin, and cells of Yoshida sarcoma (a mammary tumor) were deactivated by allicin. Similar experiments and results are described in the reference, with the perspective that *cancer cell virulence can be neutralized by fresh garlic*, and at the same time an antibody response continues intact such that the *animals become immune to untreated tumor cells*.

A further discovery is that *garlic contains a polypeptide* of unknown structure that is an inhibitor for guanylate cyclase (Reuter, Koch, and Lawson, in *Garlic*, p. 179; Lawson, in *Garlic*, p. 79). Found in several other vegetable plants, this substance has a *tumor-inhibiting property*.

Skin cancers were inhibited by topical applications of garlic oil, which contain allyl and diallyl sulfides (Reuter, Koch, and Lawson, in *Garlic*, p. 180)

The anticancer action of garlic has been explained in several ways. Thus, there is the opinion that the antibiotic substance (thiosulfinates, of which allicin is the main example) inhibit proteolytic enzymes (e.g., cathepsin) in human malignancies (Reuter, Koch, and Lawson, in *Garlic*, p. 181). Another finding is that *garlic extract inhibits pyruvate dehydrogenase*, thereby interrupting cellular respiration. (Pyruvate dehydrogenase is involved in the formation of Acetyl-CoA.)

> Enzyme inhibition may thus be generally considered as the mechanism whereby the active components in garlic exert their tumor-inhibiting effect.

With regard to the inhibiting action of garlic oil, onion oil, and diallyl sulfide on skin cancers, it has been found that these substances enhance the activity of glutathione peroxidase in epidermis cells, which is ordinarily suppressed by the presence of the tumor promoter TPA.

As to stomach cancer, the *thiosulfinates in garlic have an antimicrobial effect*, inhibiting the growth of *Fusarium moniliforme* and at the same time reducing the concentrations of carcinogenic nitrate, and preventing the formation of carcinogenic dimethylnitrosamine and other nitrosamines. In addition,

- The Ames test has been used to demonstrate that *garlic has antimutagenic properties*.
- Garlic has been found to interfere with cell division or mitosis.
- The selenium and germanium compounds present in garlic may have an anticancer effect, although it is suspected that the concentrations are too small.

Increasingly complicated mechanisms for the anticancer action of garlic and its sulfur-containing compounds are presented in the reference.

There are still other substances of interest in the *Allium* genus. Thus, there is the presence of a remarkable substance in *Allium bakeri*, a steroid called laxogenin (Reuter, Koch, and Lawson, in *Garlic*, p. 186). Another anticancer compound of interest, found in stressed garlic, is allixin.

Another interesting item is that the volatiles in garlic can repress the germination of pollen from flowers, with the effect similar to that of irradiation by gamma rays.

The aforecited section of the reference concludes with the observation that the agents in garlic responsible for its anticancer properties are allicin, allicin-derived compounds, and other yet-unidentified compounds. Further specifics are provided as follows:

1. With regard to epidemiological studies correlating garlic consumption with a decreased risk of colon cancer, the garlic was for the most part cooked. Since allicin is destroyed by cooking, the inference is that allicin is not necessary for reduced cancer risk. (We may, however, distinguish "risk" from "cure.")

2. With regard to gastric cancer, where large amounts of fresh garlic are eaten, the antibiotic effects of garlic may predominate, whereby the nitrate-reducing bacteria in the gut are affected. Garlic and its thiosulfinates (allicin) act against these bacteria and thereby reduce the amount of carcinogenic nitrosamines. It is concluded that allicin does not directly affect gastric cancer.

3. Animal studies indicate that allicin from fresh garlic greatly decreases breast cancer incidence in mice. Moreover, volatile sulfur compounds from garlic and from garlic oil both decreased liver tumor incidence in toads. Presumably allicin per se was not a factor.

4. Animal studies using diallyl sulfide and diallyl disulfide (as derived from allicin) showed positive effects against carcinogen-induced cancers. Allicin itself was not tested.

5. There is evidence from animal studies that garlic compounds other than allicin play an important anticancer role. Thus, commercial aged garlic (which contains little alliin and no active alliinase, nor allicin-derived compounds) showed a consistent decrease in carcinogen-induced tumors and DNA adducts.

The reference adds that future studies should include clinical trials with humans.

Regarding the medicinal use of garlic—even consumptive uses—it has been found that there are acute, subacute, and chronic toxicities (Koch, in *Garlic*, pp. 221–224). While absorptive poisoning by the plant itself is not suspect, the use of plant extracts, active components, or oils in highly concentrated form can be expected to have toxic effects. Thus, allicin is strongly hepatotoxic when administered in large doses over a long period. The dosage levels tested were approximately 100 mg/kg of body weight, however, equivalent to a human eating 1750 g or 500 cloves of raw garlic every day for an extended period. Oral consumption of garlic oil at levels of from 10 to 200 mg per day does not affect the erythrocytes in humans but does so in cats, causing serious anemia. Leukocytes are also noted to be changed by allicin, albeit increasing the germicidal activity.

Diallyl sulfide administered intravenously (in alcohol) at high dosages would produce heart stoppages in frogs. Rabbits affected myosis (abnormal contraction of the pupil of the eye), blood pressure drop, and increasing heart rate.

The liver and liver enzymes are adversely affected by the ingestion of *Allium* plants in large amounts. *Thus, garlic and onions can be hepatotoxic, as well as extracts of garlic—if consumed at high enough levels for a long enough time.*

Aqueous garlic extracts given to rats intraperitoneally, *increased lactate dehydrogenase activity in liver.* (This, of course, is as distinguished from other cells.)

Diphenylamine is found in onions but not garlic. Considered responsible for a blood-sugar-lowering effect, it is nevertheless questionable because of nephrotoxic (kidney-toxic) properties. An aqueous garlic extract administered to mice adversely affected weight growth and other properties, and in rats it was found to *elevate lactate dehydrogenase activities.* Garlic oil was lethal to starved rats but not to fed rats. No mutagenic effects were observed in other tests on hamsters and mice.

Appropriately, in the introduction to the aforecited chapter on "Toxicity, Side Effects, and Unwanted Effects of Garlic," the reference comments that a better term for side effects would be adverse effects (Koch, in *Garlic*, p. 221).

There have been many other books written about garlic, quite a few of which are still in print, with considerable of these concerned with culinary uses. About garlic's medicinal properties, in addition to John Heinerman's *The Healing Benefits of Garlic*, a volume for the general reader is Stephen Fulder's *The Garlic Book*. There is a section on garlic as a protective against cancer describing some of the studies where garlic or allicin has been tried (Fulder, *The Garlic Book*, pp. 99–101).

Specifically mentioned are the investigations of Dr. A.S. Weissberger of Case Western University, Cleveland, who in 1953 proposed that the sulfur in *allicin* might remove cancer cells. In experiments with mice, those injected with cancer cells and allicin lived for 6 months, whereas the control group that were injected only with cancer cells lived only 16 days.

Noting that this aroused some interest in garlic as a preventive, Fulder describes the work of Prof. Sydney Belman of the New York Medical Center. It was found that *onion and garlic oil* prevented much of the cancer that would be expected in mice injected with carcinogenic chemicals. More recently, at the M.D. Anderson Hospital in Houston TX, Professor Michael Wargovich of the Department of Medical Oncology found that three-fourths of the expected chemically induced tumors in mice could be prevented by *diallyl sulfide,* one of the several sulfides found in garlic oil.

Fulder, published in 1997, further mentions that more than 100 studies have now been carried out variously with cells, animals, and tissues which establish that garlic, garlic oil, allicin, the sulfides and other garlic compounds protect against cancer. At the same time, these substances protect against genetic changes in the DNA. *It is cautioned, however, that garlic is a preventive and not a cure.*

Fulder indicates, furthermore, that the medical folklore of Third World countries considers garlic as a cancer preventive. For instance, in China, both garlic and green tea are considered to protect against stomach and lung cancer. He cites the "designer foods" research program sponsored by the National Cancer Institute aimed at determining whether specific food components act against cancer. The food items selected for study include garlic, rosemary, licorice, and several others.

If there is no direct evidence of garlic as a cancer preventive in individuals, there is nevertheless the epidemiological statistic that *garlic-eating people have fewer cancers.* For instance, in two neighboring counties in China, the people of the one consume about six cloves per day, of the other, none. The stomach cancer incidence of the former was about 3.5 per 100,000 population, and for the latter about 40 per 100,000, or more than *10 times greater.* Also mentioned is the Iowa Women's Health Study, published in 1994 by Dr. K. Steinmetz and colleagues, wherein, of the 127 foods consumed by 41,387 women, *only garlic could be correlated with a reduced colon cancer risk.*

Fulder closes the section with the well known fact that *garlic's sulfur groups combine with toxic heavy metals in the body.* For instance, cysteine is used in conventional treatments to remove lead. A garlic preparation called *Satal* is used in Bulgaria to counteract lead poisoning. In fact, garlic is known to combine in equal weights with either lead or mercury. Garlic also acts to cleanse the body of food additives and solvents and, in the days before chemical antibiotics, served as nature's own antibiotic agent against both bacteria and fungi.

In another section of safety, Fulder comments that *garlic is extremely safe, evidenced in its daily consumption by millions of people worldwide.* As just one example, the people of Gangshan County in Shandong Province, China, eat an average of 20 g or 7 cloves of garlic each day. In studies on cholesterol reduction, the consumption was approximately 20 cloves per day over a three-month period, with no problems. Garlic oil in the amount of 200 mg, which is equivalent to 70 cloves of garlic, produces no ill effects.

Only with impossibly high doses do toxic effects enter. With rats, toxicity occurred with doses of 5 g of fresh garlic juice per kilogram of body weight, which would be equivalent to a person consuming 300 mashed cloves of garlic at one time. At these levels, the pungency of garlic injures the stomach, the same as with, say, red pepper. At very high doses, allicin is also toxic to the stomach and liver, as determined in animal studies equivalent to a person consuming 500 cloves of garlic. The pungency of garlic can irritate the skin or mouth tissues, with some people being extra sensitive. Finally, garlic slows the time for blood clotting.

Another interesting reference, more concise, is by Eric Block of the State University of New York, Albany, which appeared in the *Scientific America,* in the March 1985 issue. Titled "The Chemistry of Garlic and Onions," it says many of the same things as noted in the previous references, observing that extracts from both garlic and onions are antibacterial and antifungal as well as being *antithrombotic*—that is, they inhibit the aggregation of blood platelets into thrombi, a process that also involves fibrin.* Their therapeutic value can be traced back to the *Codex Ebers,* an Egyptian source dating back to circa 1550 B.C., which gives over 800 medicinal formulas, including 33 citations for garlic against numerous ailments, including headache, heart problems, worms, bites, and *tumors.* Mentioned also is the concoction known as *Four Thieves' Vinegar,* consisting of garlic macerated in wine, which was supposed to have made grave diggers immune to an outbreak of plague in 1721. Better known as *vinaigre des quatre voleurs,* it is still available in France. It is both mentioned and diagrammed that the method of extraction will determine the final compounds derived from both garlic and onions.

Block gives attention to the chemistry of the *onion* as well as garlic, and there is a relationship. Thus, onions contain what is named *trans-(+)-S-(1-propenyl)-L-cysteine sulfoxide,* which is a positional isomer

---

* With regard to the antithrombotic effect, this may conceivable be linked to antiangiogenesis.

of alliin. The stoichiometric formulas are the same, differing in only the position of a double bond. The compound named above turns out to be the *lacrimatory precursor,* or *LP*. It is converted by the enzyme allinase (or alliinase) into the *lacrimatory factor,* or *LF*, the substance that brings on tears when a person slices onions.

The stoichiometric formula for LF is C_3H_6SO, and it is now agreed that the structural formula can be represented as $C_2H_5CH=SO$. Named *propanethial S-oxide* (or *thiopropanal S-oxide*), there are two structural isomers, the *syn* isomer and the *anti* isomer. The former, which greatly predominates, is that where the ethyl group (C_2H_5) is nearer the oxygen atom at the end of the chain.

This is as compared with allicin, the corresponding product obtained from garlic, and whose stoichiometric formula can be written as $C_6H_{10}SSO$ or as $(C_3H_5)_2SSO$, and whose structural formula is $CH_2=CHCH_2\text{-}SS(=O)\text{-}CH_2CH=CH_2$ as indicated previously, but which can also be written as $C_3H_5SSOC_3H_5$. Thus, *there is a kind of symmetry between LF and allicin,* as if the latter was sort of a dimer of the former, doing a bit of rearranging in the hydrocarbon group, taking away an oxygen atom.

The point is, that if allicin is bioactive—say against cancer—then so may be the lacrimatory factor LF. It is in fact noted that *LF is highly reactive, as is allicin.*

The reference also states that the allinase (or alliinase) enzymes act as catalysts to produce a number of sulfur-containing side-products or by-products. These by-products include *pyruvate* and ammonia. Furthermore, there is the indication that another reactant or cofactor is involved, namely pyrodoxal phosphate, which serves to activate the principal reactant or substrate.

Interestingly, as per a reduction in blood-clotting times by *Allium*, mentioned above, and as previously stated elsewhere, *blood-clotting or coagulation disorders are somehow related to cancer formation and angiogenesis* (Boik, *Cancer & Natural Medicine*, p. 25). These disorders may involve fibrin and fibrinolysis or other factors. The same reference cites clinical tests in China using garlic preparations (Boik, *Cancer & Natural Medicine*, p. 29). In clinical tests on 57 patients with advanced carcinomas, there was a marked improvement in 13 percent and some improvement in 50 percent. Due to insufficient controls and criteria for judging improvement, however, the results were difficult to interpret. The mode of action may theoretically include a reduced angiogenesis, reduced platelet aggregation, and increased fibrinolysis.

No mention was made in any of the foregoing references about allicin or other garlic compounds as an inhibitor for lactate dehydrogenase.

8.9.2 MISCELLANEOUS

The chemical EDTA or ethylenediaminetetraacetic acid is listed as an inhibitor for L-lactate dehydrogenase. Interestingly, this chemical is also used in forensic work as a means for preserving blood samples. Whether it alters the blood DNA was a key question in the O.J. Simpson trial.

A number of other substances are listed in Anthony G. Payne's article, "Achieving Oncolysis by Compromising Tumor Cell Metabolic Processes," which was published in the December, 1996 issue of the *Townsend Letter for Doctors & Patients*. The contributing factor is said to be the *p53* gene, which ordinarily causes the production of a protein that arrests the growth of cells damaged by, say, chemicals or radiation, or else results in cell apoptosis or self-destruction. The cellular environment becomes increasingly hypoxic, that is, oxygen-deficient. *Lactic acid* or *lactate* is the principal metabolic product, but its formation has a very low heat of reaction.

Payne further notes, therefore, that malignant cells will increasingly rely on the beta-oxidation of fatty acids to produce Coenzyme A, or AcCoA, which can then enter the tricarboxylic acid cycle or citric acid cycle to be converted to carbon dioxide and water, such as occurs in normal cells (see for instance Part 1, Figure 1.4). Also noted is the conversion of amino acids as an energy source for malignant cells. (As indicated in Part 1, Figure 1.3, glutamine is probably the principal amino acid utilized, by the process of glutaminolysis.)

Payne is particularly interested in the inhibition of these alternative processes by which malignant cells may supplement their energy requirements. He emphasizes in particular the use of agents that may inhibit *hepatic fatty acid synthesis*. Also of interest are agents that may interfere with the release of lactic acid or lactate from the cell, which will further suppress anaerobic glycolysis—the main metabolic function of cancerous cells.

Among the anticancer substances or agents cited by Payne is the 10-carbon compound *limonene*, such as occurs in *lavender oil*. It is said to inhibit the formation of ubiquinone (e.g., coenzyme Q10, and so on.) in the tumor cell mitochondria, which reduces the metabolic energy available to the cell. (The Sigma catalog lists a number of coenzymes or ubiquinones, of which coenzyme Q10, which is alternatively designated ubiquinone-50, is perhaps that most generally found in the health food stores. Another version is called coenzyme Q2, or ubiquinone-10. What is called coenzyme A has many derivatives, and coenzyme B12 is a variant of vitamin B12.) Lavender, *Lavandula angustifolis* (narrow-leaved) of the family Labiatae, is listed in Hartwell.

Another anticancer agent cited is *L-hydroxycitrate*, which is said to inhibit *ATP citrate lyase*. This is the cytoplasmic (cell-plasma) enzyme that *decomposes citrate to produce AcCoA*. Maybe unfortunately, it is also said to act as an appetite suppressant.

Payne observes that *insulin drops during tumor formation*. (Thus, there is the possibility that *insulin levels might serve as an indicator for the progression or regression of cancer.* The relationship between insulin and cancer has been touched on elsewhere.) There are very likely other effects, such as interfering with the *Cori cycle,* the reconversion of metabolic products back to glucose in the liver. (The use of hydrazine or its derivatives presumably interferes with the conversion of lactic acid or lactate back to glucose, and is described as a feature of the therapy of Joseph Gold, MD, of the Syracuse Cancer Research Institute, which features hydrazine sulfate as an anticancer agent. Both Moss and Walters contain related information.) Payne further states that concentrated *garlic* extract or the exogenous introduction of insulin *will elevate the concentration levels of free or circulating insulin in the patient.*

Among the other suspected anticancer agents are exogenous *thyroid hormone* and *quercetin.* The latter is believed to interfere with the transport of lactate out of cancer cells. *Evening primrose oil* (EPO) is another, providing essential fatty acids for nutritional needs. Such acids also serve as the basis for the formation of *prostaglandins* that inhibit lypolysis.

Payne gives considerable space to *shark cartilage,* which is said to contain proteins that *inhibit tumor-produced enzymes (collagenases)* necessary for angiogenesis. (These same proteins, if relatively small, may of course be called peptides or polypeptides.) Another protein, called a *cartilage-derived inhibitor* or CDI, is said to block endothelial cell migration and proliferation. (The same issue of the *Townsend Letter* carries a letter to the editor about shark cartilage, and a response from William Lane, its principal proponent.)

Potentially of great interest, a number of compounds obtained from *yeast* appear as enzyme inhibitors as shown in Appendix Y. The form of the yeast in the main was not specified, e.g., whether baker's yeast, nutritional yeast, brewer's yeast, or whatever. (According to the Sigma catalog, under the category of Yeast, baker's yeast is the species *Saccharomycetes cerevisiae,* and torula yeast is the species *Candida utilis.*) Yeasts, of course, belong to the fungi or Mycota, and a number of fungal families are represented in the very last pages of Hartwell's *Plants Used Against Cancer.* (Also see Part 5 in the section "Medicinal Fungi and Cancer," e.g, Table 5.1.) Of particular note is the family *Saccharomycetaceae,* already mentioned and involved in fermentation, which is composed of unicellular fungi, including notably the genus *Saccharomyces.* The fungi that induce alcoholic fermentation produce an enzyme called *zymase.*

According to Appendix Y, the *yeast-derived compounds that inhibit hexokinase* are said to be dihydrogriesenin, gafrinin, geigerinin, griesenin, ivalin, o-phthalaldehyde, and vermeerin.* Yeast is also a source for *glucose 6-phosphate,* listed as another *inhibitor for hexokinase.* (This inhibiting action may be due to the fact that glucose 6-phosphate is the reaction product, e.g., see Figure 1.1.)

The various yeast-derived compounds cited in the preceding paragraph can alternatively be derived from *rabbit muscle* and are in turn listed as inhibitors for *6-phosphofructokinase.*

Also according to Appendix Y, *yeast-derived compounds* that inhibit *D-lactate dehydrogenase (cytochrome)* are EDTA, p-mercuriphenylsulphonic acid, oxalacetic acid, oxalic acid, o-phenanthroline, and pyruvic acid. (Pyruvic acid or pyruvate, being a reactant for the conversion to lactic acid or lactate as shown in Figure 1.2, would ordinarily be expected to favor the conversion rather than inhibit it.)

---

* Interestingly, some of the aforecited compounds are also derived from the genus *Geigeria* of the plant family Compositae, as found in South Africa (Watts and Breyer-Brandwijk, *The Medicinal and Poisonous Plants of Southern and Eastern Africa,* pp. 231–234). In particular, there is the compound called geigerin, which is sometimes considered toxic, as is the plant. The compound vermeerin is cited, as vermeeric acid, whose spellings reflect these South African origins. The compound vernmeerin is a dilactone, and the compound dihydrogriesenin, above, is a sesquiterpene lactone and is derived from *Geigeria. Geigeria* is not listed in Hartwell's *Plants Used Against Cancer.*

Baker's yeast is a source for 2-hydroxy-3-*butynoic acid*, which is an inhibitor for *L-lactate dehydrogenase (cytochrome).** Interestingly, *butynoic acid* per se—also called tetrolic acid—is a four-carbon organic acid, with the formula $CH_3CCCOOH$, and which is related to *butyric acid,* also named butanoic acid, $CH_3CH_2CH_2COOH$. The latter is considered an *anticancer agent producing apoptosis* (Boik, *Cancer & Natural Healing,* pp. 10, 13, 248) and is so listed in Table 8.11. The ubiquitous bacteria species *E. coli* is another source for 2-hydroxy-3-*butynoic acid,* which as noted is an inhibitor for *L-lactate dehydrogenase.*

It may be noted that *D-lactate* also serves as a source for *oxaloacetic acid and oxalic acid,* both *inhibitors for D-lactate dehydrogenase.* And since D-lactate is also the end product, a buildup of D-lactate could also suppress the further conversion of pyruvate to lactate. In further comment, since muscular or physical exercise produces lactic acid or lactate, which can in turn produce oxalate inhibitors for D-lactate dehydrogenase, then it can be inferred that *physical exercise* acts indirectly as an *inhibitor for D-lactate dehydrogenase,* and hence acts against cancer.†

Continuing further, *oxalate-bearing or oxalic acid-bearing plants*—such as *rhubarb, spinach,* and *woodsorrel*—by inhibiting *D-lactate dehydrogenase,* can be projected to be **a**nticancer agents, although there may be adverse side effects.‡ Many such oxalate-bearing plants are in fact encountered in Hartwell's compendium, e.g., the family Oxalidaceae containing the genus *Oxalis.*

Of additional interest is the fact that *glucose* itself is a source for several compounds that act as enzyme inhibitors. That is, glucose is a source for n-acetylglucosamine and glucose 6-phosphate, both of which are *enzyme inhibitors for hexokinase.*

Another natural inhibitor source of special note is the sweet potato, that is, *sweet potato roots.* Thus, sweet potato roots are listed as a source for mononucleotides and for phosphoenolpyruvic acid and pyruvic acid, all of which *inhibit L-lactate dehydrogenase.*‡ (This inhibiting effect is in spite of the fact that pyruvic acid is a reactant in the conversion to lactic acid, which ordinarily would be thought to promote the degree of reaction.) The sweet potato, of tropical origin, is the species *Ipomoea batatas* of the plant family Convolvulaceae, related to the *morning glory.* Its starchy root bears a close resemblance to the *yam,* also of tropical origin, which is the root of certain members of the genus *Dioscorea* of the plant family Dioscoreaceae. There is, moreover, a continued interest in *yams as anticancer agents* and for other purposes, as mentioned for instance in Part 3 in the section titled "Other Information about Chinese Anticancer Agents." Both plant families are represented in Hartwell's *Plants Used Against Cancer,* with the genera *Ipomoea* and *Dioscorea* listed along with several species.

The compound called *gossypol,* described in Part 2, is an *inhibitor for L-lactate dehydrogenase.* And as has been indicated in Part 2, it is known to have some undesirable side effects. Gossypol is derived from cotton or cotton-seed, of the genus *Gossypium* of the family Malvaceae, and in particular from the common species *Gossypium herbaceum.* The family, genus, and particular species are represented in Hartwell's *Plants Used Against Cancer.*

---

* *Cytochromes,* for the record, comprise several oxidoreductase *enzymes* that are found in plants and animal. They consist of iron, a protein, and a porphyrin. The last-mentioned is an iron-free or magnesium-free pyrrole derivative with a 5-membered ring structure containing nitrogen with the formula C_4H_5N. Pyrrole is formed by the decomposition of hematin and chlorophyll. Cytochromes act to catalyze intracellular oxidation—and pose the question of whether there is a relation to oxidants versus antioxidants, the latter purportedly acting as *anticancer agents.* The inference in Table Y-2 of Appendix Y is that *D-lactate dehydrogenase and L-lactate dehydrogenase serve as cytochromes.* The further inference is that these enzymes are tied in with cancer cell metabolism.

† The foregoing can be viewed as a manifestation of the *law of mass action,* whereby an overall chemical reaction or conversion consists of a forward reaction that is countered by a reverse reaction. The forward reaction rate is proportional to the concentrations of the reactants, and the reverse reaction rate is proportional to the concentrations of the products (which can also be viewed as the reactants for the reverse reaction). Therefore, the foreword reaction is favored by a buildup of reactants, and the reverse reaction is favored by a buildup of products.

‡ We distinguish between D- and L-compounds, in that the former are *dextrorotary* under polarized light, and the latter *levorotary.* However, their chemical actions or reactions, and other chemical properties, may be entirely the same. The word *dextrose,* for instance, signifies the right-handed version, and is also called *grape sugar, dextroglucose* or *D-glucose,* and may be obtained by the inversion or hydrolysis of sucrose, the familiar table sugar derived from sugar cane or sugar beets. The word *levulose* (but not levolose) denotes the left-handed version and may be obtained, along with dextrose, by the inversion of sucrose. Levulose is also called *D-fructose,* or *fruit sugar,* adding to the confusion. *Honey, and of course most sweet fruits, are natural sources of levulose.*

It may be noted that the species *Crithidia fasciculata* is a source for chemical compounds that act as enzyme *inhibitors for hexokinase*. This species is a form of lower animal life called *trypanosomes*, which are *parasites* or *flagellates*. Furthermore, the species called *Trypanosoma cruzi* is listed as furnishing a compound that acts as an *inhibitor for 6-phosphofructose*. (An information reference for such non-plant species is the multivolume *Grzimak's Animal Life Encyclopedia*.) The species *Megasphera elsidenii*, a source for 2-hydroxy-3-*butynoic* acid as an *inhibitor for D-lactate dehydrogenase*, is not further identified.

Streptococcus cremonis furnishes compounds that act as *inhibitors for L-lactate dehydrogenase. It may be speculated, therefore, that strep infections may somehow act against cancer.*

Cysteine, a nonessential amino acid, is listed as an *inhibitor for pyruvate kinase*. It is formed by the reduction of cystine, a sulfur-containing amino acid $C_4H_{12}N_2O_4S_2$ resulting from the splitting of proteins. *Yeasts*, for example, are notable sources of proteins and the amino acids, as well as for the vitamin B complex.

The *fatty acids* known as *lauric acid, myristic acid,* and *octanic acid* are further identified as *inhibitors for pyruvate kinase*. Found in vegetable oils, there is perhaps more than one reason for inclusion in the diet. *Fatty acids* are also listed as *inhibitors for L-lactate dehydrogenase (cytochrome)*.

Quercetin, a flavonoid, is again emphasized as an *inhibitor for pyruvate kinase*, as it is in Appendix A.

Vanadate compounds are derived from salts or esters formed from vanadic acid, itself considered a hydrate of vanadium pentoxide. *Vanadium* is an element of the phosphorus group, intermediate between metals and nonmetals, whose inorganic compounds may be classed as metallo-compounds. Vanadium and its compounds have long been noted to have catalytic activity toward certain organic, nonbiochemical reactions. For the case at hand, *vanadate* compounds are listed as *inhibitors for hexokinase* and *6-phosphofructokinase*. (Vanadium compounds, incidentally, are also known to act as poisons for inorganic catalysts. That is, in the catalytic refining of petroleum, vanadium compounds naturally present in the crude oil may have an adverse effect on the catalysts used.)

In further comment, many of these substances have side effects that may be undesirable. There is likely a trade-off in that these substances may at the same time act as enzyme inhibitors for still other vital body processes—the problem of selectivity.

More than this, some of these substances have in fact already been tried against cancer, with the effectiveness still in question. While there is no doubt the matter of establishing adequate dosage levels and frequencies, there is also the possibility or probability that these substances do not function perfectly as enzyme inhibitors against cancer cell metabolism.

Another constraint is that the enzyme inhibitors used should not shut down normal cell metabolism or respiration. While a certain amount of leeway may be acceptable, in the main the idea is to shut down cancer cell metabolism without severely impeding normal cell metabolism. For this reason, the preferred inhibitors would be those that mostly affect only lactate dehydrogenase, since the other enzymes are involved in both cancer cell and normal cell metabolism.

8.9.3 VITAMINS AND HORMONES AS ENZYME INHIBITORS

For the most part, vitamins are not listed as inhibitors for the enzymes involved in glycolysis. An exception is *pyridoxine* (or pyridoxin), more commonly called *vitamin B6*, which inhibits malate dehydrogenase, an enzyme involved in the tricarboxylic acid cycle (Figure 1.4). For the record, a listing is provided in Appendix Z for a number of vitamins and the particular enzymes that they inhibit. The enumeration of vitamins is based on Table 1.1 in Part 1.

Among the other inhibiting effects of vitamins are the following: the *retinoic acid form of vitamin A shows antitumor activity, vitamin B1 inhibits glucose synthesis,* and *vitamin B6 antagonists inhibit adenocarcinoma growth.* (Clinical research on Vitamin A as an anticancer agent has been underway at the University of Colorado Health Sciences Center, Denver.)

Folic acid is listed as an inhibitor for both thymidylate synthetase and dihydrofolate reductase, as previously noted in Part 1. (For instance, folic acid is prominently mentioned in the section on "Chemotherapy Drugs" and a subsection on antifolate drugs, in the section on the DNA/RNA connection and the subsections on the foregoing enzymes, and in the section on folic acid.) Conventional cytotoxic chemotherapy drugs inhibit these same enzymes and thereby interfere with DNA/RNA/protein synthesis—not only in cancer cells but in normal cells. Whether folic acid would be more selective against cancerous cells per se apparently has not been investigated, although folic acid has been used in the treatment of certain kinds of cancer, notably cervical cancer, as also mentioned in Part 1.

Interestingly, the nicotinamide form of niacin acts against *diphtheria toxin*. Conceivably, therefore, there may be yet other unsuspected benefits from nicotinamide or niacin.

Although mainstream medicine does not usually endorse vitamin therapy, an article in the March/April 1996 issue of *CA—A Cancer Journal for Clinicians* indicates otherwise. The article concerns an update on bladder cancer, by Donald L. Lamm and Frank M Torti, both MDs. The former is Professor and Chairman of the Department of Urology at the Robert C. Byrd Health Sciences Center of West Virginia University at Morgantown, and the latter is the Charles L. Spurr Professor of Medicine, Section Head of Hematology/Oncology, Chairman of the Department of Cancer Biology, and Director of the Comprehensive Cancer Center at the Bowman Gray School of Medicine of Wake Forest University in Winston-Salem NC. The authors observed a *40 percent reduction* in long-term occurrences of bladder cancer using *high doses of vitamins A, B6, C, and E*. (Lamm and Torti, p. 101). The authors also note the promise of other oral agents, namely the use of the interferon-inducer *bropirimine*, and in Japan *Lactobacillus casei* has reduced tumor recurrence.

It may be further commented that species of the genus *Lactobacillus* are used in the fermentation or conversion of sugars to produce lactic acid or lactate, as described elsewhere. This conversion is a feature of anaerobic glycolysis, that is, of cancer cell metabolism. The species of *Lactobacillus* produces the enzymes necessary for the conversion.

While the presence of bacteria may stimulate the immune system—and infections may act against cancer—there is also the possibility that *Lactobacillus* generates lactic acid or lactate in the body, independent of cancer cell metabolism. (The point that bacterial infections such as strep may act against cancer is raised within the previous section titled "An Update on Plant and Other Substances as Enzyme Inhibitors," in the subsection "Miscellaneous.") And since lactic acid or lactate is the end product of cancer cell metabolism, then a buildup of product—whatever the source—will suppress further formation. The law of mass action comes into play, whereby a buildup of reaction products suppresses the reaction. *Accordingly, it can at least be speculated that the introduction of lactic acid or lactate into the body system may act to suppress cancer.*

Inasmuch as lactic acid or lactate is a by-product of physical or muscular exercise, an interesting survey would be to determine whether athletes have markedly lower cancer rates, at least during their tenure of vigorous activity. It may be added that medical folklore pushes exercise as a means of staving off cancer.

Noted in passing is that the same article, above, describes the use of the alkylating agent *mitomycin* which, like *doxorubicin*, is an antibiotic chemotherapy agent. Although the article speaks of favorable response rates, this is not the same as cures or remissions. Another treatment described is intravesical immunotherapy using *Bacillus Calmette-Guérin* or *BCG*. (The term "vesical" refers to the bladder. Again the idea is presented about bacteria acting against cancer.)

Perhaps most interesting of all, the above article comments about the *ineffectiveness of chemotherapy* (Lamm and Torti. p. 106). *"With rare exceptions, such as Burkitt's lymphoma or choriocarcinoma in women, single-agent chemotherapy does not produce prolonged remission and is rarely curative."* (This is in line with the comments provided in Part 2 in the section on "Cancer and Anticancer Agents.") Chemotherapy agents that have been used against bladder cancer include cisplatin, notably, but also methotrexate (with folinic acid rescue), vinblastine, 5-fluorouracil, doxorubicin, and carboplatin, even the extra-toxic gallium nitrate. The article goes on to describe combination chemotherapy, in which two or more chemo drugs are used. (The acronym CMV is used to denote the combination of cisplatin, methotrexate, and vinblastine, and M-VAC denotes methotrexate, vinblastine, the antibiotic doxorubicin, and cisplatin. However, mention of CMV in turn signifies that patients rarely achieve complete responses.)

Also described are adjuvant and neoadjuvant chemotherapy, meaning that it is used following or prior to another type of treatment, namely surgery or radiation. These more extreme measures are directed in particular at cancers that may have metastasized. Depending on how the article is read or interpreted between the lines, the results may be seen as either encouraging or not encouraging.

8.9.4 VITAMIN C

In a search of MEDLINE for the five-year period 1992 to 1996, under the word combination "cancer cell metabolism," it was found that *vitamin C* was the principal concern of a paper by A. Lupulescu. Basal cell carcinomas in rats and squamous cell carcinomas in mice were induced topically by the chemical carcinogen 3-methylcholanthrene (MCA). After the administration of a daily dose of vitamin C (50 mg per kilogram of body weight) and MCA for 9 months, pronounced changes were observed as compared to the use of MCA alone. (The vitamin C dosage level would correspond to approximately 5,000 mg or units per day for a human, or about *5 g per day.*) Ultrastructural studies of the cancer cells showed *advanced cytolysis (cell destruction)* and disorganization, mitochondrial alterations (the term pertains to the minute bodies in the cell cytoplasm that are involved in metabolism), nuclear and nucleolar reduction, and increased phagolysosomes formation. (The nucleolus is the part of the cell nucleus that contains chromosomal clusters of ribosomal RNA genes and serves as the site for RNA synthesis.) "These findings demonstrate that vitamin C exerts its antineoplastic effects by increasing cytolytic and autophagic activity, cell membrane disruption, and increased collagen synthesis, and thus, *inhibits cancer cell metabolism and proliferation.*"*

It appears that Linus Pauling's advocacy of vitamin C as an anticancer agent has been scientifically and independently verified. (*Note:* For cancer, Pauling recommended a regimen of approximately 25 or 30 g per day of vitamin C—preferably without prior chemotherapy.)

It may also be mentioned, however, that vitamin C or ascorbic acid is listed in Appendix Z as an *inhibitor for urea levels,* whereas *urea itself is considered an anticancer agent* (as per Ralph Moss's *Cancer Therapy*)—and in Appendix A *urea is listed as an inhibitor for lactate dehydrogenase,* which is, as has been emphasized, a key enzyme in cancer cell metabolism.

As a further note, *vitamin C is reported to block nitrosamines,* as pertains to stomach and colorectal cancer (in *Comprehensive Biological Catalysis,* p. 212). The general subject is discussed in Part 6 in the section on "Intestinal Flora and Cancer."

These things said, it can be asked, why have massive infusions of vitamin C been inconclusive against cancer, as acknowledged, for instance, in Moss's *Cancer Therapy?*

The above search of MEDLINE also uncovered a paper by Nissler et al., which noted that *cancer cell energy metabolism is characterized by a high glycolytic rate, a rate that is maintained under aerobic conditions.* The reference did not say what the end products of the cancer cell metabolism were. That is, was the cancer cell metabolism itself anaerobic, yielding lactic acid or lactate as end products rather than carbon dioxide and water? The latter are, of course, the end products of normal cell metabolism.

The paper was concerned with the role of fructose 2,6-bisphosphate (Fru-2,6-P2), which is described as the powerful *activator* for 6-phosphofructo-1-kinase (PFK or PFK-1). It was found that concentrations of the former increase *tenfold* in Ehrlich ascites tumor cells. Very possibly, this is responsible for the *high glycolytic rate of the cancer cells.*

The paper was also concerned with the bifunctional enzyme 6-phosphofructo-2-kinase/fructose-2,6-bisphosphatase (PFK-2/FBPase-2) and its role in synthesizing and degrading the activator Fru-2,6-P2.

It was found, moreover, that PFK-2 activity is inhibited by *citrate* and *phosphoenolpyruvate,* but only weakly by glycerol 3-phosphate. (Phosphoenolpyruvate is the reaction product of step 9 and the reactant for step 10 in the glycolytic pathway presented in Figure 1.1 in Part 1.) It might be anticipated that PFK or PFK-1 is similarly inhibited, in this very complicated reactant/enzyme/product system.

8.9.5 HORMONES

Hormones also serve as enzyme inhibitors, some of which are also included in Appendix Z. With regard to glycolysis, growth hormones or their derivatives inhibit *glucose consumption* and the enzyme *pyruvate dehydrogenase.* The two effects may be interrelated. In turn, *somatostatin* inhibits the release of growth hormones and insulin. (*Insulin, incidentally, inhibits protein synthesis.*)

---

* Carried further, these processes assumably involve various enzymes and inhibitors (or promoters). As to the terms used, above, *phagolysosome* pertains to vesicles (small cavities or sacs) found within phagocytes, in which ingested material is degraded—a *phagocyte* being a specialized cell (or macrophage) that ingests and destroys foreign matter or microorganisms. The term *cytolytic* means cell-destroying, and *autophagic* indicates that the cancer cells are self-destroying. It has been noted elsewhere that *collagen* has been connected in some way or another to the formation of blood vessels in the cancerous mass—a process called angiogenesis—and this may conceivably be in either a positive or negative fashion (Boik, *Cancer & Natural Medicine,* pp. 21, 35). According to Lupulescu's study, above, *an increase in collagen synthesis evidently relates to cancer cell destruction.*

As will be seen below, *the inhibition of insulin (and growth hormones) may in turn inhibit cancer; that is, insulin (in excess) may be carcinogenic.*

Also according to Appendix Z, *glucagon inhibits glycogen synthesis. As a reminder, glycogen is formed in the liver from the lactic acid produced by anaerobic glycolysis, a feature of cancer cell metabolism. Conceivably, therefore, the inhibition of glycogen synthesis could act against cancer.*

Parathyroid hormone also acts against glycogen synthesis and can thus be viewed as an anticancer substance. Calcitonin is noted to lower glucose levels, which may or may not be advantageous in the treatment of cancer. (Calcitonin is a polypeptide thyroid hormone.)

Returning to glycolysis, estrogens inhibit glucose-6-P dehydrogenase and epinephrine inhibits phosphofructokinase, both of which are rate-controlling enzymes during glycolysis.

Progestins or *progesterones* inhibit the formation of *collagenase*, which is related to angiogenesis. Possibly, these hormones could act against the creation of blood vessels in tumors.

Thyroxine serves as an inhibitor for malate dehydrogenase, involved in the tricarboxylic acid cycle.

A search of MEDLINE under the word combination "cancer cell metabolism," mentioned above, yielded a paper by S. Golshani dealing with *insulin, growth factors,* and *cancer cell energy metabolism.* A *hexokinase*-mitochondrial acceptor theory has been developed that provides a model for the action of insulin. (Hexokinase is the first enzyme involved in the glycolysis pathway—e.g., Figure 1.1 in Part 1.) This theory unifies the metabolic effects of insulin and concludes that these follow from this hormone's stimulatory effect on *ATP synthesis.* (ATP or adenosine triphosphate is prominently involved in glycolysis, as per Figure 1.1.) It is noted that *there are similarities between the changes in cells exposed to insulin and in the mitochondria of transformed cell lines and cancer cells.* Furthermore, *this is accompanied by an increased binding of hexokinase to the mitochondria,* which are the bodies in the cell cytoplasm where metabolism, read glycolysis, occurs. This phenomenon is viewed as possibly explaining the *high rates of glycolysis* sustained by cancer cells under *aerobic conditions.* It was added that the evidence indicates that "certain growth factors and oncogenes act through stimulation of oxidative phosphorylation via promoting HK (hexokinase) binding to mitochondria."

In different words, insulin evidently promotes the binding of the enzyme hexokinase to the cell mitochondria, which stimulates the conversion of glucose via glycolysis. The paper said that this occurs under anaerobic conditions but did not specify the end products—that is, whether carbon dioxide and water were produced as in normal cells, or whether lactic acid or lactate was the end product as in cancer cells. Since the cells are said to be cancerous, it will be assumed that these particular cells per se yield principally lactic acid or lactate via anaerobic glycolysis, and the process is *catalyzed by hexokinase* and is *stimulated or promoted by insulin.*

In net sum, *(excessive) insulin can be said to cause cancer, or at least to sustain and accelerate cancer growth.* It may be noted that excess insulin production is related to hypoglycemia. Hypoglycemia is mentioned in the previous section on "Enzymes and Inhibitors for Anaerobic Glycolysis," in the cited work of Guerra et al. Here, *hypoglycemia* was found to cause neuronal injury induced via insults to the central nervous system (CNS) and is *accompanied by an increase in anaerobic glycolysis.* The latter is also a manifestation of *cancer cell activity* and is marked by *increases in alanine concentrations.* The findings of Guerra et al. may be said to confirm the theory of Golshani, above, and vice versa.*

A monograph by Aurel Lupulescu, MD, MS, PhD, of Wayne State University, whose work is cited elsewhere, notably with regard to *vitamin C as a cancer-destroying agent,* is titled *Hormones and Carcinogenesis.* His Chapter 2 is titled "Tumor Cell Cycle and Hormones," in which he has a subsection on "Cell Surface Changes During the Cell Cycle." A following section is titled "Hormonal Regulation of the Cancer Cell Cycle" and includes a subsection about the effect of steroid hormones. Lupulescu observed that *estrogens or androgens inhibit DNA synthesis,* and that *progesterone stimulates mitosis or division.* On the other hand, *androgens or estrogens induce a decrease in mitotic activity.* As to the effect of corticosteroid hormones, Lupulescu notes that it has been long known that glucorticoids have an important effect on DNA synthesis and on cell division or mitosis. For instance, it has been found that *hydrocortisone will significantly decrease DNA synthesis.* It is noted in passing also that *hydroxy urea is an inhibitor for DNA synthesis* (Lupulescu, *Hormones and Carcinogenesis,* p. 28).

---

* Another item of interest is that the presence of *antimitochondrial antibodies,* or *AMASs,* has been mentioned as an indicator for all types of cancer.

In a subsequent subsection titled "Polypeptide Hormones and the Cell Cycle," Luputescu states that adrenocorticotropic hormone (ACTH) acts oppositely, stimulating DNA synthesis *in vivo*, but inhibiting DNA synthesis in normal and tumor adrenal cells, which are attributed to cAMP levels (Lupulescu, *Hormones and Carcinogenesis*, p. 28ff). Prolactin has been observed to enhance DNA synthesis but requires the presence of insulin and glucocortinoids. Somatomedin C, a growth hormone-dependent polypeptide related to insulin, will induce DNA synthesis and cell mitosis. Insulin has been found to increase DNA synthesis, as has glucagon (albeit their other effects are generally considered offsetting). Thyroid hormones have been found to be mitogenic.

Lupulescu's Chapter 3 deals with the "Hormonal Regulation of Precancerous and Cancerous Cell Populations." The last paragraph of his chapter summary bears repeating:

> Homeostasis of precancerous and cancerous cells—the progression of precancerous cells to cancer cells—is a controllable process. Fortunately, both precancerous and cancer cells continue to be responsive cells, giving researchers a handle whereby hormones and hormone-like substances (hormonoids) can control the homeostasis and progression of precancerous cells to cancer cells. These substances can restrain the progression and maintain the precancerous cells in a latent state for years; Conversely, they can stimulate this transformation. Hence, hormones are important cellular homeostatic factors.

8.10   LACTATE DEHYDROGENASE INHIBITORS

The inhibition of lactate dehydrogenase will depend on what form of the enzyme is present and may in turn impinge on other body functions. These aspects will first be examined. The emphasis will be directed toward interfering with cancer cell metabolism, which is noted to preferentially produce lactate or lactic acid (lactic acid may be called hydrogen lactate). There is involved the anaerobic conversion of glucose to lactate, or at least pyruvate to lactate, and there is also involved the conversion of lactate back to glucose by the processes of gluconeogenesis.

8.10.1   FORMS OF LACTATE DEHYDROGENASE

The enzyme lactate dehydrogenase, or lactic dehydrogenase, designated LDH, occurs naturally in the body and exists in the form of isoenzymes, also called isozymes. Isoenzymes or isozymes are defined as enzymes that catalyze the same reaction but differ in some property or another, which may be physical, chemical, or otherwise (J. Lyndal York, in *Textbook of Biochemistry*, pp. 197–200).

Lactate dehydrogenase is described as a tetrameric enzyme, with four possibilities, but only two have been found (called subunits), which are designated *H,* for heart (myocardium), and *M,* for muscle. The reference shows how these subunits may be combined into five types, located in various parts of the body—in the myocardium (heart) and RBC (red blood cells), in the brain and kidneys, and in the liver and skeletal muscle. The end pages of the reference give the normal clinical concentration in the blood, which ranges from 60 to 120 U/ml (that is, 60 to 120 units per milliliter or cubic centimeter).*

For the record, these five types may be designated as follows:

- LDH_1 with the composition symbolized by HHHH
- LDH_2 with the composition HHHM
- LDH_3 with the composition HHMM
- LDH_4 with the composition HMMM
- LDH_5 with the composition MMMM

The first two types, in the main, are located in the myocardium and RBC, the third is in the brain and kidney, the fourth is not assigned, and the fifth is in the liver and skeletal muscle.†

---

* According to the Sigma catalog, one unit of L-lactate dehydrogenase will reduce 1.0 μmole of pyruvate to L-lactate per minute at pH 7.5 at 37° C.

† The reference also mentions that *enzymes are occasionally used as therapeutic agents*. Streptokinase, for example, prepared from a species of streptococcus, is used to clear blood clots. Asparaginase is used for some types of adult leukemia, and which acts to depress the *asparagine* requirement for tumor cells. It is remarked that *most enzymes have a short half-life in the blood, and unreasonably large amounts are required to maintain therapeutic levels.*

Whereas the M-type of lactate dehydrogenase predominates in tissues subject to anaerobic conditions, such as skeletal muscle and the liver, and the H-type predominates in aerobic tissues such as heart muscle, there are inferences to be drawn (Voet and Voet, *Biochemistry*, pp. 183, 464). *It has been advanced therefore, but not without argument, that the M-type LDH is better adapted to the reduction of pyruvate to lactate, whereas the H-type is better adapted to the reverse reaction, the oxidation of lactate to pyruvate.* Presumably, the other types may have intermediate characteristics or may be special to certain cells—say to cancer cells.*

Continuing, only the subunits H and M are known, with the two remaining subunits not yet known. Speculatively, these remaining subunits and their combinations may play a significant role, as yet undisclosed, in cancer cell metabolism.

The Sigma catalog lists both D-lactate dehydrogenase, or D-lactic dehydrogenase, and L-lactate dehydrogenase, or L-lactic dehydrogenase. The latter, L-lactate dehydrogenase, has by far the most entries. Furthermore, the various entries are categorized as to a Sigma-designated type, using Roman numerals, which in instances also correspond to an isoenzyme type. An enumeration of the different Sigma-designated types is as follows, in the order given in the Sigma catalog: Type I; II; XXXIX; V-S, LDH-5 (M_4) isoenzyme; XI; XXXVI, LDH-1 (H_4) isoenzyme; XXII; XXIV; IX, LDH-1 (H_4) isoenzyme; III; IV, LDH-1 (H_4); XV; XVII; XXV, LDH-2 (H_3M) isoenzyme; X; XVI, LDH-5 (M_4) isoenzyme; VII-S, LDH-1 (H_4) isoenzyme; XVIII; XXXV; XXIX-S; XXX-S; XXXII-S, LDH-5 (M_4) isoenzyme; VIII; XXXIII; XXXIV; XII; XIX, LDH-1 (H_4) isoenzyme; XX, LDH-2 (H_3M) isoenzyme; XXI, LDH-3 (H_2M_2) isoenzyme; XXVIII, LDH-5 (M_4) isoenzyme; XXIII; XIV; XXVII; XXXVII; isoenzyme LD4 from human liver; isoenzyme X from bovine semen. L-lactate dehydrogenase (cytochrome) is also listed, the term referring to iron-containing pigments that play a part in intracellular oxidations.

8.10.2　AEROBIC VERSUS ANAEROBIC METABOLISM IN THE BODY

The *mammalian body organs*—the brain, muscle, adipose tissue, and liver—*have different metabolic needs* (Voet and Voet, *Biochemistry*, pp. 788-792). For present purposes, muscle may be categorized as skeletal muscle and heart muscle. The brain is noted to have a remarkably high respiration rate and, under normal conditions, utilizes glucose as the fuel.

The major fuels for muscle are glucose from glycogen, fatty acids, and ketone bodies. Muscle contraction is driven by ATP hydrolysis (Voet and Voet, *Biochemistry*, pp. 606, 789, 1244), and *ultimately depends on respiration. Under conditions of high exertion,* however, *muscle contraction is anaerobic,* yielding lactic acid or lactate, producing a condition of acidity associated with fatigue.

The heart muscle is largely aerobic except for short periods of extreme exertion, when it becomes anaerobic. Thus, the heart muscle is well endowed with mitochondria, for respiration, but some types of skeletal muscle have hardly any.

The adipose tissue, consisting of cells called adipocytes, occurs throughout the body but notably under the skin, in the abdominal cavity, in skeletal muscle, around blood vessels, and in mammary glands. Not only does it provide a reservoir of high-energy fat, but it helps maintain metabolic homeostasis (metabolic stability). Adipocytes hydrolyze triacylglycerols to fatty acids and glycerol, a process that is governed by the levels of the hormones *glucagon* (a polypeptide hormone that controls glycogen metabolism), *epinephrine* (adrenaline or adrenalin), and *insulin.*

The liver is described as the body's central metabolic clearing house. Among its major functions is to serve as a "buffer" for blood glucose. It can convert glucose to glucose-6-phosphate (G6P) in a reaction catalyzed by glucokinase, which is analogous to hexokinase, the usual enzyme for conversion via the glycolytic pathway (e.g., Figure 1.1 in Part 1). However, glucokinase is not inhibited by a buildup of G6P and has a much lower affinity for glucose. That is, hexokinase has a greater tendency to form a complex with glucose than does glucokinase (Voet and Voet, *Biochemistry*, p. 447). Moreover, liver cells are permeable to glucose, whereas muscle and adipose cells are not.

---

* The arguments and representations are somewhat contradictory, for it is noted that the M-type, which predominates in muscular tissue, favors the conversion of pyruvate to lactate. But the M-type also occurs in the liver, where lactate is converted back to pyruvate, and ultimately to glucose or glycogen. As to the heart muscle, where the H-type predominates, here, for the most part, presumably we are talking about aerobic glycolysis, the conversion of glucose or glycogen to pyruvate and then to carbon dioxide and water.

The upshot of the foregoing is that the inhibition of lactate dehydrogenase should not affect normal body functions. In other words, the organs involved normally function aerobically. *The single extenuating circumstance would be that the inhibition of lactate dehydrogenase could interfere with extreme exertion or extreme muscular activity.*

The hydrolysis of ATP (adenosine triphosphate) may be represented by the following chemical/electron balance, producing ADP (adenosine diphosphate) and phosphate:

$$ATP^{4-} + H_2O \rightarrow ADP^{3-} + HPO_4^{2-} + H^+$$

Regeneration of the ATP occurs via oxidative phosphorylation in the mitochondria of slow-twitch (red) muscle fibers, and by glycolysis yielding lactate in fast-twitch (white) muscle fibers (Voet and Voet, *Biochemistry*, p. 606). (Slow-twitch muscles may also produce lactate whenever the ATP demand exceeds the oxidative flux available.) The lactate is carried by the bloodstream to the liver and reconverted to glucose by gluconeogenesis (new glucose synthesis). The glucose may be stored in the muscle as glycogen. This metabolic cycle between muscle and liver is known as the *Cori cycle.*

8.10.3 GLUCONEOGENESIS

Gluconeogenesis pertains to the formation of glucose from carbohydrate and noncarbohydrate precursors (Voet and Voet, *Biochemistry*, p. 599ff). These precursors may include not only the glycolysis products *lactate* and *pyruvate* but may include the *carboxylic acid cycle intermediates* and *most amino acids.* These latter sources are used when the liver's capacity to store glucose or glycogen is compromised, notably under fasting or starvation conditions. In other words, *if carbohydrates are not available, the body can resort to using protein as a metabolic source.* Gluconeogenesis is noted to occur in the liver and, to a lesser extent, in the kidneys.

Of first interest here is the reconversion of lactate to glucose, which can get into the esoterica of chemical reaction kinetics, of whether the same catalyst may in some way influence both forward and reverse reaction rates, and whether a catalyst may have an effect even on equilibrium.

As to the same catalysts influencing both forward and reverse reactions, gluconeogenesis—here the conversion of lactate back to glucose—involves some of the same enzymes or enzyme-catalysts as for glycolysis. That is, the one pathway is essentially the reverse of the other, and uses some of the same enzymes—but not all. Thus, the reactions catalyzed by hexokinase, phosphofructokinase, and pyruvate kinase are strongly one-way during glycolysis and must be replaced by other reactions and enzymes that favor the reverse or gluconeogenesis route. These reactions and enzyme-catalysts are spelled out in the reference and involve *biotin, a growth factor* found in yeast, for instance, and which is an essential human nutrient.

Enzymes involved in gluconeogenesis are listed in Table 8.12, along with their regulators, notably allosteric inhibitors and activators (Voet and Voet, *Biochemistry*, p. 604). These inhibitors and activators serve to reciprocally regulate both glycolysis and gluconeogenesis to prevent an uncontrolled cycling between reactants and products.

It is assumed that the starting compound for gluconeogenesis is pyruvate, rather than lactate. Thus, lactate dehydrogenase is not included in the listing. However, as previously stated, the H-type of lactate dehydrogenase favors the conversion of lactate to pyruvate.

Allosteric interactions or allosterism involves the *binding* of another substance to an active site on a *protein molecule* (Voet and Voet, *Biochemistry*, p. 241). *The binding substance may be called the ligand, and the protein may be called the receptor* (Voet and Voet, *Biochemistry*, p. 1275). That is, a *ligand* is any molecule that is bound to a macromolecule (J. Lyndal York, in *Textbook of Biochemistry*, p. 171). Moreover, the term is not limited to small organic molecules such as ATP but may include low molecular weight proteins.

Other inhibitors for gluconeogenesis are shown in Table 8.13 as obtained from Jain's *Handbook of Enzyme Inhibitors*. These inhibitors are presumed to apply to the conversion of lactate or lactic acid back to glucose or its polymer, glycogen. Note that hydrazine is listed, and hydrazine sulfate is the basis for the Gold cancer therapy and is said to inhibit the conversion of lactic acid or lactate back to glycogen or glucose, thus interfering with the cycle of cancer cell metabolism (Moss, *Cancer Therapy*, pp. 316–321; Walters, *Options*, pp. 47–54). According to both Jain and Zollner, *hydrazine also acts as an inhibitor for several other enzymes.* In other words, as is so often the case, *hydrazine is not selective as an inhibitor.*

Table 8.12 Enzymes and Regulators for Gluconeogenesis

Hexokinase—glycolysis	
Allosteric Inhibitors	Not listed
Allosteric activators	Not listed

Glucose-6-phosphatase - gluconeogenesis	
Allosteric Inhibitors	Not listed
Allosteric Activators	Not listed

Phosphofructokinase (PFK)—glycolysis	
Allosteric inhibitors:	ATP, citrate
Allosteric activators	AMP, fructose-2,6-phosphate (F2,6P)

Fructose-1,6-bisphosphatase (FBP)—gluconeogenesis	
Allosteric inhibitors	None listed
Allosteric activators	AMP, fructose-2,6-phosphate (F2,6P)

Pyruvate kinase (PK)—glycolysis	
Allosteric inhibitors	Alanine
Allosteric activators	Fructose-1,6-phosphate (F1,6P)

Pyruvate carboxylase—gluconeogenesis	
Allosteric inhibitors	None listed
Allosteric activators	Acetyl-CoA

Phosphoenolpyruvate carboxykinase (PEPCK)—gluconeogenesis	
Allosteric inhibitors	None listed
Allosteric activators	None listed

Phosphofructokinase-2 (PFK-2)	
Allosteric inhibitors	Citrate
Allosteric activators	AMP, fructose-6-phosphate (F6P), orthophosphate ion (P_i)

Fructose-1,6-bisphosphatase-2 (FBPase-2)	
Allosteric inhibitors	Fructose-6-phosphate (F6P)
Allosteric activators	Glycerol-3-phosphate (glycerol-3-P)

Source: Data from *Biochemistry*, 2nd Ed., by Donald Voet and Judith G. Voet, Wiley, New York, 1995, pp. 604–605. The order, bottom to top, is pyruvate to glucose, in the same sequence as shown in Figure 1.1 in Part 1. The forward and reverse reactions at a particular point can be independently regulated and are grouped together in the following listing. The last two enzymes listed, PFK-2 and FBPase-2, regulate the concentration of F2,P6.

The appearance of glucose as an inhibitor for gluconeogenesis is expected, since glucose is a reaction product. In similar fashion, Jain lists lactic acid as in inhibitor for lactate dehydrogenase, since lactic acid or lactate is the reaction product from the conversion of pyruvic acid or pyruvate. In other words, *the law of mass action applies.*

Table 8.13   Enzyme Inhibitors for Gluconeogenesis (from Lactate)

Adrenocochrome	Indole-2-carboxylic acid
Aminopyrine	Indole-2-carboxylic acid, methoxy-
AMP, Butyryl,-cyclic-	Indole-2-carboxylic acid,-5-methoxy-
Biguanide	Malonic acid, N-butyl ester
Butyric acid, W-phenol-	Octanoic acid
Carnitine, decanoyl-	Quabain
Diamide	PCB
Dichromate ion	Pentenoic acid, 4-
Ergotamine, dihydro-	Phenethylbiguanide
Ethanol	Phenoxybenzamine
Glisoxepide	Picolinic acid, 3-mercapto-
Glucose	Puromycin, aminonucleoside deriv.
Glutamic acid, G-hydroxy-	Pyruvic acid, methylenecyclopropane-
Glutarate, G-hydroxy-A-keto-	Quinaldic acid
Halothane	Quinolinic acid
Hydrazine	

Source: Data from M.K. Jain, *Handbook of Enzyme Inhibitors, 1965–1977*, Wiley, New York, 1982.

Jain also lists inhibitors for what is called glucose synthesis. These include indole carboxylic acid derivatives, pentanoic acid, 4-, and phenethylbiguanide, all of which are named as inhibitors for gluconeogenesis. Additionally, prostaglandin E1 and (thiamine, oxy-) are also listed.

8.10.4 THE INHIBITION OF LACTATE DEHYDROGENASE

Considering that lactate dehydrogenase (LDH) may be the most significant enzyme in cancer cell metabolism, and its inhibition may be a way to control or eliminate cancer, a search was made of MEDLINE for the five-year period 1992–1996 under the word combination "lactate dehydrogenase inhibitors." The results are encapsulated as follows, and some of the findings are striking indeed.

In a paper by Hamilton et al., it is remarked that *tumors have a greater dependence on anaerobic glycolysis for energy generation than do normal tissues*. In this regard glycolysis inhibition was studied on tumor cells *in vitro*. It was noted that the cellular ATP dropped when the cells were exposed in air to the presence of *2-deoxy glucose* or to *oxamate*, which is a known lactate dehydrogenase inhibitor. In a six-hour test, glycolysis inhibition alone did not change cell survival, but when oxamate was combined with the cytotoxic chemotherapy agent doxorubicin (Dox), the cell-killing effect was enhanced over Dox alone.

A *selective inactivating enzyme* for the M-subunit of lactate dehydrogenase was found by Watazu et al. in the form of the culture filtrate of *Penicillium citrinum* KE-1, which was isolated from soil and subsequently purified. The enzyme showed no effect on the H-subunit of LDH. The enzyme, named KE-1 proteinase, is a serine-type proteinase. (These findings are unusual in the fact that *enzyme inhibitors are most usually substances other than enzymes.*)

Investigators Haouz et al. determined a way to *lower the detection limit for L-lactate dehydrogenase* (LDH) and also L-lactate oxidase (LOD) as well as other substances such as p-chloromercuribenzoate (PCMB). Applications exist in medicine, the food industry, and the environment.

In a study by Lushchak and Lushchak, *urea* was found to competitively inhibit the reduction of pyruvate by LDH obtained from pig and *skate* muscles. [A competitive inhibitor is a substance that competes with a normal substrate (reactant) for an enzymatic binding site (Voet and Voet, *Biochemistry*, p. 356).] It was noted that *increasing the pyruvate concentration activated the enzyme* of the skate but had less effect on that of pig muscle. Activation also occurred with KCl solutions.

Urea is listed in Appendix A as an inhibitor for lactate dehydrogenase. It has been was mentioned as an anticancer agent, for instance as described in Ralph W. Moss's book *Cancer Therapy*. On the other hand, as previously observed, Appendix Z lists vitamin C or ascorbic acid as inhibiting urea levels, whereas vitamin C has also been found to be an anticancer agent.

Marmillot et al. performed *in vitro* studies on the inhibiting effect of *tubulin* on the activity of the muscle-type isoenzyme lactate dehydrogenase (LDHm or M-type LDH). However, inhibition did not occur with heart-type lactate dehydrogenase (LDHh or H-type LDH). *Tubulin is therefore selective to the M-type.* The enzyme inhibition was found to be less sensitive as the NADH concentration increased, and as the pH increased. Inhibition is apparently caused by a binding of the enzyme on to tubulin.*

In a study by Ohshita and Kido, it was determined that a *lysosomal cysteine proteinase* plays a prominent role in the lysosomal degradation of native L-lactate dehydrogenase.† L-Lactate dehydrogenase is inactivated, its subunit disappears, and the final amino acid degradation products are produced, all during an incubation with disrupted lysosomes *in vitro*. On the other hand, these enzyme inhibition processes can be suppressed by a small amount of cystatin alpha (cysteine protease inhibitor), but which does not affect the normal digestive activity of the known cysteine proteinases; that is, it does not affect cathepsins B, H, L, and J. Evidently, another cysteine proteinase is involved in inhibiting L-lactate dehydrogenase, and is naturally present in lysosomes. It can be characterized as cystatin-alpha-sensitive. *(There is the possibility that this particular lysosomal cysteine proteinase may be essential to reducing and controlling cellular lactate dehydrogenase levels, which in turn translates to cancer cell suppression.)*

Kraus et al. tested a number of *tetrazole analogs* of carboxylic substrates (reactants) and inhibitors.‡ *Lactic and pyruvic tetrazoles* proved to be *competitive inhibitors* of rabbit muscle *L-lactate dehydrogenase* in both pyruvate reduction and lactate oxidation—that is, for both the forward and reverse reactions. Lactic tetrazole is a noncompetitive inhibitor of yeast-derived L-lactate dehydrogenase, whereas pyruvic tetrazole is for the most part competitive.§ Other findings include alanine tetrazole as a weak inhibitor for D-amino acid oxidase, whereas *alanine* itself works better. Benzoic tetrazole is an inhibitor for D-amino acid oxidase and for liver alcohol dehydrogenase, and works better than benzoic acid. In general, substitution of a tetrazole ring for a carboxylic group results in decreased binding, which signifies less activity as either a reactant or an inhibitor. It can be inferred that carboxylic groups signify stronger inhibiting action.

Chaperonin, derived from the thermophilic bacterium *Thermus thermophilus*, was found to protect enzymes from heat denaturation (denaturalization, modification, degradation or decomposition) in an investigation conducted by Taguchi and Yoshida. (The genus *Thermus* consists of Gram-negative aerobic, rod-shaped or filamentous bacteria, found in hot springs, which have red, orange, or yellow coloration.) If no chaperonin is present, the denaturation is irreversible. With chaperonin present, the denaturation can be made reversible, but it also requires the addition of MgATP. The chaperonin captures the proteins produced during heat denaturation, but the proteins retain the ability to once again become enzymatically active. This ability is lost above 78° C, presumably to a loss of heat stability by the chaperonin. (There is an inference, not stated, that chaperonin might serve as an anticancer agent, if the enzymes it protects act against lactate dehydrogenase. On the other hand, it might prove carcinogenic, if it maintains or increases lactate dehydrogenase levels. The subject of *chaperonins* merges with that of *shock proteins* or *heat shock proteins,* discussed in Part 6).

---

* Tubulin is a protein that comprises the microtubules that form the supportive framework that guides the movement of organelles within a cell (Voet and Voet, *Biochemistry*, pp. 9, 1252). It is thus part of the cytoskeleton, the cell structure, and is also a major constituent of the cilia, the hairlike appendages extending from many cells.

† *Lysosomes* are single membrane-bounded organelles, which are essentially membranous bags holding hydrolytic enzymes that digest ingested materials (Voet and Voet, *Biochemistry*, p. 9). Cysteine is a nonessential amino acid, and a proteinase is a proteolytic or protein-digesting enzyme.

‡ *Tetrazole* itself is an organic compound, normally a solid, with a four-nitrogen ring structure and the formula CH_2N_4. It serves as a coupling agent in the formation of oligonucleotide chains (Voet and Voet, *Biochemistry*, p. 897).

§ A *competitive inhibitor* is a substance that competes with a normal substrate (reactant) for an enzymatic binding site (Voet and Voet, *Biochemistry*, p. 356).

Ikeda et al. isolated and characterized a substance from species of the genus *Streptosporangium*. The substance was labeled MLI and was found to inhibit lactic acid production in mutant streptococci or *Lactobacillus* species. *These inhibitory mechanisms did not result from an antibacterial effect,* since the bacterial cells were not affected—excluding *L. acidophilus.* In other words, MLI directly affected lactate dehydrogenase activity. The authors conclude that MLI may represent a new *anticariogenic* substance. (The inference of course is that the production of lactic acid may result in tooth decay, and any way to stop the oral production of lactic acid would be anticariogenic. We may carry this further, that if this stops the oral production of lactic acid, perhaps it would work against cancer cell metabolism as well.)

A reaction kinetics analysis by Holmes et al. concluded that lactate dehydrogenase catalyzes a second-order reaction, which may be expressed in terms of a ternary complex mechanism. In other words, two reactants are involved, but one of the reactants is apparently already in equilibrium with still another reactant. This is in line with most kinetic analyses, in that most (or all) reactions are considered either monomolecular at the least or bimolecular at the most, since the probability of three molecules finding each other at the exact same time is about nil. In the ternary complex mechanism, two have already found each other (to form a complex) and then react with a third. If the reacting system is heterogeneous—that is, more than one phase is involved, where the catalyst proper is generally a distinct phase—then there are such things to consider as the rate of mass transfer between phases and surface reactions. For a reacting system of many reactants and products, the reacting system may be expressed in terms of consecutive and simultaneous reactions. Such a representation is not always clear cut, however, since there is a matter of choosing whether the reactions or reaction rate equations are each to be considered independent or dependent.

Stark and Henderson performed in vitro investigations on the effects of *elastase* and *cathepsin G* on both creatine kinase and lactate dehydrogenase isoenzymes.* It is noted that the polymorphonuclear granulocyte, or neutrophil, may be a mediator of tissue-destructive events. This effect is apparently due to the release of the preformed proteolytic (protein digesting) enzymes elastase and cathepsin G. At the same time, due to a myeloperoxidase action, hypochlorous acid is released. (The prefix "myelo-" signifies *marrow,* e.g., bone marrow or spinal cord.) Elastase inactivates and fragments the creatine kinase enzymes CK-2 and CK-3, and to a lesser extent, lactate dehydrogenase isoenzyme LD-1. Cathepsin G acts only on CK-2. Both neutrophil enzymes acts against LD-3. It is noted that *hypochlorous acid* inactivates CK even at low concentrations but requires higher concentrations to inactivate LD (or LDH). After a myocardial infarction, the number of neutrophils increases, which concentrate around damaged tissue.† A conclusion reached by the authors is that neutrophils may inactivate and fragment "cardiac" enzymes that are released from tissue so damaged. (There is an inference, unstated, that traces of *hypochlorous acid,* by inactivating lactate dehydrogenase, may act as an *anticancer agent.*)

An investigation by Jurkowitz-Alexander et al. was concerned with the inhibition of *glycolytic and oxidative ATP* synthesis in what are called oligodendroglia-glioma hybrid cells (ROC-1), or hybrid glial cells, for short. The cells were found to undergo a sequence of changes involving first ATP depletion, then cell swelling and blebbing (blistering or bubbling), and lastly plasma membrane disruption and *cell death.* The morphological and biochemical changes that follow ATP depletion are affected by the presence of *polyethylene glycol,* described as a nonpermeant oncotic agent ("permeant" pertains to permeating or permeation; "oncotic" is characterized by the development of tumors). The polyethylene glycol was noted to prevent cell swelling and blebbing and to delay, but not prevent, the release of *lactate dehydrogenase* into the medium, nor did it affect the decline in ATP levels. A conclusion reached is that *osmotic cell swelling* may contribute to the loss of cell viability and is *caused by ATP depletion.* (Although polyethylene glycol is described as oncotic or cancer causing, its effect in this study was as an anticancer agent. This contradiction appears time and again, where *a substance may be either carcinogenic and anticarcinogenic, depending.*)

---

* *Creatine kinase* catalyzes the conversion between ADP and ATP, serving as a way to regenerate ATP (Voet and Voet, *Biochemistry,* pp. 370, 433, 789). Creatine and phosphocreatine are also involved, creatine itself being a white, crystalline, nitrogenous compound with the formula $C_4H_2N_3O_2$.

† The prefix "myo-" indicates muscle; the suffix "-cardial" pertains to the heart or heart region; the term "infarction" denotes a region of necrosis and hemorrhage in an organ due to obstruction of the local circulatory system; the term neutrophil pertains to a large leukocyte, that will stain with neutral dyes.

Kliachko et al. studied the temperature-caused structural and functional changes in *lactate dehydrogenase* from fish skeletal muscles. (The reminder is of shark cartilage as an anticancer agent.) As fish adapt to low and high environmental temperatures, certain changes occur in the kinetic and structural properties of lactate dehydrogenase. The LDH from fishes adapted to low environmental temperatures is more stable with respect to both *thermal and urea-induced deactivation.* (The reminder is of the treatment of cancer by *heat therapy* and of the use of *urea* as an anticancer agent, e.g., as mentioned in Moss's *Cancer Therapy.* The inference here is that both *higher temperatures and urea act as enzyme inhibitors or deactivators for lactate dehydrogenase.*)

Studies by Sharma and Schwille determined that *sodium sulfite* inhibits *oxalate production* from glycolate and glyoxylate *in vitro,* and from dichloroacetate infused intravenously into male rats. The enzymes involved were lactate dehydrogenase from rabbit muscle and as derived from rat liver. (In comment, *oxalate or oxalic acid is a known inhibitor for lactate dehydrogenase,* as is pyruvic acid for that matter, as represented in Appendix A. Presumably, therefore, in this context *sulfite may in itself be carcinogenic.* It does not appear in the list of glycolysis enzyme inhibitors of Appendix A, although sulfate is listed as an inhibitor for pyruvate kinase.)

Sulfite or sulphite is an inhibitor for many other enzymes. For the record, sulfite ion is listed in Jain's *Handbook* as an inhibitor for aryl sulfatase, enolpyruvate carboxylase, *malate dehydrogenase,* phosphoprotein phosphatase, sulfatase, sulfoacetaldehyde sulfolyase, whereas Zollner's *Handbook* lists N-acetylglucosamine, aromatic α-ketoacid dehydrogenase, arylsulphatase, creatine kinase, carbonate dehydratase, L-galactonolactone oxidase, peroxidase, sulphoacetaldehyde lyase, thiosulphate sulphurtransferase, thiosulphate-thiol sulphurtransferase.*

As to the sulfate or sulphate ion, Jain lists it as an inhibitor for ADP-glucose phosphorylase, ADPG pyrophosphorylase, aryl sulfatase, for the binding of pyridoxal phosphate, glycogen synthetase phosphatase, oxygen evolution, photophosphorylation, ADP-glucose pyrophosphorylase, ribulose-1,5-DIP carboxylase, sulfatase, the uptake of anions, 6-phosphogluconate dehydrogenase. Zollner lists acetolactate synthase, N-acetylgalactosamine-6-sulphatase, N-acetylglucosamine-6-sulphatase, arylsulphatase, arylsulphatase A, creatine kinase, glucose 1-phosphate adenyltransferase, glutamate-ammonia-ligase adenyltransferase, γ-glutamyl hydrolase, iduronate 2-sulphatase, 1L-myo-inositol-1-phosphatase, kynurenine-oxyglutarate aminotransferase, polyphosphate kinase, pyruvate kinase type L, thiosulphate sulphurtransferase, transketolase.

To round things out, Jain lists the sulfide or sulphide ion as an inhibitor for ATP sulfurylase, cysteine desulfhydrase, cytochrome C oxidase, nitrate reductase, and Zollner lists aminoacyl-histidine dipeptidase, cytochrome-c oxidase, L-galactonolactone oxidase, peroxidase, thiosulphate-thiol sulphurtransferase.

The list of enzymes that are inhibited is extensive, and the information presented seems incredibly obscurant. No doubt a similar sort of list could be found for nitrites and nitrates, and so on. *It makes one wonder, if all this kind of obscure information has been acquired about enzymes and inhibitors, then why hasn't there been more research performed on enzyme inhibitors for cancer cell metabolism?*

Investigators Smolenski et al. found that *haemodialysate and its three peptide fractions* had an effect on *lactate dehydrogenase* activity. (*Haemodialysis* or *hemodialysis* pertains to the dialysis of blood in an artificial kidney whereby the waste products are separated and removed. The blood returned or recycled to the patient would be the haemodialysate or hemodialysate.) The subjects were both healthy patients and patients treated for end-stage renal (kidney) disease. Erythrocytes (red blood cells) from the dialyzed patients showed significantly lower LDH activity than those from healthy subjects. In healthy patients, however, after incubation with haemodialysate or a peptide fraction, a significant reduction in LDH activity was observed. For the patients with end-stage renal disease, neither haemodialysate nor its peptide fractions further inhibited LDH activity in red blood cells.

Cancer was not explicitly mentioned in the foregoing reference, but it can be proposed that haemodialysate and its three peptide fractions, by *inhibiting lactate dehydrogenase activity,* are potential *anticancer agents.* Peptides or polypeptides themselves are considered to be potential anticancer agents, as discussed in Ralph Moss's *Cancer Therapy* and in Richard Walters' *Options,* for instance. In further comment, evidently there is something that occurs during the separation and removal of the waste products in the dialysis machine that causes an inhibiting effect on LDH.

---

* Note that *malate dehydrogenase* is the enzyme for Step (8) in the tricarboxylic acid cycle, as per Figure 1.4. Therefore, it can be regarded that sulfite works against respiration or aerobic glycolysis.

The differential *inhibition of lactate dehydrogenase isoenzymes* was studied by Onigbinde et al. The action of guanidinium thiocyanate (GSCN) was investigated, as used in the LD-1 assay for lactate dehydrogenase of the heart type HHHH, also called LDH_1 or H_4, as developed by the Boehringer Mannheim Corporation (BMC). An analysis of the reaction kinetics indicates that GSCN competitively inhibited LD-1 in the presence of lactate and NAD^+, but on the other hand is a noncompetitive inhibitor of LD-5, which is of the muscle type MMMM, or LDH_5 or M_4. The intermediate isoenzymes LD-2 and LD-3 showed mixed inhibition kinetics. The inhibiting effect was found to be two- to threefold smaller for LD-5 than for LD-1. On the other hand, the inhibition rate for LD-5, and for LD-2 and LD-3, was very rapid, whereas the inactivation rate for LD-5 was much slower. It was noted that the presence of lactate served to protect LD-1 but had no effect on the other enzymes. The deactivating agents were found to by both the guanidinium and thiocyanate ions, and deactivation was irreversible. The authors speculate that GSCN selectively denatures the M subunit of or LD or LDH, whereas the H subunit is less susceptible, and is further stabilized by the lactate product.*

A working group dealing with enzymes is concerned with standardizing methods for determining *enzyme catalyst concentrations in serum and plasma* at standard conditions. With regard to *glutamate dehydrogenase* or *glutaminase*, this work is embodied in a report titled "Proposal of Standard Methods for the Determination of Enzyme Catalytic Concentrations in Serum and Plasma at 37° C." Part 3 of the report is concerned with glutamate dehydrogenase. Assuming that glutamate dehydrogenase is here the same as glutaminase, this particular report evidently pertains to the processes of glutaminolysis. It may be assumed that other methods for enzyme determination have been advanced, with others in the offing, including analysis methods for the enzymes involved in anaerobic glycolysis.

Regarding lactate dehydrogenase in blood serum, Yamashiro et al. have conducted studies on a *serum factor inhibiting lactate dehydrogenase activity* in a patient's serum. *An extremely low LDH activity was found in the serum of a 70-year-old patient.* This was noticed when normal serum was incubated with the patient's serum. Interestingly, the patient's serum produced an LDH inhibition rate that was higher at 4° C than at 37° C. The patient's serum inhibited both M-subunits and H-subunits of LDH, with the M-subunit inhibited more than the H-subunit. It was found that the agent responsible was *IgG (immunoglobulin) of the lambda type*, but the mechanism remains undetermined. *(This is direct evidence that the immune system can inhibit lactate dehydrogenase isoenzymes, and in turn inhibit or block cancer cell metabolism.)*

An assay method has been developed by Shirahase et al. for determining serum levels of the lactate dehydrogenase isoenzyme LD-1. The method involves proteolysis during incubation with alpha-chymotrypsin and protein degradation. (Chymotrypsin is a hydrolytic enzyme secreted by the pancreas. It is activated in the small intestine, where it catalyzes the breakdown of proteins.) There is a cleavage of phenylalinine bonds in the A and B subunits of LD-3, LD-4, and LD-5 isoenzymes. (Phenylalanine as well as L-alanine is an inhibitor for pyruvate kinase, as per Appendix A.) A short incubation period with *alpha-chymotrypsin* completely inactivated these isoenzymes and partially inactivated LD-2. The addition of *guanidine* (mentioned previously) completed the inactivation of LD-2. However, the isoenzyme LD-1 was only affected slightly. *Normal serum levels of LD-1 in 500 healthy people were found to range from 66 to 130 U/L or units per liter, whereas serum levels of LD-2, LD-3, LD-4, LD-5 may range up to 4,000 U/L.* The results of the assay method developed correlated closely with the Roche Isomune immunochemical LD-1 method. Several common test method interferents had no effect. *(There is the strong indication that alpha-chymotropsin could serve as an anticancer agent by inhibiting lactate dehydrogenase isoenzymes, and in some instances can be enhanced by guanidine, which is somewhat*

---

* There is the possibility that guanidinium thiocyanate could serve as a lactate dehydrogenase inhibitor for one or more of the isoenzymes and thus serve as an inhibitor for cancer cell metabolism—if it is not overtly toxic in other ways. Cyanate (–OCN) of course has kinship with cyanide (–CN), which also brings to mind the Laetrile controversy, previously discussed. The guanidinium ion or group, with the chemical formula $(NH_2)_2CNH^+$, in turn has its own share of carbon-nitrogen bonds and is an analog of urea, $(NH_2)_2CO$, both acting as denaturing agents for polypeptides (Voet and Voet, *Biochemistry*, p. 112). Guanidine has the formula $(NH_2)_2C(NH)$, and may be obtained from guanine by oxidation or may be formed in other ways. Whereas the compound called *guanine*—which may be derived from guano, from mammalian liver, pancreas, and muscle, and from many plants—constitutes one of the four fundamental nucleic acid bases, along with *adenine, thymine,* and *cytosine*, as introduced in Part 1 (e.g., Voet and Voet, *Biochemistry*, p. 796). It has a nitrogen-containing ring structure akin to that of those mostly toxic compounds classed as *alkaloids*.

related to urea, a known anticancer agent. Furthermore, unhealthy patients—read cancer patients—presumably have elevated LD or LDH levels.)

In a paper by Sharma and Schwille, the conversion of glyoxalate to oxalate and glycolate was investigated *in vitro. Lactate dehydrogenase acts as a dismutase in the conversion, and is inhibited by reduced glutathione (GSH), cysteine,* and *cysteamine.* The *LDH sources were human erythrocytes* (red blood cells), *human plasma,* rabbit muscle, and rat liver. The LDH activity was assayed using glyoxalate and NADH. The activity of the LDH was thought to be regulated by the free SH-groups in the cell. The authors were interested in the possibilities for lowering oxalate production and the risk of stone formation. (*Very possibly, however, these inhibiting substances could be used to lower and control LDH, and in turn limit cancer cell metabolism.* Appendix Y lists cysteine as an inhibitor for pyruvate kinase, and Appendix A and Y list cysteamine or cystamine as an inhibitor for hexokinase. Both hexokinase and pyruvate kinase are controlling enzymes in the glycolysis pathway.)

Investigators FitzGerald et al. were concerned with the kinetics of *lactate dehydrogenase* from the lactic acid-forming bacteria species *Leuconostoc lactis* NCW1. It was found that the optimum pH for the conversion depended on the pyruvate reactant concentration. No activators were found for the enzyme, and none of the intermediates of the phosphoketolase pathway inhibited the enzyme. *It was found, however, that ATP, ADP, GTP (guanosine triphosphate), and NAD$^+$ were inhibitory.*[*] Co-metabolism of citrate and glucose did not affect the pH, but the results may have bearing on the production of diacetyl and acetoin at low pH by *Leuconostoc.*

Dunham et al. studied the structural and metabolic changes in articular (join-related) cartilage. Injuries were chemically induced by intra-articular injections of sodium iodoacetate. It was assumed that the injurious effects were produced by inhibition of the glycolytic pathway, and the study was directed at countering these effects by the use of *anti-inflammatory agents* and of potentially chondro-protective agents ("chondro-" means composed of or having to do with cartilage, e.g., a chondroma is a tumor composed of cartilage). This inhibition was greater than expected from *in vitro* investigations and affected other oxidative pathways. Moreover, the cells in close proximity to the cartilage showed virtually no inhibition. (The inference, which was not an object of the study, is that *injections of iodoacetate could serve as a localized anticancer agent by inhibiting the glycolytic pathway.* It is not apparent that any of this has anything to do with the use of shark cartilage or bovine cartilage as an anticancer agent.)

An article by Dixit et al. deals with the *inhibition of key enzymes of carbohydrate metabolism in regenerating mouse liver by ascorbic acid.* The key enzymes for carbohydrate metabolism were listed as hexokinases, phosphofructokinase, pyruvate kinase, *lactate dehydrogenase,* glucose-6-phosphate dehydrogenase, and malic enzyme. The inhibiting effect was studied in terms of the regeneration of mouse liver. All enzymes show an increase in activity during normal regeneration, but *ascorbic acid (vitamin C) reduced the activities of the enzymes in regenerating liver.* The decrease in liver weight in ascorbic acid treated animals could be correlated with its effect on these enzymes, inasmuch as the glycolytic pathway is the main source of energy for the dividing cells.

The foregoing is evidence that vitamin C inhibits not only lactate dehydrogenase but all of the key enzymes of carbohydrate metabolism—although vitamin C is not listed as an inhibitor for any of these enzymes in Appendix Z. If vitamin C indeed inhibits all of the foregoing enzymes, this can be interpreted as saying that ascorbic acid will also act against cancer cell metabolism. Whether this action might be preferential read selective is not discernible from the reported results, however, and was not an objective of the investigation.

The enzyme glucose-6-phosphate dehydrogenase (G-6-PD) is involved in the pentose phosphate pathway, generating NADPH in the process (Voet and Voet, *Biochemistry,* p. 617ff). (See the section titled Update on Glutaminolysis and the subsection on DHEA.) The malic enzyme evidently is malate dehydrogenase, which is involved in the tricarboxylic acid cycle.

Further information discloses that *G-6-PD deficiency is by far the main cause of red cell enzyme deficiency* (David J. Weatherall, in *Tropical and Geographical Medicine,* pp. 105–108). It has been

---

[*] *Guanosine* is the nucleoside form corresponding to the nucleic acid base *guanine* (Voet and Voet, Biochemistry, pp. 796, 817). As with guanine, its nitrogen-containing ring structure has a commonality with *alkaloids.*

estimated to affect *more than 100 million persons worldwide,* chiefly in Africa, the Mediterranean, the Middle East, and southeast Asia. Most of the affected individuals *show no clinical symptoms unless exposed to oxidant drugs.* Clinical symptoms include *hemolysis,* the destruction of red cells accompanied by the release of hemoglobin. The metabolic pathway is that of little oxidative energy production, the final product being lactic acid or lactate. *(This is also the main route for cancer cell metabolism.)* A deficiency in G-6-PD is described as an inherited condition, but hemolysis may be exacerbated by a number of drugs that are tabulated in the reference. These drugs include the following: aminoquinolines such as Plasmoquine; sulfones such as Avlosulfone and Promizole; sulfonamides such as Albucid and Sulamyd, Gantrisin, and Lederkyn, Midicel, Kynax; nitrofurans such as Furandantin, Furoxone, and Furacin; analgesics such as *aspirin,* acetophenetidin, and acetanilide; and such miscellany as *vitamin K, naphthalene* (moth balls), Benemid, BAL, methylene blue, acetylphenylhydrazine, phenylhydrazine, *p*-aminosalicyclic acid, quinine, quinidine, and chloroamphenicol.

A most interesting conclusion by Nelson et al. is that *copper plus ascorbate inactivates lactate dehydrogenase.* The title of the paper further asks the question, are oxygen radicals involved? This interfaces with concepts linking free radicals and oxidants with cancer. No abstract or additional information was supplied with the citation.

An article by V.I. Loushchak (or Lushchak) examines free and membrane-bound lactate as occurs in the white driving muscles of skate. Both the free (purified cytoplasmic) and membrane-bound lactate dehydrogenases were characterized in terms of pyruvate and NADH. *The membrane-bound LDH was not inhibited by high pyruvate concentrations;* contrarily, the *free or purified LDH was inhibited.* Part of the membrane-bound LDH could be released by incubation in solutions having high levels of KCl (potassium chloride) or having an alkaline pH-value. With solubilized LDH, the inactivation rate during trypsin digestion was several-fold higher than that for the membrane-enzyme. (The results may indicate several points. For one, potassium—that is, potassium chloride—may be essential for the release of membrane-bound or captive LDH. Next, a buildup of pyruvate acts as an inhibitor for LDH—although it is also a reactant and would ordinarily be expected to favor the conversion to lactate catalyzed by LDH, via the law of mass action. *Evidently, pyruvate serves as a true inhibitor, affecting or covering up the active sites of LDH. An inspection of Appendix A reveals that pyruvic acid is listed as an inhibitor for both pyruvate kinase and lactate dehydrogenase.* It may be noted that pyruvate kinase catalyzes the reaction forming pyruvate. That is, pyruvic acid or pyruvate is the product. Thus, the inhibition of the action of pyruvate kinase by pyruvic acid would normally be expected merely from the law of mass action.)

Ike et al. investigated the purification and properties of lactate dehydrogenase as prepared from the aerobic bacterium *Nocardia asteroides.* The LDH was purified by ammonium sulfate precipitation, gel filtration of Sephadex G-150, and DEAE-Sepharose column chromatography. The pH optimum was an alkaline 9.5-value, and the temperature optimum was 50° C. It was noted that the metal ions Mn^{++} (manganese), Fe^{++} (iron), Co^{++} (cobalt), Mg^{++} (magnesium), and Ca^{++} (calcium) *increased* the purified LDH activity. On the other hand, *LDH activity was completely inhibited by $CuCl_2$* (copper chloride, or more exactly, cupric chloride). Potassium chloride, ammonium sulfate, and sodium chloride were neutral, not affecting the LDH activity. (It may be noted that inorganic catalysts for organic reactions may variously involve the metals listed, and in particular iron and cobalt, as noted in the subsection "Other Bioactive Substances and Miscellaneous Agents," in the section on "Phytochemicals that May Act Against Cancer." Whether this has any bearing here may be only a coincidence. As to the inhibiting effect of copper or copper compounds, this has been previously noted in the work of Nelson et al., mentioned above. In Appendix A copper is listed as an inhibitor for both hexokinase and glutaminase. In Appendix B, both copper and cobalt are listed as inhibitors for respiration.)

Kochhar et al. denote LHD more specifically as NAD(+)-dependent D-lactate dehydrogenase. They found that there is evidence of the polypeptides Arg-235, His-303, Tyr-101, and Trp-19 at or near the active sites. ("Arg" stands for argenine, "His" stands for histamine, "Tyr" stands for tyrosine, and "Trp" stands for tryptophan.) The purified LDH source was from *Lactobacillus bulgaricus,* and its complete amino acid sequence was determined. The purified LDH used was found to a dimer of identical subunits, each containing 332 amino acid residues. The enzyme was treated with the group-specific reagents **2,3-butanedione, diethylpyrocarbonate, tetranitromethane,** and **N-bromosuccinimide,** each of which caused a complete loss of LDH activity. "The inclusion of pyruvate and/or NADH were found to reduce the inactivation rates manyfold, indicating the presence of arginine, histidine, tyrosine, and tryptophan residues at or near the active site." The loss of enzyme activity was apparently due to the modification of a single arginine, histidine, tryptophan, or tyrosine residue. (The highlighted compounds are potential anticancer agents, if they are not toxic in other ways. The quote is included, since it may not be as it appears to be. That is, pyruvate is supposedly an inhibitor for LDH as per the work of Loushchak or Lushchak, above.)

Inasmuch as the enzyme lactate dehydrogenase is not involved in normal cell metabolism, or aerobic glycolysis, its inhibition may not be critical, up to a point. On the other hand, the fact that LDH is involved in essential body processes such as occur during extreme muscular activity, and in particular that of the heart muscle under stress, may mean that its concentration cannot be reduced below certain critical limits. Moreover, one type of isoenzyme may be more essential than another.

Furthermore, cancer cells may involve a less critical form of isoenzyme. However, the particular type (or types) of lactate dehydrogenase found in cancer cell metabolism was not stated in the foregoing references. This, conceivably, is a topic for further investigation.

8.11 UPDATE ON GLUTAMINOLYSIS

As set forth in Part 1, glycolysis is not the only pathway in cell metabolism. Glutaminolysis also occurs to a limited extent, as do other amino-acid reactions. The previously described work of Eigenbrodt et al. emphasized glutaminolysis in cancer cells, but other amino acids enter into cell metabolism (Voet and Voet, *Biochemistry*, pp. 727–783). In fact, sugars other than glucose may enter into the reactions, notably *pentose* in what is called the *pentose phosphate pathway* (Voet and Voet, *Biochemistry*, pp. 599, 617ff.; Nancy B. Schwartz, in *Textbook of Biochemistry*, pp. 406–414). The term *pentose* distinguishes a five-oxygen sugar molecule from hexose, which is a six-oxygen sugar molecule, the notable example of the latter being glucose. Rather than furnishing energy as in glycolysis, the pentose phosphate pathway generates NADPH, the reduced form of nicotinamide adenine dinucleotide phosphate, and also produces ribose-5-phosphate, which is the sugar precursor for the nucleic acids. In comparing the pentose phosphate pathway vis à vis glycolysis or the glycolytic or glycotic pathway(s), the term *pentose phosphate shunt* is sometimes used.

We emphasize again that the term *anaerobic glycolysis* is here to be used to denote the conversion of glucose eventually to lactic acid or lactate, whereas *aerobic glycolysis* is the conversion or oxidation of glucose eventually to carbon dioxide and water. The distinguishing feature is that, in anaerobic glycolysis, the pyruvic acid or pyruvate intermediate is converted to lactic acid or lactate. In aerobic glycolysis, the pyruvic acid or pyruvate intermediate is converted to carbon dioxide and water via the tricarboxylic acid cycle. The details were further set forth in Part 1, in the several versions of Figure 1.

The conversion of glutamine predominates among the amino acids, and a further look at the relative significance of glutaminolysis as compared to glycolysis is at least informative, and particularly as it may also relate to glycolysis and to cancer cell metabolism. The following information is in large part based on a word search of MEDLINE under "glutaminolysis" for a recent five-year period (1992–1996).

An article by Holm et al. deals with the *utilization of nutrients by malignant tumors in humans,* in this case *colonic carcinomas.* The investigation took blood samples from an artery and the main tumor-draining vein, and these samples were used to obtain balances on the energy-yielding substrates (reactants) and amino acids. Comparisons were made against peripheral tissues. Tumor blood flow rates proved much greater than in leg tissues, in a ratio of 43.2/2.5. *The glucose net uptake and lactate release by the malignancies were at elevated rates, exceeding the peripheral tissue exchange rates 30- and 43-fold.* The ratio of lactate output to glucose consumption was 0.78 in the tumors as compared to 0.48 in leg tissues. *No differences were observed in free fatty acids and ketone balances.* It was noted that the carcinomas utilized branched-chain amino acids and serine, and in turn *alanine and particularly ammonia were released in large amounts.* Net glutamine retention varied. The summation was as follows.

It is concluded that the energy metabolism of human carcinomas relies predominantly on glucose, with fat-derived calories making no appreciable contribution. The impaired nutritive perfusion of malignant tumors appears to favor glycolysis and to limit both glucose oxidation and glutaminolysis.

A study by Meijer and van Dijken was concerned with the effects of glucose supply on myeloma growth and metabolism.* A recombinant myeloma cell line designated SP2/0 was used in a chemostat culture. It was found that lowering the glucose concentration from a figure of 25.0 units down to 1.4 units halved the cell concentration. (Which may be inferred as acting against the cancer.) Furthermore, *"Mass balances indicated that only a minor amount of glucose was utilized via the TCA cycle (tricarboxylic acid cycle) irrespective of the glucose concentration in the feed medium."* (It may be inferred that the *glucose was used in other ways, say for anaerobic glycolysis.*) The yield of cells from ATP (adenosine triphosphate) was apparently independent of the ratio of the glucose and glutamine consumption rates. A conclusion reached was that the role of glucose is to provide intermediates for anabolic reactions. (The term *anabolic* connotes constructive processes, as opposed to *catabolic* or destructive processes.) However, it is indicated that glucose may also play an indirect catabolic role during glutaminolysis by providing the pyruvate for converting glutamate to alanine and alpha-ketoglutarate. Lastly, *if the glucose concentration is low, then glutamine may be the sole energy source* for myeloma in chemostat cultures.

Petch and Butler studied the metabolism of glucose and glutamine in a culture of the antibody-secreting murine hybridoma.† The original concentrations were 20 parts glucose to 2 parts glutamine. After two days of exponential cell growth, the glucose content was reduced to 60 percent of the original concentration and the glutamine content was completely depleted. *It was found that glycolysis accounted for about 96 percent of the glucose metabolized, with about 3.6 percent fluxing through the pentose phosphate pathway, but only about 0.6 percent converted or oxidized via the TCA cycle (tricarboxylic acid cycle).* (Evidently anaerobic glycolysis prevailed, inasmuch as only 0.6 percent of the glucose was converted via the TCA cycle.) The glutamine content was partially oxidized via glutaminolysis to yield *alanine* (55%), aspartate (3%), glutamate (4%), lactate, and CO_2 (22%). Both the glucose and the glutamine contributed to the metabolic energy requirement for the cells, calculated as 59 percent for the glucose and 41 percent for the glutamine. (Inasmuch as the glucose was evidently converted to lactate, a conversion that has a very low heat of reaction, the total energy requirements were supplemented by the partial oxidation of the glutamine.)

The *human hair follicle* has been used in a study on glutaminolysis and aerobic glycolysis by investigators Kealey, Williams, and Philpott. (A *hair follicle* is the small cavity that is the source for hair growth.) For it has been observed that human hair follicles undergo these metabolic processes, which may have implications not only for skin and splanchnic (visceral) cell metabolism, but for *neoplastic or cancer metabolism* as well. Human hair follicles were maintained in supplemented Williams E medium and were observed to grow at the normal rate. The results indicated that both glucose and glutamine were largely metabolized to lactate. *"...the major fuel was glucose, and 90 percent of the glucose was metabolized to lactate, and only 10 percent oxidized. Glutamine was also an important fuel ... but this too was largely metabolized to lactate rather than oxidized."* It was noted that, rather than a fatty-acid cycle operating in the hair follicle, a glucose-glutamine cycle occurred instead, and the presence of glutamine inhibits glucose utilization.‡

In an earlier companion paper by the same three authors, in the order Williams, Philpott, and Kealey, it was reported that the metabolism of the human hair follicle had been investigated *in vitro*, and the conditions and results were essentially as outlined above. The conditions were maintained such that the glycogen and ATP (adenosine triphosphate) content, and the follicle growth rate, were the same as the values *in vivo*. Only 10 percent of the glucose utilized was oxidized to CO_2 (by aerobic glycolysis), and 40 percent of this value consisted of conversion by the pentose phosphate shunt. Whereas fatty acids and ketones were also oxidized by the hair follicles, they are poor energy substitutes for glucose and will not sustain hair growth *in vitro*. Glutamine was shown to be of significance as a fuel, with 23 percent of the uptake being oxidized. However, *64 percent of the glutamine was metabolized to lactate*, indicating

---

* Myeloma is cancer of the immune system (Voet and Voet, *Biochemistry*, p. 74).

† *Murine* refers to a mouse or rat. *Hybridoma* refers to cells that have an unlimited capacity to divide, and it results from the fusion of an antibody with a myeloma cell (Voet and Voet, *Biochemistry*, p. 74).

‡ It would appear from the above findings that *human hair follicles could simulate cancer cell behavior in testing enzyme inhibitors for, say, anaerobic glycolysis, or in testing yet other proposed anticancer agents*. In further comment, hair follicle cells are among the first to be adversely affected by conventional cytotoxic chemotherapy and can be adjudged extraordinarily sensitive to anticancer agents—more so than cancer cells per se. The criterion, of course, is for the anticancer agent to be selective, that is, not cytotoxic to vital normal cells.

that (anaerobic) glycolysis occurs predominantly, along with glutaminolysis. Evidently a glucose-glutamine cycle operates, whereas the glucose-fatty acid cycle is unimportant.

A paper by Griffiths et al. deals with the role of glutamine and glucose analogs in the metabolic inhibition of human myeloid leukemia *in vitro*. For the record, the glutamine analogs used had the chemical names L[alpha S,5S]-alpha-amino-3-chloro-4,5-dihydro-5-isoxazoleacetic acid (acivicin) and 6-diazo-5-oxo-L-norleucine (DON). Both have been shown to be cytotoxic toward a wide variety of animal and human xenografted ("xeno-" indicating strange or foreign or different) solid tumors. Human use, however, has been limited by their toxicity. An object of the investigation was to determine if the lack of success with these agents was due in part to an inefficient inhibition of glutamine metabolism. It was found that acivicin inhibited ribonucleotide biosynthesis but had little effect on energy production via glutaminolysis. (It may be inferred that the DNA/RNA/protein sequence is blocked, the usual debilitating effect of conventional cytotoxic chemotherapy agents.) As to the use of DON, it inhibited both ribonucleotide biosynthesis and glutamine oxidation. By using the glucose analog 2-deoxy-D-glucose along with the glutamine analog DON, there was an inhibition of nucleotide biosynthesis, *an inhibition of both glutaminolysis and glycolysis,* and a further reduction in cell viability. It was concluded that the preceding results support the essential role of glutamine in cell metabolism. (That is, the results support the essential role of glutaminolysis in normal cell metabolism, whereas *its inhibition acts against cancer cells.*) Furthermore, the use of DON may be more effective in the treatment of myeloid leukemia if used in combination with 2-deoxy-D-glucose. (In comment, the fact that there is an inhibition of ribonucleotide biosynthesis is a not an encouraging signal.)

Rosa et al. investigated thioglycollate and other stimuli of lymphocyte (white blood cell) metabolism and proliferation. The lymphocytes consisted of a control group (CC), a thioglycollate-injected group (TG), and a Walker 256 tumor implanted group (WT). Both nonimmune and immune inflammatory stimuli were also used. The key enzyme activities were measured for the processes of glycolysis, the pentose phosphate pathway, the Krebs cycle or tricarboxylic acid cycle, and glutaminolysis. The rates were also measured for the incorporation of [2-14C]-thymidine and [5-3H]-uridine into cultured lymphocytes. The rates of thymidine and uridine incorporation were enhanced by an average of 80 percent for lymphocytes injected with thiogallate. For tumor-implanted animals, the increased rate was even higher, about 2.4-fold over that of the controls. The *hexokinase* activity deceased by 23 percent in the TG and by 61 percent in the WT. *Glucose 6-phosphate dehydrogenase* activity was not affected by the nonimmune inflammatory stimulus. (The enzyme glucose 6-phosphate dehydrogenase is also known variously as glucose 6-phosphate isomerase or phosphoglucose isomerase or hexose phosphateisomerase. It catalyzes step two in the glycolysis sequence of Figure 1.1 and may or may not be a key or controlling enzyme, since step two is ordinarily assumed to be at equilibrium.) The activity of lymphocyte *citrate synthesis* was lowered 39 percent by thioglycollate. (Presumably the citrate is formed during the tricarboxylic acid cycle, or Krebs cycle or citric acid cycle, as per Figure 1.4 in Part 1. The inference therefore is that aerobic glycolysis is suppressed.) It was found that *glutaminase* activity was stimulated in the TG group but was not affected in the WT group. As to glutaminolysis versus glycolysis in the lymphocytes, *the presence of the Walker 256 tumor did not affect glutaminolysis but depressed glycolysis.* Furthermore, *the nonimmune inflammatory stimulus enhanced glutaminolysis but suppressed glycolysis and the tricarboxylic acid cycle.*

Citrate synthase is a key enzyme in the tricarboxylic acid cycle, or citric acid cycle or Krebs cycle, whichever it is to be called. As per Figure 1.4, it controls the first of the eight steps in the cycle, the conversion of Acetyl-CoA and oxaloacetate recycle to form citrate or citric acid, the first of the tricarboxylates or tricarboxylic acids involved (e.g., Voet and Voet, *Biochemistry*, pp. 539, 549). A number of enzyme inhibitors are listed in Jain's *Handbook*, including the following: adenosine-5′-triphosphate (ATP), carnitine derivatives, citric acid, hydroxy-citric acid, coenzyme A (CoA), 2-oxo-glutaric acid, hydroxycitrate lactone, and tricarboxybenzene.

Jain also includes the enzyme citrate synthetase (or citrate synthase, but strictly speaking there is a technical difference between synthase and synthetase, as noted in Part 1 in the section "A Detailing of Enzyme-Catalyzed Biochemical Reactions Involved in Cell Metabolism," subsection on "Glycolysis," and the subsection "Enzyme Nomenclature versus Function.") Inhibitors for citrate synthetase include ATP, CoA, fatty acids, 2-oxo-glutaric acid, lithium ion, NADH, NADPH, nucleotides, and pyrophosphate ion. Zollner's *Handbook* lists the following inhibitors for citrate synthase: citroyl-CoA, fluoroacetyl-CoA, and palmitoyl-CoA.

It is worth noting that *ATP keeps showing up as an inhibitor for various enzymes.* Some of these compounds also show up in Appendix B as affecting respiration and presumably should be avoided or used with care. Some inhibitors such as ATP, NADH, NADPH, and so on occur naturally in body chemistry and are involved in other ways in glycolysis. This illustrates the complexity of whatever is going on. It also illustrates the point that the perceived inhibiting action of some of these compounds or substances may not be a sure thing. Citrate synthase is available, as obtained variously from chicken heart, pigeon breast muscle, porcine heart, and from bacteria (Sigma catalog).

In another, earlier study by Rosa et al., metabolic and functional changes in lymphocytes and macrophages were correlated to aging.* Key enzyme activities were measured for glycolysis, the pentose phosphate pathway, the tricarboxylic acid cycle or Krebs cycle or citric acid cycle, and glutaminolysis. A comparison was made for 3-month-old versus 15-month-old rats. The test conditions and parameters were similar to those previously described in the later paper, above. It was concluded that *aging seems to reduce the capacity for glucose utilization.*

> Therefore, an impaired glucose metabolism during ageing may be one important mechanism for the alteration in lymphocyte proliferation and macrophage phagocytosis observed and also for the modification of the response to inflammatory and tumor challenges.†

In effect, as one may suspect, with age there is less potential for fighting off diseases, including cancer. Inasmuch as there is less capacity for glucose utilization, this all may correlate with the onset of diabetes and in turn be insulin and hormone related—which gets around to another paper by Rosa and associates, to follow.

In a previous paper by Rosa, Cury, and Curi, the effects of insulin, glucocorticoids and thyroid hormones were studied. As in the other papers, these effects pertained to the activities of the key enzymes involved in glycolysis, glutaminolysis, the pentose phosphate pathway, and the tricarboxylic acid cycle, also known as the Krebs cycle or citric acid cycle. The macrophages used were obtained from hormone-treated rats and those cultured for 48 hours in the presence of hormones. The maximum activities were determined for the enzymes **hexokinase, glucose 6-phosphate dehydrogenase, glutaminase,** and **citrate synthase.** It was found that *macrophage phagocytosis (the destruction of macrophages) was inhibited by dexamethasone (a glucocorticoid) and thyroid hormones but remained unchanged when insulin was added.* Moreover, changes in enzyme activity for the hormone treatment of rats produced changes similar to those found in cultures. Whereas *insulin enhanced the activity of hexokinse and citrate synthase, it reduced the activities of glucose 6-phosphate dehydrogenase and glutaminase.* Dexamethasone had similar effects except on glucose 6-phosphate dehydrogenase. Thyroid hormones raised the activities of hexokinase and glutaminase but reduced that of citrate synthase. It was concluded that insulin, glucocorticoids, and thyroid hormones affect macrophage metabolism.‡

Ahmed, Williams, and Weidemann have investigated the glycolytic, glutaminolytic, and pentose-phosphate pathways in promyelocytic cells. (Promyelocytic cells are filament-like.) Specifically, the cells involved were HL-60 and DMSO-differentiated HL60 cells.§

It was noted that the human leukemic cell line HL60 undergoes differentiation in the presence of DMSO, yielding granulocyte-like cells. The rates of glucose and glutamine metabolism were determined for both the undifferentiated and the fully differentiated cells. The rates for exogenous glucose metabolism were the same for both kinds of cells. (*Exogenous glucose is that from without the cell,* as distinguished from *indigenous.*)

---

* Macrophages are a type of large white blood cell that occurs in connective tissue and constitutes part of the cellular immune system (Voet and Voet, *Biochemistry,* p. 1207).

† *Phagocytosis* here refers to the destruction of macrophages.

‡ As to anaerobic glycolysis versus aerobic glycolysis, and glycolysis versus glutaminolysis, the effects seem somewhat offsetting. That is, if, say, the activity of hexokinase is increased, it may be offset by a decrease in the activity of glucose 6-phosphate dehydrogenase. If the activities of both hexokinase and glutaminase are enhanced, then both glycolysis and glutaminolysis will be favored, perhaps equally or nearly so. And so on. However, *any substance that will encourage macrophage metabolism may be presumed to enhance the immune system and, in this respect, serve as an anticancer agent.*

§ The acronym DMSO refers to the common chemical dimethyl sulfoxide, $(CH_3)_2SO$.

In each case, *about 75 percent of the glucose was converted to lactate.* It was found that the activities remained unaffected for the enzymes hexokinase, phosphofructokinase, pyruvate kinase, and citrate synthase. (Citrate synthase is a key enzyme in the tricarboxylic acid cycle. The other enzymes pertain to glycolysis per se, the multistep conversion of glucose to pyruvic acid or pyruvate.) The activity of the oxidative segment of the pentose phosphate pathway was enhanced for the differentiated cells, and no glycogen synthesis was detectable. It was said that these observations are consistent with lower glycogen contents, with increased activities of glucose 6-phosphate dehydrogenase and 6-phosphogluconate dehydrogenase, and with the increased oxidation of [1-14C] glucose as compared to [6-14C] glucose in the differentiated cells.

A further finding was that *glucose utilization was suppressed by exogenous glutamine, whereas glutamine utilization was enhanced by glucose in both kinds of cells.* Both effects were more pronounced in the undifferentiated cells. It was advanced that the reason that glucose utilization is suppressed in the presence of glutamine is due to an allosteric inhibition of an enzyme for a controlling step during glycolysis (e.g., the enzyme phosphofructokinase). The observation was made that glutaminase activity remained low, and in the differentiated cells was only half that in the undifferentiated cells. As to the stimulation of glutaminolysis by glucose, this may be due to the stimulation of mitochondrial glutamine transport.

The glutamine utilized in both cell types resulted in a net accumulation of glutamate, aspartate, and *alanine,* with up to 35 percent of the glutamine oxidized to CO_2. *"In contrast, almost all of the glucose utilized was converted to lactate and very little was oxidized."* It was commented that the high rates of glycolysis and glutaminolysis both before and after differentiation are not primarily for energy production. Instead, in undifferentiated cells, these processes supply reaction intermediates or substrates for the biosynthesis of nucleic acid precursors. In the case of differentiated cells, there is a synthesis of reactive oxygen intermediates or substrate that acts to maintain NADP (nicotinamide adenine dinucleotide phosphate) in a reduced state.*

The foregoing analysis may indicate why *DMSO* has been listed as an anticancer agent, as mentioned in both Moss and Walters. If so, this anticancer action is apparently tied to the production of differentiated cell types and to the maintenance of higher-than-usual levels of NADPH, the reduced form of nicotinamide adenine dinucleotide phosphate. *In other words, NADPH itself could be viewed as an anticancer agent.* More than this, the conversion of the oxidized form $NADP^+$ to the reduced form NADPH is tied in with the conversion of other forms of phosphates, such as ADP (adenosine diphosphate) to ATP (adenosine triphosphate), and to AMP (adenosine monophosphate), and so on. (Voet and Voet, *Biochemistry,* pp. 414, 474). As to AMP, consult the paragraph to follow.

Hugo et al. have studied the effects of extracellular *AMP* (adenosine monophosphate) on MCF-7 breast cancer cells. (E. Eigenbrodt, cited elsewhere, is a coauthor.) These effects were observed in a culture medium of MCF-7 breast cancer cells propagated *in vitro,* and concern cell proliferation, glycolysis, and glutaminolysis. Several adenosine derivatives were tested, and *AMP proved the most effective inhibitor of cancer cell proliferation. "In AMP-treated cells, DNA synthesis decreased, whereas RNA and protein synthesis rose normally with time."* It was further noted that, with regard to carbohydrate metabolism, *there was a drastic reduction in lactate produced.* (Lactate being the end product of anaerobic glycolysis, read cancer cell metabolism.) Whatever lactate was produced, evidently must have been from glutamine, because it was observed that there were increases in the activities of the enzymes involved in glutamine degradation and in the malate-aspartate shuttle (see, for instance, Figure 1.3 and the associated section and figures in Part 1 that deal with glutaminolysis). At the same time, actual glycolytic flux rates declined, albeit key glycolytic enzyme activities increased (an apparent contradiction). It was also noted as per the foregoing that glycolytic metabolites or intermediates such as fructose 1,6-bisphophate and pyruvate accumulated in AMP-arrested cells. The AMP-treated cells had a lowered DNA level, and malate dehydrogenase was not impaired. However, *lactate dehydrogenase was impaired, and the whole of glycolysis was inhibited.* As compensation, glutamine catabolism increased. At the same time, NAD (nicotinamide adenine dinucleotide) concentrations fell-off markedly, caused by the inhibition of P-ribose-PP synthesis via the heightened intracellular AMP levels. (The designator "P" stands for phosphate, "PP" for pyrophosphate.) The authors present a hypothetical metabolic scheme to

---

* The reduced state, incidentally, is ordinarily written as NADPH, whereas the oxidized form is written as $NADP^+$ (Voet and Voet, *Biochemistry*, p. 414).

explain the results. It includes showing how extracellular or added AMP can affect carbohydrate metabolism and cell proliferation.

In further comment, AMP overcomes the inhibition of phosphofructokinase or PFK by adenosine triphosphate or ATP (Voet and Voet, *Biochemistry*, p. 474). There may be many things going on at the same time.

The foregoing references did not always specify enzymes or an enzyme source. That is, did the enzymes occur naturally in the medium or were they added? Furthermore, were the enzymes used up or deactivated during the tests? In other tests, however, the activities of the controlling enzymes were or principal concern, and in the last-cited reference, above, *lactate dehydrogenase and its inhibition* were of paramount interest. In short, while AMP (adenosine monophosphate) occurs naturally in cell metabolism, *the extracellular addition of AMP serves as an inhibitor for lactate dehydrogenase*. Not only this, but it followed that *cancer cell proliferation is inhibited by the introduction of AMP*. Furthermore, since it is a normal component of cellular metabolism, *the presence of AMP in higher concentrations will expectedly be nontoxic to normal cells*.

Speaking of adenosine monophosphate (AMP), and of adenosine diphosphate (ADP) and adenosine triphosphate (ATP), so vital in supporting certain enzyme-catalyzed life-sustaining biochemical reactions, one can also take into account their role as enzyme inhibitors (or modulators). Similarly, some of the nicotinamide coenzymes with such acronyms as NAD, NADH, NADP, and so forth also show up as inhibitors or modulators for certain enzymes. Accordingly, a listing for several adenosine and nicotinamide derivatives is furnished in Table 8.14, as determined from Jain's *Handbook of Enzyme Inhibitors*

Table 8.14   Adinosine and Nicotinamide Derivatives as Enzyme Inhibitors

Adinosine-5′-phosphate (AMP).	Inhibits hexokinase, pyruvate kinase, PRPP amidotransferase. (Also called 5′ adenylic acid. Available from Sigma, Aldrich.)
Adenosine-5′-diphosphate (ADP)	Inhibits hexokinase, 6-phosphofructokinase, pyruvate kinase, DNA kinase, RNase (ribonuclease), PRPP amidotransferase (Obtainable from a bacterial source. Available as sodium salt. Sigma, Aldrich. *Irritant.* Check for impurities.)
Adenosine-5′-triphosphate (ATP)	Inhibits hexokinase, 6-phosphofructokinase, pyruvate kinase, **lactate dehydrogenase**, DNA kinase, RNase (ribonuclease), RNase (ribonuclease, ATP inhibited). (Obtainable from porcine, dog, and rabbit sources. Also from a bacterial source or from equine muscle preparations; the latter may contain traces of vanadium, reported to inhibit Na/K ATPase. Available as the sodium salt. Sigma, Aldrich. Check for impurities.)
Nicotinamide adenine dinucleotide (NAD)	Inhibits **lactate dehydrogenase** (NAD) (The common form of the coenzyme NAD is β-nicotinamide adenine dinucleotide, rather than the alpha- or α-version. Prepared from **yeast**. Sigma.)
Nicotinamide adenine dinucleotide in the reduced form (NADH)	Inhibits **lactate dehydrogenase**, pyruvate dehydrogenase, alpha- ketoglutarate dehydrogenase, IMP dehydrogenase. (The common form of the coenzyme NADH is β-nicotinamide adenine dinucleotide, reduced form, rather than the alpha- or α-version. Available as the disodium salt. Sigma,)
Nicotinamide adenine dinucleotide phosphate (NADP)	Inhibits dihydrofolate reductase (Also known as triphosphopyridine nucleotide or TPN. The common form of the coenzyme NADP is β-nicotinamide adenine dinucleotide phosphate rather than the alpha- or α-version. Available as the sodium salt. Sigma, Aldrich. *Irritant.*)

Source: The above information on phosphate compounds and coenzymes as inhibitors is obtained from Appendices A, B, D, C, E, and Y, and is based on Jain's *Handbook of Enzyme Inhibitors* and Zollner's *Handbook of Enzyme Inhibitors*. Most of the chemical compounds are listed in Sigma catalog and the Aldrich catalog, as noted. Items denoted in **boldface** may be of special interest.

and Zollner's *Handbook of Enzyme Inhibitors*. For the most part, the listing is concerned with the enzymes involved in anaerobic glycolysis. It may be assumed that this listing is far from complete.

The preceding raises the possibility that these compounds, which occur or are generated in the body, may be intimately connected with the processes of *cancer metabolism* as well as normal cell metabolism.

More than this, *the diminutions or excesses of these compounds may determine whether cancer cells flourish or are kept in check.* The inference, therefore, is that these compounds might be used as *anticancer agents.* Such usage might not only involve the introduction of one or more of these compounds from external sources or might merely involve the regulation of the amounts of these compounds in the body.

The above remarks are made with the qualification that body processes are rarely simple, and that all things are interrelated throughout the body, the *systemic viewpoint.* We therefore acknowledge that the body is complex beyond belief, and that biochemistry, as complicated as it seems to be, unravels only a small part. Nevertheless, there is the possibility that cancer could be held in abeyance, if not eliminated or cured entirely, by the expediency of introducing or changing the body levels of only one substance, and this in minute proportions.

It may be remarked that all the foregoing descriptive material contains a lot of information, but nobody has put it together as a means of finding a cure or cures for cancer. We can make a suggestion. First, find a cure or cures, then study the minutiae of cause and cure ad infinitum.

Clearly, the alternative or nontraditional means of cancer therapy are still an imperative. And the use of selective enzyme inhibitors for cancer cell metabolism—i.e., anaerobic glycolysis—still remains a strong possibility, especially for cancers that have metastasized.

8.11.1 DHEA, ETC.

There is considerable renewed interest at this writing in the chemical compound called DHEA, the acronym for dehydroepiandrosterone. Described as a "superhormone," it is said to be among many other things an inhibitor for glucose-6-phosphate dehydrogenase (G6PDH), an enzyme involved in the *pentose phosphate pathway.* There is the further implication that this enzyme is involved in one way or another in cancer cell metabolism and that DHEA, by being an inhibitor for G6PDH, may therefore act as an anticancer agent.*

Accordingly, some of the announced effects or side effects of decreased levels of the enzyme glucose-6-phosphate dehydrogenase or G6PDH merit attention. Thus, *it has been noted that when seemingly harmless drugs such as antimalarial agents are administered to susceptible patients, a condition of acute hemolytic anemia may ensue* (Schwartz, in *Textbook of Biochemistry,* p. 408). *This may be presumed due to a genetic deficiency of G6PDH activity in the erythrocytes* (red blood corpuscles). This particular enzyme catalyzes the coupled oxidation of glucose 6-phosphate to 6-phosphogluconate, accompanied by the reduction of NADP to NADPH. This conversion is especially vital, because the pentose phosphate pathway is the only known route for the consumption of oxygen and the concomitant production of CO_2 in red blood cells. The reference notes some of the consequences, which include a deficiency in reduced glutathione, because glutathione in the reduced state has been found necessary to maintain the integrity of the erythrocytic membrane, and a deficiency makes the red cells more susceptible to hemolysis, which can be caused by a wide variety of compounds. (*Hemolysis,* as previously indicated, is the dissolution of red blood cells with the liberation of hemoglobin.) This enzymatic deficiency may remain undetected until the administration of certain drugs, illustrating the complexity of the situation.

As to the reduction of NADP to NADPH, the latter is necessary for biosynthesis and a number of reductive processes (Voet and Voet, *Biochemistry,* pp. 622–623). The reference also observes that a plentiful supply of reduced glutathione (designated GSH) is required for erythrocyte membrane integrity.†

The reference states that, among other things, the GSH in the erythrocyte serves to eliminate hydrogen peroxide (H_2O_2) and organic peroxides. Hydrogen peroxide is a toxic product from oxidative processes,

---

* DHEA and dehydroepiandrosterone are listed in the Sigma catalog, the former in the form of a standard solution for the calorimetric determination of 17-ketosteroids in urine, and the latter in the form of dehydroisoandrosterone. The last-mentioned has several other alternate chemical names: 5-androsten-3β-ol-17-1; trans-dehydroandrosterone; DHEA or dehydroepiandrostone (as previously mentioned); 3β-hydroxy-5-androsten-17-1; prasterone.

† *Reduced glutathione* is described as a Cys- or cysteine-containing *tripeptide,* and its formation from glutathione disulfide or GSSG is catalyzed by the enzyme glutathione reductase (Voet and Voet, *Biochemistry,* p. 400ff). Among other things, *flavins* are involved (flavins being substances containing what is called the isoalloxazine ring), as are *flavoproteins* (flavin-containing proteins). There is in turn a connection with such examples as *riboflavin* (vitamin B2). *Humans are unable to synthesize flavins, so they must be obtained from the diet—although riboflavin deficiency is said to be rare in humans.*

and it reacts with the double bonds of fatty acid residues in the erythrocyte cell membrane. The products are organic hydroperoxides, which in turn react with and cleave carbon-carbon bonds in the fatty acids, further damaging the membrane. The result of a buildup of peroxides is premature cell lysis (destruction).

It is noted that peroxides are eliminated by the action of glutathione peroxidase, one of only several enzymes that have a *selenium* cofactor. In the process, glutathione disulfide or GSSG is formed, the source for reduced glutathione or GSH.*

The foregoing reference further states *that populations of African, Asian, and Mediterranean countries may have a genetic defect that results in low levels of G6PDH, whereby the administration of certain drugs such as the antimalarial agent primaquine will cause severe hemolytic anemia.* Under most conditions, there are levels of the enzyme to sustain normal functions, but such agents as primaquine stimulate peroxide formation, increasing the demand for NADPH—a demand that cannot be met. It is observed, however, that the continued use of, say, primaquine will result in the generation of new blood cells that will have higher levels of the enzyme.

Howsoever, it may be advanced that *any agent such as DHEA that inhibits G6PDH over a sustained period must be treated as suspect.* The consequences could be severe anemia.

Moreover, if an agent such as DHEA does indeed act against cancer cells in the manner indicated, it can at the same time be regarded as *nonselective,* acting against normal cells as well. Lastly, DHEA would be one of the many potential substances or compounds that lie in the public domain, and consequently there is little or no financial incentive for its further investigation purely as an anticancer agent. There are other possibilities, however. For DHEA, along with the hormone melatonin, is sometimes touted as an *anti-aging agent.*

To the list of possibilities, or suspects, can be added what is known as *HGH,* an acronym for *human growth hormone.* Otherwise, it may be referred to simply as *GH,* for growth hormone, which is also called *somatotropin* and is a *polypeptide* (Voet and Voet, *Biochemistry,* pp. 845, 1263, 1271). The reference observes that both *human insulin* and *human growth hormone* are in routine clinical use on account of their ability to synthesize proteins, as in genetic engineering (Voet and Voet, *Biochemistry,* p. 906). Also involved is the growth hormone-releasing factor or *GRF,* a polypeptide with 44 residues that originates in the hypothalamus, and the growth hormone release-inhibiting factor or *GRIF,* a polypeptide with 14 residues, and also known as *somatostatin* (Voet and Voet, *Biochemistry,* p. 1271). The latter serves to stimulate/inhibit the release of growth hormone (GH) from the adenohypophysis, otherwise known as the pituitary gland (anterior lobe).

The Sigma catalog lists melatonin, somatotropin, and somatostatin. Melatonin, incidentally, has the stoichiometric formula $C_{13}H_{16}O_2N_2$ and the chemical name N-acetyl-5-methoxytryptamine, and may be obtained from the pineal gland of cattle. Somatotropin is derived from human pituitaries and also from porcine pituitaries. Somatostatin has the amino acid makeup Ala-Gly-Cys-Lys-Asn-Phe-Phe-Trp-Lys-Thr-Phe-Thr-Ser-Cys, with the disulfide bridge: 3-14. The Sigma catalog comments that somatostatin is reported to modulate physiological functions at such sites as the pituitary, pancreas, gut, and brain. It not only inhibits the release of growth hormone but that of insulin and glucagon as well.

The reference further states that GH stimulates generalized growth and directly accelerates the growth of a variety of tissues (Voet and Voet, *Biochemistry,* p. 1251). It also induces the liver to synthesize a series of specialized polypeptide growth factors called *somatomedins,* which act to stimulate cartilage growth and have *insulin-like* properties.

It may be commented, therefore, that these things considered, and noting the complexity of the problem, the enhancement of the amount of growth hormone GH from external sources conceivably could trigger the growth also of cancer cells. The supplemental use of still other hormones can similarly be questioned, although some authorities will provide positive statistics and others negative statistics. The trouble is, no definitive answers have yet surfaced in terms of the biochemistries that may be involved, and hormone therapy finds itself in the same situation as medical folklore.

Speaking further of *glutathione* and its reactions and cycles, it has been found to be *widely distributed in plants cells as well as animal cells* (Alfred Hausladen and Ruth G. Alscher, in *Antioxidants in Higher Plants,* p. 1ff). It is most usually in the form of *tripeptide glutathione,* which is a *sulfur-containing thiol compound,* hence the acronym *GSH.* It serves as an *antioxidant,* itself being oxidized in the process.

---

* *Selenium or its compounds*—although toxic at higher levels—are considered as *anticancer agents,* at least in some quarters (e.g., Moss, *Cancer Therapy,* pp. 109–114; Walters, *Options,* pp. 41–42).

There is the supposition that the biosynthesis of glutathione from its constituent amino acids may be involved in triggering oxidative stress responses and the altered gene expression that follows. There is in fact a direct correlation between stress response and induced nuclear gene expression. The synthesis of glutathione is hypothesized to cause the production of antioxidant enzymes.

An enzyme involved is dehydroascorbate reductase (DHAR), which catalyzes the cyclic conversion between reduced glutathione and dehydroascorbate, whereby the former is reoxidized to glutathione and the latter is reduced to form ascorbate, the active form. It is further mentioned that *glutathione* and *ascorbate* play an antioxidant role along with α-tocopherol or *vitamin E*. The inference, of course, is that of anticancer agents.

In the same volume, *it is further stated that plant tissues have high concentrations of L-ascorbic acid or vitamin C* (Christine H. Foyer, in *Antioxidants in Higher Plants*, p. 31ff). Although not clearly defined, *ascorbate apparently plays a significant role in the regulation of growth, differentiation, and metabolism in plants. This role may be projected to the control of cancer in humans,* aside from its antioxidant properties. The reference further observes that the enzyme glutathione peroxidase, important in hydrogen peroxide detoxification in animals, does not for the most part occur in plant tissues. It is further stated that *L-ascorbic acid is produced in plants by the metabolism of hexose*, e.g., glucose, and the pathway branches differently in plants than in animals. *(Humans are said not to be able to synthesize their own ascorbic acid.)* It is further stated that *ascorbate is necessary for the regeneration of* α-tocopherol *or vitamin E—at least in plants.*

Another chapter in the same volume is concerned with *carotenoids* (Kenneth E.Pallett and Andrew J. Young, in *Antioxidants in Higher Plants*, p. 59ff). Carotenoids are designated as C40 isoprenoids or tetraterpenes, and *are found in all green plant tissues,* located exclusively in the *chloroplast* (a plastid or subunit within the cellular body that contains chlorophyll). They are also responsible for the *yellow to red pigmentation* in some plant tissues such as of the roots, flowers, and fruit, where they occur in what are called the *chromoplasts*, or color-giving plastids. They serve not only as auxiliary light-harvesting pigments, but also as photoprotective agents. More significantly here, they are noted as important *antioxidants*, functioning in conjunction with other antioxidants such as superoxide dismutase and ascorbate. Presumably these effects can be extended to humans as well as plants.

Pathways for the biosynthesis of carotenoids are presented, which involve the formation of an intermediate compound called phytoene, which further converts to lycopene, β-carotene, and xanthophylls. The last-mentioned is discussed in another chapter in the volume, followed by chapters on vitamin E or α-tocopherol, and on plant phenolics. The implications is of anticancer activity, with the possible exception of phenolics, some of which have been previously discussed in Part 2 as potentially or overtly toxic.

There are in fact folkloric accounts of *cures from taking large amounts of fresh carrot juice.* Sources of hearsay and anecdote: the Inst. of Noetic Sciences (Sausalito, CA), The Health Resource (Conway AR), the Kushi Inst. (Beckett MA, and sponsored by NIH), and the Cornell-Oxford-China Study ("China Project").

8.12 OBJECTIVES, MILEPOSTS, AND ROADBLOCKS

The purpose of all the foregoing is of course to find a *nontoxic* cure for cancer, all cancers. In other words, it is to find a broad-spectrum, absolute cure. There may in fact be many such substances that are curative, a fact that will expectedly also depend upon dosage level and frequency.

At the same time, it is an attempt to bring order out of chaos, to provide an underlying theory and understanding about the way in which plant or herbal substances may act against cancer—and against other ailments, for that matter.

Acknowledgment should be made that conventional medicine continues its search for a further understanding of the mechanisms involved in the cancerous condition, and which hopefully will lead to a cure or cures. This work is embodied for instance in such presentations as the *Encyclopedia of Cancer*, edited by Joseph R. Bertino and published by Academic Press at the end of 1996. In three volumes, with 163 articles, it explores the causes, potential cures, and preventive measures. The American Cancer Society keeps track of things in *CA—A Cancer Journal for Clinicians*, published bimonthly, and which has been cited elsewhere in these pages. Another source is *The Cancer Dictionary* by Robert Altman and Michael J. Sarg, MD, which also supplies information in the appendices about support organizations, cancer centers, clinical trials and cooperative groups, and drugs used. Also of note is the *Cancer Sourcebook*, edited by Frank E. Bair. The massive *Cancer Medicine*, edited by James F. Holland et al., continues into a two-volume third edition. The *Handbook of Clinical Drug Data*, 6th ed., edited by James E. Knoben and Philip O. Anderson, has a section on antineoplastic agents. (To the foregoing may be added Ralph W. Moss's commentary in *Questioning Chemotherapy.*) These are but a few out of the many, some of which have been previously listed or referenced.

As to alternative medicine and its therapies or treatments—but not "cures"—in addition to Ralph Moss's *Cancer Therapy* and Richard Walters' *Options*, others of particular interest include *Alternatives in Cancer Therapy* by Ross Pelton and Lee Overholser, and Michael Lerner's *Choices in Healing*. Moss's latest book is *Herbs Against Cancer*. A more general volume that contains a section on cancer is *Alternative Medicine: The Definitive Guide*, published by Future Medicine Publishing, which also compiled the *Alternative Medicine Yellow Pages*. In turn, the same publisher issued *An Alternative Medicine Definitive Guide to CANCER*, to which a number of prominent medical practitioners contributed.

As to carcinogens per se, there is the comprehensive *CRC Handbook of Identified Carcinogens and Noncarcinogens*, in two volumes, edited by Jean V. Soderman and published in 1982. Another, by N. Irving Sax et al. is *Cancer Causing Chemicals*, published in 1981.

It must be emphasized, however, that the cancer victim literally can't wait until a consensus is reached about the best biochemical treatment(s) [read cure(s)]. If all the pieces of the puzzle were to fit, if everything were to be known beforehand, the waiting period would be interminable. Accordingly, the methods must be adaptable to the here and now, to find something the cancer victim can utilize *immediately*, but at the same time be safe from adverse side effects. Which, incidentally, is seldom the case with conventional cancer therapies. One has to look no farther than the track record for cytotoxic chemotherapy against solid cancers.

Expectedly, no treatments or treatments so found will be patentable, nor will the commonly recognized substances used be patentable. Only if these substances are further converted to other non-natural or synthetic substances can a patent or proprietary position be obtained, which is the domain of the pharmaceutical companies.

As to U.S. government agencies or institutions, it can be argued that it is their charter to find such treatments or cures, directly or indirectly, by their own research or by supporting others, on a *nonproprietary basis*. This should involve an emphasis on a more mission-oriented sort of program, with research for the sake of research relegated to secondary importance. Research should support the mission, not the other way around.

Viewed against the dearth of unequivocal positive results so far, and considering the ancillary role of the FDA, the indication is that cancer victims will have to continue doing their own inquiries, very probably at home, albeit helped by the family and hopefully counseled by a suitably interested and broad-minded physician. The previously described testing methods are of a simplicity that potentially can be pursued by an individual on his or her own initiative, or that of the family—which, in a way of looking at it, is the object of alternative medicine, anyway. This said, it is always better to work with a qualified professional, say a physician tuned-in to alternative medicine, complementary medicine, or holistic medicine, whichever it is to be called. For one thing, bioactive substances are generally toxic, there may be adverse side effects, and there may also be allergic reactions. Read on.

For the above-stated reasons it is recommended that there be the widespread establishment of *Cancer Clinical Research Centers,* or *CCRCs,* or their equivalent, either in existing or new facilities. Directed at patients with advanced or metastasized cancer, operations would be conducted on an outpatient basis whenever possible. The direct, professional supervision and operation of each such facility would be by MDs and DOs, with appropriate technical backup from a common pool of pharmacologists, biochemists, microbiologists or molecular biologists, botanists or ethnobotanists, herbalists or naturopaths, and so on.

Of prime importance is the further development of rapid and noninvasive indicators for the progression or regression of cancer. Some of the possibilities have been mentioned, such as alanine levels, and even insulin levels, and there are very likely many more. Even tests for the vital signs may be indicative. With the new electronic age, such testing can be indirect, and correlatable to whether the cancer is growing or receding. Thus, if the treatment is not working, another substance, method, or mode can be tried.

In the clinical testing of bioactive substances, many of which can be classed as toxic or poisonous, the dosage level and frequency are critical. In the use of medicinal plants or plant substances, it may be noted that the concentration and activity of the bioactive substance(s) may vary markedly with geography, climate, season, even time of day, and with the plant part—not to mention the possibility of substitutions, unintentional or otherwise. Hence, there is the advisability of using the pure chemical or phytochemical, when possible—or an appropriate synthetic derivative.

Predictably, patterns of success will emerge, establishing the most effective substance or substances and the dosage levels and frequency. Expectedly, however, there will be variation among individuals, the manifestation of biochemical individuality.

In dealing with bioactive substances, there is not only the possibility of such immediate adverse-effects as cardiac arrest and respiration failure and of longer-term effects such as against the liver and kidneys, but also the possibility of allergic reactions. In fact, it is sometimes difficult to distinguish between toxicity and allergy—and they may even be regarded the same. Whatever, there is always the very-serious possibility of anaphylactic shock or its equivalent, to be immediately countered by quick-acting antihistamines such as Benadryl® (diphenyhydramine hydrochloride) or epinephrine (adrenalin). This emergency has been previously observed, notably in Part 7 in the section on "Immunity" and subsection on "The Immune System."

Furthermore, since these are Cancer Clinical Research Centers, their operations come under the heading of *research*, and they should be funded by the government, the same as other medical research programs, with no cost to the individual patients.

The subject of the role and importance of diet waxes and wanes. In this regard, some informative and controversial citations from yesteryear are appropriate. Thus, speaking of vegetarian diets and that sort of thing, and as noted in Part 6 in the section on "All-Meat and All-Vegetarian Diets," Vilhjalmur Stefansson, the famous explorer and chronicler of the Canadian Arctic, observed that a strictly carnivorous diet would suffice if enough fat was present, as practiced for instance by the Eskimos. No vitamin C from fruit and vegetable sources is necessary. Alternatively, a mostly (or strictly) vegetarian diet of only fruits and vegetables will also suffice, as practiced by the Hunzas of Asia. Thus, a vegetarian diet in itself will prevent scurvy (Stefansson, *Fat*, p. 171)—a fact long noted. An omnivorous or mixed diet of meat along with fruit and vegetables apparently causes the trouble. In other words, the intestinal flora adjust to one or the other, but not to both.

Stefansson was against salted meats, however, which he considered a *prime cause of scurvy* or blackleg, as it was once called. Whereas fresh meat or air-cured meat is okay, but cooked as little as possible, and then preferably *boiled*. (As indicated in Part 7 within the section "Viruses and Degenerative Diseases," in the subsection on "Rhabdoviruses," and again in the section "Viruses in Animal Products," the Navajo Indians of the American Southwest boil their mutton for a long time, don't eat poultry products, and have had a very low natural cancer incidence.) Stefansson observes also that *a high-fat diet works in the tropics in the same way it does with the Eskimos. In fact, the Eskimos dress so warmly that it is like they are always in the tropics anyway, and the same goes for the temperature levels in their dwellings.* His findings are presented in *The Fat of the Land*, first published in 1946 as *Not by Bread Alone.*

The latter half of the book goes into great detail about *pemmican*. Pemmican was prepared—notably by the Plains Indians—by pounding dried meat and storing it in rawhide (parfleche). The meat may be mixed with berries (*berry pemmican*) or not (*plain pemmican*). The meat, however, in most cases is mixed with considerable proportions of heated, liquid *fat*, which cools and congeals, and apparently enhances storage time. Moreover, *the high fat content is presumed to be life giving and life sustaining.* The subject was (and is) controversial, and Stefansson presents some conflicting views in his concluding chapter.

Along these lines, it may be mentioned that, in the late 1950s and early 1960s, a book much publicized was titled *Calories Don't Count.* It emphasized fats in the diet—and for their trouble the authors were prosecuted and convicted, if memory serves, for fraud. The scene has shifted, however, and most any kind of diet can be promoted—at least as long as the author authors don't make too much money from its promotion and sales.

It can be added that there are animal fats and vegetable fats, and both nonhydrogenated and hydro-genated vegetable fats or oils. Whereas Stefansson was speaking mainly about animal fats, a high vegetable fat diet may be something else again. For instance, he repeats the canard that *cannibalism is caused by a desire for meat and its fat content.* (Another angle is that *cannibalism is mostly a cultural matter.*) Howsoever, in these same tropical countries there are plentiful vegetable fats or oils available—e.g., from the coconut palm, and from other assorted nut sources. Still other authorities will state that the fruit from the Saharan date palm is the only diet needed (incidentally, *dried dates are 50 percent sugar*), especially along with some goat or camel milk (Langewiesche, *Sahara Unveiled*, p. 119; Norwich, *Sahara*, pp. 26, 31).

In another book, *Cancer: Disease of Civilization?*, with an Introduction by René Dubos, Stefansson further describes his initial observations in the Canadian Arctic, beginning in 1906, before the onset of civilization among the more remote Eskimos. He found that these *primitive or stone-age Eskimos did not ever contract cancer on their all-meat diet*—nor tooth problems, either. He acknowledged the same, moreover, for the Hunzas for instance, who were primarily vegetarians, and for some other more primitive societies not touched by the food habits of Western Civilization.

It can be noted that there was at one time an upbeat enthusiasm about finding the cures for cancer and other diseases via the tropical rainforests. This was exemplified in Margaret B. Kreig's *Green Medicine: The Search for Plants that Heal...*, published in 1964. There are interesting and readable accounts about the progress then being made in utilizing tropical plants and substances against disease, including background medical folklore. In a chapter on cancer, the discovery and uses of the Vinca alkaloids are prominently described, along with Jonathan L. Hartwell's ongoing and exciting work at the National Cancer Institute. (Which subsequently faded into oblivion, circa 1981, as told by Jim Duke in the foreword to Hartwell's *Plants Used Against Cancer.*) What is most arresting, however, is that the situation has hardly changed. That is, no new earth-shaking discoveries or theories are making the news, in spite of the periodic hype, and, if anything, the bright promises have proven not so bright. In a way of looking at it, a lethargy has set in. There is a lot of work going on and a lot of scurrying around, with much money being spent, but the law of diminishing returns seems to have set in.

The major media contribute their fair share of optimism and pessimism, mostly regarding the status of research within mainstream medicine. For instance, as has been previously noted, the May 18, 1998 issue of *Time* contained a special report on "Curing Cancer—the Hype and the Hope." The May 18, 1998 issue of *Newsweek* featured articles announced on the cover with "The Hope—and the Hype—Behind the Latest Breakthroughs." Perhaps "breakthroughs" should have been put in its own quotes. Anyway, rundowns were provided on the latest events making the media rounds, for instance, that what works on mice doesn't necessarily work on people, and about how the stocks of a company can literally multiply in value based on a few news items. It seems like the same refrain with a different verse. The usual disclaimer is that it will take years of further research and testing before the cure, if it is that, becomes universally available. Meanwhile, the clock continues ticking, at the rate of one cancer death per minute.

And any such high-tech curative regimens, whenever they do become available, seem to go first to those who are privileged, high-profile, and/or wealthy. Whereas the objective of alternative medicine, it would seem, is more that the curative procedures should be of a simple and low-cost nature, and be available even for home use. That is, more as things used to be.

There are, however, at least some welcome signs of a turnaround in attitudes. For instance, the *American Institute for Cancer Research,* in Washington DC, is keeping an open mind toward new approaches for treatment read cure. For another instance, the *Denison Library at the University of Colorado Health Sciences Center,* in Denver, now maintains an Indigenous Medicine Collection. It even puts out a questionnaire asking for input about using books or journals from the collection, and about one's range of interests, e.g., self-medication using herbal remedies, scientific studies on herbal remedies, natural products, active components in herbal remedies, and/or commercialization of effective herbal remedies. The questionnaire further asks about involvement in research on *noncommercialized herbal components,* about what books or journals should be added to the collection, and whether one would like to join an "herbal interest group."

An article fairly typical of changing philosophies in cancer treatment appeared in the January/February, 1996 issue of *Natural Health*. Written by Nathaniel Mead, the article describes some promising results obtained with detoxification, dietary changes, and the use of nutritional supplements and herbs, plus, sometimes, the limited use of conventional treatments. (Although there is the thought that alternative treatments should be tried before instituting conventional treatments.) In particular, the experiences were highlighted of Keith I. Block, MD, who is medical director of the Cancer Care Treatment Program at

Edgewater Hospital in Chicago, which is affiliated with the University of Illinois Medical School. Interestingly, germanium (germanium sesquioxide) is mentioned, which is a known enzyme inhibitor for a certain step or steps in the (anaerobic) glycolysis sequence. Other possibilities are explored as well. Also highlighted are the experiences of Marika Von Viczay of the ISIS Health and Rejuvenation Center in Asheville NC, and of Michael Schachter, MD, of Suffern NY.

It is emphasized, however, that no one is claiming that the treatment regimens used constitute a "cure." The disclaimer is furnished that "None of these approaches is a certain cure for cancer; there is no such thing." In fact, it is observed that the evidence seems to vary markedly, with an overall lack of hard data on survival rates. Nevertheless, a spirit of optimism persists.

Among the basic regimens presented in the above article in a blocked-in insert are diet and supplements. The latter include nutrients, *botanicals, phytochemicals,* and enzymes. The comment is added that *these substances should be taken under a doctor's prescription and care* and be *monitored for toxicity,* especially if larger doses are taken. As to conventional treatments, the following statement is made. "Most alternative doctors have no problem with many surgeries (although some are unnecessary or ill-advised), while **many vehemenently oppose chemotherapy and radiation.**" (Boldface added for emphasis.)

Elsewhere on the same page of the article it is noted that, since 1971, a trillion dollars has been spent on cancer treatment during the then 25-year span of the War on Cancer. This averages out to $40 billion per year (although the current yearly rate is much higher, a projected $100 billion per year or more). This is followed by the statement that "Few new, effective treatments have been devised for the most common cancers," according to a recent editorial in *The Journal of the American Medical Association.*

A not so encouraging signal is that not only is knowledge about native medicines being irretrievably lost, but technical expertise as well. An essay by David Ehrenfeld titled "Vanishing Knowledge" appeared in the March 1996 issue of *Harper's.* (The essay was taken from "Forgetting," which was published in the December 1995 issue of *The Sun,* Chapel Hill NC, and which also appears in Ehrenfeld's *Beginning Again: People and Nature in the New Millennium,* published by the Oxford University Press.) Ehrenfeld, a professor of biology at Rutgers University, states that *our store of knowledge about the natural world is disappearing.* Not only are we losing the ability to distinguish one plant from another, but we are losing our know-how about how plants interact between species and with the environment. In fact, hardly anyone is left in the universities who can teach this sort of information. *The trend instead is toward more "modern" fields or the use of high-tech methodologies.* The subject of comparative biochemistry, for instance, has disappeared from view, and is even laughed at. As a more specific example, Ehrenfeld cites the taxonomy of earthworms, so vital for invigorating soils. But different species play different roles, and some foreign invaders are displacing native species with potentially disastrous consequences—but practically no one is still around who can tell one worm from another.

The pharmaceutical industry gets its share of criticism in Alex Shoumatoff's *The Rivers Amazon,* published in 1978. The past reluctance of drug companies to become involved in Amazonia can be attributed to the usual reasons (Shoumatoff, *The Rivers Amazon,* pp. 76–76). For one thing, there is the risk, since it takes a great investment to locate, collect, and test a plant that may not prove commercially valuable. For instance, a lack of commercial viability may be due to a limited market. An undercurrent in the business is that a drug company must remain secretive about its efforts—so there may be more going on than suspected. And according to estimates provided in Shoumatoff's book, although dated, there is still plenty of potential in Amazonia.

Another comment that has been made is that there is a lack of commercial incentive for the development of vaccines for tropical diseases (F.Y. Liew, in *Vaccination Strategies,* p. 9). This is in addition to the formidable technical problems. *The major tropical diseases* as listed by the World Health Organization are, for the record, *malaria, schistosomiasis, leprosy, Chagas' disease* (trypanosomiasis), *African trypanosomiasis, filariasis,* and *leishmaniasis.*

Too often, however, the situation remains as has been described by Barbara Griggs in her highly readable *Green Pharmacy.* First published in 1981, and republished in 1991, Griggs describes, for example, how an herbal medicine called Bio-Strath was ignored by the medical profession, in spite of its positive results against such diseases as cancer (Griggs, *Green Pharmacy,* p. 304ff). As to the herbal trade in general, there are these who would like to see it more organized and scientifically respectable, but find it otherwise—nor is it helped by the inaccuracies of the FDA and AMA (Griggs, *Green Pharmacy,*

p. 310ff). In pages about cancer, the idea is reinforced that *Western cancer therapy is largely unsuccessful, and that traditional or herbal medicine remains the best possibility—and in the meantime much native medicinal lore has already been lost* (Griggs, *Green Pharmacy*, p. 322ff). The more things change, the more they stay the same.

REFERENCES

Academic Press Dictionary of Science and Technology, Christopher Morris Ed., Academic Press, San Diego, 1992.

Ahmed, N., J.F. Williams, and M.J. Weidemann, "Glycolytic, Glutaminolytic and Pentose-Phosphate Pathways in Promyelocytic HL60 and DMSO-differentiated HL60 Cells," *Biochem. Mol. Biol.*, 29(6), 1055–1067 (April, 1993).

Aldrich Chemical Company, *1996–1997 Catalog/Handbook of Fine Chemicals*, Milwaukee WI and St. Louis MO.

Alternative Medicine: The Definitive Guide, Compiled by the Burton Goldberg Group, Future Medicine Publishing, Puyallup WA, 1993.

Alternative Medicine Yellow Pages: The Comprehensive Guide to the New World of Health, Melinda Bonk Ed., Future Medicine Publishing, Purallup WA, 1994.

An Alternative Medicine Definitive Guide to CANCER, Future Medicine Publishing, Puyallup WA, 1997.

Altman, Robert and Michael J. Sarg, MD, *The Cancer Dictionary*, Facts on File, New York, 1992.

Atlas, Ronald M., *Microbiology: Fundamentals and Applications*, 2nd Ed., Macmillan, New York, 1984, 1988.

Antioxidants in Higher Plants, Ruth G. Alscher and John L. Hess Eds., CRC Press, Boca Raton FL, 1993.

Bailey, L.H., *The Standard Cyclopedia of Horticulture*, in three volumes, Macmillan, New York, 1900, 1914, 1928, 1942, 1947. Also see *Hortus Third*.

Banik, Allen E. and Renée Taylor, *Hunza Land: The Fabulous Health and Youth Wonderland of the World*, Whiteside Publishing Company, Long Beach CA, 1960.

Block, Eric, "The Chemistry of Garlic and Onions," *Scientific American*," 252(3), 114–119 (March, 1985).

Block, Keith I., "Who Needs a Cancer Cure, a Mouse or a Man?," *Natural Health*, September-October 1998, pp. 94–99, 164.

Boericke, William, MD, *Pocket Manual of Homœopathic Materia Medica: Comprising the Characteristic and Guiding Symptoms of All Remedies [Clinical and Pathogenetic]*, 9th Ed., with the addition of a Repertory by Oscar E. Boericke, MD, Boericke and Tafel, Santa Rosa CA, 1901, 1903, 1906,..., 1927.

Boik, John C., *Cancer and Natural Medicine: A Textbook of Basic Science and Clinical Research*, Oregon Medical Press, Princeton MN, 1995.

Brady, John, *Bad Boy: The Life and Politics of Lee Atwater*, Addison-Wesley Longman, Reading MA, 1996.

Bratman, Steven, *The Alternative Medicine Sourebook: A Realistic Evaluation of Alternative Healing Methods*, Lowell Hoiuse, Los Angeles, 1997.

Brendler, T., J. Gruenwald, and C. Jaenicke, *Herbal Remedies*, CD issued by the American Botanical Council, Austin TX.

Brock, Thomas D. and Michael T. Madigan, *Biology of Microorganisms*, 6th Ed., Prentice Hall, Englewood Cliffs NJ, 1970, 1974, 1979, 1984, 1988, 1991.

Cancer: Principles and Practices of Oncology, 5th Ed., Vincent T. DeVita, Jr., Samuel Hellman, and Steven A. Rosenberg Eds., Lippincott, Philadelphia, 1982, 1985, 1989, 1993, 1997.

Cancer Medicine, 3rd Ed., James F. Holland, Emil Frei III, Robert C. Bast Jr., Donald W. Kufe, Donald L. Morton and Ralph R. Weichselbaum Eds., in two volumes, Lea & Febiger, Philadelphia, 1973 & 1974, 1982, 1993.

Cancer Sourcebook: Basic Information on Cancer Types, Symptoms, Diagnostic Methods, and Treatments, Including Statistics on Cancer Occurrences Worldwide and the Risks Associated With Known Carcinogens and Activities, Frank E. Bair Ed., Omnigraphics, Detroit MI, 1992.

Chevallier, Andrew, *The Encyclopedia of Medicinal Plants*, DK Publishing, New York, 1996.

Clark, John, *Hunza: Lost Kingdom of the Himalaya*, Funk & Wagnalls, New York, 1956.

Colborn, T., D. Dumanoski, and J.P. Myers, *Our Stolen Future*, Dutton, Penguin Books U.S.A., New York, 1996.

The Complete German Commission E Monograph, American Botanical Council, Austin TX, 1998.

Comprehensive Biological Catalysis: A Mechanistic Reference, in four volumes, Michael Sinnott Ed., Academic Press, San Diego, 1998.

Cordell, Geoffrey A., *Introduction to Alkaloids: A Biogenetic Approach*, Wiley, New York, 1981.

CRC Handbook of Identified Carcinogens and Noncarcinogens: Carcinogenicity—Mutagenicity Database, in two volumes, Jean V. Soderman Ed., CRC Press, Boca Raton FL, 1982. Volume I. Chemical Class File. Vol. II. Target Organ File.

Crellin, John K. and Jane Philpott, *Herbal Medicines Past and Present*. Vol. II. *A Reference Guide to Medicinal Plants*. Duke University Press, Durham NC, 1990.

Critser, Greg, "Oh, How Happy We Will Be: Pills, paradise, and the profits of the drug companies," *Harper's*, 292(1753), 39–53 (June, 1996).

Davis, Wade, *Passage of Darkness: The Ethnobiology of the Haitian Zombie*, University of North Carolina Press, Chapel Hill, 1988.

Davis, Wade, *The Serpent and the Rainbow: A Harvard Scientist Uncovers the Startling Truth about the Secret World of Haitian Voodo and Zombis*, Simon and Schuster, New York, 1985. Warner Books, New York, 1987.

Dictionary of Plant Toxins, Heffrey B. Harborne, and Herbert Baxter Eds., Gerard P. Moss Asst. Ed., Wiley, Chichester, West Suffix, England, 1996.

Dixit, A., N.Z. Baqwe, and A.R. Rao, "Inhibition of Key Enzymes of Carbohydrate Metabolism in Regenerating Mouse Liver by Ascorbic Acid," *Biochem. Int.*, *26*(1) 143–151 (February, 1992).

Duke, James A., *The Green Pharmacy: New Discoveries in Herbal Remedies for Common Diseases and Conditions from the World's Foremost Authority on Healing Herbs*, Rodale Press, Emmaus PA, 1997.

Duke, James A., *Handbook of Biologically Active Phytochemicals and Their Activities*, CRC Press, Boca Raton FL, 1992.

Duke, James A., *Handbook of Phytochemical Constituents of GRAS Herbs and Other Economic Plants*, CRC Press, Boca Raton FL, 1992.

Dunham, J., S. Hoedt-Schmidt, and D.A. Kalbhen, "Structural and Metabolic Changes in Articular Cartilage Induced by Iodoacetate," *Int. J. Exp. Pathol.*, *73*(4), 455–464 (August, 1992).

Duong, see Van Duong.

Ehrenfeld, David, "Vanishing Knowledge," *Harper's*, *292*(1750), 15–17 (March, 1996).

Eigenbrodt, E., P. Fister, and M. Reinacher, "New Perspectives on Carbohydrate Metabolism in Tumor Cells," in *Regulation of Carbohydrate Metabolism*, Vol. II, Rivka Beitner Ed., CRC Press, Boca Raton FL, 1985, pp. 141–179.

Encyclopedia of Cancer, in three volumes, Joseph R. Bertino Ed., Academic Press, San Diego CA, 1996.

Enzyme Handbook, in 10 volumes, D. Schomburg and M. Salzmann Eds., Gesellschaft fhr Biotechnologische Forschung (GBF). Published by Springer-Verlag, Berlin, 1990–1995.

Enzyme Nomenclature 1978: Recommendations of the Nomenclature Committee of the International Union of Biochemistry on the Nomenclature and Classification of Enzymes, Academic Press, New York, 1979.

Felmy, Sabine, *The Voice of the Nightingale: A Personal Account of the Wakhi Culture in Hunza*, Oxford University Press, Oxford, England, 1996.

FitzGerald, R.J., S. Doonan, L.L. McKay, and T.M. Cogan, "Intracellular pH and the Role of D-Lactate Dehydrogenase in the Production of Metabolic End Products by *Leuconostoc lactis*," *J. Dairy Res.*, *59*(3), 359–367 (August, 1992).

Foulkes, Richard G., MD., "The Fluoride Connection," *Townsend Letter for Doctors & Patients*, #177, 12–16 (April, 1998).

Fulder, Stephen, *The Garlic Book: Nature's Powerful Healer*, Avery Publishing Group, Garden City Park NY, 1997

Garlic: The Science and Therapeutic Applications of Allium sativum L. and Related Species, 2nd Ed., Heinrich P. Koch and Larry D. Lawson Eds., Williams & Wilkins, Baltimore MD, 1988, 1996. See ACS Symposium Series 691.

Golshani, S., "Insulin, Growth Factors, and Cancer Cell Energy Metabolism: An Hypothesis of Oncogene Action," *Biochem. Med. Metab. Biol.*, *47*(2), 108–115 (April, 1992).

Griffiths, M., D. Keast, G. Patrick, M. Crawford, and T.N. Palmer, "The Role of Glutamine and Glucose Analogues in Metabolic Inhibition of Human Myeloid Leukemia In Vitro," *Int. J. Biochem.*, *25*(12), 1749–1755 (December, 1993).

Griggs, Barbara, *Green Pharmacy: A History of Herbal Medicine*, Viking, New York, 1981. Republished as *Green Pharmacy: The History and Evolution of Western Herbal Medicine*, Healing Arts Press, Rochester VT, 1991.

Grzimak's Animal Life Encyclopedia, in 13 volumes, Bernhard Grzimak, Editor-in-Chief, Van Nostrand Reinhold, New York, 1968, 1972–1972, 1975.

Guerra, Romera L., J.H. Tureen, M.A. Fournier, V. Makrides, and M.G. Tuber, "Amino Acids in Cerebrospinal and Brain Interstitial Fluid in Experimental Pneumococcal Meningitis," *Pediatr. Res.*, *33*(5), 510–513 (May, 1993).

Hager, Hermann et al., *Hager's Handbuch of Pharmazeutischen Praxis: fur Apotheker, Arzneimittelhersteller, Drogesten, Arzte unf Medizinalbeamte*, J. Springer, Springer-Verlag, Berlin, 1900, 1908, 1910, 1920, 1925, 1930, 1949, 1958, 1967, 1973, 1977, 1990.

Hall, Stephen S., *A Commotion in the Blood: Life, Death, and the Immune System*, Holt, New York, 1997.

Hall, Stephen S., "Vaccinating Against Cancer," *Atlantic Monthly*, *279*(4), 66–84 (April, 1997).

Hamilton, E., M. Fennell, and D.M. Stafford, "Modification of Tumour Glucose Metabolism for Therapeutic Benefit," *Acta Oncol.*, *34*(3), 429–433 (1995).

Handbook of Clinical Drug Data, 6th Ed., James E. Knoben, and Philip O. Anderson Eds., Larry J. Davis, and William G. Troutman, Asst. Eds., Drug Intelligence Publications, Hamilton IL, 1988.

Handbook of Identified Carcinogens and Noncarcinogens, see *CRC Handbook of Identified Carcinogens and Noncarcinogens*

Handbook of Microbiology, see *CRC Handbook of Microbiology*.

Handbook of Vitamins, 2nd Ed., Revised and Expanded, Lawrence J. Machlin, Ed., Marcel Dekker, New York, 1991.

Haouz, A., A. Gelosa-Meyer, and C. Burstein, "Assay of Dehydrogenases with an O_2-Consuming Biosensor," *Enzyme Microb. Technol.*, *16*(4), 292–297 (April, 1994).

Hartwell, Jonathan L., *Plants Used Against Cancer*, Quarterman Publications, Lawrence MA, 1982. Foreword by Jim Duke.

Heinerman, John, *The Healing Benefits of Garlic: From Pharoahs to Pharmacists*, Keats, New Canaan CT, 1994.

Hicks, Sam, *Desert Plants and People*, Naylor, San Antonio, 1966. Foreword by Erle Stanley Gardner.

Hoffman, E.J., "Enzyme Inhibitors for Cancer Cell Metabolism," *Townsend Letter for Doctors & Patients*, #166, 58–66 (May, 1997).

Holm, E., E. Hagmuller, U. Staedt, G. Schlickeiser, H.J. Gunther, H. Leweling, M. Tokus, and H.B. Kollmer, "Substrate Balances across Colonic Carcinomas in Humans," *Cancer Res.*, *55*(6), 1373–1378 (March 15, 1995).

Holmes, L.D., M.R. Schiller, and E.A. Boeker, "Kinetic Analysis of Lactate Dehydrogenase Using Integrated Rate Equations," *Experientia*, *49*(10), 893–901 (October 15, 1993).

Hortus Third: A Concise Dictionary of Plants Cultivated in the United States and Canada, Initially Compiled by Liberty Hyde Bailey and Ethel Zoe Bailey, Revised and Expanded by the Staff of the Liberty Hyde Bailey Hortorium at Cornell University, Macmillan, New York, 1976. Also see Bailey, L.H.

Huang, Kee Chang, *The Pharmacology of Chinese Herbs*, CRC Press, Boca Raton FL, 1993.

Hugo, F., S. Mazurek, U. Zander, and E. Eigenbrodt, "In Vitro Effect of Extracellular AMP on MCF-7 Breast Cancer Cells: Inhibition of Glycolysis and Cell Proliferation," *J. Cell Physiol.*, *153*(3), 539–549 (December, 1992).

Ike, J., P. Sangan, and M. Gunasekaran, "Purification and Properties of Lactate Dehydrogenase from *Nocordia asteroides*," *Microbios.*, *69*(279), 119–127 (1992).

Ikeda, T., T. Kurita-Ochiae, T. Takizawa, and M. Hirasawa, "Isolation and Characterization of the Substance Isolated from *Streptosporangium* Species Which Inhibits Lactic Acid Production by Oral Bacteria," *Gen. Pharmacol.*, *24*(4), 905–910 (July, 1993).

Iwu, Maurice M., *Handbook of African Medicinal Plants*, CRC Press, Boca Raton FL, 1993.

Jain, Mahenda Kumar, *Handbook of Enzyme Inhibitors (1965–1977)*, Wiley, New York, 1982.

Jurkowitz-Alexander, M.S., R.A. Altschuld, S.E. Haun, R.E. Stephens and L.A. Horrocks, "Protection of ROC-1 Hybrid Glial Cells by Polyethylene Glycol Following ATP Depletion," *J. Neurochem.*, *61*(4), 1581–1584 (October, 1993).

Kealey, T., R. Williams, and M.P. Philpott, "The human hair follicle engages in glutaminolysis and aerobic glycolysis: implications for skin, splanchnic and neoplastic metabolism," *Skin Pharmacol.*, *7*(1–2), 41–46 (1994).

Kliachko, O.S., E.S. Polosukhina, and N.D. Ozerniuk, "Temperature Causes Structural and Functional Changes in Lactate Dehydrogenase from Fish Skeletal Muscles," *Biofizika*, *38*(4), 596–601 (July/August, 1993).

Kochhar, S., P.E. Hunziker, P. Leong-Morganthaler, and H. Hottinger, "Primary Structure, Physicochemical Properties, and Chemical Modification of NAD(+)-Dependent Dlactate Dehydrogenase. Evidence for the Presence of Arg-235, His-303, Tyr-101, and Trp-19 at or Near the Active Site," *J. Biol. Chem.*, *267*(12), 8499–8513 (April 25, 1992).

Kraus, J.L., P. Faury, A.S. Charvet, and M. Camplo, "Tetrazole Isosteres of Biologically Active Acids and Their Effects on Enzymes," *Res. Commun. Pathol. Pharmacol.*, *83*(2), 209–222 (February, 1994).

Kreig, Margaret B., *Green Medicine: The Search for Plants that Heal...*, Rand MacNally, Chicago, 1964.

Lamm, Donald L. and Frank M. Torti, "Bladder Cancer, 1996," *CA—A Cancer Journal for Clinicians*, *46*(2), 93–112 (March/April, 1996).

Langewiesche, William, *Sahara Unveiled: A Journey Across the Desert*, Pantheon, New York, 1996.

Lerner, Michael, *Choices in Healing: The Best of Conventional and Complementary Approaches to Cancer*, MIT Press, Cambridge MA, 1994, 1996.

Louschak, see Lushchak.

Lupulescu, Aurel, *Hormones and Carcinogenesis*, Praeger, New York, 1983.

Lupulescu, A., "Ultrastructure and Cell Surface Studies of Cancer Cells Following Vitamin C Administration," *Exp. Toxicol. Pathol.*, *44*(1), 3–9 (March, 1992).

Lushchak, V.I., "Free and Membrane-Bound Lactate Dehydrogenase from White Driving Muscles of Skate," *Biochem. Int.*, *26*(5), 905–912 (April, 1992).

Lushchak, V.I. and L.P. Lushchak, "The Effect of Urea on the Activity of Lactate Dehydrogenase from the Muscles of Swine and Skates," *Zh. Evol. Biokhim. Fiziol.*, *30*(2), 185–191 (March/April, 1994).

Lynn, Cari, "To Save My Life," *Health* 12(6), 112–115, 139–143 (September 1998).

Mallis, Andrew, with contributing editors, *Handbook of Pest Control: The Behavior, Life History, and Control of Household Pests*, Franzak & Foster, Cleveland OH, in seven editions, 1945–1990, e.g., the 6th Ed., 1982.

Marmillot, P., T. Keith, D.K. Srivastava, and H.R. Knull, "Effect of Tubulin on the Activity of the Muscle Isoenzyme of Lactate Dehydrogenase," *Arch. Biochem. Biophys.*, *315*(2), 467–472 (December, 1994).

Mead, Nathaniel, "Breakthroughs in Cancer Research," *Natural Health*, *26*(1), 82ff. (January/February, 1996).

Meijer, J.J. and J.P. van Dijken,"Effects of Glucose Supply on Myeloma Growth and Metabolism in Chemostat Culture," *J. Cell Physiol.*, *162*(2), 191–198 (February, 1995).

Methods in Enzymology, edited by Sidney P. Colwick and Nathan O. Kaplan et al., multivolume continuing set, Academic Press, Orlando FL.

Moat, Albert G. and John W. Foster, *Microbial Physiology*, 2nd Ed., Wiley-Interscience, New York, 1979, 1988.

Moss, Ralph W., *Cancer Therapy: The Independent Consumer's Guide To Non-Toxic Treatment & Prevention*, Equinox Press, New York, 1992.

Moss, Ralph W., *Questioning Chemotherapy*, Equinox Press, Brooklyn NY, 1995.

Nabhan, Gary Paul, *The Desert Smells Like Rain*, North Point, San Francisco, 1981.

Nabhan, Gary Paul, *Gathering the Desert*, University of Arizona Press, Tucson, 1985.

Nelson, S.R., T.L. Pazdernik, and F.E. Samson, "Copper plus Ascorbate Inactivates Lactate Dehydrogenase: Are Oxygen Radicals Involved?," *Proc. West. Pharmacol. Soc.*, *35*, 37–41 (1992).

Nissler, K., H. Petermann, I. Wenz, and D. Brox, "Fructose 2,6-Bisphosphate Metabolism in Ehrlich Ascites Tumour Cells," *J. Cancer Res. Clin. Oncol.*, *121*(12), 739–745 (1995).

Norwich, John Julius, *Sahara*, Weybright and Talley, New York, 1968.

Null, Gary, Howard Robbins, Mark Tanenbaum, and Patrick Jennings, "Vitamin C in the Treatment of Cancer: Part I. Abstracts and Commentary from the Scientific Literature," *Townsend Letter for Doctors & Patients*, #166, 74–76 (May, 1997). Part II to follow.

Nussbaum, Elaine, *Recovery from Cancer: A Personal Story of Sickness and Health*, Avery Publishing Group, Garden City Park NY, 1997.

Ohshita, T. and H. Kido, "Involvement of a Cystatin-alpha-Sensitive Cysteine Proteinase in the Degradation of Native L-Lactate Dehydrogenase and Serum Albumin by Rat Liver or Kidney Lysosomes," *Eur. J. Biochem.*, 225(3), 781–786 (November 1, 1994).

Onigbinde, T.A., A.H. Wu, Y.S. Yu, M.J. Simmons, and S.S. Wong, "Mechanism of Differential Inhibition of Lactate Dehydrogenase Isoenzymes in the BMC LD-1 Assay," *Clin. Biochem.*, 25(6), 425–429 (December, 1992).

Payne, Anthony G., "Achieving Oncolysis by Compromising Tumor Cell Metabolic Processes," *Townsend Letter for Doctors & Patients*, #161, 54–57 (December, 1996).

Pelton, Ross, with Lee Overholser, *Alternatives in Cancer Therapy: The Complete Guide to Non-Traditional Treatments*, A Fireside Book, Simon & Schuster, New York, 1994.

Petch, D. and M. Butler, "Profile of Energy Metabolism in a Murine Hybridoma: Glucose and Glutamine Utilization," *J. Cell Physiol.*, 161(1), 71–76 (October, 1994).

Plotkin, David, MD, "Good News and Bad News About Breast Cancer," *Atlantic Monthly*, 277(6), 53–82 (June, 1996).

"Proposal of Standard Methods for the Determination of Enzyme Catalytic Concentrations in Serum and Plasma at 37 Degrees C. III. Glutamate Dehydrogenase (L-Glutamate: NAD(P)$^+$ Oxidoreductase (deaminating), EC 1.4.1.3., by Working Group on Enzymes, *Eur. J. Clin. Biochem.*, 330(8), 493–502 (August, 1992).

The Regulation of Carbohydrate Formation and Utilization in Mammals, Carlo M. Veneziale Ed., University Park Press, Baltimore MD, 1981. Papers from a symposium held at the Mayo Medical School, Rochester MN, July 9–11, 1981.

Regulation of Carbohydrate Metabolism, in two volumes, Rivka Beitner Ed., CRC Press, Boca Raton FL, 1985.

Rosa, L.F., A.F. de Almeida, D.A. Safi, and R. Curi, "Metabolic and Functional Changes in Lymphocytes and Macrophages as Induced by Ageing," *Physiol. Behav.*, 53(4), 651–656 (April, 1993).

Rosa, L.F., Y. Cury, and R. Curi, "Effects of Insulin, Glucocorticoids and Thyroid Hormones on the Activities of Key Enzymes of Glycolysis, Glutaminolysis, the Pentose-Phosphate Pathway and the Krebs Cycle in Rat Macrophages," *J. Endocrinol.*, 135(2), 213–219 (November, 1992).

Rosa, L.F., A.F. de Almeida, D.A. Safi, and R. Curi, "Thioglycollate stimulus modifies lymphocyte metabolism and proliferation. A comparison with lymphocyte activation by Walker 256 tumour implantation," *Cell Biochem. Funct.*, 11(4), 251–255 (December, 1993).

Rosenberg, Steven A. and John M. Barry, *The Transformed Cell: Unlocking the Mysteries of Cancer*, Putnam, New York, 1992. Avon, New York, 1993.

Roueché, Berton, *The Medical Detectives*, Washington Square Press, Pocket Books, Simon & Schuster, New York, 1980. Published also by Truman Talley Books/ E.P. Dutton, New York, and Times Books, a division of Quadrangle/New York Times Book Co., New York

Sargent, Charles Sprague, *Manual of the Trees of North America*, in two volumes, Houghton Mifflin, Boston, 1905, 1922, 1949. Dover, New York, 1961.

Sax, N. Irving, assisted by Elizabeth K. Weisburger, David Schottenfeld, Joanna Haas, Benjamin Feiner, Barry I. Castleman, and Richard J. Lewis Sr., *Cancer Causing Chemicals*, Van Nostrand Reinhold, New York, 1981.

Schaller, George B., *Stones of Silence: Journeys in the Himalaya*, Viking, New York, 1979, 1980.

Schom, Alan, *Napoleon Bonaparte*, HarperCollins, New York, 1997.

Sharma, V. and P.O. Schwille, "Oxylate Production from Glyoxylate by Lactate Dehydrogenase *in vitro*: Inhibition by Reduced Glutathione, Cysteine, Cystamine," *Biochem. Int.*, 27(3), 431–438 (July, 1992).

Sharma, V. and P.O. Schwille, "Sulfite Inhibits Oxalate Production from Glycolate and Glyoxylate *in vitro* and from Dichloroacetate Infused I.V. into Male Rats," *Biochem. Med. Metab. Biol.*, 49(2), 265–269 (April, 1993).

Shirahase, Y., Y. Watazu, N. Kaneda, Y. Uji, H. Okabe and A. Karmen, "Specific Assay of Serum Lactate Dehydrogenase Isoenzyme 1 by Proteolysis with alpha-Chymotrypsin and Protein Denaturation," *Clin. Chem.*, 38(11), 2193–2196 (November, 1992).

Shoumatoff, Alex, *The Rivers Amazon*, Sierra Club Books, San Francisco, 1978.

Sidky, H., *Hunza: An Ethnographic Outline*, Illustrated Book Publishers, Jaipur, India, 1995.

Sigma Chemical Company Catalog, *Biochemicals, Organic Compounds, and Diagnostic Reagents*, St. Louis MO, 1996–.

Smolenski, O., Z. Tabarowski, H. Miszta, and Z. Dabrowski, "Effect of Haemodialysate and Its Peptide Fractions on Lactate Dehydrogenase Activity in Erythrocytes from Healthy Subjects and Patients with End-Stage Renal Disease," *Int. Urol. Nephrol.*, 24(6), 673–678 (1992).

Solzhenitsyn, Alexander, *Cancer Ward*, Farrar, Straus and Giroux, New York, pp. 228–233).

St. George, George and the editors of Time-Life Books, *Soviet Deserts and Mountains*, Time-Life Books, Amsterdam, 1974.

Stark, J.A. and A.R. Henderson, "In Vitro Effect of Elastase and Cathepsin G from Human Neutrophils on Creatine Kinase and Lactate Dehydrogenase Isoenzymes," *Clin. Chem.*, 39(6), 986–992 (June, 1993).

Stefansson, Vilhjalmur, *Cancer: Disease of Civilization?: An Anthropological and Historical Study*, Hill and Wang, New York, 1960. Introduction by René Dubos.

Stefensson, Vilhjalmur, *The Fat of the Land*, Macmillan, New York, 1956. With Comment by Frederick J. Stare, MD, and Paul Dudley White, MD Enlarged edition of *Not By Bread Alone*, Macmillan, New York, 1946.

Stephens, Ian, *Horned Moon: An account of a Journey through Pakistan, Kashmir, and Afghanistan*, Indiana University Press, Bloomington, 1955.

Swan, Michael, *The Marches of El Dorado: British Guiana, Brazil, Venezuela*, Beacon Press, Beacon Hill, Boston, 1958.

Taguchi, H. and M. Yoshida, "Chaperonin from *Thermus thermophilus* Can Protect Several Enzymes from Irreversible Heat Denaturation by Capturing Denaturation Intermediate," *J. Biol. Chem.*, 268(8), 5371–5375 (March 15, 1993).

Textbook of Biochemistry with Clinical Correlations, Thomas M. Devlin Ed., Wiley, New York, 1982.

Tortora, Gerard J., Berdell R. Funke, and Christine L. Case, *Microbiology: An Introduction*, 2nd Ed., Benjamin/Cummings, Menlo Park CA, 1982, 1986.

Trefil, James, "Risk, Part 2: Safeguarding our cells," or "How the body defends itself from the risky business of living," *Smithsonian*, 26(9), 42–49 (December, 1995).

Tropical and Geograpical Medicine, 2nd Ed., Kenneth S. Warren and Adel A.F. Mahmoud Eds., McGraw-Hill, New York, 1984, 1990. Associate Editors: David A. Warrell, Louis H. Miller, Adel A.F. Mahmoud, Scott B. Halstead, Charles C. Carpenter, John E. Bennett, Gerald T. Keusch.

Tropical and Geographical Medicine: Companion Handbook, 2nd Ed., Adel A.F. Mahmoud Ed., McGraw-Hill, New York, 1993.

Tunáel, G., M.J.R. Nout, L. Brimer, and D. Göktan, "Toxicological, nutritional and microbiological evaluation of tempe fermentation with *Rhizopus oligosporus* of bitter and sweet apricot seeds," *International Journal of Food Microbiology*, 11, 337–344 (1990).

Tyler, Varro E., *Herbs of Choice: The Therapeutic Use of Phytomedicinals*, Pharmaceutical Products Press, New York, 1994.

Tyler, Varro E., *The Honest Herbal: A Sensible Guide to the Use of Herbs and Related Remedies*, 3rd Ed., Pharmaceutical Products Press, New York, 1992. Haworth Pess, Binghamton NY, 1993. Revised edition of *The New Honest Herbal*.

Vaccination Strategies of Tropical Diseases, F.Y. Liew Ed., CRC Press, Boca Raton FL, 1989.

Van Duong, Nguyen, *Medicinal Plants of Vietnam, Cambodia and Laos*, published by N. Van Duong, 938 26th St., Santa Monica CA 90403, (310) 828-6649, 1993.

Vitamins and Minerals in the Prevention and Treatment of Cancer, Maryce M. Jacobs Ed., CRC Press, Boca Raton FL, 1991.

Voelter, Wolfgang and Erich Schmid-Siegmann, *Peptides: Syntheses—Physical Data*, in 6 volumes, Georg Thieme Verlag, Stuttgart, 1983, Addison-Wesley, Reading MA, 1983. Vol. 1. Amino Acids. Vol. 2. Dipeptides and Amino Acids. Vol. 3. Tripeptides and Fragments. Vol. 4. Tetrapeptides and Fragments. Vol. 5. Oligopeptides and Fragments. Vol. 6. Subject Index.

Voet, Donald and Judith G. Voet, *Biochemistry*, 2nd Ed., Wiley, New York, 1995.

Walker, Morton, "Medical Journalist Report of Innovative Biologies," *Townsend Letter for Doctors & Patients*, #172, 58–64 (November, 1997).

Walters, Richard, *Options: The Alternative Cancer Therapy Book*, Avery Publishing Group, Garden City Park NY, 1993.

Watazu, Y., K. Nagamatsu, Y. Shirahase, N. Kaneda, S. Murao, and H. Okabe, "Isolation and Characterization of a Serine Proteinase, Inactivating m-Subunit of Lactate Dehydrogenase, from *Penicillium citrinum* KE-1," *Biosc. Biotechnol. Biochem.*, 58(4), 745–751 (April, 1994).

Watt, John Mitchell and Maria Gerdina Breyer-Brandwijk, *The Medicinal and Poisonous Plants of Southern and Eastern Africa: Being an Account of Their Medicinal and Other Uses, Chemical Composition, Pharmacological Effects and Toxicology in Man and Animal*, E.&S. Livingstone, Edinburgh and London, 1962.

Werbach, Melvyn, *Healing Trough Nutrition: A Natural Approach to Treating 50 Common Illnesses with Diet and Nutrients*, HarperCollins, New York, 1993.

Williams, Joseph J., *Voodoos and Obeahs: Phases of West Indian Witchcraft*, AMS Press, New York, 1970. Dial Press, New York, 1932.

Williams, R., M.P. Philpott, and T. Kealey, "Metabolism of Freshly Isolated Human Hair Follicles Capable of Hair Elongation: A Glutaminolytic, Aerobic Glycolytic Tissue," *J. Invest. Dermatol.*, 100(6), 834–840 (June, 1993).

Yamashiro, A., T. Oita, K. Hosomi, H. Sakurai, S. Kasakura, Y. Nishimura, and M. Nukina, "Studies on a Serum Factor Inhibiting Lactate Dehydrogenase (LDH) Activity in a Patient's Serum," *Rinsho. Byori.*, 40(9), 970–976 (September, 1992).

York, J. Lyndal, "Enzymes," in *Textbook of Biochemistry: With Clinical Correlations*, Thomas M. Devlin Ed., Wiley, New York, 1982.

Zollner, Helmward, *Handbook of Enzyme Inhibitors*, VCH Verlagsgellschaft mbH. Weinheim, FRG, 1989. VCH Publishers, New York.

Zollner, Helmward, *Handbook of Enzyme Inhibitors*, 2nd Ed., revised and enlarged, in two volumes, VCH Verlagsgellschaft mbH. Weinheim, FRG, 1993. VCH Publishers, New York.

Appendices

Enzymes and Inhibitors for Glycolyis, Lactate Formation, and Glutaminolysis*

Table A.1a Hexokinase or Hexosekinase

*n-Acetylglucosamine ; Adenosine-P3-glucose; Adenosine-P4-glucose; Adenosine-5'-diphosphate; Adenosine-5'-phosphate; Adenosine-5'-phosphohypophosphate; Adenosine-5'-triphosphate; **Allose**-6-phosphate; **Chromium**-ATP complex; **Copper** (Cu⁺⁺); *Cystamine, L-; ***Disulfides**; *5,5'-Dithio-Bis(2-Nitrobenzoic acid); Glucitol-6-Phosphate, 1,5-anhydro-; Glucosamine, D-; Glucosamine, n-acetyl-; Glucosamine, n-acetyl-D-; **Glucose**-1,6-diphosphate, A-; Glucose-1,6-diphosphate, A-D-; **Glucose**-6-phosphate; ***Glucose** 6-phosphate; Glucose-6-phosphate, D-; Glucose-6-phosphate, A-D-; Glucose, deoxy-; Glucose, 2-deoxy-D; Glucose, 5-thio-D; Glucose, 6-deoxy-D; *Glutathione oxidized; Glycerate, 2, 3-diphospho-; Glyceric acid, 2,3-diphospho-; Glyceric acid, 3-phospho-; **Glycerol**; Inosine-5'-triphosphate; ***Lauric acid**; **Lyxose**, D-; **Magnesium (Mg⁺⁺)**; ***Mg⁺⁺**; ***MgATP**; **Mannoheptulose**, D-; Mannoheptulose, 1-deoxy-D; **Mannose**; **Mannose**-6-phosphate; ***Myristic acid**; **Nucleotides**; *Protein inhibitor dependent on Fructose 2,6-bisphosphate; Sorbitan-6-phosphate, 1,5-; **Sorbose**-1-phosphate; Sorbose-1-phosphate, L-; Tartronic acid, 2-phospho-; Tetraiodofluorescein; **Xylose**, D-.

Table A.1b 6-Phosphofructokinase or Phosphofructokinase Inhibitors

Adenosine-5'-diphosphate; Adenosine-5'-triphosphate; Aniline naphthalene sulfonic acid, 8; Arabinose-5-phosphate, D-; *Arginine phosphate; **Caffeine** (coffee enema); ***Calcium (Ca⁺⁺)**; **Citric Acid**; **Creatine** phosphate; **Ethanol**; **Fructose** diphosphate; Fructose-1,6-diphosphate; *Fructose 2,6-disphosphate; Fructose-6-phosphate, 1-deoxy-; Fructose, 1-deoxy-; Glucitol-6-phosphate; **Glucose**-6-phosphate; **Glucose**-6-phosphate, 2,5-anhydro-; *Glutathione oxidized; Glyceric acid, 2.3-diphospho-; Glyceric acid, 3-phospho-; **Glycerol**-2,3-diphosphate; Glycerol-3-phosphate; Glycolic acid, 2-phospho-; Guanosine-3',5'-phosphate; Inosine-5'-diphosphate; **Lauric acid**; **NADH**; **Oleic acid**; **Phosphoenolpyruvate** (PEP); **Pyridoxal**-5-phosphate; **Pyrophosphate** ion; **Pyruvic acid, phosphoenol-**.

Table A.1c Pyruvate Kinase Inhibitors

Adenosine-5'-triphosphate; Adenosine, 5'-P-fluorosulfonylbenzoy; **Alanine**; **Alanine, L-**; ***Alanine, L-**; **Amino acids**; ***AMP**; **Anions**; ***ATP**; Butyric acid, phosphoenol-A-keto-; **Calcium (Ca⁺⁺)**; ***Calcium (Ca⁺⁺)**; Carbamyl phosphate; Coenzyme A, succinyl-; **Creatine** phosphate; **Diethylstilbesterol (DES)**; **Fatty acids**; ***Fatty acids**; *Glutathione oxidized; Glyceric acid, 2-phospho-; Glyceric acid, 2,3-diphospho-; **Lithium (Li⁺)**; **Phenylalanine**; **Phenylalanine, L-**; ***Phenylalanine, L-**; Phenylalanine, P-chloro-DL-; Phenylbiguanides; ***Phosphate**; Phosphoenolpyruvate; **Pyridoxal**-5-phosphate; **Pyrophosphate** ion; **Pyruvic acid**; ***Pyruvic acid**; ***Quercetin**; ***Sulphate**; Tartronic acid, 2-phospho-; **Tris**; Valeric Acid, phosphoenol-A-keto.

Table A.2 Lactate Dehydrogenase Inhibitors

Arsenite Ion; *ATP (*Steptococcus cremonus*); Butyric acid, 2-3-epoxy-; *p-Chloromercuribenzoic acid (*Streptococcus cremonis*); Chlorpromazine; ***Cibacron blue**; 3GA-dextran; Estradiol, 17-B; ***Fatty acids**; Glucosamine, D-; ***Glycerate**; *2-Hydroxy-3-Butynoic acid (*Megasphera elsdenii*); *2-Hydroxy-3-Butynoic acid (*E. Coli*); *2-Hydroxy-3-Butynoic acid (bakers yeast); **Lactate dehydrogenase inhibitor**; **Lactic acid**; ***L-Malic acid**; Mandelic acid; *Mononucleotides (sweet potato roots); **NAD**; NAD analog; ***NADH**; NADH-pyruvate adduct; NADH, pyridine analog; NADH, 5-carboxy analog;

---

* *Source:* Data from M.K. Jain, *Handbook of Enzyme Inhibitors, 1965–1977*, Wiley, New York, 1982; (*) from H. Zollner, *Handbook of Enzyme Inhibitors*, VCH, Weinheim, FRG, 1989, 1993.

Oxalic acid; *Oxalic acid; *Oxalic acid (D-lactate; yeast); *Oxaloacetic acid (D-lactate; yeast); *5-(–)Oxalylethyl-NADH; **Oxamic acid** (oxalic acid, monoamide); *Oxamic acid (oxalic acid, monoamide); *Phenylpyruvic acid; *Phosphoenolpyruvic acid (sweet potato roots); Propionic acid, 2,3, 3-epoxy-; Pyridinium bromide, 1-alkyl-3-bromoA; Pyruvate-DPN reduced adduct; **Pyruvic acid**; *Pyruvic acid (sweet potato roots); *Pyruvic acid (D-lactate; yeast); Quinoline-n-Oxide, 2-heptyl-4-hydroxy; *Reactive green 19-dextran; *Reactive red 4-dextran; **Rhein**; **Salicylic acid (aspirin)**; Salicylic acid, 4-iodoacetamido; **Serotonin**; Tartronic acid; **Urea;** Urea, methyl.

Table A.3   Glutaminase Inhibitors

*Ag⁺ (silver ion, from *E. coli*); *Albizzin; *Ammonia; Bromcresol green; Bromcresol purple; *Bromcresol purple; *Cu⁺⁺ (copper ion from *E. Coli*); *6-Diazo-5-oxo-L-norleucine (*Acinetobacter glutaminsificans*); *2,4–Dinitro-1-naphtolsulphonate; *n-Ethylmaleimide; **Flavianic acid**; *L-Glutamic acid; **Glycine**; *Hg⁺⁺ (mercury ion from *E. coli*); *Palmitoyl-CoA; *Pb⁺⁺ (lead ion from *E. coli*); *Phosphate; *Phthalfine dyes; *Stearyl-CoA.

Enzymes and Inhibitors for the Carboxylic Acid Cycle and as Affecting Respiration*

B.1 PYRUVATE DEHDROGENASE INHIBITORS

Acetaldehyde; *Acetyl-CoA (CoASH); *Acetylphosphonate; *N-(6-Amonohexyl)-5-chloro-1-naphtha-lene sulphonamide (from antagonist for calmodulin, a cell protein that binds with calcium; pea); *Buty-rophenone (calmodulin; pea): **Citric Acid**; Coenzyme A Esters, Acyl-; Coenzyme A, Acetyl-; Coenzyme A, Propionyl-; *Glyoxylic acid (pyruvate; broccoli); Growth Hormone Derivative; Guanosine-5'-triph-osphate; *Hydroxypyruvic acid (pyruvate; broccoli); *Isobutyryl-CoA; *Isovaleryl-CoA; **NADH**; *NADH; *Phenothiazine sulphonamide (from calmodulin antag.; pea); *Propionyl-CoA (CoASH); Pyru-vate Dehydrogenase Inhibitor; Valeric Acid, A-keto-iso-; *Thiamine thiazolone-pyrophosphate.

B.2 α-KETOGLUTARATE DEHYDROGENASE

Coenzyme A, succinyl-; Glutaric acid, G-hydroxy-A-keto-; **NADH**.

B.3 RESPIRATION INHIBITORS

Acetaldehyde; Acetazolamide; **Acrolein**; **Alkaloids**; Androsterone, dehydroiso-; **Anesthetics, general**; **Anesthetics, local**; *Antimycin*; *Antimycin A*; **Aromatic acids**; **Arsenate ion**; A204; Bilirubin; Bongkrekic acid; Butyric acid, A-P-chlorophenoxy-iso-; **Cadmium (Cd⁺⁺)**; Cannibinol, D9-tetrahydro-; Carnitine, 2-bromopalmitoyl-; Chlorpromazine; Cinnabarinic acid; Clofibrate; **Cobalt (Co⁺⁺)**; Coenzyme A, 2-bromopalmitoyl-; Complexing agents, metal-; **Copper (Cu⁺⁺)**; Cord factor; **Cyanide ion**; Cyclohexane, octafluoro-; Cysteine, S-(1,2-dichlorovinyl)-; Dextran sulfate; Dimycoloyl sucrose, 6. 6'-; Diphenylenei-odonium ion; Ethacrynic acid; **Fatty acids**; Feniculosin; Fuscin; Glucopyranoside, methyl-6-mycoloyl-A; **Guaiaretic acid, nordihydro (NDGA)**; Guanosine-3',5'-phosphate, dibutryl; Halothane; Helminthos-poral; HOQNO analogs; Imipramine, chlor-; **Isothiocyanates**; Lysolecithin; Methylvinyl ketone; *Mikayamycin*; Mucidin; Naphthalene dicarboxylic anhydride; Naphthoquinone, alkylhydroxy-; Nonactin homologs; **Nordihydroguiaretic acid (NDGA)**; *Oligomycin*; Ostruthin; **Papaverine**; Parathyroid hor-mone; **Phenol** derivatives; Phenol, P-nitro-; Piericidin A; **Progesterone**; Propionic acid, ethyl-BBB-trichloro-; Propionic acid, S-(1,2-dichlorovinyl)-; Protamine; Protein synthesis inhibitors; Pyrazole deriv-atives; Quinacrine; Quinazolone, 2-methyl-3-O-Tolyl-; Quinoline coccidiostats; Quinoline-N-oxide, 2-heptyl-4-hydrox; Rhodamine 6G; **Ruthenium** red; Salicylic Acid, 4-iodo-; Sarcosine, N-acyl-; SF 6847; Sporidesmin; **Sucrose**; Synthalin; Testesterone acetate, 17-nor-ethyl; Tetradifon; **Theophylline**; **Thio-cyanate ion**; Thymoquinone, dibrome-; Triethyltin; **Urea**, (+)A-(N-1-phenylethyl)-; **Vanadate ion**; Xanthothricin; **Zinc (Zn⁺⁺)**.

---

* *Source:* Data from M.K. Jain, *Handbook of Enzyme Inhibitors, 1965–1977*, Wiley, New York, 1982; (*) from H. Zollner, *Handbook of Enzyme Inhibitors*, VCH, Weinheim, FRG, 1989, 1993. Antibiotics are italicized.

Appendix C

Enzymes and Inhibitors Pertaining to Chemotherapy*

C.1 THYMIDYLATE SYNTHETASE (*THYMIDYLATE SYNTHASE)

Aminopterin; Aminopterin, deaza-; Amithopterin (methotrexate); *Arabino-UMP (*Scenedes obliquus*); Cytidine-5'-phosphate, 4-N-hydroxyde; Cytidine-5'-phosphate, 5-fluoro-2'-D; *Dihydrofolic acid (from *Streptococcus faecalis*); *5-Fluoro-2'-deoxyuridine monophosphate (dUMP; *Streptococcus faecalis*); *5-Fluoro-dUMP (from dUMP; *Streptococcus faecalis*; *Scenedes obliquus*); **Folic acid** analogs, homo-; **Folic acid** derivatives; **Folic acid,** L-tetrahydro-; **Folic acid,** 10-methyltetrahydro-; **Folic acid,** 11-methyltetrahydrohomo-; **Folic acid,** 5-methyltetrahydrohomo; Methasquin; **Pteroylglutamic acid (folic acid); Pteroylhexaglutamate; Pteroylhexaglutamate,** dihydro; Pyrimidinone deoxyribonucleotide; Quinaspar; Quinazolinyl derivatives; *Showdomycin*; Thymidylate synthetase inhibitor; *TMP (from dUMP; *Streptococcus faecalis*); *dTMP (from dUMP; *Streptococcus faecalis*); UMP, 5-mercapto-2'-deoxy-; UMP, 5'-fluoro-2'-deoxy-; **Uracil,** 5-trifluoromethyl, 6-aza-; Uridine derivatives; Uridine-5'-phosphate, 5-fluoro-; Uridine-5'-phosphate, 5-fluoro-2'-de; Uridine, 5-fluoro-2'-deoxy-; Uridylic acid, 5-fluoro-2'-deoxy-; Uridylic acid, 5-hydroxymethyl-2'-de; Uridylic acid, 5-trifluoromethyl-2'-.

C.2 DIHYDROFOLATE REDUCTASE

ADP-Phosphoribose; **Amethopterin (methotrexate); Aminopterin;** Aminopterin, isohomo; Benzylidine derivative; *1-(p-Butylphenyl)-2,2-dimethyl-4,6-diamino-1,2-dihydroxy-3-triazin (*E. coli*); Cycloguanil; *2,4-Diamino-5-(3,5 dimethoxy-4-substituted-benzyl)pyrimidines (from *E. coli*); *2,4-Diamino-6-n-butylpyrido[2,3-d]pyrimidine (*E. coli*; *S. aureus*); Folate antagonists; **Folic acid,** isohomo; **Folic acid,** 7-methyl; Isoaminopterin; Methasquin; **Methotrexate;** *Methotrexate (from *E. coli*); NADP; NADP, acetyl pyridine analog; Perimethamine; Primethamine; **Pteridine** derivatives; **Pterin,** isoamino-; **Pteroylglutamate derivative (folic acid or folate derivative);** Pyridines, 2,4-diamino-; Pyrimethamine; *Pyrimethamine (from *E. coli*; plasmodium); **Quinazoline** derivatives; **Quinazoline,** 2,4-diamino-; **Sulfa drugs;** *Tetroxoprim (from *E. coli*); Triazine derivatives; Triazines, 4,6-diamino-; **Trimethoprim;** *Trimethoprim (from *E. coli*).

C.3 DIHYDROFOLATE REDUCTASE LEVELS

Folic acid

---

* *Source:* Data from M.K. Jain, *Handbook of Enzyme Inhibitors, 1965–1977*, Wiley, New York, 1982; (*) from H. Zollner, *Handbook of Enzyme Inhibitors*, VCH, Weinheim, FRG, 1989, 1993.

Enzymes and Inhibitors for Enzymatic Changes*

D.1 IMP DEHYDROGENASE

Allopurinol, 1-ribosyl-5'-phosphate; *GMP (from IMP; *A. aerogenes*); Guanosine-3',5'-bis(diphosphate); Guanosine-5'-phosphate; Guanosine-5'-phosphate, ara-; Guanosine-5'-phosphate, 2'-deoxy-; Guanosine-5'-phosphate, 8-aza-; IMP, 6-thio-; Inosine-5'phosphate, 6-thio-; Mycophenolic acid; *Mycophenolic acid (from *Eimeria tenella*); **NADH; Nicotinamide**; Nucleotides; Purine ribosyl-5'-phosphate, 6-methy; Xanthosine-5'-phosphate; Xanthosine-5'-phosphate, ARA-Xanthosine-5'-phosphate, 2'-deoxy-; Xanthosine-5'-phosphate, 6-thio-; Xanthosine-5'-phosphate, 8-AZA-.

D.2 PRPP AMIDOTRANSFERASE

Adinosine; Adinosine-5'-diphosphate; Adinosine-5'-phosphate; Allopurinol ribonucleotide; **Guanine**; Guanosine-5'-phosphate; Nucleotides.

D.3 URIDINE KINASE

*CTP (Cytidine triphosphate, from beef erythrocytes); *UTP (Uridine triphosphate, from xanthine; beef erythrocytes)

D.4 URIDINE SYNTHESIS

Purine, 6-mercapto-

---

* *Source:* Data from M.K. Jain, *Handbook of Enzyme Inhibitors, 1965–1977*, Wiley, New York, 1982; (*) from H. Zollner, *Handbook of Enzyme Inhibitors*, VCH, Weinheim, FRG, 1989, 1993.

Appendix E

DNA Enzymes and Inhibitors*

E.1 DNA KINASE

Adenosine-3',5'-phosphate; Adenosine-5'-diphosphate; Adenosine-5'-phosphate; Adenosine-5'-phosphosulfate; Adenosine-5'-triphosphate; Adenosine-5'-triphosphate, 2'-deoxy-; Cytidine-3'-phosphate, 2'-deoxy-; Cytidine-3'-diphosphate, 2'-deoxy-; Cytidine-3'-phosphate, 2'-deoxy-; Cytidine-3'-triphosphate; Cytidine-3'-triphosphate, 2'-deoxy-; Dextran sulfate; Guanosine-5'-phosphate, 2'-deoxy-; Guanosine-5'-triphosphate; Guanosine-5'-triphosphate, 2'-deoxy-; **Heparin**; **Pyrophosphate ion**; **Silver (Ag⁺)**; Thymidine-5'-phosphate,2'-deoxy-; Thymidine-5'-triphosphate,2'-deoxy-; Uridine-5'-triphosphate.

E.2 DNA POLYMERASE

Acetic acid, phosphono-; **Acridine**, 9-amino-; **Acriflavin**; **Acrolein**; *Actinomycin D*; Adenosine dialdehyde, N6-dimethyl-; Adenosine-5'-triphosphate, arabinosy; Adenosine-5'-triphosphate, 2'-deoxy-; *Adriamycin*; *Adriamycin* octanoate; *Aphidicolin (from *Methanoccus vanielii*); *9-β-d-Arabinofuranosylcytosinetriphosphate (does not inhibit bacterial polymerase I); *Bleomycin (from *E. coli*); *Calcium elenolate; Cation (⁺); Chloroquine; *Chromomycin (from *E. coli*); Cytosine arabinoside; *Daunomycin*; *Daunomycin derivatives; Distamycin A*; *Distamycin A*(inhibits by binding to the template); *Distamycin A analogs*; DNA polymerase inhibitors; **Ellipticine**; **Ethidium bromide**; **Fluoride ion**; *Hedamycin*; Hemin; **Heparin**; Histones; *6-(p-Hydroxyphenylazo)-2-amino-4-pyrimidone (from bacterial polymerases); *6-(p-Hydroxyphenylazo) **uracil** (from bacterial polymerases); *Kanchanomycin*; **Lily extract**; *Neomycin*; Netropsin; *Netropsin (inhibits by binding to the template); Nitrosourea; Nucleotide polymers; Nucleotides; Nucleotides, poly-; Nucleotides, polyribo-; *Phosphonoacetic acid (*Herpes simplex*); Polycytidylic acid, 5-mercapto-; Polynucleotides; **Proflavin**; Propionic acid, 2-phosphono-; Pyridoxal-5-phosphate; **Pyrophosphate ion**; **Quinoline derivatives**; *Rifamycin* AF/013; *Rifamycin* AF/103; *Rifamycin;* **Sodium chloride**; **Spermidine**; **Spermine**; *Steffimycin B*; Tilorone; *5-Trifluoromethyl-2'-deoxyuridine triphosphate (*Herpes simplex*); **Ureas**, nitroso-.

E.3 DNA POLYMERASE A

CTP, 1-B-D-arabinofuranosyl- (CTP is **cytidine** triphosphate); *Novobiocin*.

E.4 DNA POLYMERASE I

Acridine derivatives; **Cytidine**-5'-triphosphate, 2'-deoxy-; *2',3'-Dideoxyguanosine 5'-triphosphate; Phenanthroline, 1, 10-.

E.5 DNA POLYMERASE II

Arabinosylcytosine triphosphate DNA, single stranded; Isocyanate, 2-chloroethyl-; Isocyanate, cyclohexyl-; Nitroso**ureas**

---

* *Source:* Data from M.K. Jain, *Handbook of Enzyme Inhibitors, 1965–1977*, Wiley, New York, 1982; (*) from H. Zollner, *Handbook of Enzyme Inhibitors*, VCH, Weinheim, FRG, 1989, 1993. Antibiotics are italicized.

E.6   DNA POLYMERASE III

Cytosine, 6-(P-tolylhydrazino)-; Cytosine, 6-(P-tolylhydrazino)iso-; *6-(p-Hydroxyphenyl)**uracil**; Pyrimidines; **Uracil derivatives**; **Uracil**, 6-(P-hydroxypenylhydrazino); **Uracil**, 6-(P-Tolylhydrazino)-; **Uracil**, 6-(P-Tolylhydrazino)-2-thio-

E.7   DNA POLYMERASE P1

DNA, single stranded

E.8   DNA POLYMERASE, A-

Cytidylic acid, oligo-; Nucleotides, poly-

E.9   DNA POLYMERASE α

*1-β-d-Arabinofuranosyl cytosinetriphosphate (from human lymphocytes); *p-Chloromercuribenzoic acid (from human lymphoid cells); *n-Ethylamide (from human lymphoid cells); *Pyridoxal 5'-phosphate.

E.10   DNA POLYMERASE β

*1-β-d-Arabinofuranosyl cytosinetriphosphate (from human lymphocytes0; *p-Chloromercuribenzoic acid (from human lymphoid cells).

E.11   DNA POLYMERASE γ

*p-Chloromercuribenzoic acid (from HeLa cells, a strain of cancer cells); *n-Ethylmaleimide (from HeLa cells); *Pyridoxal 5'-phosphate.

E.12   DNA POLYMERASE, DNA-DEPENDENT (DNA POLYMERASE)

Bleomycin; *Campthothecin*; Cytosine, arabinosyl-; Phenanthridium, 3-8-diamino-8-ethyl-; **Rhodium (Rh^{++})** propionate; Tilorone.

E.13   DNA POLERAMASE, RNA-DEPENDENT OR DNA POLYMERASE, RNA-DIRECTED (OR REVERSE TRANSCRIPTASE). ALSO SEE RNA-DIRECTED DNA POLYMERASE

Adenylic acid, polyribo-; Adenylic acid, 2'-0-alkylated-poly-; *Antibiotics*; Carbopol 934; Cytidine-5'-phosphate arabinoside; **Fagaronine**; Nucleotide, poly-; Nucleotides; Pyran copolymer; Rifamazine; *Rifamycin* analogs; *Rifamycin* derivatives; *Rifamycin* SV derivatives; Rifazone; *Sreptovaricins*.

E.14   DNA POLYMERASES (DNA-DIRECTED DNA POLYMERASES OR DNA-DEPENDENT DNA POLYMERASES)

DNA polymerase inhibitors

E.15   DNA REPAIR

Actinomycin D; **Isocyanate**, 2-cholorethyl-

E.16   DNA REPAIR, POST REPLICATION

Caffeine; Theophylline.

E.17   DNA REPAIR, REPLICATION

Progesterone

E.18   DNA REPLICATION

Cyanide ion; Ultraviolet light; Uracil, 6-(P-hydroxyphenylazo)-.

E.19   DNA SYNTHESIS

A-factor; **ACTH**; Actinobolin; *Actinomycin C3*; *Actinomycin D*; Adenine, benzyl-; Adenine-9-B-D-arabinofuranosyl-; Adenosine-N1-oxide; *Adriamycin*; *Anisomycin*; *Antibiotics*; Apurinic acid; **Asparaginase**, L-; Blasticidin S; *Bleomycin*; Bisulfan; **Camptothecin**; Chalone G1; **Chloroquine** (antimalarial drug); Chlorpromazine; *Chromomycin A3*; **Cortisol**; **Cortisol** acetate; **Cortisone**; *Coumermycin A1*; CTP, 1-B-D-arabino- (CTP, **cytidine** triphosphate); CTP, 1-B-D-arabinofuranosyl-; **Cyanide** ion; Cycloheximide; Cytidine, arabinoside; Cytosine, arabino-; Cytosine, 1-B-D-arabinofuranosyl-; Cytosine, 2,2'-anhydro-1-B-D-arabino; *Daunomycin*; Dexamethasone; **Dichromate** ion; Diphenylhydantoin; Edeine A; **Ellipticine**, 9-hydroxy-; **Emetine**; **Ethanol**; **Ethidium bromide**; Ethylenediamine tetraacetic acid (**EDTA**); *Feldamycin*; *Ficellomycin*; Flucinolone acetonide; **Folic acid**, tetrahydrohomo-; Glycine amine, diasoacetyl-; Glycine amide, diazoacetyl-; Guanine, 8-aza-; Helenalin; Histone; Imadazole carboxamide riboside; Mycophenolic acid; Nalidixic acid; Neocarzinostatin; Netropsin; *Novobiocin*; Nucleosides; Nucleotides, poly-; Orotic aldehyde derivatives; **Papaverine**; **Pentobarbital**; *Phagicin*; Phenylethyl alcohol; Phenylethyl alcohol, P-methoxy-; **Platinum (Pt^{++})** complex(es); Polyamine synthesis inhibitors; **Progesterone**; Propanolal, DL-; **Prostaglandin E1**; **Prostaglandin F1A**; Protein synthesis inhibitors; Purine, 6-chlor-8-aza-9-cyclopentyl-; *Puromycin* derivatives; Pyrazole derivatives; Pyrimidine-2-one-B-D-furanoside; Pyrimidine derivative(s); Quindine; Quinoxaline derivatives; Ribavirin; *Rifampicin*; Salicylhydrazide; Salicylhydroxamic acid; Salicylhydroxamic acid derivatives; Semicarbazones; *Sibiromycin*; Tenulin; **Theophylline**; Thioridazine; Threonine, L-O-methyl-; Thymidine; Thymidine, 5'-deoxy-; Thymidine, 5'-doxy-5'-fluoro; Trenimon; **Uracil**, 6-(P-hydroxyphenylazo)-; **Urea** derivatives; **Urea**, hydroxy-; **Urethane**, hydroxy-; Uridine, 5-fluorodeoxy-; Urinary peptides; Yoshi-864

E.20   DNA SYNTHESIS, ATP DEPENDENT

Adenosine-5'-triphosphate, 3'-deoxy-

E.21   DNA SYNTHESIS, INDUCTION

Phorbol-13-acetate, 12-O-tetradecano-

E.22   DNA SYNTHESIS, INITIATION

Cytosine arabinoside

E.23   DNA TOPOISOMERASE (ATP HYDROLYSING)

*Coumermycin A1 (from E. coli); *Nalidixic acid (E. coli); *Novobiocin (E. coli); *Oxolinic acid (E. coli)

E.24   DNA TOPOISOMERASE I

*Heparin (from mouse mammary carcinoma cells FM3A)

E.25   DNASE (DEOXYRIBONUCLEASE)

Actinomycin D; Adenyl-B, G-methylenediphosphate; DNase I inhibitor; DNase inhibitor; **Ethidium bromide**; Nucleotides; **Pentachlorophenol (PCP)**; Polyethylene sulfonate; Protein, gamma-; Ribonucleic acid, transfer-; *Sarkomycin*; U-12241.

E.26   DNASE (DEOXYRIBONUCLEASE I)

Actin; Actin, G-; Aurintricarboxylic acid; Biphenyl-2,5-dihydroxy-; Biphenyls, o-hydroxy-; *Bleomycin*; DNase I inhibitor; *2-Hydroxybiphenyl; *4-Hydroxybiphenyl (from *E. coli*).

E.27   DNASE (DEOXYRUBONUCLEASE II)

Malonic acid; **Oxalic acid.**

E.28   DNASE (DEOXYRIBONUCLEASE V)

*RNA (from *E. coli*)

Appendix F

RNA Enzymes and Inhibitors*

F.1 RNA-DIRECTED DNA POLYMERASE OR RNA-DEPENDENT DNA POLYMERASE (OR REVERSE TRANSCRIPTASE). ALSO SEE DNA POLYMERASE, RNA-DEPENDENT.

Actinomycin (inhibits by binding to template); *Adriamycin*; *Chromomycin* (inhibits by binding to template); *Cinerubin*; *Daunorubicin*; *Distamycin A* (inhibits by binding to template); **Ethidium bromide** (inhibits by binding to template); **Fagaronine** (inhibits by binding to template); *5-Mercapto-deoxyuridine triphosphate; *Olivomycin* (inhibits by binding to template); *2-Oxopropanol; *o-Phenan-throline; **Phosphate** (Rauscher leukemia virus; only the enzyme from mammalian type C viruses is affected); **Proflavin** (inhibits by binding to template); *Pyran copolymer; *Pyridoxal 5'-phosphate; *Rifamycin*; *Rifamycin derivative* AF/05; *Rifmycin derivative* AF/13; **Silicotungstic acid**; *Strepto-varicin*; *Thiosemicarbazone; *5-Tungsto-2-animoniate.

F.2 RNA POLYMERASE (DNA-DIRECTED RNA POLYMERASE OR DNA-DEPENDENT RNA POLYMERASE, OR TRANSCRIPTASE)

Acridine derivatives; *Acridine orange (inhibits by binding to template); *Actinomycin*; *Actinomycin* (inhibits by binding to template); *Actinomycin D*; Adenylic acid, poly-; *Adriamycin*; *Adriamycin* (inhibits by binding to template); **Aflatoxin B1**; **Aflatoxin G1**; **Aflatoxin G2**; Amanin; Amantin, A-; **Amatoxins**; *3'-Amino-3'-deoxyadenosine Amino acids, poly-; **Ammonium (NH₄⁺)**; *Antibiotics*; Antiviral compounds; Aurintricarboxylic acid; Biphenylacetamide, 4-; *Bleomycin*; **Camptothecin**; *Chloromycin*; **Chloroquine**; *Chromomycin A3*; *Chromomycin A3* (inhibits by binding to template); Cibachrome blue F3G; *Cibacron blue F3GA; *Cinerubin* (inhibits by binding to template); **Congo red**; **Cortisol**; Cytidine-5'-triphosphate, 6-methyl-; Cytosine arabinoside; *Daunomycin*; *Daunorubicin* (inhibits by binding to template); *3'-Deoxyadenosine; *Diacridine (inhibits by binding to template); *Distamycin*; *Distamycin A* (inhibits by binding to template); DSI; *Eosine; *Erichrome T; **Ethidium bromide**; Exotoxin; Fluorene, N-hydroxy-2-acetylamino-; Fluorenylacetamide, N-aceoxy-2-; Fluorenylacetamide, N-hydroxy-2-; Gallin; *Gallin (from *E. coli*); *Glucomannan; Gramicidin D; Guanosine-5'-triphosphate, 8-bromo-; Guanosine-5'-triphosphate, 8-keto-; *Hedamycin*; **Heparin** (bacterial); Histin; Histone(s); Jatrophone; *Kanchanomycin*; *Kanchanomycin*; **Lasiocarpine**; *Lipiarmycin*; Lomofungin; *Luteoskyrin; **Lysine**, poly-L-; Miracil D; *Netropsin (inhibits by binding to template); *Nogalamycin* (inhibits by binding to template); Nucleotides; Nucleotides, poly-; *Olivomycin* (inhibits by binding to template); *Pluramycin*; *Pluramycin A*; Polyethylene sulfonate; *Polyethylene sulfonate (bacterial); *Poly(GLU1.TYR1); *Poly(GLU3.PHE1); *Polynucleotides; **Polysaccharide**; **Prednisolone**; **Primaquine** (antimalarial drug); **Proflavin**; *Proflavin (inhibits by binding to template); Protamine; **Purine**, 6-cnlor-8-aza-9-cyclopentyl-; Ribose-5-diphosphate, D-; Ribose-5-diphosphate, D-2-deoxy-; Ribose-5-triphosphate, D-; Ribose-5-triphosphate, D-2-deoxy-; RIF amide; RIF *ampicin*; *Rifampicin*; RIF *ampicin* AF/ABDMP; RIF *ampicin* AF/103; RIF *ampicin* derivatives; RIF ampin; RIF *amycin* AF/103; *Rifamycin*; RIF *amycin* analogs; RIF *amycin* derivatives; *Rifamycin* derivatives AF05; *Rifamycin*

* *Source:* Data from M.K. Jain, *Handbook of Enzyme Inhibitors, 1965–1977*, Wiley, New York, 1982; (*) from H. Zollner, *Handbook of Enzyme Inhibitors*, VCH, Weinheim, FRG, 1989, 1993. Antibiotics are italicized.

derivatives AF13; RIF *amycin*, sepharose bound; RNA polymerase inhibitor; ***Rose bengal**; **Steroid hormones**; *Streptolydigin; **Streptovaricin (E. coli)*; *Tilorone (DNA template binding compromised); Uridine-5'-triphosphate, 5-hydroxy-; Uridine, poly-. (**Note:** As per the *American Heritage Dictionary*, the acronym RIF or prefix "rif-" is probably derived from the Italian word *riformare*, to reform.)

F.3   RNA POLYMERASE A

Cardiolipin; Exotoxin; Transcription inhibitor.

F.4   RNA POLYMERASE B

Aflatoxin; Amatoxins

F.5   RNA POLYMERASE I

Cycloheximide; *Pyridoxal 5'-phosphate (yeast); **Rifmycin derivative* AF/05; **Rifmycin derivative* AF/13.

F.6   RNA POLYMERASE I, DNA-DEPENDENT

(no entries)

F.7   RNA POLYMERASE II

Amanitin, A-; ***α-Amanitin**; Aurintricarboxylic acid; **Glycerol**; *Pyridoxal 5'-phosphate (yeast); RIF *ampicin* AF/103; RIF *amycin* SV, 3-formyl-; **Rifamycin derivative* AF/05; **Rifamycin derivative* AF/13.

F.8   RNA POLYMERASE II, DNA-DEPENDENT

Actinomycin D; **Amanitin, A-**; Ribonucleoprotein; RIF *ampicin* AF/018; RIF *amycin* AF/018.

F.9   RNA POLYMERASE III

*α-**Amanitin**; Phenanthroline, 1,10-.

F.10   RNA POLYMERASE LEVELS

Aflatoxin

F.11   RNA POLYMERASE, DNA-DEPENDENT (RNA POLYMERASE OR TRANSCRIPTASE). ALSO SEE DNA-DIRECTED RNA POLYMERASE OR DNA-DEPENDENT RNA POLYMERASE)

Actinomycin D; Adenosine-5'-triphosphate, 3'-deoxy-; **Aflatoxin B1**; **Amanitin, A-**; *Antibiotic B44P*; Benzanthracene, 7,12-dimethyl-; Cardiolipin; **Congo red**; Daunorubrin; *Distamycin*; *Distamycin A*; Exotoxin, *Bacillus thuringiensis*; Inosine derivatives; Nucleotides; Nucleotides, thiolatedpoly-; Phosphatidylglycerol; Phospholipids; Purine, 6-chloro-8-aza-9-cyclopentyl-; Pyridoxal-5-phosphate; **Quinoline**-N-oxide, 4-nitro-; RIF amazine; RIF *ampicin*; RIF *ampicin* AF/05; RIF *amycin*; RIF *amycin* derivatives; RNA polymerase inhibitor(s); *Showdomycin*; *Streptovaricin*.

F.12   RNA SYNTHESIS

Acridine; **Acrolein**; *Actinomycin D*; Adenosine, 3'-amino-3'-deoxy-; Adenosine, 3'-deoxy-; Adenosine, 5'-methylthio-; **Aflotoxin B1**; Alanosince; **Amanitin, A-**; *Anthramyxin*; Atractyloside; **Atropine**; Aurintricarboxylic acid; **Azide ion**; Basic protein from viscum album; Benzimidazole derivative; Benzimidasole, 5.6-dichloro-18-D-RIB; Benzofuroxan derivatives; **Camptothecin**; **Cholesterol**; Cordycepin; **Cortisol**; *Coumermycin A1*; Cycloheximide; Cyproterone acetate; Cytidine, 3'-deoxy-; *Daunomycin*; **Diamide**; Dinitrophenol, 2,4-; *Echinomycin*; **Emetine**; **Ethidium bromide**; Ethionine, DL-; Exotoxin, *Bacillus thuringiensis*; Fluorene, N-acetoxy-2-acetylamino-; Fluorene, N-hydroxy-2-acetyl-; Fluorene, N-hydroxy-2-acetylamino-; *Formycin*; **Germanate ion** (contains germanium) ; Guanosine-3'-phosphate; Guanosine-3',5'-bis(diphosphate); Guanosine-5'-phosphate; Guanosine-5'-phosphate, 7-methyl-; **Heparin**; Histones; Inosinic acid, polyribo-; **Interferon**; *Kasugamycin*; **Lasiocarpine**; Levallorphan; Levorphanol; Lomofungin; Luteoskyrin; Metabolic inhibitors; Methylglyoxal bis(guanylhydrazone); Maracil D; Myxin; Nebularine, 7-deaza-; Nitrosourea, 1,3-bis(2-chloroethyl)-; *Olivomycin*; **Oubain**; **Pentobarbital**; Phalloidin; Phenol, 2,4-dinitro-; POX-3; Prednesolone; Prednisolone; Prednisolone, 9A-fluoro-; Proflavin; Protein synthesis inhibitors; *Puromycin*; Quinoline, 8-hydroxy-; RIF *ampicin*; RIF *ampicin* AF/013; RIF *ampicin*-RNA polymerase complex; RNA polymerase inhibitors; RNA synthesis inhibitor; RNA synthesis pseudo-inhibitor; **Stearic acid**; *Toyokamycin*; **Trimethoprim**; Tyrocidine; **Uracil, 2-thio-; Urethane.**

F.13   RNA SYNTHESIS, CHROMOSOMAL

Amanitin

F.14   RNA SYNTHESIS, GLOBAL

Guanosine-3',5'-bis(diphosphate)

F.15   RNA SYNTHESIS, INITIATION

Benzimidazole, 5,6-dichloro-1B-D-RIB

F.16   RNA SYNTHESIS, NUCLEAR

(no entries)

F.17   RNA TRANSLATION

QB replicase, subunit I of

F.18   RNA VIRUS SYNTHESIS

Cordycepin

F.19   RNA 5'-TRIPHOSPHATASE, ACID

Phosphate, inorganic

F.20   RNASE (RIBONUCLEASE)

Adenosine-5'-diphosphate (**ADP**); Adenosine-5'-triphosphate (**ATP**); Adenosine-5'-triphosphate, 2'-deoxy; **Bentonite**; Cytidine-2'-phosphate; *Diethylpyrocarbonate; DNA; Guanosine-5'-diphosphate; *Heparin** (serum); Kethoxal; Nuclease inhibitor; Nucleotides, arabino-; Nucleotides, poly-; Poly(A)-2, poly-; Poly(styrene-maleic acid); Polyadenylic acid; Polyguanylic acid; Polycarbonate, diethyl-; Ribonuclease inhibitor; **Silver (Ag⁺)**; **Spermine**; Uridine-3'-phosphate; **Vinblastine**.

F.21   RNASE (RIBONUCLEASE A)

Heparin; Uridine **vanadate**.

F.22   RNASE (RIBONUCLEASE H)

RIF *ampicin*

F.23   RNASE (RIBONUCLEASE I)

Flavonoids; *Uridine 3'-phosphate (cyclic 2',3'-uridylate).

F.24   RNASE (RIBONUCLEASE II)

DNA

F.25   RNASE (RIBONUCLEASE REDUCTASE)

Purine thiosemicarbazone

F.26   RNASE (RIBONUCLEASE T1)

Nucleotides

F.27   RNASE (RIBONUCLEASE V)

Aurintricarboxylic acid; *Sodium chloride*.

F.28   RNASE (RIBONUCLEASE, ALKALINE)

Ribonuclease inhibitor

F.29   RNASE (RIBONUCLEASE, ATP INHIBITED)

Adenosine-5'-triphosphate (**ATP**); Adenosine-5'-triphosphate, 2'-deoxy-; Tetrazole, diaso-1-H-

F.30   RNASE (RIBONUCLEASE, MODIFIED)

Ribonuclease inhibitor

Appendix G

Proteases and Protease Inhibitors*

G.1 PROTEASE

Anesthetics, general; Antipain; Cartilage factor; Chymotrypsin inhibitor I; Guanidino acid derivatives; Leupeptin; Malic acid, poly(L)-; Ovoinhibitors; PDFA; **Pepstatin**; Protease inhibitor (black-eyed peas, bronchial secretion, lima bean, bovine cartilage, human seminal plasma, *Bacillus subtilis*, kidney bean, wheat and rye germ, potato, bee venom, guinea pig serum, Russell viper venom); Protease inhibitor, insulin specific (human serum); Protease inhibitors (synthetic arginyl- and lysyl-peptides; guanidino derivatves, TPCK, TAME, PMSF, TLCK, benzamidine, pepstatin, chymostatin, leupeptins); Proteinase inhibitor (human serum); Proteinase inhibitor, A2-;RVV inhibitor II.

G.2 PROTEASE I

Proteinase inhibitor, A2-

G.3 PROTEASE, ACID

Antipain; **Chymostatin** (bioactive peptide); Leucine Methylester, diazoacetylnor-; Leucine, diazoacetyl-DL-nor-; **Leupeptin**; **Pepstatin**; Protease inhibitor.

G.4 PROTEASE, NEUTRAL

Antitrypsin, A-; Trypsin inhibitor.

G.5 PROTEASES

Caproic acid, w-amino derivatives; Chloramphenicol; Cyclohexane carboxylic acids; Cycloheximide; Proteinase inhibitors.

G.6 PROTEASES, NEUTRAL

Clofibrate

G.7 PROTEASES, SERINE

Boronic acids, aryl-

G.8 PROTEIN DEGRADATION

Leupeptin; Protease inhibitors (tosyl-PHE- and tosyl-LYS-chloromethylketones).

* *Source:* Data from M.K. Jain, *Handbook of Enzyme Inhibitors, 1965–1977*, Wiley, New York, 1982; (*) from H. Zollner, *Handbook of Enzyme Inhibitors*, VCH, Weinheim, FRG, 1989, 1993.

G.9   PROTEIN DIGESTION

Cathepsin inhibitors

G.10   PROTEASE ASPARTIC

*Pepstatin

G.11   PROTEASE CYSTEINE

*L-trans-Epoxysuccinyl-leucylamido(4--guanido)butane; *Peptide aljehydes; *Peptidyldiazomethyl ketones.

G.12   PROTEASE METALLO

*EDTA; *o-Phenanthroline; *Phosphoramidon.

G.13   PROTEASE SERINE

*Chloromethylketone (also cysteine proteases); *Dispropyl fluorophosphate; *Peptide aldehydes; *Phenylmethylsulphonyl fluoride (also cysteine proteases); *4-Toluolsulphonylfluoride; *L-1-Tosylamido-2-phenyl(ethyl) chloromethylketone (also cysteine proteases); *N-p-Tosyl-L-lysine chloromethylketone (also cysteine proteases).

A Worldwide Selection of Anticancer Plants*

Acanthaceae	*Adhatoda vasica*: vâsâ, malabar nut. **Vasicine, acthatodine, anisotinine, betaine**, etc.
Amaryllidaceae	*Narcissus tazetta*: **narcissus, daffodil**. **Rutin**, linalool, cineol. Flowers contain narcissin, **tazettine**. Leaves contain **alkaloids**.
Anacardiaceae	*Pistacia lentiscus*: mastich, mastix, **mastic**, lenticus. Resin, masticin, mastic acid, **beta-sitosterol**, pinene, camphene.
	Rhus toxidendron. Contains urishiol, urishenol.
	Schinus spp.: molle, schinus. Brazilian pepper-tree. The triterpenes terebinthone and schinol, plus tannins, saponins, organic acids, **beta-sitosterol**.
Apocynaceae	*Acokanthera schimperi*: arrow poison tree. Acobioside A, actopectoside A, acovenoside A and B, opposide, etc. Toxic.
	Apocynum cannabinum*: Indian hemp. Plant is characterized as an extremely poisonous cardiotonic drug due to the presence of cardioactive glycosides. The **antitumor** agents are **cymarin** and **apocannoside**. Other compounds include K-strophanthin and tannins, resin, and saponins. Also lupeol, androsterol, harmelol, etc.
	Catharanthus* spp.: periwinkle. (Hartwell uses *Vinca*.) Numerous alkaloids including **ajimalicine, akummicine, vinblastine**, etc. The plant substances may be either or both carcinogenic and anticarcinogenic. That is, some compounds are presumably carcinogenic and others are anticarcinogenic, with offsetting effects.
	Nerium oleander: **oleander** (toxic). Contains cardioactive glycosides, **HCN**. Also the anticancer agents **rutin** and **ursolic acid**.
	Thevetia peruviana*: yellow oleander. The cardenolide glycoside **cerberin** is the anticancer component. Other components include the triterpene **ursolic acid**.
	Vinca minor: periwinkle. Many **alkaloids**.
Aquifoliaceae	*Ilex* spp.: **holly**. Contains the alkaloids **ilicin, caffeine**.
Araceae	*Acorus calamus*: acoron, sweet flag, calamus. Acolamone, **acorine**, acorone, camphene, camphor, choline, eugenol, etc. Oils is carcinogenic.
	Arisaema triphyllum*: jack-in-the-pulpit, Indian turnip. Contains calcium oxalate, albumin, liginin.
	Dieffenbachia purpurea*: dumbcane. **Seguine**, calcium oxalate.
	Symplocarpus foetidus: **skunk cabbage**. Contains tannins and n-hydroxytryptamine. Also calcium oxalate.

---

* *Source:* Data from *CRC Handbook of Medicinal Herbs* by James A. Duke, CRC Press, Boca Raton FL, 1985. Plant families, genera, or species **not** listed in Hartwell's *Plants Used Against Cancer* are denoted by an asterisk. There are 80 families and 212 different genera or species listed. Most appear in Hartwell. Some representative chemical compounds are listed, with most alkaloids—usually ending in "-ine"—shown in **boldface**, along with other information of potential interest. Amino acids also end in "-ine." Glycosides or glucosides, probably the second most important class of bioactive compounds, generally end in "-in." As do flavonoids. Other classes of chemical compounds tend to be characterized by still other endings or suffixes such as "-ol" for alcohols or their kin, "-one" for ketones, or "-ene" for compounds with "double bonds," etc. There are exceptions, however, and there are more classes than endings available.

Araliaceae	*Eleutherococcus* senticosus*. Coumarins, saponins.
	Hedera helix: heder, **ivy**. Saponin, **rutin, quercetin, kaempferol**.
	Panax spp.: **ginseng**. Panaxin, panaquilon, panacene, ginsenin.
Aristolochiaceae	*Aristolochia serpentaria*: Virginia snakeroot, serpentery. Contains borneol, serpentarin, **aristolochchine**, etc.
Asclepiadaceae	*Asclepias syriaca*: common **milkweed**. Latex contains cauotchonc, antitumor **beta-sitosterol**.
	Calotropis procera: arka, mudar, swallowort. Phytosterol, **stigmasterol**, calotoxin, etc.
	Cryptostegia* grandifolia: rubber vine. Contains phenolics.
	Marsdenia reichenbachii*. (*Marsdenia condurango*: **condor vine**). Contains a strychnine-like alkaloid plus condurangoglycoside.
Asteraceae* (Compositae)	*Achillea millefolium*: **yarrow**, millefolium, field hop. **Achiceine, mostchatine, stachydrine, trigonelline**. The flavonoids apigenin, artemetin, casticin, etc. Camphor compounds, etc.
	Anaphilis margaritacea: cotton-weed, sempervivum, pearly everlasting. Phytosterin, resin, tannin, etc.
	Arctium lappa: **burdock**, burdane. Leaves contain arctiol, taravasterol, etc. Roots contain polyphenolic acids; seeds contain arctiin, etc.
	Arnica montana: **arnica**. **Anthoxanthine**, tannin, flavones, ornisin, **betaine**, inulin, isoquercetrin.
	Artemisia spp.: absinthe, wormwood. Phellandrine, pinene, thujone, glucosides, lactones.
	Calendula officinalis: eliotropium, **marigold**. Calendulin, saponin, sterol.
	Chamaemelum* nobile: Roman or English camomile. One of the best-selling herbs. Contains **anticancer sesquiterpene lactones**. Also germacranolides, flavonoids.
	Chrysanthemum parthenium: feverfew, parthenion. Camphor, borneol, terpenes, esters, etc.
	Eupatorium perfoliatum: boneset. Eupatorin, tannic acid, flavonoids.
	Grindelia squarrosa: grindelia, gumweed. Organic acids, borneol, tannin, saponins.
	Lactuca virosa: wild **lettuce**. Organic acids, beta-sitosterol, squalene, and **alkaloids**, notably **hyoscyamine**.
	Lobelia inflata: **Indian tobacco, lobelia**. **Lobeline**, etc. Toxic.
	Matricaria chamomilla: German **chanomile**. Azulene, cadinene, choline, **rutin**, coumarins, etc.
	Solidago virgaurea: **goldenrod**. Pyridine, **cytisine**, plus saponin, tannin, inulin, **quercetin, rutin**, kaempferol. Toxic.
	Tanacetum vulgare: **tansy**. Contains the ketone β-thujone, plus borneol, camphene, terpenes, etc.
	Taraxacum officinale: **dandelion**. Roots contain taraxacin, inulin, glutin. Also the phytosterol taxasterol plus saponin, organic acids.
	Tussilago farfara: colt's-foot. Glucosides, organic acids, phytosterols, inulin, choline, stigmasterol, taraxesterol, kaempferol, **quercetin**.
Berberidaceae	*Berberis vulgaris*: ebsal, berberitze, barberry. **Berbamine, berberine, berberubine**, etc.
	Caulophyllum thalictroides. Contains **alkaloids** and glycosides.
	Podophyllum peltatum: **may apple**. Contains **podophyllotoxin** and **lignans** as the **anticancer** agents, plus the resin podophyllin.
Betulaceae	*Alnus glutinosa*: European **alder**, black alder. Contains taraxerol, taraxarone, etc., plus **l-ornithine**.
Bignoniaceae	*Tabebuia* spp.: **pau d'arco**, îpe roxo. Lapachol is the active ingredient. Also contains sesquiterpenes, anthraquinones.

Boraginaceae	*Borago officinalis*: **borrage**, borraga, beeplant (but not the Rocky Mountain beeplant *Cleome serrulata* of the family Capparidaceae or Capparaceae). Contains **cyanogenic** substances..
	Heliotropum europaeum: **heliotrope, herba cancri**. Alkaloids, **pyrrolizidine alkaloids**. Toxic.
	Symphatum peregrinum*. (Comfrey is *S. officinalis*.) Contains tannin, and such alkaloids as **lasiocarpine, viridiflorine, echinatrine**. The genus *Symphatum* is notorious for toxic **pyrrolizidine alkaloids**. They may also act either as carcinogens or anticarcinogens.
Bromeliaceae	*Ananas comosus*: **pineapple**. Vanillin, **bromelain**, 5-hydroxytryptamine.
Buxaceae	*Buxus sempervirens*: box, boxwood. **Buxine** alkaloids.
	Simmondsia chinensis: **jojoba**. Amino acids, flavonoids, **cyanoglucosides**. Oil is famous as a high-quality lubricant.
Caesalpiniaceae*	*Gledisia* triacanthos*: honey locust. Glycosides, tannin, hypoxysin, no alkaloids.
Caprifoliaceae	*Sambucus canadensis*: **elder, elderberry**. Organic acids, **rutin, HCN**-content.
Caricaceae	*Carica papaya*: **papaya**, pawpaw. Contains the proteolytic enzyme papain. Also an **isothiocyanate** aglycone plus sinigrin, myrosin, **carpasemine, carpaine**, etc.
Caryophyllaceae	*Agrostemma githago*: negella, cokle, raden, etc. The saponin sapotoxin A, tannin, the glycosides **cyanidin** and delphinidin. Toxic.
Chenopodiaceae	*Chenopodium ambrosioides*: payco, paico, potato. Saponins, camphol, ascaridole.
Convolvulaceae	*Rivea* corymbosa*: snakeplant. **Ergine, isoergine, penniclavine**, etc.
Cornaceae	*Cornus florida*: **dogwood**. Contains the glucoside cornin plus **kaempferol, quercetin**, etc.
Cucurbitaceae	*Citrullus colocynthis*: **cucumber**. Coumarin, eugenol, aldehydes, linallol, monoterpenes, phytosterols.
	Momordica charantia: balsam-pear, Melaõ de São. Contains the **alkaloid momordicin**.
Cycadaceae*	*Cycas* revoluta*: sago cycas. contains cycasin, etc. Both carcinogenic and anticarcinogenic.
Equisetaceae	*Equisetum*: **horsetail**. Saponin, **nicotine**, isoquercitrin, **beta-sitosterol**.
Ericaceae	*Arctostaphylos* uva-ursi*: bearberry. Arbitin, allantoin, ellagic acid, myricetin, myricitrin, etc.
	Ledum palustre: wild rosemary, marsh tea. Tannins, organic acids, ericolin, **quercetin**.
	Erythroxylum coca*: coca. **Cocaine**.
Euphorbiaceae	*Acalypha indica*. Tannins, **acalyhine**, a cyanoglucoside, **HCN**, triacetonamine. Toxic.
	Aleurites moluccana: tung, varnish tree. Bark contains tannin.
	Chamaesyce hypericifolia (or *Euphorbia hypercifolia*): **milkweed**, spurge. Contains **alkaloids**, glycosides, phorboesters, tannin.
	Euphorbia spp.: euphorbia. **Beta-sitosterol**. Both carcinogenic and anti-carcinogenic. Some species are toxic.
	Hippomane mancinella: manzanillo, manchineol. Used as arrow poison. Contains **physostigmine**, sapogenin.
	Jatropha spp.: physic-nut. **Beta-sitosterol**, stigmasterol, campesterol, etc.
	Manihot esculenta: **manioc, cassava, tapioca**, mandioca, quauhychtli. Saponin, glucosides, **HCN**.
	Mercurialis* annua: garden mercury. Contains **cyanogenetic** glucosides, **alkaloids**.
	Ricinus communis: castor bean plant. Seeds contain the toxic albumin ricin, plus **HCN, alkaloids**. Extremely toxic.
	Stillingia sulvatica: stillingia, queen's delight. **HCN** is the poisonous principle.
Fabaceae*	*Abrus precatorius*: jequirity. Root, leaves contain glycyrrhizia. Seeds
(Leguminosae)	contain abrin (extremely toxic). Also polygalactonic acid, pentosan, gallic acid, **hepaphorine**, campestrol, 5 beta cholinic acid, **trigonelline**.

Calliandra anomala: tlacoxilohxochitl, cabeza de angel. Narcotic.

Cassia spp.: **senna**, cassia. Aloe-em odin, antitumor agent. Anthraquinones are probably the purgative agent.

Cytisus scoparius: kandoul, Scotch broom. Contains **sparteine, genesteine**, scoparin, tannin.

Erythrina fusca: coral bean. Seeds contain the **alkaloid erythralin and other alkaloids.**

Genista tinctoria: woodwaxen, genista, dyer's broom. **Anagyrine, cytisine**, etc.

Indigofera tinctoria: indigo. Indigotin, indican.

Medicago sativa: **alfalfa**. Seeds contain the alkaloids **strachydrine** and **1-homo-stachydrine.**

Piscidia* piscipula: Jamaica dogwood. Contains jamaicin, **beta-sitosterol**, organic acids, tannins, and the **anticancer** agent **rotenone.**

Phaseolus spp.: bean. **Cyanogenic** glucosides.

Robinia* pseudoacacia: black locust. Contains the toxalbumin robin.

Tephrosia virginiana*: devil's shoe string. **Rotenone**, deguelin, tephrosin.

Trifolium pratense: **red clover**. Isoflavones, trypsin inhibitors, glucosides. Also pterocarpan phytoalexins, which are antiviral and antifungal.

Trigonella foenum-graecum: fenugreek. Coumarins and nicotinic acid. Plus **betaine and trigolline**. There is also a hypoglycemic action.

Gentianaceae	*Gentiana lutea*: yellow **gentian**. Contains a glucoside and the alkaloid **gentianine.**
Geraniaceae	*Geranium maculatum*: cranesbill, **geranium**, crowfoot. Tannin.
Gramineae	*Lolium temulentum*: Italian ryegrass, lolium, darnel. **Loliine, perloline, temuline**, etc.
Guttiferae	*Hypericum perforatum*: **St. John's wort**. Hypericin, tannin, **beta-sitosterol, alkaloids.**
Hamamelidaceae	*Hamamelis virginiana*: **witch hazel**. Tannin, saponin, **quercetin**, etc., plus the carcinogen safrole, eugenol.
Hippocastanaceae	*Aesculus hippocastanum*: castagno d'india, horse chestnut. Contains the glycoside aesulin. Toxic.
Iridaceae	*Crocus sativus*: **crocus, saffron**. Contains **colchicine, quercetin.**
	Iris versicolor: **flag**. Furfurol, tannin, phytosterols, organic acids, etc.
Labiatae (or Lamiaceae)	*Ajuga reptans*: oleum laurentium, bugleweed.
	Glechoma hederacea (or *Nepeta hederacea*): ground ivy. Pinene, limonene, **beta-sitosterol**, choline, etc.
	Lavandula angustifolia: **lavender**. Coumarins, flavonoids, **linalyl acetate**, linallol.
	Nepeta cataria: **catnip**. Organic acids, linonene, nerol, citronellal, geraniol. Also toxins carvacrol, saponin, tannin, thymol.
	Ociumum basilicum: **basil**. Eucalyptol, cineol, eugenol, borneol, etc.
	Rosmarinus officinalis: **rosemary**. **Ursolic acid**, tannins, borneol, camphor, thymol, etc. Also flavonoids, e.g., diosmin.
	Salvia spp.: **sage, cancer-weed**, etc. Camphene, thujene, limonene, cineol, linalool, etc.
	Stachys officinalis (or *Betonica officinalis*): betonica, cestron, bishopwort. Contains **betaine, betonicine**, organic acids.
	Thymus vulgaris: **thyme**. Thymol, linalool, borneol, **linalyl acetate**, terpinol.
Lauraceae	*Cinnamomum verum**: Ceylon cinnamon.
	Laurus nobilis: **laurel**, bay. Contains **reticuline, boldine**, etc.
	Sassafras albidum: **sassafras**. Safrole, anethole, apiole, camphor. Plus the alkaloids **boldine, cinnamolanrine**, etc. Also lignis and tannins.
Liliaceae	*Aloe barbadensis*: Mediterranean or Curacao **aloe**. Anthraquinone glycosides, e.g., aloin.

Colchium autumnale: ephemeron, colchicum, hermodactolis, autumn crocus, meadow saffron. Contains **colchicine and other alkaloids**.

Gloriosa superba: dorng-dueng, glory lily. Contains **colchicine**.

Paris quadrifolia: herb Paris, true-love. Contains the glucoside paradin, saponins.

Schoenecaulon officinale: sebadilla. **Steroid alkaloids, cebadine, veratridine**, etc.

Smilax aristolochiifolia: smilax, **China root, Mexican sarsaparillo**. Contains steroids, saponins.

Urginea maritima: **squill**. Glucoscillaron A, scillaron A, etc. Also flavonoids, e.g., **quercetin**. Plus phytosterol.

Veratrum viride: American **hellebore**. A major medicinal plant with numerous alkaloids. Alkaloids in the rhizome include alkamines, and specifically **germidine, germatrine, cevadine**, etc. Also **pseudojervine, germine, jervine, veratramine**.

Loganiaceae	*Gelsemium sempervirens*: yellow jasmine. contains the indole alkaloid **gelsemine**, etc.

Strychnos nux-vomica: nux vomica, strychnine. Contains **strychnine, brucine**, etc. There is a fine line between being useful or toxic.

Loranthaceae	*Viscum album*: European **mistletoe**. Amines, viscin, tannin, cartenoids, acetylcholine, histamine. The anticancer basis is a **protein complex**.
Lythraceae	*Lawsonia inermis*: **cypress**, henna, privet. Tannins, quinones, glucosides.
Malvaceae	*Abelmoschus moschatus*: musk **okra**, ambrette. Seeds contain ketone ambretolide, lactone of ambrettolic acid, ambrettol. Also methionine sulfoxide, phospholipids.

Gossypium spp.: **cotton, cottonseed**. Tannin, **betaine**, etc.

Hibiscus sabdariffa: kerkedeh plant, roselle. Used in the beverage called "jamaica" in Mexico. Contains hibiscrilin, phytosterols.

Malva rotundifolia: malva, malache, dwarf mallow. Organic acids, tannins.

Meliaceae	*Melia azedarach*: nimva, margosa, neem-tree, chinaberry. Leaves contain **parasine, margosine**.
Menispermaceae	*Menispermum* canadense*. Contains **dauricine, tetrandine, acutamine**, etc. (The reference makes the point that the fact that birds can eat plant seeds without ill-effects doesn't necessarily imply that humans can do the same.)
Moraceae	*Cannabis sativa*: marijuana, hemp. Cannabinoids, e.g., Δ-THC.

Humulus lupulus: **hops**. Organic acids, flavonoid glycosides, phenolics, tannins, lipids. **Also contains GLA (gamma-linoleic acid), called the "wonder cure."**

Myricaceae	*Myrica* spp.: **bayberry, wax myrtle**. Pinene, limonene, **myrcine**, linalool.
Myristicaceae	*Myristica fragrans*: **mace, nutmeg**. Safrole, eugenol, camphene, cymene, **myristicine**, etc.
Myrtaceae	*Eucalyptus* spp.: eucalyptus, blue gum tree. Contains eucalyptol (cineol) and citriodol, which acts as an **antibiotic**.

Pimenta racemosa: wild cinnamon. Eugenol, pinene, myrcene, limonene, cineol, etc.

Syzygium* aromaticum: **cloves**. Essential oil has many compounds such as 2-heptanone, 2-heptanol. Eugenol is the major component.

Oleaceae	*Chionanthus virginica*: grey beard root. Phyllerin, the aglycone phillogenin, glucosides, saponin.

Ligustrum vulgare: **privet**. Ligustrin, ligustrone, syringin.

Palmae	*Areca catechu*: kramuca, areca, betel-nut palm. **Arecoline, arecaine, arecaidine, arecolidine**, etc. Tannins.

Daemonorops draco: dragon's blood. contains dra corestinotannol.

Serenoa repens: **saw palmetto. Beta-sitosterol**.

Papaveraceae	*Argemone mexicana*: yellow thistle, wild poppy, prickly poppy. **Allocryptine, berberine, codeine, chelerythrine, morphine**, etc.

Chelidonium majus: celandine, celidonia, nipplewort. **Allocryptine, berberine, sanguinarine**, etc.

Papaver spp.: poppy, amapola. Numerous alkaloids, e.g., **thebaine, morphine, codeine**, etc.

Sanguinaria canadensis: **bloodroot**. The alkaloids α- and β-**allocryptine, berberine, chelerythrine, sanguinarine**, etc.

Pedaliaceae
: *Harpagophytum procumbens*: grapple plant, wood spider. Harpagoside, harpagide.

Phytolaccaceae
: *Phytolacca americana*: **poke**. Contains caryophyllene, **betanine**, phytolaccanin, and the active ingredient phytolaccin. Toxic.

Pinaceae
: *Juniperus* spp.: **juniper**. Contains 4-terpineol, etc. Toxic.

Piperacea
: e*Piper* spp.: **pepper**. Contains alkaloids as the active agents.

Plantaginaceae
: *Plantago major*: **plantain**, plantago. Contains aucubin as the active agent, plus resin, tannin. Also allahtoin, adenine, choline.

Polygoniaceae
: *Polygonum* spp.: knotgrass, knotweed, **bistort**, snakeweed. Glycosides, various organic acids.

Rheum officinale: Chinese **rhubarb**. Anthraquinones, **chrysophanic acid**.

Rumex spp.: **sorrel, dock**. Aanthraquinones, tannins.

Polypodiaceae
: *Dryopteris filix-mas*: male fern. Contains oleosorin, tannin, etc.

Ranunculaceae
: *Aconitum napellus*: monkshood, wolfsbane. **Aconine, aconitine, benzaconine, ephedrine**, etc. **Cancer root** from Solzhenitsyn's *Cancer Ward*. Very toxic.

Anemone pulsatilla: pulsatilla, pasqueflower. Contains anemonin.

Aquilegia vulgaris: columbine. Contains delphinidin-3,5-diglucoside, **HCN**.

Clematis vitalba: wild clematis, clematide, traveler's joy. Contains anemone, **beta-sitosterol**, etc.

Helleborus niger: black hellebore. Contains the glucosides helleborin and helleborein. Toxic.

Hydrastis canadensis: hydrastis, **goldenseal**. **Berberine, canadine, hydrastine**, etc.

Paeonia officinalis: peonia, **peony**. Organic acids, glutamine, arginine, tannin. Contains the alkaloid **peregrinine**.

Ranunculus bulbosus: bulbous **buttercup**, crowfoot. Contains ranunculin, protoanemonin, labenzyme.

Rhamnaceae
: *Frangula* * *alnus*: buckthorn. Anthraquinone glycosides.

Rhamnus purshianus: **cascara** sagrada, buckthorn. Anthracenes, O-glycosides, emodins.

Ziziphus spina-christi: jujube, syrian Christthorne, thorns. The anticancer agent is **beta-sitosterol**. Alkaloids include **amphibine A, E, F** and **mauritine A, C**.

Rosaceae
: *Agrimonia eupatoria*: agrimony. Glucosides, **alkaloids**, nicotinic acid amide.

Filipendula ulmaria: rodarum, meadow-sweet. Contains salicin.

Malus sylvestris: malum, pomi, **apple**. Seeds contain **HCN** as amygdalin or laetrile. There is also an antibacterial substance present called phloretin.

Prunus spp.: **almond, cherry, plum, peach, apricot**. Contains the **cyanoglycoside** amygdalin or latrile. The enzyme **betaglucosidase** is said to occur preferentially in tumor cells, and acts to break down the cyanoglycoside to produce HCN in the tumor.

Rubiaceae
: *Cinchona*: cinchona, Peruvian bark, **quinine** tree. Contains many quinoline **alkaloids**.

Coffea * spp.: coffee. Acetaldehydes, **caffeine, theobromine**, etc.

Rutaceae
: *Ruta graveolens*: **rue**. Arorinine, γ-**fagarine, graveoline**, etc.

Santalaceae
: *Santalum album*: white sandal, sandalwood. Contains santanols, **beta-sitosterol**, etc.

Sapindaceae
: *Bligha sapida*: African akee. Contains the hypoglycemic agents hypoglycin A and B, but too toxic to use.

Saxifragaceae
: *Hydrangea arborescens*: **hydrangea**. **Rutin**, tannin, **kaempferol, quercetin**.

Scrophulariaceae
: *Digitalis purpurea*: foxglove, digitalis. Contains cardioglucosides, e.g., digitalis, digoxin, digitoxin. **Digitoxin** has **antitumor** properties. Other compounds include the glycosides digitalein, **digitaline**, digitin, digitonin, as well as digitoxin. The seeds contain gitonin and tigonin. Still other compounds include luteolin, luteolin-7-D-glucoside, plus choline, acetylcholine, caffeic acid, etc.

	Euphrasia officinalis: eufragia, **eyebright**. Tannins, glycosides, **beta-sitosterol**.
Simarubaceae	*Quassia amara*: quassia. Contains quassin, quassinol, **beta-sitosterol**, etc.
Solanaceae	*Atropa bella-donna*: deadly nightshade, belladonna. **Hyoscamine, hyoscine**, tannin, pyridine, choline, etc. Toxic.

Euphrasia officinalis: eufragia, **eyebright**. Tannins, glycosides, **beta-sitosterol**.

Simarubaceae   *Quassia amara*: quassia. Contains quassin, quassinol, **beta-sitosterol**, etc.

Solanaceae   *Atropa bella-donna*: deadly nightshade, belladonna. **Hyoscamine, hyoscine**, tannin, pyridine, choline, etc. Toxic.

Capsicum annuum: **cayenne pepper, paprika, sweet pepper**. Contains capsaicinoids, which can be either carcinogenic or anticarcinogenic.

Datura spp.: thornapple, **Jimsonweed**, Jamestown weed. **Hyoscine, hyoscamine**. Toxic.

Hyoscyamus niger: **henbane**, black henbane, hyoscyamus. **Hyoscamine, hyoscine**.

Lycopersicon esculentum: **tomato**. Contains **tomatine**.

Mandragora officinarum: mandrake. **Atropine, belladonine, hyoscamine, scopalamine, scopine**, etc.

Methystichodendron amesianum: culebra. Contains **solanaceous alkaloids, e.g., scopalamine, atropine**, etc.

Nicotinia spp.: **tobacco. Anabasine, nicotine**, etc.

Solanum spp.: nightshade, **potato**, bittersweet, **egg plant**. Miscellaneous **solanine alkaloids, e.g., solanine**, etc. Also **glucose dulcamarine** and **glycoalkaloids**.

Withania somniferum: winter cherry, asgandh, ashwagandha. **Anahygrine, hydrine, tropine, withaninine, nicotine**, tannins, flavonoids.

Sterculiaceae   *Cola acuminata*: bitter kola, obi, kola nut. Flavoring in cola beverages. Contains **caffeine, theobromine, and other alkaloids**.

Theobroma* cacao: chocolate, cocoa. Esters, hydrocarbons, lactones, monocarbonyls, pyrazines, pyrroles, etc. Plus **theobromine and other alkaloids**.

Styracaceae   *Styrax benzoin*: gum benzoin, styrax. Contains cinnamates, organic acids.

Theaceae   *Camellia sinensis*: **green tea. Kaempferol**, quercitrin, **theophylline**, xanthine, tannin, etc.

Thymelaeaceae   *Daphne mezereum*: mezeron, laureola. contains the glycoside daphnin plus **beta-sitosterol**.

Ulmaceae   *Ulmus rubra*: **slippery elm**. Cholesterol, campesterol, **beta-sitosterol**, etc.

Umbelliferae   *Aethusa cynapium*: petite ciguë, cicuta menor. **Cynopine** is the active principle.

Anethum graveolens: **dill. Threonine, isoleucine, leucine**, lysine, methionine.

Angelica spp.: angelica. Furocoumarins, beta-phellandrine, etc. Stalks contain bergapten; seeds sontain coumarins.

Apium graveolens: apium, **celery**. Seed oil contains limonine, **selenine**.

Centella asiatica: marsh pennywort, gotu kola, fo ti tieng. Contains **sitosterol** but no glucosides, alkaloids, or saponins.

Cicuta maculata: water hemlock. **Cicutine**. Toxic

Conium maculatum: poison hemlock. Contains **coniine and other alkaloids**. Extremely toxic.

Daucus carota: **carrot. Beta-sitosterol**, acetone, asarone, choline, **HCN**, limonene.

Ferula assa-foetida: assa fetida, **asafatida**. Contains disulfides.

Foeniculum vulgare: **fennel**, finocchio. Contains organic acids, camphene, linolene.

Petroselinum crispum: celinon, apium, **parsley**. Contains the glucosides apiin and myristicin, plus apiole, etc.

Pimpenella anisum: **anise**. Contains anethole as the active agent.

Oenanthe phellandrium: phellandrio, finocchio, aquatico, water-fennel. **Phellandrine**, gallactin, mannan.

Urticaceae   *Urtica dioica*: **stinging nettle. Betaine**, choline, lecithin, phytosterins, tannin. The stinging agents are acetylcholine, histamine, and 5-hydroxytryptamine.

Verbenaceae   *Lantana camara*: tembelekan, lantana. **Lantanine, lanthanine**, sesquiterpenes.

Verbena officinalis: **vervain, verbena**. Contains the glycoside verbenalin. Also citral, geraniol, **limonene**, terpenes. Also adenosine, tannin.

Zingiberaceae   *Kaempferia galanga*. Contains carene, camphene, borneol.

Zygophyllaceae   *Larrea tridentata*: **chaparral, creosote bush, greasewood.** (Not the Rocky Moun-
                      tain region greasewood *Sarcobatus vermiculatus* of the family Chenopodiaceae.)
                      Contains **NDGA** or nordihydroguaiaretic acid.
                      Peganum harmala: **wild rue, ruta, rue.** Contains the harmala alkaloids **harmine,
                      harmaline,** etc.

Antibacterial Plant Agents

Table I.1 Antibacterial Agents of Belize

Anacardiaceae	*Spondia radlkoferi**: hog plum. Also antiviral.
Araceae	*Anthurium* schlechtendalii*: pheasant tail.
Asteraceae* (Compositae)	*Chromolaena* odorata*: hatz. Contains monoterpenes and sesquiterpenes. Also antifungal.
Bignoniaceae	*Crescentia cujete*: calabash tree, camasa. Toxic.
Bixaceae	*Bixa orellana*: annatto, achiotl. Leaves contain flavonoids; seeds contain carotenoids.
Caesalpiniaceae* (Leguminosae)	*Caesalpinia pulcherrima*: bird of paradise flower, chamolxochitl. Also antifungal.
	Senna alata*: piss a bed. Also antifungal, anti-inflammatory.
	Tamarindus indica: tamarind. Also antischistosomal (acts against the trematodes or flatworms producing bilharzia, the tropical disease caused by snails).
Caricaceae	*Carica papaya*: papaya, pawpaw. Also antifungal, scaricidal (anti-worm), may act as a cardiac depressant.
Combretaceae	*Terminalia catappa*: almond. Aerial parts contain benzenoids, coumarins, lipids, lipids, saponins, tannins.
Euphorbiaceae	*Acalypha arvensis**: **cancer herb, hierba del cancer**. Possibly anticancer. (Hartwell lists a number of species of the genus *Acalypha* as hierba del cancer or yerba del [de] cancer.)
Lamiaceae* (Labiatae)	*Ocimum basilicum*: basil. Also insecticidal, antifungal, ascaricidal (anti-worm).
Malvaceae	*Sida rhombifolia*: chichibe, atibalâ. Also antifungal.
Mimosaceae* (Leguminosae)	*Mimosa pudica*: twelve o'clock, abormidera. Also antiviral.
Musaceae	*Musa acuminata**: banana. Also antitubercular, antiulcer.
Myrtaceae	*Psidium* guajava*: guava. Also antifungal.
Poaceae* (Gramineae)	*Cymbopogon* citratus*: lemon grass. Also antifungal, analgesic.
Portulacaceae	*Portulaca oleracea*: purslane, portulaca. Contains omega-3 fatty acids, antioxidants such as alpha-tocopherol, ascorbic acid, beta-carotene, glutathione.
Rubiaceae	*Hamelia* patens*: red head. Also antifungal, analgesic.
Rutaceae	*Citrus aurantium*: sour orange, orange. Essential oil also antifungal.
	Ruta graveolens: rue, ruta. Also antitubercular. Toxic.
Verbenaceae	*Lantana camara*: wild sage, tembelekan. Contains a polycyclic triterpenoid called lantadene. Also antifungal; leaf paste is antihemorrhagic. Toxic.

Source: Data from *Rainforest Remedies: One Hundred Healing Herbs of Belize* by Rosita Arvigo and Michael Balick, Lotus Press, Twin Lakes WI, 1993. Plant families, genera, or species **not** appearing in Hartwell's *Plants Used Against Cancer* are denoted by an asterisk.

Table I.2 Some Antibacterial Agents of Latin America and Africa

Anacardiaceae	*Anacardium* humile*: caju, caju, cashew. (Shrub or small tree of central Brazil)
Asclepiadaceae	*Calotropis (Asclepias) procera*: Dead Sea fruit, mudar. Latex contains heterosides, e.g., calotropin. also contains the proteolytic enzyme calotropaine, plus calactin, calotoxin, uscharidin, uscharin, vouscharin. Poisonous. (Shrub or small tree of northern Africa and the Middle East)
Celastraceae	*Maytenus buchananii**: Umutukuza, etc.
Euphorbiaceae	*Alchornea* cordifolia*: Christmas bush. Leaves contain alchornin, bark contains traces of alkaloids. (Shrub or small tree of tropical Africa)

| Labiatae | *Ocimum suave**: umwenya, etc. Contains a volatile oil composed of phenol, mostly as eugenol. (A savanna shrub of tropical, eastern, and southern Africa) |
| Moraceae | *Chlorophora excelsa*: iroko, kamba, nkamba, etc. Contains calcium carbonate, calcium malate, a phenolic substance called chloropherine $C_{18}H_{22}O_3$, which is a derivative of recorcinol. Also antifungal. (Tree in tropical Africa) |

Source: Data from *Some Medicinal Forest Plants of Africa and Latin America*, Forest Resources Development Branch, Forest Resources Division, FAO Forestry Department, Food and Agriculture Organization of the United Nations, Rome, Italy, 1986. Plant families, genera, or species **not** appearing in Hartwell's *Plants Used Against Cancer* are denoted by an asterisk.

Table I.3 Some Antibacterial Agents in Tropical West Africa

Agavaceae* (Amaryllidaceae)	*Dracaena* mannii*: asparagus tree. Rootbark used. Active ingredients not specified. (The plant family may alternately be viewed as Liliaceae.)
Amaranthaceae	*Achyranthes aspera*: amarga, chaff tree. Seeds contain oleanoic glycoside. Leprosy.
Anacardiaceae	*Mangifera indica*: mango tree. Kernel contains mangiferin, ethylgallate, phenylpropanoids.
Aponacynaceae	*Alafia* multiflora*. Latex contains alcohol-phenol, vanillic acid.
	Tabernaemontana glandulosa*. Bark contains hydroxycoronaridine, hydroxyibogamine.
Apocynaceae	*Thevetia neriifolia*: yellow oleander. Leaves, fruit contain aucubigenol.
Asclepiadaceae	*Calotropis procera*: mudar. Latex contains calotropain (an enzyme).
Bombaceae	*Bombax malabaricum, B. buonopozense*: cotton tree. Seeds contain gallic acid, ethylgallate.
Bromeliaceae	*Ananas comosus*: pineapple. Juice contains bromelain (an enzyme). Also anthelmintic (anti-worm).
Cannabinaceae*	*Cannabis sativa*: marijuana, hemp, Indian hemp. Resin, leaves contain (Moraceae)phenols.
Capparidaceae	*Crateva religiosa*: varuna. Total extract of stembark used.
Caricaceae	*Carica papaya*: papaya, pawpaw. Fruit, seeds contain protein.
Combretaceae	*Guiera senegalensis*: n'guier. Leaves contain gallic and catechuic tannins.
	Terminalia glaucescens*, T. avicennoides*. Bark contains gallic tannins.
Compositae	*Actanthospermum* hispidum*: star bur. Leaves contain essential oil.
Connaraceae	*Cnestis* ferruginea*. Roots, leaves contain squalene, myricyl alcohol. β-sitosterol, methyl-linolenate homologues.
Cucurbitaceae	*Momordica charantia*: African cucumber, balsam pear. Aqueous extract of leaves used.
Cyperaceae	*Cyperus rotundus*: nut grass, musta. Whole plant contains obturastyrene (cinnamylphenol).
Ebenaceae	*Diospyros mespiliformis**: swamp ebony, monkey guava. Rootbark contains plumbagin. Also antifungal.
Fabaceae* (Leguminosae)	*Cassia absus*: four-leaved senna, ringworm bush, chaksu. Seeds contain chaksine, isochaksine.
Labiatae	*Ocimum basilicum*: basil, ocimum. Plant contains thymol, eugenol.
	Ocimum canum*. Plant contains camphor.
Loganiaceae	*Strychnos afzelii**. Stembark (chewing stick) contains dimeric indole alkaloids.
Lythraceae	*Lawsonia inermis*: henna, Egyptian privet, cyprus. Leaves contain lawsone, gallic acid.
Malvaceae	*Sidi acuta, S. cordifolia*: bala. Aerial parts contain cryptolepine, vasicine.
Meliaceae	*Ekebergia* senegalensis*. Stembark may contain saponin, meliacin.
	Khaya senegalensis*: dry zone mahogany. Bark contains meliacins.
Menispermaceae	*Tiliacora* funifera*. Contains funiferine.
Moringaceae	*Moringa oleifera*: horseradish tree. Roots contain athomine, pterygospermine.
Myrtaceae	*Eucalyptus globulus*: eucalyptus, blue gum tree. Leaaves contain phenol acids, essential oil. Antitubercular.
Papaveraceae	*Argemone mexicana*: prickly or Mexican poppy, yellow thistle. Leaves, stems contain berberine, sanguarine.
Piperaceae	*Piper guineense*: black or Ashanti pepper. Fruit, leaves contain piperine, amide-alkaloids (terpenes), dihydropiperine.
Polygonaceae	*Polygonum salicylifolium*, P. senegalense**. Leaves, roots, stems contain flavonoids.
Ranunculaceae	*Thalictrum rugosum**. Leaves contain thaliadanine (an alkaloid).
Salvadoraceae	*Salvadora persica*: salt bush, toothbrush tree. Leaves, twigs contain organic sulphur compounds.
Sapotaceae	*Butyrospermum* paradoxum* v. *parkii*: shea butter tree. Nut contains triterpenic alcohols.
Solanaceae	*Capsicum annuum*: capsicum, Cayenne pepper. Fruit contains capsicidin (a steroid saponin).
	Solanum nigrum (*S. nodiflorum*): nightshade. Leaves contain solanine.
	Withania somnifera: winter cherry, asgandh. Leaves contain withaferine (steroidal lactone).
Thymelaceae	*Lasiosiphon* kraussianus*. Roots contain heteroside.
Umbelliferae	*Centella asiatica*: Indian pennywort. Leaves, stems contain asiaticoside.

Source: Data from *Medicinal Plants in Tropical West Africa* by Bep Oliver-Bever, Cambridge University Press, New York, 1986. Plant families, genera, or species **not** appearing in Hartwell's *Plants Used Against Cancer* are denoted by an asterisk.

Table I.4 Chinese Antibacterial Herbs

Acanthaceae	*Andrographis* paniculata* (Chuan Xin Lian). Dried aerial parts contain deoxyandrographolide plus andrographolide, neoandrographolide, dehydroandrographolide. Acts against staph, pneumonia, strep, dysentery, typhoid. Has a sedative action and may cause dissiness and palpitations, and may act as an abortifacient.
Araceae	*Phellodendron chinense** or *P. amurense** (Huang Bai). Dried bark contains many **alkaloids**, notably **berberine** (0.6–2.5%), plus **palmatine, phellodendrine**. Active against diphtheria, streptococci, dysentery bacilli. Acts like *Coptis* of the family Ranunculaceae.
Berberidaceae	*Berberis soulieana*, B. wilsonae*, B. poiretii**, or *B. vernae** (San Ke Zhen or Xiao Yeh Gen). Root contains **berberine** plus **berbamine, palmatine, jatorrhizine, oxycanthine**. Also promotes leukocytosis, and is a choleretic.
Bile (Dan Zhi).	Mainly from pigs, cows, sheep, and chickens. Contains bile acids, biliverdin, cholesterol, lecithin. Deoxybile acid is especially active. Bile inhibits most gram-positive bacteria. Acts against bronchitis, whooping cough, TB, jaundice, hepatitis, trachoma.
Caprifoliaceae	*Lonicera japonica, L. hypoglauca*, L. confusa**, or *L. dasystala** (Jin Yin Hua). Flower bud contains luteolin, inositol, saponins, and chlorogenic acid. The last-mentioned is the main active ingredient. Active against staph, strep, pneumonia, dysentery, typhoid.
Commelinaceae	*Commelina communis** (Ya Zhi Cao). Dried aerila parts contain awobanin, flavocommelitin, flavocommelin.
Compositae	*Achillea alpina** (Chi Cao): **yarrow**. Dried aerial parts contain **alkaloids**, essential oils, and **flavonoids**. Acts against staph, pneumonia, *E. coli*, and dysentery.
	Senecio scandens* (Quian Ji Guang): **groundsel**. Dried aerial parts contain lavoxanthin, chrysanthemaxanthin, **alkaloids**. Used in treating dysentery, appendicitis, pneumonia, bronchitis. Though the toxicity is minimal, another species called *S. nemorensis* (which is listed in Hartwell) is highly toxic, causing hepatic necrosis.
	Taraxacum mongolicum, T. sinicum*, or *T. hetrolepsis** (Pu Gong Ying): **dandelion**. Dried aerial parts contain taraxasterol, taraxerol, taraxacerin, taraxacin, and vitamins A, B, D. Acts against staph, strep, typhoid, dysentery, TB, and most gram-positive bacteria. Helps protect liver functions.
Cruciferae	*Isatis indigotica*, I. tinctoria*, or *Baphicacanthus* cusi* (family unidentified), *Clerodendron cyrtophyllum** of the family Verbenaceae, *Polygonum tinctorium* of the family Polygonaceae (Da Qing Ye): woad. Dried leaf contains about one percent of the glycosides indican and isatan B. (The hydrolysis of indican yields indoxyl, which oxidizes to indigo.) Acts against staph, pneumonia, and meningitis. Also against parotitis, respiratory infections, hepatitis, dysentery, gastroenteritis. Side-effects include nausea.
Cruciferae	*Isatis tinctoria* or *I. indigotica** or *Baphicacanthus* cusia* (Ban Lan Gen). Euphorbiaceae*Acalypha australis** (Tie Xian Cai). Dried aerila parts contain the alkaloid **acalyphine** plus tannic acid and gallic acid.
	Euphorbia humifosa* or *E. supina** (Di Ji Cao). Whole plant contains tannin and gallic acid. Acts against diphtheria, staph, strep, *Pseudomonas pyocyanea*, typhoid, dysentery, *E. coli*, whooping-cough. Also acts against diphtheria toxin as well as the bacteria.
Labiatae	*Prunella vulgaris* (Xia Ku Cao): **prunella**.
	Scutellaria baicalensis, S. viscidula, S. amoena*, or *S. ikninkovii** (Huang Qin). Dried root contains baicelein, baicalin, wogonin, β-**sitosterol**. Acts against staph, cholera, paratyphoid, dysentery, diphtheria, strep, pneumonia, spirochaeta.
Leguminosae	*Sophora flavescens* (Ku Seng).
	Sophoro subprostata* (Guang Dou Gen or Shan Dou Gen). Dried root and rhizome contain about 1% alkaloids, e.g., **matrine, oxymatrine, anagyrine, methylcytisine**. Non-alkaloids include sophoranone, sophoranochromene, sophoradin, daidzen, plus the glycoside *l*-trifolirrhizin which hydrolyzes to *l*-maackinin. Also present are pterocarpin and *l*-maachlain. Highly effective against TB, staph, epidermophyton, and *Candida albicans*. Works against bronchitis, tonsillitis, and laryngitis. An **anticancer** agent. Enhances tumor immunity. Nausea, dizziness, and headaches are side-effects, as sometimes are sweating, heart palpitations, convulsions. Prevents fall in white blood cell count from radiation therapy.
Liliaceae	*Allium sativum* (Da Suan): **garlic**. Garlic bulbs contain allicin, as an essential oil. Starting out as alliin, it is hydrolyzed by the enzyme alliinase to yield allicin and diallyl disulfide. The herb acts against staph, *E. coli*, typhoid, dysentery, cholera, diphtheria, pneumonia, TB, etc. It also has **anticancer** properties, and lowers blood pressure and the concentration of low-density lipoproteins. It reduces the incidence of heart attacks.
Oleaceae	*Forsythia suspensa* (Lian Qiao): **forsythia**. Dried fruit contains forsythol, phillyroside, oleanic acid, rutoside. Acts against *Salmonella*, cholera, *E. coli*, diphtheria, plague, TB, staph, pneumonia. Enhances body immunity and liver functions. Can cause vasodilation and hypotension.

Fraxinus rhynchopylla*, F. chinensis*, F. stylosa*, F. bungeana*, or *F. paxiana** (Qin Pi): **ash tree.**
Dried bark contains the glycosides fraxin and aesculin, which hydrolyze to fracetin and aesculetin.
Acts against dysentery, staph, strep. Produces hypnotic and anti-convulsive effects. Has been used
for **rheumatic arthritis.** Also toxic, causing coma and respiratory depression.

Polygonaceae
   Polygonum cuspidatum* (Hu Zhang): **knotgrass, bistort, snakeweed, bindweed, smartweed,** etc.
Dried rhizome contains the glycosides polygonin, glucofranglin, polydatin, and emodin, plus tannins.
The leaves contain the glycosides reynoutrin, avicularin, and hyperin. Acts against staph, strep, *E.
coli,* spirochetres, and TB. Plus jaundice, hepatitis, appendicitis. Can also cause liver damage, however,
and respiratory depression.
   Polygonum orientale (Shui Hong Cao). Contains orientin, vitexin, isovitexin, isoorientin,
plastoquinone-9.

Portulacaceae
   Portulaca oleracea (Ma Chi Xian): **purslane.** Contains high concentrations of potassium salts (7.5%)
plus catecholamines, notably norepinephrine, dopamine, dopa. Also vitamins A, B1, B2, PP, C. Acts
against *E. coli, Proteus,* dysentery, typhoid. Produces vasoconstriction.

Pyrolaceae
   Pyrola decorata*, P. rotundifolia chinensis*, or *P. rotundifolia* (Lu Xian Cao): **wild lettuce,
wintergreen.** Dried whole plant contains glycosides, e.g., arbutin, homoarbutin, isohomoarbutin. Also
the substances chimapillin and monotropein. Acts against staph, dysentery, typohoid, and *Bacillus
pyrogenes.* Can increase myocardial contractility and cause an antiarrhythmic effect.

Ranunculaceae
   Coptis chinensis*, C. deltoidea*, or *C. teetoides* (Huang Lian): **goldthread.** Rhizome contains 7–9%
berberine, also **coptisine, urbenine, worenine, jatrorrhizine, columbamine.** Enhances immune
system, but larger doses cause respiratory depression or paralysis.
   Paeonia suffruticosa (Mu Dan Pi): **peony.** Dried root bark contains essential oils and glycosides, e.g.,
paeonolide, paeonoside, paeonol, paeoniflorin, astragalin, paeonin, pelargonin. Acts against *E. coli,*
typhoid, staph, strep, pneumonia, cholera, appendicitis. Also an anti-inflammatory agent,
antihypertensive.
   Paeonia veitchii* (Chi Shao): **peony.**
   Thalictrum glandulissma*, T. culturatum*, or *T. foliosum** (Ma Wei Lian or Ma Wei Huang Lian).
Contains **berberine, palmatine, jatrorrhizine, thalictrine, thalidasine, thalicarpine, saponaretin.**
Acts like *Coptis.*

Rosaceae
   Potentilla chinensis* (Wei Leng Cai): **cinquefoil, potentilla.** Whole plant contains tannin, protein,
vitamin C, Ca^{2+} salts.

Rubiaceae
   Gardenia jasminoides* (Zhi Zi): **gardenia.**
   Hedyotis diffusa (Bai Hua She She Cao).

Saururaceae
   Houttuynia cordata (Yu Xing Cao). Dried aerial parts contain an essential oil consisting mainly of
decanoylacetaldehyde which can be converted to a compound called houttuynium. Another component
is methyl-nonylketone lauric aldehyde. The leaves contain quercetrin and the flowers and fruit contain
isoquercitrin. Acts against staph, typhoid, pneumonia, bronchitis, *E. coli,* dysentery, leptospira.
Stimulates immune system.

Schizaeaceae*
   Lygodium* japonicum (Hai Jin Sha Teng): **fungus.** Spores used.

Solanaceae
   Physalis alkekengi franchetti* (Jin Deng Long): **winter cherry.** Dried calyx contains a small amount
of **alkaloids,** plus vitamin C, physalien, physalin A, B, C and hystonin. Acts against dysentery, staph.
Also tonsillitis, sore throat, laryngeal infections. Stimulates myocardial contraction and produces
vasoconstriction, causing a rise in blood pressure.
   Solanum nigrum (Long Kui): **nightshade.** Dried whole plant contains saponin-like **alkaloids.** Six
solanigirines occur, called α-, β-, γ-, δ-, ε-, ζ-solanigrine. Saponin genins include disogenin and
tigogenin. Acts against mastitis, cervitis, bronchitis, dysentery, skin infections. Side-effects include
headache, vertigo, nausea, tenesmus (urgent need to urinate or defecate).

Thymeleaeceae
   Wikstroemia indica (Liao Ge Wang). Dried root or root bark contains wikstroemin,
hydroxygenkwanin, daphnetin, and acidic resin. Acts against staph, strep, pneumonia.

Valerianaceae
   Patrinia scabiosaefolia* (Bai Jiang Cao).

Unidentified
   Sargentodoxa* cuneata (Hong Teng)

Source: Data from *The Pharmacology of Chinese Herbs* by Kee Chang Huang, CRC Press, Boca Raton FL, 1993. Plant
families, genera, and species **not** listed in Hartwell's *Plants Used Against Cancer* are denoted by an asterisk. Alkaloids
are for the most part represented in **boldface,** as are other information items of potential interest.

Antiviral Plant Agents

Table J.1 Antiviral Agents of Belize

Anacardiaceae	*Spondias radlkoferi**: hog plum. Ethanol extract from leaf and stem active against Coxsackie B4 virus, herpes simplex virus, poliovirus.
Caesalpiniaceae* (Leguminosae)	*Tamarindus indica*: tamarind.
Fabaceae* (Leguminosae)	*Piscidia* piscipula*: jabin, dogwood. Extract from dried bark and root active against poliovirus II, herpes virus type 2, influenza virus A2 [Manheim 57], Vaccinia virus.
Lythraceae	*Lagerstroemia indica**: crepe myrtle. Leaves contain steroids. Extract from entire plant acts against measles virus, adenovirus, Coxsackie B2 virus, herpes virus type 1, poliovirus 1, Semlicki-Forest virus. Bark inactive except for measles.
Minosaceae* (Leguminosae)	*Mimosa pudica*: twelve o'clock, adormidera. Contains epinephrine adrenalin.

Source: Data from *Rainforest Remedies: One Hundred Healing Herbs of Belize* by Rosita Arvigo and Michael Balick, Lotus Press, Twin Lakes WI, 1993. Plant families, genera, or species **not** appearing in Hartwell's *Plants Used Against Cancer* are denoted by an asterisk.

Table J.2 Some Antiviral Plants from Tropical West Africa

Amaryllidaceae	*Hymenocallis littoralis**: spider lily. Plant contains lycorine. Antiprotozoal, inhibits measles and coxsackie viruses.
Apocynaceae	*Allamanda* cathartica*. Bark contains plumericin, isoplumericin. Antiviral to polio virus. *Catharanthus* roseus*: Madagascar periwinkle. Roots, leaves contain α-acylindolic acid (or perivine). A$_2$ influenza virus.
Caesalpiniaceae* (Leguminosae)	*Caesalpinia pulcherrima*: pride of Barbados, chamolxochitl. Alcoholic extract from plant used. Influenza and vaccinia virus, also antibactrial. *Caesalpinia bonduc*: bonduc, physic nut. Root, stem contain α- and β- caesalpins, δ-caesalpin. Anti-vaccinia virus, anthelmintic. Hartwell lists the species as *Caesalpinia bonducella*.)
Fabaceae* (Leguminosae)	*Canavalia ensiformis**: sword or horse bean. Seeds contain xanthones, canavanin (2-amino-44-guanidinooxybutyric acid), canavalin. Influenza virus. Also bactericidal and insecticidal. *Desmodium gangeticum*: tick trefoil, vidarigandha. Roots contain flavonoids. Also antibacterial. *Milletia* barteri*. Extract from stems contains saponin. Viricidal to Newcastle disease.
Menispermaceae	*Cocculus pendulus**, and related *C. indicum**. Aerial parts contain cocculidine, picrotoxin. Newcastle disease virus.
Myrtaceae	*Syzyfium** spp. and related *S. guineense* ? (the species *S. aromatica* is not found in West Africa). Buds contain eugenin. Acts against herpes simplex virus in low concentrations.
Olacaceae*	*Olax latifolia*. Roots contain mono- and poly-unsaturated acids (or their salts). Acts against arboviruses with lipoidal envelopes.
Primulaceae	*Anagallis arvensis*: anagallis, pimpernel. Plant contains oleanane triterpenes, curcubitacins. Acts against polio virus, Newcastle disease, and herpes virus.
Rhamnaceae	*Maesopsis* eminii*. Stems contain saponoside.
Rubiaceae	*Porterandia* cladantha*. Root, stem contain saponosides. Viricidal, acts against abscesses, furunculosis, bronchitis.
Rutaceae	*Citrus* spp.: lemon, orange, grapefruit, etc. Rind contains hesperidin. Vesicular stomatitus virus.

Source: Data from *Medicinal Plants in Tropical West Africa* by Bep Oliver-Bever, Cambridge University Press, New York, 1986. Plant families, genera, or species **not** appearing in Hartwell's *Plants Used Against Cancer* are denoted by an asterisk.

Table J.3   Chinese Antiviral Herbs

Amaranthaceae	*Alternanthera philoxeroides** (Kong Xin Lian Zi Cao). Fresh aerial parts contain saponin, coumarin, tannin, and flavins. Acts against influenza, encephalitis, **rabies**.
Caprifoliaceae	*Lonicera japonica, L. hypoglauca*, L. confusa*,* or *L. dasystala** (Jin Yin Hua). Flower bud contains luteolin, inositol, saponins, and chlorogenic acid.
Commelinaceae	*Commelina communis** (Ya Zhi Cao). Dried aerial parts contain awobanin, flavocommelitin, flavocommelin. Common cold, influenza.
Compositae	*Taraxacum mongolicum, T. sinicum*,* or *T. hetrolepsis** (Pu Gong Ying): **dandelion**. Dried aerial parts contain taraxasterol, taraxerol, taraxacerin, taraxacin, and vitamins A, B, D.
Cruciferae	*Isatis indigotica*, I. tinctoria,* or *Baphicacanthus* cusi* (family unidentified), plus *Clerodendron cyrtophyllum** of the family Verbenaceae, *Polygonum tinctorium* of the family Polygonaceae (Da Qing Ye). Dried leaf contains about one percent of the glycosides indican and isatan B. (The hydrolysis of indican yields indoxyl, which oxidizes to indigo.) Acts against influenza, encephalitis. Side-effects include nausea.
	Isatis tinctoria, I. indigotica*, or *Baphicacanthus* cusia* (family unidentifed) (Ban Lan Gen). Influenza, measles.
Labiatae	*Scutellaria baicalensis, S. viscidula, S. amoena*,* or *S. ikninkovii** (Huang Qin). Dried root contains baicelein, baicalin, wogonin, β-**sitosterol**. Acts against flu.
Polygonaceae	*Polygonum cuspidatum** (Hu Zhang). Dried rhizome contains the glycosides polygonin, glucofranglin, polydatin, and emodin, plus tannins. The leaves contain the glycosides reynoutrin, avicularin, and hyperin. Can cause liver damage and respiratory depression.
Ranunculaceae	*Coptis chinensis*, C. deltoidea*,* or *C. teetoides* (Huang Lian). Rhizome contains 7–9% **berberine**, also **coptisine, urbenine, worenine, jatrorrhizine, columbamine**. Enhances immune system, but larger doses cause respiratory depression or paralysis.
Saururaceae	*Houttuynia cordata* (Yu Xing Cao). Dried aerial parts contain an essential oil consisting mainly of decanoylacetaldehyde which can be converted to a compound called houttuynium. another component is methyl-nonylketone lauric aldehyde. The leaves contain quercetrin and the flowers and fruit contain isoquercitrin. Stimulates immune system.

Source: Data from *The Pharmacology of Chinese Herbs* by Kee Chang Huang, CRC Press, Boca Raton FL, 1993. Plant families, genera, and species **not** listed in Hartwell's *Plants Used Against Cancer* are denoted by an asterisk. Alkaloids are for the most part represented in **boldface**, as are other information items of potential interest.

Appendix K

Antifungal Plant Agents

Table K.1 Antifungal Agents of Belize

Arecaceae* (Palmae)	*Cocos nucifera*: coconut, coco. The dried shell is antifungal. The species is used worldwide in folk medicine.
Asteraceae* (Compositae)	*Chromolaena* odorata*: hatz. Contains monoterpenes and sesquiterpenes.
	Neurolaena lobata: jackass bitters. Leaves contain sesquiterpenes and flavonoids. Also insecticidal.
	Pluchea symphytifolia*: santa maria. Also insecticidal.
Caesalpiniaceae* (Leguminosae)	*Caesalpinia pulcherrima*: bird of paradise flower, chamolxochitl.
	Senna alata*: piss a bed.
	Senna occidentalis*: yama bush. Seeds are cardiotoxic.
	Tamarindus indica: tamarind.
Caricaceae	*Carica papaya*: papaya, pawpaw.
Cecropiaceae*	*Cecropia* peltata*: trumpet tree. Extracts of leaves and stems are fungicidal. Toxic.
Chenopodiaceae	*Chenopodium ambrosioides*: wormseed, payco, pazote, potato. Also for intestinal parasites. Carcinogenic. Toxic.
Fabaceae* (Leguminosae)	*Piscidia* piscipula*: jabin, dogwood.
Lamiaceae* (Labiatae)	*Ocimum basilicum*: basil, ocimum.
Malvaceae	*Sida rhombifolia*: chichibe, atibalâ.
Moraceae	*Ficus radula**: fig tree. The sap is antifungal.
Myrtaceae	*Pimenta dioica**: allspice.
	Psidium guajava*: guava.
Poaceae (Gramineae)	*Cymbopogon* citratus*: lemon grass.
Rosaceae	*Rosa chinensis*: red rose, China rose, yueh-chi-hua. (Cultivated)
Rubiaceae	*Hamelia* patens*: red head.
Rutaceae	*Citrus aurantium*: sour orange, orange.
Schizaeaceae*	*Lygodium* venustum*: wire wis. Leaves treat skin fungus.
Solanaceae	*Solanum rudepannum**: susumbra. Athlete's foot (a fungus condition).
Verbenaceae	*Lantana camara*: wild sage, Bahama tea. Contains a polycyclic triterpenoid called lantadene. Toxic
	Priva lappulaceae*: mosote. Leaves also for internal infections and external infections.

Source: Data from *Rainforest Remedies: One Hundred Healing Herbs of Belize* by Rosita Arvigo and Michael Balick, Lotus Press, Twin Lakes WI, 1993. Plant families, genera, or species **not** listed in Hartwell's *Plants Used Against Cancer* are denoted by an asterisk.

Table K.2 Some Antifungal Plants from Tropical West Africa

Acanthaceae	*Hygrophyla auriculata** (*Asteracantha* longifolia*). Plant contains steroid and triterpene glycosides. Also acts agains gonorrhea.
Amaryllidaceae	*Hymenocallis littoralis**: spider lily. Plant contains lycorine. Also antitubercular.
Caesalpiniaceae* (Leguminosae)	*Haematoxylon campechianum*: logwood. Wood contains ethylgallate. Also antibacterial.
Caricaceae	*Carica papaya*: papaya, pawpaw. Seeds contain benzylisothiocyanate. Also antibacterial.
Compositae	*Bidens pilosa*: bur marigold. Leaves contain phenylheptatriyene (phototoxic polyacetylene, external use).

446

Cruciferae	*Lepidium sativum*: common cress. Plant contains glucotropeoline essential oil with senevols. Also bactericidal.
Euphorbiaceae	*Phyllanthus niruri*: tamalaka, bhumyamalaka. Roots contain glycoflavones (kaempferol 4' and eryodictyol 7-rhamnopyrosid. Also for ringworm (tinea cruris), ulcers, scabies, jaundice.
	Ricinus communis: castor oil plant. Oil produces undecylenic acid. Also antibacterial.
Fabaceae* (Leguminosae)	*Desmodium gangeticum*: tick trefoil, vidarigandha. Roots contain tannins, indole alkaloids. Also antibacterial.
Moraceae	*Chlorophora excelsa*: African oak, iroko, kamba. Wood (leaves) contains chlorophorin (phenol). Also antibiotic and acts against termites.
Palmae	*Cocos nucifera*: coco nut. Nutshell contains phenols. Also antitubercular.
Papaveraceae	*Argemone mexicana*: prickly or Mexican poppy, yellow thistle. Leaves, stems, roots contain berberine, chelerythrine. Antibacterial, antiprotozoal. Seeds contain sanguinarine (toxic).
Piperaceae	*Piper nigrum*: black pepper. Essential ois is fungicidal.
Zingiberaceae	*Alpinia speciosa**, *A. officinarum*, etc.: galangal, galanger Rhizome contains flavonoids. Also antibacterial.

Source: Data from *Medicinal Plants in Tropical West Africa* by Bep Oliver-Bever, Cambridge University Press, New York, 1986. Plant families, genera, or species **not** appearing in Hartwell's *Plants Used Against Cancer* are denoted by an asterisk.

Table K.3   Chinese Antifungal Herbs

Iridaceae	*Belamcanda chinensis* (She Gan).
Leguminosae	*Sophora flavescens* (Ku Seng).
Rutaceae	*Dictamnus dasycarpus** (Bai Xian Pi): **dittany**. Dried root bark contains the alkaloids **dictamine, skimmianine, γ-fagarine, preskimmianine, isomaculosindine**. Plus limonin, obakinone, fraxinellone, psorelen, aurapten, bergapten, and saponins and essential oils. Treats dermatitis, psoriasis, itching. Also acts against hepatitis.
Vitaceae	*Ampelopsis* (Bai Lian).

Source: Data from *The Pharmacology of Chinese Herbs* by Kee Chang Huang, CRC Press, Boca Raton FL, 1993. Plant families, genera, or species **not** listed in Hartwell's *Plants Used Against Cancer* are denoted by an asterisk. Alkaloids are for the most part represented in **boldface**, as are other information items of potential interest.

Miscellaneous Plant Agents

Table L.1 Some Other Therapeutic Agents of Belize

Amaranthaceae	*Amaranthus dubius**: amaranth. Contains lipids, triterpenes, steroids. Tea from leaves used for anemia.
Annonaceae	*Annona reticulata*: wild custard apple. Contains indole alkaloids, isoquinoline alkaloids, lactones, sesquiterpenes, diterpenes, leucoanthocyanins. Dried aerial parts in a dilute ethanol-water extract are insecticidal.
Asteraceae* (Compositae)	*Neurolaena lobata*: jackass bitters. Leaves contain sesquiterpenes and flavonoids. Malaria, amoebas, intestinal parasites.
Burseraceae	*Bursera* simaruba*: gumbolimbo. Bark extract mulluscidal.
Fabaceae* (Leguminosae)	*Desmodium adscendens**: strong back. Asthma.
	Gliricidia sepium*: madre de cacao. Contains flavonoids and carbohydrates. Insecticidal, active against *Aedes aegypti* (yellow fever mosquito).
	Piscidia piscipula*: jabin, dogwood. Extract from dried wood molluscidal.
Lamiaceae* (Labiatae)	*Hyptis verticillata*: John Charles. Leaves and stem contain lignan podophyllotoxin. Methanol extract molluscidial.
Meliaceae	*Cedrela* odorata*: cedar. Molluscicidal.
Minozaceae*	*Acacia cornigera*: cockspur. Bark for snakebite, internally and externally. Tea from thorns for asthma.
Piperaceae	*Piper amalago**: buttonwood. Contains triterpenes, steroids, proteids, alkaloids, sesquiterpenes. Molluscicidal.
Rhamnaceae	*Krugiodendron* ferreum*: ax master. Tea from bark for anemia.
Sapindaceae	*Paullinia tomentosa**: cross vine. Root extract insecticidal, molluscidal.
Simaroubaceae	*Simarouba glauca**: negrito. Contains degraded triterpenes (quassinoids, simaroubolides). Active against malaria, that is, against the parasite *Plasmodeum gallinaceum*.
Smilacaceae* (Liliaceae)	*Smilax lanceolata**: China root. Tea from roots for anemia.
Solanaceae	*Solanum rudepannum**: susumbra. Snakebite poultice. Athlete's foot (a fungus condition).

Source: Data from *Rainforest Remedies: One Hundred Healing Herbs of Belize* by Rosita Arvigo and Michael Balick, Lotus Press, Twin Lakes WI, 1993. Plant families, genera, or species **not** listed in Hartwell's *Plants Used Against Cancer* are denoted by an asterisk.

Table L.2 Some Antiprotozoal Plants from Tropical West Africa

Apocynaceae	*Alstonia boonei**: stoolwood, pattern wood. Bark contains echitamine, possibly plumeried. Acts against filariasis (Calabar swellings).
Bignoniaceae	*Newbouldia laevis*: osensenama. Bark contains harmane derivatives, harmine, harmol. Also anthelmintic.
Bixaceae	*Bixa orellana*: anatto tree, achiotl. Seed-coat contains waxy materials. Intestinal parasites.
Caricaceae	*Carica papaya*: papaya, pawpaw. Leaves contain the alkaloid carpaine. Also antitubercular.
Euphorbiaceae	*Alchornea* cordifolia*: Christmas bush. Roots contain alchornine (an alkaloid).
	Euphorbia hirta: asthma herb. Plant contains the triterpene euphorbon.
	Phyllanthus niruri: tamalaka, bhumyamalaka. Plant contains flavonoids. Also antibacterial.
Fabaceae* (Leguminosae)	*Albizia lebbeck*: woman's tongue, acacia. Pods contain saponins (the genins are triterpenoids, echinocystic acid, etc.).
Liliaceae	*Urginea indica*: Indian squill. Bulb contains scillarenin. Also inhibits rhinovirus.
Meliaceae	*Khaya senegalensis**: dry zone mahogany. Bark contains meliacin.
	*Trichilia roka**. Rootbark contains meliacins, catechuic tannins. Antimalarial.
Menispermaceae	*Chasmanthera dependens*. Root contains berberine. Trypanocidal.

	Tiliacora* funifera. Leaves contain funiferine. Antimalarial.
Mimosaceae*	*Acacia nilotica*: acacia. Leaves contain tryptamine, tetrahydroharmane.
(Leguminosae)	Acts against *Entamoeba hystolytica*.
Nymphaceae	*Nymphea lotus*: water lily, lotier odorant. Rhizomes contain nymphaeine.
Papaveraceae	*Argemone mexicana*: prickly or Mexican poppy, yellow thistle. Leaves, stems contain berberine. Also antibacterial.
Rubiaceae	*Cinchona* spp.: quinine bark., cinchona Bark contains quinine. Plasmodium, anti-amoebic.
	Mitragyna* inermis, M. stipulosa. Rootbark contains rhynchophylline.
	Pauridiantha* lyalli (not found in West Africa). Bark contains harmane derivatives, harmine, harmol.
Sapindaceae	*Paullinia pinnata**. Bark, leaves contain triterpenic saponins.
Simaroubaceae	*Brucea antidysenterica, B. guineensis*. Contins the bruceolides called bruceantin, bruceantinol, dehydrobruceins. Also antifungal.

Source: Data from *Medicinal Plants in Tropical West Africa* by Bep Oliver-Bever, Cambridge University Press, New York, 1986. Plant families, genera, or species **not** appearing in Hartwell's *Plants Used Against Cancer* are denoted by an asterisk.

Table L.3 Some Antimetazoal Plants from Tropical West Africa

Apocynaceae	*Carissa* edulis*. Twigs contain quebrachytol, cardioglycosides. Also anthelmintic, antiparasitic.
	Hunteria* umbellata (or *Polyadoa umbellata*): Erin tree. Alcoholic extract of bark used. Also acts as a smooth muscle depressant.
Capparidaceae	*Gynandropsis gynandra** : Cleome gynandra. Leaves contain glucocapparine (methyl senevol glucoside). Aamthelmintic.
Caricaceae	*Carica papaya*: papaya, pawpaw. Leaves contain the alkaloid carpaine. Seeds, latex contain carpasemin (benzylthiourea); the proteolytic enzyme papain (ascaridol) digests worms. Anthelmintic, amoebicidal.
Combretaceae	*Anogeissus* leiocarpus*. Root, stembark contain tannins.
	Quisqualis* indica: Rangoon creeper. Fruit contains sesquiterpene (santonin-like), quisqualic acid.
Ebenaceae	*Disopyros* spp.: ebony, persimmon Fruit contains plumbagin. Also insecticidal.
Euphorbiaceae	*Mallotis oppositfolius** v. *pubescens**: kamala. Leaves contain rottlerin. Tapeworms.
	Mallotus philippinensis (cultivated in West Africa): kampillaka, kampilyaka. Hairs from fruit contain rottlerin.
Fabaceae*	*Albizia lebbeck*: woman's tongue, acacia. Bark contains saponins.
(Leguminosae)	*Andira* inermis*: dog almond, wormbark. Rootbark contains n- methyltyrosine, berberine. Also anthelmintic, insecticidal.
Loganiaceae	*Spigelia* anthelmia*: pink root, wormweed. Roots, fresh leaves contain the alkaloids spigeline, spigeleine.
Mimosaceae*	*Acacia farnesiana*: cassie flower, cujf. Aerial parts contain ethylgallate, gallic acid. Also antibacterial.
(Leguminosae)	*Acacia nilotica*: acacia. Juice contains ethylgallate, flavonoids.
Polygalaceae	*Securidaca* longepedunculata*: violet tree, Senega root-tree. Roots contain saponosides. Also molluscicidal, intestinal parasites, antifungal.
Rubiaceae	*Morinda geminata**. Rootbark contains morindin (methylanthraquinone glycoside).
	Punica granatum: pomegranate. Bark contains pelletierin, tannates, friedelin. (Hartwell places this species in the family Punicaceae)
Rutaceae	*Citrus acida* (lime), *C. medica* (lemon). Rind contains the flavonoid hesperidin.
Zingiberaceae	*Alpinia galanga* and *Alpinia* spp.: galanga. Rhizome contains flavonoids.

Source: Data from *Medicinal Plants in Tropical West Africa* by Bep Oliver-Bever, Cambridge University Press, New York, 1986. Plant families, genera, or species **not** appearing in Hartwell's *Plants Used Against Cancer* are denoted by an asterisk.

Table L.4 Insecticidal/ Molluscidal Plants from Tropical West Africa

Apocynaceae	*Thevetia neriifolia*: yellow oleander. Fruit, leaves contain aucubine, which is an iridoid heteroside. Larvicidal and antibacterial.
Compositae	*Bidens pilosa*: bur marigold. Leaves contain phenylheptatriene. Insecticidal.
	Spilanthus uliginosa*: para or bresil cress. Flower-heads contain spilanthol, also called afinine (N-isobutyl-decatriene-2,6,8-amide). Larvacidal, kills anopheles, also kills cockroaches and bedbugs. (Hartwell spells the genus as *Spilanthes*.)
	Vernonia pauciflora*. Leafy twigs contain sesquiterpene lactones (as verolide and hydroxyvernolide). Termites.
Cucurbitaceae	*Momordica charantia*: African cucumber, balsam pear. Leaves contain momomordicin. Insecticidal, bacteriostatic.

Euphorbiaceae	*Euphorbia hirta*: asthma herb. Plant contains euphorbon (triterpene, quercitol). Insecticidal, also anti-amoebic and antibacterial.
	Hymenocardia acida*. Roots contain the alkaloid hymenocardine. Insecticidal.
Fabaceae*	*Afrormosia* laxiflora*: false dalbergia. Rootbark contains N-methylcytisine. Insecticidal.
(Leguminosae)	*Milletia* ferruginea*. Seeds contain rotenone, saponins. Insecticidal.
Labiatae	*Ocimum basilicum*: basil, ocimum. Leaves contain methylchavicol, eugenol. Anthelmintic, chases ants away.
Labiatae	*Ocimum canum**. Leaves contain camphor. Chases moths away.
Meliaceae	*Pseudocedrela* kotschyi*: dry zone cedar. Bark contains the phenolic lactone pseudocedrelin. Will kill goldfish.
Mimosaceae*	*Acacia nilotica*: acacia. Fruit, stembark contain tannins. Molluscidal.
(Leguminosae)	*Dichrostachys* glomerata*. Roots contain saponosides. Molluscidal.
	Pentaclethra macrophylla: oil bean tree. Root contains saponosides. Insecticidal.
	Tetrapleura tetraptera*. Fruiti contains saponosides (possibly as oleanic acid triglycoside). Insecticidal.
Pedaliaceae	*Sesamum indicum*: sesame, beniseed. Plant contains the lignan sesamine. Insecticidal.
Piperaceae	*Piper guineense*: black or Ashanti pepper. Fruit contains piperine, dihydropiperine, dihydropiperlonguminine, etc., and dihydrocubebin. Insecticidal, antibacterial.
Polygalaceae	*Securidaca* longepedunculata*: violet tree, Senega root-tree. Roots contain triterpenic saponosides. Molluscicidal.
Simaroubaceae	*Quassica* africana*. Stemwood contains quassin. Insecticidal, acts against threadworms.
Solanaceae	*Nicotinia tabacum*: tobacco plant. Juice contains nicotine, nornicotine, anabasine. Insecticidal. Also toxic to worms.
Verbenaceae	*Duranta* repens*: pigeon berry. Fruit juice contains isoquinoline (an alkaloid analog to nicotine). Insecticidal. Leaves contain flavonoids.
Zygophyllaceae	*Balanites* aegyptiaca*: soap berry tree, thorn tree, desert date. Stembark contains saponosides (the genins are dios- and yamogenins). Molluscicidal.

Source: Data from *Medicinal Plants in Tropical West Africa* by Bep Oliver-Bever, Cambridge University Press, New York, 1986. Plant families, genera, or species **not** appearing in Hartwell's *Plants Used Against Cancer* are denoted by an asterisk.

Table L.5 Anti-inflammatory Plants from Tropical West Africa

Boraginaceae	*Arnebia* hispidissima*. Flavonosides are the active constituents. Flowers contain vitexin (8β-D-glucopyranosyl-apigenin). Vitexin also occurs in the leaves of *Lophira lanceolata*.
Burseraceae	*Commiphora africana*: African myrrh, bdellium. Contains gum- resin. The resin contains essential oil com;posed of terpenoids and terpenoid glycosides; the gums contain polyholosides. In the Indian plant, *Commiphora mukal* (or *C. mukal*), the essential oil is composed of myrcene, dimyrcene, and polymyrcene. An ether extract yielded sesamin, cholesterol and other steroids such as the diterpenoids cembrene A and mululol plus fatty tetrols.
Combretaceae	*Terminalia ivorensis**: satin wood, shingle wood. Stembark is anti-Inflmmatory and contains terminolic acid, ellagic acid, sericic acid, quercetin, β-glycerrhetinic acid, and 2-8 hydroxy 18α-glycyrrhetinic acid. The wood also contains b-sitosterol, terminolic acid, and tri- and tetramethyl ellagic acid, plus laxiflorin and sitosteryl palmitate.
Convolvulaceae	*Ipomoea purpurea**, *I. pes-caprae*: goat's foot. The starchy root is commonly used by Indians for rheumatism, dropsy, and colic. The whole plant contains resins and essential oils. Compounds reported include triaconthane, pentatriaconthane, a sterol, berhenic acid and melissic, plus butyric and myistic acids. The roots also contain glycorrhetins. In Indonesia, the plant is not only used against inflammation but against **cancer**.
Cyperaceae	*Cyperus rotundus*: nutgrass, musta, cyperus. Rhizomes contain a fatty oil composed of oleic, palmitic, and linolic acids plus essential oils. The oil contains a sesquiterpenic ketone andα-cyperone. The oil from Indian tubers contains pinene, cineol, sesquiterpenoids, monoterpenic and aliphatic alcohols, β-sitosterol.
Fabaceae*	*Lonchocarpus cyanescens**. Wild indigo. Fresh leaves contain indigo, which yields indigotin. Roots
(Leguminosae)	are anti-inflammatory and contain glycyrrhetinic acid, rotenone, and lonchoterpene. The Nigerian plant, *Lonchocarpus laxiflorus**, contains the isoflavans laxiflorin and lonchoflavan plus pterocarpans.
Guttiferae	*Calophyllum inophyllum*. Flavonoids are the active constituents. Introduced from South India. Oil from the seeds applied topically. Leaves contain friedelin and the triterpenes canophyllal, canophyllol, and canophyllic acid. Heartwood contains the xanthones mesuaxanthone B and calophyllin B. Seeds contain the 4-phenylcoumarin derivatives calophylloide, inophyllolide, and calophyllic acid. Calophyllolide is the anti-inflammatory component. It is also carioactive and acts as an anticoagulant.
Periplocaceae*	*Cryptolepsis* sanguinolenta*. Roots contain the alkaloid cryptolepine.

Phytolaccaceae	*Phytolacca dodecandra**: endod, soapberry. Contains saponins (phytolaccosides), polyphenols. Saponins contain glucose or D-xylose as sugar component. The genins are phytolaccagenic acid, phytolaccagenin, jaligonic acid, and esculantic acid. In another species, the genins oleanic acid and bayogenin occur. (According to Hartwell, *Phytolaccaceae decandra* or *P. americana* is variously called poke, poleweed, poke root, or cancer-root.)
Rutaceae	*Afraegle** *paniculata*. Flavonosides are the active constituents. Stembark contains scoparone, imperatorin, xanthoxyletin. Fruit contains imperatorin, β-sitosterol, and another coumarin called xanthotoxin. The bark and fruit contain free aliphatic acids and a triacid triglyceride. The dried seeds contain lipids, plus oleic, stearic, palmitic, linoleic, linoleic, and palmitic acids. The leaves contain glucides, protides, and calcium. The coumarin xanthotoxin had anti-inflammatory properties. (Hartwell lists the genus *Aegle*, re the species *A. marmelos*, from India.)
	Zanthoxylum zanthoxyloides*: prickly ash. Rootbark contains fagaramide. Also has cardiovascular and anti-infectious properties.
Salvadoraceae	*Salvadora persica*: salt bush or toothbrush tree. Twig and roots serve as a toothbrush. Leaves and bark contain the alkaloid trimethylamine. Leaves and seeds contain a fatty oil composed of lauric, myristic, and palmitic acids. Roots contain β-sitosterol and elemental and monoclinic **sulfur**. Leaves contain the polyphenols quercetin and caffeic and ferulic acids. The rootbark contains tannins and saponins. Antibacterial action also reported.
Solanaceae	*Capsicum frutescens*: **Cayenne pepper**. Fruit contains the phenolic compound capsaicin, which is closely related to vanillin. Capsaicin or capsicin is a vanillylamide with the name 8-nonene-6 carboxylic acid. Fruits also contain vitamins C and A. Used mainly for local application. Also has antibiotic action.
	Solanum torvum*. Fruits contain sitosterol D-glucoside and the glucoalkaloid solasonine. Solasodine can be used to produce cortisone.
	Withania somnifera: winter cherry, strychnos, nightshade, ajagandha or asvagandha. Roots contain withaferine A plus steroidal lactones and withanolides, as do the leavves. **Withaferene A is a tumor inhibitor**. The plant also is also reported to have sedative and antibiotic properties.
Zingiberaceae	*Costus afer Ker-Gawl** (or *C. obliterans**, etc.): ginger lily, costus. Juice from leaves contains oxlaate, furan derivatives, and starches. Tubers yielded lanosterol, tigonenin, diosgenin. Also costugenin, anothr sapogenin related to sarmentogenin, and stigmasterol.
	Curcumo domestica or *C. longa*: **turmeric**. Oil from the rhizome is anti-inflammatory, on a par with hydrocortisone acetate and phenylbutazone. Also has an antihistamine effect.

Source: Data from *Medicinal Plants in Tropical West Africa* by Bep Oliver-Bever, Cambridge University Press, New York, 1986. Plant families, genera, or species **not** appearing in Hartwell's *Plants Used Against Cancer* are denoted by an asterisk.

Table L.6 Plasts Containing Hypoglycaemic or Antidiabetic Agents

Acanthaceae	*Hygrophila auriculta**. Roots contain lupeol (hygrosterol) and essential oil. Seeds contain steroid glycosides (phytosterols—the active principle). Leaves contain the alkaloid vasicine (peganine).
Anacardiaceae	*Anacardium occidentale*: cashew nut tree. Leaves contain quercetin and kaempferol glycosides.
	Sclerocarya* *birrea*. Leaves contain tannins and flavonoids as the active components.
Apocynaceae	*Catharanthus** *roseus*: Madagascar periwinkle. (Hartwell provides the listing under *Vinca*.) Leaves contain the hypoglycaemic alkaloids atharanthine (HCl), tetrahydroalstonine, leosine sulfate, vindoline (HCl), vinolinine. Leaves also contain anthocyanins. (The foregoing alkaloids are in addition to other alkaloids which occur, some of which are anticancer agents.)
Bignonaceae	*Tecoma stans**. Leaves contain the hypoglycaemin alkaloids tecomine and tecostanine.
Bombacaceae	*Ceiba pentranda*: silk cotton tree. Juice, roots, bark contain quercetol and kaempferol glucosides plus traces of gossypol, methylglucuronoxylan. Seeds contain β-sitosterol.
Compositae	*Centaurea perottetti**. The inflorescence (flowers) contains glycosides of the flavones apigenin, baicalein, luteolin, etc., plus the flavonols centaureidin, jadein, quercetin. Also present are β-sitosterin, β-amyrin, peptides, cnicin (centaurin, a sesquiterpenic lactone), and the alkaloid stizolphine.
Cruciferae	*Brassica oleraceae*: cabbage. Leaves contain the active principle, called vegulin, which loses its activity in about a month. Components include thioglycosides (methyl and ethyl propyldisulfides) and goitrogenic indole-myrosin glycoside (neo-glucobrassicin).
Cucurbitaceae	*Momordica charantia*: African cucumber, bitter gourd, balsam-pear. Fruit contains the following phytosterin glycosides (the active principle): charantin, momordicin, foetidin (β-sitosterol, β-D-glucoside, etc.).
	Coccinia* *grandis*. The tuberous roots produce a hypoglycaemic extract fraction containing caffeic acid, quercetin, kaempferol, β-sitosterol.

Euphorbiaceae	*Bridelia* *ferruginea*. Bark, roots, and leaves contain tannins, flavonoids, and biflavonoids, all based on apogenin and kaempferol moieties. *Phyllanthus nirui*: tamalaka, bhumyamalaka. Leaves contain the flavonoids phyllanthin and hypophyllanthin plus lignanes, quercetoside, alkaloids (norsecurinine isomers). The bark contains lupeol. *Securinega* *virosa*. Extract of seeds has hypoglycaemic action. Contains the alkaloids fluggeine, securinine, norsecurinine, virosine, etc.
Fabaceae* (Leguminosae)	*Lupinus tassilicus**. Seeds contain the alkaloids spartein and lupanine in hypoglycaemic fraction of quinolizidine alkaloids. *Macuna* *pruriens*: cow-itch. The powdered, decoated seeds contain protein, lipids, carbohydrates and the alkaloids mucinine and mucunadine, plus the soluble bases prurienine and prurienivrine. *Trigonella foenum-graecum*: fenugreek, etc. Seeds contain the hypyglycaemic alkaloid trigonelline (N-methylnicotinic acid) plus coumarin and nicotinic acid. (This species is an extensive entry in Hartwell.) *Vigna* *unguiculata*. The powdered, decoated seeds contain protein, lipids, carbohydrates. The mineral content includes calcium and phosphorus with traces of iron and vitamins.
Gramineae	*Hordeum vulgare*: barley. Germinating seeds contain hypoglycaemic principle. Must be separated from the hyperglycaemic principle (the sugars, hordenine, and vitamin B). The constituents include the alkaloids hordenine and gramine, etc., plus amylase, B vitamins, glucides, protides, lipids.
Liliaceae	*Allium cepa*: onion. Bulbs contain allyl-propyl disulfide (APDS), allicin (diallyl disulfide oxide), and methylalliin (in fresh juice, which is also bacteriostatic). Additional components are flavon glycosides, kaempferol, quercetin- and phlorglucin-derivatives. *Allium sativum*: garlic. Dried flower heads contain sulfur compounds.
Lythraceae	*Lagerstroemia speciosa**. Old leaves and ripe fruit yield the hypoglycaemic principle. The leaves contain terpenes and saponins.
Meliaceae	*Azadirachta* *indica*. Leaves contain acetylnimbin, nimbolid (lactone).
Moraceae	*Morus alba*, *M. nigra*: white and black mulberry. Leaves yield a hypoglycaemic extract fraction containing cyanidin and delphidin glucosides, rutin, moracetin (quercetin triglycoside), β-sitosterin, sitosteryl-carpate, and palmitate.
Musaceae	*Musa paradisiaca*: banana. Flowers will yield a hypoglycaemic liquid extract. the bracts contain anthocyanidins. The fruit contains hydroxytryptamine, glucides.
Myrtaceae	*Suzygium* *cumini*: jambul, Java plum. Seeds contain antimellin (a glycoside—the active principle) plus phytosterin, the alkaloid jambosine, essential oil, galli- and ellagi-tannins. The flowers and fruits contain cyanidine-2-rhamnoglucoside).
Papilonaceae* (Leguminosae)	*Phaseolus vulgaris:* kidney or haricot bean. Bean husks contain phasolon (the active principle), stigmasterin, querceturon (a glycoside: quercetin + gluconic acid), a sulfur compound, indole acetic acid oxidase inhibitor.
Periplocaceae*	*Gymnema* *sylvestre*. Leaves contain gymnemic acid, which consists of nine related glycosides.
Rhizophoraceae	*Rhizophora racemosa**: mangrove. Bark and roots contain tannins aand catechins as the active components.
Sapindaceae	*Blighia sapida*: akee apple, African akee. Fruit aryl (appendage) and seeds contain hypoglycin A (α-amino-2-methylene-L-cyclopropylpropionic acid). The seeds contain hypoglycin B (γ-glutamyl-hypoglycin A).
Scrophulariaceae	*Scoparia* *dulcis*: sweet broom weed. The whole plant contains the hypoglycaemic bitter principle called amellin. The constituents include scoparol (3'-O-methyl luteolin) and scoparoside (8-glycosyl-scopanol).
Tiliaceae	*Corchorus olitorius*: jute, molochia. A hypoglycaemic extract is produced from the leaves that is free of pectins, sugars, and fats, and which contains traces of elemental sulfur and zinc. The seeds contain the cardiac glycosides corcherosides A and B, their genin being strophanthidin olitoriside.

Source: Data from *Medicinal Plants in Tropical West Africa* by Bep Oliver-Bever, Cambridge University Press, New York, 1986. Plant families, genera, or species **not** appearing in Hartwell's *Plants Used Against Cancer* are denoted by an asterisk.

Table L.7   Chinese Antimalarial Herbs

Compositae	*Artemisia annua**, *A. apiacea*, or *A. capillares* (Huang Hua Guo): wormwood, sagebrush. Contains as the active antimalarial agent, the alkaloid **artemisinine**. Artemisinine is the source of 25 synthetic derivatives. Large doses produce severe myocardial damage.
Leguminosae	*Desmodium palchellum** (Pai Chien Cao). Dried aerial parts contain the alkaloid **bufotenine** and its methyl ester, called nigerin. Donoxime also occurs.

Saxifragaceae	*Dichroa febrifuga* (Chang Shan). Dried root contains as active ingredients the alkaloids α-, β-, γ-**dichroine** and **dichroidine**, plus 4-quinazolone. The herb is toxic.
Verbenaceae	*Verbena officinalis* (Ma bian Cao): vervain. Dried aerial parts contain the glycosides verbenalin and verbanol, plus adenosine, tannin, and essential oils. Also antibacterial and antiplasmoidal.

Source: Data from *The Pharmacology of Chinese Herbs* by Kee Chang Huang, CRC Press, Boca Raton FL, 1993. Plant families, genera, or species **not** listed in Hartwell's *Plants Used Against Cancer* are denoted by an asterisk. Alkaloids are for the most part represented in **boldface**, as are other information items of potential interest.

Table L.8   Chinese Antiprotozoal Herbs

Compositae	*Taraxacum mongolicum, T. sinicum*,* or *T. hetrolepsis** (Pu Gong Ying): **dandelion**. Dried aerial parts contain taraxasterol, taraxerol, taraxacerin, taraxacin, and vitamins A, B, D. Antispirochetic.
Leguminosae	*Sophora flavescens* (Ku Seng).
Ranunculaceae	*Coptis chinensis*, C. deltoidea*,* or *C. teetoides* (Huang Lian). Rhizome contains 7–9% **berberine**, also **coptisine, urbenine, worenine, jatrorrhizine, columbamine**. Enhances immune systems, but larger doses cause respiratory depression or paralysis.

Source: Data from *The Pharmacology of Chinese Herbs* by Kee Chang Huang, CRC Press, Boca Raton FL, 1993. Plant families, genera, or species **not** listed in Hartwell's *Plants Used Against Cancer* are denoted by an asterisk. Alkaloids are for the most part represented in **boldface**, as are other information items of potential interest.

Table L.9   Chinese Antitubercular Herbs

Moraceae (Cannabinaceae)	*Humulus lupulus* (Pi Jiu Hua): **hops**. Dried unripe fruit resins contain lupolone, humulone, isohumulone, isovaleric acid.
	Humulus scandens* (Lu Cao): **hops**. Aerial parts contain humulone, lupulone, choline, luteolin.
Unidentified	*Lysionotus* pauciflorus* (Shi Diaou Lan). Aerial parts contain organic acids, flavons, and the genin lysionotinum.

Source: Data from *The Pharmacology of Chinese Herbs* by Kee Chang Huang, CRC Press, Boca Raton FL, 1993. Plant families, genera, or species **not** listed in Hartwell's *Plants Used Against Cancer* are denoted by an asterisk. Alkaloids are for the most part represented in **boldface**, as are other information items of potential interest.

Appendix M

Some Bioactive Plants Found in the United States*

Anacardiaceae	*Rhus glabra*: smooth sumac, p. 250 (antiseptic: fruit, root, leaves) ▲
Annonaceae	*Asimina* triloba*: common pawpaw, p. 284 (insecticide, emetic, narcotic: fruit, leaves, seeds) ▲
Aquifoliaceae	*Ilex opaca*: American holly, p. 286 (malaria, epilepsy, emetic: leaves, bark, berries) ✖
Aquifoliaceae	*Ilex vomitoria**: yaupon holly, p. 232 (contains caffeine: leaves, berries) ▲
Araceae	*Arisaema triphyllum*: jack-in-the-pulpit, p. 202 (snakebite: root)
Aristolochiaceae	*Aristolochia serpentaria*: Virginia snakeroot, p. 224 (snakebite: root) ▲
Aristolochiaceae	*Aristolochia tomentosa**: Dutchman's pipe, p. 224 (**anticancer**, contains the anticancer agent aristolochic acid: leaves) ▲
Aristolochiaceae	*Aristolochia tomentosa**: Dutchman's pipe, p. 302 (snakebite: leaves) ▲
Aristolochiaceae	*Asarum canadense*: wild ginger, p. 138 (contains **anticancer** compound aristolochic acid: root)
Asclepiadaceae	*Asclepias quadrifolia**: four-leaved milkweed, p. 154 (warts: root) ▲
Asclepiadaceae	*Asclepias syriaca*: common milkweed, p. 154 (**anticancer**, warts: root, latex) ▲
Berberidaceae	*Berberis vulgaris*: common barberry, p. 236 (antibacterial, contains the alkaloid berberine: root bark) ▲
Berberidaceae	*Caulophyllum thalictroides*: blue cohosh, p. 206 (alkaloid methylcytisine, glycosides: root) ▲
Berberidaceae	*Diphylleia cymosa**: umbrella-leaf, p. 46 (**anticancer**: root) ▲
Berberidaceae	*Diphylleia sinensis**, p. 46 (**anticancer**, contains podophyllotoxin as does mayapple, snakebite, antiseptic: root) ▲
Berberidaceae	*Jeffersonia diphylla*: twinleaf, p. 46 (**anticancer**; whole plant) ▲
Berberidaceae	*Podophyllum peltatum*: mayapple, p. 46 (**anticancer**, contains podophyllotoxin: root) ✖ ▮
Betulaceae	*Alnus serrulata*: smooth alder, p. 256 (malaria: stem, bark)
Betulaceae	*Corylus americana*: American hazelnut, p. 256 (**anticancer, skin cancers**: inner bark, twig hairs)
Boraginaceae	*Cynoglossum officianale*: hound's tongue, p. 180 (**carcinogenic alkaloids**, insect bites: leaves, root) ▲
Boraginaceae	*Cynoglossum virginianum**: wild comfrey, p. 180 (leaves, root) ▲
Boraginaceae	*Echium vulgare**: viper's bugloss, p. 180 (alkaloids: whole plant) ▲
Boraginaceae	*Symphatum officianale:* comfrey, p. 180 (pyrrolizidine alkaloids: leaves, root) ▲
Cactaceae	*Opuntia humifusa*: prickly-pear cactus, p. 88 (**anticancer**: pad, fruit)
Caprifoliaceae	*Lonicera japonica*: Japanese honeysuckle, p. 298 (**anticancer, breast cancer**: bark, flowers, leaves)
Caprifoliaceae	*Triosteum* perfoliatum*: feverwort, coffee plant, p. 140 (snakebite: root, eaves)
Carophyllaceae	*Agrostemma githago*: corn-cockle, p. 148 (**anticancer**, warts: seeds) ✖
Celasteraceae	*Celastrus scandens*: American bittersweet, p. 298 (cardioactive: root bark, fruit) ✖
Cistaceae	*Helianthenum canadense*: frostweed, p. 98 (**anticancer**: whole, root)
Commelinaceae	*Tradescantia* virginiana*: spiderwort, p. 168 (**anticancer**, insect bites: whole plant)
Compositae	*Arctium lappa*: great burdock, p. 166 (**anticancer**, antiseptic, snakebite: leaves, root, seeds)
Compositae	*Arctium minus*: common burdock, p. 166 (**anticancer**, antiseptic, snakebite: leaves, root, seeds)
Compositae	*Artemisia absinthium*: wormwood, p. 220 (active principle is thujone, $C_{10}H_{16}O$, which affects nervous system: leaves) ✖
Compositae	*Artemisia annua**: annual wormwood, sweet annie, p. 222 (malaria, herbicide: leaves, seeds) ▮
Compositae	*Cacalia* atriplicifolia*: pale Indian plantain, p. 80 (**anticancer**: leaves)
Compositae	*Chamomilla* recutita*: German, Hungarian, or wild chamomile, p. 84 (**anticancer**: flower)

* *Source:* Data from *A Field Guide to Medicinal Plants* by Steven Foster and James A. Duke, Houghton Mifflin, Boston, 1990. Page numbers are cited, with **anticancer** bioactivity indicated in boldface. A few other bioactive functions or properties of interest are also noted, as well as the bioactive parts of the plant. Plant families, genera, or species **not** represented in Hartwell's *Plants Used Against Cancer* are designated by an asterisk. The symbol ✖ denotes toxic or extremely toxic or fatally toxic; ▲ denotes caution; ▮ denotes pharmaceutical use.

Compositae	*Chicorium* intybus*: chicory, p. 198 (antibiotic: root)
Compositae	*Cnicus benedictus*: blessed thistle, p. 120 (antibiotic: whole plant) ▲
Compositae	*Echinacea angustifolia*: narrow-leaved purple coneflower, p. 200 (**anticancer**, immune stimulant, snakebite, insect bites, **brown recluse spider bite**: root, whole)
Compositae	*Echinacea pallida*: pale purple coneflower, p. 200 (**anticancer**, immune stimulant, snakebite, insect bites, **brown recluse spider bite**: root, whole)
Compositae	*Echinaceae purpurea**: purple coneflower, p. 200 (**anticancer**, immune stimulant, snakebite, insect bites, **brown recluse spider bite**: root, whole)
Compositae	*Erigeron philadelphicus*: daisy fleabane, p. 164 (**anticancer**, hemorrhages: whole plant)
Compositae	*Eupatorium perfolatium*: boneset, thoroughwort, p. 78 (**anticancer**: leaves) ▲
Compositae	*Eupatorium rugosum**: white snakeroot, p. 78 (snakebite: root, leaves) ✖
Compositae	*Gnaphalium obtusifolium*: sweet everlasting, rabbit tobacco, p. 82 (**anticancer**: leaves)
Compositae	*Grindelia squarrosa*: gumweed, rosinweed, p. 122 (**anticancer**: leaves, flower)
Compositae	*Helenium* autumnale*: sneezeweed, p. 126 (NCI **anticancer** drug: flower, leaves) ▲
Compositae	*Helianthus annuus*: sunflower, p. 132 (snakebite: whole plant)
Compositae	*Hieracium venosum*: rattlesnake-weed, p. 130 (warts, snakebite: leaves, root)
Compositae	*Inula helenium*: elecampane, p. 122 (**anticancer**, rabies not mentioned: root, leaves, flower)
Compositae	*Liatris* aspera*: rough blazing-star, p. 196 (snakebite: root)
Compositae	*Parthenium integrifolium**: wild quinine, p. 78 (immune stimulant: root, leaves, top)
Compositae	*Prenanthes alba**: white lettuce, rattlesnake root, p. 80 (snakebite, dog bite: whole plant)
Compositae	*Senecio aureus**: golden ragwort, squaw-weed, p. 120 (pyrrolizidine alkaloids: leaves, root) ▲
Compositae	*Silybium marianum*: milk thistle, p. 198 (liver regeneration, contains the flavonoid silybin: whole, seeds)
Compositae	*Sonchus arvensis*: field sow-thistle, p. 128 (**anticancer**: root, sap, leaves)
Compositae	*Tanacetum vulgare*: common tansy, p. 124 (**anticancer**, antiseptic: whole plant) ✖
Compositae	*Trilisa* odoratissma*: deer's tongue, p. 196 (malaria, used as tobacco flavoring: leaves) ▲
Compositae	*Tussilago farfara*: colt's foot, p. 130 (pyrrolizidine alkaloids: leaves, flower) ▲
Compositae	*Xanthium strumarium*: cocklebur, p. 212 (rabies, malaria: leaves, root) ▲
Cruciferae	*Armoracia rusticana*: horseradish, p. 36 (**anticancer**: root) ▲
Cruciferae	*Brassica rapa*: field or wild mustard, p. 90 (**anticancer**: seeds)
Dioscoreaceae	*Dioscorea villosa**: wild yam, p. 204 (insect bites, **brown recluse spider bite**: root) ▲▋
Droseraceae	*Drosera rotundifolia*: sundew, p. 28 (warts: whole plant)
Ebenaceae	*Diospyros virginiana*: common persimmon, p. 284 (**anticancer**, warts: bark, fruit) ▲
Ericaceae	*Gaultheria procumbens**: wintergreen, teaberry, p. 26 (**anticancer**: leaves). Oil is highly toxic, absorbed through skin. ▲
Euphorbiaceae	*Euphorbia ipecacuana*: wild ipecac, p. 206 (emetic, snakebite: leaves, root) ▲
Fagaceae	*Quercus alba*: white oak, p. 228 (**anticancer**: bark) ▲
Fagaceae	*Quercus rubra*: northern red oak, p. 280 (**both anticancer & carcinogenic**, antiviral, antiseptic: inner bark) ▲
Geraniaceae	*Geranium robertianum*: herb robert, p. 146 (**anticancer**: leaves)
Gramineae	*Arundinaria* gigantea*: giant cane, p. 312 (may have ergot replacing seeds: root) ▲
Guttiferae	*Hypericum perforatum*: common St. Johnswort, p. 114 (antibacterial: leaves, flower) ▲
Hippocastanaceae	*Aesculus hippocastanum*: horsechestnut, p. 264 (malaria, lupus, prostate ailments: nuts, leaves, flowers, bark) ✖
Iridaceae	*Iris cristata**: crested dwarf-iris, p. 168 (**anticancer**: root)
Juglandaceae	*Juglans cinerea*: butternut, p. 276 (**anticancer**, antiseptic, herbicide: inner bark, nut oil)
Labiatae	*Collinsonia canadensis**: stoneroot, horse-balm, p. 112 (alkaloids: root, leaves) ▲
Labiatae	*Cunila* origanoides*: American dittany, p. 162 (snakebite: leaves)
Labiatae	*Glechoma* hederacea*: ground ivy, gill-over-the-ground, p. 192 (**anticancer**: leaves) ▲
Labiatae	*Leonurus cardiaca**: motherwort, p. 162 (conatains leonurine: leaves)
Labiatae	*Melissa officinalis*: lemon balm, melissa, p. 68 (*anticancer*: root)
Labiatae	*Mentha piperita*: peppermint, p. 188 (*herpes simplex*: leaves) ▲
Labiatae	*Mentha spicata*: spearmint, p. 188 (anticancer: leaves) ▲
Labiatae	*Salvia lyrata*: lyre-leaved sage, cancerweed, p. 192 (**anticancer**: root, leaves)
Labiatae	*Scutellaria lateriflora*: mad-dog skullcap, p. 186 (rabies, contains the flavonoid scutellarin: leaves) ▲
Labiatae	*Teucrium canadense**: germander, wood sage, wild basil, p. 162 (antiseptic: leaves)
Lauraceae	*Sassafras albidum*: sassafras, p. 278 (safrole or oil of sassafras is **carcinogenic**: leaves, twig pith, root bark) ▲
Leguminosae	*Apios americana*: groundnut, p. 158 (**anticancer**: root)
Leguminosae	*Baptisia leucophaea**: cream wild indigo, p. 116 (immune stimulant: leaves, flower) ▲
Leguminosae	*Baptisia tinctoria*: wild indigo, p. 116 (immune stimulant: root) ▲

Leguminosae	*Cercis canadensis*: redbud, p. 284 (**anticancer**: bark, flowers)
Leguminosae	*Medicago sativa*: alfalfa, p. 194 (**anticancer**: flowering plant) ▲
Leguminosae	*Telephrosia virginiana**: goat's rue, p. 118 (**both anticancer and carcinogenic**: root, leaves) ▲
Leguminosae	*Trifolium pratense*: red clover, p. 158 (**anticancer**: flower) ▲
Liliaceae	*Allium sativum*: garlic, p. 30 (**anticancer**: bulb)
Liliaceae	*Asparagus officianalis*: asparagus, p. 86 (antibiotic: root, shoots, seeds)
Liliaceae	*Erythronium americanum*: trout-lily, p. 100 (**antimutagenic**, gram-positive & gram-negative bactericide: leaves, root)
Liliaceae	*Hemerocallis fulva**: daylily, p. 134 (**breast cancer**: root, flower buds) ▲
Liliaceae	*Lilium canadense**: Canada lily, p. 134 (snakebite: root). Hartwell lists *Lilium candidum*.
Liliaceae	*Lilium philadelphicum**: wood lily, p. 134 (spider bite: root, flower)
Liliaceae	*Trillium erectum*: red trillium, wakerobin, bethroot, p. 138 (snakebite: flowers)
Liliaceae	*Veratrum viride*: American white or false hellebore, p. 104 (alkaloids: root) ✖
Liliaceae	*Yucca* glauca*: yucca, soapweed, p. 18 (**anticancer**: leaves, root) ▲
Liliaceae	*Yucca* glauca*: yucca, soapweed, p. 228 (**melanoma**, arthritis: root) ▲
Linaceae	*Linum usitatissimum*: flax, p. 178 (**anticancer**: seeds) ✖
Lobeliaceae	*Lobelia inflata*: lobelia, Indian tobacco, p. 184 (alkaloids: whole plant) ▲
Loganiaceae	*Gelsemium sempervirens*: yellow jessamine, p. 296 (**anticancer**: root) ✖
Loranthaceae	*Phoradendron serotinum**: mistletoe, p. 296 (epilepsy: leafy branch) ✖
Magnoliaceae	*Liriodendron* tulipfera**: tuliptree, p. 278 (snakebite, malaria: bark, leaves, buds)
Magnoliaceae	*Magnolia acuminata**: sweetbay, p. 282 (malaria, epilepsy: bark, leaves)
Malvaceae	*Malva neglecta*: common mallow, cheeses, p. 150 (**anticancer**, anti-TB, relative of okra: leaves, root)
Moraceae	*Cannabis sativa*: marijuana, p. 206 (gram-positive bactericide: leaves, seeds, flowering top) ▲■
Moraceae	*Humulus lupulus*: hops, p. 204 (antibiotic: fruits)
Moraceae	*Maclura pomifera*: Osage-orange, p. 282 (inedible fruit is an **anti-oxidant** and fungicide: root, fruit) ▲
Myricaceae	*Myrica cerifera*: wax-myrtle candleberry, p. 254 (oil is **carcinogenic**: leaves, fruit, root bark) ▲
Myricaceae	*Myrica gale*: sweet-gale, p. 254 (oil is antibiotic: berries, root, bark, leaves) ▲
Nymphaeaceae	*Nuphar luteum*: spatterdock, yellow pond lily, p. 88 (antagonistic alkaloids: root) ▲
Orchidaceae	*Cephalanthus* occidentalis*: buttonbush, p. 242 (malaria: bark). Hartwell lists *Cephalanthera* spp. ▲
Orobanchaceae	*Epifagus virginiana*: beech-drop, p. 224 (also called cancer root, but may not be effective as **anticancer** agent: whole plant)
Oxalidaceae	*Oxalis corniculata*: creeping wood-sorrel, p. 96 (**anticancer**: leaves) ▲
Palmae	*Serenoa repens*: saw palmetto, p. 228 (prostate disorders: fruits)
Papaveraceae	*Argemone albiflora*: prickly poppy, p. 12 (**anticancer**, alkaloids: stem, juice, seeds, leaves) ▲
Papaveraceae	*Chelidonium majus*: celandine, p. 92 (**anticancer**, warts: stem, juice, leaves) ✖
Papaveraceae	*Corydalis aurea**: golden corydalis, p. 106 (alkaloids: whole, root) ▲
Papaveraceae	*Dicentra cucullaria*, Dutchman's breeches, p. 12 (**anticancer**, alkaloids: leaves, root) ▲
Papaveraceae	*Sanguinaria canadensis*: bloodroot, p. 48 (**anticancer**, anesthetic, antiseptic: root) ✖ ■
Phrymaceae*	*Phryma* leptostachya*: lopseed, p156 (**anticancer**, boils: root)
Pinaceae	*Juniperus communis*: common juniper, p. 226 (**anticancer**: fruit) ▲
Pinaceae	*Juniperus virginiana*: eastern red cedar, p. 262 (**anticancer**, contains podophylloxin as in mayapple: fruit, leaves) ▲
Pinaceae	*Thuja occidentalis*: northern white cedar, p. 262 (**anticancer**, warts, fungus: leaves, inner bark, leaf oil) ✖
Plantaginaceae	*Plantago major*: common plantain, p. 72 (**anticancer**, antimicrobial: leaves, seeds)
Polemoniaceae	*Polemonium reptans**, p. 178 (snakebite: root)
Polygonaceae	*Rumex acetosella*: sheep-sorrel, p. 214 (**anticancer**: leaves, root) ▲
Polypodiaceae	*Adiantum capillus-veneris*: Venus maidenhair fern, p. 308 (snakebite, impetigo: whole plant)
Polypodiaceae	*Botrychium* virginianum*: rattlesnake fern, p. 310 (snakebite: root)
Polypodiaceae	*Pteridium aquilinum*: bracken fern, p. 308 (contains **carcinogens**: root) ✖
Pyrolaceae	*Chimaphila umbellata*: pipsissisewa, p. 44 (**anticancer**: leaves) ▲
Pyrolaceae	*Pyrola elliptica**: shinleaf, p. 44 (**anticancer**: whole plant)
Pyrolaceae	*Pyrola rotundfolia*: round-leaved pyrola, p. 44 (**anticancer**: leaves) ▲
Ranunculaceae	*Caltha palustris*: marsh-marigold, cowslip, p. 88 (**anticancer**: root, leaves) ▲
Ranunculaceae	*Xanthorhiza* simplicissima*: yellowroot, p. 240 (**anticancer**, contains the alkaloid berberine: root) ▲
Rhamnaceae	*Ceanothus americanus*: New Jersey tea, red root, p. 248 (snakebite, alkaloids: leaves, root)
Rosaceae	*Agrimonia purviflora**: small-flowered agrimony, p. 108 (**anticancer**: whole)
Rosaceae	*Prunus serotina*: black or wild cherry, p. 290 (contains cyanoglycosides: bark, fruit) ✖
Rosaceae	*Prunus virginiana**: chokecherry, p. 290 (contains cyanoglucosides: bark, fruit) ✖
Rosaceae	*Sanguisorba officinalis*: salad burnet, p. 160 (antibiotic: leaves, root)
Rubiaceae	*Galium aparine*: cleavers, p. 36 (**anticancer**: whole plant)

Rutaceae	*Zanthoxylum clava-herculis*: southern prickly-ash, p. 238 (**anticancer**: bark, berries)
Salicaceae	*Salix alba*: white willow, p. 286 (**anticancer**, contains salicin: bark)
Saxafragaceae	*Hydrangea arborescens*: wild hydrangea, p. 242 (contains cyanoglycosides: root, bark) ▲
Scrophulariaceae	*Pedicularis canadensis*: lousewort, wood betony, p. 106 (**anticancer**: root, leaves)
Scrophulariaceae	*Scrophularia marilandica*: figwort, p. 210 (**anticancer**: leaves, root) ▲
Scrophulariaceae	*Verbascucum thapsus*, p. 114 (**anticancer**, contains rotenone and coumarin: leaves flowering top) ▲
Scrophulariaceae	*Veronica officianalis*: common speedwell, p. 174 (antiseptic: leaves, root) ▲
Simarabaceae	*Ailanthus altissima*: tree-of-heaven, stinktree, p. 272 (malaria, contains potent antimalaria compounds: bark, root bark) ▲
Solanaceae	*Datura stramonium*: jimsonweed, p. 20 (**anticancer**: leaves, root, seeds) ✖
Solanaceae	*Datura stramonium*: jimsonweed, p. 182 (**anticancer**: leaves, root, seeds) ✖
Solanaceae	*Nicotinia tabacum*: tobacco, p. 152 (snakebite, stings: leaves) ✖
Solanaceae	*Physalis heterophylla*: clammy ground-cherry, p. 98 (**anticancer**, emetic: leaves, root, seeds)
Solanaceae	*Solanum dulcamara*: woody nightshade, p. 182 (**anticancer**, alkaloids: leaves, stem, berries)✖
Solanaceae	*Solanum nigrum*: common nightshade, p. 42 (**anticancer**: leaves, berries) ✖
Taxaceae	*Taxus canadensis**: American yew, p. 226 (**anticancer**: needles) ✖
Ulmaceae	*Ulmus rubra*: slipery elm, p. 294 (contains **anti-oxidant**: inner bark)
Umbelliferae	*Conium maculatum*: poison hemlock, p. 58 (**anticancer**: whole plant) ✖
Umbelliferae	*Daucus carota*: Queen Anne's lace, wild carrot, p. 58 (**anticancer**, bactericidal: root, seeds) ▲
Umbelliferae	*Foeniculum vulgare*: fennel, p. 110 (snakebite, bactericidal: seeds)
Umbelliferae	*Heracleum lanatum*: cow-parsnip, p. 60 (**leukemia, AIDS**, contains psoralem: root, leaves, top) ▲
Urticaceae	*Urtica dioica*: stinging nettle, p. 212 (**prostate cancer**: whole plant) ▲
Valerianaceae	*Valeriana officianalis*: valerian, p. 140 (antibiotic: root)

Anticancer Plants of the Neo Tropics

Table N.1 Anticancer/Carcinogenic Plants of Belize

Apocynaceae	*Catharantheus* roseus*: periwinkle. Contains 72 alkaloids including vincristine, vinblastine.
Caesalpiniaceae* (Leguminosae)	*Caesalpinia pulcherrima*: bird of paradise flower. Carcinogenic.
Chenopodiaceae	*Chenopodium ambrosioides*: wormseed. Carcinogenic.
Crassulaceae	*Kalanche pinnata**: life everlasting, tree of life. Rich in chemicals.
Cucurbitaceae	*Momordica charantia*: sorosi, condiamor. "The most renowned medicinal plant of Belize."
Euphorbiaceae	*Acalypha arvensis**: cancer herb, Hierba del Cancer. Inactive against colon cancer. (Called *Acalypha alopecuroidea* in Hartwell.)
Lamiaceae* (Labiatae)	*Hyptis verticillata**: John Charles. Contains the liginin podophyllotoxin.
Polypodiaceae	*Philebodium* decumanum*: bear paw fern. Cartenoids, flavonoids, steroids.
Rubiaceae	*Chiococca alba*: skunk root, zorillo. Coumarins, alkanes, carbohydrates, lignans.
Sterculiceae	*Capraria biflora*: tan chi, pasmo. Cytotoxic, contains the alkaloid biflorine.
	Guazuma* ulmifolia: bay cedar. Caffeine, tannins.

Source: Data from *Rainforest Remedies: One Hundred Healing Herbs* of Belize by Rosita Avigo and Michael Balick, Lotus Press, Twin Lakes WI 1993. Plant families, genera, or species **not** appearing in Hartwell's *Plants Used Against Cancer* are denoted by an asterisk.

Table N.2 Some Anticancer Plants of Middle America

Amaryllidaceae	*Agave cocui*: cocui.
Amaryllidaceae	*Crinum erubescens**: poison bulb.
Anardiaceae	*Rhus terebinthifolia*: quauhchichioalli.
Anacardiaceae	*Spondias purpurea**.
Annonaceae	*Annona reticulata*.
Annonaceae	*Annona squamosa*: custard apple, sugar apple, sweetsop.
Apocynaceae	*Catharanthus* roseus*: Madagascar periwinkle. (Or genus *Vinca*)
Apocynaceae	*Thevetia peruviana**.
Araceae	*Dieffenbachia seguine*: **mata del cáncer**, dicha.
Asclepiadaceae	*Asclepias curassavica*: **cancerillo**, red milkweed.
Begoniaceae	*Begonia* spp.: **begonia**.
Begoniaceae	*Begonia rotundifolia**.
Bignoniaceae	*Catalpa longissima**.
Bignoniaceae	*Jacaranda caerulea*: **cancer bush**.
Burseraceae	*Protium heptaphyllum*: tacamahaca, currucai.
Cactaceae	*Opuntia ficus-indica*: raquette, Indian fig, prickly pear.
Cactaceae	*Opuntia stricta** var. *dillenii**.
Chenopodiaceae	*Beta vulgaris* var. *cicla*: beet.
Compositae	*Ageratum conyzoides*: rompesaragüelo.
Compositae	*Ageratum houstonianum**.
Compositae	*Calendula officinalis*: eliotropium, **marigold**.
Compositae	*Egletes viscosa*: **Boton de Cancer**.
Compositae	*Gnaphalium viscosum**.
Compositae	*Helianthus annuus*: girasol.
Compositae	*Isocarpha oppositifolia*: **botón de cáncer**.

Compositae	*Mikania micrantha*: uahkoxiu.
Compositae	*Trixis radialis**.
Compositae	*Xanthium chinense**.
Cruciferaceae	*Brassica oleraceae*: **cabbage, cauliflower, Brussels sprouts**.
Cucurbitaceae	*Lagenaria siceraria**.
Cucurbitaceae	*Momordica charantia* var. *abbreviata*: balsam-pear, Melaõ de São.
Dioscoreaceae	*Dioscorea alata*: tepatli, ñame.
Equisetaceae	*Equisetum giganteum*: cola de caballo.
Euphorbiaceae	*Jatropha gossypifolia*.
Euphorbiaceae	*Pedilanthus tithymaloides*: chapolxochitl, mincapatli, flecha, etc.
Euphorbiaceae	*Ricinus communis*: castor bean plant (toxic).
Euphorbiaceae	*Tragia nepetifolia*: popox.
Fagaceae	*Quercus virginiana**: oak.
Gramineae	*Gynerium sagittatum*: caña amarga.
Gramineae	*Zea mays*: **corn**.
Labiatae	*Hyptis suaveolens*: mastranto.
Labiatae	*Mentha nemorosa*: yerba buena.
Labiatae	*Mentha spicata*: **mint**.
Lauraceae	*Cassytha filiformis*: akesbel.
Leguminosae	*Aeschynome fascicularis*: cabalpich, pega-pega.
Leguminosae	*Caesalpinia coriaria**.
Leguminosae	*Cassia occidentalis*: tlalhoaxin, ecapaatli.
Leguminosae	*Enterolobium cyclocarpum*: caro.
Liliaceae	*Allium sativum*: **garlic**.
Liliaceae	*Aloe barbadensis*: **aloe**.
Malvaceae	*Abelmoschus esculentus**: **okra**.
Malvaceae	*Abutilon abutiloides** (or *Hibiscus abelmochas*: kostuli, okra)
Malvaceae	*Bastardia viscosa*: chivatera, fistolera.
Malvaceae	*Alcea* rosea*.
Malvaceae	*Sida rhombifolia*: atabalâ, etc.
Meliaceae	*Cedrela odorata**.
Meliaceae	*Melia azedarach*: paraiso.
Meliaceae	*Trichilia hirta*: trompillo, cazabito.
Menispermeaceae*	*Cissampelos* pareira*.
Moraceae	*Cecropia peltata*: trumpet tree bois canon.
Musaceae	*Musa acuminata**.
Orchidaceae	*Vanilla inodora**: **vanilla**
Papaveraceae	*Argemone mexicana*: yellow thistle, wild poppy.
Papaveraceae	*Bocconia arborea*: cococxihuitl.
Phytolaccaceae	*Petiveria alliacea*: verveine, puante, payche, zorillo.
Piperaceae	*Pothomorphe peltata*: caisimón, pepper.
Piperaceae	*Pothomorphe umbellata**.
Plantaginaceae	*Plantago major*: plantain, plantago.
Polygonaceae	*Rumex crispus*: yellow dock.
Polypodiaceae	*Phlebodium* aureum*.
Portulaceae	*Talinum triangulare*: verdolaga de cabra.
Ranuculaceae	*Clematis dioica*: barbas de chivo.
Salvadoraceae	*Cissus erosa**.
Salvadoraceae	*Cissus sicyoides**.
Sapindaceae	*Sapindus* saponaria*.
Sapotaceae	*Chrysophyllum* cainito*.
Selaginellaceae*	*Selaginella* lepidophylla*.
Solanaceae	*Datura candida**.
Solanaceae	*Datura stramonium*: thornapple, Jimsonweed, Jamestown weed.
Solanaceae	*Solanum americanum**.
Solanaceae	*Solanum erianthum**.
Solanaceae	*Solanum melongena*: **egg plant**.
Sterculiaceae	*Melochia pyramidata*.
Tropaelaceae	*Tropaeolum majus**: chichira, hanucara, mastuerso.
Umbelliferae	*Centella asiatica*: marsh pennywort.
Verbenaceae	*Avicennia germinans*.

Violaceae	*Viola odorata*: **violet**.
Zingiberaceae	*Renealmia aromatica*.
Zygophyllaceae	*Kallstroemia maxima*: hierba de pollo.

Source: Data from *Atlas of Medicinal Plants of Middle America: Bahamas to Yucatan* by Julia F. Morton, C.C. Thomas, Springfield IL, 1981. Plant families, genera, or species **not** listed in Hartwell's *Plants Used Against Cancer* are denoted by an asterisk.

Table N.3   Some Anticancer Plants of the West Indies

Amaryllidaceae	*Hymenocallis tubiflora**: loyon dil.
Annonaceae	*Annona squamosa*: sweet sap, sugar apple.
Apocynaceae	*Catharanthus* roseus*: periwinkle. (Listed under *Vinca* in Hartwell.)
Bignoniaceae	*Jacaranda caerulea* or *J. coerulea*: **cancer bush**, horse bush.
Compositae	*Bidens pilosa*: Spanish needle.
Malpighiaceae	*Malpighia* coccigera*: myrtle.

Source: Data from *Medicinal Plants of the West Indies* by Edward S. Ayensu, Reference Publications, Algonac MI, 1978. Plant families, genera, or species **not** listed in Hartwell's *Plants Used Against Cancer* are denoted by an asterisk.

Table N.4   Some Anticancer Agents from Latin America and Africa

Anacardiaceae	*Anacardium humile**: cajù, cajú, cashew. Oil in the mesocarp (a layer enclosing the seed) contains cardol and anacardic acid. For warts. (Shrub or small tree of central Brazil)
Celastraceae	*Maytenus buchananii**: Umutukuza, etc. Stems contains maytanprine, maytanbutine, normaytansine. Fruits contain the sperimidine-type alkaloids celacinnine and celallocinine, the nicotinoyl sesquiterpene alkaloids maytoline and maytolidine. The chief secondary constituents are the group of ansa macrolide **antibiotics** represented by maytansine $C_{34}H_{46}ClN_3O_{10}$, from the stems. Maytansine is active against various tumors including B-16 melanoma, lymphatic leukemia, carcininosarcoma. Cytotoxic. Side-effects are dose limiting. Other specie contain antitumor phenoldienone triterpenes, plus a catechin and some pro-anthocyanidins. Used as a wash for **cutanaceous cancers**. (Tree of tropical Africa) Note: **The Japanese have discovered that maytensoids produced from the microsporum *Nocadia* are a more efficient source for maytensine.**
Moraceae	*Chlorophora excelsa*: iroko, etc. Wood contains calcium carbonate, calcium malate, a phenolic substance called chloropherine $C_{18}H_{22}O_3$, which is a derivative of recorcinol. Also antibacterial, antifungal. (Tree in tropical Africa)
Tiliaceae	*Luehea parvifolia**: mutamba preta. Contains tannin. External tumors. (Medium to tall tree in coastal areas of Brazil)

Source: Data from *Some medicinal forest plants in Africa and Latin America*, Forest Resources Development Branch, Forest Resources Division, FAO Forestry Department, Food and Agriculture Organization of the United Nations, Rome, Italy, 1986. Plant species **not** appearing in Hartwell's *Plants Used Against Cancer* are denoted by an asterisk.

Anticancer Plants of Africa

Table O.1 Some Traditional Plant Anticancer Agents from Africa

Apocynaceae	*Catharanthus* roseus*: Madagascar periwinkle. (Appears in Hartwell as *Vinca*.) Used in India, etc. Contains vincristine, vinblastine, vindesine.
Berbericaceae	*Podophyllum peltatum*: mandrake. Used in USA. Podophyllotoxin glycosides.
Boraginaceae	*Heliotropum indicum*: Indian heliotrope. Used in India. Contains indicine-N-oxide.
Celastraceae	*Maytenus buchananii**: bazimo, etc. Used in Africa. Contains maytensine and related compounds.
Euphorbiaceae	*Jatropha gossypiifolia*: physic nut. Used in Costa Rica. Contains jatrophone.
Simarubaceae	*Brucea antidysenterica*: kosam. Used in Ethiopia. Contains bruceantin.
Taxaceae	*Cephalotaxus* fortunei*: yew. Used in China. Contains harringtonine, homoharringtonine.
Thymelaeaceae	*Daphne mezereum*: mezerum. Used in several countries. Contains mezerein.

Source: Data from *Medicinal Plants and Traditional Medicine In Africa* by Abayomi Sofowora, Wiley, Chichester, West Sussex, UK and New York, 1982, p. 131. Plant families, genera, or species **not** appearing in Harwell's *Plants Used Against Cancer* are denoted with an asterisk.

Table O.2 Anticancer Plants of West Africa

Anacardiaceae	*Spondias mombin*
Annonaceae	*Xylopia aethiopica*
Celastraceae	*Maytenus senegalensis**
Compositae	*Vernonia amygdalina**
Cucurbitaceae	*Momordica charantia*
Euphorbiaceae	*Ricinus communis*: castor bean
Fabaceae* (Leguminosae)	*Abrus precatorius*
Labiatae	*Ocimum basilicum*
Moraceae	*Ficus asperifolia*
Musaceae	*Musa sapientum*: banana
Nyctaginaceae	*Boerhaavia diffusa*
Passifloraceae	*Adenia lobata*
Phytolaccaceae	*Hilleria latifolia*
Plumbaginaceae	*Plumbago zeylanica*: leadwort
Rutaceae	*Zanthoxylum gilletii**
Rutaceae	*Zanthoxylum xanthoxyloides**

Source: Data from *Medicinal Plants of West Africa* by Edward S. Ayensu, Reference Publications, Algonac MI, 1978. Plant families, genera, or species **not** appearing in Hartwell's *Plants Used Against Cancer* are denoted by an asterisk.

Table O.3 Some Anticancer Plants in Tropical West Africa

Anacardiaceae	*Mangifera indica*: mango tree. Whole plant contains tannins. Leaves contain the anthocyanidins as the 3-monosides of delphinidin, and as petunidin, paeonidin, cyanidin. Also leucoanthocyanins, catechic and gallic tannins, mangiferin (a flavonic heteroside), kaempferol and quercitin (both free and as glycosides). Used with success against transplantable cancers, namely adenocarcinoma and sarcoma. (p. 50)
Apocynaceae	*Rauvolfia* vomitoria, R. macrophylla, R. caffra, R. mannili*. Contain reserpine and ajmalicine (also called vincaine or δ-yohimine), the same as found in *Catharanthus* roseus* also of the family Apocynaceae, noted for antileukemic activity. (p. 37)

Convolvulaceae	*Ipomoea purpurea**, *I. pes-caprae*: goat's foot. The whole plant contains an essential oil, triaconthane, pentatriaconthane, a sterol, behenic acid, and melissic, butyric, and myristic acids. The root contains glycorrhetins. In Indonesia the plant is used against cancer. (p. 210)
Euphorbiaceae	*Euphorbia hirta*: Australian or Queensland asthma herb. Latex contains inositol, pyrogallic and catechuic tannins, and the alkaloid xanthorhamnine. Stem extracts contain **taxerol**, friedelin, β-sitossterol, myricyl alcohol, ellagic acid, hentriacontane. Others report ellagic, gallic, chlorogenic, and caffeic acids plus kaempferol, quercitol, quercitrin (as a genin of a heteroside), and a number of amino acids. The alcoholic extract of the whole plant acted as an anticancer agent against Friend luekemia virus in mice. (p. 114)
Euphorbiaceae	*Euphorbia tirucalli*: milk bush. Alcoholic and aqueous extracts from the stem reduced adenocarcinoma and sarcoma. (p. 162)
Malvaceae	*Sida cordifolia, S. acuta, S. rhombifolia*: balâ. Aerial parts noted to contain ephedrine. In the aerial and root parts the main alkaloids are ephedrin and Ψ-ephedrine. Other components are β-phenylethylamine, carboxylated tryptamines, quinazoline alkaloids, S(9)Nb-tryptophan methylester, hypaphorine, vasicinone, vasicine and vasicinol. In *S. acuta* and *S. rhombifolia* the main alkaloid is cryptolepine, originally found in the genus *Cryptolepsis* of the family Asclepiadaceae. In *S. acuta* growing in India, the alkaloids cryptolepine and ephedrine were found to occur in the roots, along with α-amyrin. An anticancer action was exhibited against human nasopharynx carcinoma (in a tissue culture), and against leukemia and sarcoma 180 in mice, as per CCNSC tests in the USA. (p. 120)
Meliaceae	*Melia azedarach*: Persian lilac, bead tree, peraiso, nimva. Extract from the leaves, bark, and seeds was slightly active against sarcoma 180 and adenosarcoma 755. (p. 182)
Papilionaceae*	*Abrus precatorius*: crab's eye, lucky bean. Contains the deadly toxic protein abrin, but has nevertheless been used to treat certain kinds of cancer. (p. 265)
Zingiberaceae	*Curcuma domestica*: turmeric. The volatile oil from the rhizome acts on **proteases** responsible for inflammation (e.g., in **arthritis**). Contains curcumol and curdione, both reported to be active against early cervical cancer. (p. 208) Note: Enzyme inhibitors for proteases are being tested as anticancer agents.

Source: Data from *Medicinal Plants in Tropical West Africa* by Bep Oliver-Bever, Cambridge Universtiy Press, New York, 1986. Plant families, genera, or species **not** appearing in Harwell's *Plants Used Against Cancer* are denoted with an asterisk.

Table O.4   Some Anticancer Plants of North Africa

Cucurbitaceae	*Cucurbita pepo*: pumpkin, gourd. The seed embryo contains an isoprenoid compound which has notable antihelminthoid properties (antiworm). It is also capable of arresting cell division, and has been used for instance against prostate cancer.
Euphorbiaceae	*Ricinus communis*: castor oil plant. Poultice of leaves for lacteral tumors. Oil for tumors. Seeds for skin diseases, leprosy, and skin cancer. Note: seeds are deadly toxic.
Liliaceae	*Colchicum autumnale*: meadow saffron, naked lady, autumn crocus. Contains the alkaloid colchicine.
Ranunculaceae	*Clematis flammula*: sweet virgin's bower. Used internally for cancer.
Umbelliferae	*Conium maculatum*: poison-hemlock. Contains five alkaloids, the most important being the highly toxic coniine. Nevertheless, weak dosages have been used against cancer.

Data *Medicinal Plants of North Africa* by Loutfy Boulos, Reference Publications, Algonac MI, 1983. Note: All plant families, genera, and species appear in Hartwell's *Plants Used Against Cancer.*

Bioactive/Poisonous Plants Found in Australia*

Anacardaceae or Mango Family
        Schinus molle: pepperina
        Toxicodendron* radicans: poison ivy
        T.* succedaeum or Rhus succedanea: scarlet rhus
Apocynaceae or Oleander Family
        Aconkanthera* oblongifolia: wintersweet
        Alamanda* cathartica: allamanda
        Catharanthus* roseus: pink periwinkle (*Vinca* in Hartwell)
        Nerium oleander: oleander
        Plumeria rubra: frangipani
        Thevetia peruviana*: yellow oleander or Cook tree
        Trachelospermum jasminoides*: star jasmine
Araceae or Arum Family
        Alocasia macrorrhiza: cunjevoir
        Anthurium* spp.: flamingo flower
        Caladium* x hortulanum: fancy-leaved caladium
        Dieffenbachia maculata*: dieffenbachia or dumb cane
        Epipremnum* aureum: pothos
        Philodendron spp.: philodendron
        Syngonium* podophyllum: syngonium
        Xanthosoma violaceum*: elephant's ear
        Zantedeschia* aethopica: arum lily or calla lily
Araliaceae or Aralia Family
        Hedera helix: English ivy
Asclepiadaceae or Asclepias Family
        Asclepias curassavica: red-head cotton bush
        Gomphocarpus* physocarpus or A. physocarpus*: balloon cotton bush
Cycadaceae* and Zamiaceae* or Zamia 'Palm' Group (Cycads)
        Macrozamia* spp. and Cycas spp.: zamia palm
Euphorbiaceae or Spurge Family
        Acalypha wilkesiana*: acalypha
        Euphorbia drummondii*: caustic creeper and red caustic creeper
        Euphorbia pulcherrima: poinsetta
        Euphorbia tirucalli: naked lady
        Euphorbia peplus: petty spurge
        Excoecaria agallocha: milky mangrove

---

* *Source:* Data from *Toxic Plants & Animals: A Guide for Australia*, edited by Jeanette Covacevich, Peter Davie and John Pearn, and published by the Queensland Museum, Brisbane, in 1987. Plant families, genera, or species **not** appearing in Hartwell's *Plants Used Against Cancer* are denoted by an asterisk.

Jatropha multifida: coral plant or physic nut
Pedilanthus tithymaloides: zigzag plant or slipper flower
Ricinus communis: castor oil plant (**ricin**)
*Sapium sebiferum**: Chinese tallow tree

Fabaceae* or Pea Family (Leguminosae in Hartwell)

Abrus precatorius: gidee gidee, crab's eyes, or jequirity bean (**abrin**)
Bauhinia spp.: bauhinia
Cassia spp.: cassia
Castanospermum australe*: black bean
Erythrina spp.: coral tree
*Lathyrus odoratus**: sweet pea
Vicia faba: broad bean
Wisteria floribunda: Japanese wisteria

Meliaceae or White Cedar Family

Melia azedarach var. *australascia**: white cedar

Myrtaceae or Myrtle Family

Eucalyptus spp.: gum tree
*Metaleuca quinquernervia**: paperbark tea-tree
Rhodomyrtus macrocarpa*: finger cherry

Ranunculaceae or Ranunculus Family

Consolidum orientalis* or *Delphinium ajacis*: larkspur
Delphinium spp.: delphinium
Ranunculus scleratus: celery buttercup

Solanaceae or Potato Family

*Brugsmansia** x *candida*: daturas, angel's trumpet
Cestrum parqui: cestrum
Physalis spp.: gooseberry and ground cherry
Solandra spp.: golden cup or chalice vine
*Solanum seaforthianum**: Brazilian nightshade
*Solanum pseudocapsicum**: Jerusalem or Madeira cherry
Solanum nigrum: blackberry nightshade

Umbelliferae or Carrot Family

Conium maculatum: hemlock

Verbenaceae or Verbena Family

Duranta repens*: duranta or golden dewdrop
Lantana camara: lantana
Vitex trifolia: vitex

Anticancer Plants of India and Pakistan

Table Q.1 Some Anticancer Plants from India

Acanthaceae	*Hygrophila auriculata**: talmalchana.
	Rhinacanthus nasutus: palakjuhi, thong pan chang.
Apocynaceae	*Catharanthus** *roseus*: Madagascar periwinkle. (*Vinca* in Hartwell.)
Asteraceae* (Compositae)	*Xanthium strumarium*: cocklebur.
Brassicaceae* (Cruciferae)	*Matthiola incana*: stock. leukoion.
Caesalpiniaceae* (Leguminosae)	*Cassia fistula*: Indian laburnum, cassia fistula.
Combretaceae	*Anogeissus** *latifolia*: dhawra, gum ghatti, axlewood.
Cucurbitaceae	*Trichosanthes dioica*: mahalcal, patola.
Ericaceae	*Gaultheria fragrantissima**: wintergreen. (*Gaultheria hispidula* is called **cancer wintergreen** in Hartwell.)
Fabaceae* (Leguminosae)	*Abrus precatorus*: jequirity.
	Indigofera aspalathoides: sivanimba.
Liliaceae	*Colchicum luteum**: golden collyrium.
	Drimia indica*: Indian squill.
Nyctaginaceae	*Boerhaavia diffusa*: hogweed, horse purslane.
	Commicarpus chinensis*.
Oxalidaceae	*Oxalis acetosella*: common wood-sorrel.
Polygonaceae	*Rumex acetosella*: sheep sorrel.
Rutaceae	*Glycosmis** *mauritiana*: jhati.
Symplocaceae	*Symplocos theaefolia*: diengpei, lodh tree.
Verbenaceae	*Vitex negundo**: nisinda, shambhalu.

Source: Data from *Medicinal Plants of India*, in two volumes, by S.K. Jain and Robert A. DeFilipps, Reference Publications, Algonac MI, 1991. Plant families, genera, and species **not** listed in Hartwell's *Plants Used Against Cancer* are denoted by an asterisk.

Table Q.2 Some Medicinal Plants of India and Pakistan

Apocynaceae	*Holarrhenia antidysenterica*: conessi bark, kurchi. Bark and seeds contain the alkaloids conessine, kurchine, and holarrhenine.
Apocynaceae	*Rauwolfia** *serpentina*: serpent wood, serpentine. The root contains six alkaloids, notably ajmaline, serpentine, and rauwolfine.
Aristolochiaceae	*Aristolochia indica**: Indian birthwort. Contains the alkaloid aristolochine.
Asclepiadaceae	*Pergularia** *extensa*: utran. A mixture of leaf juice and slaked lime applied to hard tumors.
Berberidaceae	*Berberis* spp.: Indian barberry. Contains the alkaloid berberine.
Caricaceae	*Carica papaya*: papaya, papaw. Used for warts. The digestive enzyme papain occurs in the milky juice of the unripe fruit. The glucoside caricin is found in the seeds.
Compositae	*Artimisia maritima*: wormseed. Used for skin tumors. Contains santonine.
Compositae	*Saussurea lappa*: costus. The alkaloid saussurine occurs in the root.
Compositae	*Xanthium strumarium*: cocklebur. Contains the glucoside xanthostrumarin. Decoction is a long-standing treatment for malaria.
Cucurbitaceae	*Citrullus colocynthis*: colocynth. Root powder mixed with castor oil for internal tumors. Root paste for external tumors

Euphorbiaceae	*Acalypha indica*: Indian acalypha. Contains the alkaloid acalyphine.
Euphorbiaceae	*Ricinus communis*: castor oil plant. The seeds contain the alkaloid ricine plus a deadly vegetable toxin.
Leguminosae	*Cassia tora*: foetid cassia. The leaves and seeds contain chrysophanic acid.
Loganiaceae	*Strychnos nux-vomica*: poison nut tree. Seeds contain the toxic alkaloids strychnine and brusine. Seeds in small doses have been tried or used for a wide range of disorders and diseases including gout and rabies.
Malvaceae	*Sida cordifolia*: country mallow. Contains the alkaloid ephedrine, especially in the seeds.
Nyctaginaceae	*Boerhaavia diffusa*: pigweed. contains the alkaloid punarnavine.
Salvadoraceae	*Salvadora* persicus*: tooth brush tree. Leaf poultice for external tumors.
Solanaceae	*Solanum nigrum*: black nightshade, common nightshade. Contains the toxic alkaloid solanine.
Violaceae	*Viola odorata*: violet. Tea from the leaves reported to be used for internal cancers. A leaf poultace serves for external cancers. The underground stem contains the alkaloid violine.

Source: Data from *Medicinal Plants of India and Pakistan* by J.F. Dastur, D.B. Taraporevala Sons, Bombay, 1962. Plant families, genera, or species **not** appearing in Hartwell's *Plants Used Against Cancer* are denoted by an asterisk.

Anticancer Plants of East and Southeast Asia*

Aizoaceae	*Tetragonia tetragonoides**: New Zealand spinach. Japan: decoction of dried plant.
Apocynacea	*Trachelospermum jasminoides**. China: tonic.
Aquifoliacea	*Amorphophallus** *riviera*. China: poisonous corm (underground stem) suggested for cancer.
Araliacea	*Aralia elata*: taranoki. Korea: fruits and stems. Japan: root.
Aristolochiaceae	*Aristolochia contorta*. N. China, Manchuria, Korea: root. Active constituents are allantoin, aristolochine, magnoflorine, aristolochic acid.
Betulaceae	*Betula latifolia**. Korea: bark.
	Betula platyphylla* v. *latifolia**. Korea: root bark.
Campanulaceae	*Codonopsis pilosula**. Kokonor: roots.
	Codonopsis tangshen. China: roots.
Cannabinaceae*	*Cannabis sativa*: marijuana, hemp. China, Indo-China: leaves, twigs, (Moraceae)seeds. Flowering twigs contain sesquiterpenes, cannabin, solid alcohols, hydrate of cannabin. Seeds contain protein, lipides, choline, trigonelline, xylose, inosite, acids and enzymes, phosphates, phytosterols. Resin contains cannabinol and cannabidiol, both toxic.
Caryophyllaceae	*Dianthus chinensis**. China, Indo-China: entire plant.
	Dianthus superbus*. China, Indo-China: entire plant.
	Silene aprica. Korea.
	Stellaria aquatica: alsine, chickweed. Japan: stem and leaves.
Compositae	*Carduus crispus*: fei-lein. Korea: above-ground parts when in flower. China: root.
	Taraxacum officinale: dandelion. China: poultice of macerated plant. Root contains inulin (a polysaccharide), essential oil, resinous matter, fatty acids, β-hydroxyphenylacetic acid. Plant contains saponins, choline, cerylic alcohol, arabinose (pectin sugar), and vitamins A, B, C.
Cruciferae	*Raphanus sativus*: radish. Indo-China: seeds for stomach cancer.
Dipsacaceae	*Dipsacus japonicus*. China: roots for breast cancer.
Ericaceae	*Gaultheria fragrantissima**. Indo-China: oil from leaves.
Ginkgoaceae	*Ginkgo biloba*: ginkgo. China, Japan: fruit. Kernel is antibiotic. Fruit extract is antitubercular. Seed coat contains bilobol, ginkgolic acid. Seeds contain starch, sugar, ginkgol, ginnol, asparagin, arginin, ginkgoic acid.
Guttiferae	*Garcinia morella*: t'êng-huang, gamboge. Thailand: gum resin. External cancers.
Hamamelidaceae	*Liquidambar formosana*. China: leaves and bark. Resin contains cinnamic alcohol, cannamic acid and ester, and 1-borneol. Essential oi lf the leaves contains camphene, dipentene, terpene.
Hydrocharitaceae*	*Ottelia alismoides*. China: poultice of stem and leaves.
Iridaceae	*Belamcanda chinensis*: she-kan. Manchuria, Japan, China, India: dried rhizome. Use cautiously.

---

* *Source:* Data from *Medicinal Plants of East and Southeast Asia*, compiled by Lily M. Perry with the assistance of Judith Metzger, MIT Press, Cambridge MA,1980. Plant families, genera, or species **not** listed in Hartwell's *Plants Used Against Cancer* are denoted by an asterisk.

Labiatae	*Ajuga decumbens*: isha nakasa, kiranso. China: juice from leaves for external tumors.
	*Leonurus artemesia**. Korea, Tibet, China: entire plant above ground, collected from May to August. Juice for external cancers.
	Scutellaria baicalensis. China: rootstock, rhizome. Roots contain glucose, starch, tannin, and the flavone derivatives woogonin (scutellarin) and baicalin.
Leguminosae	*Albizzia julibrissin**. China: bark, collected in spring or autumn. Lung cancer. Plant contains saponin and tannin..
	Erythrina variegata v. *orientalis*. Solomon Islands: crushed seeds. Leaves contain hydrocyanic acid (HCN). Seeds contain the alkaloids erythraline and hydrophorine, which have a curare-like action. Bark contains resins, fixed oils, fatty acids, hypaphorine, betains, choline, potassium chloride and carbonate.
	Gleditschia sinensis (*Gleditschia chinensis*): honey locust. China: seeds. Rectal cancer. Pods contain saponin; the bark contains arabinose.
	Phaseolus radiatus: ch'ih-hsiao-ton, hung-ton. China: seeds. The lima bean *Phaseolus lunatus*, a native of America, contains cyanogenetic glycosides which produce hydrocyanic acid (HCN) on contact with water in the presence of the enzyme linamarase or emulsin. This is especially so for beans growing in the wild. (Cooking is said to get rid of the HCN.)
Liliaceae	*Fritillaria* spp.: pei mu. China: dried bulb. Internal use for breast cancer. It is recommended that the plant be analyzed for anticancer agents.
Loranthaceae	*Viscum album*: mistletoe. China: dried twigs, harvested March to August. Fresh juice contains the amino acids arginine and asparagine, (-proline, cysteic acid, 1-kynurenine, hydroxylysine.
Malvaceae	*Hibiscus rosa-sinensis*: China rose. A native of the Old World, now cultivated in China: paste from leaves and flowers. Skin cancers.
Moraceae	*Ficus pumila*: Sóp. China: fruit and leaves. (Also see Cannabinaceae)
Nymphaeaceae	*Brasenia schreberi*: shun-ts'ai, shui-k'uei, junsai. China: crushed stems and leaves. Topical application for cancers.
Oleaceae	*Forsythia suspensa*: lien-ch'iao, lien-tsao (forsythia). China: dried fruits or capsules, also twigs, leaves, and roots. Also antibiotic.
Papaveraceae	*Chelidonium majus*: celandine, nipplewort. Korea: stem and leaves. Gastric cancer. Contains chelidonine, chelerythrine, protopine, homochelidonine, alliccryptopine, berberine, spartine. Toxic.
	Macleaya cordata*. China: yellow sap. Acts as a counter-poison to cancer. Leaves and flowers are insecticidal. The plant contains the alkaloids protopine, chelerythrine, homochelidonine, sanguinarine. The yellow sap is very poisonous.
Phrymaceae*	*Phryma leptostachya*. China: smashed plant. Poultice for external cancers. Also insecticidal.
Polypodiaceae	*Pyrrosia* lingua*. China: fronds.
Ranunculaceae	*Ranunculus acris*: crowfoot. China: leaves and seeds. External cancers. Also insecticidal. Toxic.
Rubiaceae	*Mussaenda hainanensis* or *hainensis*. China (Hainan): decoction of stem and leaves.
	Ophiorrhiza mungos: sarahati. Malay Peninsula. Contains tannates, alkaloids, acidic substances, methyl esters.
	*Serissa japonica**. China: stem and leaves.
Salicaceae	*Salix purpurea*: shui-yang. China: bark.
Saxifragaceae	*Dichroa febrifuga*: ch'ang shan. China south to New Guinea. Contains alkaloids, including febrifugine, which has been tested against cancer.
Scrophulariaceae	*Scrophularia buergeriana**. Korea, China, Japan: roots. Tumors and cancer of the lungs. Contains essential oi, phytosterol, phytosterolin, and oleic, linolic, palmitic, and stearic acids. Also alkaloid material, dextrose, 1-asparagine.
Umbelliferae	*Conium maculatum*: poison hemlock. China, imported into Indo-China. Used for external cancer. Contains coniine, methylconiine, conydrine, pseudoconydrine, coniciene, fixed oil. All plant parts are poisonous.

	Oenanthe javanica*. China, Indo-China: bruised plant, used as dressing.
Verbenaceae	*Vitex trifolia* v. *ovata**: garyophyllon, caryophyllon, man-ching. China, Japan: seeds and dried fruits in a decoction. Cancer of the breast.
	Vitex trifolia v. *unifoliata**: garyophyllon, caryophyllon, man-ching. China, Japan: seeds and dried fruits in a decoction. Cancer of the breast.
Violaceae	*Viola patrinii* or *patrini*: tse hoa, ti ting, violet. China: whole plant. Also used in Europe folk medicine to treat cancer.
	Viola pinnata: hu-chin-ts'ao, violet. China: whole plant. Also used in Europe folk medicine to treat cancer.
Vitaceae	*Cayratia* japonica*. China: mucilaginous root.
	Vitis labrusca: ing yu. China: root bark.
Zingiberaceae	*Alpinia galanga*. Indo-China rhizome, galanga, "galen gal." Cancer of the stomach. The rhizome contains kaempferia, galangin, a volatile oil, and galangol which yields cineole. Also pinene and eugenol.

Anticancer Plants from China

Table S.1 Some Chinese Anticancer Plants

Acanthaceae	*Acanthus ilicifolius**: sea holly. Adhatodine, anisotine, betaine, vasakin, vasicine, vasicinine, vasicnol, vasicoline, vasicolinone.
Actinidiaceae*	*Actinidia chinensis*: Chinese gooseberry
Amaryllidaceae	*Crinum asiaticum*: poison bulb. Bakonine and lycorine (an active antitumor agent).
	Lycoris radiata*: golden spiderlily. Demethylhomolycorine, 2- epigalanthamine, galanthamine, haemanthidine, hippeastrine, homolycorine, hydrolycorine, lycorenine, lycoricidine, lycoricidinol, lycorine, norpluviine, pluvine, pseudolycorine, squamigerine, tasettine, vittatine.
	Narcissus tazetta: polyanthus narcissus. Lycorine, narcitine, pseudolycorine, tazettine. Assumed to be the Biblical rose.
	Zephyranthes grandiflora*: white zephyrlily
Anacardiaceae	*Pistacia lentscus*
Apiaceae* (Umbelliferae)	*Angelica anomala**. Phellandrene. (Compositae)
	Angelica sinensis* (Compositae)
	Daucus carota: carrot. Retinoids, betasitosterol (active antitumor agent).
	Ligusticum acutilobum
Apocynaceae	*Catharanthus* roseus*: Madagascar periwinkle. Catharanthine, leurosine sulfphate, lochnerine, tetrahydroalstonine, vindoline, vindolinine. **"More than 50 alkaloids have been identified from this major medicinal plant, the most inportant plant in the anticancer armamentarium."**
	Melodinus* suaveolens. Dambonitol, deacetyloleandrin, digitoxigenin, gitosigenin, karabin, neriantin, neriocorin, neriodorin, neriodorein, nerioresin, odoroside, oleandrin, oleandrigenin, 16-acetylgitoxigenin, oleandrose, rutin, stropeside, tannic acid, uzarigenin. Contains antitumor compound adynerin.
	Rauvolfia* verticuillata: luó fú mù, one of Wong's fifty fundamental herbs. Contains reserpine, which shows both cancer-causing activity and anticancer activity., i.e., in the CA, SA, and WA tumor systems.
Araceae	*Acorus calamus*: sweet flag, calamus. Acoric acid, asarone.
	Acorus gramineus*: Chinese sweet grass
	Alocasia cucullata*
	Amorphophallus riviere*. Leviduline, levidulinase, mannose.
	Arisaema amurense*: jack-in-the-pulpit
	Pinellia ternata
Araliaceae	*Aralia elata*. Araloside A, hederagenin, choline, alpha- and beta-taralin, protocatechuic acid.
	Aralia mandschurica*: Manchurian aralia. Araloside A, B, and C.
	Eleutherococcus* senticosus: Siberian ginseng. Saponins. Anticancer effect debatable.
	Panax ginseng: Chinese or Asian ginseng. Saponins.
Arecaceae*	*Daemonorops draco*: dragon's blood. Dracoresinotannol in the form of (Palmae)benzoic and benzoyl acetic esters, resene, dracoalban. Also abietic acid, dracocarmin, dracorubin.
Aristolochiaceae	*Aristolochia contorta*. Allantoin, aristolochic acid, aristolochine, magnoflorine.
	Aristolochia molissima*. Aristolochic acid. Active antitumor agent, but too toxic.
Asclepiadaceae	*Asclepias curassavica*: West Indian ipecac, Curassavian swallowwort. Asclepiadin, calotropin and coroglaucigenin (antitumor), asclepogenin, ascurogenin, calotropagenin, clepogenin, corotoxigenin, curassavogenin, urazigenin (antitumor).
Asteraceae* (Compositae)	*Aster fastigiatus**. Arabinose, quercitol, shionone.
	Atractylodes macrocephala.* Atractylone. Anticancer reputation in China.
	Chrysanthemum morifolium: florist's chrysanthemum. Acacetin-7-rhamnoglucoside dihydrate, adenine, aminozide, borneol, choline, chrysanthemin, chrysanthenone, cosmosiin, luteolin-7-glucoside, stachydrine.

*Inula britannica**: Chinese elecampane. Inulin, flavone, caffeic acid, chlorogenic acid, isoquercitrin, quercetin, inosterols A and B.

Inula helenium: elecampane. Alantolactone, helenin, inulin.

Lactuca sativa: lettuce. Analysis provided.

*Laggers pterodonta**

Saussurea lappa: costus. Aplotaxene, camphene, alpha-costene, beta-costene, costol, kushtin, phelladrene, costunolide (antitumor).

*Senecio scandens**: ragwort. Antibiotic. Seneciphylline, senecionine (antitumor), metrorsine.

Taraxacum mongolicum: Mongolian dandelion

Tussilago farfara: coltsfoot. Sitosterol (anticancer), pectin

*Wedelia chinensis**. Alkaloids, isoflavonoids, wedelolactone.

*Xanthium sibiricum**: cocklebur

Begoniaceae	*Begonia crassirostris**
	*Begonia fimbristipula**
Berberidaceae	*Mahonia* bealei*. Also antiseptic and bactericidal.
	Mahonia fortunei*. Common anticancer plant.
Betulaceae	*Betula platyphylla**: Japanese white birch. Betulafolienetriol, betulafolienetetraol, betulin.
	*Corylus heterophylla**: Siberian hazel
Bignoniaceae	*Catalpa bungei*: Chinese catawba
Boraginaceae	*Cynoglossum officianale*: hound's tongue. Allantoin, choline, cynoglossin, consolidine, consolicine, cynoglossidine, heliosupine, heliotrine (antitumor), heliotridine, lasiocarpine (carcinogenic), platyphylline, viridiflorine. Curare-like effect on nerve endings. Consolidine and consolicine paralyze central nervous system.
	Heliotropium indicum: Indian heliotrope. Indicine-N-oxide (anticancer), acetyl indicine, indicine, indicinine.
	Lithiospermum erythrorhizon: redroot cromwell. Shikonin (bactericidal).
	*Onosma paniculatum**: onosma
Brassicaceae* (Cruciferae)	*Brassica rapa*: field mustard. Rapine. Analysis provided.
	Isatis tinctoria: dyer's woad. Quercetin, kaempferol, stachyose, manneotetrose, lupeose, cicerose, isatan.
Burseraceae	*Boswellia carteri*: frankincense
	Commiphora myrrha: myrrh
Cabombaceae* (Nymphaeaceae)	*Brasenia schreberi*: watershield. Analysis given.
Caesalpiniaceae*	*Gleditsia sinensis*: Chinese honey locust. Saponin, arabinon, gleditsin, (Leguminosae) flavonoids fisetin and fustin. Analysis given. (*Gleditschia* in Hartwell.)
Campanulaceae	*Adenophora axilliflora**: strict bellflower
	*Adenophora capillaris**: slim bellflower
	*Codonopsis pilosula**: bellflower
	*Lobelia chinensis**: Chinese lobelia. Lobeline, lobelanine, lobelanidine, isolobelanine.
Cannabinaceae* (Moraceae)	*Cannabis sativa*: hemp, marijuana. Cannabinol, cannabinin, cannabidine, cannabol, cannabinol, cannin, trigonelline, choline, eugenol, guaiacol, nicotine, piperidine, beta-resercyclic acid derivative(antibiotic, antiviral, anticancer).
Cannaceae	*Canna indica*: Indian shot
Caryophyllaceae	*Sagina* japonica*: Japanese pearlwort
Celastraceae	*Maytenus confertiflorus**. Leaves contain the antitumor agent maytensine plus dulcitol, succinic acid, syringic acid, 3-oxykojic acid, loliolide.
	*Maytenus hookeri**. Bark is used for cancer of the liver and stomach.
Chenopodiaceae	*Beta vulgaris*: beet. Argenine, betaine, histidine, isoleucine, phenylalanine, tyrosine, tyrosinase.
Chloranthaceae*	*Sarcandra* glabra*
Combretaceae	*Quisqualis* indica*: Rangoon creeper
	Terminalia chebula: myrobalan
Convolvulaceae	*Pharbitus nil*: Japanese morning glory. Angelic acid, cyanoside, pelargoniside, pharbitoside, rhamnose.
Cornaceae	*Cornus officianlis*: Japanese cornel. cornin, gallic acid, malic acid, tannic acid, tartaric acid.
Cucurbitaceae	*Melothria* indica*
	Momordica cochinchinensis: Indochinese bitter melon. Anticancer, antitumor.
	Trichosanthes kirilowii: chinese snakegourd
Cycadaceae*	*Cycas revoluta*: sago palm. Neocycasin A and B, macrozamin, cycasin.
Dipsacaceae	*Dipsacus asper*: Szechuan teasel. Lamine.
Dipterocarpaceae	*Dryobalanops aromatica*: Borneo camphor. d-borneol, camphol, camphene, sesquiterpenes.

Ebenaceae	*Diospyros ebenum*: ebony, macassar ebony. antitumor compounds alpha-amyrin acetate, betulin, betulinic acid, ursolic acid, plus bauerenol and ceryl alcohol.
Ericaceae	*Vaccinium bracteatum**: Asiatic bilberry
Eucommiaceae	*Eucommia ulmoldes*
Euphorbiaceae	*Croton tiglium*: purging croton. **"Like so many plants, this contains both cancer-causing and cancer-correcting compounds."** Phorbol (carcinogenic), phorbal 12-tiglate and 13-decanoate (anticancer), HCN, triterpenoid, oil contains poisonous resins, kernel contains crotonoside and the toxic proteins croton-globulin and croton-albumin.
	Euphorbia helioscopia: sun spurge. Butyric acid, euphorbine, phasine, saponin.
	Euphorbia lathrys: caper spurge, petroleum plant. Aesculin, betulin (antitumor), daphnetin, DOPA, euphorbetin, euphorbiasteroid, kaempferol, quercetin, taraxerol. Paste also used for melanoma.
Fabaceae* (Leguminosae)	*Abrus precatorius*: jequirity. Abraline, abrin, abrine, abrusic acid, 5 beta-cholanic acid, cycloaartenol, gallic acid, hypaphorine, precatorine, squalene, trigonelline. Abrin is deadly poisonous.
	Astragalus membranaceus*: membraneous milk vetch. Inhibits cell RNA metabolism.
	Crotalaria* assamica. Pyrrolizidine alkaloids.
	Crotalaria* ferruginea
	Crotalaria* sessiflora: narrow-leaved rattlebox. Monocrotaline. Hepatotoxic.
	Euchresta japonica
	Glycine max: soybean. Sitosterol (anticancer), stigmasterol, soybean oil.
	Glycyrrhiza uralensis*: Chinese or Manchurian licorice. Contains flavonoids, glycyrrhetic acid, glycyrrhizin.
	Phaseolus vulgaris: kidney bean. Phaseolin (fungicide).
	Sophora japonica*: Japanese pagoda tree. Antitumor alkaloids. Genestine, rutin, glucose, kaempferol glycoside, linoleic acid, quercetin, rhamnoglycoside, rhamnose, sophorabioside, sophoraflavnoside, sophorin, sophorose, sophoricoside.
	Sophora subprostata*. Antitmor alkaloids matrine and oxymatrine, antitumor agent sophajaponica, sophoradochromene.
	Trifolium pratense: red clover. Phenolic compounds daidzein, genistein, isotrifolin, isorhamnetin, pratol, pratensol, trifolin. Trifolirhizin (antifungal). Coumaric acid, hentriacontane, heptacosane, myricyl alcohol, β-sitosterol. Seeds contain trypsin and chymotrypsin inhibitors.
Flacourtiaceae	*Hydnocarpus* anthelmintica*: krabao oil tree, chalmoogra. Chalmoogra oil contains hydnocarpic acid.
Gentianaceae	*Gentiana* scabra*: gentian
Ginkgoaceae	*Ginkgo biloba*: ginkgo, maidenhair tree. Ginkgolic acid (antitubercular).
Hamamelidaceae	*Liquidambar formosana*: fragrant maple, chinese storax
	Liquidambar orientalis: Levant storax
Hypericaceae* (Guttiferae)	*Garcinia morella*: gamboge. analysis given.
Iridaceae	*Belamcanda chinensis*: blackberry lily, leopard lily. Glucoside shekanin or tectoridin, iridin.
Juglandaceae	*Juglans regia*: European walnut. Juglone (bactericidal, pesticidal, antitumor), betulin (antitumor), pyrogallol tannins. Has been used for rabies.
	Juglans mandshurica*: Manchurian walnut. Cotyledons (first leaves in whorls) are cancer cure.
Lamiaceae* (Labiatae)	*Agastache rugosa*: chinese giant hyssop
	Ajuga decumbens: bugleweed. Ecdysones cyasterone, eddyssterone, ajuglactone, ajugasterone, ajugosterone C.
	Leonurus heterophyllus*: motherwort
	Lycopus lucidus: shining water horehound
	Mentha arvensis*: cornmint, peppermint. Pulegone, menthofuran, menthofurolactone, hesperidin. Also menthol, menthone, isomenthone, carvementhone, thujone, alphapinene, limonene, beta-phellandrene, santene, piperitone, piperitonoxide, menthyl acetate, alpha-beta-hexenyl acetate, alpha-thujone, p-menthan-trans-2,5-diol, delta-menthyl pentanol, e-octanol.
	Prunella vulgaris: selfheal. Antibiotic. Caffeic acid, d-camphor, cyanidin, delphinidin, d-fenchone, hyperoside, oleanic acid, rutin, ursolic acid.
	Rabdosia* spp. Terpenes, with oridonin the main active principle. Rubescensin A and B.
	Salvia miltiorrhiza: red-rooted sage. Bactericidal. Dihydrotanshinone I, etc.
	Scutellaria baicalensis: Chinese skullcap, Baical skullcap
	Scutellaria barbata*. Root inhibits flu virus. Used for stomach cancer.
	Thymus vulgaris: thyme. Oil has carvacrol, linalol, parathymol, pinene, thymol. Also variously alpha-pinene, camphene, beta-pinene, myrcrene, alpha-phellandrene, limonene, 1,8-cinole, p-cymene, linalool, linalyl acetate, thymol, borneol, alpha terpineol.
Lardizabalaceae	*Akebia quinata*: chocolate vine. Unsaturated acids, tannins. Contains shikimic acid which is carcinogenic.

Lauraceae	*Cinnamomum camphora**: camphor tree. Azulene, bisabolene, cadinene, camphene, camphor, alpha-camphorene, carvacrol, cineole, p-cymol, eugenol, laurolitsine, d-limonene, orthodene, alpha-pinene, reticulene, safrole, salvene, terpineol.
	Laurus nobilis: bay. Methyl eugenol. Oil is bactericidal and fungicidal.
Liliaceae	*Allium sativum*: garlic. Allicin, allistatin. Bactericidal, fungicidal.
	Aloe baradensis: Barbados aloe, Curacao aloe. Barbaloin, emodin. Bactericidal.
	*Asparagus cochinchensis**: Chinese asparagus
	Asparagus officianalis: asparagus. Glycolic acid, asparagine, tyrosin, asparagin, methanethiol.
	Fritillaria verticillata: fritillary. Peimine, peimiside, peimunine, fritimine.
	Hosta plantaginea: fragrant hosta
	Ophiopogon japonicus*: lilyturf. Anticancer extracts contain beta-sitosterol, beta-sitosterol-beta-D-glucoside, stigmasterol. sugars. Glycosides ophiopogonin A, B, C, D, plus ruscogenin, etc.
	Smilax china: China root. Tannin, resin, cinchonin, sapogenins smilacin, sarsasapogenin, diosgenin. Rutin, linoleic acid.
	*Smilax glabra**: glabrous greenbrier. Antitumor hormones beta-sitosterol and stigmasterol. Glucosides.
	Tulipa edulis: tulip. Also used for rabies.
Loganiaceae	*Strychnos nux-vomica*: strychnine. Strychnine. External treatments.
Magnoliaceae	*Magnolia liliflora**: red magnolia
	Schisandra chinensis*: Chinese magnolia vine. Shizandrol lowers levels of serum glutamic pyruvic transaminase (SGPT) caused by hepatitis. Shizandrol B promotes glycogenesis.
Malvaceae	*Hibiscus mutabillis*: Chinese rose. Flowerw contain isoqercitrin, hyperoside, rutin, quercetin-4-glucoside, quercimeritrin, quercetin.
	Hibiscus rosa-sinensis: shoe flower. Flowers contain cyanidin-3-sophoroside.
	Malva verticillata: cheeseweed
Menispermaceae	*Menispermum* dauricum*: Siberian moonseed. Acutumine, acutuminine, dauricine, disinomenine, magnoflorine, menispermine, sinomenine, stepharine, tetrandine (antitumor).
Mimosaceae (Leguminosae)	*Acacia catechu*: catechu, Jerusalem thorn, black cutch. Tannin, catechin.
	Entada phaseoloides*. Unsaturated acids, raffinose, alkaloids, steroids, entagenic acid (anticancer).
Moraceae	*Ficus pumila*: creeping fig
	Morus alba: white mulberry. Analysis given.
Myrsinaceae	*Ardisia japonica**: marlberry. Isocoumarin bergenin.
Myrtaceae	*Eucalyptus globulus*: eucalyptus, blue gum tree. Bactericidal. Cineol, eucalyptol, aldehydes, alcohols,tannin, terpenes, terpineol, gallic and caffeic acids, ferulic- and gentistic-quercetol, quercitin, rutin, quercetol hyperoside and glaucoside.
Nyssaceae*	*Camptotheca* acuminata*: happy tree. Quinoline alkaloid camptothecin. Derivatives exhibit anticancer activity, especially 10-hydroxy- and 10-methoxy-camptothecin.
Oleaceae	*Forsythia suspensa*: forsythia. Phillyrin, rutin. Antibiotic.
Orchidaceae	*Pleione* bulbocodioides*. Also snakebite, TB.
Papaveraceae	*Macleaya* cordata*: plum poppy. Alpha-allocryptine, bocconine, chelerythrine (antitumor), homochelidonine, oxysanguinarine, protopine, sanguinarine (antitumor). Ethoxysanguinarine and ethoxychelerythrinatine are active anticancer agents.
Phrymaceae*	*Phryma leptostachya*: lopseed
Piperaceae	*Piper nigrum*: black pepper. Piperine. Insecticidal.
Plantaginaceae	*Plantago asiatica**: Asian plantain. Adenine, aucubin, plantagin, planteonolic acid, succininc acid. Bactericidal.
Poaceae* (Gramineae)	*Coix lacryma-jobi*: Job's tears, pearl barley. Leucine, tyrosine, arginine, histidine, lysine. Glycerides of myristic and palmitic acids.
	Imperata cylindrica: thatch grass, alang-alang. Anemonin (antitumor), arundoine, arborinolmethylethers, cylindrine, ferneol, isuarborinol, simiarenol. Viricidal.
	Miscanthus sinensis*: miscanthus
	Oryza sativa: rice. Isoleucine, leucine, lysine, phenylalanine, tyrosine, sulfur amino acids, methionine, threonine, tryptophane, valine.
	Saccharum officianarum: sugar cane
	Zeay mays: corn. Analysis given.
Polygalaceae	*Polygala* telephioides*: lesser polygala
Polygonaceae	*Polygonum cuspidatum**: Japanese knotweed. Emodin (antitumor).
	Polygonum hydropiper: water pepper, smartweed. Carvone. Flavones, quercetin, quercitrin, kaempferol, rutin, hyperoside, rhamnacin, persicarin.
	Polygonum multiflorum: climbing knotweed. Emodin and rhein (both antitumor), chrysophanic acid, chrysophanic acid anthrone, chrysarobin, chrysophanol, allantoin, lecithin, rhapontin, chelidonic acid.

Polygonum orientale: prince's feather. Beta-sitosterol, the flavone glucosides orientoside and orientin. Oxymethylanthraquinone, tannic acid, phenolic compounds, saponins.

Polypodiaceae *Dynaria* fortunei*

Pteridaceae* *Pteris multifida**: spider brake. Anticancer (hepatoma).
  (Polypodiaceae)

Ranunculaceae *Clematis chinensis*: Chinese clematis (*Clematis chinesis* in Hartwell)

*Coptis chinensis**. Alkaloids berberine, colubamine, copsine, lumicaerulic acid, palmatine, woreine. Also protoberberinium salts, epiberberine, greenlandicine, berberastine, thalifendine, osyberberine. Antiseptic.

*Paeonia lactiflora**: Chinese peony. Beta-sitosterol. The monoterpene paeoniflorigenone. Fungicidal and bactericidal.

*Thalictrum faberi**: Faber's meadow-rue. Antitumor alkaloids. e.g., thalicarpine.

Rhamnaceae *Ziziphus jujuba*: jujube, chinese date. Betulic acid, betulin (antitumor), ebelin lactone, jujubogenin, jujuboside. Flavone C-glycoside named spinosin.

Rosaceae *Duchesnea* indica*: mock strawberry. Emodin (antitumor), chrysophanic acid, phytosterols, sugar, volatile oils.

Rheum officianale*: Chinese rhubarb

Rubiaceae *Adina* pilulifera*: adina. Betulinic acid (antitumor), cinnacholic acid, morolic acid, quinovic acid.

Adina rubella*: reddish modelwood

Cinchona succiruba: chinchona bark, quinine. Quinine, quininidine. Antimalarial, etc.

Damnacanthus indicus*. Contains the glycoside asperuloside and citric acid.

Gardenia jasminoides: cape jasmine. Glycosides, e.g., crocin.

*Knoxia valerianoides**

Morinda officinalis. Morindone, morindin, rubichloric acid, alizarin alpha-methyl ether, rubiadin-1-methyl ether, morindadiol, soranjidiol, asperuloside, nordamnacanthal, wax, tannin, trihydroxy methyl-anthraquinone mono methyl ethers. Also alizarin, lucidin, morindone, nordamncanthal, rubiadin.

*Oldenlandia diffusa**. Antitumor compounds beta-sitosterol, stigmasterol, ursolic acid. Increases leukocytes (white blood cells).

Serissa foetida. Contains a glucoside and chlorogenin.

Rutaceae *Acronychia* laurifolia*. Acronycine, bauerenol, nitroacronycine. Acronycine **"possesses the broadest spectrum of *in vivo* antineoplastic activity of any plant-derived natural product."**

Boenninghausenia albiflora*. Cordell reports daphnoretin in *B. albiflora* and *B. japonica*. Exhibits antineoplastic activity in certain tests.

Citrus aurantium: sour orange. Umbelliferone (antifungal), essential oils (bactericidal and fungicidal). Contains the pyrone citrantin.

Ruta graveolens: garden rue. Arborine, furocoumarins bergapten and xanthotoxin, 2-undecanone (hirudicidal, nematicidal, vermicidal).

Scrophulariaceae *Rehmannia glutinosa*: Chinese foxglove. One of the 50 fundamental Chinese herbs. Contains the iridoid called catalpol.

*Scrophularia buergeriana**. Essential oils, phytosterol, phytosterolin, oleic-, linoleic-, palmitic- and steraic-acids, alkaloids, extrose, 1-asparagine.

*Scrophularia ningpoensis**: black figwort

Simaroubaceae *Brucea javanica*: Kosam seed. Brucamarine, brucealin, brucein A, B, C, bruceolic acid, brucenol, brusatol, kosamine, quassin, yatanine, yatanoside.

Solanaceae *Scopolia japonica*. Atropine, 1-hyoscyamine, 1-norhyoscyamine, 1-scopolamine, scopoletin (antitumor), scopoline. Betain, choline, polyphenolase.

Solanum dulcamara: bittersweet, deadly nightshade. Solanine and the glucoside dulcamarine. Glycoalkaloids present include alpha-, beta-, and gamma-soladulcine and alpha-, beta-, and gamma-solamarine.

Solanum lyratum: climbing nightshade

Taxaceae *Taxus cuspidata**: Japanese yew. *Taxus* shows good anticancer activity but apparently not due to taxol. Other compounds are beta-ecdysone, sciadopitysine, ponasterone A, quercetin, tannin. Also lariciresinol, secolariciresinol, isolariciresinol, isotaxitesinol-6-methyl ether, isotaxiresinol, sitosterol, taxusine, deacetyltaxusin. Plus lecithin, lysolecithin, cephalin, beta-sitosterol.

Theaceae *Camellia japonica**: common camellia. Camelliagenin A, B, and C, d-catechol, leucoanthocyanin. Also arabinose, camellin, rhamnose, theasaponin.

Thymelaeaceae *Aquilaria agallocha*: aloe-wood, eaglewood

Wikstroemia indica. Daphnoretin and nortrachelogenin. Also the glycoside wikstroemin.

Verbenaceae *Vitex trifolia*: Indian privet. Camphene, pinene, terpenylacetate, aucubin, agnuside, casticin, orientin, isoorientin, luteolin-7-glucoside, vitricne. Also antitubercular.

Violaceae	*Viola diffusa**: spreading violet
	Viola patrinii (*Viola patrini* in Hartwell)
Vitaceae	*Cayratia** *japonica*. Arabin, cayratinin, delphinidin-3-p-coumaroylsophoroside-5-monoglucoside.

Source: Data from *Medicinal Plants of China* by James A. Duke and Edward S. Ayensu, Reference Publications, Algonac MI, 1985. Plant families, genera, or species **not** represented in Hartwell's *Plants Used Against Cancer* are designated by an asterisk.

Table S.2   Chinese Anticancer Herbs

Apocynaceae	*Catharanthus** *roseus* (Chang Chu Hua): periwinkle. (*Catharanthus* is listed as *Vinca* in Hartwell.) The dried whole plant has over 70 alkaloids, some well-known, which notably include **vinblastine (VLB), vincristine (VCR), vinrosidine, leurosine, leurosivine, rovidine, carosine, perivine, perividine, vindoline,** and **pericalline**. A semisynthetic spin-off is **vindesine** (VDS). Called the *Vinca* alkaloids, some are very effective against blood cancer cells and lymphoma, and act against breast cancer. There is an arresting of cell division, similarly to the action of such anticancer drugs as **colchicine** and **maytensine** (or **maytansine**). The side-effects are severe, and include bone marrow depression, especially as concerns leukocytes or white blood cells.
Celastraceae	*Maytenus serrata**, *M. buchananii**, *M. hookeri**, or *M. conterliflories** (Mei Deng Mu): **cancerosa** salvidas. The fruit, bark, and rhizome contain such alkaloids as **maytensine, maytanprine, maytanbutine, maytanvaline,** and **maytanacine,** plus the compound maytansinol. **Maytensine** in particular interferes with cell division or mitosis, and inhibits the DNA/RNA/protein sequence. **Maytensine** has been found to be 20–100 times more active than the *Vinca* alkaloid **vincristine** (VCR) derived from *Catharanthus roseus*. The herb has been used variously in treating lung, breast, ovary, colon, and lung cancers, and also lymptocytic leukemia. The toxic side effects can be severe and are dose-dependent, affecting the gastrointestinal tract and sometimes the liver.
Celastraceae	*Tripterygium** *wilfordii* (Lei Gong Teng). The dried roots and leaves contain the alkaloid **wilfordine** plus other substances, notably the triptolides A, B, and C ($C_{20}H_{24}O_6$), triptonide ($C_{20}H_{22}O_6$), and tripterin ($C_{29}H_{58}O_4$). Triptolide A is the main anticancer agent, affecting leukemia cells. Toxicity is a problem, damaging the cardiovascular system and adversely affecting the CNS.
Cephalotaxaceae*	*Cephalotaxus** *fortunei*, *C. quensis*, *C. oliveri*, or *C. huaiuansis* (San Jin Shan): plum-yew tree. Twenty **alkaloids** are found in the genus. The leaves and branches of *C. fortunei* contain **cephalotaxine, epicephalotaxine, demethylcephalotaxine,** and **cephalotaxine**. Leaves of the species *C. wilsoniana* contains **wilsonine** and **epiwilsonine**. The roots and rhizomes of the species *C. harringtonia* have two groups of alkaloids, of which the first includes the well-known bioactive agents **harringtonine, homoharringtonine, isoharringtonine,** and **deoxyharringtonine,** with the second group containing **homoerythrina alkaloids**. The alkaloids act against both cancer cells and leukemia cells. Also against lymphoma. Side-effects include CNS depression and coronary constriction.
Chloranthaceae*	*Sarcandra** *glabra* (Zhong Jie Feng). The dried whole plant contains glucosides and essential oils, plus fumaric acid and succinic acid, and substances called CI,CII,CIII, and CIV. The essential oil and substance CII are active against cancer. Used against solid tumors of the pancreas, stomach, esophagus, rectum, bladder, colon, lungs, and thyroid. May be taken in tablet form or injected intravenously or intramuscularly.
Compositae	*Eupatorium formosanum** (Taiwan Pei Lan): boneset. The plant contains sesquiterpene lactones, notably eupaformonin, eupaformosanin, michelenolide, costunolide, parthenolide, and **santamarine**. These lactones have the α-methylene-γ-lactone moiety. Inhibit Walker-256 carcinoma and Ehrlich ascites tumor growth. Act as an enzyme inhibitor for **phosphofructokinase** (in the glycolysis pathway) and glycogen synthetase, by reacting with the critical SH groups of these enzymes.
Labiatae	*Rabdosia** *rubescens* (Dong Ling Cao). The dried aerial parts contain terpenes plus essential oils and tannic acid. The active agents are **rubescensine B**, and oridonin and **ponicidine**. Used in treatment of esophageal cancer and breast cancer. Rubescensine B is also used against liver cancer. May cause nausea and diarrhea. Tablets or intravenous or muscular injections may be prescribed.
Leguminosae	*Crotalaria** *sessiflora* or *C. assamica* (Ye Bai He or Nung Gi Li). The dried whole plant contains alkaloids which act against leukemia. Clinical trials show activity against skin cancer, cervical cancer, and rectal cancer. The alkaloid **monocrotaline A** inhibits the DNA/RNA/protein sequence. Vitamin C, glycyrrhizic acid, and glucoronic acid may be effective against toxicity.
Nyssaceae*	*Camptotheca** *acuminata* (Xi Zhu): tree of joy. The fruit has the alkaloids **camptothecine, hydroxyl-camptothecine, methoxylcamptothecine,** and **venoterpine**. Apparently the first and third are the active anticancer agents, affecting various cancers including leukemia, and cervical, liver, and lung cancers. Also cancers of the stomach, rectum, colon, and bladder. Side effects include bone marrow depression.

Simarubaceae	*Brucea antidysenteria* or *B. javanica* (Ya Dan Zi). The species *B. antidysenteria* contains the quassinoid derivative bruceantin. Bruceantin acts against lymphocytic leukemia cells, and also against lymphoid leukemia cells, Lewis lung carcinoma, and B-16 melanocarcinoma. The primary action is against protein synthesis.
Stylopsidae	*Mylabris* phalerata* or *M. cichoorii* (the **beetle** Ban Sao, order Coleoptera). The dried body contains cantharides, e.g., the anticancer agent cantharidin. Acts against hepatoma and against esophageal, anus, lung, and breast cancers. **Has a stimulating effect on bone marrow and white blood cell count.** Thus it can be used to offset the anti-immune effects of conventional cytotoxic chemotherapy. Tablets are effective, but have the side effects of nausea and urinary irritation.
Zingiberaceae	*Curcurma zedoaria, C. aromatica,* or *C. kwangiensis** (E Zhu): turmeric. The dried rhizome has fifteen different chemicals in the essential oil, including curserenone, curcumenol, and curdione. The latter two are the anticancer agents. Act against cervical cancer. Intravenous or direct injection causes no kidney or liver damage. Oral doses may cause dizziness and nausea, or even shock. Also used for ovarian, skin, and genital cancers, for lymphoma and hepatoma, and for thyroid cancer, gastric cancer, and lung cancer.

Source: Data from *The Pharmacology of Chinese Herbs* by Kee Chang Huang, CRC Press, Boca Raton FL, 1993. Plant families, genera, or species **not** listed in Hartwell's *Plants Used Against Cancer* are denoted by an asterisk. Alkaloids are for the most part represented in **boldface**, as are other information items of potential interest.

Table S.3   Other Chinese Anticancer Herbs

Actinidiaceae*	*Actinidia* chinensis* (Teng Li Gen). Root and fruit contain **alkaloids** and **vitamin C**. Act against mouse S-180, stomach, esophageal cancer.
Apocynaceae	*Allamanda* cathartica* (Yuan Xi Huang). Contains allamandin. Acts against P-388 leukemia.
Araceae	*Arisaema consanguineum*, A. heterophyllum*,* or *A. amurense** (Nan Xing). Rhizome contains saponins, β-**sitosterol**. Acts against mouse S-180, and cervix and esophageal cancers.
Araliaceae	*Aralia chinensis** (Jia Mu): **spikenard**. Bark contains saponins, essential oils. Acts against alimentary tract, gall bladder cancers.
Caryophyllaceae	*Vaccaria* pyramidata* (Liu Xin Zi): **cowherb**. Seeds contain saponins, alkaloids. Acts against esophageal, stomach cancers.
Compositae	*Elephantopus elatus*, E. Scaber,* or *E. mollus* (Di Dan Tou): **elephant's foot**. Contains elephantopin, molephantinin, deoxoelphantopin. Acts against P-388 lymphocytic cancer, ascites cells. *Rhaponticum* uniflorum* (Lour Lu). Contains essential oils. Acts against liver, stomach, breast cancers. *Senecio campestris** (Gou Shi Cao): **ragwort**. Contains **alkaloids**. Acts against mouse L-1210 leukemia.
Cycadaceae*	*Cycas* revoluta* (Tie Shu Yie): **sago palm.** Leaf contains glucosides, choline. Acts against stomach, liver, lung, uterus, nose cancers.
Ericaceae	*Pieris* multifida* (Feng Wei Cao): **pieris**. Whole plant contains flavonoids. Acts against uterus and bladder cancers.
Gekkonidae	*Gekko* chinensis* (Tian Long): **gekko**, a lizard of the suborder Sauria. Whole body contains toxin. Acts against esophagus, stomach, lung cancers.
Gramineae	*Coix lachryma* (Yi Yi Ren): hatomugi, **coix grain**. Seed contains α,β-**sitosterol**, fat, amino acids. Acts against mouse A-180, Yoshida sarcoma, Ehrlich ascites cells, lung and cervix cancers, and chorionic epithelioma.
Inorganic salts	Sal ammoniac (Lu Sha). Composed of ammonium chloride plus NaCl and $MgCl_2$ as contaminants. Acts against esophageal cancer.
Iridaceae	*Iris pollasii** var. *chinensis** (Ma Lian Zi): **Iris**. Contains irisquinone. Acts against cervix, mouse U-14, liver, lymph, and Ehrlich cancers.
Juglandaceae	*Juglans regia* (He Tao Shu Zhi): **walnut**. Branch and unripe fruit skin contain tannin, glucosides. Act against mouse S-37 cells and solid tumors.
Labiatae	*Prunella vulgaris* (Xia Ku Cao): **prunella**. Flower petal contains saponins, **alkaloids**. Acts against mouse S-180, cervix cancer-14, and thyroid, breast, liver cancers. *Salvia chinensis** (Shi Jian Chuan): **cancer weed**. Whole plant contains **sitosterol** and amino acids. Acts against mouse S-180. *Salvia przewalskii** (Tan Seng): **sage**. Contains przewaquinone A, B. Acts against mouse tumors. *Scutellaria barbata** (Ban Zhi Lian): **skullcap**. Whole plant contains **alkaloids, flavonoids**. Acts against mouse S-180, Ehrlich ascites cells.
Leguminosae	*Gleditschia sinensis* (Zao Ci): **honey locust**. Needle (thorn) contains **flavonoids**. Acts against mouse S-180, and alimentary tract, breast, cervix cancers.

Psoralea corylifolia (Bu Gu Zhi): **scurf-pea**. Seed contains furocumarin, psoralen, corylifolinin, bavachinin, etc. Acts against mouse S-180. Ehrlich ascites cells, bone, lung cancers. Treats neurosis, impotence.

*Sophora alopecurosides** (Ku Don Zi). Contains **sophocarpine, sophoridine**. Acts against U-14, S-37, S-180 cancer cells.

*Sophora subprostrata** (Shan Dou Gen): **wild indigo**. Contains **matrine, dauricine, anagyrine**. Acts against mouse S-180, leukemia, liver cancers. Also antimicrobial.

Liliaceae   *Asparagus cochinensis** (Tian Dong): **asparagus**. Root contains β-**sitosterol**. Acts against mouse S-180 leukemia, lung cancer.

Iphigenia indica* (Shan Ci Gu). Tuber rhizome contains **colchicine**. Acts against mouse S-180, Walker sarcoma, and breast, thyroid, esophagus cancers.

Lobeliaceae   *Lobelia chinensis** (Ban Bian Lian): **lobelia**. Contains **alkaloids**, glucosides, saponins. Acts against mouse S-180, and liver, stomach, intestinal cancers.

Malvaceae   *Gossypium hiersutum**, *G. herbaceum*, or *G. arboreum* (Mian Hua Gen): **cottonseed**. Root contains cottonphenol, $MgSO_4$. Acts against mouse S-180, Walker sarconma, and lung, liver, stomach, esophagus, larynx cancers.

Malvaceae   *Hibiscus mutabilis* (Fu Rong Yie): **hibiscus**. Leaf contains **flavonoids**. Acts against stomach, breast, lung cancers.

Menispermaceae   *Stephania tetranda** (Han Fang Ji). Contains **tetrandine, fangchinoline**. Acts against Walker-256 carcinoma.

Moraceae   *Ficus pumila* (Bi Li Guo): **fig**. Fruit contains β-**sitosterol**, glucosides. Acts against cervix, breast, prostate, testes, colon cancer.

Palmae   *Livistona* chinensis* (Kui Shu Zi). Seed contains tannin, phenols. Acts against chorionic epithelioma, esophageal cancer.

Polygonaceae   *Polyganum bistorta* (Cao He Che): **bistort, snakeweed**. Rhizome contains β-**sitosterol**, tannin. Acts against mouse S-180.

Polyganum orientale (Shui Hong Hua). Fruit contains β-**sitosterol** glucosides. Acts against stomach, intestine, liver cancers.

Polygonum perfoliatum (Gang Ban Gui). Whole plant contains cardiac glucosides. Act against esophagus, gastrointestinal, prostate cancers.

*Rumex japonica** or *R. crispus* (Yang Ti Gen): **yellow dock**. Root contains **emodin**. Acts against leukemia and malignant lymphoma.

Polyporaceae   *Polyporus umbellatus** (Zhu Ling): **fungus**. Contains zhu-ling polysaccharides. Acts against S-180 cells, provides **immunostimulation**.

Ranunculaceae   *Ranunculus ternatus** (Mao Zhua Cao): **crowfoot**. Root contains amino acids, organic acids. Acts against mouse S-180, Sarcoma-37, Ehrlich ascites cells, lymphoma, thyroid cancer.

Semiaquilegia adoxoides* (Tian Kui Zi). Contains **alkaloids**. Acts against lymphoma, and prostate, lung, and bladder cancers.

Rosaceae   *Duchesnea* indica* (She Mei): **Indian strawberry**. No components listed. Acts against mouse S-180, Ehrlich ascites cells, thyroid, liver cancers.

*Galium spurium** var. *echinospermen** (Zhu Yin Yin): **cleavers**, etc. Contains saponin. Acts against leukemia, breast cancer.

*Oldenlandia chrysotricha** (Shi Da Chuan). Whole plant contains α,β-**sitosterol**. Acts against U-14 cervix cancer.

Rubiaceae   *Adina* rubella* (Shei Yiang Mei Gen). Root contains β-**sitosterol**, salicylic acid. Acts agains cervical, lymph, gastrointestinal cancers. (Also classified in the plant family Naucleaceae.)

*Oldenlandia diffusa** (Bai Hua She-She Cao). Contains asperuloside, palderoside, desacetylasperuloside, oldenlandoside. Acts against malignant tumors, stimulates reticuloendothelial system.

Rutaceae   *Zanthoxylum nitidum** (Liang Mian Chen): **prickly ash**. Contains **nitidine chloride**. Antileukemic, acts against lung cancer.

Selaginellaceae*   *Selaginella* doederleinii* (Shi Shang Bai). Leaf contains **alkaloids**, sterol saponins, skikimic (shikimic?) acid. Acts against malignant hydatid (cystic) moles, chorionic epithelioma (pertaining to outer fetal membrane).

Simarubaceae   *Ailanthus altissima* (Chen Gen Bi). Contains quassin, saponin. Acts against mouse S-180, cervix, intestinal cancers.

Solanaceae   *Solanum lyratum* (Bai Ying): **nightshade**. Contains **alkaloids**. Acts against uterus, liver cancers.

Solanum nigrum (Long Kui): **nightshade**. Contains **alkaloids**, saponins. Acts against stomach, liver, ascites cancers.

Testudinidae*	*Chinemys** (*Geoclemys**) *reevesii* (Gui Ban): water **tortoise**, of the order Chelonia. The abdominal plate of the water tortoise contains gelatin, Ca^{2+}, and phosphorus. Acts against lymphoma and liver cancer, enhances cancer immunity.
Thymelaeaceae	*Daphne genkwa* (Yuan Hua): **mezereum**. Contains guidilatichin. Antileukemic.
Valerianaceae	*Patrinia heterophylla** or *P. scabra** (Mu Tom Hui). Contains essential oil. Acts against leukemia, cervix cancer.
Vitaceae	*Ampelopsis brevipedunculata** (Yie Pu Tao Teng). Root and branch contain **flavonoids**, phenols. Acts against mouse S-180, alimentary tract and urinary tract cancers, and malignant lymphoma.
Unidentified	*Dyosma** *pleiantha* (Pa Jiao Lian). Contains podophyllotoxin, deosypodophyllotoxin, **isopicropodophyllodine**. Acts against TLX-5 cancer cells, nasopharynx cancer.
	Ganoderma* *lucidum* (Ling Zhi Cao). contains pollysaccharides Gl-1. Gl-2, Gl-3. Acts against S-180 cells.
	Hirudo* *nipponica* (Shui Zhi). Contains anticoagulant substances. Acts against ovarian, cervix, stomach, esophagus cancers.
	Lasiosphaera* *nipponia* (Ma Bo). Contains cavacin, uric acid. Acts against larynx and lung cancers.

Source: Data from *The Pharmacology of Chinese Herbs* by Kee Chang Huang, CRC Press, Boca Raton FL, 1993. Plant families, genera, or species **not** listed in Hartwell's *Plants Used Against Cancer* are denoted by an asterisk. Alkaloids are for the most part represented in **boldface**, as are other information items of potential interest.

Table S.4 A Chinese Pharmacopoeia of Anticancer Agents

Actinidiaceae*	*Actinidia** *chinensis* (Teng Li). Contains **actinidine**.
Apocynaceae	*Catharanthus** *roseus* (Chang Chun Hua): **periwinkle. Cytotoxic.** (Listed as *Vinca* in Hartwell)
Araceae	*Amorphophallus rivieri** (Ju Ruo).
	Arisaema consanguineum* (Tian Nan Xing).
	Pinellia ternata (Ban Xia).
Araliaceae	*Panax ginseng* (Ren Shen): **ginseng.**
Aristolochiaceae	*Aristolochia mollissima** (Xun Gu Feng).
Balsaminaceae	*Impatiens balsamina* (Ji Xing Zi): garden balsam, **touch-me-not.**
Bombaceae	*Bombax mori** or *Bombyx mori** (Jiang Can).
Bovidae	*Bos** *taurus domesticus* (Niu Huang): **bull's gallstone** (powdered).
Bufonidae	*Bufo** *bufo gargarizans* (Chan Su): **toad** skin. Contains **bufotenine.**
Caryophyllaceae	*Dianthus superbus** (Qu Mai).
	Vaccaria* *segetalis* (Wang Bu Liu Xing): **cowherb.**
Celastraceae	*Tripterygium wilfordii.*
Compositae	*Atractylodes macrocephala** (Bai Zhu).
	Carthamus tinctorius (Hong Hua): **crocus.**
	Eclipta* *prostrata* (Han Lian Cao).
	Senecio integrifolius* (Kou She Cao).
	Xanthium sibiricum* (Cang Er Zi): **cocklebur.**
Cruciferae	*Isatis tinctoria* (Qing Dai): **indigo**, isatis, woad.
Cucurbitaceae	*Trichosanthes kirilowii* (Gua Lou or Gua Lou Ren).
Gentianaceae	*Gentiana scabra** (Long Dan Cao): **gentian.**
Gramineae	*Coix lachryma-jobi* (Yi Yi Ren): **coix grain**, hatomugi..
Hypocreaceae	*Cordyceps** *sinensis* (Dong Chong Xia Cao): caterpillar **fungus.**
Iridaceae	*Iris pallasii** (Ma Lin Zi).
Juglandaceae	*Juglans regia* (Hu Tao Ren): **walnut.**
Labiatae	*Moschus** *moschiferus* (She Xinag). Also *Moschosma.*
	Prunella vulgaris (Xia Ku Cao): **prunella, selfheal.**
	Rabdosia* *rubescens.*
	Salvia chinensis* (Shi Jian Chuan): **sage.**
	Salvia multiorhiza (Dan Chen): **sage.**
	Scutellaria baicalensis (Huang qin): **skullcap.**
	Scutellariae barbatae* (Ban Zhi Lian): **skullcap.**
Leguminosae	*Crotalaria sessiflora* (Ye Bai He): **rattlebox.**
	Gleditschia sinensis (Zao Jiao): **honey locust.**
	Glycyrrhiza uralensis* (Gan Cao): **licorice.**
	Psoralea coryfolia (Bu Gu Zhi).
	Sophora flavescens (Ku Shen).
	Sophora subprostrata* (Shan Dou Gern).
Liliaceae	*Asparagus cochinchinensis** (Tian Men Dong): **asparagus.**
	Smilax chinensis (Tu Fu Ling): **China root.**

Lobeliaceae	*Lobelia chinensis** (Bab Bian Lian). **Lobelia.**
Malvaceae	*Gossypium herbaceum* (Mian Hua Gen): **cottonseed.**
Menispermaceae	*Stephania tetranda** (Han Fang Ji).
Moraceae	*Ficus pumila* (Xue Li Shi): **sóp.**
Nyssaceae*	*Camptotheca* acuminata* (Xi Shu): **tree of joy. Cytotoxic.**
Oleaceae	*Ligustrum lucidum** (Nu Zhen Zi): **privet.**
Orchidaceae	*Cremastra variabilis** (Shan Ci Gu).
Polygonaceae	*Rheum tanguticum** (Da Huang): **rhubarb.**
Polyporaceae	*Polyporus umbellatus** (Zhu Ling): a **fungus** called **agaric.**
Ranunculaceae	*Paeonia abovata** (Chat Shao): **peony.**
	*Ranunculus teratus** (Mao Zhua Cao): **crowfoot.**
Rosaceae	*Chaenomeles* lagenaria* (Mu Gua).
	Duchesnea indica* (She Mei): **Indian strawberry.**
Rubiaceae	*Gardenia jasminoides* (Zhi Zi): **gardenia.**
	*Oldenlandia diffusa** (Bai Hua She She Cao).
	Rubia cordifolia (Qian Cao Gen): **madder.**
Rutaceae	*Phelodendron amurense* (Huang Bai): **phelodendron.**
	*Zanthoxylum nitidum** (Liang Mian Zhen): **prickly ash.**
Saururaceae	*Houttuynia cordata* (Yu Xing Cao).
Saxifragaceae	*Dichroa febrifuga* (Chang Shan).
Simarubaceae	*Ailanthus altissima* (Feng Yen Cao).
	Bruceae javanica (Ya Dan Zi).
Solanaceae	*Solanum lyratum* (Shu Yang Quan): **nightshade.**
	Solanum nigrum (Long Kui): **nightshade.**
Stylopside	*Mylabris* phalerata* (the **beetle** Ban Mao, order Coleopta). Dried body.
Valerianaceae	*Patrinia scabiosaefolia** (Bai Jiang Cao).
Zingiberaceae	*Curcuma zedoaria* (E Zhu): **seduer.**
Unidentified	*Hirudo* nipponica* (Shu Zhi).
	Manis pentadactyla* (Chuan Shan Jia). *Manisuris* belongs in Gramineae.
	Ostrea gigas* (Mu Li): **oyster.** *Ostrya** (hornbeam or ironwood) belongs in Cupiliferae* or Carpinaceae*.
	Polistes mandarinus* (Lu Feng Fang).

Source: Data from *Cancer & Natural Medicine: A Textbook of Basic Science and Clinical Research* by John Boik, Oregon Medical Press, Princeton MN, 1995, 1996, pp. 220–223. Plant families, genera, or species **not** in Hartwell's *Plants Used Against Cancer* are denoted by an asterisk.

Table S.5   Some Promising Chinese Anticancer Agents

Araliaceae	*Acanthopanax** spp. (Wu Jia Pi, Ci Wu Jia).
	Panax ginseng (Ren Shen): **ginseng.**
Bufonidae	*Bufo* bufo gargarizans* (Chan Su): **toad skin.** Contains **bufotenine.**
Carophyllaceae	*Pseudostellaria* heterophylla* (Tai Zi Shen).
Compositae	*Arctium lappa* (Niu Bang Zi): **burdock.** Contains lignans.
	*Atractylodes macrocephala** (Bai Zhu).
	Carthamus tinctorius (Hong Hua): **crocus.**
	Echinacea purpurea: **echinacea, coneflower.**
	Tanacetum parthenium: **feverfew.**
Cruciferae	*Isatis tinctoria* (Qing Dai): **indigo,** isatis, woad. Contains indirubin.
Cucurbitaceae	*Gynostemma* pentaphyllum* (Jiao Gu Lan): **güsser tee.**
Ericaceae	*Vaccinium myrtillus*: **bilberry.** Contains anthocyanins.
Hippocastanaceae	*Aesculus hippocastanum*: **horse chestnut.** Contains escin.
Labiatae	*Salvia multiorrhiza* (Dan Shen): **sage.**
	Scuttellaria baicalensis (Huang Qin): **skullcap.**
Leguminosae	*Astragalus membranaceus** (Huang Qi): **gum traganth, milk-vetch.**
	*Glycyrrhiza uralensis** (Gan Cao): **licorice.**
Liliaceae	*Allium sativum*: **garlic.** Contains thiol (sulfur) compounds.
	Aloe vera: **aloe vera** gel.
Linaceae	*Linum usitatissimum*: **flax seed.** Contains lignans.
Polygonaceae	*Rheum palmatum* (Da Huang): **rhubarb.**
Polyporaceae	*Ganoderma* lucidum* (Ling Zhi): **fungus.**
Ranunculaceae	*Paeonia lactiflora** (Chi Shao and Bai Shao): **peony.**

Rhamnaceae	*Ziziphus jujuba* (Da Zao): **kola, cola.** Contains **alkaloids.**
Rosaceae	*Crataegus* oxycantha* (Shan Zha): **hawthorn.** Contains anthocyanins.
Scrophulariaceae	*Picrorrhiza kurroa* (Hu Huang Lian).
Solanaceae	*Lycium barbarum** (Gou Qi Zi).
Theaceae	*Camellia sinensis*: **green tea.** Contains polyphenols.
Umbelliferae	*Angelica sinensis* (Dang Gui): **angelica.**
	Bupleurum chinense* (Chai Hu): **thoroughwax.**
	Ligusticum chuanxiong* (Chuan Xiong): **bladder-seed.**

Source: Data from *Cancer & Natural Medicine: A Textbook of Basic Science and Clinical Research* by John Boik, Oregon Medical Press, Princeton MN, 1995, 1996, pp. 177–181. Plant families, genera, or species **not** in Hartwell's *Plants Used Against Cancer* are denoted by an asterisk.

Table S.6　Some Less-Promising Chinese Anticancer Agents

Acanthaceae	*Andrographis* paniculata* (Chuan Xin Lian).
Actinidiaceae*	*Actinidia* chinensis* (Teng Li). Contains **actinidine.**
Amaranthaceae	*Achyranthes bidentata** (Miu Xi).
Araliaceae	*Panax pseudoginseng** (San Qi).
	Panax quinquefolium* (Xi Yang Shen): **American ginseng.**
Aspergillaceae	*Aspergillus* oryzae*: **fungus.** Contains the proteolytic enzyme **brinase.**
Berberidaceae	*Berberis aquifolium**: **Oregon grape, barberry.**
	Epimedium sagittatum* (Yin Yang Huo).
Bombaceae	*Bombax mori** or *Bombyx mori* (Jiang Can).
Boraginaceae	*Symphytum* spp.: **comfrey.** Contains **pyrrolizidine alkaloids.**
Campanulaceae	*Codonopsus pilosula** (Dang Shen).
Compositae	*Artemisia argyi** (Ai Ye): **wormwood, sagebrush.**
	Artemisia capillaris (Yin Chen Hao): **wormwood, sagebrush.**
	Eclipta* prostrata (Han Lian Cao): **false daisy.**
	Eupatorium cannabinum: **hemp agrimony.**
Convolvulaceae	*Cuscuta australis** (Tu Si Zi): **dodder.**
Gingkoaceae	*Gingko biloba*: **gingko.**
Hypocreaceae	*Cordyceps* sinensis* (Dong Chong Xia Cao): caterpillar **fungus.**
Iridaceae	*Crocus sativus*: **saffron.**
Labiatae	*Leonurus heterophyllus** (Yi Mu Cao): **motherwort.**
Laminariaceae	*Laminaria* spp. (Kun Bu), *Sargassum** spp. (Hai Zao): brown **algae.**
Lauraceae	*Cinnamomum cassia* (Rou Gui): cassia, **cinnamon.**
Leguminosae	*Cassia angustifolia, C. acutifolia* (Fan Xie Ye): **senna.**
	Cassia tora and *C. obtusifolia** (Jue Ming Zi): **foetid cassia.**
	Polygonatum odoratum (Yu Zhu): **Solomon's seal.**
	Psoralea coryfolia (Bu Gu Zhi): **scurf-pea.**
	Sophora flavescens (Ku Shen).
	Sophora subprostrata* (Shan Dou Gen).
Liliaceae	*Allium bakeri* (Xie Bai): **garlic, onion,** etc.
	Paris formosana* (Quan Shen): **herb Paris.**
	Ruscus aculeatus: **butcher's block.**
Loranthaceae	*Viscum album* (Sang Ji Sheng): **mistletoe.**
Magnoliaceae	*Magnolia salicifolia** (Xin Yi Hua): **magnolia.**
Malvaceae	*Altheae officinalis*: **marsh mallow.**
Moraceae	*Cannabis sativa*: **marijuana, hemp, hashish.**
	Humulus lupulus: **hops.**
Myrtaceae	*Eugenia caryophyllata* (Ding Xiang): **cloves.**
Palmae	*Serenoa repens*: **saw palmetto.**
Papaveraceae	*Corydalis turtschaninovii** (Yan Hu Suo): **corydalis.**
Piperaceae	*Piper kadsura** (Hai Feng Tang): **pepper.**
	Piper wallichii* (Shi Nan Teng): **pepper.**
Plantaginaceae	*Plantago* spp.: **psyllium seeds.**
Polygonaceae	*Polygonum cuspidatum** (Hu Chang): **knotweed,** etc.
	Polygonum multiflorum (He Shou Wu): **knotweed,** etc.
	Rumex crispus: **yellow dock.**
Polypodiaceae	*Scolopendrium subspinipes* mutilans** (Wu Gong): **polypody.**
Ranunculaceae	*Coptis chinensis** (Huang Lian): **goldthread.**

	Hydrastis canadensis: **goldenseal**, orangeroot.
Rhamnaceae	*Rhamnus frangula*: alder **buckthorn**.
	Rhamnus purshiana: **cascara** sagrada.
Rosaceae	*Agrimonia pilosa* (Xian He Cao): **agrimony, harvest lice**.
Rubiaceae	*Rubia cordifolia* (Qian Cao Gen): **madder**.
Schisandraceae*	*Schisandra* chinensis* (Wu Wei Zi).
Solanaceae	*Capsicum annuum*: **Cayenne pepper**.
	Solanum indicum (Huang Shui Qie): **nightshade**.
Typhaceae	*Typha angustifolia* and *T. latifolia* (Pu Huang): **bullrush, cattail**.
Umbelliferae	*Angelica dahurica** (Mu Xiang or Tian Xian Teng, or Ma Dou Ling): **angelica**.
	*Peucedanum praeruptorum** (Qian Hu): **hog-fennel**.
	Glehnia littoralis* (Bei Sha Shen).
Verbenaceae	*Vitex negundo** (Huang Jing Zi).
Zingiberaceae	*Curcuma aromatica* (Yu Jin or E Zhu).
Other	(The following are also cited in Huang's *The Pharmacology of Chinese Herbs*.)
Hirudinea	*Hirudo* nipponia* (Shui Zhi): **leech**, of the class Hirudinea.
Oligochaeta	*Pheretima* aspergillum* (Di Long): **earthworm**, of the class Oligochaeta.
Scorpionidae	*Buthus* martensi* (Qian Xie): **scorpion**. Contains katsutoxin.
Viperidae	*Agkistrodon* acutus* (Bai Hua She): **copperhead, moccasin**, a pit viper of the subfamily Crotalinae.

Source: Data from *Cancer & Natural Medicine: A Textbook of Basic Science and Clinical Research* by John Boik, Oregon Medical Press, Princeton MN, 1995, 1996, pp. 248–253. Plant families, genera, or species **not** in Hartwell's *Plants Used Against Cancer* are denoted by an asterisk.

Table S.7   Chinese Plants/Organisms as Immunostimulants

Amaranthaceae	*Achyranthes bidentata** (Niu Xi). Contains polysaccharides.
Araliaceae	*Acanthopanax* spp.* (Wu Jia Pi, Ci Wu Jia). Contains polysaccharides.
	Panax ginseng (Ren Shen): **ginseng**. Contains dammarane-type saponins.
	*Panax pseudoginseng** (San Qi). Contains dammarane-type saponins.
	*Panax quinquefolium** (Xi Yang Shen): **American ginseng**. Contains dammarane-type saponins.
Aristolochiaceae	*Aristolochia debilis** (Mu Xiang or Tian Xian Teng, or Ma Don Ling).
Boraganaceae	*Symphytum* spp.: **comfrey**. Contains **pyrrolizidine alkaloids**.
Campanulaceae	*Codonopsis pilosula* (Dang Shen).
Caryophyllaceae	*Pseudostellaria* heterophylla* (Tai Zi shen). Contains polysaccharides.
Compositae	*Atractylodes macrocephala** (Bai Zhu).
	*Echinacea purpurea**: **Echinacea, coneflower**. Contains polysaccharides.
	Eclipta prostrata* (Han Lian Cao): **false daisy**.
	Eupatorium cannabinum: **hemp agrimony**. Contains polysaccharides.
	Eupatorium perfoliatum: **boneset**. Contains polysaccharides.
Convolvulaceae	*Cuscuta australis* (Tu Si Zi).
Cruciferae	*Isatis tinctoria* (Qing Dai): **indigo**, isatis, woad.
Cucurbitaceae	*Gynostemma* pentaphyllum* (Jiao Gu Lan). Contains dammarane-type saponins.
Hypocreaceae*	*Cordyceps* sinensis* (Dong Chong Xia Cao): caterpillar **fungus**.
Lauraceae	*Cinnamomum cassia* (Rou Gui).: cassia, **cinnamon**.
Leguminosae	*Astragalus membranaceus** (Huang Qi): **gum traganth, milk-vetch**.
Liliaceae	*Paris formosana** (Quan Shen): **herb Paris**. Contains glycosides.
Malvaceae	*Altheae officinalis*: **marsh mallow**. Contains polysaccharides.
Oleaceae	*Ligustrum lucidum** (Nu Zhen Zi).
Plantaginaceae	*Plantago* spp.: **psyllium seeds**. Contains polysaccharides.
Polygonaceae	*Polygonum odoratum** (Yu Shu): **Solomon's seal**.
	Rheum palmatum (Da Huang): **rhubarb**.
Polyporaceae	*Ganoderma* lucidum* (Ling Zhi): **fungus**.
Rhamnaceae	*Ziziphus jujuba* (Da Zao): **kola, cola**. Contains dammarane-type saponins, and **alkaloids**.
Scrophulariaceae	*Picrorrhiza kurroa* (Hu Huang Lian).
Solanaceae	*Lycium barbarum** (Gou Qi Zi). Contains polysaccharides.
Umbelliferae	*Angelica sinensis* (Dang Gui): **angelica**.
	*Bupleurum chinense** (Chai Hu): **thoroughwax**.
	*Ligusticum chuanxiong** (Chuan Xiong).

Source: Data from *Cancer & Natural Medicine: A Textbook of Basic Science and Clinical Research* by John Boik, Oregon Medical Press, Princeton MN, 1995, 1996, pp. 70–75. Plant families, genera, or species **not** in Hartwell's *Plants Used Against Cancer* are denoted by an asterisk.

Table S.8   Chinese Plants that Raise cAMP Levels

Acanthaceae	*Andrographis* paniculatai* (Chuan Xin Lian).
Actinidiaceae*	*Actinidia* chinensis* (Teng Li). Contains **actinidine**.
Labiatae	*Salvia multiorrhiza* (Dan Shen).
Polyporaceae	*Polyporus umbellatus** (Zhu Ling).
Ranunculaceae	*Aconitum carmichaeli** (Fu Zi).
Rhamnaceae	*Ziziphus jujuba* (Da Zao): **kola, cola**. Contains **alkaloids**.
Rubiaceae	*Coffea* spp.: **coffee**. Contain **caffeine**.
Umbelliferae	*Cnidium monnieri* (She Chuang Zi).

Source: Data from *Cancer & Natural Medicine: A Textbook of Basic Science and Clinical Research* by John Boik, Oregon Medical Press, Princeton MN, 1995, 1996, p. 216. Plant families, genera, or species **not** in Hartwell's *Plants Used Against Cancer* are denoted by an asterisk.

Table S.9   Chinese Plants that Lower cAMP Levels

Scrophulariaceae	*Rehmannia glutinosa* (Shu Di Huang).
Testudinidae*	*Chinemys* (Geoclemys) reevesii* (Gui Ban). Abdominal plate of the water **tortoise**, of the order Chelonia.

Source: Data from *Cancer & Natural Medicine: A Textbook of Basic Science and Clinical Research* by John Boik, Oregon Medical Press, Princeton MN, 1995, 1996, p. 216. Plant families, genera, or species **not** in Hartwell's *Plants Used Against Cancer* are denoted by an asterisk.

Chemical Taxa of Medicinal Plants*

T.1 TERPENES AND RELATED COMPOUNDS

T.1.1 TERPENE COMPOUNDS; SESQUITERPENE LACTONES

Apiaceae*/Umbelliferae

Anatheum graveolens: dill. Carvone, dillapiol.

Carum copticum*. Thymol, p-thymol, carvicrol, terpenene.

Coriandrum sativum: coriander. Linalool.

Crithmum maritimum.: sea fennel, cardo. Dillapiol, phellandrene.

Cuminum cyminum: cumin. Ketone/cryptone.

Daucus carota: **carrot**. Carotol, pinene, cymol, geranylacetate, sesquiterpene, daucol, bizabolol, asaron, sabinene, α-pinene, geraniol, terpene esters, carophyllene, geranyl, trans-iso-asarone.

Foeniculum vulgare: fennel. Fenchone, estragole, fenchone, anethol,

Libanotis transcaucasica.* Geraniol, phellandrene, sesquiterpenes, bisabolol.

Petroselinum crispum: selinon. Myristicine, apiol, pinenes, allyltetramethoxybenzene.

Araceae

Acorus calamus: sweet flag, calamus, acoron, vacha. Asarone, camphor, calamene, geranylacetate, geraniol, camphene, asaron, pinene, sesquiterpenes.

Aristolochiaceae

Asarum europaem: asarum. Sesquiterpenealcohols, trans-isoeugenolmethylether, unknown phenylpropane.

Asiasarum heterotropoides. Eucarvone, methyleugenol, safrole.

A. sieboldii. Cineol, eucarvone, safrole, methyleugenol.

Asteraceae/Compositae—I. Terpenes

Achillea aspenifloia. Prochamazulenes.

A. ageratum: agaeraton. Prochamazulenes.

A. clypeolata. Prochamazulenes.

A. depressa. Prochamazulenes.

A. grandiflora. Prochamazulenes.

A. microphylla. Prochamazulenes.

A. millefolium: yarrow. Azulenes, prochamazulenes.

A. nobilis. Prochamazulenes.

A. odorata. Prochamazulenes.

A. stricta. Prochamazulenes.

A. setacea. Prochamazulenes.

---

* *Source:* Data from *Infraspecific Chemical Taxa of Medicinal Plants* by Péter Tétény, Chemical Publishing Co., New York, 1970. Plant family headings are in **boldface**. Plant families, genera, or species **not** listed in Hartwell's *Plants Used Against Cancer* are denoted by an asterisk. Plant families, genera, and species which **are** listed in Hartwell are underlined for emphaisis. The order of presentation is in the main alphabetical. The abbreviation ORP stands for optical rotatory power. Most alkaloids are in **boldface**, as are some other compounds or items of potential interest.

A. tanacetifolia*. Prochamazulenes.

Artemisia absinthium: absinthe, wormwood. Thujone, thujylalcohol, myrcene, sabinene, isothujyl Ac, cadinene (azulenes), s-guajazulene, proartemazulene, various azulenes.

A. arborescens: artemisia, mugwort. Azulenes, thujene, thujone, thujylalcohol, borneol, camphor, **arborescine**.

A. austriaca*. Cineol, thujone, camphor, aldehydes, azulenes.

A. balchanorum*. Linalool, geraniol, citral.

A. cina*. Cineol, camphor.

A. dracunculus*. Sabinene, pinene, methylchavicol.

A. ferganensis*. Sesquiterpene-alcohol, terpenes, camphor, cineol.

A. herba-alba*. Camphor, camphene, thujone, phenols, sesquiterpenes.

A. lercheana*. Camphor, borneol.

A. macrocephala*. Guajazulenes.

A. pallens*.

A. porrecta*. Cineol, camphor, thujone, linalylbiturate.

A. santolinifolia*. Cineol, phenols, thujone, thujylalcohol.

A. scoparia*. Scoparylene, eugenol, pinene, cadinene, pinene, agropyrenes, pinene, myrcene.

A. scopariioides*. Eugenol.

A. sieversiana*. Pinene, cineol, myrcene, sesquiterpenes, azulenes, borneo, camphor, cineol.

A. terrae-albae*. Camphor, cineol, artemisiaketone.

A. tridentata. Cineol, camphor, artemisol, pinene, **methacroleine**, thujone, camphene.

Chrysantheum cinerariaefolium*. **Pyrethrines**.

C. vulgare*. Camphor, thujone, borneol, cineol, isothujone, umbellulone, monoterpene hydrocarbons, monoterpene ester, sesquiterpene derivatives, artemisiaketone, chrysantemum epoxide, α-pinene, β-pinene, γ-terpinene.

Matricaria chamomilla: chamomile. Azulenes, prochamazulenes, bisabolols, farnesol.

Asteraceae/Compositae—II. Sesquiterpene lactones

Ambrosia acanthicarpa*. Confertiflorin, chamissonin, artenovin.

A. ambrosioides*. Damsin, franserin, hispidulin.

A. artemisiifolia. Coronopilin, psilostachyin, aartemisiifolin, cumanin, peruvin.

A. chamissonis*. Sequiterpene lactones.

A. confertiflora*. Confertiflorin, desacetylconfertiflorin, other germacranolides, psilostachyin, psilostachyin C.

A. cumanensis*. Cumanin, psilostachyin. psilostachyin B, psilostachyin C, ambrosin, coronopilin, damsin.

A. dumosa*. Coronopilin, ambrosiol, burrodin, apulodin.

A. peruviana*. Psilostachyin C. tetrahydroambrosin, peruvin, peruvinin.

A. psilostachya*. Coronopilin, ambrosiol, psilostachyin, damsine, 3-hydroxydamsin, cumanin, parthenin.

Artemisia brevifolia*. Santonin.

A. coerulescens*. Santonin, β-santonin.

A. cina*. Santonin.

A. gallica*. Santonin.

A. kurramensis*. Santonin, α-, β-, γ-santonin.

A. maritima: sea wormwood. Santonin, 1-β-santonin, **pseudosantonine**, α- or β-santonin.

A. tenuisecta*. Santonin.

Cnicus benedictus: carducellus, cardo benedictus. Cnicin, benedictin.

Chrysantheum parthenium: feverfew. Parthenolide, santamarin.

Gaillardia pulchella*. Helenalin, pulchellin, puchellin B, C, D, gaillardin.

Helenium amarum*. (Hartwell lists this genus in the index, but has the wrong page number. Moreover, it does not appear in Compositae, where it should.) Tenulin, aromaticin, amaralin.

H. autumnale*: sneezeweed. Helenalin, dehydromexicanin.

H. mexicanum*. Helenalin, mexicanins.

Iva axillaris*. Ivaxillarin, anhydro-ivaxillarin, axivalin, ivaxilin.

I. microcephala*. Ivalin, microcephalin, pseudoivalin.

Parthenium hysterophorus: absynthe batarde. Parthenin, hysterin, ambrosin.

Petasites albus*. Petasins, furoeremophilanes.

P. hybridus: pestilence weed. Petasol, **petasines**, eremophilanes, sesquiterpenes, furoeremophilanes, petasin.

Xanthium strumarium: burweed, cocklebur.

Burseraceae

Bursera* *microphylla*. Terpenes.

Cannabiaceae/Cannabinaceae* (Moraceae)

Cannabis sativa: hemp, marijuana. Tetrahydrocannabinol/cannabidiol, cannabinol.

Humulus lupulus: hops. Myrcene, farnasene, ocimene, caryophyllene, posthumulene, β-selinene.

Chenopodiaceae

Chenopodium ambrosioides: payco, potato. Ascaridol, pinene, phellandrene. pinocarvone, aritasone.

C. botrys*. Ascaridol, esther.

C. integrifolium*. Ascaridol, p-cymol, limonene.

C. schraderianum*. Ascaridol.

C. suffruticosum*. ORP laevo- or dextrarotatory.

Roubieva multifida*. Ascaridol, p-cymol, phellandrene, anethol, limonene, carveol.

Cupressaceae* (Pinaceae)

Chamaecyparis obtusa*. Hinoki A, one diterpene, sabinene, chamene, terpinene-4-ol.

Juniperus virginiana: red cedar. Cedrene, cedrol, thujopsene.

Libocedrus* *bidwillii*. Rumen-like depentene, isophyllocladene.

Thujopsis* *dolabrata*. (*Thuja* is in Hartwell.) Carvacrol, thujaplicines, isopropylphenol.

Cyperaceae

Cyperus rotundus: musta, cyperus, angular rush. Cyperol, cyperene, cyperone.

Dipterocarpaceae

Dipterocarpus* *appendiculatus*. Caryophyllene, humulene.

D.* *baudii*. Gurjunene, calarene.

D.* *geniculatus*. Humulene, caryophyllene, aromadendrene.

D.* *grandiflorus*. Alloaromadendrene, gurjunene, humulene.

D.* *obtrusifolius*. Humulene, cyperene.

D.* *turbinatus*. Calarene, humulene, gurjunene.

D.* *warburgii*. Alloaromadendrene, copaene, caryophyllene, humulene, cyperene.

D.* *zeylanicus*. farnesane, caryophyllene, humulene.

Ericaceae

Ledum palustre: wild rosemary, marsh tea. Myrcene, ledol, palustrol, p-cymol, sesquiterpenes, p-cresol, p-cymol, pinene, germacrone.

Erythroxylaceae

Erythroxylum* *monogynum*. Bisabolene, cadinene, pinene, monogynol, diterpenes.

Geraniaceae

Pelargonium roseum*: geranio. Citronellol, geraniol, menthone.

Gramineae

Bothriochloa* *decipiens*. Extremely variable in variations.

B.* *glabra*. Variable.

B.* *insculpta*. Variable races.

B.* intermedia. Extremely variable in composition.

B.* ischaemum. Variable in composition.

Cymbopogan* coloratus. Citral, geraniol, geranyl Ac, camphene, sesquiterpenes.

C.* connatus. perillaalcohol, unknown aldehyde, phellandrene, carvone,.

C.* flexuosus. Citral, geranylsalycylate, cineol.

C.* martinii. Geraniol, perillaalcohol, menthdienols.

C.* nardus. Citronellal, geraniol, terpenes, alcohols, camphene, dipentene.

Elyonurus* viridulus. Citral a and b, camphene, pinene, sesquiterpenes.

<u>*Vetiveria zizanioides*</u>: sevya, ucira. ORP range –22° to +45°.

Grimaldiaceae*

Grimaldia* fragrans

Lamaceae*/<u>Labiatae</u>

<u>*Agastache formosana**</u>. Pulegone, isomenthone.

Elsholtzia* ciliata. Elsholtziaketone, naginataketone, isovaleric A.

E.* oldhami. Elsholtziaketone, dehydroelsholtziaketone, naginataketone.

<u>*Galeopsis ladanum**</u>. Acetylharpaagid.

<u>*Hyptis suaveolens*</u>: mastranto. Sabinene, sesquiterpenes, menthol.

<u>*Hyssopus officinalis*</u>: hyssop.

<u>*Lavandula angustifolia**</u>. Linalylacetate.

Majorana* hortensis. Sabinene hydrate, geraniol, eugenol.

<u>*Mentha aquatica*</u>: menta. Linalyl. linalool, limonene, carvone, menthofurane, cineol, isopinocamphene.

M. arvensis*. Pulegone, isomenthone, menthone, menthol, menthofuran, carvone, piperitone, Δ-3-octanone, Δ3-octanonol, limonene, ethylamylcarbinol.

M. canadensis*. Pulegone, menthone.

<u>*M. longifolia.*</u> Pulegone, menthofurane, carvone, piperitone, piperitone-oxide, piperitenone-oxide, hydrocarbons, dihydrocarveol, limonene, linallol, piperitol, menthol, linalool.

<u>*M. pulegium*</u>: pennyroyal. Pulegone, isopulegone.

<u>*M. rotundifolia*</u>: mente. Pulegone, carvone, limonene, piperitenone oxide, neisoisopulegol, piperitenone, isopiperitenone.

M. sachalinensis*. Menthol, menthone.

M. satureioides*.Menthol, pulegone, menthenone, menthone.

<u>*M. spicata*</u>: mint. Carvone, pulegone, menthone, piperitenone oxide, piperitenone, cineol, piperitone, limonene, isopulegone, linallol, carvacrol.

Monarda* fistulosa. Carvacrol, thymol, p-cymene, cineol, sabinene, -cymene, terpinolene, -terpineol.

M.* mexicana. Thymol, cineol, -bornyl.

M.* punctata. Thymol, cymene, cineol, carvacrol.

Mosla* carvonifera. Carvone, carvacrol, thymol.

M.* chinensis. Carvacrol, carvacryl Ac, borneol.

M.* formosana. Dillapiol, caryophyllene, carvacrol.

M.* grosseserrata. Methyluegenol, methylchavicol, **myristicine**, methylisoeugenol.

M.* hadai. Carvacrol, γ-terpinene.

M.* hirta. Thymol, carvacrol.

M.* lanceolata. Cineol, geranyl, citral, dihydrocarvone, sabinol.

M.* linaloolifera. d-Linalool, limonene, 1-linallol, caryophyllene.

M.* punctulata. Thujone, **elemicine**, methyleugenol, bisabolene, asarone.

M.* tenuicaulis. Thymol, thymol-methylether.

<u>*Nepeta cataria*</u>: catnip. Citral, citronellal, nepetalic acid, carvacrol, citrenellol, geraniol, nepetalactone.

N. mussinii*. Menthol or aldehyde, citral (?), epinepetalactone.

N. transcaucasica*. Geranyl acetate, citronellol, citral.

Ocimum basilicum: basil. linalool, methylcinnamate, methyl chavicol, terpinene, ocimene, camphor, eugenol.

O. canum*. Citral, camphor, methylcinnamate.

O. gratissimum*. Citral, bisabolene, eugenol, ocimene, thymol.

O. menthafolium*. Citral, methylchavicol, camphor, anethol.

O. sanctum*. Aldehydes (citrale), eugenol, methylchavicol, chavibetol, cineol.

O. viride*. Citral, thymol, phenols.

Origanum vulgare: origanum, oregano, wild marjoram. Thymol, carvacrol, linalyl Ac/phenols, sesquiterpenes.

Perilla* frutescens. Perillaaldehyde, piperitone, naginataketone, elsholtziaketone, citral, perillaketone, dillapiol, caryophyllene, egomaketone, isoegomaketone.

Pogostemon plectanthoides*. Menthol, aromadendrene, caryophyllene, cadinene, guajol.

Prunella vulgaris: prunella. Camphor.

Rosmarinus: rosemary.

Salvia apiana.* Cineol, camphor-borneol.

S. officinalis: salvia, sage. Thujone.

S. sclarea: cleere eye. Linalyl Ac, linalool.

Satureja abyssinica*. Pulegone, isomenthone, citral, limonene, menthone.

S. biflora*. Pulegone, citral, mentone, camphor.

S. odora*. Pulegone, lippione, piperitenone oxide, piperitone oxide.

Thymus armeniacus*. Limonene,camphor, geraniol, linalool, thymol.

T. austriacus*. Terpineol, borneol, thymol.

T. eriophorus*. Citronellol, citral.

T. fedtschenkoi*.

T. froelichianus*. Linallol, terpineol, nerolidol, borneol, eucalyptol, thymol, terpinyl Ac.

T. hadzhievii*. Citral, camphor, borneol, geraniol, linalool.

T. karamarianicus*. Citral, borneol, camphene, carvacrol.

T. karjagini*. Citral, camphor, borneol, geraniol, linalool.

T. kjapazi*.

T. kotschyanus*. Citronellal, thymol, linalylacetate, limonene, borneol, citral, camphor.

T. marschallianus*. citral, borneol, terpineol, phenols, thymol, p-cymene, geraniol, linalool, nerolidol, eucalyptol..

T. nigricus*. Citronellol, linalool.

T. oenipontanus*. Linalool, geraniol, borneol, citral, thymol, carvacrol, geranyl Ac, neryl Ac.

T. polytrichus*. Linalool, terpineol, borneol, thymol, carvacrol.

T. pulegioides*. Citral, carvacrol, thymol, phenols, borneol.

T. serpyllum*. Carvacrol, p-cymene, γ-terpene, thymol, linalool, linalacetate, myrcene, sesquiterpene, caryophyllene, cineol, geraniol, borneol, citral.

T. serrulatus*. Carvacrol, thymol, linalool.

T. sudeticus*. Borneol, citral, thymol, geranyl Ac.

T. tiflisiensis*. Citral, camphor, borneol, linalool, geraniol.

T. transcaucasicus*. Linalool, geranylacetate, terpinene, thymol.

T. trautvetteri*. Geraniol, citronellol, citral.

T. vulgaris*. Citral, p-cymol, thymol/carvacrol, cineol, linalool, terpinene, borneol, phenol, p-cymene, carvacrol, linalyl Ac, terpineol, terpenyl Ac, terpinyl-4, terpinene, bornyl Ac.

Lauraceae

Aniba* rosaeodora. 1-linallol, dl-linallol.

Cinnamomum camphora: camphor tree. Camphor or cineol, borneol, safrole, sesquiterpene, sesquiterpene alcohol, linalool.

C. glandiuliferum*. Cineol, terpineol, camphor.

*C. molle**. Camphor.

*C. parthenoxylon**. Cineol, cadalene, terpineol, phellandrene.

<u>*C. zeylanicum*</u>.: malabathrom, cinnamon. Caryophyllene, eugenol, benzyl benzoate.

*Litsea** zeylanica. Ocimene, bycyclicsesquiterpenes, terpinene, alcohol.

<u>*Persea gratissima*</u>: avocado. d-α-Pinene, methylchavicol.

Myoporaceae*

*Myroporum** deserti. Sesquiterpenes.

Myristicaceae

<u>*Myristica fragrans*</u>: mace, nutmeg. Geraniol, linallol, terpinolene, safrole, camphor, eugenol.

Myrtaceae

*Baeckea** gunniana. Pinene, cineol, baeckol, eudesmol.

*Backhousia** angustifolia. Dehydroangustione, angustifolionol, angustione.

*B.** citriodora. Citral, citronellal.

*Blepharocalyx** tweediei. Terebenthene, australene.

*Calythrix** tetragona. Pinenes, sesquiterpenes, citronellol, citronellylformate.

*Eucalyptus amygdalina**. Cineol, piperitone.

*E. andreana**. Piperitones.

*E. andrewsi**.

*E. camaldulensis**. p-Cymol, phellandrine, cineol, pinene.

*E. citriodora**. Citronellal, citronellylesther, citronellol, hydrocarbons.

*E. dives**. Piperitone, phellandrene, cineol.

*E. flocktoniae**. Torquatone.

*E. numerosa**. Phellandrene, piperitone, piperitolesther, Cineol.

*E. oleosa**. Cineol, pinenes.

*E. ovalifolia**. Phellandrene, sesquiterpenes, cineol, pinene.

*E. pauciflora**. Pinene, phellandrene.

*E. piperita**. Piperitone, cineol, eudesmol, phellandrene.

*E. punctata**. Cineol.

*E. racemosa**. Cineol, piperitone, phellandrene, cryptone.

*E. radiata**. Cineol, terpinene, β-phellandrene, α-phellandrene, eudesmol.

*E. sparsifolia**. Eudesmol.

*E. spathulata**. Torquatone.

*E. tereticornis**. Phellandral, p-cymane, cuminal, cineol, α-pinene.

*E. viminalis**. Cineol, benzaldehyde, α-phellandrine.

*Leptospermum** citratum. Citral, citronellal, d-γ-pinene, γ-terpinene, citronellol, geraniol.

*L.** lanigerum. Eudesmene, α-pinene, darwinol.

*L. *liversidgei*. Citral, α-pinene, citronellal, geraniol.

<u>*Melaleuca alternifolia**</u>. α–Pinene, cineol, pinenes, terpinene, terpinolene, terpineol-4, p-cymene.

*M. ericifolia**. α-Terpinol, cineol, terpenes, linalool, sesquiterpenes.

<u>*M. leucadendra*</u>: cajeput. Cineol, eugenolmethylether.

*M. linariifolia**. Cineol, alsohol (borneol?), terpinene, terpinenol, terpenes.

*M. quinquenervia**. Cineol, nerolidol, linallol, limonene, viridiflorol.

Pinaceae

<u>*Abies balsamea*</u>: pitch tree. Δ^3-Carene.

*A. concolor**. Δ^3-Carene, camphene, β-pinene.

*A. lasiocarpa**. Δ^3-Carene, limonene, phellandrene.

*A. pindrow**. Terpineol, terpineol-nonylate, sesqiterpene alcohol, Δ^3-carene, depentene, cadinene, bornyl Ac.

<u>*Picea abies*</u>: pine. Cadinene, borneol-bornyl-Ac, camphene, limonene.

*P. engelmanni**. Camphor, borneol-bornyl-Ac, myrcene, limonene, δ-cadinene.

*P. pungens**. Bornyl-Ac, limonene.

Pinus contorta*. β-phellandrene, Δ³-carene.

P. elliottii. α-Pinene, β-pinene, phellandrine.

P. khasya. α-Pinene, β-pinene, longifolene, phellandrine.

P. longfolia.Δ³-Carene, longifolene, pinene.

P. montezumae. dl-α-Pinene, limonene, Δ³-carene.

P. monticola. Limonene, pinenes, Δ³-carene.

P. muricata. α-Pinene, Δ³-carene, sabinene, terpinolene.

P. michoacana. α-Pinene, β-pinene.

P. nigra. ORP range –10° to –48°.

P. palustris: sarala. Various ORP (optical rotatory power).

P. pinaster: pinaster, wild pine. ORP range –90° to –16°. α-Pinene, β-pinene.

P. pityusa. 1-α-Pinene, Δ³-carene.

P. ponderosa Various ORP. Limonene, terpinolene, cadinene, longifolene, β-pinene, Δ³-carene.

P. pseudo-strobus. α-Pinene, limonene, longifolene.

P. radiata. dl-α-Pinene, 1-β-pinene, α-pinene, β-pinene, camphere.

P. silvestris: pisa, colofinia. Various ORP. Pinene, Δ³-carene,limonene, 1-β-phellandrine, pinenes.

P. washoensis. Δ³-Carene, 1-β-pinene.

Pseudotsuga menzieslii. Sabinene.

Podocarpaceae*

Dacrydium biforme. Phyllocladene, biformene, myrcene, β-terpene.

D. colonsoi. Phyllocladene, cadinene, pinene.

D. laxifolium. Phyllocladene, kaurene.

Podocarpus macrophyllus. Phyllocladene, isophyllocladene, kaurene.

P. spicatus. Kaurene, oxyterpene, phyllocladene.

P. totara. Totarene, rimuene, kaurene, isokaurene, phyllocladene.

Rutaceae

Boronia ledifolia*. Sesquiterpenes, terpenes (oxygenless), methyl-n-heptyl-, nonylketone.

B. pinnata*. Terpenes, sesquiterpenes, citronellol, citronellylesssther, **elemicine**, safrole.

B. thujona*. α- and β-thujone, safrole.

Citrus aurantifolia: vijapura. Furfurol, borneol, geraniol, cineol, camphene, p-cymol.

C. hystrix. Citral, citronellol, terpenes, citronellal.

C. limon: lemon. Citral, linalool, pinene, terpinene, octanal, octanol.

C. paradisi. Terpinol-4, α-terpineol.

C. reticulata. Mandarin orange. Thymol, thymilmethylether, ocimene, pinene, terpineol-4, sabinene, terpineol, nonanol, octanal, linallol, nonyl Ac.

C. sinensis: orange. Ocimene, citronellal, γ-terpineol, linallol, gerianial, neral.

Geifera parviflora*. Linallol, geijerene, azulenes, camphene, limonene.

Murraya koenigii*. Caryophyllene, cadinene, cadinol, sabinene, pinene, dipentene.

Poncirus trifliata*. Limonene, myrcene.

Ruta graveolens: rue. Methyl-n-nonylketone.

Zanthoxylum budrunga. Sabinene, α-terpinene, β-phellandrene, δ-terpinene, α-phellandrine, pinene.

Taxodiaceae*

Cunninghamia lanceolota. β-Pinene, phellandrine.

Sciadopytis verticillata. Kaurene, isophyllacladene, phyllocladene.

Valerianaceae
(see **Pseudoalkaloids**)
Verbenaceae

Lantana camara. Caryophyllene, phellandral, linalool, cadinene, pinene, dipentene, cineol, terpinene, cymene.

*Lippia alba**. piperitone, lippione, pinene, dihydrocarvone, limonene, lippion, citral, cineol.

*L. seriphioides**. Thymol (?), phenol, citral, geraniol.

Zingiberaceae

Alpinia galanga: galanga, "Galen Gal." Cinnamic A methylester, campher-cineol, sesquiterpenes.

*A. nutans**. Camphor, camphene, pinenes, cineol.

Elettaria cardamomum: cardamon, cardamomum, amomum. Cineol, limonene, linalool-1-Ac, linalool, linalyl Ac.

T.1.2 TERPENOIDS (TRITERPENES, STEROIDS, SAPONINS, CARDENOLIDS)
Agavaceae* (**Amaryllidaceae**)

*Agave aurea**. Hecogenin, 9-dehydrohecogenin, tigogenin, manogenin.

*A. brandegeei**. Hecogenin, tigogenin, manogenin, sapogenin.

*A. caerulata**. Sapogenins, hecogenin, tigogenin, gitogenin.

*A. funkiana**. Tigogenin, manogenin, smilagenin, yuccagenin, mexogenin, samogenin.

*A. marmorata**. Smilagenin, chlorogenin, sapogenins.

*A. nelsoni**. Manogenin, tigogenin, hecogenin.

*A. promontorii**. Manogenin, tigogenin, sapogenins.

*A. roseana**. Tigogenin, hecogenin, sapogenin.

*A. sobria**. Manogenin, gitogenin, hacogenin, tigogenin, sapogenins.

*Furcraea guatemalensis**. Tigogenin, sarsasapogenin.

Yucca alifolia*. Smilagenin, tigogenin, gitogenin, chlorogenin.

Y. de-smetiana*. Tigogenin, sapogenin.

Y. filamentosa*. Gitogenin, tigogenin, smilagenin, gitogenin.

Y. gloriosa*. Smilagenin, gitogenin, tigogenin.

Y. recurvifolia*. Smilagenin, gitogenin, tigogenin.

Y. schidigera*. Sarsasapogenin, manogenin.

Amaranthaceae

*Alternanthera denticulata**. Saponins.

*Celosia cristata**. Saponins.

Apiacae*/Umbelliferae

Hydrocotyle asiastica*. Centelloside, indocentoic A, asiaticoside, madecassoside, brahmozide, brahminozide, thankuniside, isothankuniside.

Apocynaceae

Acanthera schimperi*. Acovenoside, ouabain.

Cerbera manghas*. Cardenolids.

C. venenifera*. Tanginin, tangiferin, cardenolids, tanginoside.

*Strophantus sarmentosus**. Sarmutoside, musaroside, sarveroside, panstroside, sarmentocymarin, sarnovide, cardenolids.

Asclepiadaceae

Parquetina nigrescans*. Nigrescigenin, strophantidol, strophantigenin, convallatoxin.

Sarcostemma viminale*. Cardenolids, metaplexigenins, vimolin, sarcostins.

Betulaceae

Alnus glutinosa:, erle, alder. Taraxerol, taracerone, lupeol, glutinone, β-sitosterol.

*A. viridis**. Taraxerol, taraxerone, taraxerylacetate, alnincanone.

Convolvulaceae

*Ipomoea hederacea**. Sterin components.

Cruciferae

*Erysimum canescens**. Glycosides, erysimoside, erycanoside, helveticoside, digitoxose, erysimin, erysimoside, cheirotoxin.

Cucurbitaceae

Citrullus colocynthis: cucumber. Cucurbitacins.

*C. lanatus**. Sterine components.

Cucumis sativus: cucumis edulis, cucumber. Cucurbitacins.
Cucurbita pepo: cucurbita. Cucurbitacins.
Lagenaria siceraria*: gourd. Cucurbitacins.

Cyperaceae

Carex* arenaria. Saponins.

Dioscoreaceae

Dioscorea composita*. Diosgenin, yamogenin.
D. deltoidea*. Sapogenins.
D. humilis*. Sapogenins.
D. pusilla*. Saponins.
Tamus communis: bryony. Diosgenin, sapogenins.

Dipsacaceae

Succisa inflexa*. Saponins.

Ericaceae

Agauria* salicifolia. Agauriolic acetate, agauric A, agaurolene, morolic A.

Euphorbiaceae

Euphorbia hirta: milkweed. Taraxerone, taraxerol, friedelin, β-amyrin, β-sitosterin, hentriakontan.

Fabaceae*/Leguminosae

Trigonella* foenum-graecum. Diosgenin, tigogenin, gitogenin.

Geraniaceae

Geranium sanguuineum: gotsgnad, **herba cancri**. Saponins, sterins.

Gramineae

Miscanthus* sinensis. Sterin components.

Liliaceae

Bowiea volubis*. Bevoside A, bevosides.
Ruscus aculeatus: brusco, hedionda. Ruscogenin, neoruscogenin.
Urginea maritima: squill. Scillirosidin, scillarenin.

Moraceae

Antiaris toxicaria*. α-, β-antiarin.

Polemoniaceae

Phlox* paniculata. Sterin components.
Polemonium coeruleum: polemonia. Saponins.

Rosaceae

Potentilla rupestris: quinquefolium. Tormentoside.
Hydrocotyle* asiastica. Centelloside, indocentoic A, asiaticoside, madecassoside, Brahmozide, brahminozide, thankunoside, isothankuniside.

Scrophulariaceae

Digitalis cariensis*. Digoxin, lanatoside, acetyldigitoxin, glucofucoside, gitorosides.
D. lanata*. Cardenolides, lanatosides A, B and C.
D. mertonensis*. Acetyldigitoxin, digitoxin, gitoxin, lanatoside E, strospeside, verodoxin.
D. purpurea: foxglove. Cardenolides, digitoxin, gitoxin, strospeside, gitaloxin, purpurea-glycoside A.

Solanaceae

Browallia demissa: Botonera. Saponins, sterine components.
Cestrum parqui: palqyui. Gitogenin, digitogenin, steroids, sapogenins, sterins.
C. nocturnum*. Sapogenins.
Iochroma* coccinea. Sterin components.
Nicandra* physaloides. Sterin components.
Physalis ixocarpa*. Sterin components.
Solanum tripartitum*. Sterins, diosgenin, saponins.
Withania somnifera: strychnos, asgandh, winter cherry. Somnirol, somnitol, unsaturated lactone, withanon, unknown withanolide, withaferin A, withanolides.

Verbenaceae

Lantana camara. Lantadene A and B, cardenolids.

Zygophyllaceae

Tribulus terrestris: chi-li. **Tigogenine,** sapogenins, disogenin, gitogenin, ruscogenin.

T.1.3 PSEUDOALKALOIDS

Buxaceae

Buxus microphylla*. Cyclomicrobuxin, cyclobuxomirein, cyclomirosin, cyclobux-ophyllin, suffrobuxin, cyclobuxoviridin, cycloboxosuffrin

Sarcococca* pruniformis. Epipachysamin A, kurchetin, 5-α-pregnane, pregn-5-ene.

Liliaceae

Veratrum album: hellebore. **Protoveratrine, protoveratrine A and B, vera-troylzygadenine, germine, geralbine, jervine.** Also veratramin, **zygacine.**
V. viride: American hellebore, green hellebore. **Germidine, germitrine, neoger-mitrine, protoveratrine, protoveratridine, neogermbudine, germbudine.**

Ranunculaceae

Aconitum napellus: monkshood. **Aconitine.**
A. soongoricum*. **Aconitine, songorine, acetyl-songorine.**

Solanaceae

Lycpersicon esculentum: **tomato. Tomatidin,** soladulcidin, unknown **steroid alka-loid.**
Solanum alatum*. Solasonin, ssonin, smargin, solamargin.
S. atropurpureum*. β-solanigrin, **steroid alkaloids, solasodine.**
S. boerhaavii*. **Solasonine,** solamargin, **tomatine.**
S. capsicastrum*. Solanocapsin, **steroid-alkaloids.**
S. carolinense*. **Steroid alkaloids,** solamargin, solasonin, **solasodine,** diosgenin, tigogenin, soladulcidin, tigogenin.
S. cornutum*. Solasonin, solamargin, β-solamargin, solasodin, diosgenin, unknown **steroid alkaloid,** sapogenin.
S. douglasii*. Solamargin, **steroid alkaloids.**
S. dulcamara: bittersweet, **cancer plant,** dulcamara, climbing nightshade, woody nightshade. Sdulcidin, tomatidenol, smarin, ssodine. ssonin, β-smargin, tigogenin, diosgenin.
S. gila*. **Steroid alkaloids.**
S. gracile*. **Solasodine, steroid alkaloid,** solamargin.
S. haematocarpum*. **Tomatidin,** solasonin, solamargin.
S. nigrum: nightshade. Solasonin, solomargin, β-solomargin, tigogenin, unknown sapogenin, **steroid alkaloids, solasodine.**
S. luteum*. Smargin, ssonin, **steroid alkaloids,** svillin.
S. macrocarpum*. Solasonin, **steroid alkaloids.**
S. melongena: **egg plant. Steroid alkaloids,** solasonin.
S. nitidibaccatum*. **Tomatidin,** solasonin, solamargin, solasodin, diosgenin.
S. nodiflorum*. **Solasodine, steroid alkaloid,** tigogenin.
S. radicans*. **Steroid alkaloids.**
S. rostratum*. Solamargin, solasonin, **solasodine,** diosgenin.
S. sinaicum*. **Steroid alkaloids, solasodine,** diosgenin.
S. sisymbrifolium: revienta cabello, putuy, yuá. **Steroid alkaloids.**
S. stoloniferum*. **Tomatin, solanin,** chaconin.
S. tomatillo*. **Tomatidin,** demissidin, diosgenin.
S. torvum*. **Steroid alkaloids.**
S. vernel*. **Solanin,** chaconin, **steroid alkaloids.**

Valerianaceae

Nardostachys jatamansi: spikenard. ORP range +31° to −7.4°.
Valeriana wallichii*. ORP range −13° to −56° or +7° to +19°. Maalioxide, ar-curcumene, patchoulenes.

T.2　OTHER COMPOUNDS CONNECTED WITH ACETATE METABOLISM

T.2.1.1　DERIVATIVES OF RESORCIN AND OF ORCELLINIC ACID

Aspergillaceae* (the fungi family **Moniliaceae**)

Aspergillus terreus*. **Geodine, erdine, geodoxine**, asterric acid.

Cladoniaceae*

Cladonia* chlorophaea. Novochlorophaeic A, G-L usnic A, FPC A, graic A, cryptochlorophaeic A, merochlorophaeic A..

C.* furcata. Atranoric A, FPC A.

C.* impexa.

C.* nemoxyna.

C.* pityrea. FPC A, homosecicaic A.

C.* squamosa. Squamatic A.

C.* tenuis.

Lecanoraceae*

Haematomma* puniceum.

Lecanora* caesiorubella. Monoacetyl PC A, norST A, PC A.

L.* epanora. Rgysocarpic A, pannarin, epanorin, U A.

L.* pallida. NorST A.

Ochrolechia* tartarea. LE A, E A, G A.

Rinodina* oreina. PC A, gyrophoric A.

Parmeliaceae (Lichens)

Anzia* opuntiella. Divaricatic A, sekikaic A.

A.* ornata. Sekikaic A, divaricatic A.

Asahinea* chrysantha. α-collatic A.

Cetraria ciliaris*. Alectoronic A, O A, PLI A.

C. crispa*. FPC A, 1-PLI A, alloPLI A, d-PLI A, LI A.

C. islandica*. Allo-PLI A, d-PLI A, U A, FPC A, PLI A, d,1-U A.

Parmelia arnoldii*. Alectoronic A, SL A/P.

P. bolliana*. LE A, AT, U A, G A, PLI A.

P. borreri*. LE A, AT, U A, G A, AT/P

P. conspersa*. SL A, FPC A, PC A, ST A.

P. caperata*. CA A, **caperine, caperidine**.

P. cetrarioides*. Imbricaric A, perlatolic A, collatolic A.

P. furfuracea*. Physodic A, O A, AT.

P. isidiata*. ST A, norST A, SL A, FPC A.

P. stenophylla*. SL A, FPC A.

P. tinctorum*.

Parmeliopsis ambigua*. U A, AT.

Peltigeraceae*

Peltigera* horizontalis. Scabrosin A and B.

P.* malacca. Dolichorrhizin.

P.* scrabosa. Scabrosin A and B, dolichorrhizin.

Rocellaceae*

Rocella* portentosa. Lecanoric A, rocellic A, protocetraric A.

R.* fuciformus. Acetylportentol, rocellic A, portentol.

Strictaceae*

Lobaria* pulmonaria. NorST A and G A, squamatic A.

Usneaceae (Lichens)

Ramalina* carpathica. Ramalinic A, eveernic A.

R.* farinacea. PC A, norST A, SL A, hypoPC A.

R.* scopulorum. ST A, SL A.

R.* siliquosa*. PC A, A, U A, ST A, hypoPC A.

Thamnolia* vermicularis. Thamolic A, SQ A, béomycetic A.

Usnea comosa*. U A, SQ A, thamnolic A, SL A, norST A.

U. confusa*. U A, SL A, PC A.

U. dasypoga*. U A, SL A, usnaric A, Tc A, barbatolic A.

U. kushiroensis*. U A. norST A, SL A, ST A.

U. longissima*. U A, B A, barbatolic A, evernic A, diffractaic A, SL A, FPC A, (AT).

U. montis-fuji*. U A, SL A, AT.

U. orientalis*. ST A, SL A, psoronic A.

U. roseola*. U A, B A, diffractaic A, unknown rosaceous substance.

U. rubescens*. U A, norST A, SL A, ST A.

U. rubicunda*. U A, norST A, SL A, ST A.

T.2.1.2 PHLOROGLUCINS
Aspidiaceae* (Polypodiaceae)

Dryopteris assimilis*. desASP, paraASP, ASP. base X, flavASP, phloropyron.

D. carthusiana*. ASP, flavASP, base X, ASPol (paraASP?), albASP, flavASP Ac ASP.

D. cristata*. ASP, ASPol, desASP, albASP, paraASP, flavASP.

D. dilatata*. Phloroglucins, ASP/albASP, aspidin, paraASP.

D. fragrans*. albASP, unknown phloroglucid.

D. maderensis*. ASP acetylASP, desASP, albASP, base X.

D. villarii*. paraASP, ASP.

Aspleniaceae* (Polypodiacea)

Asplenium rhizophyllum*. Phenolics (phloroglucins?)

T.2.1.3 RANUNCULINS
Helleboraceae* (Ranunculaceae)

Helleborus corsicus*. Ranunculin.

Ranunculaceae

Anemone vitifolia*. Ranunculin.

Clematis vitalba: wild clematis, clematide. Ranunculin.

Myosurus* minimus. Ranunculin.

Ranunculus aconitifolius*. Ranunculin.

R. aquatilis: ranunculis, strumis. Ranunculin.

R. auricomus*. Ranunculin, protoanemonin.

R. baudotii*. Ranunculin.

R. cincinnatus*. Ranunculin.

R. ficaria*. Ranunculin.

R. lanuginosus: batrachion, ranculus, strumus. Ranunculin.

R. lingua*. Ranunculin.

R. sardous*. Ranunculin.

T.2.1.4 QUINONES
Caesalpiniaceae* (Leguminosae)

Cassia tora: foetid cassia. Rubrofuzarin, chrysophanal, obtusifolin.

Liliaceae

Aloe ferox: Aloes do Cabo. Aloin, aloinoside A and B.

A. marlothii*. Aloin, homonataloin.

Myrsinaceae

Ardisia crenata*. 3-alkyl-2-hydroxy-5 methoxy Benzoquinone.

A. quinquegona*. Rapanone.

Myrsine seguinii*. Rapanone, embelin.

Polygonaceae

Rheum palmatum: rawend, rhubarb. Anthraquinones, rhein, chrysophanic A, emodin, aloe-emodin.

Rumex confertus*. Chrysophanol, emodin.

R. conglomeratus*. Emodin, chrysophanol.

R. crispus: yellow dock. Physcion, emodin, chrysophanol, oxy-methylanthraquinone.

Sphaerioidaceae*

Phoma* terrestris. Phomazarin.

T.3 PHENYLPROPANE DERIVATIVES AND FLAVONOIDS

3.1.1 SIMPLE PHENOLICS AND PHENYLPROPANE COMPOUNDS
Dipterocarpaceae

Shorea robusta: sal. Homobrenzcatechin, dimethoxypropylbenzol, p-cymol, **naphthalines**, alkoxyls.

Ericaceae

Artctostaphylos* uva-ursi. **Methylarbutine**.

Lamiaceae*/Labiatae

Ocimum sanctum: epipertron. Methylchavicol, chavibetol, cineol, eugenol, aldehydes.

Thymus drucei*. Phenols.

Lauraceae

Cinnamomum bodinieri*. Safrole, etc.

C. cecidodaphne*. Methyleugenol, safrole, elemicin, myristicin.

C. culilawan*. Safrole, methyleugenol, eugenol.

C. glanduliferum*. Safrole, **myristicine, elemicine**.

C. kiamis*. Cinnamic aldehyde, eugenol.

C. loureirii: cinnamon. Cinnamic aldehyde, eugenol.

C. pedunculatum*. Safrole, eugenol, methyleugenol.

C. sintok*. Eugenol, methyleugenol, safrole..

C. tamala: patra, malabathron. Eugenol, cinnamic aldehyde, safrole.

C. zeylanicum: malabathron, malabar leaf, cassia, cinnamon. Cinnamic aldehyde, safrole, eugenol.

Ocotea pretiosa*: cujumary-rana. Safrole, methyleugenol, camphor, safrol.

Lycopodiaceae

Lycopodium annotinum*. p-Hydroxy benzoic A, vanillic A,

L. clavatum*. Vanillic A, syringic A

L. sabinaefolium*. Syringic A.

Monimiaceae*

Doryphora* sassafras. Safrole, methyleugenol.

Myrtaceae

Backhousia* myrtifolia. Elemicin, isoelemicin, eugenolmethylether, isoeugenolmethylether.

Melaleuca bracteata*. Methyleugenol, methyisoeugenol, elemicin, eugenol.

Syzygium* aromaticum. eugenol, eugenin, eugenone.

Piperaceae

Piper betle: betel pepper. **Allylbrenzcatechine**, chavicol, chavibetol, eugenol.

Rutaceae

Zieria* smithii. Safrole, zierone, methyleugenol.

3.1.2. COUMARINS AND STILBENES
Apiaceae/Umbelliferae

Ammi majus: ameus, ameos, ameu. Xanthotoxin, imperatorin, isopimpinellin, marmesin, bergaptene, coumarins.

Angelica archangelica: archangel, angelica. Archangelicin, archangin, unknown coumarin, umbelliprenin, imperatorin, bergaptene, xanthotoxol, xanthotoxin, osthenol, archangelin, prangolarin.

A. dahurica*. Byak-angelicol, isoimperatorin, oxypeucedanin hydrate.

A. saxicola*. Angelicin, calcicolin, oroselol.

A. sylvestris: angelica, angelika root. Oxypeucedanin, isoimperatorin, oxypeucedanin hydrate.

Laser trilobum*. Silerin, oxypeucedanin, prangenin, sesquiterpenelactons.
Pastinaca sativa: parsnip, wild parsnip. Pastinacin, xanthotoxol, xanthotoxin, isopimpinellin, bergaptene, imperatorin.

Fabaceae (Leguminosae)

Derris* scandens. Warangalone, chandelone.

Guttiferae/Hypericaceae*

Calophyllum inophyllum: tacamahaca, palo maria, tamanou. Calophyllic Ac, calophyllic A, inophyllolid, calophyllolid, inophyllic A.

Lauraceae

Aniba* firmula. 4-Methoxyparacotoin, 5,6-dihydrokawain, **4-methoxyphenylcoumaline**, anibin.

Myrtaceae

Eucalyptus clavigera*. Stilbenes.
E. dalrympleana*. Stilbenes.
E. glaucescens*. Stilbenes.
E. kondininensis*. Stilbenes.
E. longicornis*. Stilbenes.
E. melliodora*. Stilbenes.
E. papuana*. Stilbenes.
E. rugosa*. Stilbenes.
E. salmonophloia*. Stilbenes.
E. sideroxylon*. Stilbene-glucosides, rhapontin, piceid, astringin.
E. smithii*. Stilbenes.

Pinaceae

Pinus radiata*. Pinosylvin.

Rubiaceae

Galium mollugo*. 6-Methoxy-7-coumarin.

Rutaceae

Phebalium* drummondii. Imperatorin oxide racemic.
Ptelea* trifoliata. Isopimpinellin, phellopterin, byakangelicin.

Solanaceae

Capsicum annuum.: Cayenne pepper. **Capsaicine**.
C. baccatum: capsicum, Cayenne, bird pepper. **Capsaicines**.
C. frutescens: Cayenne pepper. **Capsaicine**.
C. pubescens*. **Capsaicine**.

3.2 Flavonoids

Apiaceae*/Umbelliferae

Daucus carota: **carrot**. Carotene, carotenoids, syanidin (?) diglucosides.

Asteraceae*/Compositae

Helichrysum bracteatum*. Quercetin, apigenin, antochlor.
Hymenoxys* scaposa. Flavonol-7-glycosides, flavonole-3-glycosides, etc.
Solidago virgaurea: **goldenrod**. Quercitrin, rutin, astragalin, chlorogenic A, isochlorgenic A.
Thelesperma* simplicifolium. Flavonoid components (antochlors).

Corynocarpaceae*

Corynocarpus* laevigatus. **Leucocyanidin**.

Cupressaceae*(or Cupressineae*)

Chamaecyparis* obtusa: white cedar, cypress. sotetsuflavone, taxifolin.

Ericaceae

Lyonia* ovalifolia. Astilbin, quercetrin.
Pieris* japonica. Asebotin, phloridzin.

Eupomatiaceae*

Eupomatia* laurina. Quercetin.

Eupteleaceae*

Euptelea* polyandra. Quercetin, kaempferol.

Fabaceae*/Papilionaceae* (Leguminosae)

Baptisia leucophaea*. Phenolic compounds.

Lathyrus luteus*. Quercetin, caffeic A.

L. sphaericus*. **Cyanidin**, unknown flavonoid.

Lotus* corniculatus. Unknown phenol, sinapic A.

L.* pedunculatus. Quercetin, sinapic A.

Pongamia glabra: chiravilvra, karanda, hoàng-bá. Kanugin, desmethoxykanugin, karanjin, pongapin, gamatin, pinnatin.

Pterocarpus indicus: chandana, red sandalwood. Pterocarpin, homopterocarpin, angolensin, formononetin.

Trifolium israeliticum*: trefoil, clover. Biochanin A, genistein.

T. lappaceum*. Genestein, formononetin, biochanin A.

T. pilulare*. Genistein, formononetin.

T. subterraneum*. Biochanin A, genistein, kaempferol, daidzein, formononetin, quercetin.

Fumariaceae* (Papaveraceae)

Dicentra formosa*. Kaempferol, quercetin.

Gramineae

Agropyron intermedium*. Flavonoids.

Grossulariaceae*

Carpdetus* serratus. Leucodelphinidin, **leucoanthocyanidins**.

Hamamelidaceae

Hamamelis japonica*. **Leucoanthocyanins**, myricetin, quercitin.

Hypericaceae* (Guttiferae)

Hypericum perforatum: St. John's wort. Quercetin.

Juglandaceae

Juglans regia: **walnut**. Hyperin, quercetin-3-galactoside, kaempferols, kaempferol-3-arabinosid, quercetin, **cyanidin**, caffeic A.

Lamiaceae*/Labiatae

Teucrium chamaedrys: **germander**. Scutellarin.

Lardizabalaceae

Akebia trifoliata*. Quercetin, kaempferol.

Lemnaceae

Lemna perpusilla*. Apigenin-7-glycoside.

Liliaceae

Allium douglasii*. Flavonoid-like components.

Smilax glyciphylla*. Glyciphyllin, dihydrochalcones.

Magnolicaceae

Magnolia grandiflora*. Quercetin, kaempferol.

Liriodendron* tulipifera. Rhamnetin.

Malvaceae

Hoheria* sexstylosa. **Leucocyanidin, leucoanthocyanins**.

Meliaceae

Dysoxylum spectabilis*. **Leucoanthocyanins**.

Menispermaceae

Cissampelos* pareira. Quercetin, luteolin, kaempferol.

Menispermum* canadense. Luteolin, apigenin.

Mimosaceae* (Leguminosae)

Acacia dealbata*. Mearnsitrin.

A. mearnsii*. Mearnsitrin.

Mniaceae*

Mnium* affine. Chemovars.

Monimiaceae*

Laurelia* novae-zealandiae. **Leucoanthocyanins**.

Myrtaceae

Eucalyptus angophoroides*. Myricetin, astringin, ellagic A, rhapontin.

E. apodophylla*. Ellagic A.

E. caliginosa*. Myricetin.

E. camaldulensis*. Ellagic A, quercetin, polyphenol compounds.

*E. confertiflora**. Myricetin, ellagic A.
*E. cornuta**. Ellagic A, quercetin.
*E. dalrympleana**. Astringin, rhapontin, kaempferol.
*E. eugenioides**. Renantherin.
*E. fibrosa**. Myricetin.
*E. glaucescens**. Astringin, rhapontin, delphinidin, **cyanidin**, quercetin.
*E. kondininensis**. Rhapontin, chlorogenic A.
*E. leucoxylon**. Quercetin, ellagic A, gallic A.
*E. melliodora**. Quercetin, ellagic A.
*E. obliqua**. Leucodelphinidins.
*E. odorata**. Leucodelphinidin.
*E. oleosa**. Ellagic A, engelitin.
*E. ovata**. Myricetin.
*E. papuana**. Myricetrin, ellagic A, pelargonidin, quercetin.
*E. phaecotricha**. Delphinidin, ellagic A.
*E. risdonii**. Delphinidin, quercetin.
*E. rugosa**. Quercetin, ellagic A, astringin.
*E. salmonophloia**. Aromadendrin, astringin, rhapontin.
*E. sideroxylon**. **Leucocyanidin**, ellagic A, quercetin, gallic A.
*E. sieberi**. Myricetin, ellagic A.
*E. smithii**. Astringin.
*E. tereticornis**. Myricetin.
*E. watsoniana**. Myricetin.
*Psidium** guaiava. **Leucoanthocyanins**, ellagic A, diglycosides.

Pinaceae

Picea abies: pine, spruce. Fluorescence with blue (chlorogenic A?) or yellow (flavonglycosides?) spot.
*Pinus nigra**: pine. Pinobanksin.
*P. strobus**. Pinocembrin.
*Pseudotsuga** menziesii. Flavone constituents (taxifolin?).

Polygonaceae

*Fagopyrum** esculentum. Rutin, glycosides.
*F.** tataricum. Glycosides, rutin.
Polygonum hydropiper: water-pepper. Rhamnasin, persicarin, persicarin-7-methy-laether, rutin, one quercetinglycoside, rhamnasinbisulphate, quercetrin, hyperin.
P. persicaria: persicary, arsmart. Hyperin, avicularin, quercetrin.
Rumex acetosa: garden sorrel. Hyperin, rutin, quercetrin.

Polypodiaceae

*Pityrogramma**triangularis**. Flavonoid aglycones, ceroptene pigment.

Rosaceae

Geum urbanum: benedicte, auencia, avenes, geum. **Leucoanthocyanins**.
*Malus zume**. Phloridzin, sieboldin.
*Pyrus betulifolia**. Apigenin, luteolin.
*P. calleryana**. quercetin, chrysoeriol.
*P. pashia**. Luteolin, apigenin, flavonglycosides.
*P. phaeocarpa**. Luteolin, catechin.

Rubiaceae

*Galium mollugo**. Hesperidin, asperuloside, chlorogenic A.

Rutaceae

*Evodia** micrococca. Pinoresional dimehtyl ether, sesamin.
*Melicope** ternata. Meliternin, meliternatin, ternatin, narangin, xanthoxyletin.

Simarubaceae

*Harrisonia** perforata. Quercetin, myricetin, **cyanidin**.

Taxodiaceae*

*Cunninghamic** lanceolata. Sotetsuflavone.

<u>Theaceae</u>

> *Camellia sinensis*: **green tea**. Flavonoids, Ca-oxalate.

<u>Winteranaceae</u>

> *Drymys* brasiliensis*. Apigenin.
> *D.* confertifolia*. Dihydroquercetin, apigenin.
> *D.* granadensis*. dihydroquercetin.
> *D.* lanceolata*. Apigenin, luteolin.
> *D.* piperita*. Quercetin, dihydroquercetin, apigenin, luteolin.
> *D.* winteri*. Dihydroquercetin.
> *Pseudowintera* axillaris*. Quercetin, apigenin, kaempferol.

T.4   ALKALOIDS

T.4.1   PROTOALKALOIDS; ANOMALIC ORGANIZED PEPTIDES
<u>Agaricaceae</u> (Fungi)

> *Amanita phalloides*: ~ fly agaric. **Phalloidine, amanitines, α-amanitine**, toxins.
> *Iocyble* xanthomelas*. **Muscarine, alkaloids**.

<u>Clavicipitaceae*</u>/<u>Hypocreaceae</u> (Fungi)

> *Claviceps paspali**: ~ ergot. Lysergic A derivatives, hydroxyethylamide, lysergic A amide, methylcarbinol amide, **ergotamine**.
> *C. purpurea*: ergot, spurred rye. **Ergotamine, ergotoxine, ergometrine, ergocristine, ergocryptine**, lysergic A derivatives, **isolysergic-alkaloids, clavinic alkaloids.**

<u>Convolvulaceae</u>

> *Ipomoea violacea**. Lysergic and isolysergic A amide, **clavinic alkaloids**.

<u>Ephedraceae*</u>

> *Ephedra* distachya*. **Alkaloids, ephedrine, pseudoephedrine.**
> *E.* gerardiana*. **Alkaloids, ephedrine.**
> *E.* intermedia*. **Alkaloids, pseudoephedrine, ephedrine.**
> *E.* nebrodensis*. **Alkaloids, pseudoephedrine, ephedrine.**

<u>Equisetaceae</u>

> *Equisetum arvense*: horsetail. **Nicotine, metoxypiridine, palustrine, alkaloids.**

T.4.2   ALKALOIDS PROPER
<u>Amaranthaceae</u>

> *Alternanthera denticulata**. Alkaloids.

<u>Amaryllidaceae</u>

> *Amaryllis* bella-donna*. **Ambelline, lycorine, caranine, bellamarine, amaryllidine, belladine, galanthamine, lycorenine.**
> *Leucojum* aestivum*. **Galanthamine, lycorine, isotacettine.**
> *Pancratium* maritimum*. **Lycorine, tacettine, haemanthidine.**

<u>Apiaceae*</u>/<u>Umbelliferae</u>

> *Prangos pabularia**. Alkaloids.

<u>Apocynaceae</u>

> *Aspidosperma* australe*. **Aspidospermine, olivacine, guatambuine.**
> *A.* cuspa*. **Aspidopermine.**
> *A.* nigricans*. **Uleine, dihydrouleine.**
> *A.* pyricollum*. **Aspidospermine, uleine, olivacine, guatambuine, apparicine,** dasycarpidone.
> *A.* quebracho-blanca*. **Yohimbine, aspidospermine, querbrachacidine**, yohimboic A, **quebrachamine, quebrachine.**
> *Catharanthus* roseus*. Alkaloids.
> *Rauvolfia* canascens*. **Deserpidine.**
> *R.* ligustrina*. **Reserpine, reserpinine, deserpidine.**
> *R.* serpentina*: snakeroot. **Ajmaline, serpentine, serpentinine, rauvolfinine.**

R.* vomitoria. **Ajmaline, sarpagine, ajmaline, alstonine, reserpine, raumitorine, rescinnamine, rauvomitine, reserpiline, seredine.**
Vinca major: periwinkle. **Reserpinine, kajdine, carapaunabine.**
V. minor: periwinkle. **Vincamine, isovincamine.**
Voacanga* thouarsii. **Dregamine, voakamine.**

Asteraceae*/Compositae
Anthemis tinctoria: cotila, amarusca. Alkaloids.
Gnaphalium luteo-album: pate-di-tchèt. Alkaloids.
Nardosmia* laevigata. **Plataphylline, renardine, senecionine, seneciphylline.**
Senecio platyphyllus*. **Plataphylline, seneciphylline,** heliotridane, **sarracine.**
S. riddellii*. **Riddelliine, retrorsine.**
Siegesbeckia orientalis: si-tzian'-tsao. Alkaloids.
Vittadinia* triloba. Alkaloids.

Berberidaceae
Berberis asiatica: Indian barberry, Indian lycium. **Berberine, oxyacanthine, palmatine.**
B. laurina*. **Berberine, hydrastine, berberastine.**
B. thunbergii*. **Magnoflorine, isotetrandrine.**
Nandina* domestica. **Nandinine, nantenine, menisporine, protopine.**

Caesalpiniaceae* (Leguminosae)
Crotalaria* anagyroides.: ~ rattlebox. **1-Methylene pyrrolidine, senecionine.**
C.* retusa. **Monocrotaline, monocrotaline-N-oxide.**
C.* spectabilis. **Monocrotaline, spectabiline.**

Caryophyllaceae
Gypsophila paniculata*. Alkaloids.
Melandrium* album. Alkaloids.

Celasteraceae
Catha* edulis. **Cathine, cathinine, cathidine, d-nor-isophedrine, d-nor-pseudoephedrine (cathine).**

Chenopodiaceae
Anabasis* aphylla. **Anabasine,** unkown alkaloids.
Beta vulgaris: beet. **Betacyanines, betaxanthines.** Also **betacyanic glycosides.**
Girgensohnia* oppositifolia. **Girgensonine, methylpiperideine.**
Salsola kali: glass-worte. **Salsoline.**
S. paletzkiana*. Alkaloids.
S. richteri*. **Salsoline, salsolidine.**

Crassulaceae
Sedum acre: ~ stonecrop. **Sedamine, nicotine, sedridine, sedinine.**

Erythroxylaceae
Erythroxylum coca*. **Cocaine, cinnamylcocaine, tropacocaine, cuscohygrine.**

Euphorbiaceae
Croton flavens*. **Norsinoacutine, flavinantine, salutaridine, sinocutine.**
C. sparsiflorus*. **Sparsiflorine, crotsparine, pronuciferine.**
Phyllanthus discoides*. **Allosecurinine, phyllanthine, phyllantidine.**
Securinega* suffruticosa. **Securinine, suffruticodine, suffruticonine, securine, allosecurinine, dihydrosecurinine.**
S.* virosa. **Hordenine, virosecurinine, norsecurinine, dihydronorsecurinine.**

Fabaceae*/Papilionaceae* (Leguminosae)
Baptisia leucophaea*. Alkaloids.
Cytisus monspessulanus*. **Cytisine, N-methylcytisine, monspessulanine, lupanine, methylcystisine.**
C. nigricans*. **Calycotomine, sparteine.**
C. supinus*. **Lupanine, sparteine, anagyrine.**
Galega* officinalis. **Galegine, peganine, chinasolon-4, anagyrine, hydroxygalegine.**

Genista aetnensis*. **Sparteine, retamine.**
G. hispanica*. **Sparteine, retamine.**
G. pumila*. **Retamine, sparteine, lupanine, cytisine.**
Sparteum* junceum. **Spartein, cytisine.**
Thermopsis* fabacea. **Cytisine, methylcytisine, anagyrine, sparteine, lupanine, pachycarpine, thermopsine.**
Th.* caroliniana. **Lupanine, anagyrine, cytisine.**
Ulex* europaeus. **Anagyrine, cytisine.**

Geraniaceae

Geranium sanguineum: gotsgnad, **herba cancri.** Alkaloids.

Gramineae

Lolium perenne: darnell. **Perloline.**
Phalaris* arundinacea. **Hordenine, methoxy-methyltriptamine, gramine, dimethyltriptamine.**

Hernandiaceae

Gyrocarpus americanus*. **Pheanthine, magnocurarine, o-desmethylphaeanthine.**

Himantandraceae*

Galbulimima* belgraveana. **Himgaline, himbadine, himbacine, himandridine.**

Lauraceae

Cryptocarya* bowiei. **Cryptaustoline, cryptowoline.**
Ocatea rodiaei*. **Sepeerine, ocotine, norrodiasine, dirosine, octeamine, ocotanine, demerarine, ocodemerine.**

Lobeliaceae

Lobelia inflata: lobelia. Alkaloids.

Loganiaceae

Gelsemium elegans*: ~ jasmine. **Koumidine, koumine, koumicine, sempervirine.**
Strychnos colubrina. **Strychine, brucine.**
S. henningsii*. **Strychnine, brucine, diaboline, henningsoline, henningsamine, rindline.**
S. ignatii*. **Strychnine, brucine.**
S. nux-vomica: yettie kolindoo, nux vomica. **Brucine, strychnine.**

Lycopodiaceae

Lycopodium annotinum*. **Obscurine, annotine, acrifoline.**
L. clavatum: lycopode. **Clavatine, clavatoxine, clavolonine, lycodine, lopholine.**
L. saururus*. **Pillijanine, saururine, sauroxine.**

Menispermaceae

Cissampelos* pareira. **Hayatine, hayatinine, 1-curine, d-isochondrodendrine.**

Monimiaceae*

Daphnandra* micrantha. **Micranthine, daphnandrine, daphnoline.**

Nyctaginaceae

Heimerliodendron* brunonianum. Alkallids.

Oxalidaceae

Oxalis corniculata: **Indian sorrel, yellow oxalis.** Alkaloids.

Papaveraceae

Argemone platyceras: cardosanto. **Protopine, allocryptopine, platycerine.** Nophenolic bases.
A. pleicantha*. **Berberine, allocryptopine, cryptopine, bisnorargemonine, protopine, munitagine.**
A. sanguinea*. **Berberine, allocryptopine.**
A. squarrosa*. **Allocryptopine, muramine, berberine.**
Chelidonium majus: celidonia, celandine. Alkaloids.
Eschscholtzia* californica. **Allocryptopine, chelerythrine, sanguinarine.**

Glaucium flavum: mekone, pavot, glaucum, poppy. **Aurotensine, glaucine, corydine, norcorydine, chelidonine, norchelidonine.**

Papaver argemone: argemonia, argemone. **Rhoeadine, protopine, rhoeagenine.**

P. bracteatum*. **Isothebaine, oripavine, bracteine, thebaine, bractamine,** orientalinone, **salutaridine, alpinigenine.**

P. dubium*. **Aporheine, berberine, aporheidine, rhoeagenine, rhoeadine, protopine, allocryptopine.**

P. fugax*. **Mecambrine, armepavine, floripavine, pronuciferine.**

P. glaucum*. **Rhoeadine, glaupavine, coptysine, glaudine, glaucamine, papaverrubine B.**

P. lateritium*.

P. nudicaule*. **Nudaurine, amuronine, amuroline, muramine, amurine, protopine, rhoeadine, coptysine, sanguinarine.**

P. orientale. **Thebaine, isothebaine, oripavine, glaucidine, laudanine, protopine, narcotine.**

P. pavonium*. **Roemeridine, α-allocryptopine, rhoeadine,** unknown alkaloid, **protopine, allocryptopine.**

P. persicum*. **Coptysine, mecambrine, armepavine.**

P. rhoeas: poppy, amapola. **Rhoeadine, morphine, papaverine,** unknown alkaloids, **protopine, coptisine, thebaine.**

P. somniferum: opium poppy. **Morphine, codeine, thebaine, papaverine, narcotine, narceine.**

Ranunculaceae

Thalictrum dasycarpum*. **Magnoflorine, berberine, thalicarpine.**

T. foliolosum*. **Berberine, magnoflorine, palmatine.**

T. minus*. **Thalicmine, thalicmidine, magnoflorene, thalictuberine, thalicrine, berberine.**

Rosaceae

Sanguisorba minor: **pimpernel. Alkaloids.**

Rubiaceae

Cinchona calisaya. **Quinidine.**

C. ledgeriana*. **Cinchonidine, quinidine.**

C. micrantha*. **Chinchonine, cinchonidine.**

C. officinalis: Peruvian bark, cinchona. **Quinine, cinchonine, cinchonidine.**

C. pubescens*.

Crucianella* angustifolia. **Alkaloids.**

Mitragyna* parvifolia. **Rotundifoline, isorotundifoline, rhyncophylline, isorhynchophylline. akuammigine, pteropodine, isopteropodine, speciophylline, mitraphylline, isomitraphylline, uncarine F, isoajmalicin, hirsutine, dihydrocorynantheine,** pteropodinex. **akuammine.**

M.* speciosa. Rotundifoline, isorotundifoline, speciofoline, mitraphylline, isomitraphylline, speciophylline, rhynchophylline, isorhynchophylline.

Rutaceae

Flindersia* dissospermia. **Maculine, dictamnine, flindersiamine.**

F.* maculosa. **Maculine, dictamnine, maculosidine, kokusaginine, flindersiamine, maculosine.**

Sapindaceae

Dodonaea viscosa*. **Alkaloids.**

Solanaceae

Atropa belladoona: belladona, deadly nightshade. **Hyoscyamine, hyoscine, cuscohygrine.**

Browallia viscosa*. **Alkaloids.**

Datura arborea: floripondio. **Alkaloids.**

D. ferox*. **Hyoscyamine, hyoscine, meteloidine.**

D. metel: thornapple. **Hyoscyamine, meteloidine, hyoscine.**

D. sanguinea*. **Atropine, hyoscine, hyoscyamine.**
D. stramonium: Jimsonweed, Jamestown weed, thornapple. **Hyoscine, hyoscamine, meteloidine.**
Duboisia* hopwoodii. **Nicotine, nornicotine.**
D.* leichhardtii. **Hyoscyamine, hyoscine, norhyoscyamine.**
D.* myoporoides. **Hyoscine, hyoscamine,** tropane bases, **nicotine, nornicotine.**
Physalis ixocarpa*. Alkaloids.
Solanum aculeatissimum*. Alkaloids.
S. atropurpureum*. Alkaloids.
Withania somnifera: strychnos, asgandh, winter cherry. **Nicotine.**

T.5   ISORHODANIDOGENES

Brassicaceae*/Cruciferae

Arabis* hirsuta. Glucohirsutin, other isorhodanidogenes.
A.* holboelli. Isorhodanidogene.
Brassica juncea: pai-chieh-tzu. **Isothiocyanate,** sinigrin, gluconapin (**crotonyl-isothiocyanate**).
B. napus: rape, **turnip. Isothiocyanates.** Glucobrassicin, neoglucobrassicin.
B. nigra: sinapsis, **mustard.** Sinigrin, isorhodanidogenes.
B. oleracea: **cabbage.** Rhodanidogenic glucosides.
B. rapa: rape, **turnip. Isothiocyanates.**
Capsella bursa-pastoris: **shepherd's purse.**
Iberis* sempervirens. Glucoiberin, glucoibervirin.

Capparidaceae

Crataeva roxburghii*. Glucotropeolin, glucocapparin.

Euphorbiaceae

Putranjiva* roxburghii. Glucochlearin, glucoputranjivin, **phenyl-isothiocyanate, 2-methylbutyl-isothiocyanate.**

Liliaceae

Allium falcifolium*. Allylsulfide radical.

Limnanthaceae*

Limnanthes* douglasii. **Glucolimnanthine.**

Plant Families Listed in Hartwell and Cordell*

Acanthaceae quinazoline alkaloids (p. 253): branche ursine, vasa, sahachara, caricature plant, vrisha. **Vasicine, febrifugine, rutaecarpine, arborine.**

Aceraceae: striped maple **cancer** bush (*Acer pensylvanicum* or *striatum*), polecat tree

ACTINIDIACEAE (p. 848): **β-Skytanthine** and **actinidine** from *Actinidia* * *polygama* (p. 848)

Aizoaceae: doca, turuna, toston

Alangiaceae monoterpene alkaloids (p. 656): ankota, ramatha

Alismaceae: alisma, damasonium, lyron or liron

Amaranthaceae: aspamarga, chaff tree, amaranta, Hierba del **cancer** de Mexico (*Gomphrena decumbens*)

Amaryllidaceae (p. 4, 533–553): maguey, maguei, century plant, poison bulb, narcissus, daffodil, St. John's amaryllis. **Lycorine, galanthamine, crinine, tazettine, narciclasine, montanine. Galanthamine** has been used in the treatment of **myasthenia gravis** and other diseases of the nervous sytem.

Anacardiaceae: beladeur, cashew, cashew-nut tree, cashew nut, maranon, frankincense, mastich, mastix, mastic, turpentine, shumac, sumac, poison ivy, rhus

Annonaceae aporhine alkaloids (p. 389), monoterpene alkaloids (p. 656), phenylated indole alkaloids (p. 618), proterberberine alkaloids (p. 472): sweetsop, sugar apple. For **alkaloids** see Monimiaceae.

ANCISTROCLADACEA (p. 219). **Ancistrocladidine, ancistrocladine, ancistrocladisine** from the genus *Ancistrocladus*.

Apocynaceae (p. 4), monoterpene alkaloids (p. 848), monoterpene indole alkaloids (p. 574, 656, 659–661, 665, 674, 678, 681, 684, 691–692, 697–698, 702, 734, 736, 740, 744–747, 758, 761, 771, 775–777, 781–782, 785, 790–791, 798–799, 800, 807): oleander, jasmine tree, *Vinca*.**Vinca alkaloids** (p. 795), **vincadine** (p. 791), **vincaleukoblastine** (p.785, 789–90), **vincamine** (p. 658). **Anticancer agents** include **camptothecine** from *Camptotheca* * *acuminata*; **leurocristine** from *Catharanthus* * *roseus*; and **vincaleukoblastine** from *Catharantheus* * *roseus*. The genera *Holarrhena, Funtamia* *, *Malouetia**, and *Chonemorphia** contain **steroidal alkaloids** (p. 904). These include **funtamine, irehine, kurchessine, connessine.** Hallucigenic **N,N-dimethyltryptamine** in

---

* This listing includes the names of all 214 of the plant families—comprising 1,430 genera and circa 3,000 species—that appear in Jonathan A. Hartwell's *Plants Used Against Cancer*, Quarterman Publications, Lawrence MA, 1982. Of these, the particular plant families which are indexed in Geoffrey A. Cordell's *Introduction to Alkaloids*, Wiley, New York, 1982, are in **boldface**, followed by page numbers and other information. Information of special note is also highlighted in **boldface**.

Plant families in Cordell but **not** Hartwell are **capitalized and in boldface**. It may be noted that 70 plant families are in boldface, that is, appear in both Hartwell and Cordell. In other words, about one-third of the plant families represented in Hartwell appear in Cordell. There are 12 other plant families that appear in Cordell but not in Hartwell. The total number of plant families in Cordell is therefore 82.

Each plant family listed in Cordell is known to have at least one species which contains alkaloids. Furthermore, it is understood that not all of the species within an alkaloid-containing family will contain alkaloids, with the exception of the plant family Papaveraceae, where all the species contain alkaloids.

Representative common specie names are included as found in Hartwell.

Some of the specific alkaloids found in a particular plant family are listed separately in **boldface**, as appear in Cordell. It is noted that Cordell lists about 660 genera and species in an Organism Index, most of which are plants.

Plant genera or species **not** found in Hartwell are denoted by an asterisk.

leaves of *Prestonia* amazonia* (p. 577). **Yohimbine** from *Rauvolfia*, Amsonia*, Vallesia*, Aspidosperma*, Catharanthus** (p. 684). **Oncinotine** from *Oncinotis* nitida* (Fig. 1, p. 931). **Tricanthine** from *Holarrhena mitis** (p. 954).

Aquifoliaceae purine alkaloids (p. 953): holly, American holly, black elder. The leaves of *Ilex paraguensis* make a tea called mate, which is drunk for instance in Paraguay, and may contain up to 2 percent **caffeine** (p. 953).

Araceae: acoron, calamus, calmus, sweet flag, aaron, aron, odorless vanilla, dragonwort, dracontium, skunk cabbage

Araliaceae: tarano, spikenrd, hedera, ivy, **ginseng**

Aristolochiaceae: clematis, birthwort, guaco, aristolochia, aristologia, asarum. **Aristolochic acid** may be regarded as an **alkaloid** (p. 6, 421)

Asclepiadaceae (p. 273), phenanthroindolizidine alkaloids (p. 567): **cancerillo** (*Asclepias curassavica*), milkweed, arka, mudar, swallow wort, asclepias, **condurango**, condor vine. **Cryptoline** occurs in the two Belgian Congo species *Cryptolepsis triangularis* and *C. sanguinolenta* (p. 273). **Quindoline** also occurs in the latter. The genus *Tylophora* is found in eastern and southern India and contains **tylophorine** and **tylophorinine**. Other alkaloid-containing genera of Asclepiadaceae include *Atitoxicum*, Vencetoxicum*, Cyananclus*, and *Pergularia**. Other alkaloids isolated include **tylophorinidine, tylocrebrine, isotylocrebine, and pegularinine.** The condor vine is designated variously in Hartwell as of the genus *Marsdenia, Equatoria*, or *Gonolobus*. None are cited in Cordell.

Balsaminaceae: jewelweed, touch-me-not

Basellaceae: Yedra del pais, Ulluco

Begoniaceae: begonia

Berberidaceae aporphine-benzyl isoquinoline dimers (p. 410), bisbenzylisoquinoline alkaloids (p. 354), phthalideisoquinoline alkaloids (p. 496), proterberine alkaloids (p. 472, 485). The alkaloid **berberine** (p. 7, 473, 483) is noted to have **anticancer** and **antibiotic** properties. The alkaloid **taspine** occurs in *Leontice* albert*i and *Caulophyllum robustum.* **Pakistanamine** from *Berberis* baluchistanica** (p. 410). **Petaline** from the Lebanese plant *Leontice leontopetalum* (p. 333).

Betulaceae: erle, alder, alnus, birch, hazelnut

Bignoniaceae: catalpa, calabash, caroba, **cancer** bush (*Jacaranda caerulea*), patala, **pau d'arco**

Bixaceae: achiotl

Bombacaceae: baobab, cotton-tree

Boraginaceae pyrrolizidine alkaloids (p. 118): bugloss, buglosse, borrage, hound's tongue, wild comfrey, comfrey, heliotropum, beggar lice. Pyrrolizinde alkaloids are in the genera *Heliotropum, Echium, and Trachelanthus** (p. 118). The somewhat-similar alkaloids include **supinidine, heliotrodine, retronecine,** and **platynecine**. The genus *Symphytum*, or comfrey, evidently contains these particular pyrrolizidine alkaloids, and is listed in Cordell.

Bromeliaceae: pineapple, pina, Spanish moss

Bursericeae: myrrh, frankincense, thus, tus, incense, olibanum, bdeilium, balsam

Buxaceae steroidal alkaloids (p. 904): box or boxwood, bouis, buis, **jojoba. Terminaline** occurs in *Pachysandra* terminalis* (p. 904). *Buxus* steroidal alkaloids are noted to have **antimalarial** and **antitubercular activity** (p. 907). Examples are **cycloprotobuxine, cyclovirobuxine, cyclobuxine, buxamine, cyclobuxidine** (p. 909).

Cactaceae tetrahydroisoquinoline alkaloids (p. 319), tyramine alkaloids (p. 278): peyote, mescal, prickly pear. The drug called peyote is from the plant species *Lophophora williamsii* found in the Chihuahuan Desert of Texas and Mexico. The alkaloids are **anhalonine** and the well-known hallucigen **mescaline**, with the latter also found in the cactus genus *Trichocereus*.

CALYCANTHACEAE (590), bisindole alkaloids. **Calycanthine.**

Campanulaceae (p. 82): lobelia, (campanula), rampion, Indian tobacco. **Codonopsine** from *Codonopsis* clematidea* (p. 82). **Lobinaline** from *Lobelia cardinalis** (p. 145). **Lobeline** from *Lobelia inflata* or Indian tobacco (p. 146). Action similar to nicotine.

Cannaceae: canna

Capparidaceae: cappero, caper, caparis, varuna

Capfrifoliaceae: elder, elderberry

Caricaceae (p. 211): papaya, pawpaw. **Carpaine** from the leaves of *Carica papaya* or papaya tree (p. 211). Cardioactive, amoebicide.

Caryophyllaceae: soapwort, wort, chickweed

Celastraceae macrocyclic peptide alkaloids (p. 937), **maytansinoids** (p. 948–949), phenethylamine alkaloids (p. 287), sesquiterpene alkaloids (p. 856, 863–864), spermidine alkaloids (p. 931): bittersweet, **cancerosa** (*Maytenus ilicifolia*). **Antileukemic** or **anticancer** alkaloids **maysine, maytanprine, maytansine, maytine, maytoline** from fruit of the genus *Maytenus (p. 948)*. **Pleurostyline** from *Pleurostylia* africana* (Fig. 1, p. 931).

CENTROSPERMAE (p. 311). **Betalain.**

CEPHALOTAXACEAE (p. 528), *Cephalotaxus* alkaloids. **Cephaline, cephalotaxine, cephalotax-inone.** The cephalotaxine alkaloids are obtained from the Japanese plum-yew *Cephalotaxus har-ringtonia* and include **harringtonine** and **homoharringtonine.** They display strong **antitumor** activity, notably **antileukemic** activity. Similar alkaloids occur in *Schelhammera* spp. and *Phelline comosa* of the family Liliaceae.

Chenopodiaceae (p. 147, 207), anabasine alkaloids (p. 143), simple tryptoamine alkaloids (p. 577): salt-bush, beets, spinach. **Girgenshohnine** from *Girgensohnia* oppositiflora* (p. 147). **Piperidine alkaloids** with short aliphatic side chains from *Nanophyton* erinaceum* (p. 207). *Atriplex spinacia* or *A. olericea*, but more usually called *Spinacia oleracea*, and more familiarly known as spinach, contains **phenylalanine-tyrosine alkaloid precursors** (p. 275). **n-Methyltryptamine** or **dipterine** from *Girgensohnia* diptera* and *Arthrophytum* leptocladum* (p. 577).

Cistaceae: ladanum

Clethraceae: white alder

Combretaceae: almond, myrobalan, citrinum

Compositae (p. 4), diterpene alkaloids (p. 868), pyrrolizidine alkaloids (p. 118), simple quinoline alkaloids (p. 237): yarrow, millefolium, angelica, chamomile, burdock, arnica, absinthe or worm-wood, artemisia, mugwort, daisies, marigold, century plant, corn-flour, knapweed, endive, chicory, Echinacea or coneflower, fleabane, plantain, elecampane, lettuce, wild lettuce, prickly lettuce, manzaanilla, Senecio or groundsel, goldenrod, sow thistle, lechuguilla, dandelion, tansy, globe thistle, sunflower. The pyrrolizidine alkaloid **Senecionine** occurs in *Senecio* (p. 128). **Echinopsine** from *Echinops* (p. 237). The diterpene alkaloids **vetchine, atisine, garryine** from *Inula* (p. 868). (The genus *Echinacea*, a folkloric **anticancer** agent and remedy for many other ailments, is not mentioned in Cordell though it is listed in Hartwell. The fact that it is not cited in Cordell does not necessarily mean that it contains no alkaloids. Howsoever, the plant is not considered toxic.)

Connaraceae: awennade

Convolvulaceae ergot alkaloids (p. 631): sweet potato (genus *Ipomoea*), dodder, bindweed. **Cly-moclavine, chanoclavine-1** from the seeds of *Ipomoea violacea** and *Rivea* corymbosa* (p. 631).

Cornaceae:dogwood, red willow

Crassulaceae (p. 145): sedum or stonecrop. Piperidine alkaloids from *Sedum acre* (p. 145). Sedum alkaloids from *Sedum* (p. 181).

Cruciferae spermidine alkaloids (p. 931): mustard, turnip, cabbage, rape, nasturtium, cress, water-cress, radish, erisimum, krambe (cauliflower, broccoli). **Spermidine, spermine, putrescine** (p. 930). **Lunarine** from *Lunaria biennis** (Fig. 1, p. 931). Alkaloids occur in cabbage leaves, tomato juice, apples, spinach and in the leaves of wheat, maize, pea, black currant, and tobacco.

Cucurbitaceae: melon, cucumber, gourd (squash, pumpkin, zucchini)

Cyperaceae (p. 82), harmala alkaloids (p. 612): papyrus, rush, cyperus. **Brevicolline** from *Carex* brevicollis* (p. 82).

DIONCHOPHYLLACEAE (p. 219), naphthalene-isoquinoline alkaloids from *Triphyophyllum peltatum.*

Dioscoreaceae (p. 201): yam. **Dioscorine** from *Dioscorea hispida.*

Dipsacaceae: teasel

Dipterocarpaceae: camphora, sal

Droseraceae: sundew

Ebenaceae: ebony, persimmon

Elaeagnaceae: oleaster, wild olive

Elaeocarpaceae (p. 222): maqui. **Elaeocarpine, isoelaeocarpine, elaeocarpidine, elaeokanine** from the genus *Elaeocarpus*.

Equisetaceae spermidine alkaloids (p. 931): horsetail. **Palustrine** from *Equisetum* (Fig. 1, p. 931)

Ericaceae: heather, wintergreen, wild rosemary, cranberry

Erythroxylaceae: chuchuhuasha, jiba

ESCALLONIACEAE (p. 868), diterpene alkaloids from the genus *Anopterus*.

Eucommiaceae: no common names listed

Euphorbiaceae (p. 144, 197, 218, 304, 379, 684, 846): **Yerba del cancer,** spurge, Euphorbium, chickweed, cassava, mandioca, castor. **Astrophylline, astrocasine, adenocarpine, isoorensine** from *Astrocasia* phyllanthoides* (p. 144). **Ricinine** from *Ricinus communis*, native to India (p. 197). **Porantherine** from *Poranthera* corymbosa* (p. 218). **Securinine** from the genus *Securinega** (p. 304). Proaporphine alkaloids, e.g., **pronuciferine** from *Croton linearis** (p. 379). **Yohimbine** from the genus *Alchornea** (p. 684). **Alchorneine** and the guanidine alkaloid **pterogynine** from *Alchornea** (p. 846).

Fagaceae: oaks (genus *Quercus*)

Filicineae: fern, burcus or burkus

Flacourtiaceae spermidine alkaloids (p. 931): chaulmoogra. **Homaline** from *Homalium pronyense* (Fig. 1, p. 931)

FUMARIACEAE (p. 509, 367, 488), benzophenanthridine alkaloids, cularine-type, and protopine alkaloids. **Fumaricine, fumariline** from *Fumaria officinalis* (p. 503). **Cularine** from *Dicentra* and *Corydalis* (p. 367). **Reticuline, protopine** from *Dicentra spectabilis* (p. 488).

Garryaceae diterpene alkaloids (p. 868): cuauchichic. **Garryine** from *Garrya*.

Gentianaceae monoterpine alkaloids (pp. 850–852): centauria, centory, gentian, buckbean. **Gentianine, gentianidine** from *Gentiana*.

Geraniaceae geraniol (pp. 824–825): geranium, crowfoot, herb Robert

Gesneriaceae: medallita

Gingkoaceae: *Ginko biloba* (nuts)

Gnetaceae phenethylamine alkaloids (p. 284): Indian abutua. **Ephedrine** or "Ma Huang"—known to Chinese physicians for five millenia—is obtained from the aboveground parts of *Ephedra equisetina*.

Gramineae 1,4-benzoxazin-3-one alkaloids (p. 269), plants for ergot growth (p. 622), purine alkaloids (p. 276)): grama grass, rye, barley, rice, millet, sugar cane, sorghum, wheat (genus *Triticum*), trigo, corn, maiz. **Gramine** and **hordenine** occur in *Hordeum vulgare* or barley (p. 276, 575). The pyrrolizidine alkaloids **laburnine, laburnum,** and **festucine** occur in *Festuca** or fescue (p. 118). The alkaloid ***trans*-zeatin** occurs in *Zea mays* and is a stimulator for cell division (p. 955).

Guttiferae: St. John's wort

Haloragidaceae: millefolium

Hamamelidaceae: witch hazel, storax, styrax, liquid amber

Hernandiaceae aporphine-benzylisoquinoline dimers (p. 410): hernandaline. **Thalicarpine.**

HIMANTANDRACEAE (pp. 224–225). **Himbacine, himbosine.**

Hippocastanaceae: castagno d'india.

Humiriaceae: uchy

Hydrophyllaceae: espino

Hymenophyllaceae: doradilla

ICACINACEAE (p. 850, 665), monoterpene alkaloids, monoterpene indole alkaloids. **Cantleyine** from *Cantleya corniculata*, **10-methoxycamptothecine** and **9-methoxycamptothecine** from *Mappa foetida*. (The alkaloid **camptothecine**, which exhibits very high **antitumor** activity, is derived from the rare Chinese ornamental tree *Camptotheca acuminata*.)

Iridaceae: crocus, saffron, iris, fleur de Lis, blue flag

Juglandaceae: butternut, black walnut, walnut

Julianiaceae: chalalactii, cuachocolate

Juncaceae: flos iunci, ceperum, ciperus

Labiatae sesquiterpene alkaloids (p. 866): laburnine hyssop, deadnettle, espic, lavender, horehound, mint, horsement, Yerba buena, pennyroyal, peppermint, mentha, catnip, ground ivy, marjoram, sweet marjoram, origanum, oregano, rosemary, **cancer-weed** (*Salvia lyrata*), salvia, sage, clary.

calamint, betonica, germander, c(h)amadreos, polion, thyme or time. **Guaipyridine, patchouli pyridine** from *Pogostemon patchouli**.

Lardizabalaceae: akebi

Lauraceae (p. 4, 148): aporphine alkaloids (p. 389), proaporphine alkaloids (p. 379), protoberberine alkaloids (p. 472): camphora, camphor, camphor tree, cassia, cinnamon, oleum, petra, bayberry, lauri, laurel, bay tree, sassafras. The proaporphine alkaloids **pronuciferine, glaziovine, linearisine, oreoline** (p. 379). For **alkaloids** also see Monimiaceae.

Lecythidaceae: nichula, janiparandiba

Leguminosae (p. 4, 157, 169, 221, 584), N-cinnamoyl piperidine alkaloids (p. 144), diterpene alkaloids (p. 882), *Erythrina* alkaloids (p. 450, 462), harmala alkaloids (p. 611), monoterpene alkaloids (p. 847), *Ormosia* alkaloids (p. 165–166), piperidine alkaloids (pp. 213–214), purine alkaloids (p. 955), pyrrolizidine alkaloids (p. 118), quinolizidine alkaloids (p. 153, 163), simple tryptamine derivatives (pp. 577–579), tetrahydroisoquinoline alkaloids (p. 319): jequirity, gum arabic, acacia, peanut, devil's claws, gum tragacanth, indigo, wild indigo, senna, cassia, redbud, chickpea, peas, broom or broomweed, frijolillo, licorice, lentil, lenticula, lupine, alfalfa, melilot, sweet clover, lima beans, red-spotted beans, bean, green peas, sandalwood, **cancer bush** (*Sutherlandia frutescens*), tamarind (India), red clover, field clover, trefoil, honeysuckle, clover, fenugrecum, linseed, vetch, pulse. **Stachydrine** in alfalfa or *Medicago sativa* (p. 80). Pyrrolizidine alkaloids which appear in *Crotaliaria** species include **1-methylenepyrrolizidine** (p. 118). The quinolizidine alkaloids called lupin akaloids are found in *Cystisus scoparius* or broom, in *Laburnum* anagyroides* or laburnum, and in *Lupinus* or lupins. Examples are **lupinine, angustifoline, sparteine, matrine, cytisine. Lupinine** occurs in *Lupinus luteus*. Other alkaloids are **pohakuline** and **ormosanine** (p. 185). Hallucigenic**N, N-Dimethyltryptamine** from the seeds and pods of *Piptadenia perigrina** (p. 577). Used as snuff by Indians. **5-Hydroxytryptamine** or **serotonin** from *Mucuna pruriens* (p. 579). β-**Carboline** (p. 611). **Chaksine** from *Cassia lispidula** (p. 847). (The indolizidine alkaloid **swainsonine** is not listed in Cordell, neither are the plant genera where it is found, namely the genus *Swainsona** of Australia, and *Astragalus* and *Oxytropis** of the American West, otherwise known as milkvetch and locoweed or crazy weed. **Swainsonine** has been under study in Japan as an **anticancer** agent, as noted in Part 4.)

Lemniaceae: duckwood

Lentibulariaceae: butterwort

Liliaceae (p. 4), colchicine-type alkaloids (p. 522), homocrythrina alkaloids (p. 531), phenethylisoquinoline alkaloids (p. 518), steroidal alkaloids (p. 895): onions, cepa, cebolla, garlic, leek, aliumaloe, ephemeron, colchicum, lily, sarsaparilla, squilla, hellebore. **Colchicine** from *Colchicum autumnale* (p. 522). **Schelhammeridine** from *Schelhammera** (p. 518, 531). **Vericine** from *Frittillaria* (p. 895). Alkaloids similar to the **Cephalotaxus alkaloids** of the family Cephalotaxaceae occur in *Schelhammera* spp. and *Phelline comosa* (p. 529).

Linaceae: flax, linseed

Loasaceae: zazalic de chietlano

Lobeliaceae lobelia alkaloids (p. 146, 181): lobelia. **Lobeline, Lobinaline**from *Lobelia* (p. 181).

Loganiaceae (p. 4), monoterpene alkaloids (p. 574, 656, 662, 684, 697, 721, 726), *Strychnos* alkaloids (p. 721, 726), yohimbinoid derivatives (p. 684): quisuar, jasmine, gelsenium.

Strychnine (p. 656, 721), **loganin** (p. 814, 828). **Yohimbine** from *Gelsemium, Strychnos* (p. 684). The genus *Strychnos* consists of climbing shrubs and small trees as found variously in Africa, Asia, and South America (p. 721). The *Strychnos* alkaloids **strychnine** and **brucine** occur in the Asian species *S. ignatii** and *S. nux vomica*. The group of *Strychnos* alkaloids called **curare** or **Calabesh curare** are found in the South American species *S. toxifera** and *S. castelneana** (p. 726). These liana or vines are the sources for the poison used by South American Indians on their arrows, for instance along the Orinoco River in Venezuela (p. 355). Also see Menispermaceae.

Loranthaceae: mistletoe, viscum

Lycopodiaceae *Lycopodium* alkaloids (p. 170): lycopode, musco clavato, ground pine.

Lycopodine (p. 3, 138, 170–176).

Lythraceae (p. 150), Lythraceae alkaloids (p. 150), **lythranidine** (pp. 150–151), **lythranine** (p. 150), **lythrine** (p. 138, 150): **Yerba del cancer**, cyprus, oleum, privet, henna

Magnoliaceae: canelo

Malpighiaceae harmala alkaloids (p. 611): nanchi, malti. β-**Carboline**.

Malvaceae quinazoline alkaloids (p. 253): cannabis, hemp, hibiscus, mallow, marsh mallow, wild mallow, holyhoke, althea, cotton, cottonseed, okra, China rose, malbas, malva, bala. **Vasicine, februgine, rutaecarpine, arborine** (p. 253).

Marantaceae: no common names listed

Melastomaceae: tompillo

Meliaceae: priyangu, African or Lagos mahogany

Menispermaceae (p. 4), bisbenzylisoquinoline alkaloids (p. 319), *Erythrina* alkaloids (p. 450), hasubanan alkaloids (p. 466), proaporphine alkaloids (p. 339), protoberberine alkaloids (p. 472), protostephanine alkaloids (p. 462): patha. **Tiliacorine** and **tiliacorinine** occur in *Tiliacora racemosa* (p. 364) (Note: The genus *Tilia* ocurs in the family Tiliaceae). Another bisbenzylisoquinoline alkaloid called **tetrandine** has displayed **antitumor** activity (p. 357, 365) Tetrandine occurs in the Japanese plant *Stephania tetrandra* and in the roots of *Cyclea peltata*. A similar alkaloid (an optical antipode of tetrandine) called **phaeanthine**, isolated from the bark of *Phaenthus ebracteotatus*, shows **antitubercular** activity. The azaflouranthine alkaloids **imeluteine** and **rufescine** have been isolated from the stems of *Abuta imene* and *A. rufescens*, as has **norrufescine** (p. 421). The proaporphine alkaloids **pronuciferine, glaziovine, linearisine, oreoline** (p. 379). The alkaloids called **tubocurare** are obtained from the fruit of *Chondrodendrom* tomentosum* (p. 356). A specific alkaloid in the mixture is **tubocurarine**. The preparation is stored in a tube and used to poison arrows by the Indians of the upper Amazon and Colombia. Also see Loganiaceae.

MONIMIACEAE (p. 389, 329), aporphine, proaporphine alkaloids. **Glaucine, bulbocapnine, laureline, nuciferine, isothemaine, stephanine, apoglaziovine.** The proaporphine alkaloids **pronuciferine, glaziovine, linearisine, oreoline** (p. 379).

Moraceae spermidine alkaloids (p. 931): hemp, Indian hemp, cannabus, fig, ficus, hops, Osage orange, mulberry. **Cannabisativine** from *Cannabis sativa* (Fig. 1, p. 931).

Moringaceae: ben, ben nut

Musaceae: banana

Myricaceae: myrtle, bayberry, meadow fern

Myristicaceae: nutmeg, muscata

Myrsinaceae: vidango kernal

Myrtaceae: myrtine 143 eucalyptus, cloves, myrtle, myrta

Nyctaginaceae: maravilla, cazabito

Nymphaeaceae proaphorphine alkaloids (p. 379), sesquiterpene alkaloids (p. 861): lotus, water lily, pond lily. The proaporphine alkaloids **pronuciferine, glaziovine, linearisine, oreoline** (p. 379). The *Nuphar* alkaloid **deoxynupharidine** from *Nuphar japonicum** (p. 861). A number of sulfur-containing alkaloids, including **thiobinupharidine**, from *N. luteum*.

Nyssacaceae monoterpene indole alkaloids (p. 656, 665): black gum tree. **Camptothecine** from the Chinese ornamental tree *Camptotheca* acuminata* (p. 665). Exhibits **antitumor** activity.

Ochnaceae: Yerba de san, martin

Oleaceae: lian-tsai, white ash, ash, jasmine, privet, olive. **Cantleyine** from *Jasminum* (p. 850).

Onagraceae: noha, mutun, Yerba del gople, hishi, trapa

Ophioglossaceae: moonwort, Herba lunaria, adders-tongue

Orchidaceae (p. 204), 1-phenyltetrahydroisoquinoline alkaloids (p. 328), sesquiterpene alkaloids (p. 856): pai-chi, **cancer weed** (*Goodyera pubescens*), testiculus, foolstones, rasna, green or odorless vanilla. **Shihunine** from the Chinese orchid *Dendrobium* lolohense* (p. 204). **Cryptostyline** from *Cryptostylis* fulva* (p. 328).

Orobanchaceae: sqaw root, **cancer root** (*Conopholis americana, Epifagus virginiana*)

Osmundaceae: osmund, buckthorn

Oxalidaceae: wood sorrel, shamrock, sheep sorrel, sorrel. **Oxaline** (p. 606).

Palmae (p. 197): coco, coconut, palm, date, dactili, **saw palmetto. Palmatine, arecoline, guvacine.**

Papaveraceae (p. 4, 82), aporphine alkaloids (p. 388–389), benzophenanthridine alkaloids (p. 509), ochotensane alkaloids (p. 502), phthalideisoquinoline alkaloids (p. 496), proaporphine alkaloids (p. 379), protoberberine alkaloids (p. 472), protopine alkaloids (p. 485), tetrahydroisoquinoline alkaloids (p. 319): yellow thistle, prickly poppy, Mexican poppy thistle, celidonia, celandine, nipple-wort, celandine, glaucium, poppy, amapola, opium, papaver, bloodroot, sanguinaria. **San-**

guinarine, chelerythine, nitidine display cytotoxic and **antitumor** activity (p. 515). **Sanguinarine** for instance is found in *Sanguinaria canadensis* or bloodroot. **Pyrrolidinoisoquinoline macrostomine** from *Papaver macrostomum** (p. 82). **Laudanosoline** from *Papaver somniferum* or opium (p. 333). **Papaverine** and **papaveraldine** from *P. somniferum* (p. 333, 338), and **sanguinarine, chelerythrine, chelidonine, nitidine** (p. 514). The species *Chelidonium majus*—variously called celidonia, celandine, swallowwort, or nipplewort—has a long history in the treatment of **tumors**, as does *Sanguinaria canadensis* or bloodroot. The former, especially, has extensive entries in Hartwell—not to mention *Papever somniferum* or the opium poppy. **Protopine** from *Chelidonium majus* (p. 488). In particular, extracts from *Chelidonum majus* have been used to treat gastric cancer, warts, papillomas, and condylomas (p. 515).

Passifloraceae: maracuja roxo

Pedaliaceae: sesame

Penaeaceae: sarcocolla

Phytolaccaceae spermidine alkaloids (p. 932): pau d'alho, pokeweed, **cancer-root** (*Phytolacca americana* or *decandra*), poke, poke-root, Yyamolin, **Yerba de cancer** (genus *Rivina*). **Codonocarpine** from *Codonocarpus australis** (Fig. 1, p. 931).

Pinaceae (p. 206): balsam, fir, cedar, cypress, juniper, savin, sabina, larch, pine, spruce, pine nuts, resin, turpentine, colophonia, arbor vitae. **Pinidine** from *Pinus sabiniana**.

Piperaceae (p. 146, 183,197): pepper, piper. **Piperidine** (p. 8, 147, 178–183), **piperine** (p. 146).

Plantaginaceae monoterpene alkaloids (p. 847): **cancer root** (*Plantago cordata*), plantago, ribwort, plantain, llanten, psylium, fleabane, fleawort. **Arenaine** from *Plantago arenaria*.

Plumbaginaceae: leadwort, **Yerba del cancer** (*Plumbago europaea*), loco

Polemoniaceae: polemonia

Polygalaceae: snakeroot

Polygonaceae: yellow dock, unero, sourdock, bistorta, knotgrass, smartweed, persicary, sanguinaria, rhubarb, sorrell, sheep sorrel, dock, sour dock, horse sorrel, sour sorrel

Polypodiaceae: polypodium, bracken

Portulacaceae: portulaca, purslane

Potamogetonaceae: water-caltrop, water chestnut, saligot

Primulaceae: anagallis, pimpernel, sowbread, cowslip

Proteaceae tropane alkaloids (pp. 96–97): huinque. **Bellendine** from *Bellendena* montana*. **2-Methylbellendine** from *Darlingia* ferruginea*.

Punicaceae (p. 201): pomegranate. (Not further identified in Cordell.)

Pyrolaceae: pippsisewa, pipsissewa, wintergreen

Rafflesiaceae: hypocistis, cistus

Ranunculaceae (p. 4), anthanilic acid-derived alkaloids (p. 236), aporphine-benzylisoquinoline alkaloids (p. 410), bisbenzylisoquinoline alkaloids (p. 349), diterpene alkaloids (p. 868), protopine alkaloids (p. 485): wolfsbane, monkshood, columbine, black snakeroot, squawroot, crowfoot, clematis, leather flower, virgin's bower, black hellebore, hellebore, golden seal, liverwort, nigella, peony, buttercup, figwort. **Damascenine** from *Nigella damascena* (p. 236). **Thalicarpine** from *Thalictrum dasycarpum* (p. 411). *Aconitum* and **aconitine** (p. 868 ff).

Resedaceae: woad, wild wood, reseda

Rhamnaceae macrocyclic peptide alkaloids (p. 937), **maytansinoids** (p. 949), piperidine alkaloids (p. 214): New Jersey tea, lycium, buckthorn, cascara, kola, jujube. **Ziziphine** from *Ziziphus* (p. 937). **Antibiotic** properties.

Rhizophoraceae: mangrove

Rosaceae diterpene alkaloids (p. 868, 872): agrimony, agrimonia, quince, strawberry, fragola, avens, herba Robertus, tormentill, cinquefoil. sweet almond, almond, bitter almond, amygdala, cherry, plum, peach, wild cherry, apple, pear, rose, bramble, pimpernel, saxifrage, ninebark

Rubiaceae (p. 4), cinchona alkaloids (p. 707), harmala alkaloids (p.611), macrocyclic peptide alkaloids (p. 937), monoterpene alkaloids (p. 574, 656, 658, 661, 665, 673, 684, 707–709, 713, 789), oligomers of tryptamine (p. 591–597), prenylated indole alkaloids (p. 618), purine alkaloids (p. 953), ipecac alkaloids from the root of the Brazilian plant *Cephaelis ipecacuanha* (p. 560): hepatica, ipecac, Peruvian bark, cinchona, cleavers, goosegrass, crosswort, **cancerillo** (*Psychotria*). **Quinine, emetine.** What is known as coffee is obtained from the seeds of *Coffea arabica* and other members of the genus *Coffea*, and the alkaloid is of course **caffeine** (p. 953). Coffee is sometimes mentioned as an **anticancer** agent, perhaps due to the presence of the alkaloid caffeine. **Yohimbine** from the bark of the tree *Corynanthe* yohimbe* of the Cameroons and French Congo (p. 684). β-**Carboline** (p. 611).

Rutaceae (p. 4), acridine alkaloids (p. 264–269), anthranilic acid-derived alkaloids (p. 236), benzo[c]phenanthridine alkaloids (p. 509), canthin-6-one alkaloids (p. 619), carbizole alkaloids (p. 614), cinnamic acid alkaloids (p. 288), harmala alkaloids (p. 611), protoberberine alkaloids (p. 472), protopine alkaloids (p. 485), quinazoline alkaloids (p. 253): vilva, orange, lime, lemon, grapefruit, citrus, citron, rue, ruta, prickly ash. **Evoprenine, aeronycine, meliopicine** (p. 264). **Rutaecarpine** and **evodiamine** have been isolated from the Chinese drug *Evodia* rutaecarpa* and from *Zanthoxylum* (p. 257, 259). **Cusparine** and **galipene** from *Cusparia** and *Galipea** (p. 238). **4-Quinolones** with long alkyl side chains have been isolated from *Ruta graveolens*, or rue (and from several fungi including *Pseudomonus aeruginosa*). The quinazoline alkaloids **vasicine, harman, harmine, harmaline** occur with furoquinolines and acridones (p. 253). **Murrayanine, heptaphylline, mahanimbine, girinimbine** from *Murrayaya koenigii* or Indian curry leaf (p. 614). **Canthin-6-one** from *Pentaceras* australis* and *Zanthoxylum* (p. 619)

Salicaceae: poplar, willow

Salvadoraceae: ark, tooth brush tree

Santalaceae: toadflax, sandalwood, sandal

Sapindaceae purine alkaloids (p. 953): kokalende, winter cherry, baloon vine, quahmecatl. **Caffeine** from *Paulinia cupana*, native to Brazil and Uruguay. The dried paste from the crushed seeds is called guarana, and is used to make a beverage.

Sapotaceae: mamey, buckthorn, madhuka

Saururaceae: Yerba del manza, Apache beads

Saxifragaceae quinazoline alkaloids (p. 253): alumroot, maple leaf, hydrangea, saxifrage. **Vasicine, februgine, rutaecarpine, arborine** (p. 253). **Febrifugine** is found in the Chinese drug *Dichroa febriguga* (p. 257).

Scrophulariaceae monoterpene alkaloids (p. 847): snapdragon, foxglove, digitalis, mudwort, toadflax, linaria, lousewort, rue, figwort, mullein. **Cantleine, bakankoside, gentianine, gentioflavine** from *Antirrhinum majus* (p. 847).

Simarubaceae canthin-6-one alkaloids (p. 619): quassia, simaruba. **Canthin-6-one**.

Solanaceae (p. 4, 80, 99), steroidal alkaloids (p. 900), tropane alkaloids (p. 94): belladonne, deadly nightshade, solanum lethale, belladonna, capsicum cayenne pepper, red pepper, thornapple, Jamestown weed (Jimsonweed), henbane, tomato, mandrake, tobacco, strychnos, nightshade, bittersweet, dulcamara, solanum, potato, Irish potato, white potato, winter cherry. **Hyoscyamine** in (p. 4), toxicity of plants (p. 94). **Hyoscyamine**, of which the optically-inactive form is otherwise known as **atropine**, is the most common tropane alkaloid, and is found in the *Datura* species (p. 94). Another source is *Hyoscymus muticus*, a native of Egypt, but now cultivated in Southern California. **Scopolamine** and **hyoscyamine** found in *Scopolia tangutica**(p. 115). **Solanidine** and **solanidine** alkaloids, **solanine** (p. 903), **solanum** alkaloids (p 72). **Pyrrolidine** in *Nicotinia tabacum* (p. 80). **N-Methylpyrrolidine** in tobacco as well as in the deadly nightshade *Atropa belladona*. **Cuscohygrine** in *Atropa belladonna* and the genus *Datura*.

Stemonaceae: no common names listed

Sterculiaceae macrocyclic peptide alkaloids (p. 937), purine alkaloids (p. 953), simple quinoline alkaloids (p. 240): **una de gato** (cat's claw), bitter kola, obi, bandhuli. Cola or Kola is obtained from the cotyledons (first leaf of a whorl) from various cola trees of the genus *Cola*, and has a high **caffeine** content (p. 953). Cocoa is obtained from the seeds of *Theobromo cacao*, and contains **theobromine** (p. 953). Adouétines from *Waltheria* americana* (p. 937).

Styracaceae: benzoin, storax, styrax

Symplocaceae: lodhra, lodh tree

Tamaricaceae: myrica, tamarisk

Taxaceae: talisa

Theaceae purine alkaloids (p. 953): green tea, **tea**. Tea is made from the leaves and leaf buds of *Camellia sinensis*, and the main alkaloid is **caffeine** along with smaller amounts of **theobromine** and **theophylline** (p. 953). Interestingly, tea is sometimes noted as an **anticancer** agent.

Theophrastaceae: siempreviva

Thymelaeceae: lignin aloe, aloe wood, gnidian berry, laureola,leatherwood

Tiliaceae: tilo, tilia.

TRICHOLOMATACEAE (p. 954). **Deoxyeritadenine** occurs in *Leontinus edodes* and has hypocholesterolemic properties.

Tropaeolaceae: chichira, hanucara, mastuerso

Typhaceae: totora, cat-tail flag

Ulmaceae: elms

Umbelliferae (p. 208): cicuta, ameudill, anetum, angelica, apium, celery, jareta, careum, caraway, water hemlock, hemlock, poison hemlock, conium, coriander, coriandrum, cumin, carrot, ammoniacum, ammoniac, rosemary, fennell, galbanum, sagapenum, cow parsnip, myrrh, opoponax, wild parsnip, parsnip, parsley, anise. **Coniine** from *Conium maculatum* or poison hemlock. Also **N-methylconiine, γ-coniine, conhydrine, pseudoconhydrine.**

Urticaceae (p. 147, 579): parietaire, nettle, stinging nettle, urtica, ortie

Valerianaceae: nardum, nard, nardus, spica, valeriana, valerian

Verbenaceae: white mangrove, dwarf mulberry, **cancer plant** (*Lippia cuneifolia*), oregano, verbena, vervain, agnos. **Verbenalin** (p. 811).

Violaceae: violet, bonewort, sweet violet, violeta, viola, pansy

Vitaceae: caro, amomum, Virginia creeper, American ivy, grapes, wild grapes, raisins, currants

Vochysiaceae: cachimbo de jaboty

Winteranaceae (Canellaceae): no common names listed

Zingiberaceae: grains of paradise, galanga, amomum, cardamomum, costus, turmeric, zedoary, conopia, ginger

Zygophyllaceae quinazoline alkaloids (p. 253): guaiacum, jarilla, **chaparral or ceosote weed** (*Larria tridenta*), wild rue, rue, ruta, abrojo. **Vasicine, februgine, rutaecarpine, arborine.** Occur with harman alkaloids in *Peganum harmala*.

Bioactive/Toxic Plants Found in the United States

Table V.1   Poisonous Plants from the Western United States

Anacardiaceae	*Toxicodendron* rydbergii*: poison ivy
Apiaceae*	*Cicuta maculata*: water hemlock
(Umbelliferae)	*Conium maculata*: poison hemlock
	Daucus carota L.: wild carrot
Apocynaceae	*Apocynum androsaemifolium**: spreading dogbane
	Apocynum cannabinum: hemp dogbane
Asclepiadaceae	*Asclepius fascicularis**: Mexican whorled milkweed
	A. incarnata: swamp milkweed
	A. labriformas*: Labriform milkweed
	A. subverticillata*: western whorled milkweed
Asteraceae*	*Conyza canadensis**: horseweed
(Compositae)	*Grindelia squarrosa*: curlycup gumweed. Used by Indians.
	Gutierrezia* sarothrae: broom snakeweed
	Hemizonia* pungens: spikeweed
	Senecio jacobaea: tansy ragwort. **Alkaloids.**
	S. riddellii*: Riddell groundsel. **Pyrrolizidine alkaloids.**
	S. vulgaris: common groundsel
	Tanacetum vulgare: common tansy. Used as medicine.
	Tetradymia* canescens: gray horsebrush
	Xanthium strumarium: common cocklebur
	Xylorhiza* glabriuscula: woodyaster. Selenium indicator.
Boraginaceae	*Amsinckia* intermedia*: coast fiddleneck
	Cynoglossum officianale: houndstongue
Cannabaceae*	*Cannabis sativa*: marijuana
(Moraceae)	
Chenopodiaceae	*Halogeton* glomeratus*: halogeton. Oxalates.
	Kochia* scoparia: kochia. High nitrate.
	Sarcobatus* vermiculatus: greasewood. Oxalates.
Clusiaceae*	*Hypericum perforatum*: common St. Johnswort
(Guttiferae)	
Compositae (see Asteraceae)	
Cucurbitaceae	*Coccinia* grandis*: ivy gourd. Used as medicine.
Equisetaceae	*Equisetum hyemale*: scouringrush
Euphorbiaceae	*Eremocarpus* setigerus*: turkey mullein
	Euphorbia esula: leafy spurge
	Ricinus communis: castorbean
Fabaceae*	*Astragalus bisculatus**: twogrooved milkvetch. Selenium.
(Leguminosae)	*Lupinus wyethii**: Wyeth lupine
	Oxytropis* sericea: silky crazyweed
	O.* lambertii: Lambert crazyweed
	Thermopsis* rhombifolia: goldenpea
Iridaceae	*Iris missouriensis**: Rocky Mountain iris
Juncaginaceae*	*Triglochin* maritimum*: seaside arrowgrass
Lamiaceae*	*Salvia reflexa**: lanceleaf sage. Nitrates.
(Labiatae)	

Leguminosae (see Fabaceae)	
Liliaceae	*Zigadenus* * *paniculatus*: foothills death camus
	Z. * *venenosus*: meadow deathcamus
	Lily Family contains enzyme inhibitors.
Papaveraceae	*Argemone polyanthemos* *: annual pricklypoppy
Poaceae*	*Sorghum halepense* *: Johnsongrass. Cyanides.
(Gramineae)	
Ranunculaceae	*Delphinium geyeri* *: Geyer larkspur
	D. nuttallianum *: low larkspur
	D. occidentale *: tall larkspur
	Ranunculus acris: tall buttercup
	R. repens: creeping buttercup
	R. testiculatus *: bur buttercup
Scrophulariaceae	*Digitalis purpurea*: foxglove
	Kickxia * *elatine*: sharppoint fluvellin, cancerwort
Solanaceae	*Datura innoxia*: sacred datura. Hallucinogenic.
	D. discolor *: small datura
	D. stramonium: Jimsonweed, Jamestown weed
	Hyoscyamus niger: black henbane
	Physalis virginiana *: Virginia groundcherry
	P. wrightii *: Wright groundcherry
	Solanum dulcamara: bitter nightshade
	S. elacagnifolium *: silverleaf nightshade
	S. nigrum: black nightshade
	S. rostratum *: buffalobur
	S. sarrachoides *: hairy nightshade
	S. triflorum *: cutleaf nightshade
Umbelliferae (see Apiaceae)	
Zygophyllaceae	*Larrea tridentata*: creosotebush. Medicine and antiseptic
	Peganum harmala: African rue, wild rue. **Harmala alkaloids**

Source: Data from *Weeds of the West*, Tom D. Whitson Ed., published by the Western Society of Weed Science in cooperation with the Western United States Land Grant Universities Cooperative Extension Services, College of Agriculture, University of Wyoming, Laramie, January 1991. Plant families, genera, or species **not** found in Jonathan L. Hartwell's *Plants Used Against Cancer* are denoted by an asterisk. Specific notations as may be found in the reference are added, with alkaloids shown in **boldface**.

Table V.2   Poisonous Plants from the Tallgrass Prarie

Amaryllidaceae	*Agave lecheguillo* *: lechuguilla
Apiaceae (or	*Cicuta maculata*: spotted waterhemlock
Umbelliferae)	*Conium maculatum*: poison hemlock
Apocynaceae	*Apocynum cannabinum*: hemp dogbane
Asclepiadaceae	*Asclepias latifolia*: broadleaf milkweed
Asteraceae*	*Actinea* * *adorata*: bitterweed, actinea
(Compositae)	*Aplopappus heterophyllus* *: rayless goldenrod
	Eupatorium rugosum *: white snakeroot
	Gutierrezia * *sarothrae*: broom snakeweed
	Senecio longilobus *: threadleaf groundsel
	Xanthium spp.: cocklebur
	Xylorrhiza * *parryi*: woody aster
Campanulaceae	*Lobelia cardinalis* *: cardinal flower
Chenopodiaceae	*Halogeton* * *glomeratus*: halogeton
Clusiaceae*	*Hypericum perforatum*: St. Johnswort
(Guttiferae)	
Compositae (see Asteracea)	
Crucifereae	*Stanleya* * *pinnata*: prince's plume
Equisetaceae	*Equisetum arvensi*: common horsetail
Euphorbiaceae	*Croton texensis* *: Texas croton
Fabaceae*	*Astragalus mollissimus* *: woolly loco

(Leguminosae)	*Astralagus wootoni**: wooton loco
	Crotalaria* sagittalis: arrow crotalaria
	Lupinus argentus*: silvery lupine
	Oxytropis* lambertii: lambert crazyweed
Fagaceae	*Quercus gambellii*: Gambel oak, encino. Tannic acid in leaves and acorns.
Gramineae	*Claviceps purpurea*: ergot, spurred rye. Fungus sclerotia replaces seed kernel. **Ergot alkaloids. "Ergotoxine."**
Hippocastanaceae	*Aesculus arguta**: Texas buckeye
Juncaginaceae*	*Triglochin* maritima*: arrowgrass
Leguminosae (see Fabaceae)	
Liliaceae	*Zigadenus* nuttalli*: Nuttall death camus
Ranunculaceae	*Delphinium virescens**: plains larkspur
Rosaceae	*Prunus virginiana**: common chokecherry. Cyanides in leaves.
Solanaceae	*Solanum nigrum*: black nightshade
Umbelliferae (see Apiaceae)	

Source: Data from *Poisonous Grassland Plants*, Section 4 of a Series *Pasture and Range Plants*, Phillips Petroleum Company, Bartlesville OK, 1957, 1959. Plant families, genera, or species **not** found in Jonathan L. Hartwell's *Plants Used Against Cancer* are denoted by an asterisk. Specific notations as may be found in the reference are added, with alkaloids shown in **boldface**.

Table V.3   Poisonous Plants from the Eastern United States

Amaryllidaceae	*Amaryllis* spp.: amaryllis. **Alkaloids.**
	Galanthus* nivalis: snowdrop. **Alkaloids.**
	Narcissus spp.: daffodils, jonquils. Oxalates.
Anacardiaceae	*Rhus* spp.: poison ivy, oak, sumac. Urushiol phenolics.
Apocynaceae	*Apocynum cannabinum*: dogbane, Indian hemp. Cardiac glycosides.
	Nerium oleander: oleander. Cardiac glycosides ~ digitalis.
	Vinca spp.: periwinkles. **Alkaloids, vincamine.**
Aquifoliaceae	*Ilex* spp.: hollies. Saponin glycosides.
Araceae	*Arisaema triphyllum*: Jack-in-the-pulpit. Oxalates.
	Dieffenbachia spp.: dumbcane. Oxalates.
	Symplocarpus foetidus: skunk cabbage. Oxalates.
Araliaceae	*Aralia spinosa**: Hercules' club, devil's walking stick. Unknown.
	Hedera helix: English ivy. **Steroids,** saponic glycosides.
Asclepiadaceae	*Asclepias* spp.: milkweeds. Cardiac glycosides.
Berberidaceae	*Caulophyllum thalictroides*: squaw root. Saponins, **Alkaloids.**
	Podophyllum peltatum: mayapple. Podophyllins: **anticancer/antimitotic.**
Bignoniaceae	*Compsis* radicans*: trumpet vine. Unknown.
Boraginaceae	*Echium vulgare**: blue devil, blue thistle. **Pyrrolizidine alkaloids.**
Buxaceae	*Buxus sempivirens*: boxwood or common box. **Buxine alkaloids.**
Campanulaceae	*Lobelia* spp.: lobelia, Indian tobacco. **Lobelia alkaloids** ~ nicotine.
Cannabinaceae* (Moraceae)	*Cannabis sativa*: marijuana, hemp. Tetrahydrocannabinol phenolics.
Caprifoliaceae	*Sambucus canadensis*: elderberry. **Alkaloids,** cyanoglycosides: lvs, rts. *Symphoricarpos** spp.: coralberry, snowberry. Saponins.
Caryophyllaceae	*Argostemma githago*: corn cockle. Sapogenic glycosides.
	Saponaria officinalis: soapwort, bouncing bet. Sapogenic glycosides.
Celastraceae	*Celastrus* spp.: bittersweet. Unknown.
	Euonymus* spp.: euonymous. Cardiotonic glycosides, **alkaloids.**
Compositae	*Eupatorium rugosum**: white snakeroot. Tremetol.
	Helenium* autumnale: sneezeweed, bitterweed. Glycosides.
	Senecio spp.: groundsels. **Pyrrolizidine alkaloids.**
	Xanthium strumarium: cocklebur. Hydroquinone.
Convolvulaceae	*Convolvulus* spp.: bindweed. Toxic and **hallucinogenic** substances.
	Ipomoea purpurea*, *I. tricolor**: morning glories. LSD-like toxins.

Cruciferae	*Brassica* spp.: wild mustard. Glycosides.
Ericaceae	*Kalmia** spp.: mountain laurel. **Terpenoids**, andromedotoxin.
	Leucothoe* spp.: dog laurel, sweet bells. Andromedotoxin.
	Pieris* japonica: Japanese andromeda. Andromedotoxin.
	Rhododendron* spp.: rhodendrons and azaleas. Andromedotoxin.
Euphorbiaceae	*Aleurites fordil**: tung-oil tree, tung nut. Saponins.
	Cnidoscolus* stimulosus: tread-softly. Unknown.
	Euphorbia spp.: spurge. **Diterpenoids phorbal, ingenol:** carcinogenic.
	Ricinus communis: castor bean. Ricin proteins (water-soluble).
Fumariaceae*	*Corydalis* spp.: fumatory. **Alkaloids.**
(Papaveraceae)	*Dicentra* spp.: dutchman's breeches, bleeding heart. **Protopine.**
Guttiferae	*Hypericum perforatum*: St. John's wort. Hypericin: photosensitive.
Hippocastanaceae	*Aesculus* spp.: buckeyes, horsechestnuts. Glycosides aesculin, aescin.
Iridaceae	*Iris* spp.: irises. Unknown.
Labiatae	*Glechoma* hederaceae*: ground ivy, creeping charlie. Unknown.
Leguminosae	*Baptisia* spp.: false indigo. **Alkaloids.**
	Cassia spp.: senna. Cathartics.
	Gymnocladus* diocica: Kentucky coffee tree. **Cytisine alkaloids.**
	Laburnum* anagyroides: golden chain. **Cytisine alkaloids.**
	Lathyrus spp.: sweet pea. Amines: cause lathyrism.
	Lupinus spp.: lupines. **Simple alkaloids.**
	Robinia* pseudo-acacia: black locust. Toxic proteins (phytoxins).
	Wisteria spp.: wisteria. Toxic glycosides and lectins.
Liliaceae	*Colchicum autumnale*: autumn crocus. **Colchicine alkaloids.**
	Convallaria* majalis: lily-of-the-valley. Cardiac glycoside convallarin.
	Hyacinthus* orientalis: garden hyacinth. Unkown.
	Melanthuim* virginicum: bunch flower. Unknown.
	Ornithogalum* umbellatum: star of Bethlehem. Cardiac glycosides.
	Scilla spp.: squill. Cardiac glycosides.
	Veratrum viride: Eastern false hellebore. **Steroid (veratrum) alkaloids.**
	Zigadenus* spp.: death camus. **Steroid alkaloids.**
Linaceae	*Linum usitatissimum*: flax. Cyanogenic glycosides.
Loganiaceae	*Gelsemium sempervirens*: yellow or Carolina jessamine. **Alkaloids.**
	Spigelia* marilandica: pinkroot, Indian pink. **Spigiline alkaloid.**
Loranthaceae	*Phoradendron serotinum**: mistletoe. Amines.
Meliaceae	*Melia azedarach*: chinaberry. Resins.
Menispermaceae	*Menispermum* canadens*: Canada moonseed. **Alkaloids.**
Moraceae	*Morus* spp.: mulberries. Unknown ~ Osage orange.
Nyctaginaceae	*Mirabilis jalapa*: four-o'clock. Unknown.
Oleaceae	*Ligustrum vulgare*: privet. Glycosides.
Papaveraceae	*Papaver* spp.: poppies. **Isoquinoline (opium) alkaloids.**
	Sanguinaria canadensis: bloodroot. **Opium alkaloids.**
Phytolaccaceae	*Phytolacca americana*: poke, pokeweed. Saponic glycosides, mitogens.
Polygonaceae	*Rheum rhaponticum*: rhubarb. Oxalates, anthraquinone glycosides.
Ranunculaceae	*Aconitum* spp.: monkshood, wolfsbane. **Aconitine (diterpene alkaloid).**
	Actaea spp.: baneberry, doll's- eyes. Unknown.
	Anemone spp.: windflowers. Protoanemonin glycoside.
	Caltha paluste or *C. palustris*: marsh marigold, cowslip. Protoanemonin.
	Clematis spp.:clematis, virgin's bower. Protoanemonin.
	Delphinium spp.: larkspur. Akaloids.
	Helleborus niger: Christmas rose. Glycosides.
	Hydrastis canadensis: golden seal. **Isoquinolines hydrastine, berberine.**
	Ranunculus spp.: buttercup, crowfoot. Protoanemonin.
Rhamnaceae	*Rhamnus cathartica*: buckthorn. Anthraquinone or anthracene glycosides.

Rosaceae	*Prunus serotina*: wild cherry, black cherry. Amygdalin: seeds, twigs, lves. *Rhodotypos* scandens*: jetbead. Organic cyanides (amygdalin).
Scrophulariaceae	*Digitalis purpurea*: foxglove. Cardiac glycosides.
Simarubaceae	*Ailanthus altissima*: tree-of-heaven. Unknown.
Solanaceae	*Atropa belladona*: belladonna, deadly nightshade. **Atropine.**
	Datura stramonium: jimsonweed. **Alkaloids.**
	Hydrocyamus niger: henbane. **Tropane alkaloids (hallucinogenic).**
	Lycopersicon esculentum: tomato. **Solanine alkaloids: leaves, stems.**
	Nicotiana tabacum: tobacco. **Nicotine.**
	Physalis spp.: ground cherry, Chinese lantern. **Solanidine alkaloids.**
	Solanum spp.: nightshades **solanine alkaloids.**
Thymelaeaceae	*Daphne mezereum*: flowering mezereon **diterpenoids (carcinogenic).** Umbelliferae *Cicuta maculata*: water hemlock. Cicutoxin.
	Conium maculatum: poison hemlock. **Coniine alkaloids.**
	Pastinaca sativa: wild parsnip. Furanocoumarin.
Urticaceae	*Laportea* canadensis*: wood nettle. Skin irritants.
	Urtica dioica: stinging nettle. Histamine, acetylcholine, serotonin, formate.
Verbenaceae	*Lantana camara*: lantana. **Triterpenoids.**
Vitaceae	*Pathenocissus quinquefolia*: Virginia creeper. Unknown.

Source: Data from *Poisonous and Medicinal Plants* by Will H. Blackwell, Prentice-Hall, Englewood Cliffs NJ, 1990. Plant families, genera, or species **not** found in Jonathan L. Hartwell's *Plants Used Against Cancer* ar⁻ denoted by an asterisk. Specific notations as may be found in the reference are added, with alkaloids shown in **boldface.**

Antitumor Phytochemicals*

*Abrin (cytotoxic)
Aceratioside (cytotoxic)
Acetic acid-ethyl ether
1-Acetoxychavicol
1-Acetoxyeugenol
15-Acetoxyrudmollin (antileukemic)
Acobioside-A
Acofrioside-L
Acolongifloriside-G
Acolongifloriside-H
Acolongifloriside-K
Acoschimperoside-P
Acoschimperoside-Q
Acospectoside-A
Acovenoside-A
Acridone
Adynerin
Agrimoniin
Alanine
Alatolide
*Alkannin
Allamandin (antileukemic, cytotoxic)
*Allicin
*Allyl-isothiocyanate
*Aloe-emodin (also antileukemic)
Amaralin
Amygdalin (cyanogenic)
Amyrin
alpha-Amyrin (cytotoxic)
*Anacardic acid
Anacardol
Anacrotine
*Anemonin
*Anethole

(trans-Anethole is a sweetener)
alpha-Angelicalactone
Angustibalin
16-Anhydrogitoxigen
Anopterine
*Apigenin
Apocannoside
Arctiopicrine
*Aristolactam-IA (antileukemic, cytotoxic)
*Aristolochic acid (also carcinogenic?)
*Aristolochic acid-I (antileukemic, cytotoxic)
Armepavine
*Arnebin
Arnicolide-A
Aromadendrin
Artemisetin
Artemisiifolin
1-Asparaginase (also antileukemic)
Astragalin (antileukemic)
beta-Alantone
Atractylon (esophagus)
*Aucubigenin
Autumnolide (cytotoxic)
Baileyin (cytotoxic)
Barringtogenol-C-21-angelate
Benzoic acid-ethyl ether
3-O-Benzoyl-ursolic acid (cytotoxic)
Berberine
Berberine chloride (HIV-RT-inhibitor)
Bersaldegenin-3-acetate
Bersaldegenin-1-3-5-orthoacetate
Bersamagenin-1-3-5-orthoacetate
Berscillogenin

---

* *Source:* Selected from *Handbook of Biologically Active Phytochemicals and Their Activities* by James A. Duke, CRC Press, Boca Raton FL, 1992. Entries which are also pesticides are denoted by an asterisk, as indicated in the reference. As a means for comparing frequency of occurrence, alkaloids—presumably the most bioactive—are for the most part shown in **boldface**, as are other items of potential interest. Other properties are set forth in parens, such as being cytotoxic or cell-toxic, or being antileukemic, or as inhibiting HIV-RT, the acronym used to denote the AIDS virus HIV, that is, the retrovirus that affects T lymphocytes in the immune system. Some compounds which are not anticancer agents, but which have unusual properties or uses, are isolated in parens. For the full range of compounds and information, consult the reference, which also supplies sources.

Bersenogenin
Betuoin (cytotoxic)
Betulinic acid (cytotoxic)
Bhilawanol
Biochanin-A
Biscatechin
(1)-Bisparthenolidine
Bouvardin
Bowman-Birk-Inhibitor (BBI)
Brickellin (cytotoxic)
*Bromelain (also antiplaque, proteolytic)
Bruceanic acid (cytotoxic)
Bruceanic acid-D (antileukemic, cytotoxic)
Bruceanol (antileukemic)
Bruceantarin
*Bruceantin (also antileukemic, cytotoxic)
*Bruceantinol (antileukemic)
Brucein-A
*Bruceine (also antileukemic)
Bruceoside (antileukemic)
*Brusatol (antileukemic)
Bufotalidin acetate
*Bullatacin (antileukemic, cytotoxic)
Burseran (cytotoxic)
Butenolide-B (esophagus)
*Caffeic acid
*Caffeine
Calmodulin
Calotropin (cardioactive)
Camelliin-B
*Camphor
*Camptothecin (also antileukemic)
*Canthine-6-one (antileukemic, cytotoxic)
Capsaicin (also carcinogenic)
beta-Carotene
*Carpaine
Carpesterol (cytotoxic)
*Carvone
Casearin
Casimiroedine (antileukemic)
*Catechin (also carcinogenic)
d-Catechin
*Catechol (also carcinogenic)
Cedrene
Celsioside-C
Centaureidin
*Cepharanthine (colon)
Cesalin
Chamanetin (antileukemic, cytotoxic)
Chaparrinone
*Chelerythrine
Chelidimerine
*Chlorogenic acid
*Chlorophyll
Choline (antialszheimeran)

*Chrysin
Chrysoeriol
Chrysosplenol-B (cytotoxic)
Chrysosplenol-C (cytotoxic)
*Chrysosplenol-D (cytotoxic)
Chrysosplenol-E (cytotoxic)
Chrysosplenol-F (cytotoxic)
Chrysosplenol-G (cytotoxic)
Cicutoxin (antileukemic)
*Cinnamaldehyde
*trans-Cinnamaldehyde (also sweetener)
*Cinnamic acid
3-O-Cinnamoyl-ursolic acid (cytotoxic)
*Cirsilineol
*Cirsimaritin
Cissampareine
*Citral (teratogenic)
Citric acid
Citrinin
Cleomiscosin-A (antileukemic)
*Cnicin
Cocculinin
Cocslinine
Coixenolide
Colchiceine-amide
*Colchicine (cytotoxic)
Colchicine amide (breast, cervix, liver, lymph)
Colubrinol
Colubrinol acetate (also antileukemic)
*Columbamine chloride (HIV-RT-inhibitor)
Concavalin-A
*Conessine
Conoduramine
Conodurine
Convallatoxin (also cardiotonic)
Coptisine
(Coriatin is antischizophrenic)
Coroglaucigenin
Corydine (CNS-depressant)
Corytuberine (CNS-suppressant)
*Costulonide (cytotoxic)
Costunolide
*p-Coumaric acid
*Coumarin
*o-Cresol
*p-Cresol
Crinamine
Crispatine
Crotepoxide
3-O-Crotonyl-ursolic acid (cytotoxic)
*Cryptopleurine (cytotoxic)
Cryptowolline (cytotoxic)
*Cucurbitacin (cytotoxic)
Cucurbitacin-B (cytotoxic)

(Cucurbitacin-E is antihepatotoxic but cyto-
toxic)
Cucurbitacin-F (cytotoxic)
Cucurbitacin-I
Cucurbitacin-I (also antileukemic)
Cucurbitacin-J
Cucurbitacin-K
Cucurbitacin-L
alpha-Curcumene
*Curcumin
Curcumol
Curdione
*Curine
1-Curine
Curzerone
Cycasin (also antiaging, carcinogenic)
Cycleadrine
Cycleaneonine (stomach)
Cycleanine (cytotoxic)
Cycleapeltine
Cycloprotobuxine
Cycloshikonin
*Cymarin
*Cynaropicrin
Cysteine
Daidzin
Damsin (cytotoxic)
Damsinic acid
Daphnoretin
Datiscocide
Daucosterol
Deacetylconfertiflorin
Deacetyleupaserrin (cytotoxic)
gamma-Decalactone
Decan-1-AL
Dehydroailanthinone (cytotoxic)
Dehydroailanthion (cytotoxic)
Dehydroanhidropicropodophyllin
Dehydrobruceantarin
Dehydrobruceantin
Dehydrobruceantol
Dehydroemetine
Dehydroheliotridine (also antileukemic)
*cis-Dehydromatricarea ester
3-dehydronobilin
*Delphinidin
Demecolcine
3'-Demethylpodophyllotoxin
Deoxyelephantopin
Deoxyharringtonine (also antileukemic)
Deoxypodophyllotoxin (cytotoxic)
Desgalactotigonin
Desglucouzarin
5'-Desmethoxy-beta-peltatin-methyl ether
3-Desmethylcolchicine (also antileukemic)

N-Desmethylthalidasine
N-Desmethylthalistyline
Desmethyltylophorinine
Desoxypodophyllotoxin
Diacetylmonocrotaline
*Diallyl-disulfide
*Diallyl-sulfide
3,4-Dicaffeoylquinic acid
2,3-Dicarboxy-6,7-dihydroxy-1-(3',4'-
dihydroxy)-phenyl-1,2-(–)-dicentrine
Dichamanetin (antileukemic)
Dichroidine
*Dichroine
Dichroside-C
Dichroside-D
Digallic acid (antileukemic, HIV-RT-inhib)
*3,5-Di-O-galloylshikimic acid (AIDS, HIV-
RT)
Digiferruginol (antileukemic)
Digitonin
Digitoxin (also cardiotonic)
Diglucoacoschimperoside-N
Diglucoacoschimperoside-P
Digoxin (also cardiotonic)
Dihydrocoumarin
Dihydrocucurbitacin-B
25,26-Dihydrophysalin-C
25,26-Dihydrophysalin-D
(Dihydroquercetin-3-acetate is sweetener)
*Dihydroquercitin
Dihydroshikonin
Dihydrovaltrate (cytotoxic)
4-(3,4-Dihydroxy-benzoyl-oxy-methyl)-
phenyl-beta-D-glucopyranoside
[15,19-Dihydroxylabda-8(9)-13(14)E-dien-
17-AL-6alpha-O-alpha-L-arabino-
pyranoside is a sweetener]
1,3-Dihydroxy-2-methoxymethyl-
anthraquinone (antileukemic)
3,5-Dihydroxy-4-methoxybenzoic acid-
methyl ester (cytotoxic)
3,3'-Diindolymethane
1,11-Dimethoxycanthin-6-one (antileukemic)
N-(3,4-Dimethoxycinnamoyl)-delta-3-
pyridin-2-one (antileukemic)
*3-(3,3-Dimethylallyl)-5-(3-acetyl-2,4-dihy-
droxy-5-methyl-6-methoxybenzyl)-phlo-
racetophenone (also antileukemic, antimelanomic, cytotoxic)
(+)-Dimethylisolariciresinol-2-alpha-xylo-
side
O,O-Dimethylliensinine
(3,3'-Dimethylquercetin is antipolio)
Di-O-caffeoyl-quinic acid

Diosmetin
Diphyllin (antileukemic, cytotoxic)
Dircin (antileukemic)
Diuvaretin (antileukemic, cytotoxic)
Dulcitol
(Dumbcain is proteolytic)
Echinatine-N-oxide
Eicasanol
Eicosapentaenoic acid
Elabunin (antileukemic, cytotoxic)
Elagnin
Elephantin (cytotoxic)
Elephantopic (cytotoxic)
*Ellagic acid (also anticataract, antiHIV)
Ellagitannin
***Ellipticine** (also antileukemic, cardiotoxic)
Emargeinatine-A (antileukemic, cytotoxic)
Emarginatine-B (cyctotoxic)
***Emetine** (also antileukemic, cytotoxic)
*Emodin
*Enmein
*Ent-clerodane (antileukemic)
3-Epebercillogenin
*(–)-Epicatechin
Epicatechin gallate
2-Epicucurbitacin-B
10-Epieupatoroxin (cytotoxic)
(–)-Epigallocatechin gallate
Epitulipinolide
1,10-Epoxynobilin
Epoxyshikoccin
Eremantholide (cytotoxic)
*Eriodyctyol
Eriofertin
Eriofertopin
Erioflorin (cytotoxic)
Erioflorin acetate (cyctotoxic)
Erioflorin methacrylate (cytotoxic)
Erucic acid
(**Erythrine** is strychnine antidote)
Esculin
(Ergoside is sweetener)
Estragole (also carcinogenic)
Estrogens (breast, prostate)
6-Ethoxychelerythrine
Ethoxysanguinarine
*Ethylgallate
Etoposide
*Eugenol
Eugenol-methyl-ether
Eupachlorin (cytotoxic)
Eupachlorine acetate
Eupachloroxin (cytotoxic)
Eupacunin (cytotoxic)
Eupaformonin (cytotoxic)

Eupahyssopin
Euparotin (cytotoxic)
Euparotin acetate
Eupaserrin (cytotoxic)
Eupatin
Eupatocunin (cytotoxic)
Eupatolide
Eupatolitin (also antihepatotoxic)
Eupatoretin
Eupatorin (cytotoxic)
*Eupatoriopicrin (cytotoxic)
Eupatoroxin (cytotoxic)Eupatundin (cyctotoxic)
(Euperfolin is an immunostimulant)
(Euperfolitin is an immunostimulant)
Fabacein
***Fagaronine** (also antileukemic, HIV-RT inhibitor)
(***Fagaronine** chloride is an HIV-RT inhibitor)
Fastigilin-A
Fastigilin-C (cytotoxic)
*Ferulic acid
trans-Ferulic acid
Fiber
Formononetin (also abortifacient)
N-formyldesacetylcolchinine
Fraxinol
Fulvine
(*Fulvoplumierin is antiHIV, cytotoxic)
Fumaric acid (also antihepatocarcinogenic)
Galangin
Gallic acid
Geiparvarin
Genistein (also antileukemic, abortifacient)
Genkwadaphnin (antileukemic)
*Geraniol
*Geranylgeraniol
*Gingerol
Gitoxigenin
Glaucarubolone
Glucaric acid
Glutathione (also anticytotoxic)
(Glycerol is anticataract, anti-earwax, anti-Meniere's)
Glycine
Glycitein
Oglycoflavone-C-glycoside
*Glycyrrhetic acid
*Glycyrrhizic acid
*Glycyrrhizin (also antihepatic, but pancreaprotective, sweetener)
Gnidicin (cytotoxic)
Gnididin (cytotoxic)
Gnidilatidin (antileukemic)

Gniditrin (cytotoxic)
Goniothalamicin (antileukemic)
(Gossypin is anticataract)
*Gossypol (also male contraceptive)
(*Gossypol acetic acid is HIV-RT inhib)
*Grandinol
Grosheimin
d-Guatambuine (antileukemic)
Guattegaumerine (antimelanomic)
(Gypsogenic acid is hepatoprotective)
Hainanensine
Hainanolide (also antileukemic)
(**Harmeline** is antiparkinsonian, hallucino-
    genic, phototoxic)
Harringtonine (also antileukemic)
Hayatine
(*HCN antidote is amyl nitrate)
Hecogenin glycoside
*Hederasaponin-C
*Helenalin (cytotoxic/cytoprotective)
Heliamine
Heliotrine (also antileukemic)
Heliotrine-N-oxide
Hellebrigenin-3-acetate
Hellebrigenin-3,5-acetate
Hellebrin
(Hernandulcin is sweetener)
*Hesperetin
3',4',5,6,7,7-Hexamethoxyflavone
Hippocaesculin
Hispidulin (also antihepatotoxic)
(Hispiduloside is anticataract)
(**Histamine** is antimeniere's, radioprotective)
Histone
(Hodulcin is sweetness supressor)
*Homograndinol
Homoharringtonine (also antileukemic,
    tachycardic)
Homoisomelodienone (cytotoxic)
*Honokiol (also anticariogenic, Ca-blocker,
    CNS-depressant)
Huangshanine
*p-Hydroxybenzoic acid
16-beta-Hydroxybersaldegenin-1-acetate
16-beta-Hydroxybersaldegenin-3-acetate
*(+)-8-16-beta-Hydroxybersaldegenin-
1,3,5-ortho-acetate
10-Hydroxycamptothecin (also antileuke-
    mic)
4-Hydroxycinnamic acid
3-Hydroxydamsin
12-Hydroxydaphnetoxin
7-Hydroxy-6-hydromelodienol (also anti-
    melanomic, cytotoxic)
1-Hydroxy-2-hydroxymethylanthraquinone

(antileukemic)
9-Hydroxyparthenolide
*5-Hydroxy-3',4,6',7,8-pentamethoxyflavone
Hydroxytoluene
4,8-Hydroxywithanoline-E
Hymenoflorin
Hymenoxin
(**Hyoscamine** is antiparkinsonian, cardio-
    tonic, psychoactive, sedative)
(**Hyoscamine** sulfate is antimanic, antipar-
    kinsonian)
*Hypericin (antileukemic, antiHIV)
*Hyperoside (also antiflu)
Imperatorin
Incanumine (cytotoxic)
Indicine
Indicine-N-oxide (antileukemic, antimela-
    nomic, but hepatotoxic)
Indirubin (antileukemic)
Indole (also carcinogenic)
Indole-3-acetic acid
Indole-3-acetonitrile
3,3'-Indoyl-dimethane
Ingenol-3,20-dibenzoate (cytotoxic)
beta-Ionone
Ipolearoside
Irisquinone
Isoacteoside (antileukemic, cytotoxic)
Iboccharin
*Isobruceine-B
Isochamanetin (antileukemic, cytotoxic)
*Isochlorogenic acid
Isochondodendrine
Isocucurbitacin-B
*Isodonal
*Isoeugenol (cytotoxic)
Isofraxidin (antileukemic)
Isoharringtonine (antileukemic)
*Isoimperatorin
Isoliensinine (cytotoxic)
Isoliquiritigenin
Isoplumericine
*Isorhamnetin (also hepatoprotective)
Isovaleric acid-ethyl ester
Isouvaretin (antileukemic, cytotoxic)
Isovitexin
Ivasperin
Jaconine
Jasmone
Jatroham
Jatrophatrione (cytotoxic)
(***Jatrorrhizine** chloride is HIV-RT-inhib)
*Juglone
Justicidin (antileukemic, cytotoxic)
Kaempferol (also mutagenic, teratologic)

Kaempferol-3-O-beta-D-glucopyranoside (antileukemic)

Kalbetorine

Khasianine (cytotoxic but hepatoprotective)

Lanatoside-A (also antiflu)

Lanatoside-B (also antiflu)

Lanatoside-C (also antitachycardic)

Lanosterol

*Lapachol

Lasiocarpine (carcinogenic, hepatotoxic)

Lasiocarpine-N-oxide

Lasiodiplodin (antileukemic)

Laudanosine (also convulsant)

*Lawsone

Leukemin-E

Leurosine (also hypoglycemic)

Liatrin (cytotoxic)

Licocoumarone

Licoflavanone

(**Lidocaine** is anti-tennis-elbow, antitinnitic)

*Limonene

*d-Limonene (also breast cancer)

*Linalool (also tumor promoter)

Linoleic acid (also hepatoprotective)

(gamma-Linolate is anti MS)

alpha-Linolenic acid (see Rudin's The Omega-Three Phenomenon for more information)

gamma-Linolenic acid (also antialcoholic, antiMS, antiobesity)

Lipiferolide (cytotoxic)

*Liriodenine** (cytotoxic)

(**Lobeline** sulfate is antismoking)

Loline

Lomatiol

Lupeol (antirheumatic, cytotoxic)

*Luteolin

Luteolin-7-O-beta-glucoside

Lychnostatin-1 (cytostatic)

Lychnostatin-2 (cytostatic)

Lycobetaine (also antileukemic)

Lycopene

*Lycorine (also antipolio, cytotoxic)

(Macin is proteolytic)

Macrocliniside-C

*Magnolol (also anticariogenic, Ca-blocker, CNS-depressant)

Mallotochrome

Maltol

Matrine (CNS-inhibitor)

(+)-Matrine

Maysenine

Maysine

Maytanacine

Maytanprine

Maytansine (also antileukemic, antimelanomic)

Maytansinol

Maytanvaline

Maytenfolic acid (antileukemic)

Maytenfoliol (antileukemic)

Melampodinin-A

Melinonine

Melodorinol (also antimelanomic, cytotoxic)

Melidorinol acetate (also antimelanomic)

Methionine

9-Methoxycamptothecin (antileukemic, antimelanomic)

10-Methoxycamptothecin (also antiherpetic, antiplaque)

*1-Methoxycanthin-6-one

*5-Methoxycanthin-6-one

Methoxydihydronitidine

9-Methoxyellipticine (antileukemic, CNS-depressant)

Methoxyharringtoneine

N-(3-Methoxy-4,5-Methylenedioxycinnamoyl)-delta-3-pyridin-2-one (antileukemic, cytotoxic)

N-(3-Methoxy-4,5-Methylenedioxyhydrocinnamoyl)-delta-3-pyridin-2-one (antileukemic, cytotoxic)

p-Methoxyphenol

5-Methoxypsoralen (also carcinogenic?)

*8-Methoxypsoralen (also carcinogenic)

O-Methyl-atheroline

N-Methyldemecolcine

(*O-Methylellipticine** is HIV-RT-inhib)

24-Methylene-cycloartanol

7-Methyl-eriodictyol ether

(*Methyleugenol is strychnine antidote)

O-Methyl fagaronine

*Methyl gallate (antileukemic)

(*O-Methylpsychotrine** sulfate is HIV-RT-inhib)

(3-Methylquercietin is antipolio)

(*Methyltaboganate is ant repellant)

O-Methylthalbrine

O-Methylthalicberine

O-Methylthalmethine

4-Methylthiocanthin-6-one (cytotoxic)

N-Methyltyramine

(Mexicain is proteolytic)

Mezerein (also antileukemic, cytotoxic)

Michelenolide

Micromelin (cytotoxic)

*Mimosine** (antimelanomic)

(*Miricetin is saccharomycide)

(Mogroside is sweetener)

Molephantin (cytotoxic)

Molephantinin (also antileukemic, cytotoxic)
alpha-Momorcharin (also abortifacient)
(Monellin is anorexic, and a sweetener)
*Monocrotaline (also antileukemic, cardiodepressant, hepatoxic)
alpha-Monolinolein
Monoterpenyl-magnolol
Montanin (antileukemic, cytotoxic)
Montanic acid-monoglyderide
*Morin
Morindaparvin-A (antileukemic)
Morindaparvin-B (antileukemic)
Mucilage
Multiradiatin (cytotoxic)
beta-Myrcene
*Myricetin
Myristic acid
*Myristicin
Nagilactone
Nagilactone-B
Nagilactone-C
Nagilactone-D
Nagilactone-E
Naringenin
*Narigin
Neferine
(Neohesperidin-dihydrochalcone is sweetener)
Neojusticin-A (antileukemic)
Nepetin (also anticataract)
Nepetrin (also anticataract, radioprotective)
*Neriifolin (cardiotonic/cardiotoxic, cytotoxic)
(*Nerylacetate is antiflu)
Niacin
Nicotinamide
Nitidine (also antileukemic)
(*Nitidine chloride is HIV-RT inhib)
Nobilin
*Nordihydroguaiaretic acid or NDGA
Normaysine
Normaytancyprine (antileukemic)
(+)-Nortrachelogenin (antileukemic, CNS-depressant)
Obamegin
(*Obovatol is anticariogenic)
(–)-Odorinol (antileukemic)
Oenothein-A
*Oenothein-B (also antiHIV)
Oleandrigenin
Oleandrigenin-3-rhamnoside
Oleandrin (also cardiotonic)
Oleanic acid (also anticariogenic, antifertility, cardiotonic)
Oleic acid

*Olivacine (also antileukemic)
Onopordopicrin
Opposide
*Oridonin (esophagus)
(Gamma-Orzanol is antiPMS)
(Osladin is sweetener)
Oubagenin
Ovatifloin
Oxopurpureine
*Oxycanthine (cytotoxic)
Oxyayanin-A (cytotoxic)
Oxygen
Oxylycorine (liver, stomach)
Oxymatrine
Oxynitidine
Oxypeucedanin
Oxytylocrebrine
Pabulenol
Palmilycorine
3-O-Palmitoyl-ursolic acid (cytotoxic)
Pancratistatin
Pantothenic acid
(*Papain is teratogenic)
*Parillin
*Parthenin
*Parthenolide
*Pectin
Pectolinarigenin
Pelargonidin
Pellotine
*alpha-Peltatin
*beta-Peltatin
*beta-Peltatin-A-methyl ether
cis-1,8-Pentadecadiene
(Z)-1,8-Pentadecadiene
1-Pentadecene
4',5,6,7,8-Pentamethoxyflavone
(Perillaldehyde-oxime is sweetener)
*Perivine
Peucedanin
Phantomolin (cytotoxic)
*Phebalosin
Phenethylisothiocyanate
*Phenol (also carcinogenic, CNS-depressant)
(Phenylalanine is antiparkinsonian)
*2-Phenylethyl-isothiocyanate
Phenylpropionic acid
*Phloroglucinol
Phyllanthoside (also antimelanomic, cytotoxic)
(*Phyllodulcin is sweetener)
Physalin-B (also abortifacient)
Physalin-D (also abortifacient)
(*Physostigmine is antialzheimeran)
Phytic acid

Phytohaemagglutinin
Phytol
*Piceatannol (antileukemic)
(*__Pilocarpine__ is Alzheimerigenic)
Pilocereine
Piperonal
Piplertine dimer (antileukemic, cytotoxic)
Pleniradin
*Plenolin (cytotoxic)
*Plumbagin (also antileukemic, cytotoxic)
__Plumericine__ (cytotoxic)
*Podolide (cytotoxic)
*Podophyllotoxin (also antileukemic,
abortifacient)
Polycarpol
Ponicidin (esophagus)
__Pretazettine__ (antileukemic, HIV-RT inhib)
(*Procyanidin is antiHIV)
3-O-Propionyl-ursolic acid (cytotoxic)
Propyl gallate (also sunscreen)
Proscillaridin-A (also antiflu, cardiotonic)
Prostglandin (also cytoprotective)
Prostglandin-A1
Prostglandin-E1
Prostglandin-F2 (also abortifacient)
*Protoanemonin (also antileukemic)
Provincialin (cytotoxic)
Pseudohypericin (antileukemic)
*Pseudolaric acid-A (antileukemic,
abortifacient, cytotoxic)
Pseudolaric acid-B (antileukemic,
abortifacient, cytotoxic)
Pseodlycorine (antileukemic)
*Psoralen (also photocarcinogenic)
Psorospermin (antileukemic)
(PUFAs are antiacne, antiMS)
*Pulegone (hepatotoxic)
(*Punicacortein is antiAIDS, HIV-RT inhib)
(*Punicalagin is antiHIV)
(Punicalin is antiAIDS, HIV-RT inhib)
Pycnogenol
(__Pyridoxine__ is antianemic, anti-carpal-tun-
nel, antischizophrenic)
(*Pyrogallol is antilupus, CNS-active)
Quassimarin (antileukemic, cytotoxic)
(Quercetagetin is HIV-RT inhib)
__Quercetin__ (also antiflu, cytotoxic, HIV-RT
inhib)
Quercetin-3-O-beta-D-glucoside
*Quercitrin (also anticataract, cardiotonic,
CNS-depressant)
Quercitrin-3-D-beta-glycoside
(Quinine ascorbate is antismoking)
Radiatin (cytotoxic)
(Rebaudioside is sweetener)

__Reserpine__ (also antiRaynaud's, __hepatopro-__
__tective__)
Retusin (cytotoxic)
Rhamnetin
(Rhamnocitrin is antiplaque)
*Rhein (cytotoxic, also __proteinase__ inhib)
Rhodexin-B
Riboflavin
Robinetin
Robinin
Rosmanol (also antihepatotoxic)
Rosmaridiphenol
*Rosmarinic acid
Rosmariquinone
*Rotenone (also convulsant)
Rubescensin-A (also antihepatomic)
Rubescensin-B (also antihepatomic)
Rubescensine (esophagus, liver)
(Ruboside is sweetener)
Rudmollin (antileukemic)
*__Rutin__ (also capillariprotective)
*Safrole (also hepatotoxic)
Saikosaponin (also antileukemic, CNS-
depressant)
*__Salicylic acid__
Sanguidimerine
(*Sanguin-H-11 is antiAIDS, HIV-RT inhib)
*__Sanguinarine (also cardiotonic)__
Santamarine
(Saposhnikovan-A is immunostimulant)
Scillaren-A (also cardioactive)
*Scillarenin (also antirhinovirus, cardio-
tonic)
Scilliglaucosidin (also cardiac)
*Scilliroside
(__Scopolamine__ is antimanic, antiMeneire's,
antiparkinsonian, cardiodpressant,
CNS-depressant, psychoactive)
*Scopoletin (also CNS-stimulant, hypogly-
cemic)
Scutellarein
Secocepharanthine
Secoisolariciresinol
__Selenium__ (depressant, also antidote for mer-
cury)
__Senecionine__ (hepatotoxic)
__Senecionine-N-oxide__
__Seneciphylline__ (hepatotoxic)
Sergeolide (antileukemic, cytotoxic)
Serine
(Serotonin is teratogenic)
*__Serpentine__ (also carcinogenic)
__Sesbanine__ (antileukemic)
Seselidiol (cytotoxic)
Shikoccidin

Shikoccin
*Shikonin
(Siamenoside-1 is a sweetener)
(Sideritoflavone is anticataract)
Simalikalactone-D (antileukemic)
*Simplexin (antitmor?, abortifacient)
Sinapic acid
*Sinigrin
*beta-Sitosterol (also antileukemic)
beta-Sitosterol-D-glucoside (also
CNS-stimulant, hypoglycemic)
beta-Sitosterol-beta-D-glucoside (also
antileukemic, hypoglycemic)
*Solamargine (cytotoxic)
beta-Solamarine
Solapalmatenine
Solaplumbin
Solasodine (cytotoxic, also hepatoprotective,
teratogenic)
*Solasonine (cardiodepressant/cardiotonic)
Somalin (also cardioactive)
Sophocarpine
Sophorajaponocin
*Soyasaponin (also hepatoprotective)
Spectabiline (also antileukemic, hepato-
toxic)
Spruceanol (antileukemic, cytotoxic)
*Squalene
Steganacin
Steganangin
Steganol
Steganone
Stephavanine
(*Steviolbioside is sweetener)
(*Stevioside is sweetener)
Stigmasterol (antihepatotoxic, sedative,
estrogenic)
Strophanthidin (also cardiac)
(Stropanthin-G is antiflu)
k-Strophanthoside
(Suavioside is sweetener)
(Sugaroside is sweetener)
(*Sulfur is antiacne)
Supinine
Swainsonine (antimelanomic, antimeta-
static, immunoregulator)
Synephrine
Tagitinin-F
(*Tannic acid is antiHIV, cytotoxic)
(*Tannin is hepatoprotective)
Taspine
Taxifolin (hepatoprotective)
Taxodione (cytotoxic)
Taxodone (cytotoxic)

Taxol (breast, lung, prostate, also antimela-
nomic)
Tectochrysn
Teniposide
Testosterone (breast, carcinogenic)
(*Tetragalloylquinic acid is antiAIDS, HIV-
RT inhib)
Tetrandine (lung, hepatotoxic)
d-Tetrandine
l-Tetrandine
alpha-Tetraol
Thalidasine
Thalifaberine
(Thaumatin is sweetener)
(Thioctic acid is Amanita antidote)
alpha-Thujaplicin
Thymidine (also antileukemic, methotrexate
antidote?)
(*Thymol is sprout inhibitor)
(Tigloidine is antiparkinsonian, CNS-
depressant, sedative)
Tigogenin
Tigogenin-glycoside
*Tingenone
(Tochibanan-A is immunostimulant)
(Tochibanan-B is immunostimulant)
Tochopherol (also antiarteriosclerosis, anti-
cataract, anticoronary, antilupus, antiMD,
antiMS, antioxidant)
(Toddaculine is sunscreen)
(*alpha-Tomatine is antifeedant)
*Trewiasine (also antifeedant)
Trichosanthin (also abortifacient)
Tricin (also antileukemic, estrogenic)
(*1,3,4-Tri-O-galloylquinic acid is antiAIDS,
HIV-RT inhib)
(*3,4,5-Tri-O-galloylshikimic acid is anti-
AIDS, HIV-RT inhib)
Trigonelline (cervix, liver, hypocholester-
olemic, hypoglycemic)
3',5,7-Trihydroxy-3,4'-dimethoxyflavone
Trilobolide
N-(3,4,5-Trimethoxycinnamoyl)-delta-3-
pyridin-2-one (antileukemic, cytotoxic)
(5,7,4'-Trihydroxy-8-methoxyflavone is anti-
flu)
(2-beta,3-beta-27-Trihydroxyolean-12-ene-
23,28-dicarboxylic acid is antieczemic,
antiMS)
Trilobine
N-(3,4,5-Trimethoxycinnamoyl)-delta-3-
pyridin-2-one (antileukemic, cytotoxic)
Trioxalen
Triptolide (also antileukemic, cytotoxic)
Triptonide

(Troxerutin is antihemorrhoidal, anti-Raynaud's, antiulcer, antivaricosity, capillariprotective)

(Tryptophan is carcinogenic, insulinotonic)

Tubeimoside

Tubulosin

Tubulosine (cytotoxic)

Tulipinolide (cytotoxic)

*ar-Turmerone

(Tutin is antischizophrenic, convulsant)

Tylocrebrine (also antileukemic)

Tylophoridine

Tyophorine (also antileukemic, antirhinitic, cardiodepressant/cardiomyostimulant)

Tylophorinine (also antileukemic)

Tyrosine (also antidepressant)

(Ubiquinone is immunostimulant)

(Ukonan-A is immunostimulant)

*Umbelliferone (also sunscreen)

Ursiniolide

Urrsolic acid (also antileukemic, CNS-depressant, cytotoxic, hepatoprotective)

1-Usnic acid

Uvaol (cytotoxic)

Uvaretin (cytotoxic)

Uvaricin

Uzarigenin (cytotoxic)

Valeopotriates (CNS-depressant, cytotoxic, sedative)

Valtrate (cytotoxic)

*Vanillin

Vatamine (antileukemic, cytotoxic)

Vatine (antileukemic, antihepatotomic, cytotoxic)

Vernodalin (cytotoxic)

Vernolepin

Vernolide (cytotoxic)

Vernomenin (cytotoxic)

Vinblastine (also antiHodgkin's, antiKaposi's, antileukemic, antilymphomic, antimitotic, immunosuppressant, teratogenic)

Vincristine (also antiKaposi's, antileukemic, immunosuppressant, teratogenic)

Vindesine (also antiadenocarcinoma, anti-Hodgkin's, antileukemic, antilymphomic, antimelanomic, antimiotic)

Vinleurosine

Vinrosidine (also antileukemic)

Vismione

(Vitamin K is coagulant)

Vitexin-2"-O-rhamnoside

Voacamine (also cardiotonic, CNS-depressant)

Voacorine (cardiotonic, CNS-depressant)

Wikstromol

Withacnistrin

*Withaferin

*Withaferin-A (antiadenocarcinomic, **antiarthritic**, antimiotic)

*Withanolide-E (also antifeedant)

Woodforin-C

Woodforin-D

*Xanthotoxin (cytotoxic)

Xanthotoxol (also antinicotinic)

(Xylitol is anticariogenic?, antiplaque?)

(**Yohimbine** is antiatherosclerotic)

Yuanhuacine (antileukemic, abortifacient)

Zaluzanin-C

(*Zinc is antiacne?, antidote for cadmium, anti-impotence, antiviral?, immunosuppressant)

(Zingibain is proteolytic)

Ziniolide (cytotoxic)

Agents that Affect Angiogenesis*

X.1 INHIBIT MAST CELL GRANULATION

Araliaceae	*Acanthopax** spp. (wu jia pi, ci wu jia)
Compositae	*Tanacetum parthenium**: feverfew, tansy. Inhibits release of histamine from mast cells.
Ginkgoceae	*Ginko biloba* extract. Inhibits release of histamine from mast cells.
Hesperidin	A flavonoid which inhibits release of histamine from mast cells (Sigma; Aldrich).
Labiatae	*Scutellaria baicalensis* (huang qin). Contains flavonoids which inhibit the release of histamine from mast cells.
Leguminosae	*Glycyrrhiza* spp. (gan cao): licorice. Inhibits release of histamine from mast cells.
Liliaceae	*Aloe vera* gel. Inhibits release of histamine from mast cells.
Magnoliaceae	*Magnolia salicifolia** (xin yi hua). Inhibits release of histamine from mast cells.
Proanthocyanidins	Contain flavonoid-like compounds which reduce histamine levels.
Quercetin	A flavonoid which inhibits release of histamine from mast cells (quercetin dihydrate: Sigma; Aldrich).
Scrophulariaceae	*Picrorrhiza kurroa* (hu huang lian): katuka, rohini.
Umbelliferae	*Peucedanum** *praeruptorum* (qian hu): sulfur-root, as used in veterinary medicine. Contains coumarins which inhibit the release of histamine from mast cells.
Unidentified	*Centipeda minima* (shi hu sui). Contains flavonoids and sesquiterpene compounds. Inhibits release of histamine from mast cells. More effective than extracts from *Citrus* spp. (family Rutaceae), *Magnolia* spp. (family Magnoliaceae), *Scutellaria* spp. (family Labiatae), and *Glycyrrhiza* spp. (family Leguminosae). According to the *Academic Press Dictionary of Science and Technology* (Christopher Morris Ed., Academic Press, San Diego CA, 1992), the species of *Centipeda* are anaerobic bacteria. In spite of the similarity in names, centipedes cannot be found under any such classification, but instead belong to the anthropod class Chilopoda (cf., J.G.E. Lewis, *The Biology of Centipedes*, Cambridge University Press, Cambridge, England, 1981). The particular species remains unresolved.
Unidentified	*Ganoderma** *lucidum* (ling zhi). Inhibits release of histamine from mast cells.

X.2 INHIBIT THE PRODUCTION OF PLATELET ACTIVATING FACTOR (PAF)

Docosahexaenoic acid	
	Found in fish oil. Also called DHA. Available in matrix of beaded agarose (Sigma).
Ginkgoceae	*Ginkgo biloba* extract.

---

* *Source:* Data from *Cancer & Natural Medicine* by John Boik, Oregon Medical Press, Princeton, MN, 1995, pp. 22–30. Plant families, genera, or species **not** appearing in Hartwell's *Plants Used Against Cancer* are denoted with an asterisk. Chinese names where given appear in parens. For further medicinal details, consult the reference. Other citations are from the Sigma catalog *Biochemicals, Organic Compounds, and Diagnostic Reagents*, Sigma Chemical Company, P.O. Box 14508, St. Louis MO 63178-9916, and from the Aldrich catalog, the *Catalog/Handbook of Fine Chemicals*, Aldrich Chemical Company, P.O. Box 355, Milwaukee WI 53201-9358.

Labiatae   *Leonuris heterophyllus** (yi mu cao). The active ingredient is prehispanolone.
Leguminosae   *Glycyrrhiza uralensis** (gan cao): licorice.
Piperaceae   *Piper kadsura** (hai feng tang): pepper. Active ingredient is kadsurenone.
                    *Piper wallichi** (shi nan teng): pepper. Active ingredient is kadsurenone.
Umbelliferae   *Bupleurum chinense** (chai hu).

X.3   INHIBIT FIBRIN PRODUCTION OR STIMULATE FIBRINOLYSIS

Brinase   Proteolytic enzyme from *Aspergillus oryzae** (of the fungus family Moniliaceae).
Bromelain   Protease enzyme from pineapple (Sigma; bromelain inhibitor also available: Sigma).
Compositae   *Carthamus tinctorius* (hong hua): crocus.
                    *Artemisia argyi** (ai ye): artemisia, wormwood, mugwort, absinthe.
                    *Attractylodes macrocephala** (bai zhu).
Fucaceae   *Sargassum* spp. (hai zao): brown algae.
Labiatae   *Salvia multiorrhiza* (dan shen): sage, cancerweed.
Laminariaceae   *Laminaria* sp. (kun bu): brown algae.
Liliaceae   *Allium sativum* (da suan): garlic.
Oligochaeta   *Pheretima** aspergillum* (di long): earthworm, of the class Oligochaeta.
Polypodiaceae   *Scolopendra subspinipes** mutilans (wu gong). Listed as *Scolopendrium* in Hartwell.
Ranunculaceae   *Paeonia lactiflora** (chi shao and bai shao): peony.
Solanaceae   *Capsicum annuum*: Cayenne pepper.
Unidentified   *Hirudo** nipponia (shui zhi).
                    *Bathus** matensi (quan xie).
Viperidae   *Agkistrodon** acutis (bai hua she): copperhead, moccasin, a pit viper of the subfamily Crotalinae.
Zingiberaceae   *Curcuma longa* (jiang huang): turmeric.

X.4   INHIBIT VASCULAR PERMEABILITY

Hippocastanaceae   *Aesculus hippocastanum*: horse chestnut, Castagno d'india. Active ingredient is apparently the saponin called escin.
Liliaceae   *Ruscus aculeatus*: butcher's broom, brusca, brusco, hedionda.
Omega-3-fatty acids Octanoyl-N-methyl glucamide is known as Omega-8 (Sigma).
Papaveraceae   *Corydalis turtschaninovii** (yan hu suo). Most species have tubers. Also listed under the family Fumariaceae*.
Proanthocyanidins
Umbelliferae   *Angelica sinensis* (dang gui)
                    *Bupleurum chinense** (chai hu).

X.5   DECREASE TISSUE COPPER LEVELS OR INHIBIT FIBRONECTIN SYNTHESIS

Berberidaceae   *Epimedium sagittatum** (yin yang huo).
Cysteine   Nonessential amino acid (available as D-, DL-, and L-cysteine: Sigma; Aldrich).
Labiatae   *Salvia multiorrhiza* (dan shen): sage, cancerweed.

X.6   ANTIANGIOGENIC SUBSTANCES

Cartilage extract   Contains collagen inhibitors (bovine cartilage powder available from Sigma; shark cartilage from any number of sources).
Genestein   An isoflavone which serves as an inhibitor of tyrosine protein kinase, with the chemical name 4',5,7-trihydroxyisoflavone (Sigma).
Gold thiomalate   A compound of gold, sulfur, and malic acid. Gold sodium thiomalate monohydrate, for example, is also called sodium aurothiomalate monohydrate (Aldrich).

Hydrocortisone and heparin complexes (hydrocortisone: Sigma; Aldrich; heparin: Sigma).

Interferon-alpha	A cytokine, also designated as IFN-α (Sigma). Called Anti-Human IFN-α.
Magnoliaceae	*Magnolia lilifora** (xin yi hua). Contains the lignan magnosalin. Less effective than hydrocortisone.
Penicillamine-D	Copper chelator (Sigma; Aldrich).
Platelet factor IV	Binds heparin (Sigma).
Protamine	Any of a group of simple proteins which hydrolyze to form amino acids (Sigma). Binds heparin.
SCM-chitin	Derivative of chitin, a polysaccharide. From crab shells (Sigma; Aldrich). Also found in insect exoskeletons, such as from the molting of cicada of the species *Cryptotympana atrata* (chan tui).
Thiol compounds	E.g., glutathione and as found in *Allium* spp.: garlic, onion. Glutathione and derivatives (Sigma; Aldrich).
Vitamin A	Also known as retinol (Sigma; Aldrich). IRRITANT. Inhibits growth of endothelial cells *in vitro* and inhibits angiogenesis in the CAM assay, possibly due to the inhibition of collagen synthesis.
Vitamin D3	Also known as cholescalciferol (Sigma; Aldrich). HIGHLY TOXIC. Metabolites of vitamin D3 include 1,25-dihydroxyvitamin D3 (1,25-diOHD3), the active metabolite in humans, which may also promote the effect of vitamin A. Active in CAM assay.

Update on Enzymes and Inhibitors Involved in Anaerobic Glycolysis*

Table Y.1a Hexokinase or Hexosekinase

*n-Acetylglucosamine (from **glucose**; MgATP); **Allicin**; *L-cystamine; **Dihydrogriesenin** (yeast); *Disulfides; Disulfiram; *5,5'-Dithio-bis(2-nitrobenzoic acid); **Gafrinin** (yeast); **Geigerinin** (yeast); *Glucose 6-phosphate (**glucose; yeast**); *Glutathione oxidized (MgATP); **Griesenin** (yeast); 4',5',7-Hydroxy-3,6-methoxyflavonone; 4-Hydroxypentenal; 2-(p-Hydroxyphenyl)-2-phenylpropane (*Crithidia fasciculata*); **Ivalin** (yeast); *Lauric acid; Merlasoprol (*Crithidia fasciculata*); *Mg⁺⁺ (MgATP); *MgATP (glucose); *Myristic acid; **o-Phthalaldehyde** (yeast); *Protein inhibitor dependent on Fructose 2,6-bisphosphate; **Quercetin**; **Vanadate** oligomers; **Vermeerin** (yeast).

Table Y.1b 6-Phosphofructokinase or Phosphofructokinase Inhibitors

Agaric acid ; *Arginine phosphate; Aurintricarboxylic acid; *Ca⁺⁺; Decavanadate; **Dihydrogriesenin**; *Fructose 2,6-disphosphate; **Gafrinin**; **Geigerin**; **Geigerinin**; *Glutathione oxidized; **Grieseni**; Hydroxycitrate; **Ivalin**; 3-mercaptopicolinic acid (*Trypanosoma cruzi*); Mono**vanadate**; **o-Phthalaldehyde**; Triethylphosphine gold; **Vanadate**; **Vermeerin**.

Table Y.1c Pyruvate Kinase Inhibitors

*ADP; *L-Alanine; *AMP; *ATP (from ADP); *Ca⁺⁺; Cysteine (PEP, only PK of some tumor cell lines); *Fatty acids; *Glutathione oxidized; **Lauric acid; Myristic acid; Octanic acid**; *L-Phenylalanine; *Phosphate; *Pyruvic acid(from phosphenolpyruvate); *Quercetin; Succinyl-CoA; *Sulphate.

Table Y.2 Lactate Dehydrogenase Inhibitors

Inhibitors for D-Lactate Dehydrogenase (Cytochrome)
> EDTA (yeast); **p-Mercuriphenylsulphonic acid** (yeast); *Oxalacetic acid (D-lactate; yeast); *Oxalic acid (D-lactate; yeast); **o-Phenanthroline** (yeast); *Pyruvic acid (D-lactate; yeast)

Inhibitors for D-Lactate Dehydrogenase
> *2-Hydroxy-3-**butynoic** acid(*Megasphera elsdenii*); *5-(–)Oxalylethyl-NADH.

Inhibitors for L-Lactate Dehydrogenase (Cytochrome)
> *Fatty acids; *Glycerate; *2-Hydroxy-3-**butynoic** acid (**bakers yeast**); *L-Malic acid; *Oxalic acid; *Phenylpyruvic acid.

Inhibitors for L-Lactate Dehydrogenase
> **Allicin**; *ATP (NAD; *Streptococcus cremonis*); P1-N6-(4-Azidophenylethyl)adenosine-P2-[4-(3-azidopyridino)butyl]diphosphate; Ca²⁺/EDTA complex (EDTA); *p-Chloromercuribenzoic acid (pyruvate; *Streptococcus cremonis*); *Cibacron blue 3GA-dextran; Diethyldithiocarbamate; **Disulfiram; Gossypol; Gossypol** acetic acid (pyruvate); 1,6-Hexanediol; *2-Hydroxy-3-**butynoic** acid (*E. Coli*); 4-Hydroxypentenal; Methyl **parathion**; *Mononucleotides (sweet potato roots); *NADH; *5-(–)Oxalylethyl-NADH ; *Oxamic acid; *Phenylpyruvic acid; *Phosphoenolpyruvic acid (sweet potato roots); *Pyruvic acid (sweet potato roots); *Reactive green 19-dextran; *Reactive red 4-dextran.

Note: A cyctochrome is defined as an an electron-carrying iron porphyrin pigment protein present in all animal and plant cells, usually in the mitochondria, and is involved in respiration.

---

* *Source:* Data from H. Zollner, *Handbook of Enzyme Inhibitors*, in two volumes, VCH, Weinheim, FRG, 1993.; (*) from H. Zollner, *Handbook of Enzyme Inhibitors*, VCH, Weinheim, FRG, 1989. The information denoted by an asterisk (*) appears in Appendix A. Items in **boldface** may be of special interest.

Vitamins and Hormones as Enzyme Inhibitors*

Vitamins	Chemical name	Formula
Vitamin A	Retinol	$C_{19}H_{24}\text{-}CH_2OH$

Retinol inhibits β-glucuronidase
Retinoic acid inhibits estrogen sulfotransferase, glutamate dehyrogenase, metaplasia; shows **antitumor activity**. (The term "-metaplasia" signifies abnormal development.)
β-Retinoic acid inhibits hyperplasia (atrophy).
13-cis-Retinoic acid inhibits **carcinogenesis**.
Vitamin A topical application **inceased incidence of rous sarcomas** in chickens
Vitamin A acid (retinoic acid) inhibits alcohol dehydrogenase.

Vitamin B1	Thiamine hydrochloride	$C_{12}H_{18}Cl_2N_4OS$
	Thiamin chloride	

Thiamine derivatives inhibit **glucose synthesis**, transketolase (from yeast), phosphodiesterase (from snake venom), thiamine triphosphatase, thymidylate kinase.
Thiamine antagonists inhibit acetylcholinesterase.

Vitamin B2	Riboflavin	$C_{17}H_{22}N_4O_6$
	Lactoflavin; Vitamin G	

Inhibits Daminoacid oxidase, FAD pyrophosphylase, galactonolactone dehydrogenase, glutamate racemase, riboflavin synthetase.
*Inhibits cytochrome-B5 reductase.

Vitamin B6	Pyridoxin	$C_8H_{11}NO_3$

Inhibits alanine racemase, **malate dehydrogenase**, pyridoxamine pyruvate transami.
Vitamin B6 antagonists inhibit **adrenocarcinoma** growth.
*Inhibits alanine racemase, pyridoxamine-pyruvate aminotransferase.

Vitamin B12	Cobalamine;	$C_{63}H_{90}N_{14}O_{14}PCo$
	cyanocobalamin	

Cobalamin analogs inhibit ethanolamine deaminase. (Ethanolamine is an industrial solvent which selectively absorbs the acid gases CO_2 and H_2S.)
Cobalamin derivatives inhibit ribonucleotide reductase.
Hydroxy-cobalamin inhibits diol dehydratase.

---

* *Source:* Data from M.K. Jain, *Handbook of Enzyme Inhibitors, 1965–1977*, Wiley, New York, 1982; (*) from H. Zollner, *Handbook of Enzyme Inhibitors*, VCH, Weinheim, FRG, 1989, 1993. The list of vitamins is according to Table 1.1 of Part 1. The list of hormones is from D. Voet and J.G. Voet, *Biochemistry*, New York, 1990, p. 1142.

Note: the Zollner reference in the main does not include hormones as enzyme inhibitors. Items that may be of particular interest are in **boldface**.

Folic acid	Pteroylglutamic acid (PGA)	$C_{14}H_{11}N_6O_2$-$(C_5H_7NO_3)_n$-OH
	Folacin; Vitamin Bc; Vitamin M	where n = 1-7
		$C_{19}H_{19}N_7O_6$ for n = 1

Inhibits **thymidylate synthetase**.

Pteroylglutamate derivative inhibits **dihydrofolate reductase**.

*Both pteroyl-α-glutamic acid and pteroyl-γ-glutamic acid inhibit 5-methyltetrahydropteroyltriglutamate-homocysteine methyltransferase.

Niacin	Nicotinic acid	$(C_5H_4N)COOH$
	3-Pyridinecarboxylic acid	

Inhibits catecholase, D-aminoacid oxidase, fatty acid synthesis, lipolysis, nicotinamide deaminase, NMN aminhydrolase, phenol oxidase, tributyrinase.

Nicotinic acid derivatives inhibit accumulation of nicotinic acid, lipolysis.

Nicotinamide inhibits ADPR polymerase, cytochrome P-450 reductase, **diphtheria toxin**, IMP dehydrogenase, NAD glycohydrolase, NAD nucleosidase, NADase, nucleoside pyrophosphatase, mixed function oxidation, cAMP phosphodiesterase, poly ADPR synthesis, prostaglandin A1 metabolism, T-RNA methylase, xanthine oxidase, 6-phosphogluconate dehydrogenase.

***Nicotinamide** inhibits NAD ADP-ribosyltransferase, NAD(P)nucleosidase, unspecific monooxygenase.

Pantothenic acid		$HOCH_2C(CH_3)_2CH(OH)CO$-$NHCH_2CH_2COOH$
		or N(α,γ-dihydroxy-β,β-dimethylbutyryl)β-alanine $C_9H_{17}NO_5$

Vitamin C	Ascorbic acid	$CO\ (COH)_3CHOHCH_2OH$
	Antiscorbutin	$C_6H_8O_6$

Inhibits adenylate cyclase, Na,K-ATPase, catalase, catechol O-methyltransferase, ferredoxin-NADP reductase, glucose-6-P dehydrogenase, lipase, fatty acid oxygenase, peroxidase, CAMP phosphodiesterase, tyrosinase, **urea levels**.

Abscorbic acid derivatives inhibit ascorbate-2-sulfate sulfohydro, dehydro-ascorbic acid.

L-ascorbic acid inhibits β-acetylhexosaminidase.

*Ascorbate inhibits o-aminophenol oxidase, catalase, β-glucuronidase, GTP cyclohydrolase I, hydroxymethylglutaryl-CoA reductase, lactoylglutathione lyase.

Vitamin D	Calciferol	$C_{28}H_{44}O$

Vitamin D2 inhibits ATPase.

Vitamin E	α-Tocopherol	$C_{14}H_{17}O_2\ (C_5H_{10})_3\ H$
	5,7,8-Trimethyltocol	

Inhibits arachidonate peroxidation, Na,K-ATPase, **glutamate dehydrogenase**, fatty acid oxygenase.

Tocopherol analogs inhibit phosphodiesterase.

*Inhibits lipoxygenase.

Vitamin K	Phthiocol	$C_{11}H_8O_3$
	1,4-Naphthoquinone, 2-hydroxy-3-methyl-	

Vitamin K1 inhibits incorporation of glucosamine.

2-chloro-Vitamin K1 inhibits prothrombin levels.

Vitamin K3 inhibits aniline hydroxylase.

Hormones	Origins
Polypeptides	
Corticotropin-releasing factor (CRF)	Hypothalmus
Corticotropin analogs inhibit adenylate cyclase.	
Gonadotropin-releasing factor (GnRF)	Hypothalmus
Human chorionic gonadotropin inhibits release of A-amylase.	
Thyrotropin-releasing factor (TRF)	Hypothalmus
Inhibits growth hormone biosynthesis.	
Growth hormone-releasing factor (GRF)	Hypothalmus
Growth hormone inhibits glucose consumption.	
Growth hormone derivative inhibits pyruvate dehydrogenase.	
Somatostatin	Hypothalmus
Inhibits accumulation of cAMP, cAMP levels, parathyroid hormone action, release of CCK, release of **growth hormone**, release of **insulin**.	
Adrenocorticotropic hormone (ACTH)	Adenohypophysis (pituitary)
Inhibits DNA synthesis in adrenal tumor cells; inhibits replication in adrenocortical cells.	
ACTH analogs inhibit adenylate cyclase, fatty acid synthesis.	
ACTH derivatives inhibit lipolytic action, cAMP synthesis, corticosterone synthesis, and ACTH activity.	
Follicle-stimulating hormone (FSH)	Adenohypophysis
Lutinizing hormone (LH)	Adenohypophysis
Leuteinizing hormone inhibits cholestrol synthesis.	
Luteinizing hormone inhibits sterol synthesis.	
Chorionic gonadotropin (CG)	Placenta
Thyrotropin (TSH)	Adenohypophysis
Inhibits inteferon action.	
Somatotropin (see **growth hormone**)	Adenohypophysis
Met-enkephalin	Adenohypophysis
Leu-enkephalin	Adenohypophysis
Enkephalin inhibits neuronal firing.	
β-Endorphin	Adenohypophysis
Inhibits acetylcholine turnover.	
Has opiate-like activity in mice.	
Endorphin inhibits CAMP formation.	

Vasopressin   Neurohypophysis

    Forms conductance channels across planar bylayer.

    Inhibits carbon dioxide synthesis.

Oxytocin   Neurohypophysis

    Oxytocin analog antagonizes oxytocin action on uturus and mammary gland.

    Oxytocin analogs inhibit binding to oxytocin recepter, uturus contraction.

    Oxytocin derivatives inhibit binding of oxytocin, oxytocin effects.

Glucagon   Pancreas

    Inhibits contraction of dog paillary muscle, **fatty acid synthesis, glycogen synthesis,**
    vasoconstriction in dog artery.

Insulin   Pancreas

    Inhibits lypolysis, adenylate cyclase, binding of NSILA, CAMP levels, cathepsin D,
    incorporation of thymidine, lipase, PEP carboxykinase synthesis, phosphorylase,
    protein kinase, **protein synthesis**.

Gastrin   Stomach

Secretin   Intestine

Cholecystokinin (CCK)   Intestine

Gastric inhibitory peptide (GIP)   Intestine

    Gastric secretion inhibitor blocks secretion of acid.

Parathyroid hormone   Parathyroid

    Inhibits ATP-P_i exchange, **glycogen synthesis, respiration**.

    Analogs inhibit bovine enzyme; adenylate cyclase.

Calcitonin   Thyroid

    Lowers calcium, **glucose**, phosphate and potassium levels.

Somatomedins   Liver

    Inhibits binding to insulin receptor, NSILA binding.

Steroids

Glucocorticoids   Adrenal cortex

    Glucocorticoid receptor inhibitor inhibits binding to DNA.

Mineralocorticoids   Adrenal cortex

    Corticosteroids inhibit binding of calcium, collagen synthesis, prostaglandin synthesis,
    release of prostaglandins.

Estrogens (gonads include testes and ovaries)   Gonads and
                                                                adrenal cortex

    Estradiol, stilbesterol, methyltestosteron, and stilbesterol inhibit bile acid metabolism.

Estrogens inhibit binding of estradiol, cortisone reduction, **glucose-6-P dehydrogenase**, steroid D4-5B-reductase, steroid NAG transferase.

Androgens   Gonads and
                                                                                  adrenal cortex

Derivatives bind to specific proteins. The resulting complex migrates into the prostate cell nuclei where they appear to regulate gene transcription.

Derivatives inhibit aromatase in the human placenta.

Progestins or Progesterones   Ovaries and placenta

Inhibits aldehyde dehydrogenase, amylase, **induction of collagenase** (which is modulated by cAMP), DNA repair and replication, DNA synthesis.

*Inhibits aldehyde oxidase, cholesterol acyltransferase, retinol fatty-acyltransferase.

Vitamin D or Calcifero   Diet and sun

Vitamin D2 inhibits ATPase.

Amino Acid Derivatives

Epinephrine   Adrenal medulla

Inhibits adenylate cyclase, CA-ATPase, uturus contaction, drug metabolism, lipgenesis, PE N-methyl transferase, **phosphofructokinase**, release of β-glucuronidase, release of tyrosine A-KG transminase.

Norepinephrine

Inhibits binding of penoxybenzamine in aorta, permeability of water, pigmentation, serotonin levels, tryptophan levels, tryptophan 2,3-dioxygenase, tyrosine hydroxylase, tyrosine transaminase.

Triiodothyronine (T_3)   Thyroid

Inhibits protein synthesis, secretion of prolactin.

Thyroxine (T_4)   Thyroid

Inhibits alcohol dehydrogenase, glutamate dehydrogenase, glutamic dehydrogenase, lipid peroxidation, **malate dehydrogenase**, oxidative phosphorylation, thyroid transaminase.

L-thyroxine inhibits nicotinamide deaminase, cAMP phophodiesterase, triglyceride levels.

Index